FIRST AID™

Q&A FOR THE USMLE STEP 1

Third Edition

SENIOR EDITORS

Tao Le, MD, MHS
Associate Clinical Professor
Chief, Section of Allergy and Clinical Immunology
Department of Medicine
University of Louisville

James A. Feinstein, MD
Clinical Instructor, Section of General Pediatrics
The Children's Hospital Colorado
Research Fellow
Primary Care Research Program
University of Colorado School of Medicine

EDITORS

Mark W. Ball, MD
Resident
The James Buchanan Brady Urological Institute
The Johns Hopkins Hospital

Annie Dude, MD
Resident
Department of Obstetrics and Gynecology
Duke University Medical Center

Rebecca L. Hoffman, MD
Resident
Department of General Surgery
Hospital of the University of Pennsylvania

Mark Robert Jensen
University of Rochester School of Medicine
Class of 2012

Kimberly Kallianos
Harvard Medical School
Class of 2012

Cesar Raudel Padilla
University of Rochester School of Medicine
Class of 2012

Lauren Rothkopf, MD
Masters in Public Health candidate
Temple University College of Health Professions and Social Work

James Yeh, MD
Resident
Department of Medicine
Cambridge Hospital, Cambridge Health Alliance

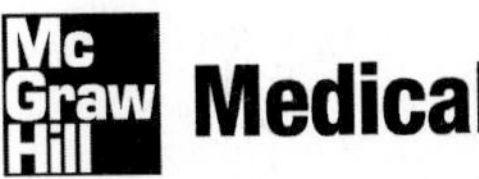

New York / Chicago / San Francisco / Lisbon
Milan / New Delhi / San Juan / Seoul / Singap

The McGraw·Hill Companies

First Aid™ Q&A for the USMLE Step 1, Third Edition

5 6 7 8 9 0 QVS/QVS 17 16 15

ISBN 978-0-07-174402-7
MHID 0-07-174402-9
ISSN 1932-5207

NOTICE

Medicine is an ever-changing science. As new research and clinical experience broaden our knowledge, changes in treatment and drug therapy are required. The authors and the publisher of this work have checked with sources believed to be reliable in their efforts to provide information that is complete and generally in accord with the standards accepted at the time of publication. However, in view of the possibility of human error or changes in medical sciences, neither the authors nor the publisher nor any other party who has been involved in the preparation or publication of this work warrants that the information contained herein is in every respect accurate or complete, and they disclaim all responsibility for any errors or omissions or for the results obtained from use of the information contained in this work. Readers are encouraged to confirm the information contained herein with other sources. For example and in particular, readers are advised to check the product information sheet included in the package of each drug they plan to administer to be certain that the information contained in this work is accurate and that changes have not been made in the recommended dose or in the contraindications for administration. This recommendation is of particular importance in connection with new or infrequently used drugs.

This book was set in Electra LH by Rainbow Graphics.
The editors were Catherine A. Johnson and Cindy Yoo.
The production supervisor was Jeffrey Herzich.
Project management was provided by Rainbow Graphics.
Quad/Graphics was printer and binder.

This book is printed on acid-free paper.

DEDICATION

To the contributors to this and future editions, who took time to share their knowledge, insight, and humor for the benefit of students, residents, and clinicians.

and

To our families, friends, and loved ones, who supported us in the task of assembling this guide.

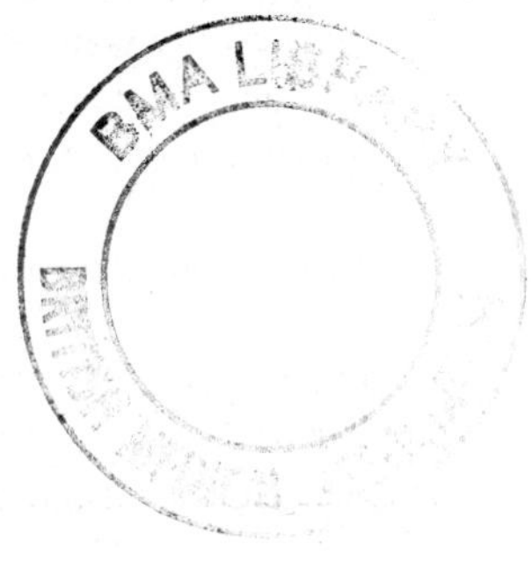

CONTENTS

AUTHORS

KIRSTEN AUSTAD
Fellow
Edmond J. Safra Center for Ethics
Harvard University

EIKE BLOHM
Johns Hopkins University School of Medicine
Class of 2012

BENJAMIN CAPLAN, MD
Resident
Department of Family Medicine
Boston University

PO-HAO CHEN
Harvard Medical School
Class of 2012

LAUREN DE LEON, MD
Intern
Department of Internal Medicine
The Alpert Medical School of Brown University

PHILIP EYE
Boston University School of Medicine
Class of 2012

JIM GRIFFIN, MD
Resident
Department of Surgery and Surgical Oncology
Johns Hopkins Hospital

JOHN HEGDE
Harvard Medical School
Class of 2012

EMILY HEIKAMP
Johns Hopkins University School of Medicine
Class of 2014

THOMAS ROBERT HICKEY, MD
Resident
Department of Anesthesiology
Brigham and Women's Hospital

HENRY R. KRAMER, MD
Resident
Department of Medicine
Massachusetts General Hospital

THOMAS LARDARO
Johns Hopkins University School of Medicine
Class of 2012

KATHERINE LATIMER
Johns Hopkins University School of Medicine
Class of 2012

JOSEPH LIAO
Boston University School of Medicine
Class of 2012

JERRY LOO
University of Southern California Keck School of Medicine
Class of 2012

AYA MICHAELS, MD
Resident
Department of Radiology
Brigham and Women's Hospital

SOMALA MUHAMMED, MD
Resident
Department of General Surgery
Baylor College of Medicine

BEHROUZ NAMDARI, MD
Resident
Department of Psychiatry
Duke University Medical Center

TASHERA PERRY, MD
Resident
Department of Obstetrics and Gynecology
The University of Illinois at Chicago School of Medicine

CHRISTOPHER ROXBURY
Johns Hopkins University School of Medicine
Class of 2012

NEEPA SHAH
Boston University
Class of 2012

BETHANY STRONG
Harvard Medical School
Class of 2012

SEENU SUSARLA, MD, DMD, MPH
Resident
Department of Oral & Maxillofacial Surgery
Massachusetts General Hospital

JEFFREY TOSOIAN
Johns Hopkins University School of Medicine
Class of 2012

JACKSON VANE, MD
Resident
Department of Pediatrics
University of California, Irvine School of Medicine

DANIEL J. VERDINI, MD
Resident
Department of Internal Medicine
University of Nevada School of Medicine at Reno

MARC E. WALKER
Harvard Medical School
Class of 2012

PREFACE

With the third edition of *First Aid Q&A for the USMLE Step 1,* we continue our commitment to providing students with the most useful and up-to-date preparation guides for the USMLE Step 1. This new edition represents an outstanding effort by a talented group of authors and includes the following:

- Almost 1000 high-yield USMLE-style questions based on the top-rated *USMLERx Qmax Step 1 Test Bank* (www.usmlerx.com)
- Concise yet complete explanations to correct and incorrect answers
- Questions organized by general principles and organ systems
- Seven full-length test blocks simulate the actual exam experience
- High-yield images, diagrams, and tables complement the questions and answers
- Organized as a perfect complement to *First Aid for the USMLE Step 1*

We invite you to share your thoughts and ideas to help us improve *First Aid Q&A for the USMLE Step 1*. See How to Contribute, p. xiii.

Louisville Tao Le
Denver James A. Feinstein

ACKNOWLEDGMENTS

This has been a collaborative project from the start. We gratefully acknowledge the thoughtful comments and advice of the medical students, international medical graduates, and faculty who have supported the authors in the continuing development of *First Aid Q&A for the USMLE Step 1*.

For support and encouragement throughout the project, we are grateful to Thao Pham, Louise Petersen, Selina Franklin, Jonathan Kirsch, and Vikas Bhushan. Thanks to our publisher, McGraw-Hill, for the valuable assistance of their staff. For enthusiasm, support, and commitment to this challenging project, thanks to our editor, Catherine Johnson. For outstanding editorial work, we thank Mary Dispenza and Emma D. Underdown. A special thanks to Rainbow Graphics for remarkable production work.

Louisville Tao Le
Denver James A. Feinstein

HOW TO CONTRIBUTE

This edition of *First Aid Q&A for the USMLE Step 1* incorporates hundreds of contributions and changes suggested by faculty and student reviewers. We invite you to participate in this process. We also offer paid internships in medical education and publishing ranging from three months to one year (see next page for details). Please send us your suggestions for:

- Corrections or enhancements to existing questions and explanations
- New high-yield questions
- Low-yield questions to remove

For each entry incorporated into the next edition, you will receive a $10 gift certificate, as well as personal acknowledgment in the next edition. Diagrams, tables, partial entries, updates, corrections, and study hints are also appreciated, and significant contributions will be compensated at the discretion of the authors.

The preferred way to submit entries, suggestions, or corrections is via our blog:

www.firstaidteam.com

Alternatively, you can email us at: firstaidteam@yahoo.com. All entries become property of the authors and are subject to editing and reviewing. Please verify all data and spellings carefully. In the event that similar or duplicate entries are received, only the first entry received will be used. Include a reference to a standard textbook to facilitate verification of the fact. Please follow the style, punctuation, and format of this edition if possible.

INTERNSHIP OPPORTUNITIES

The First Aid Team is pleased to offer part-time and full-time paid internships in medical education and publishing to motivated medical students and physicians. Internships may range from three months (e.g., a summer) up to a full year. Participants will have an opportunity to author, edit, and earn academic credit on a wide variety of projects, including the popular *First Aid* and *USMLERx* series. Writing/editing experience, familiarity with Microsoft Word, and Internet access are desired. For more information, e-mail a résumé or a short description of your experience along with a cover letter to **firstaidteam@yahoo.com**.

SECTION I

General Principles

- Behavioral Science
- Biochemistry
- Embryology
- Microbiology
- Immunology
- Pathology
- Pharmacology

CHAPTER 1

Behavioral Science

QUESTIONS

1. Researchers investigating the development of the idiopathic inflammatory myopathies (IIMs) such as polymyositis read that vitamin D may act as an immunomodulator that reduces the development and severity of autoimmune diseases. Given that many Americans are vitamin D deficient, the researchers design an observational study to assess the impact of vitamin D supplementation on IIM symptom severity. Subjects are surveyed at time 0 and after two years, and the results are listed in the chart. Which equation represents the chance of symptom improvement in subjects who took vitamin D supplements relative to subjects who did not take vitamin D supplements?

	Vitamin D supplement taken	Vitamin D supplement not taken
Symptoms improved	50	60
Symptoms not improved	300	400

Reproduced, with permission, from USMLERx.com.

(A) (50 / 300) / (60 / 400)
(B) (50 / 350) / (60 / 460)
(C) (50 / 460) / (60 / 300)
(D) (60 / 400) / (50 / 300)
(E) (60 / 460) / (50 / 350)

2. A 16-year-old boy is brought to the pediatrician by his mother because of excessive daytime sleepiness. She states that over the past six months she has received numerous phone calls from the boy's school informing her that her son sleeps throughout all of his afternoon classes and is often difficult to arouse at the end of class. The patient reports that occasionally when he wakes up in the morning he cannot move for extended periods. He says that sometimes when he laughs at jokes or becomes nervous before a test, he feels as if he cannot move his legs. He admits that he has even fallen to the floor because of leg weakness while laughing. Which of the following is the best choice for treating this patient?

(A) Chloral hydrate
(B) Hydroxyzine
(C) Modafinil
(D) Prochlorperazine maleate
(E) Zolpidem

3. A 52-year-old woman is being treated by a male psychiatrist for depression stemming from her recent divorce. Recently, the patient has been coming to her appointments dressed up and wearing expensive perfumes. She has also started to flirt with the doctor. The patient's demeanor and appearance had initially reminded the psychiatrist of his aunt. He is uncomfortable with the patient's new behavior patterns and tells her so. She becomes very angry and storms out of the office, canceling all remaining appointments on her way out. Which of the following behaviors is an example of negative transference?

(A) The doctor seeing the patient as his aunt
(B) The doctor telling the patient he is uncomfortable
(C) The patient being angry with the doctor
(D) The patient dressing up for appointments
(E) The patient flirting with the doctor

4. A 28-year-old woman presents to her primary care physician because of depressed mood. She states that she has been depressed for as long as she can remember and feels bad about herself almost all of the time. She states that her only happy moments were during her honeymoon two years ago, and during a ski trip in college when she felt "on top of the world." She confides that for a couple weeks last month she felt life was no longer worth living. At that time, she was having extreme difficulty

sleeping, a complete loss of energy, and a lack of appetite. A review of the patient's history shows that during the past two years she has seen a physician for complaints of stomach upset, fatigue, headaches, and an unintentional 3.6-kg (8-lb) weight gain. Physical examination and results of laboratory tests are within normal limits. Which of the following is an adverse effect the patient may experience during the course of the treatment of this illness?

(A) Agranulocytosis
(B) Anorgasmia
(C) Arrhythmia
(D) Polyuria
(E) Stevens-Johnson syndrome

5. A 6-year-old girl is brought to the pediatrician by her mother because of fecal incontinence. The mother says this behavior usually occurs at school. According to Freud, which stage of psychosexual development has this child failed to progress through?

(A) Anal stage
(B) Genital stage
(C) Latency stage
(D) Oral stage
(E) Phallic stage

6. A 20-year-old man became very agitated at a party, and as a result was brought to the emergency department. In the waiting room he is belligerent and uncooperative. A physical examination reveals fever, tachycardia, horizontal nystagmus, hyperacusis, and pupils that are 3 mm in diameter bilaterally. Which of the following substances is most likely causing the behavioral changes and physical findings exhibited by this patient?

(A) Alcohol
(B) Amphetamines
(C) Cocaine
(D) Lysergic acid diethylamide
(E) Nicotine
(F) Phencyclidine

7. The figure below is a common representation used in studying the characteristics of a test's results. Using the letters in the figure, which of the following accurately describes the prevalence of the disease?

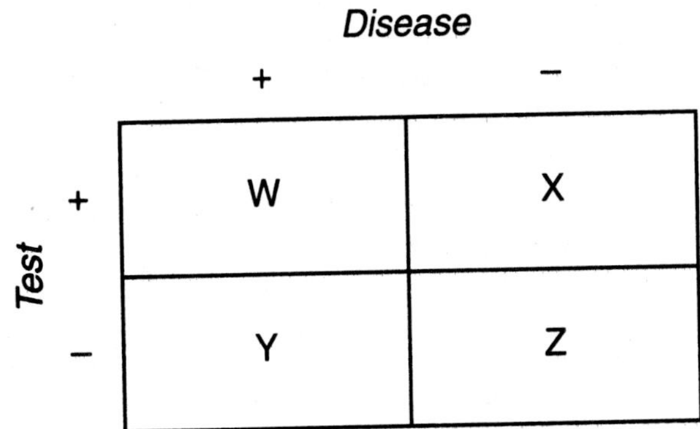

Reproduced, with permission, from USMLERx.com.

(A) (W+X) / (W+X+Y+Z)
(B) (W+Y) / (W+X+Y+Z)
(C) W / (W+X+Y+Z)
(D) W / (X+Y+Z)
(E) W / (X+Z)

8. A 75-year-old man is recovering in the hospital from a left-sided below-the-knee amputation. Three days after the surgery, the patient suddenly develops chest pain and shortness of breath that last for 20 minutes. His pain medication is increased, which improves the pain but not the shortness of breath. X-ray of the chest is negative for a pulmonary embolus, so the medical team decides to monitor him expectantly. The next day, a similar episode of shortness of breath and chest pain occurs. The patient then sustains cardiac arrest and dies. Autopsy reveals multiple pulmonary emboli. The family threatens to sue for malpractice for mismanaged postoperative care. Which of the following is necessary to prove malpractice?

(A) A patient directly suffers harm
(B) A physician's presence at the time of injury
(C) Intent to harm
(D) Proof beyond reasonable doubt
(E) Use of standard procedures

9. A 2-month-old boy is brought to the emergency department with respiratory insufficiency and failure to thrive. The pregnancy and perinatal course were uneventful. Generalized hypotonia, tongue fasciculations, and flaccid paralysis are noted on physical examination. His hospital stay is complicated by the development of tracheobronchomalacia and respiratory insufficiency that necessitates mechanical ventilation. Despite these efforts, the patient dies of respiratory complications. Muscle biopsy shows denervation and panfascicular atrophy. A genetics consult yields the pedigree shown in the image. Which of the following diseases is most consistent with this patient's presentation and the pedigree shown in the image?

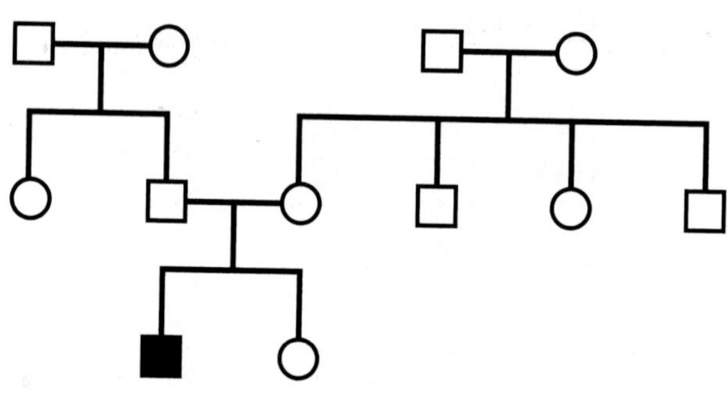

Reproduced, with permission, from USMLERx.com.

(A) Becker muscular dystrophy
(B) Duchenne muscular dystrophy
(C) Kugelberg-Welander disease
(D) Spinal muscular atrophy, type II
(E) Werdnig-Hoffmann disease

10. A new screening test for the development of mitral regurgitation in the setting of rheumatic fever is created. A study of 1000 patients with a history of *Streptococcus pyogenes* infection and a diagnosis of rheumatic fever is performed using this test, which has 90% sensitivity and 85% specificity. The prevalence of mitral regurgitation in this population is estimated to be 40%. What is the positive predictive value of this test?

(A) 8%
(B) 20%
(C) 80%
(D) 85%
(E) 93%

11. A 66-year-old man presents to his primary care physician with a complaint of erectile dysfunction. His past history is significant for hypertension, type 2 diabetes mellitus, peripheral vascular disease, and coronary artery disease status postmyocardial infarction. His current medications are propranolol, captopril, aspirin, lovastatin, metformin, fluoxetine, and sublingual nitroglycerin. On further questioning, he admits to wanting a prescription for sildenafil. Which of his medications is unsafe to take with sildenafil?

(A) Aspirin
(B) Captopril
(C) Fluoxetine
(D) Lovastatin
(E) Metformin
(F) Nitroglycerin
(G) Propranolol

12. A 17-year-old girl presents to her primary care physician with a complaint of missed menses. A urine pregnancy test confirms that she is pregnant. She returns to the office two weeks later asking for recommendations on obtaining an abortion. She explains that she works, lives with her husband, and is not ready for a child. She decides that she does not want to notify anyone, and says she has chosen not to talk with her parents for many months. Her doctor understands that he must abide by her wishes because she is emancipated. Which of the following makes this patient emancipated?

(A) Age 17 years is considered an adult
(B) Full-time work
(C) High school diploma
(D) Living separately from her parents
(E) Marriage

13. A group of scientists decides to conduct a study addressing the long-term effects of maternal alcohol consumption on their infants after conception. Two hundred women, including those who suffer from alcoholism and those who do not, are recruited into the study when they present for their first primary care visit. A medical history is taken on alcohol use, prenatal care, nutritional status, and smoking behaviors; these are measured monthly during the pregnancy. The researchers follow the women's pregnancies until term, after which they devote their attention to the health and behaviors of the offspring. Which of the following is the most appropriate statistic the researchers will be able to calculate as a result of their study?

    (A) Attributable risk of offspring abnormalities in mothers who smoke
    (B) Odds ratio of offspring abnormalities in mothers who consume alcohol during pregnancy
    (C) Prevalence of alcohol consumption during pregnancy
    (D) Proportion of all offspring abnormalities that are due to alcohol consumption during pregnancy
    (E) Relative risk of offspring abnormalities in mothers who consume alcohol during pregnancy

14. An 11-year-old girl is brought to the pediatrician with complaints of back pain. On physical examination, a right thoracic scoliotic curve is noted. The pediatrician mentions to the parent that the development of adolescent idiopathic scoliosis is due to the girl being at peak height growth velocity. Peak height velocity is associated with a certain Tanner stage; what other physical attributes would one expect to occur in this girl at the same time?

    (A) Elevation of the breast papilla only, and no pubic hair
    (B) Enlargement of the breast and areola with a single contour, and darker, coarse, curled pubic hair
    (C) Mature breast, and adult quantity and pattern of pubic hair that extends to the thighs
    (D) Projection of the areola and papilla (with separate contours), and adult-type pubic hair limited to the genital area
    (E) Small breast buds with elevation of breast papilla, and sparse, straight, downy hair on the labial base

15. A 10-year-old Hispanic boy is admitted for bone marrow transplantation as treatment for acute myelogenous leukemia. The doctor wants to enroll the patient in a clinical trial for a new pain medication, but both the parents speak only Spanish. The consent form is in English, and the physician has a limited knowledge of Spanish. What is the physician's best option for obtaining consent from this patient?

    (A) Explain the study to the whole family in Spanish, to the best of the physician's ability
    (B) Have a Spanish-speaking employee of the hospital translate for the patient
    (C) Have the parents sign the English form after discussing the study via an interpreter
    (D) Obtain a translated consent form and discuss the study via an interpreter
    (E) The boy speaks English, so the parents' consent will not be required

16. A 70-year-old man comes into his doctor's office for a routine check-up. His past medical history is significant for a heart attack, for which he takes a daily baby aspirin and a β-blocker. He practices safe habits and always wears his seat belt while driving. His health has been "great" for the past few years, although he is concerned about his wife because she recently suffered a mild stroke. He denies any visual loss or motor or sensory weakness. The patient's physical examination is unremarkable. Which of the following is the leading cause of death among people age 65 years or older?

    (A) Heart disease
    (B) Malignancy
    (C) Motor vehicle crashes
    (D) Stroke
    (E) Suicide

17. A 54-year-old man with a history of poorly controlled hypertension complains of new-onset headaches. His mother passed away at an early age due to a stroke, and his father died of a myocardial infarction. When asked why he does not take better care of his blood pressure, he states that he is so busy with work and with the church that, by the end of the day, he often forgets to take his pills. He states that he "feels fine, anyway." What ego defense mechanism is this patient using?

    (A) Denial
    (B) Displacement
    (C) Projection
    (D) Rationalization
    (E) Repression

18. A 3-year-old girl presents for her regular checkup. Her mother reports that she is fully toilet trained, and that she can dress and undress with minor assistance. She speaks in full sentences, can name four colors, and can copy a simple circle drawing. What other milestone would this child most likely have reached since her last visit one year ago?

    (A) Engages in cooperative play
    (B) Has imaginary friend(s)
    (C) Hops on one foot
    (D) Reads
    (E) Rides a tricycle
    (F) Stacks five blocks

19. A retrospective cohort study is examining birth complications in women with diabetes. The study determines that babies are more likely to be born large for gestational age (LGA) if the mother has diabetes. The relative risk for the study is calculated to be 4. Which of the following accurately describes this relative risk?

    (A) The incidence rate of diabetes among mothers with LGA babies is four times that of non-LGA mothers
    (B) The incidence rate of LGA among women with diabetes is four times that of women without diabetes
    (C) The incidence rate of LGA among women without diabetes is four times that of women with diabetes
    (D) The odds of diabetes among mothers with LGA babies is four times that of non-LGA mothers
    (E) The odds of LGA among women with diabetes is four times that of women without diabetes

20. A 45-year-old man presents to a psychiatrist at his wife's prompting. He is an English professor at the University of Virginia and regularly wins accolades for his well-organized and articulate lectures. In the past three months, he has become convinced that his wife is having an affair with a co-worker, despite her protests to the contrary. His wife recently discovered that he hired a private investigator to track her whereabouts. He is very defensive when the counselor questions his suspicions about his wife. Mental status examination reveals a well-dressed, middle-aged man without hallucinations or other mood disturbances. His speech is normal and displays an appropriate affective range. Which of the following is the most likely diagnosis?

    (A) Antisocial personality disorder
    (B) Avoidant personality disorder
    (C) Delusional disorder
    (D) Schizoid personality disorder
    (E) Schizophrenia
    (F) Schizophreniform disorder

ANSWERS

1. **The correct answer is B.** This prospective, observational study is a cohort study. Therefore, the likely unit of measure is the relative risk, which is the risk of a health outcome with a given exposure versus the risk of a health outcome without the exposure. In this case, the relative "risk" of a health outcome is really the relative chance of improvement of symptoms. To calculate the relative "risk," first calculate the chance of improvement with vitamin D supplementation by dividing the number of subjects receiving supplementation whose symptoms improved (50) by the total number of subjects taking vitamin D; this is 50/350. Then calculate the chance of improvement without vitamin D supplementation by dividing the number of subjects not receiving supplementation whose symptoms improved by the total number of subjects not taking vitamin D; this is 60 / 460. The ratio of these values is the relative risk: (50 / 350) / (60 / 460).

   Answer A is incorrect. This value does not appropriately calculate the relative risk with vitamin D supplementation. The value is equivalent to the odds ratio, which is the measure typically used to analyze a retrospective, case-control study.

   Answer C is incorrect. This value does not appropriately calculate the relative risk with vitamin D supplementation. It does not represent any commonly used measure of analysis.

   Answer D is incorrect. This value does not appropriately calculate the relative risk with vitamin D supplementation. Instead, the value is essentially equivalent to the inverse of a calculation for odds ratio, which is not a measure used in data analysis.

   Answer E is incorrect. This value does not appropriately calculate the relative risk of vitamin D supplementation. The value instead calculates the chance of improvement without vitamin D supplementation relative to the chance of improvement with vitamin D supplementation. This is the inverse of what the question asked.

2. **The correct answer is C.** This patient exhibits some of the classic symptoms of narcolepsy, including daytime sleepiness, cataplexy, and sleep paralysis. Cataplexy is defined as brief episodes of bilateral weakness brought on by strong emotions such as laughing or fear, without alteration in consciousness. Sleep paralysis is an episode of partial or total paralysis that occurs at the beginning or end of a sleep cycle. Patients are often aware that they are awake, but may suffer from frightening hallucinations known as hypnagogic when they occur at sleep onset, and hypnopompic when they occur on awakening. Modafinil is an amphetamine derivative used to treat attention deficit/hyperactivity disorder and narcolepsy. Patients suffering from cataplexy and sleep paralysis may also benefit from the initiation of tricyclic antidepressants or selective serotonin reuptake inhibitors.

   Answer A is incorrect. Chloral hydrate is a nonbenzodiazepine hypnotic that is used for sedation and insomnia. This patient does not need help sleeping.

   Answer B is incorrect. Hydroxyzine is a nonselective antihistamine that is used in the treatment of anxiety, pruritus, nausea/vomiting, sedation, and insomnia.

   Answer D is incorrect. Prochlorperazine maleate is a typical antipsychotic used in the treatment of nausea, vomiting, anxiety, and psychosis.

   Answer E is incorrect. Zolpidem is a nonbenzodiazepine hypnotic that is used in the treatment of insomnia.

3. **The correct answer is C.** Transference occurs when a patient projects feelings from his or her personal life onto a doctor; countertransference takes place when the doctor projects feelings onto the patient. These feelings can be either positive or negative. The patient's anger at the doctor when her sexual advances are rebuffed is an example of negative transference.

Answer A is incorrect. The doctor being reminded of his aunt by this patient is an example of countertransference.

Answer B is incorrect. The doctor telling the patient that he is uncomfortable is not an example of countertransference or transference.

Answer D is incorrect. The patient dressing up for appointments is positive transference.

Answer E is incorrect. The patient flirting with the doctor is positive transference. In its most extreme form, positive transference can take the form of sexual desire.

4. **The correct answer is D.** This patient has a history of at least one major depressive episode and at least one hypomanic episode without the presence of mixed or manic episodes, a history consistent with bipolar II disorder. Treatment for this disorder is a mood stabilizer, most commonly lithium. A common adverse effect of this therapy is nephrogenic diabetes insipidus, in which the principal cells of the renal collecting duct are unable to respond to ADH secreted by the posterior pituitary. As a result, the patient will be unable to concentrate urine and will thus experience frequent urination.

   Answer A is incorrect. Agranulocytosis is a toxicity associated with clozapine, an atypical antipsychotic. This medication is generally used in treatment of schizophrenia, but may be used in cases of mania that are unresponsive to first-line drugs such as lithium. Although the patient did have a history of a hypomanic episode, there is no indication for clozapine as a first-line treatment for bipolar II disorder.

   Answer B is incorrect. Anorgasmia is a common adverse effect of selective serotonin reuptake inhibitors. This class of medication, which includes fluoxetine, paroxetine, sertraline, and citalopram, is commonly used in the treatment of major depression. Although this patient has a history of feeling depressed, she also has a history notable for a hypomanic episode. A major depressive episode is diagnosed if the patient has 5/9 symptoms for at least two weeks, including Sleep changes, loss of Interest (anhedonia), Guilt, Energy loss, Concentration changes, Appetite changes, Psychomotor abnormalities, and Suicidal thoughts (**SIG E CAPS**). One of the symptoms has to be depressed mood or anhedonia. Major depressive disorder is diagnosed after a major depressive episode without a history of mania, hypomania, or mixed episodes (when criteria for both manic and major depressive episode are simultaneously present for at least one week), and is further specified by modifiers such as recurrent, chronic, or postpartum onset.

   Answer C is incorrect. Arrhythmias are a well-known adverse effect of the tricyclic antidepressants. This class of medications, which includes imipramine, clomipramine, and amitriptyline, work to block the reuptake of norepinephrine and serotonin. They are commonly used medications in the treatment of major depression, obsessive compulsive disorder, and fibromyalgia. However, the patient in this case has a clinical history most consistent with bipolar II disorder, and thus a mood stabilizer such as lithium should be used rather than an antidepressant, which could lead to further manic episodes in this patient.

   Answer E is incorrect. Stevens-Johnson syndrome is a well-known adverse effect of carbamazepine, an anti-epileptic drug that is sometimes used to treat bipolar disorder. Although this patient has a medical history consistent with bipolar II disorder, first-line treatment is generally with a different mood stabilizer such as lithium, as this medication has been proven effective, is cheaper, and has a relatively less severe adverse-effect profile.

5. **The correct answer is A.** The proper stage sequence of Freud's psychosexual theory is oral, anal, phallic, latency, and genital. Freud's theories of psychosexual development associate pleasure with certain bodily functions. Freud believed that between the ages of 18 months and 3 years, children are preoccupied with anal functions. Encopresis is fecal incontinence and can range from mild to severe.

   Answer B is incorrect. Freud's genital stage encompasses adolescents to adults and is characterized by the desire to achieve sexual gratification.

Answer C is incorrect. Freud's latency stage encompasses the ages of 6-12 years and is characterized by a suppression of sexual desire.

Answer D is incorrect. Freud's oral stage encompasses birth to the age of 18 months. Freud believed that children of this age gain satisfaction from oral functions.

Answer E is incorrect. Freud's phallic stage encompasses the ages of 3-5 years and is most commonly known as the oedipal phase. Freud believed that at this stage children begin to develop sexual fantasies.

6. **The correct answer is F.** This patient has taken phencyclidine, or PCP. Patients with PCP intoxication show signs of belligerence, impulsiveness, fever, psychomotor agitation, vertical and horizontal nystagmus, tachycardia, ataxia, homicidality, psychosis, and delirium. On withdrawal, patients may demonstrate a recurrence of intoxication when the PCP, which was trapped in an ionized form in the acidic gastric lumen, is reabsorbed in the alkaline duodenum. PCP users will have normal or small pupils. Death can result from a variety of causes, including respiratory depression and violent behavior.

   Answer A is incorrect. Patients presenting with acute alcohol intoxication will show symptoms of disinhibition, emotional lability, slurred speech, ataxia, coma, and blackouts. On withdrawal, they will demonstrate a tremor, tachycardia, hypertension, malaise, nausea, seizures, delirium tremens, tremulousness, agitation, and hallucinations.

   Answer B is incorrect. Patients presenting with amphetamine intoxication will display psychomotor agitation, impaired judgment, pupillary dilation, hypertension, tachycardia, euphoria, prolonged wakefulness and attention, cardiac arrhythmias, delusions, hallucinations, and fever. On withdrawal, they will show a post-use "crash" that includes depression, lethargy, headache, stomach cramps, hunger, and hypersomnolence.

   Answer C is incorrect. Patients presenting with acute cocaine intoxication will show symptoms of euphoria, psychomotor agitation, impaired judgment, tachycardia, pupillary dilation, hypertension, hallucinations, paranoid ideations, angina, and sudden cardiac death. On withdrawal, they will show a post-use "crash" that includes severe depression, hypersomnolence, fatigue, malaise, and severe psychological craving.

   Answer D is incorrect. Patients presenting with acute lysergic acid diethylamide intoxication will display marked anxiety or depression, delusions, visual hallucinations, flashbacks, and pupillary dilation.

   Answer E is incorrect. Patients presenting with acute nicotine intoxication will show symptoms of restlessness, insomnia, anxiety, and arrhythmias. On withdrawal, they will have symptoms of irritability, headache, anxiety, weight gain, craving, and tachycardia.

7. **The correct answer is B.** The prevalence is the number of individuals with a disease in a given population at a given time. Prevalence is estimated by test results but is not a measure of a test's validity. In the chart shown, the prevalence can also be determined by calculating the number of true-positive plus false-negative results divided by the total number of patients.

   Answer A is incorrect. This term represents the incidence of positive test results.

   Answer C is incorrect. This represents true-positive results divided by the total number of patients. This would be the percent of true-positive results of all tested, but it is not used very often.

   Answer D is incorrect. This represents true-positive results divided by the total number of patients tested less those with true-positive results, and would not be a meaningful calculation.

   Answer E is incorrect. This represents the number of true-positive results over the total number of patients without disease. This would not be a meaningful calculation.

8. **The correct answer is A.** Malpractice suits require that the patient prove dereliction, damage, and direct harm by a physician with whom there was an established relationship. Direct harm is a concept that the injury is causally related to the actions of the physician. This is also known as proximal cause, and in many cases is the most difficult aspect to prove, as a temporal relationship does not necessarily imply a causal relationship.

   Answer B is incorrect. It is not necessary for the doctor to have been present at the time of injury, but there must be an established relationship between the physician and patient.

   Answer C is incorrect. Intent is not a factor in malpractice proceedings. These proceedings are civil lawsuits, not criminal. As such, when intent or gross misconduct is proven, additional punitive damages may be assessed against the physician.

   Answer D is incorrect. As malpractice suits are civil rather than criminal proceedings, the plaintiff is required only to prove "more likely than not" that the actions of the defendant led to damages.

   Answer E is incorrect. Proof of malpractice requires dereliction, or deviation from standard procedure, that leads to the injury in question.

9. **The correct answer is E.** Spinal muscular atrophy (SMA) is one of the most common autosomal-recessive diseases, affecting approximately one in 10,000 live births. It has a carrier frequency of approximately one in 50 and is characterized by symmetric proximal muscle weakness due to the degeneration of the anterior horn cells of the spinal cord. SMA is classically divided into three subtypes based on age of onset and clinical severity. Type I SMA (Werdnig-Hoffmann disease), the most severe, is characterized by the onset of significant muscle weakness and hypotonia in the first few months of life, and the inability to sit or walk. Manifestations may even occur in utero with reduced fetal movement. Fatal respiratory failure usually occurs before the age of 2 years. Muscle biopsy demonstrates large numbers of atrophic fibers that involve entire fascicles (panfascicular atrophy). Unlike SMA types II and III, this patient's disease developed at an early age, so early milestones were not achieved. This is not the case in the less severe forms of SMA.

   Answer A is incorrect. BMD involves the same genetic locus that is affected in DMD, but its occurrence is less common. It follows a more indolent course, with onset often occurring in late childhood.

   Answer B is incorrect. Duchenne muscular dystrophy (DMD) and Becker muscular dystrophy (BMD) are both characterized by defects in the 427-kDa protein dystrophin, encoded on the Xp21 region. DMD is the most common form of muscular dystrophy, with an incidence of about one in 3500 live births. Onset typically occurs after infancy and before the age of five. The clinical course is characterized by progressive muscle weakness and wasting that lead to wheelchair dependence by 10-12 years of age. Early motor milestones are met in patients with BMD and DMD.

   Answer C is incorrect. Type III spinal muscular atrophy, or Kugelberg-Welander disease, is characterized by the onset of proximal muscle weakness after the age of 2 years, the ability to walk independently until the disease progresses, and survival into adulthood.

   Answer D is incorrect. Type II spinal muscular atrophy is characterized by the onset of proximal muscle weakness before 18 months of age, the ability to sit but not to walk unaided, and survival beyond 4 years of age.

10. **The correct answer is C.** Positive predictive value (PPV) is the probability that a positive test result is truly positive. It can be calculated by taking the number of true-positive results and dividing it by the total positive results. Since the prevalence is 40%, the number of positive patients will be $0.4 \times 1000 = 400$ and the number of negative patients will be $1000 - 400 = 600$. The number of true-positives can be found by multiplying the sensitivity by this total, giving us $0.9 \times 400 = 360$. The number of false-positives can be found by multiplying the specificity by the total negative patients

and subtracting that product from the total negatives, or 600 – (0.85 × 600) = 90. Then, 360 / (360 + 90) = 0.8, or 80%. Remember: PPV and negative predictive value change with prevalence in a population, so the estimated prevalence must be taken into account when calculating the number of true-positives and true-negatives.

Answer A is incorrect. Dividing the number of false-negative results by the total negative results would give an answer of 8%.

Answer B is incorrect. Dividing the number of false-positive (rather than true-positive) findings by the total positive results would give an answer of 20%.

Answer D is incorrect. Switching the values for sensitivity and specificity would give an answer of 85%.

Answer E is incorrect. The negative predictive value is 93%.

11. **The correct answer is F.** As is common for many older patients, this man is taking several prescription medications. Though a couple of his prescriptions should be used with caution with sildenafil (captopril and propranolol), the only one that might significantly interact with sildenafil is sublingual nitroglycerin. Nitroglycerin is used for prompt relief of an ongoing attack of angina precipitated by exercise or emotional stress. Nitrates relax vascular smooth muscle by their intracellular conversion to nitrite ions and then to nitric oxide, which in turn activates cGMP and increases the cell's cGMP level. Elevated cGMP ultimately causes vascular smooth muscle relaxation. This is the same mechanism sildenafil uses to cause smooth muscle relaxation and increased blood flow into the corpus cavernosum at a certain level of sexual stimulation. Using these drugs together can lead to severe hypotension and cardiovascular collapse.

    Answer A is incorrect. Aspirin and sildenafil have no known dangerous interactions.

    Answer B is incorrect. Captopril and sildenafil have no known dangerous interactions, though the combination may increase the risk of hypotension-related adverse effects. However, the captopril is probably contributing to his erectile dysfunction.

    Answer C is incorrect. Fluoxetine and sildenafil have no known dangerous interactions. However, the fluoxetine is probably contributing to his erectile dysfunction.

    Answer D is incorrect. Lovastatin and sildenafil have no known dangerous interactions.

    Answer E is incorrect. Metformin and sildenafil have no known dangerous interactions.

    Answer G is incorrect. Propranolol and sildenafil have no known dangerous interactions, though the combination may increase the risk of hypotension related adverse effects. However, the propranolol may be contributing to his erectile dysfunction.

12. **The correct answer is E.** Emancipation is a legal definition through which minors become independent of their parents and are free to make medical decisions for themselves. A minor, which is a legal condition defined by age, can generally acquire emancipation through court order or marriage. These situations usually suggest that the minor will be financially independent of his or her parents. This patient is married and is therefore emancipated.

    Answer A is incorrect. While this patient has many adult responsibilities, 18 years is the legal age of consent and adulthood.

    Answer B is incorrect. Full-time work suggests that the patient is financially independent, but taken alone it is not proof of emancipation.

    Answer C is incorrect. A high school diploma does not provide emancipation. Even though a minor becomes the primary decision maker after high school graduation, he or she is not necessarily financially independent of the parents.

    Answer D is incorrect. A teenager may state he or she has separated from the parents, but unless the courts have approved a legal separation, merely saying she is "separated" from her parents is not enough; legally the parents are still financially responsible for the child until he or she turns 18.

13. **The correct answer is E.** The study described here is a cohort study, because it includes a group with and a group without a given risk factor (fetal exposure to alcohol) and then looks at whether the risk factor changes the chances of offspring getting the disease (abnormalities). The study is prospective, because the group members are looked at before the disease (abnormality) develops in the offspring. Relative risk can be calculated from the results of a cohort study by comparing the rate of disease in the group with the risk factor to the rate of disease in the group without the risk factor.

Answer A is incorrect. Attributable risk can be calculated from the results of a cohort study and describes the proportion of disease that is due to the risk factor under study. Although smoking behavior of the women is being recorded, the study is not designed to look at the impact of this risk factor on fetal abnormality; the rate of smoking in the two groups of women is unknown, and thus we do not know whether there are sufficient numbers of women in the "exposed" and "unexposed" groups when it comes to tobacco.

Answer B is incorrect. An odds ratio is similar to relative risk, but it is calculated from the results of a case-control study, not from a cohort study. Because birth abnormality is a relatively rare outcome, the odds ratio from a case-control study would likely closely approximate the actual relative risk.

Answer C is incorrect. Prevalence is a measure of how many cases of a given disease exist in a population that is at risk for that disease. This is not the best answer in this case, because there are no data to judge whether this group of 200 women represents the true prevalence of alcoholism during pregnancy in the community.

Answer D is incorrect. The statistic described in this answer is the population attributable risk (PAR), which helps us understand, in a given population, how much less common a disease (fetal abnormality) would be if a given risk factor (alcohol consumption during pregnancy) were completely eliminated. To calculate PAR, the attributable risk is multiplied by the prevalence of the risk factor in the population, which would not be known in this study.

14. **The correct answer is B.** Tanner stage 3 is the stage when most girls experience peak height velocity. Peak height velocity occurs approximately one year after the initiation of breast development. Also, pubic hair becomes dark and curly during this stage.

Answer A is incorrect. This description corresponds to Tanner stage 1.

Answer C is incorrect. This description corresponds to Tanner stage 5.

Answer D is incorrect. This description corresponds to Tanner stage 4.

Answer E is incorrect. This description corresponds to Tanner stage 2.

15. **The correct answer is D.** Obtaining informed consent from the patient means that the patient understands the risks, benefits, and alternatives to the study, and that the doctor relays to the patient pertinent matters about the plan of care. For the non-English-speaking patient, the consent is translated into the appropriate language and discussed with him/her through an interpreter. This allows the patient (or in this case, his parents) freedom to read and process the consent and to discuss it later. Whereas this option may not be possible for every language or reasonable for every study, it is appropriate in this non-emergent situation.

Answer A is incorrect. With limited knowledge of Spanish, the doctor will unlikely be able to address all the important issues delineated in the consent form.

Answer B is incorrect. Having someone other than an interpreter translate will be invading patient privacy, incomplete, and not perfectly accurate/reliable.

Answer C is incorrect. In a non-emergent setting, the best approach is to allow the patient/family to view a translated copy of the consent and consider all their options in an unbiased manner. The use of an interpreter, however, would be invaluable in an emergent setting.

Answer E is incorrect. The patient is too young to give consent (<18 years).

16. **The correct answer is A.** Heart disease is the leading cause of death among the elderly (65 years old and older), as well as the leading cause of death if all ages are combined. The patient is at a particularly high risk for subsequent cardiac events due to his previous history of myocardial infarction. Other major risk factors for cardiac events are high blood pressure, hypercholesterolemia, and diabetes mellitus.

    Answer B is incorrect. Cancer is the second most common cause of death. It ranks after heart disease, but before stroke.

    Answer C is incorrect. Motor vehicle crashes, and accidents in general, are leading causes of death. However, they are the most common cause of death among children (1-14 years old) and adolescents (15-24 years old) and not among the elderly.

    Answer D is incorrect. Stroke is the third most common cause of death among the elderly, behind heart disease and then cancer.

    Answer E is incorrect. Suicide is not the leading cause of death in the elderly. It is a common cause of death among adolescents.

17. **The correct answer is A.** The mechanism of denial is when one fails to recognize the obvious implications or consequences of a thought, act, or situation. This ego defense mechanism is often seen in patients with recently diagnosed HIV or cancer.

    Answer B is incorrect. Displacement is a defense mechanism whereby ideas and feelings that a patient wishes to avoid are transferred to another person or object; for example, a patient who yells at the nurse because he is angry at news he has just received from the doctor.

    Answer C is incorrect. Projection is the process of attributing one's thoughts or impulses, usually ones that are unacceptable or undesirable, to another person.

    Answer D is incorrect. Rationalization produces a more socially acceptable and apparently more or less logical explanation for an act or decision actually produced by unconscious impulses. This patient's assertion that he "feels fine, anyway" may be a form of rationalization, but the primary ego defense mechanism that he is using is denial.

    Answer E is incorrect. Repression is the unconscious exclusion of a painful or anxiety-provoking thought, impulse, or memory from awareness.

18. **The correct answer is E.** This is a typical well-child visit. Other milestones reached at approximately this age include stacking nine blocks, riding a tricycle, and beginning to engage in group play. Riding a tricycle at 3 years is easy to remember because a tricycle has three wheels. The number of blocks stacked between ages 2 and 4 years is about three times the child's age in years; that is, a 2-year-old can stack six blocks, whereas a 3-year-old can stack nine blocks.

    Answer A is incorrect. Engaging in cooperative play is achieved between 4 and 5 years of age.

    Answer B is incorrect. Imaginary friends are typically present between 4 and 5 years of age.

    Answer C is incorrect. Hopping on one foot is typical of a 4-year-old child.

    Answer D is incorrect. Reading is most often learned at 5-6 years of age and older.

    Answer F is incorrect. Children at 2 years of age can usually stack six blocks, whereas children at 3 years can stack nine blocks.

19. **The correct answer is B.** A retrospective cohort study includes a group of subjects who had a certain condition or received a certain treatment at some time in the past and compares their outcomes to those of another group (a control group) made up of subjects who did not have this condition or receive the treatment. In this study the risk factor is the presence of diabetes in the mothers and the outcome is LGA babies. The incidence of LGA births in women with diabetes is four times that in women without diabetes. Relative risk is

defined as the incidence rate of some outcome in those exposed to a risk factor divided by the incidence rate of those not exposed. This definition gives the factor at which the incidence rate of LGA among women with diabetes is larger than the incidence rate of LGA among women without diabetes.

Answer A is incorrect. This choice describes the correct type of risk analysis but describes the relationship in reverse.

Answer C is incorrect. This choice reverses the findings of the study, which shows that the incidence of LGA is four times more in women with diabetes.

Answer D is incorrect. This choice incorrectly uses odds rather than incidence rates and also describes the relationship of the findings of the study in reverse.

Answer E is incorrect. This choice describes an odds ratio for a case-control study. A case-control study evaluates the presence of risk factors in people with and without a disease. Although this is the opposite of a cohort study, the results are still reported in terms of disease presence with respect to risk factors; that is, the presence or absence of disease is categorized in the group with risk factors and compared to the group without risk factors. The difference, however, is that odds are used rather than incidence. The incidence rate is a percentage (eg, 50 out of 100). Odds are calculated by dividing those with disease by those without (50 to 50, or 1 to 1).

20. **The correct answer is C.** Delusional disorder is diagnosed following one month of nonbizarre delusions that are usually focused around a particular topic, in this case, the fidelity of the patient's wife. The delusions are not attributable to another psychiatric disorder such as schizophrenia. Delusional disorder does not markedly impair the person's functioning in daily activities. The ramifications are limited to the delusional content.

Answer A is incorrect. Cluster B personality disorders include antisocial, borderline, histrionic, and narcissistic types. Patients with antisocial personality disorder show a disregard for and often violate the rights of others. These individuals often have a criminal history. This is the only personality disorder with an age limit (18 years). Minors with similar behavior are classified as having conduct disorder.

Answer B is incorrect. Cluster C personality disorders are characterized by anxiety and include avoidant, obsessive-compulsive, and dependent personality types. Individuals with avoidant personality disorder are sensitive to rejection, are socially inhibited, and have overwhelming feelings of inadequacy.

Answer D is incorrect. Patients with schizoid personality disorder exhibit voluntary social withdrawal (unlike avoidant patients) and have limited emotional expressions. They lack strange beliefs and thoughts of the schizotypal personality disorder.

Answer E is incorrect. Schizophrenia is a chronic psychiatric condition. It affects 1% of the population and usually begins before age 25. The *Diagnostic and Statistical Manual of Mental Disorders*, Fourth Edition, specifies the active phase of the disease and requires that at least two of the following symptoms be present during a one-month period: delusions, hallucinations, disorganized speech, grossly disorganized or catatonic behavior, and negative symptoms (eg, flat affect, lack of motivation, or poverty of speech). Moreover, signs of the disturbance must be present for at least six months, such as one of the above symptoms in an attenuated form (eg, magical thinking, social withdrawal, or other negative symptoms).

Answer F is incorrect. Schizophreniform disorder is similar to schizophrenia except that its symptoms have lasted between one and six months. In contrast, patients with schizophrenia must have had symptoms for longer than six months.

CHAPTER 2

Biochemistry

QUESTIONS

1. A 6-year-old boy presents to his pediatrician with skin lesions all over his body. For several years he has been very sensitive to sunlight. Neither the boy's parents nor his siblings have the same skin lesions or sun sensitivity. Biopsies of several of the boy's lesions reveal squamous cell carcinoma. Which mutation would one expect to see in this patient's DNA?

    (A) Methylation of the gene
    (B) Missense mutation in the gene
    (C) Nonsense mutation in the middle of the gene
    (D) Point mutation within the enhancer region
    (E) Point mutation within the operator region
    (F) Point mutation within the promoter region
    (G) Thymidine dimers

2. A metabolic process is pictured below. Which intermediate in this process inhibits the rate-limiting enzyme of glycolysis and activates the rate-limiting enzyme of fatty acid synthesis?

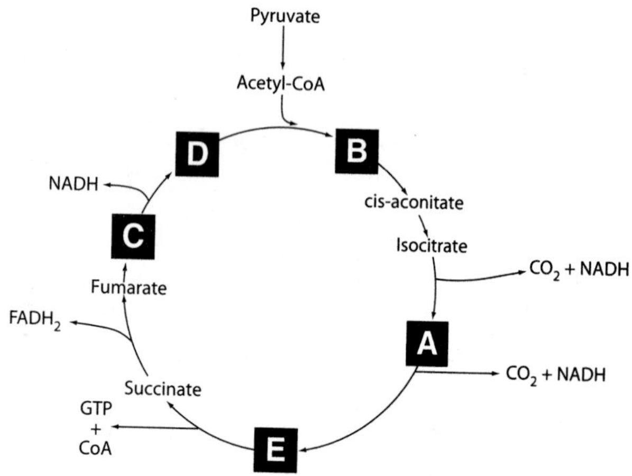

Reproduced, with permission, from USMLERx.com.

    (A) A
    (B) B
    (C) C
    (D) D
    (E) E

3. A 54-year-old woman complains of fatigue, difficulty climbing stairs, and weight loss. Her medical history is notable for hypertension. She takes no medications. Her skin is moist and she has a prominent stare. The patient's vital signs are:

    Heart rate: 112/min
    Blood pressure: 143/90 mm/Hg
    Respiratory rate: 14/min
    Oxygen saturation: 98% on room air

    Laboratory tests reveal markedly elevated levels of a specific hormone. What is the first molecule produced within a cell in response to this hormone?

    (A) Carbohydrate
    (B) DNA
    (C) Fatty acid
    (D) Protein
    (E) RNA

4. A 35-year-old man presents to the physician with arthritic pain in both knees along with back pain. He states that the pain has been present for months. In an effort to obtain relief, he has taken only aspirin, but this has been of little benefit. The patient is afebrile, and his slightly swollen knee joints are neither hot nor tender to palpation; however, the pain does restrict his motion. The cartilage of his ears appears slightly darker than normal. No tophi are present. A urine specimen is taken for analysis of uric acid content and turns black in the laboratory while standing. A defect in which of the following is the most likely underlying cause of the patient's condition?

    (A) α-Ketoacid dehydrogenase
    (B) Galactokinase
    (C) Homogentisic acid oxidase
    (D) Orotate phosphoribosyl transferase
    (E) Phenylalanine hydroxylase

5. A patient who is a carrier of sickle cell trait presents to the clinic. The single base-pair mutation for sickle cell anemia destroys the MstII restriction enzyme recognition site represented by an asterisk in the image. The restriction enzyme-binding sites are shown as arrows on the map. DNA from this patient is treated with MstII and run on an electrophoresis gel. The DNA is then hybridized with a labeled probe that binds to the normal gene in the position shown on the map. In the Southern blot shown in the image, which lane represents the patient?

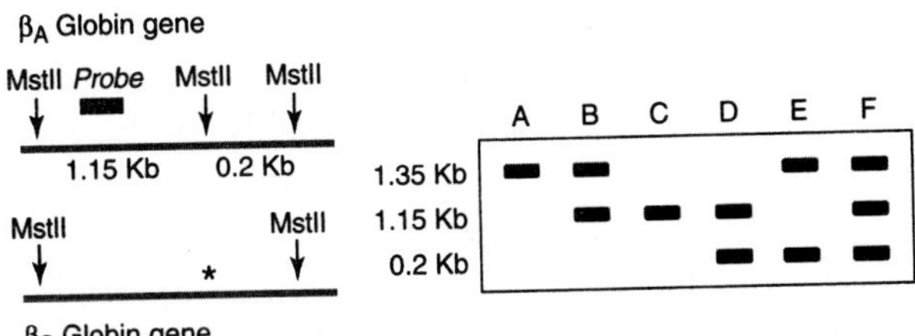

Reproduced, with permission, from USMLERx.com.

(A) A
(B) B
(C) C
(D) D
(E) E
(F) F

6. A 57-year-old woman visits her primary care physician. Laboratory studies reveal an LDL of 194 mg/dL and HDL of 41 mg/dL. Her physician begins therapy with a drug that inhibits production of mevalonic acid. Which of the following is a common side effect of this therapy?

(A) Hepatomegaly without elevations in aspartate aminotransferase or alanine aminotransferase
(B) Muscle injury clinically similar to myositis
(C) Spontaneous abortion of a pregnancy
(D) Suicidality and homicidality in patients with bipolar disorder
(E) Tonic-clonic seizures

7. A nucleic acid fragment is added to four different tubes along with a polymerase, a radiolabeled primer, and deoxynucleotides. Each tube also contains one of the four bases as dideoxynucleotides. The four tubes are then run on electrophoresis gel and visualized by autoradiography. For which of the following purposes would the described laboratory technique be utilized?

(A) To amplify DNA fragments
(B) To create an allele-specific oligonucleotide probe
(C) To decipher the order of nitrogenous bases in the human genome
(D) To determine the base pairing of a segment of DNA with a DNA probe
(E) To determine the base pairing of a segment of RNA with a DNA probe
(F) To establish the presence of a given protein
(G) To show the presence of a specific antibody in plasma

8. A 45-year-old white woman presents to her physician complaining of several months of worsening shortness of breath. Previously she was told she had asthma because she was having intermittent episodes of wheezing combined with a productive cough and difficulty catching her breath. She used to run two miles every morning but can no longer walk more than 10 city blocks without stopping. She has never smoked. On physical examination she is using her accessory muscles to assist with respiration. Pulmonary examination is notable for an increased decreased FEV_1/FVC ratio, decreased air movement with each breath, and increased resonance upon percussion. X-ray of the chest is shown in the image. Which of the following is the most likely underlying cause for this patient's disease?

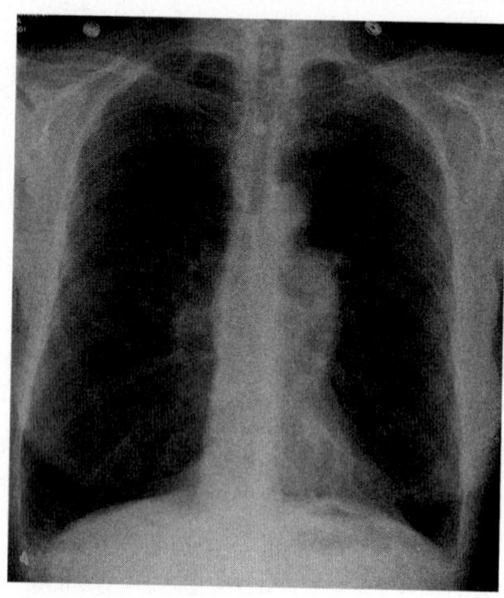

Courtesy of Dr. James Heilman.

(A) A genetic mutation resulting in deficient levels of a protease
(B) A genetic mutation resulting in deficient levels of a protease inhibitor
(C) A mutation in the *p53* gene
(D) A mutation of the *CFTR* gene, which encodes a regulated chloride channel
(E) Airway inflammation, airflow obstruction, and bronchial hyperresponsiveness

9. As increased intracellular calcium is detrimental to the cell, calcium homeostasis is tightly regulated both across the cell membrane and within the cell via sequestration in the endoplasmic reticulum and mitochondria. In which of the following ways does increased intracellular calcium concentration cause the most cell damage?

(A) Enzyme activation
(B) Free radical generation
(C) Increased membrane permeability
(D) Inhibition of glycolysis
(E) Inhibition of oxidative phosphorylation

10. A scientist working in a research laboratory has been examining different agonists of serotonin receptor 1B (5-HT_{1B}), a G-protein-coupled receptor. Compound A has a much higher affinity for 5-HT_{1B} than compound B. Both compounds have a higher affinity for the receptor than serotonin. Which of the following describes the relationship between compound A and compound B when considering the guanine-nucleotide exchange activity of 5-HT_{1B}?

(A) K_m for the exchange reaction with compound A is higher than that with compound B
(B) K_m for the exchange reaction with compound A is lower than that with compound B
(C) K_m values with compounds A and B are the same
(D) The maximum reaction rate with compound A is greater than that with compound B
(E) The maximum reaction rate with compound B is greater than that with compound A

11. A mother brings her 6-month-old son to the pediatrician. She has noticed that he seems "afraid of light" and, after some Internet research, she is concerned that he might be an albino. Laboratory analysis reveals uroporphyrin in his urine. The child most likely has which of the following conditions?

(A) Deficiency of coproporphyrinogen oxidase
(B) Deficiency of porphobilinogen deaminase
(C) Deficiency of uroporphyrinogen decarboxylase

(D) Inhibition of ferrochelatase and δ-aminolevulinic acid dehydrase
(E) Overexpression of porphobilinogen deaminase

12. A 48-year-old woman of Mediterranean descent presents because of fatigue, arthralgias, discomfort in her right upper abdominal quadrant, and polyuria. Laboratory tests are remarkable for elevated glucose level, elevated bilirubin, low hemoglobin, elevated reticulocytes, and increased transferrin saturation. Cardiac testing shows moderate restrictive cardiomyopathy. She frequently has required blood transfusions throughout her life. Which hereditary disorder does this patient most likely have?

    (A) Absence of the hemoglobin α-chain
    (B) Absence of the hemoglobin β-chain
    (C) Mutation resulting in increased absorption of dietary iron
    (D) Mutations in the gene encoding ankyrin
    (E) Mutations resulting in copper accumulation

13. A 52-year-old man with a 12-year history of poorly controlled diabetes mellitus presents to his physician complaining of changes in his vision. Physical examination reveals opacities on the lens of the eye similar to those seen in this image. Which enzyme most likely contributed to this complication?

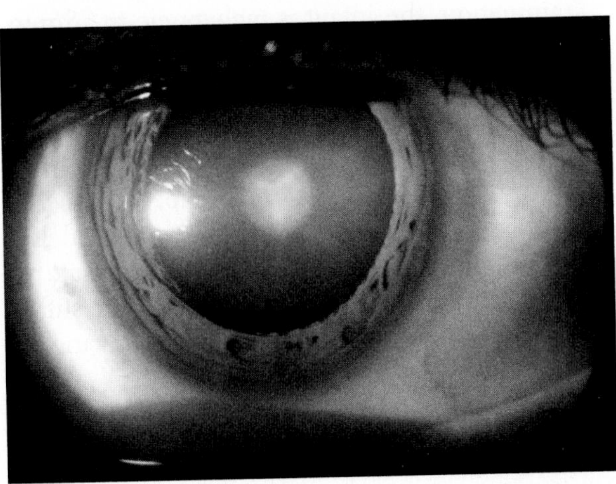

Courtesy of Dr. Rakesh Ahuja.

    (A) 3-Hydroxy-3-methylglutaryl coenzyme A reductase
    (B) Adenosine deaminase
    (C) Aldose reductase
    (D) Galactose-1-phosphate uridyltransferase
    (E) Hexokinase
    (F) Insulin-like growth factor

14. Acquired mutation in the *p53* gene is the most common genetic alteration found in human cancer (> 50% of all cancers). A germline mutation in *p53* is the causative lesion of Li-Fraumeni familial cancer syndrome. In many tumors, one *p53* allele on chromosome 17p is deleted and the other is mutated. What type of protein is encoded by the *p53* gene?

    (A) Caspase
    (B) DNA repair enzyme
    (C) Membrane cell adhesion molecule
    (D) Serine phosphatase
    (E) Telomerase
    (F) Transcription factor
    (G) Tyrosine kinase

15. A segment of DNA is isolated and added to a mixture of four deoxynucleotides, two specific oligonucleotide sequences, and heat-stable DNA polymerase. The mixture is then heated to denature the DNA, cooled, and reheated in a number of cycles. Which of the following laboratory techniques does this describe?

    (A) Enzyme-linked immunosorbent assay
    (B) Gel electrophoresis
    (C) Northern blot
    (D) Polymerase chain reaction
    (E) Sequencing
    (F) Southern blot
    (G) Western blot

16. A 32-year-old woman presents to her physician for the third time in six months. She has been feeling very tired and depressed, and has come to talk about starting antidepressants. She also complains of a 4.5-kg (10-lb) weight gain over the past three months. During her physical examination the physician notices that she is wearing a sweater and a coat, despite the room being at a warm temperature. Problems with the thyroid are suspected, and a biopsy is performed (see image). This woman may have a human leukocyte antigen subtype that also increases her risk of which disease?

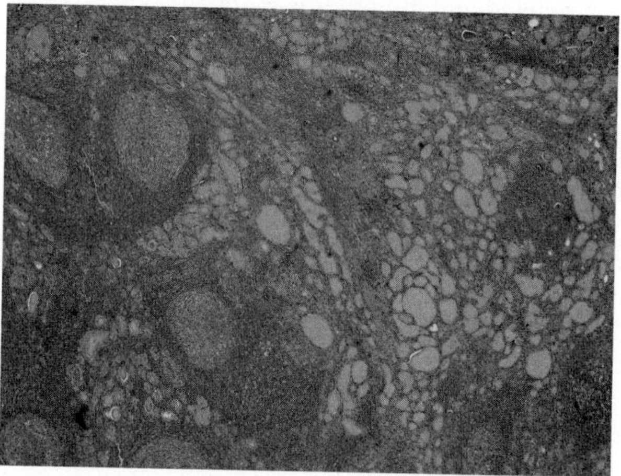

Reproduced, with permission, from USMLERx.com.

(A) Multiple sclerosis
(B) Pernicious anemia
(C) Psoriasis
(D) Steroid-responsive nephrotic syndrome

17. A 65-year-old woman who has been in the hospital for three weeks receiving cefotaxime to treat *Klebsiella* pneumonia develops a urinary tract infection. Urine cultures are positive for *Enterococcus faecium*. Treatment with vancomycin is attempted but is unsuccessful. Which of the following aided in this microorganism's ability to persist despite vancomycin treatment?

(A) Alteration of microorganism's gyrase
(B) Methylation of microorganism's rRNA at a ribosome-binding site
(C) Microorganism's ability to produce β-lactamase
(D) Mutation in terminal amino acid of microorganism's cell wall component
(E) Mutation in the microorganism's penicillin-binding protein

18. A 2-year-old boy presents to the pediatrician with fever, facial tenderness, and a green, foul-smelling nasal discharge. The patient is diagnosed with sinusitis, and the physician notes that he has a history of recurrent episodes of sinusitis. X-ray of the chest is ordered because of the fever; it reveals some dilated bronchi and shows the heart situated on the right side of his body. A congenital disorder is diagnosed. Which other finding would this patient be most likely to have?

(A) Defective chloride transport
(B) Elevated blood sugar
(C) Infertility
(D) Reactive airway disease
(E) Tetralogy of Fallot

19. A 5-day-old boy is brought to the emergency department after a tonic-clonic seizure at home. The infant is the product of a full-term, uneventful pregnancy, and was normal until two days prior to presentation. The mother reports irritability and poor feeding at home, and the infant was difficult to rouse this morning before suffering the seizure. On physical examination, the infant is tachypneic to 75/min, has icteric sclerae, and has poor muscle tone throughout. Laboratory studies show the following levels: plasma ammonia, 300 μmol/L (normal = 10-40 μmol/L); blood urea nitrogen, 1.5 mg/dL; and creatinine, 0.4 mg/dL. A plasma amino acid analysis fails to detect citrulline. Urine amino acids demonstrate elevated orotic acid levels. This patient suffers from a deficiency of which of the following enzymes?

(A) α-Galactosidase A
(B) Aldose B
(C) Galactose 1-phosphate uridylyltransferase
(D) Lysosomal α-glucosidase
(E) Ornithine transcarbamylase

20. A 42-year-old woman presents to her physician with generalized itching. Physical examination reveals scleral icterus. Laboratory tests show:

Total bilirubin: 2.7 mg/dL
Conjugated bilirubin: 2.4 mg/dL
Alkaline phosphatase: 253 U/L
Aspartate aminotransferase: 36 U/L
Alanine aminotransferase: 40 U/L

What is the most likely mechanism underlying this patient's jaundice?

(A) Absence of UDP-glucuronyl transferase
(B) Decreased levels of UDP-glucuronyl transferase
(C) Extravascular destruction of the patient's RBCs
(D) Intrahepatic or extrahepatic biliary obstruction
(E) Intravascular destruction of the patient's RBCs

21. A 5-year-old boy was playing outside during recess when he began to experience difficulty breathing. He was brought to his physician, because his symptoms seemed to be getting worse. On examination, the physician notes that the boy is struggling to breathe and hears diffuse wheezing bilaterally. The boy's heart rate is 98/min, respiratory rate is 24/min, and oxygen saturation is 90%. His medical history is significant only for seasonal allergies and mild eczema. Which type of medication will alleviate this patient's respiratory symptoms?

(A) β_1 Antagonist
(B) β_1 Agonist
(C) β_2 Agonist
(D) Histamine$_1$ agonist
(E) Histamine$_2$ agonist

22. An 8-month-old boy is brought to the pediatrician by his parents because he has recently lost the ability to crawl or hold his toys. On examination the patient is tachypneic and breathing with considerable effort; the liver is palpable five finger widths below the right costal margin. X-ray of the chest reveals cardiomegaly. He has a difficult time sitting upright and cannot squeeze the physician's fingers or the ring of his pacifier with any noticeable force. Despite a number of interventions, the child's symptoms continue to worsen until his death two weeks later. On autopsy, it is likely that this patient's cells will contain an accumulation of which of the following substances?

(A) Glucose
(B) Glycogen
(C) Oxaloacetate
(D) Pyruvate
(E) Urea

23. After consumption of a carbohydrate-rich meal, the liver continues to convert glucose to glucose-6-phosphate. The liver's ability to continue this processing of high levels of glucose is important in minimizing increases in blood glucose after eating. What is the best explanation for the liver's ability to continue this conversion after eating a carbohydrate-rich meal?

(A) The hepatocyte cell membrane's permeability for glucose-6-phosphate
(B) The high maximum reaction rate of glucokinase
(C) The high maximum reaction rate of hexokinase
(D) The high Michaelis-Menten constant of hexokinase
(E) The low Michaelis-Menten constant of glucokinase

24. A 30-year-old man is diagnosed with type I familial dyslipidemia. Recent laboratory studies show an elevated triglyceride level but normal LDL and HDL cholesterol levels. Which of the following explains the pathophysiology of this disease?

(A) Apolipoprotein E deficiency
(B) LDL cholesterol receptor deficiency
(C) Lipoprotein lipase deficiency
(D) VLDL cholesterol clearance deficiency
(E) VLDL cholesterol overproduction

25. A 59-year-old woman with history of morbid obesity, hypercholesterolemia, and diabetes mellitus presents to the emergency department with complaints of substernal chest pain lasting two hours. An ECG reveals ST elevations in the lateral leads. The troponin level at admission is extremely elevated, and a creatine kinase-myocardial bound test is pending. Which of the following is a key cell mediator in the pathogenesis of an atherosclerotic plaque?

(A) γ-Interferon
(B) Complement
(C) Interleukin-6
(D) Natural killer cells
(E) Platelet-derived growth factor

26. A 53-year-old man presents to his physician, because he has blood in his urine and some low back pain. A gross specimen of kidneys from a patient with the same condition is shown in the image. Which of the following also is associated with this disorder?

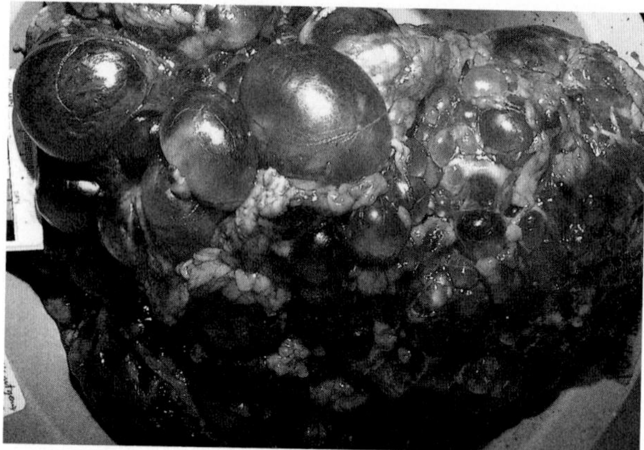

Reproduced, with permission, from USMLERx.com.

(A) Astrocytomas
(B) Berry aneurysm
(C) Ectopic lens
(D) Optic nerve degeneration
(E) Squamous cell carcinoma

27. At a routine check-up, a 7-year-old boy is found to have osteoporosis. The patient is tall and thin with pale skin, fair hair, and flushed cheeks. He has arachnodactyly, pes cavus, and bilaterally dislocated lenses, and demonstrates developmental delay with mild mental retardation. His mother is told that her child might benefit from folic acid supplementation. Which is the most appropriate test to confirm the diagnosis?

(A) Enzymatic assay for the enzyme HGPRT
(B) Genetic studies demonstrating a mutation in type I collagen
(C) Genetic studies indicating >200 copies of the CGG trinucleotide repeat on the X chromosome
(D) Nitroblue tetrazolium test
(E) Nitroprusside cyanide test

28. A 6-year-old boy is brought to his pediatrician's office by his parents, who report that the child has been unusually thirsty for the past week. He also has increased urinary frequency and has wet the bed three times in the past two weeks. A random blood glucose level is 215 mg/dL. The pediatrician suspects that the child has type 1 diabetes mellitus caused by autoimmune destruction of insulin-producing pancreatic β cells. Which of the following is the transporter for glucose to enter pancreatic β cells?

(A) GLUT 1
(B) GLUT 2
(C) GLUT 4
(D) Simple diffusion

29. Hemoglobin consists of four polypeptide subunits: two α subunits and two β subunits. The arrangement of these subunits shifts between a taut and relaxed conformation, resulting in changes in hemoglobin's oxygen affinity. At a given partial pressure of oxygen, which of the following will decrease hemoglobin's affinity for oxygen?

(A) Decreasing the partial pressure of carbon dioxide
(B) Increasing the amount of 2,3-bisphosphoglycerate in RBCs
(C) Increasing the number of oxygen molecules bound to a hemoglobin from one to three

(D) Increasing the pH by moving from peripheral tissue to lung
(E) The presence of excess carbon monoxide

30. A 15-year-old boy presents with prolonged fatigue and mild jaundice following a serious infection. Blood tests reveal hemoglobin of 10.5 g/dL and an elevated reticulocyte count. A peripheral blood smear reveals Heinz bodies. Which of the following best describes the normal action associated with this patient's metabolic defect?

(A) To generate glucose-6-phosphate in all cells
(B) To generate glucose-6-phosphate in RBCs only
(C) To generate mucopolysaccharides
(D) To regenerate reduced nicotinamide adenine dinucleotide phosphate in all cells
(E) To regenerate reduced nicotinamide adenine dinucleotide phosphate in RBCs only

31. Hyperparathyroidism is a common manifestation of several distinct genetic disorders that predispose to endocrine gland neoplasia and cause hormone excess syndromes. Which of the following is a consequence of parathyroid hormone?

(A) Increase calcium absorption in the small intestine
(B) Inhibit the production of 1,25-dihydroxyvitamin D
(C) Promote calcium excretion in the renal tubules
(D) Stimulate further secretion of parathyroid hormone
(E) Stimulate phosphate reabsorption in the renal tubules

32. A 22-year-old woman presents to the hospital with severe abdominal pain, abdominal distention, and ileus, along with peripheral neuropathy. Her boyfriend notes that she has been acting strange lately, and that she "seems like a different person." Which of the following enzymes is deficient in this patient?

(A) Adenosine deaminase
(B) Homogentisic acid oxidase
(C) Lysosomal α-1,4-glucosidase
(D) Ornithine transcarbamylase
(E) Porphobilinogen deaminase

33. A 2-year-old boy is brought by his parents to the emergency department after the discovery of blood in a wet diaper. The physician palpates an abdominal mass in the right flank. CT of the abdomen reveals a large tumor invading the right kidney; the gross specimen is shown in the image. Cytogenetic analysis of the tumor cells reveals a deletion of chromosome 11p. Which of the following is the most likely diagnosis?

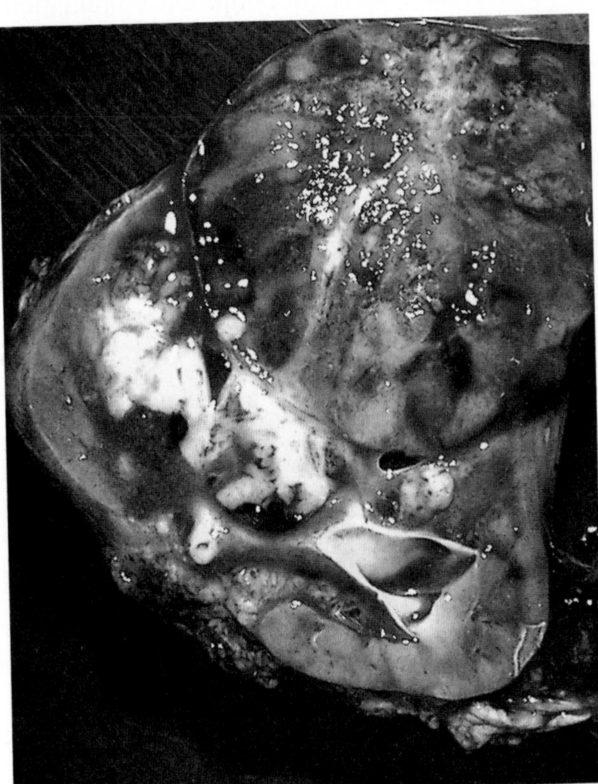

Reproduced, with permission, from USMLERx.com.

(A) Adrenocortical adenoma
(B) Neuroblastoma
(C) Renal cell carcinoma
(D) Transitional cell carcinoma
(E) Wilms tumor

34. A 6-year-old boy is diagnosed with a worsening ataxic gait and a cardiac dysrhythmia. His uncle also has this condition, but his symptoms did not appear until he was 12 years of age. What is the molecular mechanism of this disease?

    (A) Unstable repeats affect protein folding
    (B) Unstable repeats affect protein splicing
    (C) Unstable repeats cause an amino acid substitution
    (D) Unstable repeats impede protein translation
    (E) Unstable repeats result in a truncated protein

35. A 3-month-old child is brought to his pediatrician's office for a check-up. On examination, the physician notices that he has a social smile, but does not hold his head up on his own or make noises. The infant also has pale skin, eczema, odd odor, and hyperreflexia. What is the most appropriate treatment for the condition the infant most likely has?

    (A) A diet low in isoleucine and leucine
    (B) A diet low in phenylalanine
    (C) A diet low in tyrosine
    (D) A high-protein diet
    (E) Recombinant enzyme therapy

36. A 63-year-old man who is an alcoholic is brought into the emergency department by his daughter. She states that the patient's memory has been very poor, and he constantly creates elaborate yet untrue stories. Physical examination reveals ataxia and bilateral horizontal nystagmus. Wernicke-Korsakoff syndrome, caused by a water-soluble vitamin deficiency, is suspected. Which of the following conditions is also a result of a water-soluble vitamin deficiency?

    (A) Increased erythrocyte hemolysis
    (B) Neonatal hemorrhage
    (C) Night blindness
    (D) Osteomalacia
    (E) Pellagra

37. A term child is delivered by spontaneous vaginal delivery without complications. Upon physical examination the child has bilateral hip dislocations, restricted movement in shoulder and elbow joints, and coarse facial features. Laboratory studies show that the activities of β-hexosaminidase, iduronate sulfatase, and arylsulfatase A are deficient in cultured fibroblasts, but are 20 times normal in the patient's serum. The primary abnormality in this disorder is associated with which of the following organelles?

    (A) Golgi apparatus
    (B) Lysosomes
    (C) Ribosomes
    (D) Rough endoplasmic reticulum
    (E) Smooth endoplasmic reticulum

38. Patients with albinism appear white-pink (skin color), have white hair, and have nonpigmented or blue irises. In many cases, these individuals may have melanocytes, but lack melanin in their skin. What is the most useful advice to give to a guardian of a child diagnosed with albinism?

    (A) To avoid foods with lactose
    (B) To avoid foods with phenylalanine
    (C) To avoid strenuous activity
    (D) To give growth hormone to help the child grow to a normal height
    (E) To wear clothing and sunscreen that protect from the sun when outside

39. A 65-year-old African-American man presents to his physician because of jaundice. He says that in the past few months he has not had much of an appetite and has lost 13.6 kg (30 lb). Physical examination is notable for a gallbladder that is palpable. What set of characteristics is expected in this patient?

Choice	Type of hyperbilirubinemia	Urine bilirubin	Urine urobilinogen
A	conjugated	↑	normal
B	conjugated	↑	↓
C	unconjugated	↑	↓
D	unconjugated	↓	↑
E	unconjugated	↓	↓

Reproduced, with permission, from USMLERx.com.

(A) A
(B) B
(C) C
(D) D
(E) E

40. A 3-year-old boy recently developed weakness of his lower extremity and uses his arms to stand up even though his lower legs appear quite muscular. Laboratory tests reveal a creatine kinase level of 20,000 U/L. A DNA test confirms the working diagnosis. What is the function of the altered gene product in this patient?

(A) Exocytosis of acetylcholine at the neuromuscular junction
(B) Linking actin filaments to laminin
(C) Promoting actin-myosin cross-bridge cycling
(D) Receptor for acetylcholine
(E) Release of calcium from the sarcoplasmic reticulum

41. A 55-year-old man is found unresponsive and breathing rapidly in his apartment. His daughter found him while stopping by to visit. She stated that she was concerned after he told her on the phone that he was "drowning his sorrows," having been fired from his job earlier that day. He has no significant medical history other than moderate hypertension, for which he takes a β-blocker. Relevant laboratory findings are:

Na^+: 135 mEq/L
K^+: 4.5 mEq/L
Cl^-: 95 mEq/L
HCO_3^-: 9 mEq/L
Glucose: 40 mEq/L
Serum pH: 6.8
Lactate: 9.5 mmoL/L

What metabolic process induced this patient's current condition?

(A) Decreased levels of glycerol 3-phosphate
(B) Elevated pyruvate levels
(C) Inappropriate induction of gluconeogenesis
(D) Overproduction of reduced nicotinamide adenine dinucleotide
(E) Thiamine deficiency

42. A 78-year-old man with asthma presents to his primary care physician for an annual checkup. The physician performs a physical examination and orders routine blood work, which reveals a macrocytic anemia. Subsequent laboratory tests show an elevated serum methylmalonic acid level. A peripheral blood smear is shown in the image. If this patient's vitamin deficiency is not corrected, what neurological symptoms is he most likely to experience?

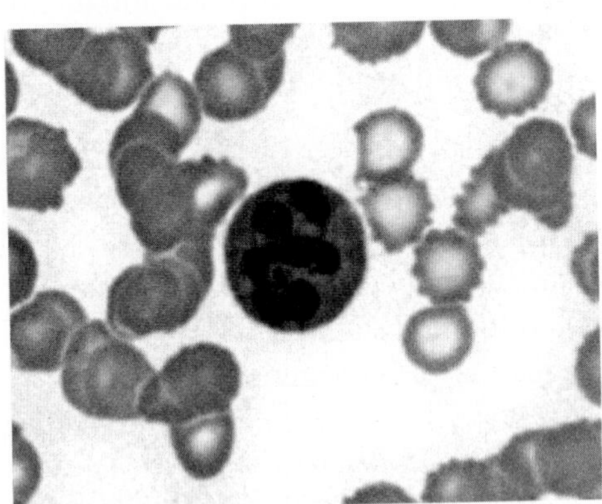

Reproduced, with permission, from USMLERx.com.

(A) Confusion and confabulation
(B) Deficiency in this vitamin does not cause neurological symptoms
(C) Dysarthria and diplopia
(D) Paresthesias and ataxia
(E) Syncope and lethargy

43. A young woman currently being treated for HIV is brought to the emergency department because of a headache and cyanosis of her nail beds and lips. She also reports feeling dizzy. The resident on call immediately places her on supplemental oxygen and draws blood for arterial blood gas analysis. While drawing the blood, he notes that the arterial blood has a dark brown color. Blood gas analysis reveals a pH of 7.39, partial oxygen pressure of 96 mm Hg, partial carbon dioxide pressure of 35 mm Hg, and oxygen saturation of 82% on room air. What enzyme is primarily responsible for preventing this condition in the normal adult?

(A) ATPase
(B) Flavin adenine dinucleotide reductase
(C) GTPase
(D) Lactase
(E) Nicotinamide adenine dinucleotide reductase
(F) Pyruvate kinase

44. A mass is felt in the groin of an infant girl during a physical examination. Surgical resection shows that it is a testicle. The baby is diagnosed with testicular feminization syndrome. In this syndrome, androgens are produced but cells fail to respond to the steroid hormones because they lack appropriate intracellular receptors. After binding intracellular receptors, steroids regulate the rate of which of the following?

(A) Initiation of protein synthesis
(B) mRNA degradation
(C) mRNA processing
(D) Protein translation
(E) Transcription of genes

45. The wife in an Ashkenazi Jewish family brings her 1-year-old daughter to the pediatrician. Her previous pregnancy was uneventful and resulted in a full-term healthy girl who is now 4 years old. Her younger daughter, however, has demonstrated a progressive series of behaviors over the first year of life. Her motor skills have diminished and she demonstrates an increased startle reaction. Physical examination is notable only for the ocular findings shown in the image. Deficiency of which enzyme is responsible for this disease?

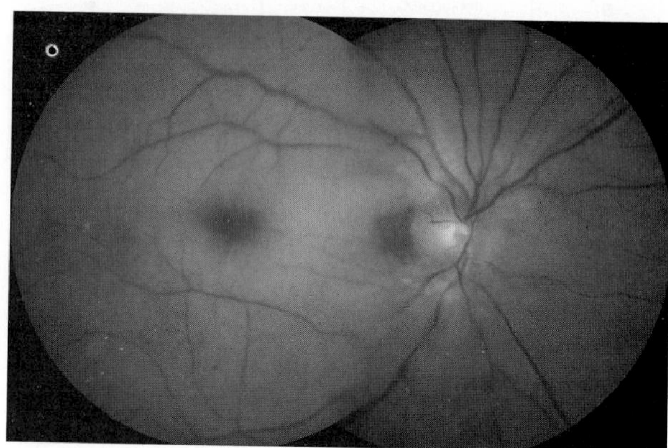

Reproduced, with permission, from USMLERx.com.

(A) α-Galactosidase A
(B) Arylsulfatase A
(C) Hexosaminidase A
(D) Iduronate sulfatase
(E) Lysyl hydrolase

46. A pediatrician examines a baby with a deficiency in fructose metabolism. Upon administration of a fructose bolus, the child becomes symptomatic and blood glucose levels begin to decrease. Which of the following will also occur after the administration of a fructose bolus in this patient?

(A) A fall in serum phosphate levels
(B) A rise in cellular ATP levels
(C) A sustained rise in serum fructose levels
(D) An increase in the serum pH
(E) Large amounts of fructose in the urine

47. A 28-year-old African-American man is receiving primaquine therapy for treatment of malaria, which he contracted while visiting Asia. He presents to his physician after noting blood in his urine. Physical examination is significant for scleral icterus, and urinalysis shows hemoglobinuria. A peripheral blood smear shows spherocytes, bite cells, and Heinz bodies. Which of the following is the most likely diagnosis?

(A) Alkaptonuria
(B) Cystinuria
(C) Glucose-6-phosphate dehydrogenase deficiency
(D) Hereditary fructose intolerance
(E) Hereditary spherocytosis
(F) Lactase deficiency

48. A neonate born at 28 weeks' gestation is having difficulty breathing. On physical examination, the neonate's heart rate is 120/min, blood pressure is 100/60 mm Hg, and respiratory rate is 55/min. He has nasal flaring and subcostal retractions. Which of the following components is deficient in this infant?

(A) Dipalmitoyl phosphatidylcholine
(B) Elastase
(C) Functional cilia
(D) Phosphatidylglycerol
(E) Sphingomyelin

49. A group of scientists at a pharmaceutical company are conducting in vitro experiments to investigate the effects of an antineoplastic drug. Under the microscope, it appears that with treatment, the majority of the cells are arrested at a stage in which their chromosomes are aligned in the vertical axis of the cells. Which antineoplastic agent has a mechanism of action similar to the one described?

(A) 5-Fluorouracil
(B) Cyclophosphamide
(C) Etoposide
(D) Methotrexate
(E) Vincristine

50. A 28-year-old woman is trying to conceive a child. She has a nephew with fragile X syndrome (a genetic disorder characterized by trinucleotide repeat expansion) and she would like to assess her risk as a carrier for the disease. Blood is drawn, and DNA is extracted and cut by restriction enzymes that flank the CGG repeat region. The DNA is then treated with a labeled probe that binds the affected region of the gene. The woman is found to carry one normal X chromosome and one X chromosome with some expansion of the CGG sequence. However, the number of CGG repeats in this X chromosome is not sufficient to alter phenotype. Which lane on the Southern blot represents this woman's genotype?

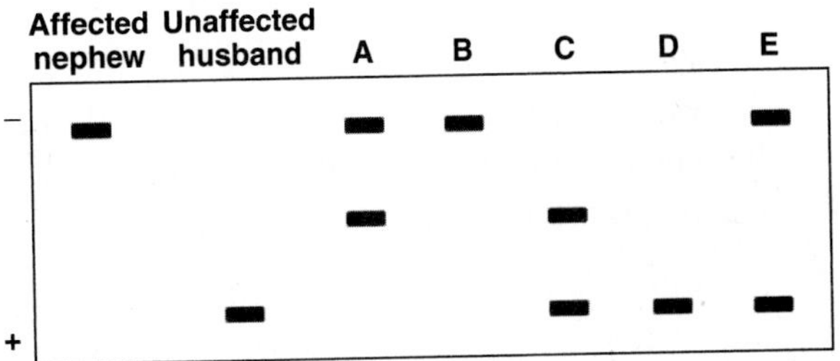

Reproduced, with permission, from USMLERx.com.

(A) A
(B) B
(C) C
(D) D
(E) E

ANSWERS

1. **The correct answer is G.** This patient has xeroderma pigmentosa, an autosomal recessive disease characterized by a defect in excision repair. This disease results in an inability to repair thymidine dimers that can form in the presence of ultraviolet light. This can lead to the development of skin cancer and photosensitivity.

   Answer A is incorrect. Methylation of a particular gene does not cause xeroderma pigmentosum.

   Answer B is incorrect. A missense mutation does not cause xeroderma pigmentosum.

   Answer C is incorrect. A nonsense mutation does not cause xeroderma pigmentosum.

   Answer D is incorrect. A mutation in the enhancer region of a gene does not cause xeroderma pigmentosum.

   Answer E is incorrect. A mutation in the operator region of a gene does not cause xeroderma pigmentosum.

   Answer F is incorrect. A mutation in the promoter region of a gene does not cause xeroderma pigmentosum.

2. **The correct answer is B.** Citrate, formed from oxaloacetate and acetyl CoA by the enzyme citrate synthase, inhibits phosphofructokinase and allosterically activates acetyl CoA carboxylase. Citrate synthase regenerates a molecule of CoA and is an important regulator of the tricarboxylic acid cycle. It is inhibited by adenosine triphosphate.

   Answer A is incorrect. α-Ketoglutarate is not an important regulator of the tricarboxylic acid cycle, but it is an important intermediate in protein metabolism.

   Answer C is incorrect. Malate is not an important regulator of the tricarboxylic acid cycle, but it is important in the malate shuttle.

   Answer D is incorrect. Oxaloacetate is not an important regulator of the tricarboxylic acid cycle, but it is important in glyconeogenesis.

   Answer E is incorrect. Succinyl-CoA down-regulates its own synthesis by inhibiting the enzyme responsible for dehydrogenation of α-ketoglutarate.

3. **The correct answer is E.** Characteristic symptoms of hyperthyroidism include tachycardia, heat intolerance, weight loss, weakness, tremulousness, and diarrhea. This patient also displays another symptom of elevated thyroid hormone levels, exophthalmos. Thyroid hormone enters target cells through carrier-mediated transport or possibly diffusion, and binds to nuclear receptors. The hormone-receptor complex then binds DNA and acts as a transcription factor, regulating the transcription of genes. Transcription results in the production of RNA, specifically messenger RNA.

   Answer A is incorrect. Carbohydrate is produced by the joining of sugar molecules during cellular metabolism; for example, glycogen is produced from the linkage of glucose molecules by glycogen synthase.

   Answer B is incorrect. DNA binding occurs when the thyroid hormone molecule enters the nucleus and binds on nuclear receptors. However, this leads to the transcription of RNA from DNA, not production of new DNA or DNA replication.

   Answer C is incorrect. Fatty acid is synthesized from acetyl-coenzyme A (CoA) in the cell cytoplasm via the action of acetyl-CoA carboxylase and other enzymes.

   Answer D is incorrect. Protein may be produced from the RNA template but is not the first molecule produced in response to thyroid hormone.

4. **The correct answer is C.** The patient has alkaptonuria, a condition corresponding to the one described in the stem. A deficiency of the enzyme homogentisic acid oxidase leads to deposition of homogentisic acid in the joints and cartilage, giving them a dark color (ochronosis) and resulting in degenerative changes. Clas-

sically, the urine of these patients turns black on contact with air or when the urine is made alkaline. The associated defect is on chromosome 3.

Answer A is incorrect. A deficiency in α-keto-acid dehydrogenase causes maple syrup urine disease, a metabolic disorder of autosomal recessive inheritance that affects the metabolism of branched-chain amino acids (leucine, isoleucine, and valine) and causes the urine of affected patients to smell like maple syrup. The urine does not, however, turn black upon standing. The disease is not classically associated with arthritis in middle-aged individuals.

Answer B is incorrect. A deficiency in galactokinase causes galactosemia and galactosuria, but is otherwise a fairly benign condition and would not present with any of the symptoms seen in this patient. Other symptoms would be cataracts in affected children, owing to the accumulation of galactitol, a by-product of galactose metabolism when galactokinase is not present.

Answer D is incorrect. Orotate phosphoribosyltransferase is an enzyme involved in pyrimidine synthesis. Deficiencies in this enzyme or in orotidine 5′-monophosphate decarboxylase (an enzyme involved in the same pathway and located on the same chromosome) cause a very rare disorder called hereditary orotic aciduria. Symptoms include poor growth, megaloblastic anemia, and orate crystals in urine. Treatment involves cystidine or uridine to bypass this step in pyrimidine synthesis and also to negatively downregulate orotic acid production.

Answer E is incorrect. A congenital deficiency of phenylalanine hydroxylase causes phenylketonuria. This enzyme converts phenylalanine to tyrosine, and a deficit of this enzyme leads to a deficiency of tyrosine and a build-up of phenylketones in the urine. It is associated with mental retardation and with the presence of phenylketones in the urine (which do not classically turn black upon standing).

5. **The correct answer is B.** Lane B represents the Southern blot of a heterozygous carrier of sickle cell anemia. The β-A-globin gene results in a 1.15-kb fragment of DNA cut by the MstII restriction enzyme. The β-S-globin gene results in a 1.35-kb band because the single base-pair mutation responsible for sickle cell anemia eliminates an MstII restriction site. A heterozygote will have two bands indicating one normal allele with an intact MstII site (two fragments), and a mutant allele with a missing MstII site (one fragment).

   Answer A is incorrect. The band in lane A is from a sickle cell anemia patient with two copies of the β-S-globin gene. This gene results in a 1.35-kb band because the single base-pair mutation responsible for sickle cell anemia eliminates an MstII restriction site.

   Answer C is incorrect. The band in lane C is from an unaffected patient with two copies of the β-A-globin gene. The gene results in a 1.15-kb fragment of DNA cut by the MstII restriction enzyme.

   Answer D is incorrect. The bands in lane D could not result from any patient. The labeled DNA probe does not bind to the 0.2-kb DNA fragment and therefore would not be visualized on the Southern blot.

   Answer E is incorrect. The bands in lane E could not result from any patient. The labeled DNA probe does not bind to the 0.2-kb DNA fragment and therefore would not be visualized on the Southern blot.

   Answer F is incorrect. The bands in lane F could not result from any patient. The labeled DNA probe does not bind to the 0.2-kb DNA fragment and therefore would not be visualized on the Southern blot. A heterozygote will have two bands indicating one normal allele with an intact MstII site (two fragments), and a mutant allele with a missing MstII site (one fragment).

6. **The correct answer is B.** This patient was started on an 3-hydroxy-3-methylglutaryl coenzyme A (HMG CoA) reductase inhibitor (statin), which prevents the conversion of HMG CoA to mevalonic acid, the rate-limiting step in cholesterol biogenesis. HMG CoA is

formed from three acetyl CoA molecules and is a precursor to sterols and ketone bodies. Muscle pain or injury resembling myositis has been known to occur with statins. Although the mechanism is unknown, it may be related to a decrease in muscle tissue synthesis of ubiquinone, a coenzyme used in muscle cell metabolism.

Answer A is incorrect. Another common side effect of statins is transient elevation of transaminases. Alanine aminotransferase and aspartate aminotransferase elevations are usually seen within 12 weeks after the onset of therapy and may be persistent. No studies have demonstrated an adverse affect of this transaminitis. Hepatomegaly, however, is not a known side effect.

Answer C is incorrect. The teratogenicity of statins is unknown. Fetal toxicity has been demonstrated at high enough concentrations to adversely affect the mother, but the consequence of standard doses is unknown. Statins have not been shown to induce spontaneous abortions.

Answer D is incorrect. Statins have also been implicated as causes of irritability and depression, specifically in patients with major depression, but this relationship has not been confirmed. Homicidality is not caused by statins.

Answer E is incorrect. Seizures are not a common side effect of statin therapy.

7. **The correct answer is C.** Sequencing is a laboratory technique that uses dideoxynucleotides to randomly terminate growing strands of DNA. Gel electrophoresis is used to separate the varying lengths of DNA. The DNA sequence can then be read based on the position of the bands on the gel.

Answer A is incorrect. Polymerase chain reaction (PCR) is a laboratory technique used to produce many copies of a segment of DNA. In the procedure, DNA is mixed with two specific primers, deoxynucleotides and a heat-stable polymerase. The solution is heated to denature the DNA and then cooled to allow synthesis. Twenty cycles of heating and cooling amplify the DNA more than a million times. Dideoxynucleotides are not used in PCR techniques.

Answer B is incorrect. Allele-specific oligonucleotide probes are short, labeled DNA sequences complementary to an allele of interest. These probes can be used to detect the presence of disease-causing mutations.

Answer D is incorrect. In a Southern blot procedure, DNA is separated with electrophoresis, denatured, transferred to a filter, and hybridized with a labeled DNA probe. Regions on the filter that base-pair with the labeled DNA probes can be identified when the filter is exposed to film that is sensitive to the radiolabeled probe.

Answer E is incorrect. In a Northern blot procedure, RNA is separated by electrophoresis, denatured, and transferred to a filter. RNA is hybridized to a labeled radioactive DNA probe. The hybridized RNA/DNA strand is radioactive and visualized when the filter is exposed to film.

Answer F is incorrect. In a Western blot procedure, protein is separated by electrophoresis and labeled antibodies are used as a probe. This technique can be used to detect the existence of an antibody to a particular protein.

Answer G is incorrect. Enzyme-linked immunosorbent assay (ELISA) is an immunologic technique used to determine whether a particular antibody is present in a patient's blood. Labeled antibodies are used to detect whether the serum contains antibodies against a specific antigen precoated on an ELISA plate.

8. **The correct answer is B.** This patient has α_1-antitrypsin deficiency, a genetic disease characterized by a deficiency in the serine protease inhibitor α_1-antitrypsin. This protein normally functions to inhibit neutrophil elastase in the lung. When deficient, there is overabundant activity of elastase, which destroys elastin and collagen in the alveolar walls, progressing to emphysema. Most patients with α_1-antitrypsin deficiency are homozygous for the Z allele. Clinically, α1-antitrypsin deficiency can affect the lung, liver, and less com-

monly the skin. In the lung, the most common manifestation is early onset panacinar emphysema, which is more prominent at the lung bases than apices. Slowly worsening dyspnea is the most common symptom, although patients may initially complain of cough, sputum production, or wheezing. As in this case, patients who present early complaining of episodes of wheezing and productive cough may be told they have asthma. Although treatment for asthma may initially improve symptoms, it does not slow the progression of the disease. Her x-ray of the chest shows a pattern typical for this disease; hyperinflated lungs, a flattened diaphragm, and hyperlucent lungs due to decreased lung markings (it is difficult to see at this resolution due to the overlying breast tissue, but we expect that the lung markings would be especially absent at the bases). α_1-Antitrypsin deficiency can also cause cirrhosis of the liver and panniculitis of the skin.

Answer A is incorrect. α_1-Antitrypsin deficiency is characterized by low levels of a protease inhibitor. This leads to elevated activity of the protease elastase and increased destruction of elastin.

Answer C is incorrect. Mutations in the tumor suppressor gene *p53* lead to uncontrolled cellular proliferation. Such mutations are commonly seen in the lung cancers associated with smoking (small cell and squamous cell), and they have been found in many non-small cell types. This patient's history and x-ray findings do not suggest cancer.

Answer D is incorrect. Mutations in the gene encoding the cystic fibrosis transmembrane conductance regulator (CFTR) on chromosome 7 lead to the disease cystic fibrosis (CF). CF is a multisystem disease that affects the respiratory tract, digestive tract, sweat glands, and reproductive tract. This patient does not present with symptoms characteristic of CF.

Answer E is incorrect. Airway inflammation, airway obstruction, and bronchial hyperresponsiveness are characteristic of asthma. While this patient's presentation mimicked that of asthma, her history, physical exam, and radiographic findings are more consistent with emphysema.

9. **The correct answer is A.** Calcium is maintained in high concentrations outside of the cell and in discrete compartments within the cell (eg, in mitochondria). Free intracellular calcium can activate several enzymes the cumulative effect of which is to induce significant cell injury. A few important enzyme classes include ATPases, which decrease the ATP supply; phospholipases, which decrease membrane stability; endonucleases, which induce DNA damage; and several proteases, responsible for protein breakdown.

   Answer B is incorrect. Free radical generation is a common mechanism of cell injury, but calcium excess does not induce free radical generation.

   Answer C is incorrect. Activation of proteases and phospholipases induces the breakdown of necessary components of cell membranes.

   Answer D is incorrect. ATP depletion, resulting from the activation of ATPases, can contribute to the inhibition of glycolysis.

   Answer E is incorrect. Inhibition of oxidative phosphorylation is an effect of ATP depletion caused by enzyme activation. Although this may contribute to cell damage, it is not the best answer. The enzyme activation resulting from calcium excess is the root cause of the cell damage, and thus would be the primary insult responsible for the majority of cell damage.

10. **The correct answer is B.** G-protein coupled receptors exist in an equilibrium between their active and inactive states that is dependent on whether ligand is present, and the affinity of the ligand for the receptor. When active, these receptors catalyze guanine-nucleotide exchange (GTP for guanosine diphosphate) of their associated G proteins. The Michaelis-Menten constant (K_m) for any enzyme-catalyzed reaction is inversely proportional to the affinity of the enzyme for its substrate. Therefore, the K_m for compound A will be lower than that for compound B because compound A has a higher

affinity for the receptor than compound B. The maximum rate of reaction (V_{max}) will be reached at a lower concentration of A than it would for B, although the V_{max} is unchanged.

Answer A is incorrect. The K_m of compound A will be lower than that of compound B.

Answer C is incorrect. Given that compounds A and B have different affinities for the receptor, their Michaelis-Menten constant values cannot be the same.

Answer D is incorrect. V_{max} is directly proportional to the enzyme concentration, and is unaffected by the concentration of substrates or competitive inhibitors.

Answer E is incorrect. V_{max} is directly proportional to the enzyme concentration, and is unaffected by the concentration of substrates or competitive inhibitors.

11. **The correct answer is C.** This individual suffers from porphyria cutanea tarda. The porphyrias are diseases resulting from enzymatic deficiencies in heme biosynthesis, and porphyria cutanea tarda is the most common form. This disorder is caused by deficiency of uroporphyrinogen decarboxylase, the hepatic enzyme that catalyzes the formation of coproporphyrinogen III from uroporphyrinogen III. Lack of this enzyme results in uroporphyrin accumulation in the urine (giving the urine a tea-colored appearance) and uroporphyrinogen accumulation systemically. This compound absorbs light and releases heat, causing extreme photosensitivity.

Answer A is incorrect. Hereditary coproporphyria is a disease due to the deficiency of coproporphyrinogen oxidase, the enzyme that catalyzes the formation of protoporphyrinogen from coproporphyrinogen III. Coproporphyrinogen III accumulates in the urine. Patients with this condition tend to be photosensitive.

Answer B is incorrect. Acute intermittent porphyria is caused by a deficiency in porphobilinogen deaminase (also called uroporphyrinogen 1 synthetase), the enzyme that catalyzes the formation of pre-uroporphyrinogen from porphobilinogen. Lack of this enzyme causes porphobilinogen and δ-aminolevulinic acid to accumulate in the urine. Patients with acute intermittent porphyria are not photosensitive, but they do experience symptoms of painful abdomen, polyneuropathy, and psychological disturbances. They also have pink coloration of their urine.

Answer D is incorrect. Ferrochelatase and δ-aminolevulinic acid (ALA) dehydrase are sensitive to inhibition by lead. Thus, lead poisoning leads to an accumulation of coproporphyrin and ALA in the urine. Lead poisoning is a problem seen in children who live in old houses with chipped paint (lead was used in paint manufacturing until the 1970s). Ingestion of large quantities of lead can cause lines on the gingiva and epiphyses of long bones, encephalopathy, erythrocyte basophilic stippling, abdominal colic, sideroblastic anemia, and neuropathy leading to foot and wrist drops. It is not associated with photosensitivity. The first line of treatment is dimercaprol and EDTA to bind up the free lead in the serum.

Answer E is incorrect. Porphobilinogen deaminase deficiency, not excess, results in acute intermittent porphyria. One would expect to find δ-aminolevulinic acid and porphobilinogen in the urine and no photosensitivity.

12. **The correct answer is B.** This woman suffers from β-thalassemia major, the most severe form of β-thalassemia, in which the β-chain is absent. Clinically β-thalassemia major manifests as severe hemolysis and ineffective erythropoiesis. These individuals are transfusion dependent and frequently develop iron overload. The consequences of iron overload due to transfusion dependency or secondary hemochromatosis are described in the stem. These manifestations are due to iron deposition in various tissues including the pancreas, heart, and skin. β-Thalassemia is more common among Mediterranean populations, whereas β-thalassemia is more common among Asian and African populations.

Answer A is incorrect. This answer describes the most severe form of α-thalassemia, a disease in which a fetus is unable to make any functional hemoglobin aside from the γ_4-tetramer (Hb Bart). Clinically α-thalassemia manifests as congestive heart failure, anasarca, and intrauterine fetal death.

Answer C is incorrect. This answer describes hereditary hemochromatosis, a disease caused by iron overload due to an intrinsic defect in the body's ability to control the absorption of iron. Clinically this disease manifests in a manner similar to that of secondary hemochromatosis. However, the laboratory picture in hereditary hemochromatosis is not characterized by hemolysis.

Answer D is incorrect. This answer describes hereditary spherocytosis, a disease in which mutations in either the ankyrin or spectrin gene contribute to instability of the RBC plasma membranes. This condition is characterized by extravascular hemolysis. Clinically this disease manifests as gallstones, anemia, jaundice, and splenomegaly. The definitive treatment is splenectomy, thus obviating any need for chronic blood transfusion.

Answer E is incorrect. This answer describes Wilson disease, a disease in which failure of copper to enter the circulation in the form of ceruloplasmin results in copper accumulation in the liver, brain, and cornea. Clinically this disease manifests as parkinsonian symptoms, Kayser-Fleischer rings, asterixis, and dementia.

13. **The correct answer is C.** Aldose reductase catalyzes the breakdown of glucose into sorbitol. Sorbitol is then metabolized to fructose, a process that is relatively slow. In patients with hyperglycemia, as would be present in this patient with poorly controlled diabetes, sorbitol accumulation with the cells of the lens leads to a rise in intracellular osmolality, causing water movement into the cells. This results in cellular swelling and osmotic damage. It also leads to a decrease in intracellular myoinositol, interfering with cellular metabolism. Swelling of lens fiber cells can lead to rupture and cataract formation. Inhibition of aldose reductase could decrease sorbitol accumulation in the lens and thus prevent cataract formation. No drug is currently approved to inhibit aldose reductase, but aldose reductase inhibitors such as epalrestat and ranirestat are currently being tested.

Answer A is incorrect. 3-Hydroxy-3-methylglutaryl coenzyme A (HMG CoA) reductase catalyzes the conversion of HMG CoA into mevalonate and eventually into cholesterol. Inhibition of this enzyme is commonly affected by statin drugs to reduce cholesterol levels, but it would not help prevent the development of cataracts.

Answer B is incorrect. Adenosine deaminase inhibition would result in problems in the purine salvage pathway. Disrupting this pathway would result in excess ATP and dATP via feedback inhibition of ribonucleotide reductase. This excess ATP prevents DNA synthesis and thus affects lymphocyte development. Congenital deficiency of this enzyme results in severe combined immunodeficiency. Inhibition of this enzyme would not prevent the development of cataracts.

Answer D is incorrect. Galactose-1-phosphate (G-1-P) uridyltransferase is important in the breakdown of galactose; it catalyzes the formation of glucose-1-phosphate from G-1-P. Hereditary deficiency of this enzyme leads to hepatosplenomegaly, mental retardation, jaundice, and cataract formation. Inhibition of this enzyme in an adult would certainly not prevent the development of cataracts.

Answer E is incorrect. Hexokinase is the enzyme that catalyzes the first step in the catabolism of glucose, converting glucose to glucose-6-phosphate. It is stimulated by insulin. Inhibition of hexokinase would not prevent the development of cataracts in this patient. Congenital hexokinase deficiency is a rare autosomal recessive condition that results in severe hemolysis. Inhibition of hexokinase would likely have a similar, albeit less severe, result.

Answer F is incorrect. Insulin-like growth factor (IGF) is a product synthesized in the liver that mediates many of the physiologic effects of growth hormone (GH). Its name refers to a high degree of structural similarity to insulin, and it is even capable of binding to the insulin receptor directly, although with lower affinity than insulin. Its effects include increased protein synthesis, and IGF levels are especially high during puberty. Inhibition of IGF would not help prevent the development of cataracts.

14. **The correct answer is F.** The *p53* gene protein product is a transcription factor that regulates apoptosis. It acts as a cell-cycle regulator, preventing cells from undergoing division. Mutations in *p53* cause uncontrolled cell division, leading to various types of tumors. Another example of a cell-cycle regulator is the retinoblastoma gene.

    Answer A is incorrect. The *p53* gene product is involved in apoptosis induced by DNA damage and other stimuli, but it is not a caspase protein.

    Answer B is incorrect. *p53* is involved in cell cycle regulation but not direct DNA repair activity. DNA repair products are produced by genes such as *BRCA1* (chromosome 17) and *BRCA2* (chromosome 13), among others.

    Answer C is incorrect. Membrane cell adhesion products are produced by the *APC* gene found on chromosome 5. Mutations in the *APC* gene lead to colon cancer.

    Answer D is incorrect. *p53* is not a G-protein product. G proteins such as *ras* can be involved in oncogenesis. Mutations in *ras* can lead to cancer in the lungs, pancreas, and colon as well as leukemia.

    Answer E is incorrect. DNA polymerase is unable to replicate at the end of chromosomes (telomeres), resulting in the loss of DNA with each replication cycle. Telomerase is an enzyme that adds repeats onto the 3′ends of chromosomes to protect them from being recognized as broken or damaged DNA. Although most normal somatic cells do not express enough telomerase to prevent telomerase attrition with each cell division, telomerase is often reexpressed in cancer cells. However, *p53* is not involved in the process of adding nucleotides to telomeres.

    Answer G is incorrect. Tyrosine kinase products play a role in cell signaling through phosphorylation. The *p53* gene product is not a tyrosine kinase.

15. **The correct answer is D.** This question describes the polymerase chain reaction (PCR). PCR is a laboratory technique used to produce many copies of a segment of DNA. In the procedure, DNA is mixed with two specific primers, deoxynucleotides and a heat-stable polymerase. The solution is heated to denature the DNA and then cooled to allow synthesis. Twenty cycles of heating and cooling amplify the DNA over a million times.

    Answer A is incorrect. Enzyme-linked immunosorbent assay (ELISA) is an immunologic technique used to determine whether a particular antibody is present in a patient's blood. Labeled antibodies are used to detect whether the serum contains antibodies against a specific antigen precoated on an ELISA plate. This is not the technique described above.

    Answer B is incorrect. Gel electrophoresis uses an electric field to separate molecules based on their sizes.

    Answer C is incorrect. Northern blots are similar to Southern blots except that in Northern blotting, mRNA is separated by electrophoresis instead of DNA. This is not the technique described above.

    Answer E is incorrect. Sequencing is a laboratory technique that utilizes dideoxynucleotides to randomly terminate growing strands of DNA. Gel electrophoresis is used to separate the varying lengths of DNA. The DNA sequence can then be read based on the position of the bands on the gel. This is not the technique described above.

    Answer F is incorrect. In a Southern blot procedure, DNA is separated with electrophoresis, denatured, transferred to a filter, and hybridized with a labeled DNA probe. Regions on the filter that base-pair with the labeled DNA probes can be identified when the filter is exposed to film that is sensitive to the radiolabeled probe. This is not the technique described above.

Answer G is incorrect. In a Western blot procedure, protein is separated by electrophoresis and labeled antibodies are used as a probe. This technique can be used to detect the existence of an antibody to a particular protein.

16. **The correct answer is B.** This woman has symptoms of Hashimoto thyroiditis, an autoimmune disorder resulting in hypothyroidism (also known as myxedema), although there may be a transient hyperthyroidism at the very onset of disease when follicular rupture occurs. It is a type IV hypersensitivity associated with autoantibodies to thyroglobulin, thyroid peroxidase, and the thyroid-stimulating hormone receptor itself. The most common presenting symptoms of Hashimoto thyroiditis are those seen in this patient, as well as constipation and dry skin. Histologic characteristics include massive infiltrates of lymphocytes with germinal cell formation. Hashimoto thyroiditis is associated with the DR5 human leukocyte antigen subtype, as is pernicious anemia, a disease that leads to vitamin B_{12} deficiency caused by atrophic gastritis and destruction of parietal cells.

    Answer A is incorrect. Multiple sclerosis is associated with the DR2 human leukocyte antigen subtype. It is not associated with Hashimoto thyroiditis.

    Answer C is incorrect. Psoriasis is associated with the B27 human leukocyte antigen subtype. It is not associated with Hashimoto thyroiditis.

    Answer D is incorrect. Steroid-responsive nephrotic syndrome is associated with the DR7 human leukocyte antigen subtype. It is not associated with Hashimoto thyroiditis.

17. **The correct answer is D.** Vancomycin is a glycopeptide antibiotic that is effective in fighting only gram-positive bacteria. It binds tightly to a cell wall precursor that contains the terminal amino acid sequence D-ala D-ala and prevents cell wall synthesis. Resistance to vancomycin is transferred via plasmids and encodes enzymes that convert the D-ala D-ala peptide bridge to D-ala D-lac, preventing vancomycin from binding. Vancomycin resistance is much more common with *Enterococcus faecium* than with *Enterococcus faecalis*. High-dose ampicillin, often in combination with gentamicin, is generally first-line treatment in urinary tract infections due to vancomycin-resistant *Enterococcus*.

    Answer A is incorrect. Microorganisms become resistant to quinolones through the alteration of their gyrase.

    Answer B is incorrect. Microorganisms become resistant to macrolides through the methylation of its rRNA at a ribosome-binding site.

    Answer C is incorrect. β-Lactamases are enzymes produced by microorganisms that cleave β-lactam antibiotics, deactivating them. To overcome resistance, β-lactams are usually given with β-lactamase inhibitors such as clavulanic acid, tazobactam, and sulbactam.

    Answer E is incorrect. β-Lactam antibiotics bind to penicillin-binding proteins (enzymes that synthesize peptidoglycan, a major component of bacterial cell walls), preventing cell wall synthesis by the microorganism. Microorganisms such as methicillin-resistant *Staphylococcus aureus* and penicillin-resistant *Streptococcus pneumoniae* have alterations in their penicillin-binding proteins that result in low affinity and thus resistance to these β-lactams. β-Lactam antibiotics include penicillins, cephalosporins, monobactams, and carbapenems (not vancomycin).

18. **The correct answer is C.** Kartagener syndrome, or immotile cilia, is caused by a defect in dynein that prevents effective movement of cilia. The full syndrome is characterized by sinusitis, bronchiectasis, situs inversus, and male infertility. Cilia play an important role in moving mucus along the airway and clearing debris; the absence of this function contributes to the pulmonary findings of the syndrome. Cilia are also very important for leukocyte movement and phagocytosis. Infertility is present in most patients due to immotile cilia.

Answer A is incorrect. Defective chloride transport is the cause of cystic fibrosis. Cystic fibrosis frequently causes bronchiectasis, but it is not associated with situs inversus.

Answer B is incorrect. Patients with diabetes are predisposed to developing chronic fungal sinusitis. However, the bronchiectasis and situs inversus are not consistent with diabetes.

Answer D is incorrect. Mucus plugging in reactive airway disease can cause atelectasis at the lung bases. An x-ray film of the chest of a patient with reactive airway disease would likely reveal hyperinflated lungs with areas of atelectasis, not bronchiectasis.

Answer E is incorrect. Tetralogy of Fallot is a congenital heart defect, but it is not associated with infections or cardiac inversion. Patients with this condition develop early cyanosis because of the malformed right-to-left shunt. The four components of the tetralogy are (1) ventricular septal defect, (2) overriding aorta, (3) infundibular pulmonary stenosis, and (4) right ventricular hypertrophy.

19. **The correct answer is E.** This child is suffering from an inherited form of hyperammonemia as a result of a defect in ornithine transcarbamylase (OTC). In the urea cycle, OTC combines carbamoyl phosphate and ornithine to make citrulline. When OTC is deficient, excess carbamoyl phosphate enters the pyrimidine synthesis pathway to cause increased orotic acid in the blood, which distinguishes OTC deficiency from other urea cycle disorders. A defect in OTC causes an excess of ammonia in circulation, which leads to mental retardation, seizures, and ultimately death. Some patients with OTC deficiency also exhibit a very low blood urea nitrogen, but this is not enough to make a conclusive diagnosis. Unlike the rest of the urea cycle disorders that are autosomal recessive, deficiency of OTC is X-linked.

Answer A is incorrect. Fabry disease is caused by mutations in the α-galactosidase A gene, resulting in the accumulation of ceramide trihexoside. Patients classically have angiokeratomas, hypohidrosis, corneal and lenticular opacities, acroparesthesias, and vascular disease of the kidney, heart, and brain. Laboratory results show diminished α-galactosidase A activity in plasma, leukocytes, or cultured fibroblasts. Enzyme replacement therapy is now available for patients, and renal transplant and long-term hemodialysis are mainstays of treatment.

Answer B is incorrect. Hereditary fructose intolerance is caused by the inability of aldose B to split fructose 1-phosphate, resulting in its accumulation along with inhibition of glucose production. Patients are usually asymptomatic until they begin ingesting food containing fructose, sucrose, or sorbitol after weaning from breastfeeding. Symptoms include nausea, vomiting, pallor, sweating, and trembling with fructose ingestion; continued ingestion can lead to seizure and coma.

Answer C is incorrect. Absent function of galactose-1-phosphate uridylyltransferase in galactosemia results in the accumulation of galactose and galactose-1-phosphate. Galactose-1-phosphate has direct toxic effects on renal, hepatic, and neuronal cells. The disorder is characterized by onset of clinical symptoms within the first few days of life: vomiting, diarrhea, failure to thrive, and hypotonia. Patients who undergo early galactose restriction may still have developmental delays, ataxia, and apraxia. Laboratory findings include an elevated blood galactose level, low glucose, and galactosuria.

Answer D is incorrect. Pompe disease is caused by absent function of lysosomal α-glucosidase, characterized by generalized hypotonia, muscle weakness, and hypertrophic cardiomegaly. Patients usually have cardiorespiratory failure by 1 year of age with the early onset form of the disorder. Laboratory findings include significantly elevated serum creatinine kinase.

20. **The correct answer is D.** This patient has obstructive jaundice, causing her pruritus and scleral icterus. In this situation conjugated bilirubin cannot be excreted, and its levels are therefore elevated in the serum. The unconju-

gated bilirubin level, however, is not elevated. Alkaline phosphatase is usually elevated in cases of obstructive jaundice.

Answer A is incorrect. This is seen in Crigler-Najjar syndrome type I, which leads to kernicterus and is diagnosed during childhood. Extremely high levels of unconjugated bilirubin would be expected in this case.

Answer B is incorrect. This is seen in Gilbert syndrome, which does not have any clinical consequence. This syndrome is more common in men, the jaundice is typically associated with stress or exercise, and alkaline phosphatase levels are normal.

Answer C is incorrect. Extravascular hemolysis (eg, hereditary spherocytosis) would lead to increased levels of unconjugated bilirubin. Hemoglobinuria would not be observed in these patients.

Answer E is incorrect. Intravascular hemolysis (eg, due to mechanical injury to RBCs, defective cardiac valves, toxic injury to RBCs) would lead to an increase in unconjugated bilirubin, which is not the case in this patient. Also, levels of alkaline phosphatase would not be elevated in a patient with increased RBC destruction. Hemoglobinuria would be expected in these patients.

21. **The correct answer is C.** This patient is experiencing an acute asthma attack. Treatment is targeted at relieving bronchoconstriction and inflammation. This patient should be treated with a β_2 agonist such as albuterol. When activated with an agonist, the β_2 receptor will cause bronchodilation.

Answer A is incorrect. β_1 Blockers inhibit sympathetic stimulation of β_1 receptors by epinephrine. β_1 Blockers reduce the effect of excitement/physical exertion on heart rate and force of contraction; they also add to the dilation of blood vessels, some opening of bronchi, and also reduction of tremor.

Answer B is incorrect. β_1 Agonists work on the heart more than the lungs. Activation of β_1-receptor agonists leads to inotropy (increased heart contraction) and chronotropy (increased heart rate).

Answer D is incorrect. Activation of histamine$_1$ receptors results in pruritus, bronchoconstriction, and increased nasal and bronchial mucus production. Histamine$_1$-receptor antagonists are primarily used in the treatment of seasonal allergy symptoms.

Answer E is incorrect. Activation of histamine$_2$ receptors leads to increased gastric acid production. Therefore, histamine$_2$-receptor antagonists such as cimetidine are used in the treatment of gastroesophageal reflux disease.

22. **The correct answer is B.** This patient has Pompe disease, a glycogen storage disorder. Pompe disease is an autosomal recessive disease that is characterized by a deficiency or defect in lysosomal α-1,4-glucosidase. This enzyme is necessary for the dissolution of the polymer linkages in glycogen. In its absence, glycogen accumulates to toxic levels in both the cytoplasm and lysosomes.

Answer A is incorrect. Glucose is stored as glycogen in the cells and is also present in blood. However, hyperglycemia is not responsible for the symptoms observed in this patient.

Answer C is incorrect. Oxaloacetate is the first intermediate in the Krebs cycle. It is regenerated with each turn of the cycle but is not present in excessive amounts in the cell.

Answer D is incorrect. Pyruvate is a component of the cellular respiration pathway and an intermediate in gluconeogenesis. It is not stored in cells in any significant quantity.

Answer E is incorrect. Disorders of the urea cycle lead to nitrogen accumulation in the body and result in progressive lethargy and coma. They do not cause the myopathy seen in this patient.

23. **The correct answer is B.** Glucokinase catalyzes the initial step of glycolysis, which is the phosphorylation of glucose to glucose-6-phosphate. In most other tissues, this process is catalyzed by hexokinase. Both enzymes are found in the liver. Glucokinase has a higher Michaelis-Menten

constant and a higher V_{max} than hexokinase; it thus has a low affinity for glucose but large capacity of activity. Importantly, it is not inhibited by glucose-6-phosphate, as is hexokinase.

Answer A is incorrect. The hepatocyte cell membrane is permeable to glucose, which is trapped in the cell after phosphorylation to glucose-6-phosphate.

Answer C is incorrect. Hexokinase has a high affinity (low Michaelis-Menten constant, K_m) for glucose and processes glucose to glucose-6-phosphate at lower levels of glucose. At higher glucose levels, hexokinase is overwhelmed (low V_{max}), and sufficient substrate is available for glucokinase to process the excess glucose despite its higher K_m.

Answer D is incorrect. Hexokinase has a relatively low Michaelis-Menten constant.

Answer E is incorrect. Glucokinase has a relatively high Michaelis-Menten constant.

24. **The correct answer is C.** Type I dyslipidemia (or familial lipoprotein lipase deficiency) is caused by a deficiency of lipoprotein lipase. This enzyme exists in capillary walls of adipose and muscle tissue and cleaves triglycerides into free fatty acids and glycerol. The enzyme is activated by apolipoprotein C-II, which is found on VLDL cholesterol and chylomicrons. Type I dyslipidemia is characterized by an accumulation of triglyceride-rich lipoproteins in the plasma. Deficiency in apolipoprotein C-II produces a similar result.

Answer A is incorrect. VLDL cholesterol remnants are removed from the circulation by apolipoprotein E receptors. Thus, apolipoprotein E deficiency (dysbetalipoproteinemia) results in an elevated VLDL cholesterol, triglyceride, and cholesterol levels. Often this disorder manifests with other conditions that cause hyperlipidemia such as diabetes. Xanthomas are often present.

Answer B is incorrect. LDL cholesterol receptor dysfunction is characteristic of familial hyperbetalipoproteinemia, also known as type II hyperlipidemia. In these cases, plasma LDL cholesterol levels rise, which causes an increase in plasma cholesterol; triglyceride levels remain normal.

Answer D is incorrect. Mixed hypertriglyceridemia (type V) is a dyslipidemia characterized by extremely high triglyceride levels and visibly foamy plasma. Unlike type I, type V is characterized by elevated VLDL cholesterol levels and is thought to be related to a VLDL cholesterol clearance problem.

Answer E is incorrect. VLDL cholesterol overproduction is another characteristic of type V dyslipidemias, as well as type IIb combined hyperlipidemia.

25. **The correct answer is E.** Following endothelial injury, the subendothelial space accumulates lipoproteins. Next, chemical modification (eg, glycation or oxidation) of lipoproteins occurs that recruits monocytes to the vessel wall. Monocytes are converted to macrophages upon entry into the subendothelial space, and unregulated macrocytosis of modified LDL cholesterol occurs, yielding foam cells. At this point, various cell mediators, most notably platelet-derived growth factor, tumor necrosis factor, and interleukin-1, recruit platelets and smooth muscle to the intimal lining, where proliferation and production of extracellular matrix leads to the development of a fibrous plaque.

Answer A is incorrect. γ-Interferon is secreted by T-helper cells and stimulates macrophages. This mediator does not play a prominent role in the pathogenesis of atherosclerotic plaque.

Answer B is incorrect. Complement defends against gram-negative bacteria and is activated by IgG or IgM in the classic pathway, and activated by molecules on the surface of microbes in the alternate pathway. Complement has not been shown to be an active participant in the pathogenesis of atherosclerotic plaque.

Answer C is incorrect. Interleukin-6 (IL-6) is secreted by T-helper cells and macrophages, and is responsible for stimulating the production of acute-phase reactants and immunoglobulins. IL-6 does not play a prominent role in the pathogenesis of atherosclerotic plaque.

Answer D is incorrect. Natural killer cells are a form of cytotoxic lymphocytes and constitute a major component of the innate immune system. These cells play a major role in the host rejection of both tumors and virally-infected cells, and do not play a prominent role in the pathogenesis of atherosclerotic plaque.

26. **The correct answer is B.** This patient has adult polycystic kidney disease, an autosomal dominant condition characterized by massive bilateral cysts in the kidneys, asymptomatic hepatic and pancreatic cysts, mitral valve prolapse, and berry aneurysms. All disease manifestations are believed to be secondary to abnormal epithelial cell differentiation, most likely caused by a mutation in the polycystic genes. The renal cysts eventually progress to end-stage renal disease. Berry aneurysms tend to increase in size with age, thus increasing the risk of rupture and intracranial hemorrhage.

Answer A is incorrect. Astrocytomas are seen in patients with tuberous sclerosis, an autosomal dominant disorder affecting the tuberin and hamartin proteins, which regulate cellular growth and differentiation.

Answer C is incorrect. Ectopic lens is seen in Marfan syndrome, an autosomal dominant connective tissue disorder associated with slender body habitus and aortic dissection.

Answer D is incorrect. Optic nerve degeneration can be seen in Leber hereditary optic neuropathy, a condition in which patients develop a rapid loss of central vision.

Answer E is incorrect. Increased incidence of squamous cell carcinoma is seen in patients with xeroderma pigmentosum, an autosomal recessive disease caused by a deficiency in DNA repair of thymine dimers.

27. **The correct answer is E.** Homocystinuria is an autosomal recessive condition caused by deficiencies of various enzymes involved in the pathway that converts methionine to cysteine. This results in the accumulation of homocysteine, which is then excreted in urine. In this condition, cysteine becomes an essential amino acid. Clinically, homocystinuria is manifested by mental retardation, osteoporosis, tall stature, kyphosis, lens subluxation, and atherosclerosis (causing premature stroke and myocardial infarction). Diagnosis is based on a positive nitroprusside cyanide test. Marfan syndrome is the primary differential diagnosis. Clinical features of homocystinuria, such as ectopia lentis, tall and thin body habitus, and chest and spinal deformities, are similar to the features found in patients with Marfan syndrome. However, generalized osteoporosis, arterial and venous thrombosis, premature atherosclerosis, changes in hair, and the disorders of mental development are absent in patients with Marfan syndrome.

Answer A is incorrect. Lesch-Nyhan syndrome is an X-linked recessive condition caused by a defect in the purine salvage pathway due to the absence of HGPRT (hypoxanthine guanine phosphoribosyl transferase), which converts hypoxanthine to inosine monophosphate and guanine to guanosine monophosphate. As a result, excess uric acid accumulates and causes hyperuricemia and gout. Patients also present with mental retardation, self-mutilating behavior, aggression, and choreoathetosis.

Answer B is incorrect. Osteogenesis imperfecta is an autosomal dominant disorder caused by a variety of gene defects that result in abnormal synthesis of type I collagen. Clinically, it is characterized by multiple fractures occurring with minimal trauma ("brittle bone disease"), blue sclerae due to the translucency of connective tissue over the choroid, hearing loss due to abnormal middle ear bones, and dental imperfections due to lack of dentition.

Answer C is incorrect. Fragile X results from an expansion of the CGG trinucleotide repeat on the FMR-1 locus of the X chromosome. Methylation of these trinucleotide repeats will result in nonproduction of the FMR-1 protein, resulting in a phenotype that includes mental retardation, an elongated face, protruding ears, macro-orchidism, and low muscle tone. While children suffering from fragile X might exhibit the same developmental delays and mild retardation as the child in this vignette, they will not have pes cavus, arachnodactyly, and dislocated lenses, and folic acid supplementation will not help them.

Answer D is incorrect. Chronic granulomatous disease is an X-linked recessive condition caused by a lack of reduced nicotinamide adenine dinucleotide phosphate oxidase activity within neutrophils. As a result, neutrophils can ingest bacteria but cannot kill them due to a defective oxidative burst. Patients present with a marked susceptibility to opportunistic infections with bacteria, especially *Staphylococcus aureus*, *Escherichia coli*, and *Aspergillus*. Diagnosis is confirmed with a negative nitroblue tetrazolium test.

28. **The correct answer is B.** Glucose enters pancreatic β cells via GLUT 2 channels. GLUT 2 transporters are insulin-dependent glucose channels that are present on pancreatic β cells when glucose levels are low.

Answer A is incorrect. GLUT 1 transporters are found in RBCs and the brain. GLUT 2 transporters are found in pancreatic β cells, liver, and kidney.

Answer C is incorrect. GLUT 4 transporters are found in adipose tissue and skeletal muscle.

Answer D is incorrect. Glucose cannot simply diffuse across membranes; it requires transporters.

29. **The correct answer is B.** 2,3-Bisphosphoglycerate (BPG) promotes oxygen unloading by binding to a pocket formed by the two α subunits. It can bind only when they are close together, such as in the taut form. It is essential to add inosine to stored blood for transfusions to prevent the loss of 2,3-BPG. Any change that enhances the taut form of hemoglobin will decrease hemoglobin's affinity for oxygen.

Answer A is incorrect. Hemoglobin carries oxygen better when it is in the relaxed form, which has a higher affinity for oxygen. Conversely, the taut form of hemoglobin has a lower affinity for oxygen. The taut form is stabilized by the processes that result in increased oxygen unloading, including binding of carbon dioxide, low pH, and increased levels of 2,3-BPG in RBCs. Therefore, by decreasing the partial pressure of carbon dioxide, one increases hemoglobin's affinity for oxygen.

Answer C is incorrect. Binding of oxygen molecules is the major cause of the shift of hemoglobin from its taut structure to the relaxed form. The oxygen molecule disrupts the weak polar bonds and "opens up" the molecule for more oxygen to bind.

Answer D is incorrect. The Bohr effect comes from an increase in protons, which subsequently stabilize the taut form of hemoglobin preferentially. In addition, an increase in protons means an increase in carbon dioxide because of the bicarbonate buffer present in blood. Remember, though, that increasing the pH means a decrease in protons.

Answer E is incorrect. Carbon monoxide stabilizes the relaxed form of hemoglobin so that the dissociation curve shifts dramatically to the left; thus oxygen cannot be unloaded.

30. **The correct answer is D.** Glucose-6-phosphate dehydrogenase (G6PD) deficiency often manifests in young adulthood or adolescents after a serious infection. Genetic mutation variants have been described, including the common G6PDA and G6PD Mediterranean, both of which are X-linked. Normal G6PD generates reduced nicotinamide adenine dinucleotide phosphate (NADPH) from oxidized nicotinamide adenine dinucleotide phosphate ($NADP^+$), which is used to reduce glutathione. Reduced glutathione is used to detoxify oxidizing agents. Oxidizing agents are found at times of infection, as with certain drugs such as primaquine, and with ingestion of fava beans (called favism when symptomatic).

Answer A is incorrect. Glucose-6-phosphate is generated from glucose by hexokinase in all cells. High levels of glucose are processed by glucokinase in liver cells and pancreatic B cells.

Answer B is incorrect. Glucose-6-phosphate is generated from glucose by hexokinase in all cells.

Answer C is incorrect. Hunter disease is an X-linked mucopolysaccharidosis that results from a deficiency of mucopolysaccharide breakdown. It is not associated with this patient's presentation.

Answer E is incorrect. The conversion of glucose-6-phosphate (G6P) to 6-phosphogluconate (6PG) is the first step in the pentose-phosphate pathway (also known as the hexose-monophosphate shunt). This particular step produces NADPH (reduced $NADP^+$), which is used to maintain a reduced pool of glutathione. It is also used to synthesize fatty acids and steroids, to generate the cytochrome P450 (CYP450) enzyme system, and in phagocytosis. 6PG can be converted to ribose-5-phosphate for use in DNA synthesis. These processes occur in all cells, but deficiency of G6P has the greatest effect on RBCs, which have no alternate means of reducing oxidizing toxins.

31. **The correct answer is A.** Parathyroid hormone (PTH) plays a key role in the regulation of calcium and phosphate balance. When the serum calcium level falls, PTH is rapidly released from the parathyroid glands and acts to restore serum calcium levels to normal through the following mechanisms: (1) increasing calcium absorption in the small intestine; (2) promoting calcium reabsorption in the renal tubules; (3) inhibiting phosphate reabsorption in the renal tubules; (4) inhibiting the further release of PTH as part of a negative feedback loop; and (5) stimulating the production of 1,25-dihydroxyvitamin D. Primary hyperparathyroidism is one of the most common forms of hypercalcemia, whereby a parathyroid adenoma spontaneously produces excess PTH, leading to hypercalcemia and hypophosphatemia. Secondary PTH is caused by excess PTH in response to renal failure or other situations like 1,25-dihydroxyvitamin D deficiency (rickets or osteomalacia), in which low calcium and high phosphate levels detected by the body lead to excess PTH production.

Answer B is incorrect. PTH stimulates the production of 1,25-dihydroxyvitamin D, which in turn increases calcium and phosphate absorption from the gut. It does not inhibit 1,25-dihydroxyvitamin D production.

Answer C is incorrect. PTH promotes calcium reabsorption in the renal tubules, not calcium excretion.

Answer D is incorrect. PTH inhibits the further release of PTH as part of a negative feedback loop; it does not induce further release of PTH.

Answer E is incorrect. PTH inhibits phosphate reabsorption in the renal tubules and, in fact, promotes phosphate excretion. Think "**PTH**": **P**hosphate **T**rashing **H**ormone.

32. **The correct answer is E.** Deficiency of porphobilinogen deaminase (also known as uroporphyrinogen I synthetase) causes acute intermittent porphyria (AIP), a disease characterized by acute attacks of gastrointestinal, neurologic/psychiatric, and cardiovascular symptoms. A deficiency in porphobilinogen deaminase leads to a deficiency in heme synthesis, in turn causing a build-up of intermediary products such as aminolevulinic acid and porphobilinogen, which cause the symptoms of the disease. Age at onset is almost always after puberty, it is more common in women, and symptoms often are precipitated by drugs that induce heme-containing CYP450. Because of the intermittent nature of attacks, AIP can be difficult to diagnose. These patients often will present with urine that turns a dark color when exposed to air.

Answer A is incorrect. A deficiency in adenosine deaminase (ADA) can cause severe combined immunodeficiency disorder. It presents with recurrent viral, bacterial, fungal, and protozoal infections. ADA normally functions to convert adenosine to inosine in the purine salvage pathway. Deficiency of this enzyme causes an excess of ATP and dATP that imbalances nucleotide synthesis through negative feedback, thus preventing DNA synthesis and decreasing lymphocytes. ADA deficiency would not be associated with the symptoms seen in this patient, nor would it become clinically apparent at the age of 22 years.

Answer B is incorrect. Congenital deficiency of homogentisic acid oxidase, an enzyme in the degradative pathway of tyrosine, results in a disease called alkaptonuria. This deficiency leads to the accumulation of homogentisate, forming polymers that cause urine to darken on standing. This disease is generally innocuous but may cause arthritis with darkening of the joints. It would not be associated with the systemic symptoms described in this patient.

Answer C is incorrect. Lysosomal α-1,4-glucosidase deficiency causes a rare glycogen storage disease called Pompe disease, which is transmitted in an autosomal recessive manner. It presents with cardiomegaly along with weakness and hypotonia in the first six months of life. It is often fatal by age 2 years. Pompe disease would not be associated with the symptoms seen in this patient.

Answer D is incorrect. Ornithine transcarbamylase deficiency, an X-linked disorder, is the most common genetic deficiency of the five enzymes of the urea cycle. Failure to synthesize urea, and therefore break down ammonia, leads to hyperammonemia during the first weeks of life and can lead to mental retardation. Treatment includes limiting protein intake in the diet and administering compounds like phenylbutyrate, which help bind to amino acids and promote their excretion. This disorder would not present with the symptoms seen in this patient, nor would it normally present at age 22 years.

33. **The correct answer is E.** The patient is a young boy presenting with an abdominal mass involving the kidney. The most common renal tumor in young children is Wilms tumor, which accounts for approximately 6% of pediatric malignancies. Wilms tumor typically presents with a palpable mass, and about 25% of patients present with gross or microscopic hematuria. It is an embryonal neoplasm that tends to occur between ages 1 and 3 years, with most cases occurring before the age of 7 years. Wilms tumor is often associated with the deletion of *WT1*, a tumor suppressor gene located on chromosome 11p.

Answer A is incorrect. Adrenocortical adenomas are usually asymptomatic and are often incidentally found at autopsy or on CT. They are usually smaller tumors, nodular lesions <2.5 cm in diameter. They rarely cause pathology.

Answer B is incorrect. Neuroblastoma is the most common extracranial solid tumor in children. They can present retroperitoneally, often involving the adrenal medulla, as they arise from the neural crest cells; they would not typically be of renal origin. Neuroblastoma is associated with the *N-myc* oncogene, located on chromosome 2p.

Answer C is incorrect. Renal cell carcinoma is the most common renal cancer in adults. It usually presents in older adults after the fifth decade of life and is uncommon in children.

Answer D is incorrect. Transitional cell carcinoma can involve any part of the urothelium. In the kidney, it usually involves the renal pelvis. Transitional cell carcinoma accounts for 5%-10% of primary renal tumors.

34. **The correct answer is D.** This child and his uncle appear to have Friedreich ataxia, a trinucleotide repeat disease. Like other trinucleotide repeat diseases, illness occurs because the unstable microsatellite regions on certain chromosomes have triplet codons that expand, typically worsening from generation to generation (and often making the age of onset earlier for each successive generation). These regions of massively expanded triplet repeats (most commonly between 600 and 1200 in Friedreich ataxia) cause a decrease in the product of a gene, frataxin, at the translation stage.

Answer A is incorrect. The triplet repeats in Friedreich ataxia typically do not affect protein folding because the gene product does not usually get to that stage.

Answer B is incorrect. The triplet repeats in Friedreich ataxia typically do not affect protein splicing.

Answer C is incorrect. The triplet repeats in Friedreich ataxia typically do not cause a substitution, such as that which occurs in sickle cell disease.

Answer E is incorrect. The triplet repeats in Friedreich ataxia typically do not contain a stop codon.

35. **The correct answer is B.** The clinical vignette strongly suggests phenylketonuria (PKU). PKU results most commonly from a deficiency of phenylalanine hydroxylase, the first enzyme in the breakdown pathway for phenylalanine. The product of this reaction is tyrosine, a nonessential amino acid in healthy patients. Infants with PKU have inappropriately high blood phenylalanine levels. High phenylalanine levels are neurotoxic, so this may lead to mental retardation if untreated. Other symptoms include hypopigmentation (due to impaired melanin synthesis), musty odor, eczema, and hyperreflexia. Treatment includes a diet low in phenylalanine with tyrosine supplementation (since it is now essential). It is most effective if instituted before the child is 3 weeks old. Most infants in North America are currently routinely screened for PKU.

Answer A is incorrect. A diet low in the branched-chain amino acids leucine and isoleucine is used to treat patients with maple syrup urine disease. These patients lack a branched-chain dehydrogenase, and thus have inhibited breakdown of leucine, isoleucine, and valine. Infants with this disorder would have an odd smell to their urine. They can have severe central nervous system defects. They do not typically have pale skin, as branched chain amino acids, unlike phenylalanine, are not involved in the melanin synthesis pathway.

Answer C is incorrect. A diet low in tyrosine would cause harm to a patient with PKU, who cannot make this amino acid.

Answer D is incorrect. A high-protein diet would not be recommended in a patient with PKU, as it would lead to high levels of amino acids including phenylalanine. High-protein diets may be used in therapy of some of the glycogen storage diseases. In particular, high protein plus creatinine supplementation may be recommended in McArdle disease, a glycogen storage disease that primarily affects skeletal muscle. This disease causes painful muscle cramps and myoglobinuria with strenuous exercise.

Answer E is incorrect. Recombinant enzyme therapy has not been developed for PKU. This technology has been used to develop a treatment for the adult-onset form of Gaucher disease, a lysosomal storage disorder. This disorder is characterized by hepatosplenomegaly, aseptic necrosis of the femur, and bone crisis.

36. **The correct answer is E.** Pellagra is caused by vitamin B_3 (niacin) deficiency. Patients classically present with diarrhea, dermatitis, and dementia (and beefy glossitis). Other water-soluble vitamins include riboflavin (B_2), niacin (B_3), biotin, folate, and cobalamin (B_{12}).

Answer A is incorrect. Increased erythrocyte hemolysis is the result of vitamin E deficiency, which results in increased fragility of RBCs. Vitamin E is an antioxidant that protects RBCs from hemolysis. It is fat-soluble.

Answer B is incorrect. Neonatal hemorrhage is due to vitamin K deficiency. Vitamin K catalyzes γ-carboxylation of glutamic acid residues on various proteins concerned with blood clotting. It is a fat-soluble vitamin.

Answer C is incorrect. Night blindness is a consequence of vitamin A (retinol) deficiency. Vitamin A is a constituent of visual pigments and is a fat-soluble vitamin.

Answer D is incorrect. Osteomalacia is due to vitamin D deficiency. Vitamin D is a fat-soluble vitamin.

37. **The correct answer is A.** This patient suffers from I-cell disease, which is caused by a failure of addition of mannose-6-phosphate by GlcNAc phosphotransferase on the Golgi apparatus. Without mannose-6-phosphate, lysosomal enzymes cannot be properly directed for inclusion into lysosomes and will instead be excreted by the cell. Thus lysosomal enzymes,

including hexosaminidase, iduronate sulfatase, and arylsulfatase A, will be found in the extracellular, but not intracellular, space. I-cell disease is characterized by skeletal abnormalities, restricted joint movement, coarse facial features, and severe psychomotor impairment. Death usually occurs in the first decade of life.

Answer B is incorrect. Although lysosomes may be abnormal in I-cell disease, that abnormality results from defective trafficking of intracellular proteins caused by an abnormal Golgi apparatus, not from an intrinsic lysosomal abnormality. This is proven by the finding that cultured cells from patients with I-cell disease are capable of incorporating lysosomal enzymes if properly tagged with mannose-6-phosphate.

Answer C is incorrect. Ribosomes are primarily responsible for ensuring the proper matching of messenger RNA with transport RNA, therefore ensuring protein synthesis. The ribosomes of patients with I-cell disease are not abnormal.

Answer D is incorrect. Rough endoplasmic reticulum (RER) typically translates proteins meant for extracellular use. The RER in I-cell disease is not abnormal.

Answer E is incorrect. Smooth endoplasmic reticulum (SER) is the site of cell lipid synthesis and processing of protein. The SER of patients with I-cell disorder is not abnormal and does not play a role in the addition of 6-mannose-phosphate.

38. **The correct answer is E.** Patients with congenital albinism have problems producing melanin. This can be due to a deficiency in the tyrosine (precursor to melanin) transporters or a deficiency in the tyrosinase enzyme. Either way, patients will have generalized decreased pigmentation in the skin, eyes, and hair. Without aggressive photoprotection, most albinism patients will eventually develop skin cancer. The other major problems are ocular, as the lack of melanin causes poor development of the retinal pigment epithelium. The lack of pigment in the iris also causes problems. Nystagmus, strabismus, and impaired visual acuity are a few of the many ophthalmologic problems such patients can have.

Answer A is incorrect. Lactose intolerance is not associated with albinism.

Answer B is incorrect. Children with phenylketonuria should avoid foods with phenylalanine.

Answer C is incorrect. Avoiding strenuous activity may be useful for patients with certain rare cardiac diseases, but is not necessary for children with albinism.

Answer D is incorrect. Patients with Turner syndrome will be very short at full growth (<5 feet tall) unless GH is given in childhood. Children with albinism have normal growth and development.

39. **The correct answer is B.** The patient most likely has pancreatic adenocarcinoma that is located at the head of the pancreas, leading to obstruction of the common bile duct. Weight loss, painless jaundice, and a palpable gallbladder (Courvoisier sign) can occur in pancreatic cancer. The obstruction from the growing tumor results in conjugated hyperbilirubinemia, increased urine bilirubin levels, and decreased urine urobilinogen levels. The majority of bilirubin results from the breakdown of heme groups in senescent RBCs. After cellular release, bilirubin binds to albumin, which delivers the molecule to the liver. Hepatocellular uptake and glucuronidation in the endoplasmic reticulum generate conjugated bilirubin, which is water soluble and excreted in the bile. Gut bacteria deconjugate the bilirubin and degrade it to urobilinogens. The urobilinogens are excreted in the feces, with some reabsorption and excretion into urine. Based on this metabolic schema, the laboratory values in obstructive liver disease become evident. Failed excretion of conjugated bilirubin leads to a direct bilirubinemia. Failure of urobilinogen production by gut flora leads to low levels of urine urobilinogen. The urine bilirubin level is elevated secondary to the increased plasma concentration of direct bilirubin, which undergoes renal excretion.

Answer A is incorrect. Conjugated hyperbilirubinemia, increased urine bilirubin levels, and normal urine urobilinogen levels can be seen in patients with hepatocellular jaundice. The urine urobilinogen level is normal because, unlike in obstructive jaundice, gut bacteria have the opportunity to synthesize urobilinogen. The clinical presentation and physical findings presented here supports a diagnosis of pancreatic adenocarcinoma, not hepatocellular jaundice.

Answer C is incorrect. Unconjugated hyperbilirubinemia, increased urine bilirubin levels, and decreased urine urobilinogen levels can occur with hepatocellular disease if there is also concurrent conjugated hyperbilirubinemia. However, a pure obstructive condition is not characterized by unconjugated hyperbilirubinemia.

Answer D is incorrect. Unconjugated hyperbilirubinemia, decreased urine bilirubin levels, and increased urine urobilinogen levels is a classic pattern seen in hemolytic jaundice. In this case the bilirubin level rises due to increased heme turnover and may overwhelm the liver's ability to conjugate it. These features would not be seen in obstructive liver disease. Patients with certain diseases that increase RBC turnover, such as sickle cell disease, spherocytosis, and glucose-6-phoshate dehydrogenase deficiency, may have hemolytic jaundice. The clinical presentation and physical findings here point to a diagnosis of pancreatic adenocarcinoma, not hemolytic jaundice.

Answer E is incorrect. Unconjugated hyperbilirubinemia, decreased urine bilirubin, and decreased urine urobilinogen are very unlikely to occur simultaneously in any given condition.

40. **The correct answer is B.** This boy suffers from Duchenne muscular dystrophy, an X-linked recessive disorder caused by a frameshift mutation that deletes the dystrophin gene and causes accelerated muscle breakdown (increases creatine kinase). Dystrophin normally links actin filaments to a group of transmembrane glycoproteins in the extracellular space, including laminin. The legs look muscular, but are actually pseudohypertrophic due to massive interstitial fibrosis.

    Answer A is incorrect. Dystrophin has no involvement with signaling at the neuromuscular junction.

    Answer C is incorrect. Actin-myosin cross-bridge cycling is promoted by calcium binding to troponin C, which causes a conformational change that allows tropomyosin to move so that actin-myosin cycling can occur.

    Answer D is incorrect. Dystrophin is not an acetylcholine receptor.

    Answer E is incorrect. The ryanodine receptor and the dihydropyridine receptor are involved in the control of exocytosis of calcium from the sarcoplasmic reticulum.

41. **The correct answer is D.** This patient presents with altered mental status, hyperventilation, and lactic acidosis with hypoglycemia. This presentation is consistent with ethanol-induced hypoglycemia. Oxidation of ethanol produces the reduced form of nicotinamide adenine dinucleotide (NADH) in the liver via two key enzymes: alcohol dehydrogenase and acetaldehyde dehydrogenase. A high ratio of NADH to oxidized nicotinamide adenine dinucleotide (NAD) induces pyruvate metabolism to lactic acid, which leads to lactic acidosis. Note the anion gap and the high lactate level. This elevated NADH / NAD ratio limits the supply of pyruvate needed for gluconeogenesis, hence hypoglycemia ensues.

    Answer A is incorrect. Glycerol 3-phosphate levels are increased (rather than decreased) as a result of the low pyruvate levels. Incidentally, it is important to understand that this leads to increased very low density lipoprotein levels and hyperlipidemia.

    Answer B is incorrect. Pyruvate is not overproduced; rather, it is metabolized to lactate.

    Answer C is incorrect. Gluconeogenesis is inhibited (note the low glucose level) during lactic acidosis as a result of the pyruvate conversion to lactic acid.

Answer E is incorrect. Thiamine (vitamin B_1) deficiency can cause lactic acidosis, because it is a cofactor in the pyruvate dehydrogenase complex; this causes pyruvate accumulation, which induces lactic acid production. However, this patient has not been drinking for a long time, so he is less likely to be vitamin B_1 deficient.

42. **The correct answer is D.** Vitamin B_{12} is a necessary cofactor in the regeneration of folate for methyl group donation in DNA synthesis. For this reason, vitamin B_{12} and folate deficiencies each present with megaloblastic anemia and hypersegmented neutrophils, as all blood cell lines are affected by the defect in DNA synthesis. However, only vitamin B_{12} deficiency increases serum methylmalonic acid levels and impairs myelin synthesis. This myelin defect primarily impacts the posterior and lateral spinal columns, causing paresthesias and impaired proprioception. Thus, neurologic abnormality in the context of megaloblastic anemia is a USMLE-favorite hint that vitamin B_{12}, rather than folate, is deficient.

Answer A is incorrect. Confusion, confabulation, and ataxia are typical of Wernicke-Korsakoff syndrome, a disorder of thiamine (vitamin B_1) deficiency typical in alcoholics.

Answer B is incorrect. Folate and vitamin B_{12} deficiencies present similarly, but folate deficiency does not manifest with an elevated methylmalonic acid level or neurologic problems. In the absence of increased serum methylmalonate levels, therefore, the physician would diagnose folate deficiency, and no neurologic symptoms would be expected.

Answer C is incorrect. Concurrent onset of dysarthria (defective articulation) and diplopia may indicate that a transient ischemic episode or cerebrovascular accident has occurred. These symptoms are not typical of any vitamin deficiency.

Answer E is incorrect. Syncope may be a sign of vasovagal stimulation, low blood pressure, arrhythmia, and other cardiovascular disorders. Lethargy is a sign of decreased consciousness. Neither of these symptoms is typically associated with a vitamin deficiency.

43. **The correct answer is E.** This patient is suffering from methemoglobinemia, in which symptoms typically develop as the percentage of circulating hemoglobin that is instead methemoglobin rises above 3%. Methemoglobin contains Fe^{3+} (as opposed to the Fe^{2+} of circulating hemoglobin) and is formed by nonoxygen oxidizing agents. One such agent known to cause this is dapsone, which is used for toxoplasmosis prophylaxis in HIV-positive patients. The Fe^{3+} of methemoglobin is unable to bind oxygen, and so cannot deliver it to the cells of the body and the patient becomes cyanotic. Nicotinamide adenine dinucleotide reductase (NADH) converts Fe^{3+} into Fe^{2+} by simultaneously oxidizing NADH to the oxidized form of nicotinamide adenine diphosphatase, and so oxygen-carrying capacity is restored. This system may be overwhelmed in the presence of oxidizing agents such as dapsone. Of note, the arterial blood gas of patients with methemoglobinemia will show a normal partial oxygen pressure of because the level of dissolved oxygen is normal; it is only the level of hemoglobin-bound oxygen that is reduced, hence, reduced oxygen saturation. The patient may be acidotic secondary to lactic acidosis from an oxygen deficit at the tissue level.

Answer A is incorrect. ATPase, the enzyme responsible for releasing a phosphate group from ATP, is not responsible for converting methemoglobin to hemoglobin. It is involved in many other reactions in the body and is often used to provide energy for an energetically unfavorable but necessary reaction.

Answer B is incorrect. Flavin adenine dinucleotide ($FADH_2$) reductase is not responsible for converting methemoglobin to hemoglobin, but instead returns $FADH_2$ to its reduced form so that it can accept electrons in the Krebs cycle.

Answer C is incorrect. GTPase, the enzyme responsible for releasing a phosphate group from GTP, is not responsible for converting methemoglobin to hemoglobin. It is used in many second messenger pathways and can help provide energy for an energetically unfavorable but necessary reaction.

Answer D is incorrect. Lactase, the enzyme responsible for cleaving lactose into its monosaccharide constituents, is not responsible for converting methemoglobin to hemoglobin.

Answer F is incorrect. Pyruvate kinase, the enzyme responsible for converting phosphoenolpyruvate to pyruvate at the end of glycolysis, is not responsible for converting methemoglobin to hemoglobin.

44. **The correct answer is E.** Steroid hormones enter cells and bind to receptor proteins. The receptor-hormone complex binds to specific response elements, or the regulatory region of DNA, and activates gene transcription.

Answer A is incorrect. Steroid hormones do not regulate the initiation of protein synthesis.

Answer B is incorrect. Steroid hormones do not regulate mRNA degradation.

Answer C is incorrect. Steroid hormones do not regulate mRNA processing.

Answer D is incorrect. Steroid hormones regulate gene transcription, not translation.

45. **The correct answer is C.** Tay-Sachs disease results from a deficiency of hexosaminidase A activity. This disorder is inherited as an autosomal recessive trait and has a carrier frequency of 1:25 in the Ashkenazi Jewish population. Findings include loss of motor skills, increased startle reaction, macular pallor, and a cherry-red spot on the macula (as shown in the image). Diagnosis is confirmed by the quantification of hexosaminidase level in isolated WBCs in the blood. Future at-risk pregnancies can be monitored via prenatal diagnosis by either amniocentesis or chorionic villus sampling.

Answer A is incorrect. Fabry disease occurs in α-galactosidase A deficiency. This disease is characterized by symptoms of peripheral neuropathy, cardiovascular, and renal disease.

Answer B is incorrect. Arylsulfatase A deficiency characterizes metachromatic leukodystrophy, a syndrome that consists of central and peripheral demyelination, ataxia, and dementia.

Answer D is incorrect. Hunter syndrome is a lysosomal storage disease that is characterized by developmental delay, aggressive behavior, and airway obstruction. It is due to a deficiency of iduronate synthase.

Answer E is incorrect. Mutations in lysyl hydroxylase have been found in certain forms of Ehlers-Danlos syndrome. These mutations reduce the content of hydroxylysine in collagen and reduce the content of collagen cross-links. These defects are believed to decrease the tensile strength of collagen and account for the symptoms of Ehlers-Danlos syndrome.

46. **The correct answer is A.** This patient has fructose intolerance caused by a deficiency in aldolase B. Aldolase B catalyzes the reaction in which fructose-1-phosphate is metabolized to dihydroxyacetone-phosphate and glyceraldehyde. If there is a deficiency in aldolase B, the reactant fructose-1-phosphate accumulates in the liver. This depletes the liver's stores of free phosphate, which inhibits the production of glucose through gluconeogenesis and causes a fall in cellular ATP levels. The common preceding event to the drop in glucose and ATP levels is a decrease in free phosphate levels.

Answer B is incorrect. ATP will not be increased, because much of the free phosphate needed to combine with adenosine diphosphate to form ATP is already bound to fructose.

Answer C is incorrect. When a patient with aldolase B deficiency is challenged with fructose, glucose levels will fall and a lactic acidosis will ensue. Therefore the pH will decrease, not increase.

Answer D is incorrect. Rough endoplasmic reticulum (RER) typically translates proteins meant for extracellular use. The RER in I-cell disease is not abnormal.

Answer E is incorrect. In aldolase B deficiency fructose can be converted to fructose-1-phosphate and become trapped intracellularly. Thus there should not be a significant rise in urinary fructose excretion as occurs in fructokinase deficiency.

47. **The correct answer is C.** Glucose-6-phosphate dehydrogenase (G6PD) deficiency is characterized by acute episodes of hemolytic anemia following administration of certain medications, infection, or ingestion of fava beans. G6PD is the first and rate-limiting enzyme of the pentose phosphate pathway, which produces two reducing equivalents that keep glutathione in its reduced state. Reduced glutathione is necessary to detoxify peroxides and free radicals that can accumulate within RBCs and cause damage to various cellular structures. Heinz bodies are small round inclusions seen within RBCs that comprise hemoglobin and other protein precipitates. G6PD deficiency is most common in people who are black, people of Mediterranean descent, and people from tropical Africa and Asia.

    Answer A is incorrect. Alkaptonuria is a rare genetic disorder in which patients present with urine that darkens on exposure to air. These patients cannot breakdown the amino acid tyrosine, which results in the accumulation of a by-product called homogentisic acid. Homogentisic acid builds up in the skin and connective tissues and is excreted in the urine, causing the dark color. Patients typically have a good prognosis, although many suffer from arthritis as well as heart disease and kidney/prostate stones.

    Answer B is incorrect. Cystinuria is caused by a defect in an amino acid transporter in the renal tubules. This is an inherited defect that affects the absorption of four amino acids: cystine, ornithine, lysine, and arginine. Cystine kidney stones can form as a result of excess cystine in the urine. This disorder is not associated with the jaundice or hematologic abnormalities seen in this patient.

    Answer D is incorrect. Hereditary fructose intolerance is an autosomal-recessive inherited disease due to a deficiency of aldolase B, which causes an accumulation of fructose-1-phosphate. The decrease in available phosphate leads to inhibition of gluconeogenesis and glycogenolysis. Patients present with jaundice, cirrhosis, hypoglycemia, and scleral icterus. Hepatosplenomegaly is often seen on physical examination. It is usually diagnosed in early childhood, when children are weaned from formula to regular table food.

    Answer E is incorrect. Hereditary spherocytosis is caused by a variety of molecular defects in genes that code for spectrin, ankyrin, protein 4.1, and other RBC membrane proteins. The structural defect makes the RBCs more fragile and they take on a spherical shape, hence the name "spherocytes." Spherocytes are recognized as abnormal and destroyed in the spleen, resulting in severe anemia and splenomegaly. Splenectomy curbs the anemia; however, the RBCs will continue to be spherical in shape.

    Answer F is incorrect. Lactase deficiency can be due to either an inherited intolerance or an age-dependent acquired intolerance of the sugar lactose. Acquired lactase deficiency (decreased expression with increased age) is more common in Africans and Asians. Patients present with osmotic diarrhea, abdominal cramps, and bloating.

48. **The correct answer is A.** At 28 weeks, this neonate's lungs have not had the opportunity to fully develop, and are deficient in dipalmitoyl phosphatidylcholine, also known as surfactant. Surfactant, synthesized by type II pneumocytes, is essential in stabilizing air-expanded alveoli by decreasing surface tension, thus preventing lung collapse during expiration. Surfactant is usually made most abundantly after the 35th week of gestation. The most common way to determine lung maturity is by the lecithin:sphingomyelin ratio of the amniotic fluid. If this ratio is >2.0, then the risk of developing neonatal respiratory distress syndrome (NRDS) is significantly decreased.

    Answer B is incorrect. Elastase is an endogenous proteolytic enzyme in the lung that is normally broken down by antitrypsin. In patients with α_1-antitrypsin deficiency, there is an increased level of elastase, which leads to lung tissue destruction and emphysema. Liver cirrhosis also occurs as a result of the increased level of elastase in the liver.

Answer C is incorrect. Cilial dysfunction may result in decreased mucus clearance from the lungs and may predispose patients to recurrent respiratory infections. In Kartagener syndrome, cilia are immotile because of a dynein arm defect. This results in infertility, bronchiectasis, and recurrent sinusitis.

Answer D is incorrect. This neonate has signs and symptoms consistent with NRDS secondary to his prematurity. NRDS is caused by a deficiency of dipalmitoyl phosphatidylcholine, not phosphatidylglycerol. Phosphatidylglycerol is a compound measured in amniotic fluid to determine fetal lung maturity, and is used in conjunction with the lecithin:sphingomyelin ratio.

Answer E is incorrect. Sphingomyelin is found primarily in the brain and nervous tissue. Although it is measured to help in determining fetal lung maturity, deficiency of sphingomyelin does not lead to NRDS.

49. **The correct answer is E.** The cells described above are in metaphase of the mitosis (M) phase of the cell cycle, which is characterized by chromosomes migrating and lining up in the middle of the cell. In metaphase, the nuclear envelope has disintegrated and the mitotic spindle moves into the nuclear area. The chromosomes then become arranged in the plane of the spindle equator. Vincristine acts by binding to tubulin and blocking formation of microtubules, which are required to form the mitotic spindle.

Answer A is incorrect. 5-Fluorouracil acts in the synthesis (S) phase of the cell cycle. It works by complexing to folic acid, which inhibits thymidylate synthesis and therefore DNA synthesis. In the S phase the chromosomes are not vertically aligned in the cell

Answer B is incorrect. Cyclophosphamide is an alkylating agent, a class of cell cycle-nonspecific antineoplastic drugs. By permanently cross-linking DNA strands, cyclophosphamide causes breaks in double-stranded DNA during cellular repair efforts, leading to apoptosis.

Answer C is incorrect. Etoposide acts in the growth 2 (G_2) and synthesis (S) phases of the cell cycle, by inhibiting topoisomerase II and thereby inhibiting DNA synthesis. In the G_2 and S phases, the chromosomes are not vertically aligned in the cell.

Answer D is incorrect. Methotrexate acts in the synthesis (S) phase of the cell cycle. It binds to dihyrofolate reductase and thereby inhibits formation of purine nucleotides and thymidylate so that DNA synthesis cannot take place. In the S phase the chromosomes are not vertically aligned in the cell.

50. **The correct answer is C.** Fragile X syndrome is a complex genetic disorder that most closely follows an X-linked dominant pattern of inheritance. It is caused by a trinucleotide repeat expansion (CGG). The disease is characterized by mental retardation and physical features such as macroorchidism (large testicles), long face, large mandible, and large, everted ears. The number of CGG repeats in patients with the full mutation average around 230-4000. In the normal population, this sequence repeats an average of 29 times. Patients with premutations have from 52 to 230 repeats and lack the disease phenotype. Differences in the size of CGG repeats can be shown on a Southern blot. Shorter fragments of DNA migrate more rapidly through a gel toward the positive electrode. Therefore, patients with full mutations (who have longer strands of DNA) will have a "sluggish" band that stays toward the top of the gel, the normal population will show a band at the bottom of the gel, and patients with a premutation will have a band in the middle. Lane C would best represent the Southern blot of a woman who carries a premutation for fragile X and one normal X.

Answer A is incorrect. Lane A on the Southern blot shows two bands. The band at the top of the gel represents a large fragment of DNA and an amplification of the CGG region to a full-blown mutation. The band at the middle of the gel represents a medium-sized fragment of DNA or a premutation.

Answer B is incorrect. Lane B represents a patient with the full fragile X mutation. The DNA band is located at the top of the gel and represents a large fragment of DNA and an amplification of the CGG region to a full-blown mutation.

Answer D is incorrect. The DNA band on lane D represents a patient with no trinucleotide repeat expansion.

Answer E is incorrect. Lane E on the Southern blot shows two bands. The band at the bottom of the gel represents a short fragment of DNA and thus a normal-sized CGG repeat region. The band at the top of the gel represents a large fragment of DNA and an amplification of the CGG region to a full-blown mutation.

CHAPTER 3

Embryology

QUESTIONS

1. A physician is asked to evaluate a 5-year-old girl who has developed a mass in her neck. During the interview, he learns that the mass appeared within the past few months and has been enlarging; however, it causes no pain or discomfort. The mass is in the midline of the neck just inferior to the hyoid bone. Laboratory tests reveal a triiodothyronine level of 150 ng/dL, a thyroxine level of 8.0 μg/dL, and a thyroid-stimulating hormone level of 1 μU/mL. A CT scan of the neck is performed and the doctor recommends surgery. Which of the following is the most likely diagnosis?

   (A) Branchial cleft cyst
   (B) Dermoid cyst
   (C) Ectopic thyroid gland
   (D) Enlarged pyramidal lobe of the thyroid
   (E) Lipoma
   (F) Thyroglossal duct cyst

2. A 5-year-old girl is brought to her pediatrician because her mother says she is frequently bumping into stationary objects while playing. Visual field examination shows bilateral peripheral vision defects. CT of the head reveals calcifications in the pituitary fossa. Which of the following is the most likely origin of this child's brain tumor?

   (A) Adenohypophyseal lactotrophs
   (B) Fourth ventricle neuroectoderm
   (C) Rathke pouch
   (D) Vascular endothelium
   (E) Ventricular lining

3. A 6-week-old boy is brought to the clinic because of fever. Urinalysis is positive for WBCs. Physical examination reveals the boy's urethral opening to be displaced to the ventral (inferior) aspect of the penis. Which of the following is the embryologic cause of this congenital abnormality?

   (A) Abnormal expansion of the ureteric bud
   (B) Abnormal positioning of genital tubercle
   (C) Failure of the mesonephric (wolffian) duct to regress
   (D) Incomplete fusion of urethral (urogenital) folds
   (E) Patency of the processus vaginalis

4. Ensuring adequate maternal intake of a specific nutrient is especially important in reducing the incidence of the congenital anomaly shown in the image. A deficiency of this nutrient, when present in an adult, is associated with which of the following conditions?

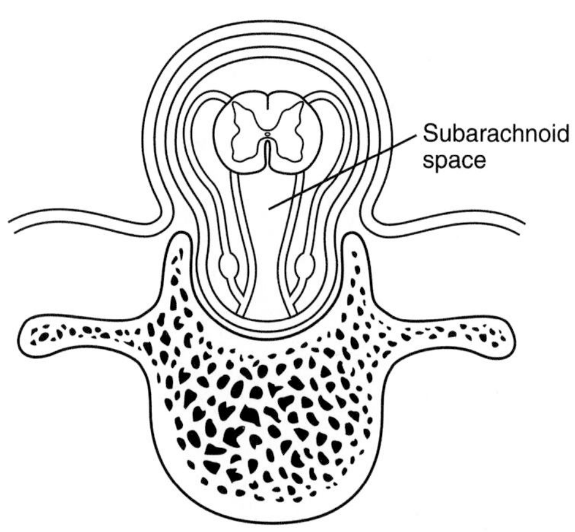

Reproduced, with permission, from USMLERx.com.

   (A) Confabulation and anterograde amnesia
   (B) Diarrhea, dermatitis, and dementia
   (C) Megaloblastic anemia
   (D) Megaloblastic anemia with neurologic symptoms
   (E) Microcytic anemia
   (F) Polyneuritis and cardiac pathology
   (G) Swollen and bleeding gums, easy bruising, and poor wound healing

5. A 1-year-old girl presents to the pediatrician because of increasing neuromuscular irritability and tetany over the past few weeks. She has also had recurrent viral and fungal infection since birth, and was born full term. Results of physical examination are within normal limits. X-ray of the chest reveals the absence of a thymic shadow. Thorough laboratory testing reveals a T-lymphocyte deficiency. What other findings are most likely in this child?

   (A) Elevated parathyroid hormone levels
   (B) Enlarged thymus gland
   (C) Enlarged thyroid gland
   (D) Low serum calcium levels
   (E) Low serum phosphorus levels

6. A 13-month-old child is brought to the emergency room after his parents found blood in his stool. They state that he did not appear distressed at the time, although he now displays some tenderness to abdominal pressure. Other than this tenderness, there are no significant findings on physical examination. After performing radionuclide imaging using ^{99m}Tc pertechnetate, the doctor makes a diagnosis and recommends surgery to correct the problem. What is the probable source of this child's condition?

   (A) Blockage of the intestine due to folding of the distal ileum into the proximal colon
   (B) Breakdown of the stomach mucosal barrier, with erosion of the underlying mucosa
   (C) Damage to the intestinal epithelium due to ingestion of coins
   (D) Ectopic gastric epithelium in a persistent omphalomesenteric duct
   (E) Incomplete bowel rotation resulting in obstruction of the superior mesenteric artery

7. The x-ray shown in the image is from a child with a congenital condition. Which of the following is the most common cause of death in infants with this condition?

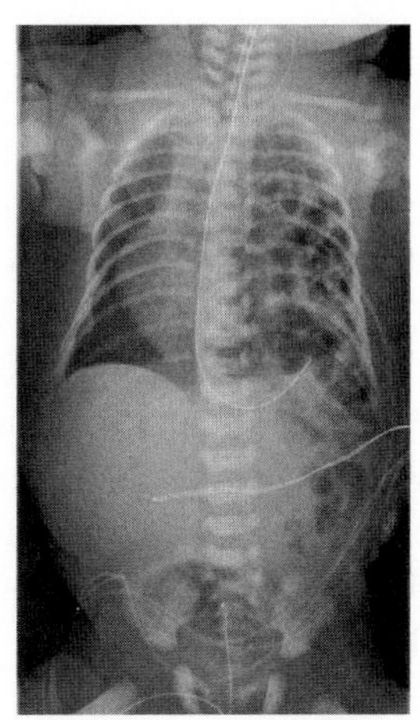

Reproduced, with permission, from USMLERx.com.

   (A) Cardiac tamponade
   (B) Coarctation of the aorta
   (C) Diaphragmatic eventration
   (D) Mediastinal shift
   (E) Pulmonary hypoplasia

8. A 5-month-old girl is brought to the emergency department by her parents because she is "turning blue." She is cyanotic, weak, and dyspneic. Her parents state that she has experienced similar episodes in the past, but never this severe. Physical examination reveals the lungs are clear to auscultation, with no wheezing, rales, or rhonchi. Cardiac examination reveals a regular rate and rhythm, normal S_1, single S_2, a grade III rough systolic murmur at the left sternal border in the third intercostal space, and a palpable right ventricular lift. Echocardiography demonstrates unusual positioning of the aorta, which overrides both the left and right ventricles in the long axis view. In this condition, the primary developmental defect occurs in which portion of the primitive heart?

   (A) Bulbus cordis
   (B) Conal septum
   (C) Left and right horns of the sinus venosus
   (D) Primitive atria
   (E) Primitive ventricle

9. Spermatogenesis, the process of forming spermatozoa, occurs in the seminiferous tubules of the testes. As the cells proceed through the different stages of spermatogenesis, they contain varying numbers of chromosomes and varying amounts of DNA. A laboratory investigator is observing, under the microscope, cells undergoing this process. He has focused on a group of cells that recently gained an acrosome and tail. Which of the following best describes the amount of DNA and the number of chromosomes that exist in those cells?

(A) 23, 1n
(B) 23, 2n
(C) 46, 1n
(D) 46, 2n
(E) 46, 4n

10. During embryonic development of the urinary system, a portion of the bladder extends into the umbilical cord. Failure of this vestigial structure to degenerate may lead to which of the following complications?

(A) Bladder exstrophy
(B) Bladder adenocarcinoma
(C) Meckel diverticulum
(D) Polycystic kidney disease
(E) Renal agenesis

11. A 4-year-old boy is brought to the pediatrician by his mother, who says that he has been having problems eating. She says he quickly becomes full and often vomits following a meal. When questioned, the boy says his stomach hurts when he eats. The mother says that the boy ate well up until about six months ago, when the current problems began; he experienced no abnormal vomiting as an infant. X-ray of the abdomen is remarkable for a distended, air-filled stomach that narrows at the level of the proximal duodenum and then dilates again in the distal duodenum. Which of the following developmental abnormalities is most likely responsible for this patient's condition?

(A) Abnormal rotation of the ventral pancreatic bud around the duodenum
(B) Failure of duodenal recanalization
(C) Failure of the midgut to return to the abdominal cavity after physiological midgut herniation
(D) Hypertrophy of the pyloric muscles
(E) Incomplete separation of the esophagus and laryngotracheal tube

12. A 16-year-old pregnant girl has not received prenatal care. At 17 weeks, she noted some painless vaginal spotting (bleeding) which prompted her to seek medical attention. On arrival at the hospital, pelvic examination showed fetal parts in the cervical os and the patient was told that a miscarriage was inevitable. The products of conception as delivered are shown in the image. What is the most likely pathogenesis of this condition?

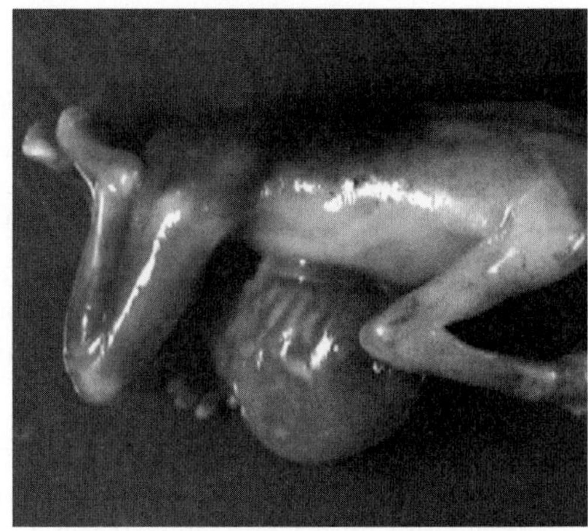

Reproduced, with permission, from USMLERx.com.

(A) Ethanol toxicity
(B) Malrotation
(C) Maternal folate deficiency
(D) Omphalomesenteric vessel occlusion
(E) ToRCHeS infection

13. Immediately following delivery, a newborn is observed to have multiple abnormalities, including a small lower jaw, abnormal feet, and hands that are clenched into fists. Treatment is started for a congenital heart condition. The survival of a patient with this condition is most similar to that of a person affected by which of the following genetic abnormalities?

(A) An F508 deletion in the *CFTR* gene
(B) CAG tandem repeats
(C) CGG tandem repeats
(D) Trisomy of chromosome 13
(E) Trisomy of chromosome 21

14. A neonate is found to have a congenital heart defect. Physical examination reveals that the patient is not cyanotic, but a harsh holosystolic murmur is heard at the left lower sternal border. No other murmurs are heard on auscultation. From which of the following congenital heart defects is this neonate most likely suffering?

(A) Atrial septal defect
(B) Tetralogy of Fallot
(C) Transposition of the great arteries
(D) Truncus arteriosus
(E) Ventricular septal defect

15. A scientist creates a model of fetal circulation in order to study blood flow during this stage of development. During one experiment, he measures the partial oxygen pressure in various fetal vessels. His results are as follows:

Vessel A: 20 mm Hg
Vessel B: 27 mm Hg
Vessel C: 35 mm Hg
Vessel D: 12 mm Hg

The vessel labeled C will develop into which structure in the adult?

(A) Falciform ligament
(B) Ligamentum teres hepatis
(C) Ligamentum venosum
(D) Medial umbilical ligament
(E) Median umbilical ligament

16. A baby boy dies several hours after birth. He was born with wrinkled skin, deformed limbs, and abnormal facies. The mother's pregnancy was complicated by oligohydramnios. Which of the following embryologic processes most likely failed in this child?

(A) Development of the ureteric buds
(B) Closure of the rostral neural tube
(C) Formation of the tracheoesophageal septum
(D) Migration of neural crest cells to the distal colon
(E) Recanalization of the duodenum

17. A 34-year-old man complains of dry mouth and difficulty swallowing. He has no other complaints. Physical examination is begun in the head and neck region. The eye examination is grossly benign. The nasal sinus appears unremarkable. The patient's oral cavity is then examined. To enable evaluation of the palatal elevation, the patient is asked to "say ah." The muscles used to perform palatal elevation are derived from which of the following embryologic structures?

(A) Branchial arches 1 and 2
(B) Branchial arches 3 and 4
(C) Branchial arches 4 and 6
(D) Branchial clefts 1 and 2
(E) Branchial pouches 3 and 4

18. A child has a unilateral notch of the upper lip (see image). What is the most likely etiology of this lip malformation?

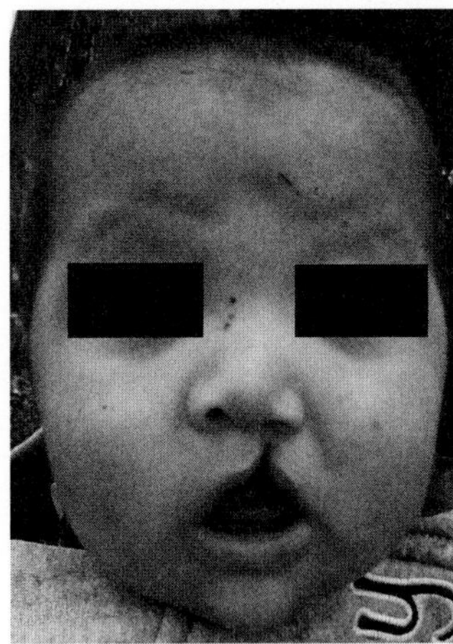

Courtesy of Dr. James Heilman.

(A) Abnormal fusion of the maxillary and medial nasal processes
(B) Altered development of the third and fourth branchial pouches
(C) Flaws in the mandibular and maxillary bones
(D) Incomplete development of the third pharyngeal arch

19. A 3-week-old boy presents to his pediatrician because his mother has noticed that he "looks yellow." On questioning, she elaborates that the jaundice began several days after birth and has been associated with dark urine and clay-colored stools. Laboratory studies show a direct bilirubin level of 5.0 mg/dL and a total bilirubin level of 5.5 mg/dL. Which of the following is characteristic of the most likely diagnosis?

(A) Caused by a genetic mutation in a promoter region
(B) Caused by deficiency in uridine 5'-diphosphoglucuronosyltransferase
(C) Commonly treated with phototherapy
(D) Inherited in an autosomal dominant pattern
(E) Untreated, it leads to cirrhosis by six months of age

20. Over the course of embryologic development, the predominant location of hematopoiesis changes several times. When the uterine fundus is palpable above the umbilicus, where is the main location of hematopoiesis in the fetus?

(A) Bone marrow
(B) Liver
(C) Pancreas
(D) Thymus
(E) Yolk sac

ANSWERS

1. **The correct answer is F.** The thyroid gland originates as the thyroid diverticulum on the floor of the pharynx. It descends into the neck during development, but remains connected to the tongue by the thyroglossal duct. The thyroglossal duct eventually disappears, leaving a small cavity (the foramen cecum) at the base of the tongue. The pyramidal lobe of the thyroid can be thought of as the caudal part of the duct. Occasionally, part of the duct epithelium persists in the neck and may form cysts. Thyroglossal duct cysts are usually painless or slightly tender and appear in the midline of the neck. They often appear over or just below the hyoid, but may appear anywhere between the base of the tongue and the thyroid. If a normal thyroid gland is present, surgery to remove the thyroglossal duct cyst is recommended to prevent infection. In this case, the presence of a normal thyroid is demonstrated by normal triiodothyronine, thyroxine, and thyroid-stimulating hormone (TSH) levels and is confirmed by CT scan.

   Answer A is incorrect. Branchial cleft cysts can also occur in the neck but are not always in the midline. Unlike thyroglossal duct cysts, they are often associated with fistulas or sinus tracts.

   Answer B is incorrect. Dermoid cysts are the second most common cause of midline neck masses, after thyroglossal duct cysts. They tend to be more superficial than thyroglossal duct cysts and more mobile relative to underlying structures.

   Answer C is incorrect. Ectopic thyroid glands are often seen in the presence of a thyroglossal duct cyst. An ectopic thyroid gland occurs when the thyroid fails to descend during development; in contrast, ectopic thyroid tissue may occur along the path of the thyroglossal duct in the presence of a normal thyroid gland. Unlike this patient, who has normal thyroid levels, about one third of patients with an ectopic gland are hypothyroid. A CT scan is usually performed to confirm the presence of a normal thyroid gland before surgery is performed on a thyroglossal duct cyst.

   Answer D is incorrect. Hypertrophy of the pyramidal lobe of the thyroid is not the most likely cause of midline neck swelling in a young child. Furthermore, hypertrophic thyroid tissue would most likely alter thyroid hormone and TSH levels.

   Answer E is incorrect. Lipomas may cause neck swelling, but the location of this mass and the age of the patient make a thyroglossal duct cyst much more likely. Lipomas tend to be very superficial, with poorly defined edges.

2. **The correct answer is C.** The visual-field defect described is a bitemporal hemianopia, typically caused by lesions in the sella turcica impinging on the optic chiasm. In children the most common tumor in this location is a craniopharyngioma, derived from the remnants of Rathke pouch. This embryologic structure buds from the roof of the mouth to form the anterior pituitary. Bitemporal hemianopia is typically accompanied by severe headaches and poor pituitary function. Treatment includes surgery, radiotherapy, or both.

   Answer A is incorrect. Pituitary adenomas, derived from secretory cells of the adenohypophysis, can cause bitemporal hemianopia and headaches, as they are also sella turcica tumors. However, they are more common in older patients, and are unlikely in a child. Also, pituitary adenomas tend to secrete pituitary hormones. The three most common forms of pituitary adenoma are prolactinomas (which are derived from lactotrophs and secrete prolactin, causing galactorrhea and amenorrhea), growth hormone-secreting tumors (somatotrophs, causing acromegaly), and ACTH-producing tumors (corticotrophs, causing Cushing disease). In this case, the only data making this an incorrect answer are the patient's age and the lack of secretory action.

   Answer B is incorrect. Medulloblastoma arises from primitive neuroectoderm in the fourth ventricle. It does not cause the visual symptoms seen in this patient, but the tumor may compress the fourth ventricle to cause hydrocephalus and symptoms consistent with increased intracranial pressure such as morning headache and vomiting. An additional, specific sign of this posterior fossa tumor is a head tilt. Treatment consists of surgery, chemotherapy, and radiation. When in doubt, remember that medulloblastoma is the most common malignant brain tumor in children.

Answer D is incorrect. Hemangioblastomas are vascular tumors of the central nervous system that usually occur in the cerebellum and spinal cord and thus would be unlikely to cause the visual field defects described in this case. Symptoms include cerebellar ataxia, motor weakness, and sensory dysfunction. Hemangioblastomas can occur sporadically or in patients with von Hippel-Lindau disease, which is an autosomal dominant disease in which patients develop cerebellar and retinal hemangioblastomas, pancreatic cysts, and pheochromocytomas.

Answer E is incorrect. Ependymomas form from the cells lining the ventricles and most often occur in the fourth ventricle. Like medulloblastomas, ependymomas can block the flow of cerebrospinal fluid and cause hydrocephalus. These patients, however, do not have the visual disturbances of the patient in this vignette.

3. **The correct answer is D.** This vignette describes a urinary tract infection in an infant with hypospadias, a congenital abnormality in which the urethra opens on the ventral (inferior) aspect of the penis. It occurs as a result of a failure of the urethral folds (also known as the urogenital folds) to fuse fully. Infants with hypospadias should undergo surgery to prevent urinary tract infections.

   Answer A is incorrect. The ureteric bud develops into the upper urinary system (collecting duct, calices, renal pelvis, and ureters) and is unrelated to the lower urinary system. Its abnormal expansion is not associated with known urogenital anomalies.

   Answer B is incorrect. Abnormal positioning of the genital tubercle may result in epispadias, a condition in which the urethral opening is located on the dorsal (superior) surface of the penis. This condition is less common than hypospadias and is associated with exstrophy of the urinary bladder.

   Answer C is incorrect. The mesonephric (wolffian) duct develops into the seminal vesicles, epididymis, ejaculatory duct, and ductus deferens in the male. Regression of this duct might lead to an absence of these reproductive structures rather than hypospadias.

   Answer E is incorrect. Patency of the processus vaginalis allows fluid to flow from the peritoneum into the tunica vaginalis, resulting in a hydrocele of the testes. This would not cause hypospadias, an abnormality in which the urethra opens on the ventral surface of the penis.

4. **The correct answer is C.** The image shows a meningomyelocele, a neural tube defect in which the meninges and spinal cord herniate through a defect in the spinal canal. Folate, if given to a mother early in pregnancy, lowers the risk of developing neural tube defects (spina bifida occulta, meningocele, or meningomyelocele). In the adult, folate deficiency produces a megaloblastic anemia without neurologic symptoms. Folate deficiency is seen in alcoholics, pregnant women, patients with hemolytic anemia, and those taking drugs such as methotrexate that inhibit folate metabolism. Folate can be found in uncooked vegetables and fruits. A deficiency of vitamin B_{12} also causes a megaloblastic anemia, but produces neurologic symptoms as well. Such symptoms include distal neuropathy and loss of position sense due to demyelination of the posterior and lateral columns of the spinal cord and of the peripheral nerves.

   Answer A is incorrect. Confabulation and anterograde amnesia, chronic neurologic sequelae of thiamine (vitamin B_1) deficiency, are seen in Wernicke-Korsakoff syndrome. This is commonly seen in alcoholics.

Answer B is incorrect. Diarrhea, dermatitis, and dementia are characteristic of pellagra, caused by a deficiency of niacin (vitamin B_3).

Answer D is incorrect. Megaloblastic anemia with neurologic symptoms is a result of vitamin B_{12} (cobalamin) deficiency. Typically, neurologic symptoms result from demyelination of the posterior and lateral columns of the spinal cord and of peripheral nerves. Symmetric numbness or burning in the extremities and loss of position sense are common. Unlike folate deficiency, this is not associated with congenital neural tube defects. Cobalamin deficiency can manifest as dementia as well.

Answer E is incorrect. Microcytic anemia is caused by iron deficiency as well as lead poisoning and the thalassemias.

Answer F is incorrect. Polyneuritis and cardiac pathology are signs of beriberi, which results from thiamine (vitamin B_1) deficiency.

Answer G is incorrect. Scurvy is a disorder of swollen and bleeding gums, easy bruising, and poor wound healing seen in vitamin C (ascorbic acid) deficiency. Vitamin C is an essential cofactor for the hydroxylation of proline and lysine residues. Hydroxyproline and hydroxylysine allow crosslinking of collagen, giving connective tissue adequate tensile strength.

5. **The correct answer is D.** This child has DiGeorge syndrome, which is associated with defective development of the third and fourth pharyngeal pouches. These structures typically give rise to the thymus and parathyroid glands. Their absence explains the typical T-lymphocyte immunodeficiency and hypoparathyroidism seen in these patients, and evidenced by the hypocalcemia in this case. Most patients also display congenital cardiac defects.

   Answer A is incorrect. With hypoparathyroidism from underdeveloped parathyroid glands, a decreased parathyroid hormone level would be expected.

   Answer B is incorrect. DiGeorge syndrome is characterized by thymic hypoplasia, not hyperplasia.

   Answer C is incorrect. DiGeorge syndrome can less frequently involve the clear cells of the thyroid gland, but would not be expected to cause an enlarged thyroid.

   Answer E is incorrect. With hypoparathyroidism, an increased serum phosphorus level is anticipated.

6. **The correct answer is D.** The child has a Meckel diverticulum, which describes the persistence after birth of part of the omphalomesenteric duct (vitelline duct or yolk stalk). Meckel diverticulum is usually found in the mid to distal ileum, and may end blindly or connect to the umbilicus. It is described by the "**rule of 2s**": It is about **2** inches long, is located **2** feet proximal to the ileocecal valve, occurs in about **2**% of the population in a **2**:1 male:female ratio, often presents before **2** years of age (60% of cases), and may contain **2** types of epithelium (gastric or pancreatic). Ectopic gastric epithelium is present in about half of cases and can cause ulcers and painless bleeding, but does not generally cause severe pain unless inflammation occurs. In the half of Meckel diverticulum patients with no ectopic gastric epithelium, there is no bleeding. ^{99m}Technetium (^{99m}Tc) pertechnetate is absorbed preferentially by gastric mucosa, and thus may be used to detect ectopic gastric mucosa in the diverticulum.

   Answer A is incorrect. Intussusception is the telescoping of the distal ileum into the proximal colon. It usually presents in the first two years of life, and a Meckel diverticulum may predispose to this condition. However, intussusception typically has an abrupt and severe presentation, with paroxysmal bouts of screaming, vomiting, diarrhea, and bloody bowel movements occurring within 24 hours of onset. A sausage-shaped mass in the abdomen may be palpable on physical exam.

   Answer B is incorrect. Breakdown of the mucosal barrier of the stomach and erosion of the underlying mucosal epithelium describes the pathology of a peptic ulcer. Peptic ulcers may present at any age, but are more common in patients 12-18 years than in very young children. Additionally, it is not diagnosed by ^{99m}Tc-pertechnetate scanning, but would be diagnosed by endoscopy.

Answer C is incorrect. Ingestion of foreign objects occurs frequently in young children and may cause mechanical damage to the intestinal lining. However, these tears are not detected with ^{99m}Tc-pertechnetate scanning.

Answer E is incorrect. Abnormal or incomplete rotation of the intestine as it returns to the abdomen after physiologic herniation can trap and twist loops of bowel; twisting of these loops (volvulus) can result in obstruction of circulation and potentially lead to gangrene of the affected segment of intestine. Most affected infants present within the first three weeks of life with bile-containing vomit or bowel obstruction. Bloody stool is not a principal sign of malrotation or volvulus.

7. **The correct answer is E.** Pulmonary hypoplasia is the most common cause of death in infants born with congenital diaphragmatic hernia. When the pleuroperitoneal folds fail to fuse with the other components of the diaphragm during development, a hole is created that allows bowel into the thorax. The physical compression of the bowels on the lung buds then prevents full development of the respiratory system (pulmonary hypoplasia). This leads to a common presentation of dyspnea and cyanosis and, unless it can be repaired surgically, eventually leads to death.

   Answer A is incorrect. Cardiac tamponade is most frequently associated with a pericardial effusion. This is not a common complication of congenital diaphragmatic hernia.

   Answer B is incorrect. Cardiac abnormalities such as ventriculoseptal defects, vascular rings, and coarctation of the aorta are associated with congenital diaphragmatic hernias; however, they are not the most common cause of death.

   Answer C is incorrect. Eventration of the diaphragm is a disorder in which all or part of the diaphragmatic muscle is replaced by fibroelastic tissue. The weakened hemidiaphragm is displaced into the thorax, which can compromise breathing. Similarly to congenital diaphragmatic hernias, this can also cause pulmonary hypoplasia, although usually not as severe.

   Answer D is incorrect. Mediastinal shift does occur in congenital diaphragmatic hernia, as the bowel invades the thorax and pushes the mediastinum to the right. However, this in itself is not a cause of death.

8. **The correct answer is B.** This patient has tetralogy of Fallot (TOF). TOF is the most common congenital cyanotic lesion and is characterized by four congenital cardiac abnormalities: (1) pulmonary stenosis, (2) ventricular septal defect (VSD), (3) overriding (right-arched) aorta, and (4) right ventricular hypertrophy (due to outflow blockage). The severity of the condition is determined by the degree of cyanosis, which is, in turn, most dependent on the degree of pulmonary stenosis. In the most severe cases patients are cyanotic at birth, but most infants with TOF present at 4-6 months of age with recurrent bouts of hypoxemia and cyanosis. The primary developmental defect is an abnormal anterior and cephalad displacement of the conal septum, resulting in an enlarged aorta and obstructed pulmonary artery.

   Answer A is incorrect. The bulbus cordis becomes the smooth parts of the left and right ventricles, which are not primarily involved in this lesion.

   Answer C is incorrect. The left horn of the sinus venosus gives rise to the coronary sinus. The right horn of the sinus venosus gives rise to the smooth part of the right atrium. Neither of these structures is primarily involved in this lesion.

   Answer D is incorrect. The primitive atria become the trabeculated parts of the left and right atria, which are not primarily involved in this lesion.

   Answer E is incorrect. The primitive ventricle becomes the trabeculated parts of the left and right ventricles, which are not primarily involved in this lesion.

9. **The correct answer is A.** Spermiogenesis is the series of post-meiotic morphologic changes that marks the final maturation of the sperm. Spermatids are the 23, 1n cells that result from secondary spermatocyte meiosis II completion. They undergo morphologic changes to become mature sperm that include acrosome, head, neck, and tail.

   Answer B is incorrect. Secondary spermatocytes are 23, 2n cells that result from primary spermatocytes completing meiosis I. Each primary spermatocyte forms two secondary spermatocytes, each going on to form two spermatids.

   Answer C is incorrect. At no point during male gametogenesis is there a haploid cell with 46 chromosomes.

   Answer D is incorrect. Both primordial germ cells in the testes, which are dormant until puberty, and type A spermatogonia, which develop at puberty, are 46, 2n cell types. A type A spermatogonium perpetuates itself to provide a constant supply of sperm cells; it also differentiates into type B spermatogonia.

   Answer E is incorrect. Primary spermatocytes are 46, 4n cells that result from the DNA replication of type B spermatogonia.

10. **The correct answer is B.** The portion of the bladder that extends into the umbilical cord is the allantois, an extraembryonic cavity within the body stalk that projects onto the cloaca (the future bladder), and regresses prior to birth as the bladder descends into the pelvis. It gives rise to the urachus, which later degenerates into a fibrous structure running along the anterior abdominal wall extending to the umbilicus known as the median umbilical ligament. Failure of the urachus to completely degenerate (persistent urachus) results in a number of clinical complications, depending on the degree of patency of the urachus. A totally patent urachus creates a fistulous urinary tract between the bladder and the umbilicus. At other times, only the umbilical end, the bladder end, or the central urachal region remains patent, which gives rise to urachal cysts. These cysts are potential sites of bladder adenocarcinomas.

    Answer A is incorrect. Bladder exstrophy is a congenital developmental anomaly resulting from failure of the abdominal wall to close during embryogenesis. This causes the posterior bladder wall to protrude through the lower abdominal wall. It is not a complication of a patent urachus.

    Answer C is incorrect. Meckel diverticulum is the most frequent congenital anomaly found in the gastrointestinal tract, and it is caused by persistence of the omphalomesenteric duct. It is often asymptomatic but can present with rectal bleeding, volvulus, intussusception, and obstruction. Meckel diverticulum can be remembered by the "**rule of 2s**": found in **2**% of the population, commonly presents around age **2** years, measures **2** inches long, can be found **2** feet from the ileocecal valve, and often contains **2** types of epithelia (gastric and pancreatic).

    Answer D is incorrect. Polycystic kidney disease is a hereditary disease characterized by bilateral development of multiple cysts in the renal parenchyma, ultimately leading to renal failure. There are two forms of polycystic kidney disease: adult autosomal dominant (ADPKD) and childhood autosomal recessive (ARPKD). They are caused by distinct genes. ADPKD has been mapped to the *PKD1* and *PKD2* genes, which code for the integral membrane proteins polycystin-1 and polycystin-2, respectively. ARPKD is caused by mutations in the *PKHD1* gene, which codes for a large protein called fibrocystin. Neither ADPKD nor ARPKD is a complication of a patent urachus.

    Answer E is incorrect. Ectopic kidney is a condition that arises from development of a kidney at an unusual anatomic location. Most ectopic kidneys are found either within the pelvis or just above the pelvic brim. Functionally, these kidneys are normal; however, the ureter may kink, leading to urinary flow stagnation that predisposes to recurrent bacterial infections. Ectopic kidney is not a complication of a patent urachus.

11. **The correct answer is A.** This patient most likely has an annular pancreas. Normally the ventral bud of the pancreas rotates around the duodenum to fuse with the dorsal bud. The ventral bud forms the uncinate process and part of the head of the pancreas, and the duct of the ventral bud becomes the main pancreatic duct. Rarely, a bifid ventral bud grows around the duodenum in both directions, forming a ring. Especially in the setting of inflammation or malignancy, this ring can block movement of food through the duodenum; such blockage causes epigastric pain, postprandial fullness, nausea, and vomiting. Onset of symptoms can occur any time between infancy and adulthood, or not at all. Blockage is also associated with the "double-bubble sign" in the radiograph: the stomach is dilated proximal to the blockage point and the duodenum is dilated distal to it.

Answer B is incorrect. During normal development, the lumen of the duodenum is obstructed by overgrowth of endothelial cells and then restored as these cells recede. Failure of this process results in duodenal atresia. The signs and symptoms of duodenal atresia are very similar to those seen with an annular pancreas, but they always present within hours after birth. Vomit containing bile and the radiographic double bubble sign are indicative of duodenal atresia in an infant.

Answer C is incorrect. Physiological midgut herniation occurs at the beginning of the sixth week of embryogenesis, when the midgut herniates into the proximal umbilical cord. Normally, it returns to the abdomen during the tenth week. Failure to return to the abdomen results in omphalocele, in which a portion of the newborn's abdominal contents remain outside the abdomen, covered by the umbilical cord epithelium. This condition requires immediate surgical repair.

Answer D is incorrect. Hypertrophy of the pyloric muscles results in blockage of the digestive pathway. Infants with congenital hypertrophic pyloric stenosis generally present with nonbilious projectile vomiting soon after birth.

Answer E is incorrect. Incomplete separation of the esophagus and laryngotracheal tube results in a tracheoesophageal fistula. In its most common form, the tracheoesophageal septum is deviated posteriorly and the esophagus ends in a blind pouch connected to the trachea. The fetus cannot swallow amniotic fluid and polyhydramnios may occur during pregnancy. Newborns appear healthy at first and swallow normally, but quickly begin regurgitating fluid through the nose and mouth and enter respiratory distress. The defect can be repaired surgically with high success rates.

12. **The correct answer is B.** The patient has an omphalocele, which results from failure of closure of the anterior abdominal wall. In this midline abdominal wall defect, the herniated viscera are covered by a membrane consisting of the amniotic membranes, Wharton jelly, and peritoneum. Between 50% and 70% of children with omphalocele have additional congenital anomalies (including cardiac defects and genitourinary malformations such as bladder exstrophy), which are also thought to be related to ventral closure defects. The pathogenesis of omphalocele is believed to be sporadic defective closure of the abdominal wall secondary to malrotation of the midgut derivatives during the 10th week of embryonic development. Alternative theories include abnormal persistence of the primitive body stalk and the failure of body wall closure secondary to incomplete lateral body wall migration. The incidence of omphalocele is 1:5000 live births, and it is most commonly associated with extremes of maternal age (<20 or >40 years of age). It may be associated with a chromosomal abnormality if there is only herniation of the small bowel or the liver.

Answer A is incorrect. Ethanol toxicity is not associated with abdominal wall defects. Ethanol exposure during embryogenesis is associated with fetal alcohol syndrome, which includes mental retardation and a typical facies characterized by a smooth philtrum, thin upper lip, and small palpebral fissures.

Answer C is incorrect. Maternal folate deficiency is not associated with abdominal wall defects. Folate deficiency has been associated with a number of neural tube defects, including anencephaly and spina bifida. A myelomeningocele would be located at the posterior side (superior if using fetal terminology).

Answer D is incorrect. Omphalomesenteric vessel occlusion and consequent ischemia is believed to be the cause of gastroschisis, another congenital abdominal wall defect. This condition is a full-thickness defect in the abdominal wall, and there is no protective membrane with a variable amount of herniation of the intestines and parts of other abdominal organs. Unlike omphalocele, gastroschisis herniation occurs to the right of the umbilicus, and is rarely associated with other congenital anomalies. Children with this defect should be given a warm moist occlusive dressing and receive immediate surgical intervention.

Answer E is incorrect. The **ToRCHeS** infections include **To**xoplasmosis, **R**ubella, **C**ytomegalovirus (CMV), **He**rpesvirus/HIV, and **S**yphilis. Congenital infection with one of the ToRCHeS viruses is not associated with abdominal wall defects. Instead, common manifestations include fevers, hepatosplenomegaly, jaundice, poor feeding, and intrauterine growth restriction. Other specific signs include chorioretinitis, cataracts, and neural deafness (rubella); intracranial calcifications (toxoplasmosis); rhinitis, "blueberry-muffin" skin lesions, and interstitial keratitis (syphilis); cerebral calcifications (CMV); and vesicular skin lesions (herpes simplex virus).

13. **The correct answer is D.** This newborn has Edwards syndrome, or trisomy 18. Affected children are born with clenched fists, "rocker-bottom" feet, micrognathia (a small lower jaw), congenital heart disease, and mental retardation. The survival rate of <1 year is similar to that of trisomy 13 (Patau syndrome), from which it should be distinguished. Trisomy of chromosome 13, or Patau syndrome, is characterized by a constellation of findings including mental retardation, microphthalmia, microcephaly, cleft lip/palate, abnormal forebrain structures, polydactyly, and congenital heart disease.

Answer A is incorrect. F508 deletion in the *CFTR* gene is the most common cause of cystic fibrosis. Patients with cystic fibrosis have frequent pulmonary infections, impaired mucous clearance, and poor growth secondary to pancreatic involvement. Survival can extend into the fourth and fifth decades in these patients.

Answer B is incorrect. CAG tandem repeats are found in Huntington disease, among others. Huntington is asymptomatic until the patient's third or fourth decade and is caused by degeneration of the caudate and putamen. Patients present with gradually worsening choreiform (dance-like) movements, but not the birth defects found in this patient.

Answer C is incorrect. This is fragile X syndrome. Associated with CGG tandem repeats, this syndrome is characterized by mental retardation, a large jaw, and large testes. Children with fragile X syndrome typically survive beyond one year of age.

Answer E is incorrect. Down syndrome can cause mental retardation and characteristic physical findings that include microgenia (a small chin), macroglossia, epicanthal folds, and a round face, but clenched fists and "rocker-bottom" feet are classic for trisomy 18. The survival of a child affected by Down syndrome is approximately 50 years.

14. **The correct answer is E.** This individual is most likely suffering from a VSD. Infants with VSDs are generally not cyanotic at birth, but can become cyanotic if a large defect is left untreated. The majority of small VSDs involving the membranous portion of the septum resolve on their own. With larger defects involving the muscular portion of the septum, higher pressures in the left ventricle initially cause a shunt of blood from the left ventricle to the right ventricle during systole. Over time, due to the volume and pressure overload on the right-sided circulation, the child will develop increased resistance in the pulmonary circulation (termed pulmonary hypertension), which increases the pressure in the right ventricle to a point at which the shunt reverses

and blood flows from the right ventricle to the left through the VSD. This shunt reversal is termed Eisenmenger syndrome. As described in the vignette, these children present early with a harsh holosystolic murmur at the left lower sternal border. The intensity of the murmur is inversely proportional to the size of the defect.

Answer A is incorrect. Atrial septal defect (ASD) is a communication between the right and left atria. Patients may remain asymptomatic or manifest symptoms of right-sided heart failure, depending on the size of the defect. Cyanosis may occur if there is a patent foramen ovale with right-to-left shunting, but is not systematically seen. On exam, patients with ASD have an ejection systolic murmur with fixed splitting of S_2.

Answer B is incorrect. Tetralogy of Fallot is characterized by pulmonary artery stenosis, right ventricular hypertrophy, an overriding aorta, and a VSD. Infants with cardiac defects are typically cyanotic at birth. The pulmonary artery stenosis reduces the caliber of the outflow tract, causing the pressure in the right ventricle to be unusually high. As a result, deoxygenated blood is shunted from the right to the left side of the heart through the VSD.

Answer C is incorrect. Transposition of the great arteries is a congenital defect in which the pulmonic artery exits from the left ventricle and the aorta exits from the right ventricle. In this defect there are essentially two closed circuits with no way for oxygenated blood to reach the systemic circulation outside of the patent ductus arteriosus (PDA). Efforts to keep the PDA open are necessary to keep the baby alive so it can be taken to the operating room to have the defect corrected. Neonates with this condition are typically cyanotic at birth, have shortness of breath, and feed poorly. Since the defect is so severe, it is typically discovered in the first week of life.

Answer D is incorrect. Truncus arteriosus is a congenital defect in which there is a large VSD and a common trunk that eventually separates into the aorta and pulmonary arteries. Due to the anatomy there is significant mixing of deoxygenated blood with oxygenated blood, causing cyanosis in the neonate. The cyanosis is not as pronounced as in transposition of the great arteries, and greatly depends on the anatomy of the individual's defect.

15. **The correct answer is B.** The vessel labeled C is most likely the umbilical vein, which has the highest oxygen saturation level in the fetus. It carries blood enriched in oxygen from the placenta to the fetus. Its oxygen saturation is typically between 30 and 35 mm Hg. Soon after birth, the umbilical vein becomes dysfunctional as the neonate makes the transition from fetal circulation to that found in adult anatomy. In place of this vein is a fibrous structure, the ligamentum teres hepatis, or the round ligament of the liver. It extends from the umbilicus to the transverse fissure of the liver, where it joins the ligamentum venosum, thus effectively separating the liver into its right and left lobes. Recanalization of this vein occurs under the pathologic condition of portal hypertension associated with liver cirrhosis.

Answer A is incorrect. The falciform ligament is a developmental remnant of the ventral mesentery of the fetus, thus it is a peritoneal fold enclosing the round ligament of the liver anteriorly and the ligamentum venosum posteriorly.

Answer C is incorrect. The ligamentum venosum is a fibrous structure that is derived from the ductus venosus in the fetal circulatory system. The ductus venosus is a shunt that conducts oxygen-rich blood from the umbilical vein into the inferior vena cava. It may be associated with the round ligament of the liver, coursing through the fissure that demarcates the boundaries between the left and caudate lobes of the liver. Most often, it is found attached to the left branch of the portal vein in the porta hepatis.

Answer D is incorrect. There are two medial umbilical ligaments in the adult. They course longitudinally on the deep surface of the anterior abdominal wall underneath the medial umbilical folds. The medial umbilical ligaments represent vestigial remnants of the fetal umbilical arteries. The paired umbilical arteries have a very low oxygen saturation level (vessel D), as they carry blood depleted of oxygen from the fetus back to the placenta.

Answer E is incorrect. The median umbilical ligament is a single ligament that runs longitudinally on the deep surface of the anterior abdominal wall between the medial umbilical ligaments in the adult, extending from the apex of the bladder to the umbilicus. It is a vestigial remnant of the embryonic urachus.

16. **The correct answer is A.** The presentation described here is consistent with Potter syndrome, one cause of which is bilateral renal agenesis. The renal parenchyma (except for the nephrons) is derived from the ureteric bud (recall that the nephrons arise from mesoderm surrounding the ureteric bud). A failure of ureteric bud maturation would result in a fetus without kidneys. An absence of kidneys would lead to oligohydramnios, as the fetus would be unable to excrete urine into the amniotic sac. This, in turn, would lead to compression of the fetus by the uterine wall, causing limb deformities, abnormal facies, and wrinkly skin. Death would occur shortly after birth unless an appropriate kidney donor could be found.

    Answer B is incorrect. Anencephaly may result from a failure of the rostral neural tube to close. Anencephalic infants are born with a marked reduction in fetal brain tissue and usually an absence of the overlying skull. These infants are unable to swallow amniotic fluid in utero, so their mothers' pregnancies are usually marked by polyhydramnios (too much amniotic fluid) rather than oligohydramnios (too little).

    Answer C is incorrect. Failure of development of the tracheoesophageal (TE) septum is the cause of a TE fistula. There are several variants of TE fistula, the most common of which is a blind upper esophagus with the lower esophagus having an anomalous connection to the trachea. TE fistulas commonly result in polyhydramnios rather than oligohydramnios, and they are unlikely to cause the other findings in this infant.

    Answer D is incorrect. This describes the defect in Hirschsprung disease, which manifests as severe constipation and an inability to pass meconium. Hirschsprung disease would not account for the symptoms described in this scenario.

    Answer E is incorrect. A failure of duodenal recanalization may give rise to duodenal atresia. Duodenal atresia is associated with Down syndrome, and it is often marked by a "double bubble" sign on abdominal radiographs. Duodenal atresia would result in polyhydramnios rather than oligohydramnios.

17. **The correct answer is B.** The muscles that elevate the palate are derived from branchial arch 3 (the stylopharyngeus) and branchial arch 4 (the levator veli palatini). These are innervated by cranial nerves IX and X, respectively.

    Answer A is incorrect. The first branchial arch generates "**M**" muscles: muscles of **M**astication (te**M**poralis, **M**asseter, **M**edial and lateral pterygoids) and the **M**ylohyoid. The second arch gives rise to "**S**" muscles: **S**tapedius, **S**tylohyoid, and facial expression muscles. None of these muscles is involved in palatal elevation.

    Answer C is incorrect. Although branchial arch 4 does give rise to the levator veli palatini, branchial arch 6 gives rise to the intrinsic muscles of the larynx (except the cricothyroid, which is a fourth arch derivative). These muscles are not involved in elevating the palate.

    Answer D is incorrect. The first branchial cleft gives rise to the external auditory meatus, and the second, third, and fourth clefts are obliterated during development. The clefts are formed from ectoderm and could not give rise to muscles, which are derived from mesoderm.

    Answer E is incorrect. Branchial pouch 3 gives rise to the thymus (ventral wings) and inferior parathyroid glands (dorsal glands), and the fourth branchial pouch gives rise to the superior parathyroids. These are not involved in palatal elevation. Remember that pouches give rise to endoderm-derived tissue, and arches give rise to mesoderm-derived tissue such as muscle. Use the mnemonic "**CAP**" to remember that **C**lefts, **A**rches, and **P**ouches give rise to ecto-, meso-, and endoderm, respectively.

18. **The correct answer is A.** This child has a cleft lip, which is most often caused by failure of the maxillary prominence to fuse with the medial nasal prominence. Cleft lip may occur unilaterally or bilaterally and represents the most common congenital malformation of the head and neck. This commonly occurs with a cleft palate.

    Answer B is incorrect. Abnormal development of the third and fourth branchial pouches gives rise to DiGeorge syndrome, which results in thymic aplasia and failure of parathyroid development.

    Answer C is incorrect. The mandibular and maxillary bones are typically normally developed in a cleft lip. Abnormal development of these bones typically causes various facial dysostoses.

    Answer D is incorrect. The third pharyngeal arch forms the hyoid bone, stylopharyngeus muscle, and glossopharyngeal nerve, which are not altered in a simple cleft lip.

19. **The correct answer is E.** The patient is presenting with congenital extrahepatic biliary atresia. Descriptions of a pure elevation in direct (conjugated) bilirubin strongly suggest an obstructive etiology, as the liver is able to effectively conjugate bilirubin but fails to excrete it into the small intestine. The absence of bilirubin in the small bowel results in acholic stools, whereas increased renal excretion of conjugated bilirubin causes a darkening of the urine. Congenital extrahepatic biliary atresia occurs when the developing bile ducts close completely and fail to recanalize. Surgical therapy of biliary atresia involves anastomosis of the small bowel directly to intrahepatic bile ducts, a maneuver known as Kasai's procedure, which is appropriate for the 10% of patients with limited disease. Liver transplantation continues to be the best chance of survival for the remaining patients.

    Answer A is incorrect. Gilbert syndrome is a benign disorder caused by a mutation in the promoter region of uridine 5′-diphosphoglucuronosyltransferase, leading to diminished expression of the gene. Patients with Gilbert syndrome develop a mild unconjugated hyperbilirubinemia but usually are asymptomatic and have a normal life expectancy.

    Answer B is incorrect. Crigler-Najjar syndrome type 1 is caused by a complete deficiency in uridine 5'-diphosphoglucuronosyltransferase, the hepatic enzyme necessary to conjugate bilirubin. This disorder produces a severe unconjugated (indirect) hyperbilirubinemia that causes death within the first few years of life. The patient in this case, however, has a conjugated hyperbilirubinemia, suggesting an obstructive cause and ruling out Crigler-Najjar syndrome.

    Answer C is incorrect. Physiologic jaundice refers to the mild unconjugated (indirect) hyperbilirubinemia that affects nearly all newborns because of the greater turnover of neonatal RBCs and the decreased bilirubin clearance in the first few weeks of life. The peak total serum bilirubin occurs between 72 and 96 hours of age and resolves within the first few weeks of life. Often phototherapy is used to hasten resolution. This patient has a severe conjugated hyperbilirubinemia that cannot be explained by normal neonatal physiologic jaundice.

    Answer D is incorrect. Biliary atresia is a rare condition whose cause is not entirely known; it is not inherited in an autosomal dominant pattern. Hereditary spherocytosis is an example of an autosomal dominant condition that can cause jaundice and hyperbilirubinemia secondary to hemolytic anemia. This autosomal dominant condition is due to mutations in spectrin or ankyrin causing RBC membrane defects that make the cells more fragile to hemolysis. Peripheral blood smears show small RBCs without central pallor, and diagnosis can be confirmed with the osmotic fragility test. Unlike this case, hereditary spherocytosis usually presents later in life, with a mixed hyperbilirubinemia and normal stools.

20. **The correct answer is B.** The uterine fundus is palpable above the umbilicus at 20 weeks' gestational age. Another landmark to keep in mind is that the uterine fundus is palpable above the pubic symphysis at 12 weeks' gestational age. The liver is the predominant site of hematopoiesis at weeks 6-30 of gestation.

    Answer A is incorrect. The bone marrow is the predominant site of hematopoiesis beginning around week 28 and remains so throughout adult life.

    Answer C is incorrect. The pancreas produces insulin, glucagon, and digestive enzymes. It plays no role in hematopoiesis.

    Answer D is incorrect. The thymus is the site of early development of the immune system; it is not a site of hematopoiesis.

    Answer E is incorrect. The yolk sac is the predominant site of hematopoiesis between fetal weeks three and eight.

CHAPTER 4

Microbiology

QUESTIONS

1. A 30-year-old sexually active woman presents with a painful vesicle on her external genitalia and bilateral inguinal lymphadenopathy. A Tzanck smear from the vesicle is negative, and a Venereal Disease Research Laboratory assay is also negative. Which of the following medications would be most appropriate for this patient?

   (A) Acyclovir
   (B) Ceftriaxone
   (C) Foscarnet
   (D) Ribavirin
   (E) Vancomycin

2. A 51-year-old man living near St. Louis, Missouri presents to his primary care physician with recent-onset productive cough, pleuritic chest pain, and a fever of 39.1°C (102.4°F). He recently returned from a business trip to Phoenix, Arizona. A sample of the man's purulent sputum is sent for analysis, which reveals yeast cells up to 15 µm in diameter. The pathologist is able to identify several dividing yeast organisms. Direct fluorescent antibody staining (see image) is notable for large, broad-based budding from mother cells. What fungal species is responsible for this man's illness?

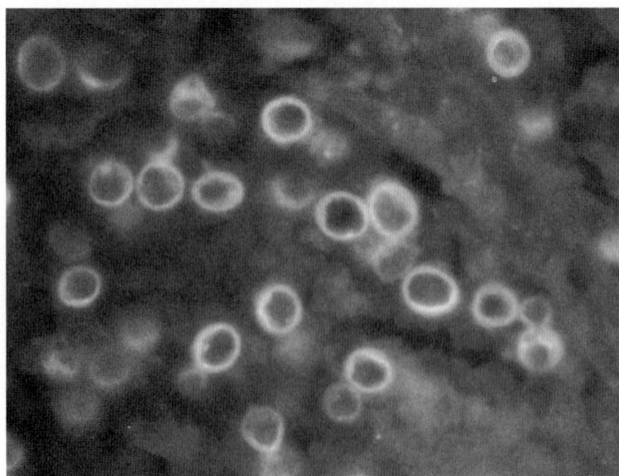

Courtesy of Dr. William Kaplan, Centers for Disease Control and Prevention.

   (A) *Blastomyces dermatitidis*
   (B) *Coccidioides immitis*
   (C) *Cryptococcus neoformans*
   (D) *Histoplasma capsulatum*
   (E) *Paracoccidioides brasiliensis*

3. A 17-year-old boy visits his physician with complaints of recurrent bouts of dizziness, palpitations, and joint pain. He went on a summer hiking trip in eastern Massachusetts about six months ago but does not recall getting a tick bite and notes no rashes. The ECG is shown in the image. What is the most likely diagnosis of this patient's symptoms?

   (A) Brugada syndrome
   (B) Chagas disease
   (C) Hypertrophic cardiomyopathy
   (D) Lyme disease
   (E) Third-degree heart block

4. A 30-year-old woman complains of a nonproductive cough that has developed over the past 10 days. She reports feeling achy, and having a sore throat and headaches. X-ray of the chest demonstrates patchy bilateral interstitial infiltrates. After work-up, the patient is diagnosed with *Mycoplasma pneumoniae* pneumonia. Which of the following is associated with the causative organism?

   (A) Growth on buffered charcoal yeast extract media
   (B) IgM cold agglutinins
   (C) Phyocyanin production
   (D) Polysaccharide capsule
   (E) Reticulate bodies

5. A homeless 37-year-old woman with HIV infection comes to the clinic with a four-week history of worsening hemiparesis, visual field deficits, and cognitive impairment. The patient's CD4+ count is 22/mm^3. MRI shows several hyperintensities on T2-weighted images that do not enhance with contrast and are not surrounded by edema. A lumbar puncture shows a normal opening pressure, and cerebrospinal fluid analysis shows a mildly elevated protein level and the presence of myelin basic protein, with a mild mononuclear pleocytosis. Which of the following entities is most likely responsible for this patient's clinical picture?

(A) Cortical tuberculoma
(B) Cytomegalovirus encephalitis
(C) JC virus
(D) Primary central nervous system lymphoma
(E) Toxoplasmosis

6. A family who recently emigrated from Romania brings their 7-year-old child to the pediatrician with complaints of conjunctivitis and periorbital swelling. The child has had coughing with a runny nose and high fever for three days. Small lesions with blue-white centers are seen in his oral cavity. Which of the following is the most likely cause of this child's symptoms?

(A) Diphtheria
(B) Pertussis
(C) Roseola
(D) Rubella
(E) Rubeola

7. A 5-year-old girl is brought to her pediatrician because of an eight-day history of a painful rash confined to her flank. Physical examination reveals the crusted lesion shown in the image. Which of the following describes the mechanism of action of the treatment for this lesion?

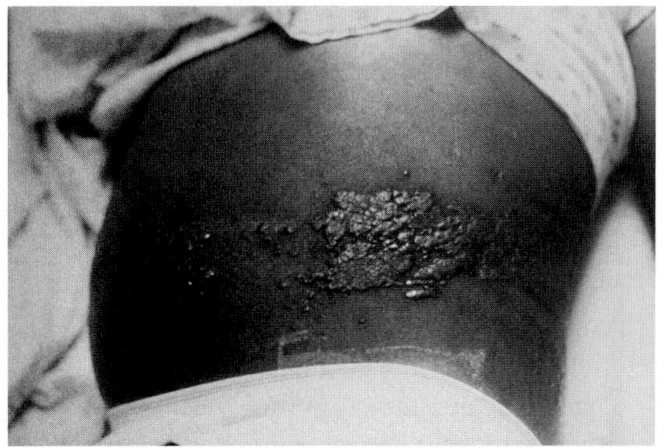

Courtesy of the Centers for Disease Control and Prevention.

(A) Inhibition of cell wall synthesis
(B) Inhibition of DNA polymerase
(C) Inhibition of genome uncoating
(D) Inhibition of nucleoside reverse transcriptase
(E) Inhibition of protein synthesis

8. A 38-year-old man comes to the emergency department complaining of cyclic fevers and headaches. The fevers began about one week ago; two weeks ago the patient returned from a trip to Africa. Physical examination reveals hepatosplenomegaly. Imaging of the brain shows signs of significant cerebral involvement. Which of the following parasites most likely caused this patient's symptoms?

(A) *Plasmodium falciparum*
(B) *Plasmodium malariae*
(C) *Plasmodium ovale*
(D) *Plasmodium vivax*
(E) *Plasmodium knowlesi*

9. A 15-year-old boy presents to the pediatrician with a two-day history of fever and headache. The patient is unable to touch his chin to his chest when asked to do so. He also asks that the lights in the room be turned down. In addition to performing a lumbar puncture to obtain cerebrospinal fluid (CSF), the physician begins empiric treatment. The CSF is sent for analysis and culture. The patient's condition improves over the next week. In the meantime, bacterial and fungal culture results are negative. Which of the following is the most likely result of the CSF analysis?

Choice	Pressure	Lymphocyte count	Protein	Sugar
A	normal	normal	normal	normal
B	normal	normal	normal	↑
C	normal or ↑	↑	normal	normal
D	↑	↑	↑	↓
E	↑	↓	↑	↓

Reproduced, with permission, from USMLERx.com.

(A) A
(B) B
(C) C
(D) D
(E) E

10. Oncogenic viruses act through a variety of mechanisms. Some introduce oncogenes directly into host cells, while others force cells to repeatedly undergo cycles of proliferation that eventually become unregulated. Still others introduce oncogenic potential by manipulating chromosomal structure through deletions or translocations. Which of the following viruses causes neoplasia by inactivating tumor suppressor genes such as *p53* and *Rb*?

(A) Epstein-Barr virus
(B) Hepatitis C virus
(C) Human immunodeficiency virus
(D) Human papillomavirus
(E) Human T-cell lymphotropic virus type 1

11. Influenza virus type A usually produces a mild, self-limited febrile illness in the general population. However, worldwide epidemics have occurred at different times in history due to rapid changes in viral genetic makeup. Which of the following is the most important reason why these sporadic worldwide epidemics occur?

(A) Antigenic drift
(B) Antigenic shift
(C) Hemagglutinin develops the ability to destroy a component of mucin, becoming more infectious
(D) Neuraminidase develops the ability to attach to sialic acid receptors, becoming more infectious
(E) RBCs agglutinate with certain strains

12. A 66-year-old woman who recently emigrated from Mexico comes to the physician because she has begun to have seizures. A test for anticysticercal antibodies is positive. A T1 weighted, non-contrast MRI of the head is shown in the image below. Which of the following organs or tissues is most likely to have similar lesions?

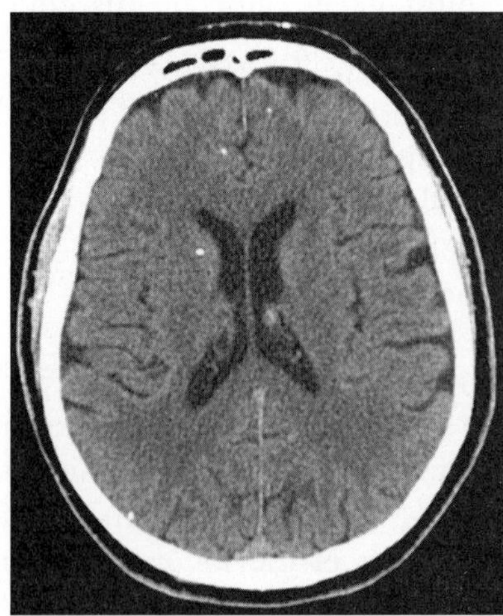

Courtesy of Dr. Per-Lennart Westesson, University of Rochester Medical Center.

(A) Bladder
(B) Bone
(C) Kidney cortex
(D) Skeletal muscle
(E) Small bowel

13. A young girl living in rural New Mexico is brought to her pediatrician with complaints of fever, cough, and fatigue for the past two weeks. The physician notices that the patient is having intermittent bouts of many coughs in a single breath, followed by a deep inspiration. The parents report that this pattern of coughing had started in the past two days. The physician informs them that their daughter will most likely recover with only supportive care. However, she wants to confirm his diagnosis. A throat swab is sent for culture for a specific organism. Which of the following culture media will be used?

(A) Bordet-Gengou medium
(B) Charcoal yeast extract with iron and cysteine
(C) Chocolate agar with factors V and X
(D) Loeffler medium
(E) Thayer-Martin medium

14. A worried mother brings her infant to the emergency department because he appears to be unable to swallow and continues to choke on his formula. On physical examination, the physician notes generalized muscle weakness. On further questioning, the patient's mother says that she recently started sweetening the baby's food with honey. Which of the following is a characteristic of the organism most likely responsible for this infant's symptoms?

(A) Production of IgA protease
(B) Production of exotoxin A
(C) Production of lecithinase
(D) Production of lipopolysaccharide
(E) Production of spores that can only be killed by autoclaving

15. A 27-year-old woman presents to her physician complaining of fever, chills, and flu-like symptoms. A sputum culture at 25°C (77°F) is shown in the image. Which of the following is most likely to be elicited on further questioning?

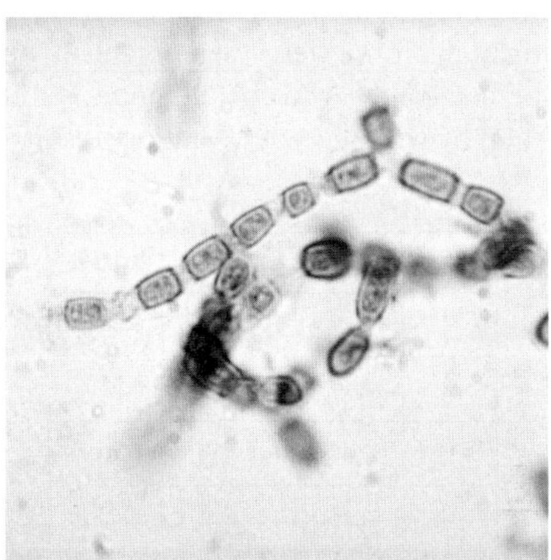

Courtesy of Dr. Hardin, Centers for Disease Control and Prevention.

(A) A recent trip to Namibia
(B) A recent trip to New Mexico
(C) A recent trip to Ohio
(D) Recent hiking in wooded areas
(E) Recent work in her large rose garden

16. At birth, a newborn is noted to be unresponsive to verbal stimulation from the doctors, nurses, and his parents. A routine physical examination of the child reveals a split S_2 heart sound with an accentuated P_2 component. The newborn has bounding pulses with a wide pulse pressure. After a week the newborn's parents notice that he has developed shortness of breath and respiratory distress. What pathogen did the mother contract during her pregnancy that could explain the newborn's current condition?

(A) Cytomegalovirus
(B) Herpes simplex virus 2
(C) Rubivirus
(D) *Toxoplasma gondii*
(E) *Treponema pallidum*

17. A 45-year-old man presents to the clinic complaining of several weeks of vague abdominal discomfort and early satiety. The physician orders upper GI endoscopy as part of his workup. During the study, mucosal rigidity and hyperplasia are seen in the stomach, and a biopsy is taken from the affected area. Microscopic analysis of the biopsy specimen shows sheets of atypical lymphocytes. The organism believed to be associated with this condition is best described by which set of laboratory results?

Choice	Urease	Catalase	Oxidase
A	negative	negative	negative
B	negative	negative	positive
C	negative	positive	negative
D	negative	positive	positive
E	positive	negative	negative
F	positive	positive	negative
G	positive	positive	positive

Reproduced, with permission, from USMLERx.com.

(A) A
(B) B
(C) C
(D) D
(E) E
(F) F
(G) G

18. A 36-year-old man comes to the physician because he is experiencing abdominal pain, vomiting, and a non-bloody diarrhea. He last ate chicken and rice about four hours ago at a Chinese restaurant. He has no other symptoms. Which of the following treatments should this man receive?

(A) Bismuth subsalicylate, metronidazole, and amoxicillin
(B) Ciprofloxacin
(C) Erythromycin
(D) Prompt replacement of water and electrolytes; tetracyclines shorten the disease's course
(E) Supportive care only, without antibiotics

19. A 65-year-old man with a history of viral hepatitis presents to his primary care physician with complaints of early satiety, a 4.5-kg (10-lb) weight loss over three months, upper abdominal pain, and yellowing of his eyes. The patient says he has lived in Rochester, New York (upstate) for his entire life, has not traveled outside of the country, and received two blood transfusions in the early 1970s following an automobile accident. Work-up reveals extensive macronodular cirrhosis with a 2-×2-cm mass in his liver. Which of the following viral infections is most likely to result in this patient's current presentation?

(A) Cytomegalovirus
(B) Hepatitis A
(C) Hepatitis C
(D) Hepatitis E
(E) HIV

20. A neonate with purulent umbilical discharge for one day presents with fever, irritability, and diffuse flushing. One day later she is covered in large, fluid-filled blisters that rupture easily, leaving raw red areas beneath. Blood cultures are taken, which within 24 hours grow an organism that is subsequently Gram stained with the results shown below. The skin symptoms observed in this case are due to the involvement of which of the following intercellular structures?

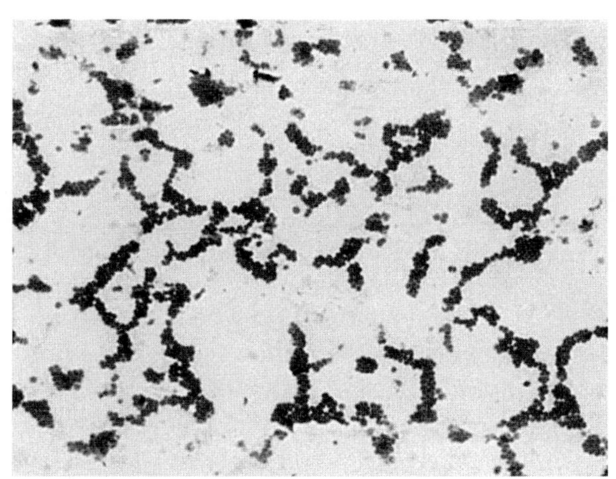

Courtesy of Dr. Richard Facklam, Centers for Disease Control and Prevention.

(A) Desmosomes
(B) Gap junctions
(C) Hemidesmosomes
(D) Intermediate junctions
(E) Tight junctions

21. A 5-year-old boy develops diarrhea after eating at a fast-food restaurant. The following day, his mother notices that he seems lethargic and brings him to the urgent care center. His blood pressure is 150/90 mm Hg. Laboratory tests show a hemoglobin level of 9 g/dL, platelet count of $40,000/mm^3$, and creatinine level of 2.8 mg/dL. What is the most likely cause of this patient's condition?

(A) *Campylobacter*
(B) *Escherichia coli*
(C) Rotavirus
(D) *Shigella*
(E) *Vibrio cholerae*

22. A 32-year-old man presents to his doctor with painful urination and a purulent urethral discharge. The discharge material is cultured, and a sample from the culture is stained with Giemsa and is shown in the image. Which of the following is the treatment of choice for this infection?

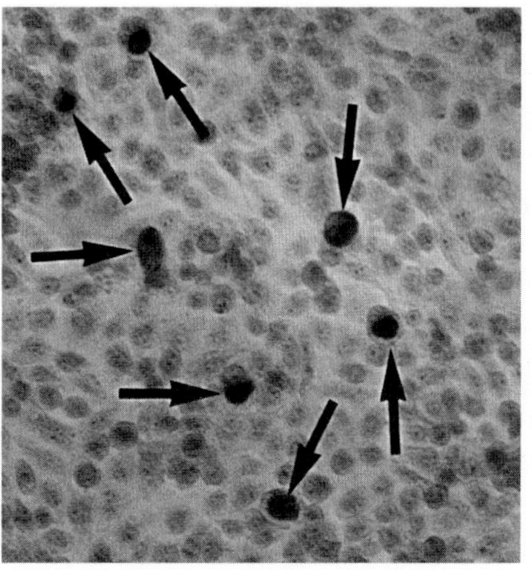

Courtesy of Drs. E. Arum and N. Jacobs, Centers for Disease Control and Prevention.

(A) Azithromycin
(B) Ceftriaxone
(C) Fluconazole
(D) Penicillin
(E) Vancomycin

23. A 47-year-old woman comes to the clinic complaining of fever and malaise. She reports having severe headaches associated with some nausea and vomiting, over the past few days. Her urine has been exceptionally dark for the past few days. The patient is mildly jaundiced with scleral icterus. Based on these symptoms the physician suspects hepatitis B and draws blood for serologic testing for hepatitis B markers. If the patient had unprotected intercourse during this infection, the presence of which of the following would be most concerning for her partner?

(A) Hepatitis B e antibody
(B) Hepatitis B e antigen
(C) Hepatitis B surface antibody
(D) IgG hepatitis B core antibody
(E) IgM hepatitis B core antibody

24. A 1-year-old girl presents to the emergency room because of a three-day history of coughing attacks that are occasionally followed by episodes of vomiting. Her parents are especially concerned because sometimes she becomes blue after an episode. She has markedly injected sclera but no discharge. She is afebrile and has no other symptoms. Laboratory tests show a WBC count of 25,000/mm^3 with marked lymphocytosis. A bacterial infection is diagnosed. Which of the following is a result of the exotoxin produced by the organism causing this child's symptoms?

    (A) Blocked release of acetylcholine into the synaptic cleft
    (B) Formation of a pore in the plasma membrane
    (C) Inactivation of elongation factor 2, a protein involved in translation
    (D) Inhibition of G proteins to increase cAMP
    (E) Release of lipopolysaccharide-lipid A

25. A 50-year-old man develops profuse, nonbloody, watery diarrhea while working as an aid worker in Bangladesh. He arrived in the area two days ago. A stool smear shows no WBCs. His mucous membranes are dry, and his skin shows signs of tenting. He subsequently develops electrolyte abnormalities that lead to cardiac and renal failure. What is the mechanism of action of the exotoxin produced by the most likely causative organism?

    (A) Cleaves host cell rRNA
    (B) Directly acts as an adenylate cyclase
    (C) Inactivates elongation factor 2
    (D) Permanently inactivates G_i
    (E) Permanently activates G_s

26. A biotechnology company is developing a small protein to block the cascade by which allergens can cause shock. Patients often die from vasodilation and massive edema; therefore, the new protein could lead to a life-saving drug. Which of the following molecules is the most promising target to block the anaphylactic pathway?

    (A) γ Interferon
    (B) IgE surface receptors
    (C) Hageman factor
    (D) C5a
    (E) Interleukin-1
    (F) Nitric oxide

27. A 30-year-old man from Mexico comes to the physician because of a two-day history of a fever of 38.8° C (101.8° F), a sore throat, and shortness of breath. On physical examination, the patient is found to have cervical adenopathy and a thick, gray, tissue-like material covering his tonsils. Which of the following types of culture should be used to determine the organism infecting this patient?

    (A) Löwenstein-Jensen agar
    (B) Bordet-Gengou agar
    (C) Chocolate agar with factors V and X
    (D) Loeffler medium, blood agar, and tellurite plate
    (E) Thayer-Martin media

28. A 12-year-old boy presents to the emergency room five days after returning from a camping trip in Virginia. He complains of a fever, headache, and muscle aches for several days, and recently developed a rash on his wrists, palms, and legs that has since spread to his trunk, as seen in the image. Which of the following is the most appropriate treatment?

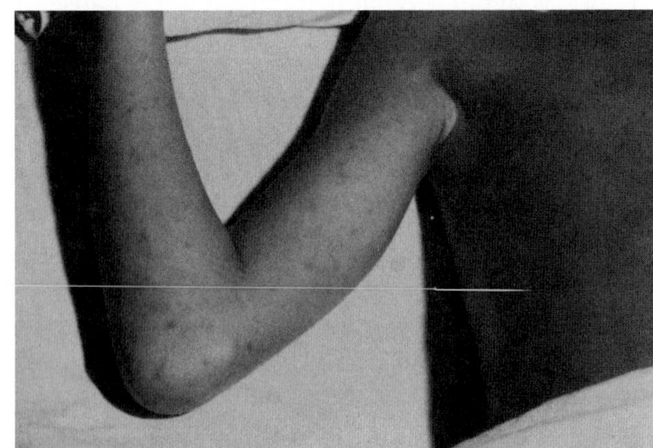

Courtesy of the Centers for Disease Control and Prevention.

    (A) Ceftriaxone
    (B) Doxycycline

(C) Gentamicin
(D) Nystatin
(E) Penicillin

29. A 53-year-old obese man with poorly controlled noninsulin-dependent diabetes mellitus presents with fever to 39.6°C (103.2°F), jaundice, hypotension, and acute onset of right upper quadrant pain. Right upper quadrant imaging shows multiple gallstones and cholecystitis. Urgent cholecystectomy is performed, and subsequent gall bladder fluid and blood cultures grow aerobic, nonlactose-fermenting, oxidase-positive, gram-negative rods. Blood tests show:

Hematocrit: 29%
WBC count: 14,700/mm^3
Platelet count: 76,000/mm^3
International Normalized Ratio: 3.2
D-dimer: 8500 ng/mL
Fibrinogen levels: low

Microscopic inspection of peripheral blood smear shows schistocytes and multiple helmet cells. Clinically, there is no evidence of active bleeding. What is the most appropriate treatment for this patient's coagulopathy?

(A) Amoxicillin
(B) Aztreonam
(C) Fresh frozen plasma
(D) Vancomycin
(E) Vitamin K

30. A 16-year-old girl complains of abnormal vaginal discharge as well as itching, tenderness, and burning in the vulvovaginal area. On examination there is vulvar and vaginal erythema and colpitis macularis. Results of a wet mount examination are shown in the image. Which additional symptom would most likely be seen in this patient?

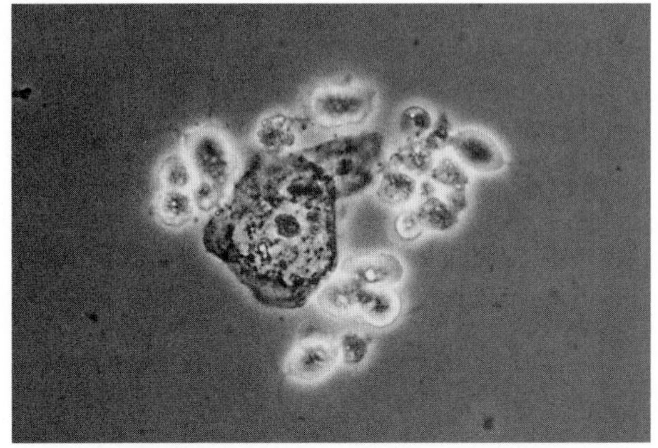

Courtesy of the Centers for Disease Control and Prevention.

(A) Bloody and foul-smelling vaginal discharge
(B) Pelvic pain
(C) Profuse, frothy vaginal discharge
(D) Thick, white, cottage cheese-like vaginal discharge
(E) Thin, gray-white, fishy-smelling vaginal discharge

31. A 40-year-old man goes on a camping vacation with his family. One day after swimming in a freshwater lake near the campsite, he develops nausea and vomiting and starts to behave irrationally. His family takes him to the emergency department, where blood samples are taken and a spinal tap is performed. He is diagnosed with a rapidly progressing meningoencephalitis and dies shortly thereafter. Which of the following protozoa was most likely the cause of the man's illness?

(A) *Cryptosporidium* species
(B) *Entamoeba histolytica*
(C) *Leishmania donovani*
(D) *Naegleria fowleri*
(E) *Plasmodium falciparum*

32. A mother brings her 12-year-old daughter to an outpatient clinic. The child complains of aching pain localized to the joints of the extremities. The mother recalls her daughter was sick with a sore throat about a month ago, but recovered completely without medical attention. The girl is admitted to the hospital for further examination and testing. A tissue biopsy is taken, and the abnormal results are seen in the image. Given the most likely diagnosis, what finding would be expected in this patient on cardiac physical examination as an adult?

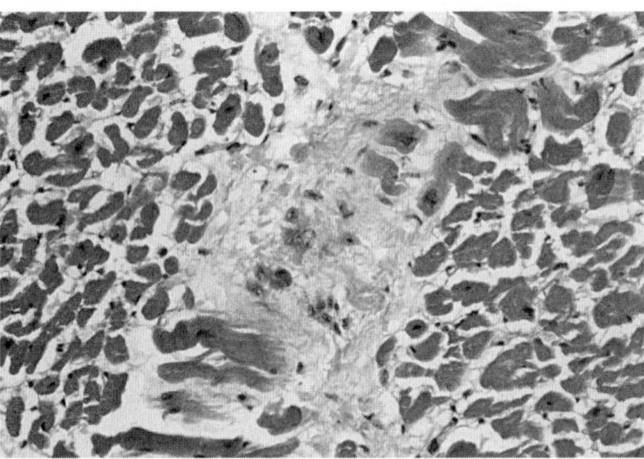

Courtesy of Dr. Ed Uthman.

(A) A friction rub heard throughout the precordium
(B) A harsh crescendo-decrescendo early systolic murmur heard at the right upper sternal border with radiation to the carotids
(C) A late diastolic murmur heard best at the apex
(D) A midsystolic click heard best at the apex
(E) An S_4 gallop heard at the apex

33. A 23-year-old man from Kenya presents with night sweats, fevers, oliguria, and a large submandibular mass. Biopsy of the mass shows an aggressive tumor with sheets of lymphocytes staining positive for CD20, as well as very high levels of nuclear *c-myc* with interspersed macrophages. What is the mode of transmission of the virus associated with this malignancy?

(A) Blood products
(B) Fecal-oral transmission
(C) Mosquito bites
(D) Saliva and respiratory secretions
(E) Sexual contact

34. While hospitalized for treatment of an episode of aspiration pneumonia, a 45-year-old man begins to have episodes of severe non-bloody diarrhea and lower abdominal pain. Temperature is 38°C (100.4°F). CT of the abdomen and pelvis with oral and intravenous contrast demonstrates marked diffuse colonic thickening (see image). What is the pathophysiology of the most likely cause of this patient's condition?

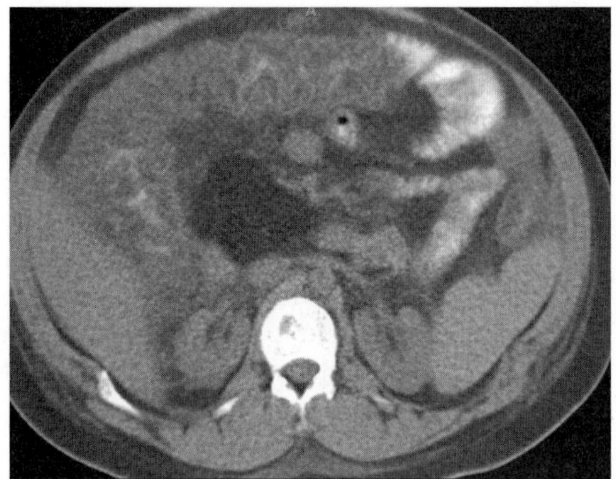

Reproduced, with permission, from USMLERx.com.

(A) Directly damages the microvilli of the enterocytes but does not invade
(B) Produces an exotoxin that can induce cytokine release and cause hemolytic uremic syndrome
(C) Produces an exotoxin that increases the secretory activity of enterocytes
(D) Produces an exotoxin that kills enterocytes
(E) Produces both heat-stable and labile toxins that promote secretions in the intestines

35. A 56-year-old man presents with sharp substernal pain radiating to his back and arms. The patient is seated and leaning forward. He states that the pain is less severe in this position, and worsens when he lies down and takes a deep breath. He recently recovered from a febrile illness. On physical examination a scratchy,

leathery sound is heard at the left lower sternal border. An ECG shows diffuse ST-segment elevation. Which of the following describes the microorganism that is the most likely cause of this condition?

(A) Catalase- and coagulase-positive cocci
(B) Double-stranded, linear, enveloped, icosahedral DNA virus
(C) Double-stranded, segmented RNA virus
(D) Positive, single-stranded, helical RNA virus
(E) Small, naked, single-stranded RNA virus

36. A 28-year-old man complains of increasing muscle weakness and numbness that began in his legs and feet three days ago and that now involves his arms and hands. The patient reports recently experiencing a self-limited episode of gastroenteritis. Which organism is commonly associated with this patient's neurologic symptoms?

(A) α-Hemolytic, encapsulated, gram-positive cocci that produce an IgA protease
(B) Comma-shaped, oxidase-positive, gram-negative bacteria that can be grown at 42°C
(C) Non-lactose-fermenting, oxidase-positive, gram-negative, aerobic bacilli
(D) Rod-shaped, gram-positive, spore-forming anaerobe that produces a heat-labile toxin
(E) Spiral-shaped bacteria with axial filaments, visualized using dark-field microscopy

37. An otherwise healthy 15-year-old boy sustains a deep puncture wound in his left heel while playing in a junkyard. Four days later, his father brings him to the emergency department because the boy has become lethargic and has developed shaking chills. He refuses to bear weight on his left foot. The patient's temperature is 39.7°C (103.4°F). Physical examination shows a warm, swollen, and extremely tender area around the puncture wound. A specimen through uninfected tissue is obtained via percutaneous needle biopsy. A Gram stain of this sample is most likely to show which of the following?

(A) Acid-fast bacilli
(B) Catalase-negative, gram-positive cocci in chains
(C) Coagulase-negative, gram-positive cocci in clusters
(D) Coagulase-positive, gram-positive cocci in clusters
(E) Oxidase-negative, gram-negative bacilli

38. A 28-year-old woman presents to her primary care physician complaining of a generalized body rash, especially on the inside of her wrists and ankles, and lesions on her genitals (see image). Physical examination reveals generalized lymphadenopathy and a mild fever. Which of the following could be used to confirm the diagnosis?

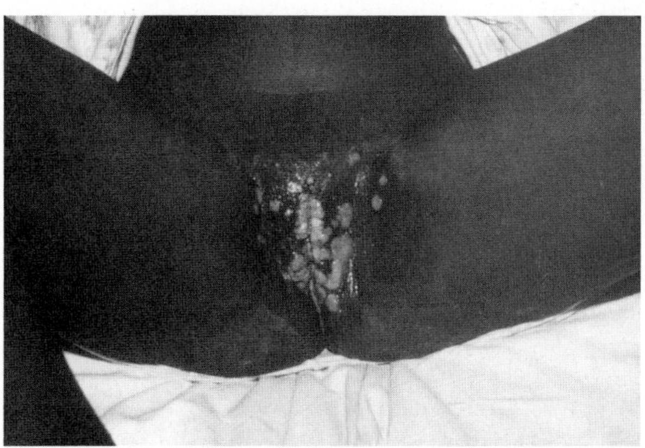

Courtesy of Dr. J. Pledger, Centers for Disease Control and Prevention.

(A) Culture on Thayer-Martin agar
(B) Tzanck preparation
(C) Venereal Disease Research Laboratory test
(D) Weil-Felix reaction
(E) Ziehl-Neelsen stain

39. A 43-year-old HIV-positive man presents to his physician complaining of recent-onset abdominal pain and diarrhea, along with an increased level of general fatigue and occasional night sweats. Physical examination is significant for a fever of 37.8°C (100.1°F), bilateral cervical adenopathy, and a weight loss of 4.5 kg (10 lb) compared to his last physician's visit. A blood sample is taken, which when cultured shows the presence of nonbranching bacilli that stain positively for Ziehl-Neelsen stain. His CD4+ cell count is 50/mm^3. Which of the following is the most worrisome for causing the patient's recent symptoms?

(A) *Actinomyces israelli*
(B) *Mycobacterium avium-intercellulare*
(C) *Mycobacterium marinum*
(D) *Mycobacterium tuberculosis*
(E) *Nocardia asteroides*

40. An 8-day-old infant has developed fever, irritability, decreased level of consciousness, apnea, and a full anterior fontanelle. Prenatal laboratory tests results are not available, as the infant's mother received no prenatal care and delivered at home at 36 weeks' gestation. What routine prophylactic intrapartum antibiotic could the mother have been treated with in order to eradicate the likely cause of the infant's illness?

(A) Fluconazole
(B) Metronidazole
(C) Moxifloxacin
(D) Penicillin
(E) Vancomycin

ANSWERS

1. **The correct answer is B.** The differential diagnosis of a genital ulcer in a sexually active patient should include primary syphilis (though these ulcers are usually painless), genital herpes, and chancroid. Because the Tzanck smear (which looks for multinucleated giant cells typical of herpes infection), is negative, as is the VDRL test for syphilis, chancroid becomes most likely. Chancroid is a bacterial infection caused by *Haemophilus ducreyi*, which presents typically as a painful genital ulcer with associated inguinal lymphadenopathy. It is typically treated with ceftriaxone given as a one-time, 250-mg, intramuscular injection, or with azithromycin as a single 1000-mg dose.

   Answer A is incorrect. Acyclovir is an antiviral agent used to treat herpes infections. It is activated by viral thymidine kinase, whereupon it inhibits the herpes viral polymerase. It can be used to treat herpes simplex virus types 1 and 2, varicella-zoster virus, and Epstein-Barr virus infections.

   Answer C is incorrect. Foscarnet inhibits viral DNA polymerase without the need of activation by thymidine kinase. It is used to treat cytomegalovirus (CMV) retinitis, but it can also be used to treat acyclovir-resistant herpes simplex virus.

   Answer D is incorrect. Ribavirin is used to treat respiratory syncytial virus. It functions by inhibiting inosine monophosphate dehydrogenase, thus blocking the synthesis of guanine nucleotides.

   Answer E is incorrect. Vancomycin is a bactericidal antibiotic used for multidrug-resistant gram-positive organisms such as *Staphylococcus aureus* and *Clostridium difficile*. It functions by binding to mucopeptide precursors, preventing formation of the bacterial cell wall.

2. **The correct answer is A.** This patient is suffering from a fungal pneumonia. In USMLE-style questions, students are often asked to differentiate between candidate yeast species based on the location where the patient acquired the illness and/or the morphology of the organism. In this case, one cannot reach a conclusion based on location. The man lives near the Mississippi River basin (where histoplasmosis and blastomycosis are endemic), and he has recently traveled to the Southwest (where coccidioidomycosis is endemic). Only paracoccidioidomycosis (endemic to Central and South America) can be eliminated as a likely answer by location. Rather, the morphology of the yeast is the key to reaching the correct conclusion. In the lower-right portion of the image, an example of broad-based budding can be seen, which is most consistent with blastomycosis. A common mnemonic regarding the appearance of ***Blastomyces*** is that it is a **B**ig, **B**road-**B**ased, **B**udding organism.

   Answer B is incorrect. The distinguishing morphologic feature of *Coccidioides immitis*, which is endemic to the southwestern United States, is its tendency to form large (up to 70 µm in diameter) spherules filled with endospores.

   Answer C is incorrect. Unlike the other answer choices, *Cryptococcus neoformans* most commonly causes fungal meningitis (with pneumonia as the second most common manifestation) in the immunocompromised. Like *Blastomyces*, it is a budding organism, but is distinguishable morphologically by a thick capsule that may be visualized with India ink stain.

   Answer D is incorrect. *Histoplasma capsulatum*, which is endemic to the Mississippi and Ohio River valleys, is unique among the answer choices in that it can live as an intracellular pathogen. Microscopic evaluation of a lesion can show numerous small (1-5 µm) yeast forms within an individual macrophage.

   Answer E is incorrect. *Paracoccidioides brasiliensis*, which is endemic to rural Latin America, is often described as having a captain's-wheel or Mickey-Mouse-head appearance. This is due to several smaller daughter cells that are simultaneously budding from a single mother cell.

3. **The correct answer is D.** Lyme disease is caused by infection with the spirochete *Borrelia burgdorferi*, and is transmitted by the bite of the *Ixodes* tick. Initially, the disease presents with constitutional symptoms such as fever and malaise, as well as a rash surrounding the bite site. However, the bite site often goes unnoticed, and erythema chronicum migrans is not necessarily present in every case. Early disseminated disease presents four-six weeks after the initial infection and is characterized by cardiac and neurologic abnormalities. Cardiac abnormalities include myocarditis, arrhythmias, and conduction disturbances. Lyme arthritis is a late-stage finding, occurs in about 60% of patients months to years later, and is associated with pain and swelling of large joints, most often in one or both knees. Lyme disease is most prevalent in the northeast Atlantic Coast states, but cases have been reported throughout the United States.

   Answer A is incorrect. Brugada syndrome is a conductive heart disease that usually affects young men and carries an increased risk of sudden cardiac death. The disease has been associated with sodium ion channel abnormalities. The typical ECG pattern is a right bundle-branch block and ST-segment elevation on leads V_1-V_3.

   Answer B is incorrect. Chronic Chagas disease usually manifests during its earliest phase with arrhythmias (eg, heart block and ventricular tachycardia). Dilated cardiomyopathy, megacolon, and megaesophagus occur later in the course of the disease. The disease presents acutely after the transfer of *Trypanosoma cruzi* (found in the southern United States, Mexico, and Central and South America) by the reduviid bug (also called the kissing bug). Transmission is associated with a hardened red area or chagoma. This is followed by fever, malaise, lymphadenopathy, tachycardia, and meningoencephalitis that resolve within one month. The patient's ECG tracing is classic for Mobitz type II heart block. Chagas disease would be a rare diagnosis in the northern United States.

   Answer C is incorrect. Hypertrophic cardiomyopathy is the most common cause of death in young athletes in the United States. It is characterized by an asymmetric hypertrophic, nondilated left ventricle. Histopathologically, the myocardial architecture is disorganized and scarred. The typical ECG shows repolarization changes or frank hypertrophy.

   Answer E is incorrect. Classic third-degree heart block is "complete," which means that the atria and the ventricles beat independently of each other, with the P waves and the QRS waves bearing no relation to one another. Severe bradycardia is usually present, and sudden death is a possibility. This condition is usually treated with a pacemaker.

4. **The correct answer is B.** The gradual onset of her symptoms, together with the radiologic findings of diffuse interstitial infiltrates, suggests atypical pneumonia. Atypical pneumonia is caused most commonly by *Mycoplasma pneumoniae*, *Legionella pneumophila*, *Chlamydia pneumoniae*, and viruses; however, IgM cold agglutinin production is seen only with *Mycoplasma* infection.

   Answer A is incorrect. Culture on buffered charcoal yeast extract medium is performed to diagnose *L pneumophila* pneumonia. *L pneumophila* causes atypical pneumonia that is seen most commonly in older individuals who smoke and abuse alcohol. Although *Legionella* is transmitted through environmental water sources, infection does not imply aspiration.

   Answer C is incorrect. Phyocyanins, a product of *Pseudomonas aeruginosa*, lead to the blue-green color of the organisms. *Pseudomonas* can cause pneumonia but typically in patients who have cystic fibrosis or are severely immunocompromised.

   Answer D is incorrect. Polysaccharide capsules are a characteristic of *Streptococcus pneumoniae* and other organisms including certain strains of *Haemophilus influenzae*, *Neisseria meningitidis*, and *Escherichia coli*. *S pneumoniae* is the cause of typical lobar pneumonia, which is characterized by sudden onset of fever, chills, cough, and pleuritic pain. X-ray of the chest usually shows focal lung consolidation rather than diffuse infiltrates, as seen in this case.

Answer E is incorrect. Reticulate bodies are the intracellular form of *Chlamydia* species, including *C pneumoniae*. *C pneumoniae* can cause atypical pneumonia that presents similarly to *Mycoplasma* pneumonia. It is difficult to distinguish between the two based on symptoms and presentation, so treatment usually is designed to cover both organisms. *Mycoplasma* infection, however, is much more common.

5. **The correct answer is C.** The clinical picture and imaging are consistent with progressive multifocal leukoencephalopathy (PML) secondary to reactivation of latent JC virus infection, which can occur with CD4+ counts <50/mm^3. It typically presents with rapidly progressive focal neurologic deficits without signs of increased intracranial pressure. Ataxia, aphasia, and cranial nerve deficits also may occur. Lumbar puncture is nondiagnostic and frequently demonstrates mild elevations in protein and WBCs. Cerebrospinal fluid (CSF) analysis can reveal the presence of myelin basic protein, which is due to demyelination caused by the JC virus. PML typically presents as multiple nonenhancing T2-hyperintense lesions. When it is suspected, stereotactic biopsy is required for definitive diagnosis, but a positive CSF polymerase chain reaction for JC virus is diagnostic in the appropriate clinical setting. Histology of the lesions shows nuclear inclusions in oligodendrocytes. Although there is no definitive treatment, clearance of JC virus DNA can be observed with response to highly active antiretroviral therapy.

Answer A is incorrect. Uncommon in the developed world, but presenting with increased risk in homeless and HIV patients, cortical tuberculomas are caseating foci within the cortical parenchyma occurring from previous hematogenous mycoplasma bacillemia. The clinical presentation may be similar to that of the current patient; however, presentation would include enhancing nodular lesions on imaging and elevated protein and low glucose on CSF examination.

Answer B is incorrect. CMV encephalitis can mimic the appearance of PML, but would be associated with enhancing periventricular white matter lesions in cortical and subependymal regions. CMV encephalitis also is associated typically with more systemic signs and symptoms. Polymerase chain reaction analysis of CSF would be positive for CMV, and histologic exam shows giant cells with eosinophilic inclusions in both the cytoplasm and the nucleus.

Answer D is incorrect. Central nervous system (CNS) lymphoma typically affects those with CD4+ cell counts <50/mm^3. MRI will demonstrate one or more enhancing lesions (50% are multiple and 50% are single) that typically are surrounded by edema, and can produce a mass effect. CNS lymphoma can present with polymerase chain reaction findings positive for Epstein-Barr virus on CSF.

Answer E is incorrect. Space-occupying lesions due to toxoplasmosis infection represent the most common cause of cerebral mass lesions in HIV-infected patients, and typically present with multiple enhancing lesions on MRI. The lesions typically are located at the corticomedullary junction, and are surrounded by edema that frequently produces a mass effect and distinguishes its appearance from PML. Positive *Toxoplasma* serologies can assist in diagnosis, and clinical improvements will result from treatment with sulfadiazine/pyrimethamine or trimethoprim/sulfamethoxazole.

6. **The correct answer is E.** Rubeola, also called measles, is a relatively rare illness in the United States because of the ubiquity of the measles/mumps/rubella (MMR) vaccine. It presents with the prodrome described in this patient. The rash that spreads from head to toe over a three-day period develops one or two days after the appearance of Koplik's spots, which are red oral lesions with blue-white centers.

Answer A is incorrect. Diphtheria is an illness virtually unknown in the United States because of the prevalence of the diphtheria/tetanus/pertussis (DTaP) vaccine. It is caused by *Corynebacterium diphtheriae* and is characterized by a membranous pharyngitis.

Answer B is incorrect. Pertussis, or whooping cough, is also rare due to widespread vaccinations. It is a respiratory infection of children that characteristically produces coughing spasms followed by a loud inspiratory whoop.

Answer C is incorrect. Roseola is a febrile disease of very young children that begins with a high fever and progresses to a rash similar to measles. Infants and young children are most at risk. It is believed to be caused by human herpesvirus 6.

Answer D is incorrect. Rubella, also known as German measles, is a less severe viral exanthem. Many infections are subclinical, but rubella can cause severe birth defects when infection occurs during the prenatal period.

7. **The correct answer is B.** Based on the dermatomal and unilateral distribution of this rash, the patient most likely has shingles. This is a focal reactivation of a prior varicella-zoster virus (VZV) infection. Most patients who develop shingles have a two- to three-day prodrome of pain, tingling, or burning in the involved dermatome, followed by the development of a vesicular rash. The treatment of choice for herpesvirus infections is acyclovir, ganciclovir, and (for VZV specifically) famciclovir, which work by inhibiting viral DNA polymerase.

   Answer A is incorrect. Bacteria, not viruses, have cell walls. Inhibition of cell wall synthesis is accomplished by the penicillin family of antibiotics.

   Answer C is incorrect. The antiviral medication amantadine, used only in the treatment of influenza A virus infection, works by inhibiting viral genome uncoating in the host cell.

   Answer D is incorrect. Nucleoside reverse transcriptase inhibitors are first-line medications for treating HIV infection.

   Answer E is incorrect. Inhibition of protein synthesis is achieved by five types of antibiotics: chloramphenicol & clindamycin, linezolid, erythromycin, tetracycline & doxycycline, and the aminoglycosides. Doxycycline is the main treatment for both *Rickettsia rickettsii* (Rocky Mountain spotted fever) and *Borrelia burgdorferi* (Lyme disease) infections. The rash of Rocky Mountain spotted fever is typically petechial and begins around the wrists and ankles, although it may begin on the trunk or diffusely. The rash of Lyme disease may be solid red or may form a ring or multiple rings with a bulls-eye appearance.

8. **The correct answer is A.** Four members of the *Plasmodium* genus of protozoa commonly infect humans and cause malaria. All are spread by the female *Anopheles* mosquito; diagnosis is made through a blood smear. The species that causes cerebral involvement is *P falciparum*, which is almost entirely responsible for the severe cases of disease that proceed to coma and death.

   Answer B is incorrect. *Plasmodium malariae* infection causes a 72-hour cyclic fever. *P malariae*, however, does not cause cerebral malaria.

   Answer C is incorrect. *Plasmodium ovale* infection causes a 48-hour cyclic fever. A unique feature of *P vivax* and *P ovale* organisms is that they can form hypnozoites that can remain dormant in the liver for long periods, only to resurface later. However, *P ovale* does not cause cerebral malaria.

   Answer D is incorrect. *Plasmodium vivax* infection causes a 48-hour cyclic fever. A unique feature of both *P vivax* and *P ovale* organisms is that they can form hypnozoites that can remain dormant in the liver for long periods, only to resurface later. However, *P vivax* does not cause cerebral malaria.

   Answer E is incorrect. *Plasmodium knowlesi* is a simian malaria parasite that primarily infects macaques, although it has been reported to infect humans in southeast Asia. There are reports of cerebral involvement in monkeys, and of isolated fatal human cases.

9. **The correct answer is C.** These lab results and the clinical presentation (fever, headache, nu-

chal rigidity, and photophobia) are typical of viral meningitis. Because the cultures are negative, a viral cause should be considered. This patient would have recovered without complications with only symptomatic support. Viral aseptic meningitis usually is caused by enteroviruses and runs a milder course than bacterial meningitis.

Answer A is incorrect. This profile does not suggest meningitis. However, because the clinical presentation strongly suggests meningitis, it is not likely that the CSF analysis would be completely normal.

Answer B is incorrect. In this profile, only the CSF sugar level is elevated. This does not suggest bacterial meningitis, in which sugar levels would decrease. This profile may suggest systemic hyperglycemia, such as in uncontrolled diabetes.

Answer D is incorrect. This is a typical profile of fungal or mycobacterial meningitis. Note that it is the same profile as that of bacterial meningitis, except the increase in WBCs is due to lymphocytes, not neutrophils. Fungal and mycobacterial meningitis also have a more subacute presentation than has bacterial meningitis.

Answer E is incorrect. This is a typical profile of bacterial meningitis, in which neutrophils predominate over lymhocytes.

10. **The correct answer is D.** Human papillomavirus (HPV) causes carcinoma (usually cervical) by inactivating tumor suppressor genes such as *p53* and *Rb* through the actions of viral proteins E6 and E7, respectively.

    Answer A is incorrect. Epstein-Barr virus (EBV) is associated with Burkitt lymphoma (a B-lymphocyte lymphoma) and nasopharyngeal carcinoma. The t(8;14) translocation is consistently associated with Burkitt lymphoma, but the translocation alone is not responsible for the neoplasm and is not found in nasopharyngeal carcinomas. The other factors that determine oncogenesis of EBV remain unclear.

    Answer B is incorrect. Both hepatitis C (HCV) and hepatitis B virus (HBV) infections are associated with an increased risk of developing hepatocellular carcinoma. The liver has a high regenerative potential, but if this process is overused, the chance of an oncogenic mutation occurring during the regeneration of cells increases.

    Answer C is incorrect. HIV as a direct oncogenic agent is being intensely researched, but it is already known that immune suppression and dysregulation caused by HIV infection give rise to lymphomas and Kaposi sarcoma.

    Answer E is incorrect. Human T-cell lymphotropic virus causes adult T-cell leukemia, and although the mechanism of oncogenesis remains unclear, there is some evidence that integration into the host genome at locations near cellular growth genes may play a role.

11. **The correct answer is B.** Influenza virus has both hemagglutinin (HA) and neuraminidase (NA) molecules on its surface. These two molecules are responsible for the ability of the virus to be absorbed and penetrate the host cells. After a human is infected with the influenza virus, that person will be immune to infection by the same virus because of antibodies created against HA and NA. If either HA or NA is changed, as can be the case if two different influenza viruses infect the same cell and exchange RNA, antigenic shift can occur. This creates a new virus that has never been exposed to the human immune system before, with potentially catastrophic consequences. This type of mixing is most commonly thought to be between a human and an avian strain mixing in an intermediary porcine host, thus leading to the term "avian flu."

    Answer A is incorrect. Antigenic drift describes mutations that can occur in hemagglutinin and neuraminidase, making them less antigenic to the preexisting antibodies in the human host. Since this results in small changes in viral toxicity, it will lead to a slightly different strain, but it is not likely to lead to a global epidemic.

    Answer C is incorrect. Hemagglutinin has the ability to attach to sialic acid receptors, which activates fusion of the virus to the cell. All infectious influenza viruses have this molecule.

Answer D is incorrect. Neuraminidase has the ability to destroy neuraminic acid, a component of mucin. This helps break down the barrier to the upper airways and aids in infectivity.

Answer E is incorrect. RBCs agglutinate in the presence of hemagglutinin; hence the name. This does not affect the infection rate of the influenza virus.

12. **The correct answer is D.** The image shows multiple lesions throughout the brain parenchyma and subarachnoid space, which are characterized by ring-shaped regions of low T1 intensity consistent with calcification. This appearance is most consistent with the nodular calcified stage of neurocysticercosis and is seen only in individuals with long-standing, chronic infection from endemic areas. Although this patient's presentation is highly suspicious for malignancy, the image provided and laboratory data confirm a diagnosis of neurocysticercosis, which is caused by infection with *Taenia solium*, a pork tapeworm. It is the most common parasitic infection of the CNS worldwide, and is particularly endemic to Central and South America, Eastern Europe, and some parts of Asia. After humans ingest the tapeworm's eggs, the eggs hatch and the larvae invade the wall of the small intestine and disseminate hematogenously. Cysticerci may be found in any organ, but are most commonly found in the brain, muscles, skin, and heart. Since we know that this patient is already suffering from cysts in her brain, the most likely additional location would be her muscles. Fortunately, the disease rarely results in death and patients are often asymptomatic; however, when the disease does result in neurologic sequelae, specific symptoms depend on the location of the cysts. Cysticercosis is treated with administration of albendazole.

   Answer A is incorrect. Although the cysticerci may be found in virtually any organ, they almost never involve the urinary bladder. Schistosomiasis is a parasite that commonly invades the bladder.

   Answer B is incorrect. Bone is an extremely unlikely source for cysticerci due to its relatively low blood flow.

   Answer C is incorrect. The kidney can be a location for cysticerci but is much less likely than cysts involving muscle tissue.

   Answer E is incorrect. While the small bowel is the site of infection of primary hosts like the pig, secondary hosts (humans) do not develop an adult tapeworm infection.

13. **The correct answer is A.** This patient is presenting with a classic case of whooping cough caused by *Bordetella pertussis*. The initial phase is characterized by flu-like symptoms for the first one-two weeks. During this time, erythromycin is an effective treatment. The second phase, the paroxysmal stage, is marked by bouts of multiple coughs in a single breath followed by a deep inspiration (the classic whooping cough). Treatment during this phase does not change the disease course, so only supportive care is indicated and the infection ought to pass in otherwise healthy individuals. In the United States, the diptheria/tetanus/pertussis (DTaP) vaccine is supposed to be given to all infants and protects them against diphtheria, tetanus, and pertussis. Infants who are not vaccinated are at risk for infection. *B pertussis* can only be cultured on Bordet-Gengou medium.

   Answer B is incorrect. Charcoal yeast extract when buffered with increased levels of iron and cysteine is used to culture *Legionella pneumophila*.

   Answer C is incorrect. Chocolate agar with factor V and X is used to culture *Haemophilus influenzae*.

   Answer D is incorrect. Loeffler medium is needed to culture *Corynebacterium diphtheriae*.

   Answer E is incorrect. Thayer-Martin medium is used to culture *Neisseria gonorrhoeae*.

14. **The correct answer is E.** This describes all spore-forming bacteria, which include *Bacillus anthracis*, *Bacillus cereus*, and *Clostridium*.

However, only *Clostridium botulinum* produces the symptoms seen in this baby and also fits the mode of transmission. *C botulinum* causes botulism via the production of a heat-labile toxin that inhibits the release of acetylcholine into the neuromuscular junction. Infants may initially become constipated and then develop generalized muscle weakness ("floppy baby"). The organism is spread through the ingestion of contaminated canned or bottled food. Additionally, fresh honey has been shown to harbor the organism.

Answer A is incorrect. IgA protease is produced by some bacteria so they can cleave secretory IgA and colonize mucosal areas; *Neisseria gonorrhoeae, Neisseria meningitidis, Streptococcus pneumoniae,* and *Haemophilus influenzae* are the most well known. However, none of these are typically transmitted via food, namely honey.

Answer B is incorrect. Exotoxin A is produced by *Pseudomonas aeruginosa* as well as some *Streptococcus* species. Exotoxin A has been associated with toxic shock syndrome and scarlet fever. However, none of these organisms produce the symptoms seen in this case or is transmitted by honey ingestion.

Answer C is incorrect. Lecithinase is produced by *Clostridium perfringens* and is responsible for the development of gas gangrene, cellulitis, and diarrhea. This organism is associated with contaminated wounds, which is not a part of this baby's history.

Answer D is incorrect. Lipopolysaccharide, also called endotoxin, is produced by gram-negative bacteria and *Listeria*. It is highly antigenic and can cause sepsis in severe infections. However, generalized muscle weakness is not characteristic of sepsis.

15. **The correct answer is B.** This patient's history and sputum culture are suggestive of coccidioidomycosis, a fungal infection caused by the inhalation of *Coccidioides immitis* or *Coccidioides posadasii*. These organisms are found in soil in dry areas of the southwestern United States, Mexico, and Central and South America. Coccidioidomycosis is the second most common fungal infection in the US. About 60% of these infections cause no symptoms, and in the remaining 40% of cases, the symptoms can range from mild to severe. Severe forms of the infection can present with blood-tinged sputum, loss of appetite, weight loss, a painful red rash on the legs, and change in mental status. Cultures from sputum samples or biopsy show a dimorphic fungus seen as hyphae at 25°C (77°F) and spherules filled with endospores at 37°C (98.6°F). Treatment with amphotericin B or fluconazole is usually required only in severe, disseminated disease.

Answer A is incorrect. In a patient with fever, chills, and flu-like symptoms who has recently returned from Namibia, there is concern for infection by *Plasmodium* species, which cause malaria. Malaria is transmitted by the female *Anopheles* mosquito. The time course and pattern of symptoms depend on the *Plasmodium* species with which the patient is infected. Treatment is tailored to the geographic area of infection and the *Plasmodium* species involved; agents include chloroquine, hydroxychloroquine, and atovaquone-proguanil. Malarial infection would be evident on a blood smear.

Answer C is incorrect. Sickness after travel to the Mississippi and Ohio River valleys is suggestive of histoplasmosis. Although histoplasmosis typically does not present symptomatically, some patients experience a flu-like illness with fever, cough, headaches, and myalgias. Histoplasmosis can result in lung disease resembling tuberculosis (TB) and widespread disseminated infection affecting the liver, spleen, adrenal glands, mucosal surfaces, and meninges. On microscopy, histoplasmosis appears as spherules filled with endospores, as opposed to the hyphae and spherules observed in the sputum of those with coccidiomycosis.

Answer D is incorrect. Recent hiking in wooded areas carries the risk of contracting tick-borne illnesses, such as those carried by the *Ixodes* tick: *Babesia microti*, a protozoon that causes babesiosis; *Borrelia burgdorferi*, a spirochete that causes Lyme disease; and *Ehrlichia chaffeensis*, a rickettsial bacterium that causes erlichiosis. None of these organisms appears as hyphae on microscopy.

Answer E is incorrect. A wound while gardening, such as a thorn prick, can cause inoculation with *Sporothrix schenckii*. This fungus can be found in various environments, including sphagnum moss, decaying vegetation, hay, and soil. When *S schenckii* is introduced into the skin, it causes a local pustule or ulcer with nodules along the draining lymphatics (ascending lymphangitis). *S schenckii* is a dimorphic fungus, existing as hyphae at 25°C (77°F) and as a budding yeast form at 37°C (98.6°F). Itraconazole or potassium iodide is used for treatment. On microscopy, one would not expect to see spherules.

16. **The correct answer is C.** All five answers are part of **ToRCHeS** (**To**xoplasmosis, **R**ubella, **C**ytomegalovirus, **He**rpesvirus/HIV, and **S**yphilis) infections, the group of infections for which every newborn is tested. If the mother becomes infected during pregnancy, the pathogens can cross the placenta and infect the fetus. Rubivirus causes rubella in adults. The virus crosses the placenta in the first trimester and causes congenital abnormalities that range from deafness to cataracts to cardiovascular abnormalities. The abnormal heart exam findings in this newborn are classic for a patent ductus arteriosus (PDA) with delayed symptoms of heart failure. A PDA is the most common cardiovascular abnormality seen in congenital rubella syndrome. A PDA results from the failure of the ductus arteriosus to close in the first days of life. This results in a left-to-right shunt from the aorta to the pulmonary artery. In a substantial shunt, deoxygenated blood returning from the body to the heart bypasses the lung via the PDA to the aorta. Because blood is shunted, there is a widening of pulse pressure (the difference between systolic and diastolic). A split S_2 sound occurs in PDA because of the increased flow through the pulmonary artery. The S_2 sound is a composite of two distinct heart valves. Normally, the aortic valve closes just before the pulmonary valve. When the pulmonary valve is forced to stay open longer than the aortic valve, such as "physiologic split" and, in this case, a large PDA, we hear the split S_2 sound.

Answer A is incorrect. Congenital CMV infection is marked most commonly by petechial rashes, jaundice, hepatosplenomegaly, and sensorineural hearing loss. Cardiovascular abnormalities are not features of congenital CMV infection.

Answer B is incorrect. Congenital herpes infection most often either affects skin, eyes, and mouth or presents as localized CNS infection. Symptoms usually develop within four weeks of birth. CNS symptoms can include temperature instability, respiratory distress, poor feeding, and lethargy. Herpes simplex virus type 2 is also one of the most common causes of neonatal encephalitis.

Answer D is incorrect. Congenital toxoplasmosis infection most often is asymptomatic initially. The class triad of symptoms that develop include chorioretinitis, hydrocephalus, and intracranial calcifications. Early symptoms can include a maculopapular rash, jaundice, and hepatomegaly. Most complications develop if the infection is not treated soon after birth.

Answer E is incorrect. Newborns with congenital syphilis normally are asymptomatic at birth. When symptoms develop, the babies often have hearing problems (based on cranial defect VIII) and cutaneous lesions that normally appear on the palms and soles first. More serious symptoms include anemia, jaundice, and hepatomegaly. Patent ductus arteriosus is not found with congenital syphilis.

17. **The correct answer is G.** This patient is likely presenting with a mucosa-associated lymphoid tissue (MALT) lymphoma. This type of indolent lymphoma is believed to be associated with infection by the organism *Helicobacter pylori*. *H pylori* is commonly identified by the presence of urease, catalase, and oxidase. Eradication of the infection with antibiotics and proton-pump inhibitors is often sufficient to cause regression of the lymphoma.

Answer A is incorrect. This pattern is seen in benign flora such as the lactobacilli.

Answer B is incorrect. This pattern would be commonly seen in streptococcal species such as *Streptococcus pneumoniae*.

Answer C is incorrect. This pattern of results is commonly seen in facultative anaerobes such as *Escherichia coli*.

Answer D is incorrect. This pattern represents *Pseudomonas aeruginosa*, an opportunistic lung pathogen.

Answer E is incorrect. This represents a pattern common of true anaerobes in the *Bacteroides* family.

Answer F is incorrect. This pattern is seen in *Proteus mirabilis*, a common cause of urinary tract infection.

18. **The correct answer is E.** Food poisoning is the major cause of illness in this patient, and the most likely cause in this case is preformed exotoxin from *Bacillus cereus* secreted into the gastrointestinal (GI) tract. These exotoxins are fast acting, so the symptoms of food poisoning (nausea, vomiting, diarrhea) are usually rapid in onset (within four-eight hours of ingestion). Other major causes of food poisoning resulting in nonbloody diarrhea include *Staphylococcus aureus*, *Clostridium perfringens*, and enterotoxigenic *Escherichia coli*, which cause traveler's diarrhea. These organisms are typically found in specific types of food, and *B cereus* is found in reheated rice. Because the food poisoning in *B cereus* infection is caused by preformed enterotoxins, antibiotic treatment will not help and supportive care is recommended.

Answer A is incorrect. Bismuth subsalicylate, metronidazole, and amoxicillin are used to treat *Helicobacter pylori* infection, which does not result in the symptoms seen in this patient.

Answer B is incorrect. Fluoroquinolones can be used to treat severe *Shigella* infection, which causes a bloody diarrhea.

Answer C is incorrect. *Campylobacter jejuni* enterocolitis can be treated with erythromycin or ciprofloxacin. Infection with this organism is not associated with eating reheated rice and would typically result in bloody diarrhea. Moreover, an invasive process by the organism would likely take >4 hours to produce symptoms.

Answer D is incorrect. *Vibrio cholerae* causes large-volume, watery diarrhea. Treatment involves prompt replacement of water and electrolytes. Although antibiotics are not needed for treatment, tetracyclines have been shown to reduce the course of the disease. However, there is nothing about this patient's history to suggest that he has been exposed to cholera. Rather, the history indicates a food-related cause.

19. **The correct answer is C.** This patient presents with classic symptoms of hepatocellular carcinoma. Approximately 10%-30% of people infected with HCV will develop cirrhosis of the liver. Approximately 1%-5% of these patients develop hepatocellular carcinoma. HCV is transmitted via blood or blood transfusions and, rarely, by sexual contact. This patient is more likely to have HCV infection due to his lack of travel, history of blood transfusion prior to the availability of sensitive screening methods, and extensive macronodular cirrhosis. Up to 90% of HCV-related hepatocellular carcinomas occur in patients with cirrhosis. Onset of hepatocellular carcinoma occurs on average 30 years after initial infection with HCV.

Answer A is incorrect. In the immunocompetent host, CMV infection is often asymptomatic, or it may produce a mononucleosis syndrome. Disease manifestations are more common in the immunocompromised host, and include CMV colitis and CMV retinitis. Patients with symptomatic CMV infection may have subclinical transaminitis; however, there is no association with chronic hepatitis.

Answer B is incorrect. Hepatitis A is transmitted via the fecal-oral route and causes an acute self-limited GI infection. It may rarely result in fulminant hepatic failure requiring liver transplantation, but it does not cause a chronic hepatitis or cirrhosis.

Answer D is incorrect. Hepatitis E is transmitted via the fecal-oral route and has been linked to fatalities in pregnant women. It does not cause chronic hepatitis except very rarely in patients who have previously received solid organ transplants.

Answer E is incorrect. HIV is transmitted via bodily fluids and causes the death of CD4+ T lymphocytes, resulting in an immunocompromised state and increased susceptibility to opportunistic infections. It does not cause hepatitis.

20. **The correct answer is A.** The image shows gram-positive cocci in clusters. Staphylococcal scalded skin syndrome (SSSS) is caused by the release of two exotoxins (epidermolytic toxins A and B) from *Staphylococcus aureus*. Desmosomes (also called "macula adherens") are responsible for binding epithelial cells to one another to form a coherent whole. The exotoxins that are released bind to a molecule within the desmosome called desmoglein 1, thereby disrupting cell adhesion. In SSSS, the epidermis separates at the stratum granulosum due to the binding of exotoxins to desmosomes in this layer. Clinically, this results in bullous lesions and a positive Nikolsky sign.

    Answer B is incorrect. Gap junctions are circular intercellular contact areas that permit the passage of small molecules between adjacent cells, allowing communication to facilitate electrotonic and metabolic function.

    Answer C is incorrect. Hemidesmosomes are present on the basal surface of epithelial cells adjacent to the basement membrane, and serve to connect epithelial cells to the underlying extracellular matrix.

    Answer D is incorrect. Intermediate junctions lie deep to tight junctions, comprised of actin filaments forming a continuous band around the cell, providing structural support just below tight junctions.

    Answer E is incorrect. Tight junctions are located beneath the luminal surface of simple columnar epithelium (eg, intestinal lining) and seal the intercellular space to prevent diffusion between cells.

21. **The correct answer is B.** This boy is suffering from the classic hemolytic-uremic syndrome (HUS) caused most often by the endotoxin of *Escherichia coli* O157:H7 contracted from undercooked beef. This disease is caused by endothelial injury and platelet aggregation that lead to the classic triad of microangiopathic hemolytic anemia, thrombocytopenia, and acute renal injury. Up to 75% of cases of classic HUS occur as a result of infection with *E coli* O157:H7.

    Answer A is incorrect. *Campylobacter* infections can cause diarrheal illnesses and have been implicated in the development of Guillain-Barré syndrome, but would not be expected to cause HUS.

    Answer C is incorrect. Rotavirus is a common cause of infantile gastroenteritis. It is caused by a double-stranded virus (reovirus). It is typically spread throughout daycare centers but does not cause HUS.

    Answer D is incorrect. *Shigella* is known to cause bloody diarrhea. It can cause HUS, but this is less common than *E coli*-induced HUS.

    Answer E is incorrect. *Vibrio cholerae* causes massive watery diarrhea by secreting cholera toxin. *Vibrio* infections are not implicated in classic HUS. This bacterium is generally associated with contaminated water sources rather than ill-prepared food.

22. **The correct answer is A.** These symptoms are typical of urethritis. The most common causes of urethritis in males are *Chlamydia trachomatis* and *Neisseria gonorrhoeae*. The image shows intracellular inclusions consistent with infection by *C trachomatis*. While they may be difficult to differentiate, *C trachomatis* infection induces a predominantly immunologic reaction, with only a few polymorphonuclear leukocytes (PMNs), while *N gonorrhoeae* induces predominantly nonimmunologic inflammation, with a PMN-rich infiltrate. The antibiotic of choice for chlamydia urethritis is azithromycin (macrolide) or doxycycline (tetracycline).

Answer B is incorrect. Ceftriaxone is an effective treatment for gonorrhea, but the cephalosporin class of antibiotics is relatively ineffective against *Chlamydia trachomatis*.

Answer C is incorrect. Fluconazole inhibits fungal steroid synthesis. It is used in the treatment of fungal infections, such as *Candida albicans*.

Answer D is incorrect. Penicillin has been shown to suppress chlamydial multiplication. However, it does not eradicate the organism and thus is not the best treatment for this type of infection. Penicillin is the treatment of choice for syphilis.

Answer E is incorrect. Vancomycin has not been shown to be effective in the treatment of chlamydial infection. It is used to treat drug-resistant *Staphylococcus aureus* and *Clostridium difficile*.

23. **The correct answer is B.** HBV is transmitted via parenteral, sexual, or maternal-fetal routes. Of the markers listed, only hepatitis B e antigen (HBeAg) signifies active viral replication, and would therefore make transmission of HBV to a partner more likely. HBeAg and hepatitis B core antigen (HBcAg) are antigenic markers of the virus core. They can be detected two-four months after exposure.

    Answer A is incorrect. Hepatitis B e antibody (HBeAb) is an antibody directed against HBeAg. Its presence indicates low transmissibility. HBeAb can be detected five months after exposure to HBV and one month after the detection of HBeAg.

    Answer C is incorrect. Hepatitis B surface antibody (HBsAb) provides immunity to HBV infection. It can be detected in former carriers of HBV or in patients immunized with the HBV vaccine.

    Answer D is incorrect. IgG HBcAb is an indicator of chronic disease.

    Answer E is incorrect. Hepatitis B core antibody (HBcAb) is produced in response to hepatitis core antigen (HBcAg). IgM is an indicator of recent disease, given that IgM is the first antibody produced in response to an antigen.

24. **The correct answer is D.** This patient likely has pertussis, or whooping cough, which is caused by the gram-negative rod *Bordetella pertussis*. This organism has four virulence factors, including pertussis toxin. The A subunit of this exotoxin inhibits membrane-bound $G\alpha_i$ proteins, which ultimately results in the accumulation of cAMP. The effects of this accumulation include histamine sensitization, increased insulin synthesis, lymphocytosis, and inhibition of phagocytosis.

    Answer A is incorrect. The botulinum toxin released by *Clostridium botulinum* prevents the release of acetylcholine into the synaptic cleft, resulting in muscle weakness and paralysis.

    Answer B is incorrect. The alpha toxin of *Staphylococcus aureus* binds to the plasma membrane of host cells, forming a pore in the membrane that allows ions and small molecules to enter the cell. This leads to cell swelling and eventual lysis. Streptolysin O of *Streptococcus pyogenes* functions in a similar manner.

    Answer C is incorrect. The exotoxin of *Corynebacterium diphtheriae* functions via the inactivation of elongation factor 2, causing pharyngitis and the formation of a pseudomembrane in the throat. *Pseudomonas aeruginosa* exotoxin A also works via this mechanism.

    Answer E is incorrect. Lipopolysaccharide-lipid A is an endotoxin released only by gram-negative bacteria, with the exception of *Listeria monocytogenes*, a gram-positive bacteria responsible for meningitis in neonates and immunosuppressed patients. Endotoxins are a normal part of the bacterial membrane released upon lysis of the cell.

25. **The correct answer is E.** *Vibrio cholerae* causes watery stools, often called "rice-water" stool. This illness is not accompanied by abdominal pain, but the symptoms are due to dehydration, which leads to electrolyte imbalances. Cholera toxin binds to the GM1 entero-

cyte receptor via the pentameric B subunit. Once inside the cell, the toxin must undergo cleavage of the active, A1 component, which goes on to constitutively activate the G_s protein through ADP ribosylation. This results in high cyclic AMP levels, which activate the CFTR (cystic fibrosis transmembrane conductance regulator) channel, leading to a large efflux of chlorine and other ions into the GI lumen. This results in extremely watery diarrhea accompanied by electrolyte imbalances.

Answer A is incorrect. This is a characteristic of Shiga toxin, which typically leads to bloody diarrhea.

Answer B is incorrect. *Bacillus anthracis* produces a toxin that acts as an adenylate cyclase (edema factor) but is not associated with severe watery diarrhea.

Answer C is incorrect. Diphtheria toxin and exotoxin A from *Pseudomonas* inactivate elongation factor 2, but neither is a likely cause of watery diarrhea.

Answer D is incorrect. *Bordetella pertussis* produces an exotoxin that increases cAMP levels by inactivating the inhibitory G_i. However, pertussis causes whooping cough, not severe watery diarrhea.

26. **The correct answer is B.** Anaphylactic shock is a life-threatening disorder that occurs when an allergen overactivates mast cells and basophils, leading to widespread release of histamines, serotonins, and other compounds stored in the granules of these immune cells. These compounds lead to vasodilation and leaky capillaries. The crosslinking of IgE receptors present on these cells causes the activation of these cell types. By blocking this cross reaction, the anaphylactic pathway can be stymied.

    Answer A is incorrect. γ Interferon is produced by T lymphocytes and, among other functions, activates tumoricidal macrophages.

    Answer C is incorrect. Endotoxin can directly activate Hageman factor, activating the coagulation cascade and leading to disseminated intravascular coagulation (DIC). However, the mechanism of shock through anaphylaxis is not related to DIC.

    Answer D is incorrect. The C5a component of the complement cascade, activated by endotoxin, functions in neutrophil chemotaxis. This is not the mechanism involved in anaphylaxis.

    Answer E is incorrect. The cytokine interleukin-1, released by macrophages activated by endotoxin, causes fever. Fever is absent in anaphylaxis.

    Answer F is incorrect. Nitric oxide, released by macrophages activated by endotoxin, causes hypotension (shock). However, this is not the mechanism of anaphylactic shock.

27. **The correct answer is D.** Loeffler medium, blood agar, and tellurite plate are used to culture a throat swab from patients with suspected *Corynebacterium diphtheriae* infection. This organism causes symptoms of pseudomembranous pharyngitis (thick gray membrane) and lymphadenopathy. A possible complication of this disease is the extension of the membrane into the larynx and trachea, resulting in airway obstruction. Rapid treatment with diphtheria antitoxin, penicillin, or erythromycin and the DTP vaccine is indicated in this patient

    Answer A is incorrect. Löwenstein-Jensen agar is used to culture *Mycobacterium tuberculosis*, the bacterium that causes TB.

    Answer B is incorrect. Bordet-Gengou agar is used to culture *Bordetella pertussis*, the etiologic agent responsible for whooping cough.

    Answer C is incorrect. Chocolate agar with factors V and X is used to culture *Haemophilus influenzae*. This organism typically causes upper respiratory infections but is not responsible for pseudomembranous pharyngitis.

    Answer E is incorrect. *Neisseria gonorrhoeae* is cultured on Thayer-Martin media. This bacterium can cause gonorrhea, septic arthritis, neonatal conjunctivitis, and pelvic inflammatory disease.

28. **The correct answer is B.** This patient presents with Rocky Mountain spotted fever (RMSF) caused by *Rickettsia rickettsii*, a small, gram-negative bacterium carried by the American dog tick (*Dermacentor variabilis*). Despite its name, RMSF is more common in the southeastern United States than in the Rocky Mountains. Patients often present first with severe headache, fever (>38.9°C or >102°F), and myalgias followed by a petechial rash on the palms and soles (or wrists and ankles) that spreads to the trunk. The Weil-Felix assay reaction is the classic test for rickettsial disease. The treatment of choice for adults with RMSF is doxycycline; chloramphenicol is also used but has more significant adverse effects.

    Answer A is incorrect. Cephalosporins (ceftriaxone) are not effective against *Rickettsia rickettsii*. They are generally used to treat neonatal/infant sepsis or gonorrhea, as well as bacterial meningitis.

    Answer C is incorrect. Aminoglycosides (gentamicin) are not effective against *Rickettsia rickettsii*. Aminoglycosides are effective against many gram-negative bacteria and some strains of *Staphylococcus aureus*. It is also used as broad-spectrum therapy when combined with a penicillin or metronidazole.

    Answer D is incorrect. Nystatin is used in the treatment of fungal infections such as oral candidiasis.

    Answer E is incorrect. Penicillin is not effective against *Rickettsia rickettsii*. Penicillin is still the treatment of choice for syphilis. Other derivatives that are used more frequently include oxacillin, cloxacillin, dicloxacillin, and amoxicillin when *Staphylococcus* and *Streptococcus* species prove sensitive.

29. **The correct answer is B.** This patient has leukocytosis and Charcot's triad (fever, jaundice, right upper quadrant pain), along with the ominous sign of hypotension, a clear clinical picture of cholecystitis. In addition, he has *Pseudomonas aeruginosa* sepsis and DIC. Gram-negative rod sepsis is the clear cause of this patient's DIC, and antipseudomonal coverage with aztreonam is most appropriate. Aztreonam is a β-lactamase-resistant monobactam that interferes with cell wall biosynthesis by binding to penicillin-binding protein 3. Aztreonam is a potent antipseudomonal agent indicated for pseudomonal sepsis.

    Answer A is incorrect. Amoxicillin is an aminopenicillin antibiotic that interferes with cell wall synthesis. Although amoxicillin has an extended spectrum compared with penicillin (covering *Haemophilus influenzae*, *Escherichia coli*, *Listeria*, *Proteus*, *Salmonella*, and *Enterococci*), it does not provide antipseudomonal coverage.

    Answer C is incorrect. Use of fresh frozen plasma (FFP) is reserved for patients with coagulopathy and signs of active, life-threatening bleeding. Although provision of FFP will temporarily reverse some of this patient's laboratory signs of DIC (elevated International Normalized Ratio, decreased fibrinogen), treatment of the underlying cause (ie, *Pseudomonas* sepsis) is most important.

    Answer D is incorrect. Vancomycin is an antibiotic used for serious multidrug-resistant, gram-positive infections. Major uses are for methicillin-resistant *Staphylococcus aureus* and moderate to severe *Clostridium difficile* infections. Its mechanism of action is to inhibit cell wall mucopeptide formation by binding the D-ala-D-ala portion of cell wall precursors.

    Answer E is incorrect. Coagulopathy caused by warfarin overdose is reversed by pharmacologic administration of vitamin K. This patient's coagulopathy is caused by *Pseudomonas* sepsis, so vitamin K therapy plays no role here.

30. **The correct answer is C.** Trichomoniasis is caused by *Trichomonas vaginalis*. Symptoms include a profuse, frothy discharge that is associated with vulvovaginal pruritus, tenderness, and burning. The vulva and vagina are frequently inflamed. The cervix and vagina may develop small, red, punctate lesions, causing the classic "strawberry" appearance. Diagnosis is made by wet mount, on which small, pear-shaped, flagellated organisms can be seen moving around.

Answer A is incorrect. Bloody and foul-smelling vaginal discharge suggest a vaginal foreign body.

Answer B is incorrect. Pelvic or lower abdominal pain with an abnormal, foul-smelling vaginal discharge is suggestive of pelvic inflammatory disease, which can involve the endometrium, fallopian tubes, ovaries, and peritoneum. Fever, nausea, and vomiting may be present. The typical organisms involved are *Neisseria gonorrhoeae* and *Chlamydia trachomatis*.

Answer D is incorrect. *Candida* species typically cause intense pruritus and a thick, odorless, white, cottage cheese-like vaginal discharge. Erythema, edema, dysuria, and urinary frequency may be present. Budding yeasts and hyphae are seen on a wet mount.

Answer E is incorrect. Bacterial vaginosis typically presents with an unpleasant fishy-smelling discharge that is thin, gray-white, and homogeneous. Pruritus and inflammation are unusual in bacterial vaginosis, thus the term "vaginosis" rather than "vaginitis." On a wet mount, one will see clue cells that are formed from bacteria-coated epithelial cells.

31. **The correct answer is D.** *Naegleria fowleri* presents with a rapidly progressing meningoencephalitis that can progress to coma or death within six days. Other symptoms include nausea, vomiting, and irrational behavior. Transmission occurs through swimming in freshwater lakes. Microscopic analysis will reveal amebas in the spinal fluid. Unfortunately, there is no treatment for *N fowleri*.

    Answer A is incorrect. *Cryptosporidium* species infection presents with severe diarrhea in HIV-positive patients and mild watery diarrhea in HIV-negative patients. *Cryptosporidium* species are transmitted via cysts in water (fecal-oral transmission). Microscopically, acid-fast staining cysts are found. Unfortunately, there is no treatment available for *Cryptosporidium* species infection; however, in healthy patients, cryptosporidiosis is self-resolving.

    Answer B is incorrect. *Entamoeba histolytica* infection presents with bloody diarrhea (dysentery), abdominal cramps with tenesmus, and pus in the stool. It can also cause right upper quadrant pain and liver abscesses. *E histolytica* is transmitted via cysts in water (fecal-oral transmission). On microscopy, one observes amebas with ingested RBCs. Treatment for *E histolytica* infection includes metronidazole and iodoquinol.

    Answer C is incorrect. *Leishmania donovani* infection presents with hepatomegaly and splenomegaly, malaise, anemia, and weight loss. *L donovani* is transmitted via the sandfly. Microscopically, macrophages containing amastigotes are observed. Sodium stibogluconate is used to treat *L donovani* infection.

    Answer E is incorrect. The *Plasmodium falciparum* parasite is responsible for causing malaria. It is spread by the *Anopheles* mosquito. Diagnosis of *Plasmodium falciparum* infection is made through a blood smear.

32. **The correct answer is C.** This image of the mitral valve reveals Aschoff's nodule, which is pathognomonic for rheumatic fever. Rheumatic fever is caused by group A streptococci. Years after a bout of rheumatic fever, rheumatic heart disease can develop due to calcification of warty vegetations on fibrotic healing, most commonly on the mitral valve. As a result, it most commonly causes mitral stenosis, which in mild disease causes a late diastolic murmur heard best at the apex. In the US, the incidence of this mitral stenosis secondary to rheumatic fever is low given the widespread use of antibiotics. However, rheumatic mitral stenosis is prevalent in immigrant populations.

    Answer A is incorrect. A friction rub heard throughout the precordium would correspond to pericarditis, an inflammation of the pericardial sac that leads to friction with an expanding and contracting myocardium. It is not a long-term complication of rheumatic fever. Rather, a friction rub may be associated with malignancy, uremia, active infections such as viral or tuberculous, and other rare causes.

Answer B is incorrect. Aortic stenosis is represented by a harsh crescendo-decrescendo early systolic murmur heard best at the right upper sternal border with radiation to the carotids. Rheumatic heart disease can lead to calcification of the aortic valve, which leads to aortic stenosis, but for unclear reasons, this occurs much less frequently than on the mitral valve. An aortic stenosis murmur in a middle-aged woman should raise the suspicion for a calcified bicuspid aortic valve (remember the "fish mouth").

Answer D is incorrect. A systolic click heard best at the apex corresponds to mitral valve prolapse, which is a relatively common and benign finding in middle-aged women. It occurs when an abnormally thickened mitral valve leaflet displaces into the left atrium during ventricular systole. It is not related to rheumatic heart disease. It may lead to mitral regurgitation and ultimately valve surgery may be required, but typically it is followed by a cardiologist with serial exams and echocardiography.

Answer E is incorrect. An S_4, which is heard best at the apex and is associated with concentric left ventricular hypertrophy, is indicative of either chronic extensive afterload (ie, from uncontrolled hypertension) or long-standing aortic stenosis. It also can be caused by diastolic heart failure because the left ventricle is not as compliant as it should be. The exam finding is due to turbulent blood flow caused by blood filling a stiff ventricle. An S_4 is not associated with rheumatic heart disease.

33. **The correct answer is D.** This patient has Burkitt lymphoma, a lymphoma endemic to Africa. Clinically, Burkitt lymphoma often presents with "B symptoms" (fever, night sweats, weight loss), signs of tumor lysis syndrome such as oliguria, and solitary jaw masses. Histopathologically, Burkitt lymphoma typically assumes a "starry sky" appearance with sheets of lymphocytes interspersed with occasional macrophages. The cytogenetic abnormality associated with Burkitt lymphoma is a t(8;14) translocation in which the oncogene *c-myc* is placed under the expression of the immunoglobulin heavy chain enhancer. There is a strong association between Burkitt lymphoma and Epstein-Barr virus (EBV). In endemic regions, children are typically infected with EBV by the age of three years, compared with infection during adolescence in other regions. EBV, the cause of infectious mononucleosis, is spread by saliva and respiratory secretions.

Answer A is incorrect. HBV and HCV are spread by blood-borne contacts. Although these viruses are associated with hepatocellular carcinoma, there is no association between HBV or HCV and Burkitt lymphoma.

Answer B is incorrect. Hepatitis A virus (HAV) is transmitted by the fecal-oral route. There is no association between HAV and Burkitt lymphoma.

Answer C is incorrect. Arboviruses and flaviruses can be transmitted through mosquito bites. These viruses cause tropical diseases such as dengue fever and yellow fever, but not Burkitt lymphoma.

Answer E is incorrect. Viruses such as HIV, herpes simplex virus type 2, and human herpesvirus type 8 are spread by sexual contact. None of these pathogens is associated with Burkitt lymphoma.

34. **The correct answer is D.** This patient's constellation of symptoms and prior hospitalization points toward pseudomembranous colitis. *Clostridium difficile* proliferation causes the severe non-bloody diarrhea associated with pseudomembranous colitis by producing an exotoxin that kills enterocytes. Antibiotic treatments suppress the normal flora of the GI tract, allowing *C difficile* to multiply. Clindamycin was the first antibiotic associated with *C difficile* gastroenteritis and is used often to treat anaerobic infections above the diaphragm, such as aspiration pneumonia. However, many antibiotics have been implicated since then, especially cephalosporins and ampicillin. Always consider *C difficile* in patients with gastroenteritis and recent antibiotic use.

Answer A is incorrect. This describes how the Norwalk virus can cause gastroenteritis characterized by nausea, vomiting, and diarrhea that resolves spontaneously within 12-24 hours.

Answer B is incorrect. This describes the exotoxin produced by *Shigella* species, which can cause a bloody and mucus-rich diarrhea.

Answer C is incorrect. This describes the exotoxin produced by *Vibrio cholerae*, which causes a large volume of watery diarrhea devoid of RBCs or WBCs (sometimes called rice-water stool). It is not associated with prior antibiotic use.

Answer E is incorrect. This describes *Escherichia coli*, which causes the abrupt onset of profuse watery diarrhea.

35. **The correct answer is E.** The patient presents with classic signs and symptoms of pericarditis, including precordial chest pain. This pain is relieved when leaning forward and worsens with inspiration. On physical exam the patient has a pericardial friction rub, which accounts for the scratchy, leathery sound heard during both systole and diastole. Classic ECG findings include diffuse ST-segment elevation and depression of the PR segment. Pericarditis is frequently preceded by a viral upper respiratory infection. Although many viruses may cause pericarditis, coxsackie B is the most common cause of inflammation of the pericardial membrane. Coxsackievirus is a picornavirus, the smallest of the RNA viruses. They are positive, single-stranded, naked, icosahedral RNA viruses.

Answer A is incorrect. *Staphylococcus aureus* is a gram-positive, catalase-positive, and coagulase-positive bacterium. Infection with *S aureus* may lead to acute bacterial endocarditis from seeding secondary to bacteremia. The bacterium rarely causes pericarditis.

Answer B is incorrect. This describes the structure of Herpesviridae. Herpesvirus is characterized by multinucleated giant syncytial cells with intranuclear inclusion bodies. Members of this family include CMV and Epstein-Barr virus. Both cause a mononucleosis syndrome in young adults similarly characterized by fever and pharyngitis. Both cause pericarditis only rarely.

Answer C is incorrect. Reoviridae is the only double-stranded RNA virus. Members of this family include rotavirus, which is responsible for diarrhea in children, and reovirus, which causes Colorado tick fever.

Answer D is incorrect. This answer choice describes the structure of Coronaviridae. Coronavirus (CoV) is a common virus that causes a self-limited cold-like syndrome. SARS-CoV, however, has been identified as the cause of severe acute respiratory syndrome.

36. **The correct answer is B.** Guillain-Barré syndrome (GBS) is a common cause of acute peripheral neuropathy that results in progressive weakness over a period of days. Laboratory abnormalities associated with GBS include elevated gamma-globulin, decreased nerve conduction velocity indicative of demyelination, and albuminocytologic dissociation (CSF shows increased protein concentration with normal cell count in the setting of normal glucose). Although one third of patients report no history of an infection, the other two thirds will have recently experienced an acute GI or influenza-like illness prior to developing the neuropathy. The most common epidemiologic associations involve infections with *Campylobacter jejuni*, a comma-shaped, oxidase-positive, gram-negative bacterium that can be grown at 42°C. *C jejuni* causes a gastroenteritis that often presents with bloody diarrhea. Although a recent history of *C jejuni* enteritis is epidemiologically linked with GBS, the infection does not directly cause GBS. The proposed mechanism of GBS is that a preceding infection incites an immune response that cross-reacts with peripheral nerve components, leaving them susceptible to damage also.

Answer A is incorrect. *Streptococcus pneumoniae* is an α-hemolytic, encapsulated, gram-positive coccus that produces an IgA protease. Pneumococcal pneumonia can result in bacteremia, meningitis, osteomyelitis, or septic arthritis, but is not associated with the development of GBS syndrome.

Answer C is incorrect. *Pseudomonas aeruginosa* is a non-lactose-fermenting, oxidase-positive, gram-negative, aerobic bacillus that can cause otitis externa, urinary tract infection, pneumonia, and sepsis in immunocompromised hosts. It is not associated with GBS syndrome or other neurologic conditions.

Answer D is incorrect. *Clostridium botulinum* is a rod-shaped, gram-positive, spore-forming, anaerobe that produces a heat-labile toxin that inhibits acetylcholine release at the neuromuscular junction, causing flaccid paralysis. Botulism, therefore, does not lead to sensory findings, and is not associated with increased CSF protein on lumbar puncture.

Answer E is incorrect. *Treponema pallidum*, the causative agent of syphilis, is a spiral-shaped bacterium with axial filaments, visualized using dark-field microscopy. Tertiary syphilis causes sensory deficits rather than muscle weakness and is preceded by a painless chancre and maculopapular rash. Neurologic findings develop after years, not weeks, of untreated infection.

37. **The correct answer is D.** This teenager most likely has osteomyelitis secondary to a contiguous focus of infection, such as bites, puncture wounds, and open fractures. Most of these cases are caused by *Staphylococcus aureus*, a gram-positive, coagulase-positive coccus that occurs in clusters. This organism expresses receptors for bone matrix components, such as collagen, which help it to attach to and infect bone. When compared to hematogenous osteomyelitis, continguous-focus infections are more likely to also include gram-negative and anaerobic bacteria.

Answer A is incorrect. Acid-fast bacilli such as *Mycobacterium tuberculosis* are found in patients with TB. Infection of the bone by TB is known as Pott disease, but its usual presentation is vertebral osteomyelitis.

Answer B is incorrect. *Streptococcus* species are catalase-negative, gram-positive cocci. Group A streptococci can cause cellulitis, necrotizing fasciitis, and streptococcal toxic shock syndrome. Group B streptococci are a common cause of neonatal bacterial meningitis. Group D streptococci (*Enterococcus*) are a frequent cause of urinary tract infections and subacute bacterial endocarditis.

Answer C is incorrect. *Staphylococcus epidermidis* is a coagulase-negative, gram-positive coccus that grows in clusters. It is common skin flora. It can be a cause of osteomyelitis, but this is more common after implantation with orthopedic appliances.

Answer E is incorrect. *Salmonella* species are oxidase-negative, gram-negative bacilli. *Salmonella* osteomyelitis is often associated with patients who have sickle cell disease.

38. **The correct answer is C.** The patient is now in the secondary stage of a syphilis infection, characterized by wart-like lesions known as condylomata lata, generalized rash, and systemic symptoms such as lymphadenopathy, weight loss, and fever. The fluorescent treponemal antibody absorption (FTA-ABS) test, the Venereal Disease Research Laboratory (VDRL) test, and the rapid plasma reagin test approach 100% sensitivity for detecting syphilis.

Answer A is incorrect. Thayer-Martin agar is used to culture *Neisseria gonorrhoeae*.

Answer B is incorrect. Tzanck preparation using Giemsa stain reveals multinucleated giant cells indicative of herpes simplex virus (HSV) or vesicular stomatitis virus infection. Although HSV can cause genital lesions, they are usually painful and come in clusters.

Answer D is incorrect. The Weil-Felix reaction assay tests for antirickettsial antibodies. This test would be positive if the patient were infected with *Rickettsia rickettsii* (Rocky Mountain spotted fever). Rocky Mountain spotted fever can also present with a rash on the palms and soles but would not present with genital lesions.

Answer E is incorrect. Ziehl-Neelsen stain is used to stain acid-fast mycobacteria such as *Mycobacterium tuberculosis*.

39. **The correct answer is B.** The first step in answering this question is to recognize that Ziehl-Neelsen stain is what is used for the acid-fast test. The presence of acid-fast rods in the blood indicates that this man has a disseminated mycobacterial infection. In order of prevalence, the three main candidate organisms in patients with HIV are: (1) *M avium-intracellulare* (MAC), (2) *Mycobacterium tuberculosis*, and (3) *Mycobacterium kansasii*. Disseminated MAC infection can present with generalized symptoms (such as fatigue, night sweats, fever, and weight loss) as well as organ-specific symptoms, and occurs when the patient's CD4+ cell count has dropped to <50/mm^3. It can include gut pain (from mycobacterial enteritis), pulmonary symptoms, or adenopathy. Although *M tuberculosis* infection is frequently seen in HIV-infected patients, it is rare to recover it from blood cultures.

    Answer A is incorrect. *Actinomyces israelii* is a bacterial pathogen with a fungal-like morphology. Unlike *Nocardia*, it is not acid-fast.

    Answer C is incorrect. *Mycobacterium marinum* is a species native to fresh-water and salt-water environments. It is a rare cause of cutaneous wound infection in anglers, swimmers, and aquarium owners. It is not commonly associated with disseminated infection in immunocompromised patients.

    Answer D is incorrect. *M tuberculosis* could be a causative agent for the symptoms found in this patient, except that his CD4+ count is <50/mm^3, which makes infection with *M avium-intracellulare* most likely.

    Answer E is incorrect. *Nocardia* is eliminated as the correct answer by the given morphology of the observed bacteria. Although *Nocardia* can stain weakly acid-fast, they demonstrate a branching filamentous morphology that resembles fungal hyphae.

40. **The correct answer is D.** This infant is showing signs of neonatal sepsis and meningitis. The most common cause of neonatal sepsis and meningitis is group B *Streptococcus* (GBS), which frequently colonizes the genitourinary tract of women and can be passed to the infant during delivery. Penicillin G would have provided adequate coverage for the mother's likely colonization with GBS.

    Answer A is incorrect. Fluconazole, an antifungal agent that interferes with fungal ergosterol synthesis, would not have been an appropriate antibiotic for GBS prophylaxis. Fluconazole has good coverage against fungal infections.

    Answer B is incorrect. Metronidazole, a disruptor of nucleic acid structure, would not have been an appropriate antibiotic for GBS prophylaxis. Metronidazole has good activity against protozoans and anaerobic organisms.

    Answer C is incorrect. Moxifloxacin, a DNA gyrase inhibitor, would not have been an appropriate antibiotic for GBS prophylaxis. Fluoroquinolones have good coverage against gram-negative and select gram-positive organisms, and are often used to treat urinary tract infections and community-acquired pneumonia. Additionally, fluoroquinolones are a class C substance, as they have the potential to cause teratogenic or embryocidal effects. Giving fluoroquinolones during pregnancy is not recommended unless the benefits justify the potential risks to the fetus.

    Answer E is incorrect. Vancomycin, a cell wall synthesis inhibitor, would not have been an appropriate antibiotic for GBS prophylaxis in this case. While vancomycin has good coverage against GBS, its use is reserved for cases of known resistance. Vancomycin could have been used if the mother were known to harbor GBS that was resistant to other first-line antibiotics, or had an allergy that prevented the use of other agents.

CHAPTER 5

Immunology

QUESTIONS

1. A 48-year-man with chronic renal failure underwent a cadaveric renal transplant. The operation was a success, and the transplanted kidney started producing urine "on the operating table." However, one week later, the patient's creatinine level begins to rise and his urine output drops. He does not experience dysuria, and urinalysis shows no bacteria or crystals. A biopsy taken from the transplanted kidney shows a cellular infiltrate. Which of the following would most likely be found on the surface of the cells responsible for this patient's current condition?

   (A) CD20
   (B) CD27
   (C) CD34
   (D) CD4
   (E) CD8

2. An infant boy experiences multiple bacterial, viral, and fungal infections during his first year of life. He has also been suffering diarrhea since birth. Tests are performed to determine the likely cause of his symptoms. Serum calcium levels are normal, and the patient's white blood cells change nitroblue tetrazolium from clear to bright blue; however, his B- and T-lymphocyte counts are very low. What is a possible mechanism accounting for his symptoms?

   (A) Defective interleukin-2 receptors
   (B) Failure of the third and fourth pharyngeal pouches to descend
   (C) Inability of helper T lymphocytes to switch classes
   (D) Lack of NADPH oxidase activity
   (E) X-linked tyrosine kinase defect

3. A 45-year-old woman presents to her family physician with complaints of two months of joint stiffness and pain that is worst in the morning. Physical examination reveals swelling of the left metacarpophalangeal joints and of the wrists bilaterally. She is diagnosed with a condition associated with the release of proinflammatory cytokines. Which of the following opposes the action of cytokines?

   (A) Interferon-γ
   (B) Interleukin-7
   (C) Transforming growth factor-β
   (D) Tumor necrosis factor-α
   (E) Tumor necrosis factor-β

4. The image depicts a cell that is activated by bacterial products, upregulates costimulatory molecules, and migrates to the draining lymph node. Which of the following types of cells is shown in this image, and of which type of immune cell is it a specialized form?

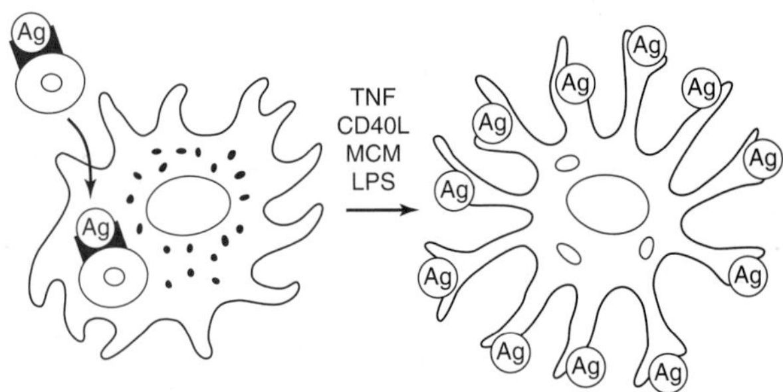

Reproduced, with permission, from USMLERx.com.

   (A) Kupffer cell, dendritic cell
   (B) Kupffer cell, macrophage
   (C) Langerhans cell, dendritic cell
   (D) Langerhans cell, macrophage
   (E) Microglia, dendritic cell

5. To assess the risk of erythroblastosis fetalis during the future pregnancy of an Rh-negative woman, a clinician sends a sample of serum for detection of anti-Rh blood group antibodies. The laboratory performs an indirect Coombs test by mixing the patient's serum with Rh-positive RBCs and then adding an anti-IgG antibody. In doing so, the laboratory technician observes agglutination of the RBCs. After receiving this test result, the clinician would be correct to conclude which of the following?

(A) The laboratory performed the test incorrectly; it should have mixed the patient's serum with Rh-negative rather than Rh-positive RBCs
(B) The patient has had previous pregnancies and all of her children are Rh-negative
(C) The patient is currently pregnant with an Rh-positive fetus
(D) The presence of anti-Rh antibodies in the patient's serum suggests that she has been pregnant with an Rh-positive fetus
(E) The results of the test cannot be used to determine the Rh status of a current fetus; the results only assess the presence of antibodies in the mother. To determine fetal Rh status, direct typing of fetal blood must be done.

6. A 68-year-old woman has been hospitalized for three days after an exacerbation of emphysema. Her clinical course progresses well until the fourth hospital day, when she develops shortness of breath, fatigue, and cough productive of yellow sputum. Her oxygen saturation drops by 10%, and she is started on vancomycin and gentamicin via rapid infusion. Thirty minutes after the initiation of antibiotics, the patient develops erythema of the face and neck, itchiness, and hypotension. The patient has no known drug allergies and has not been treated with vancomycin prior to this hospitalization. Which of the following is the mechanism of this reaction?

(A) Binding of antibody-complement to target cells
(B) Cross-linking of IgE by Fc receptors on mast cells
(C) Deposition of antibody-drug immune complexes
(D) Release of cytokines by activated T lymphocytes
(E) Release of histamine by mast cells

7. A 1-year-old child whose parents just emigrated from Mexico presents to the emergency room with stridor. The child is in obvious distress and is drooling. Examination of the pharynx reveals a cherry-red mass at the base of the tongue. The vaccine that could have prevented this child's illness contains two parts: purified bacterial capsule and mutant diphtheria toxoid. Which of the following characteristics of the causative organism makes necessary the addition of the diphtheria toxoid to the vaccine?

(A) Attachment pili
(B) Gram-negative rod
(C) IgA protease
(D) Polyribitol-ribose phosphate capsule
(E) Protein A

8. A type B blood group, Rh-positive recipient mistakenly receives a kidney from a type A blood group, Rh-negative donor. Which of the following best describes the mechanism of transplant rejection that is most likely to ensue in this recipient?

(A) Pre-formed recipient antibodies
(B) Macrophages
(C) Pre-formed donor antibodies
(D) Donor T lymphocytes
(E) Recipient T lymphocytes

9. A 3-year-old boy is admitted to the hospital with aspergillosis. He has had multiple admissions for viral and fungal infections previously. His serum calcium level is 7.8 mg/dL. Biopsy of one of this patient's lymph nodes would most likely reveal which of the following abnormalities?

(A) Decreased number of follicles
(B) Hypocellular paracortex
(C) Hypocellular medullary sinuses
(D) Enlarged follicles throughout the entire lymph node
(E) Increased number of the medullary cords

10. A 60-year-old postmenopausal woman presents with fatigue, mild jaundice, and tingling in the lower extremities. Laboratory studies show elevated serum levels of homocysteine and methylmalonic acid, and mild thrombocytopenia. A peripheral blood smear supports the diagnosis. In which of the following disorders would a peripheral blood smear be similar to the one seen in this case?

(A) Acute blood loss
(B) Anemia of chronic disease
(C) Iron deficiency anemia
(D) Pernicious anemia
(E) Pyridoxine deficiency

11. The image below depicts a series of steps in an immunologic activation pathway. This pathway is most important for which activity of the immune system?

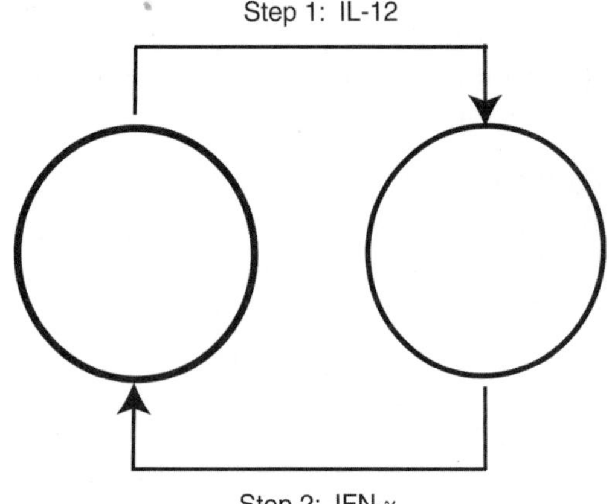

Reproduced, with permission, from USMLERx.com.

(A) Antigen presentation and destruction of intracellular pathogens
(B) Defense against parasites by eosinophils
(C) Immediate allergic hypersensitivity reaction
(D) Neutrophil chemotaxis

12. A 35-year-old woman presents to the clinician with symptoms suggestive of an autoimmune etiology. A biopsy is sent for immunofluorescent staining, and the results indicate the presence of anticentromere antibodies. Which of the following symptoms is this patient most likely experiencing?

(A) Episodic palpitations, sweating, and headaches with no apparent trigger
(B) Intermittent ischemia of fingers and toes associated with pallor and pain
(C) Joint pain, dry eyes and mouth
(D) Urethritis
(E) Widespread tightening of the skin

13. A 10-month-old boy is brought to the pediatrician by his parents because of fever, cough, and difficulty breathing. A profile of the patient's immunoglobulin isotypes shows low IgA, low IgG, and markedly elevated IgM levels. The number of T and B lymphocytes is normal. Which of the following is the most likely etiology of the increased level of IgM in this patient?

(A) A defect in DNA repair enzymes
(B) A defect in LFA-1 adhesion proteins on phagocytes
(C) A defect in the CD40 ligand on CD4 T helper cells
(D) Failure of interferon-γ production
(E) Failure of the thymus and parathyroid glands to develop

14. A 40-year-old man presents to his physician with numbness and tingling on the dorsal surface of his right hand and forearm, and raised "varicose veins" that are firm to the touch along the same distribution. He also complains of weight loss. His serum creatinine level is 2.0 mg/dL. He has no previous medical history of significance. An immune complex disease is suspected, and assays for autoantibodies inside neutrophils are conducted. What diseases are associated with the identification of anti-myeloperoxidase and anti-proteinase-3 antibodies, respectively?

(A) Kawasaki disease, Buerger disease
(B) Microscopic polyangiitis, Wegener granulomatosis
(C) Polyarteritis nodosa, Buerger disease
(D) Takayasu arteritis, Wegener granulomatosis

(E) Takayasu arteritis, Buerger disease
(F) Temporal arteritis, Wegener granulomatosis

15. A 24-year-old woman presents with a four-month history of fever, night sweats, and weight loss. X-ray of the chest reveals enlarged mediastinal lymph nodes. The biopsy of one such lymph node is shown in the image. From which of the following cell types is the cell with the bilobed nucleus derived?

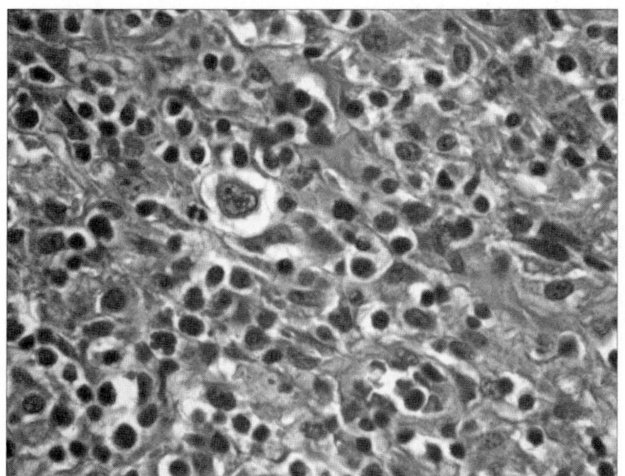

Reproduced, with permission, from USMLERx.com.

(A) B lymphocyte
(B) Fibroblast
(C) Macrophage
(D) Neutrophil
(E) T lymphocyte

16. Patients who share similar clinical symptoms and disease pathology may nevertheless present differently based on age at disease onset. How does the presentation of the disease evident in the image differ between juvenile and adult-onset disease?

(A) Juvenile rheumatoid arthritis is simply the presence of rheumatoid arthritis that begins before the age of 21 years
(B) Patients with juvenile rheumatoid arthritis are less likely to have systemic symptoms, but the likelihood of high levels of serum rheumatoid factor is the same
(C) Patients with juvenile rheumatoid arthritis are more likely to have large-joint involvement, but the likelihood of concurrent systemic symptoms is the same
(D) Patients with juvenile rheumatoid arthritis are more likely to have systemic symptoms and high levels of serum rheumatoid factor
(E) Patients with juvenile rheumatoid arthritis are more likely to have systemic symptoms and large-joint involvement

17. A 6-month old boy is noted at his well-child visit to have very poor growth and weight gain since his last visit. His mother states that he was hospitalized for pneumococcal pneumonia, and has had several bad colds with purulent nasal discharge since he was born. His physician suspects an immunodeficiency, and laboratory results indeed reveal deficiency of a complement protein. Which of the following antibodies functions in the same manner as the missing complement protein in this child?

(A) IgA
(B) IgD
(C) IgE
(D) IgG
(E) IgM

18. A 29-year-old intravenous drug user has suffered from recurrent pneumonias, fungal infections in the axillae, and a recent ear infection. He now presents with a cough and painful swallowing. Physical examination reveals a patchy, white oral lesion. Cells with which of the following markers are most likely to be deficient in this patient?

(A) CD4
(B) CD8
(C) CD20
(D) CD40
(E) CD56

19. A 2-year-old girl with a lifelong history of malabsorptive and foul-smelling diarrhea, weakness, and general failure to thrive has just undergone a small intestine biopsy (see image). Her parents believe her problems began at 6 months of age, when she started eating solid foods, but have significantly worsened over the past few months. The only recent change in her diet is that she eats a bowl of cereal every morning with her parents before they go to work. She tried a dairy-free diet a month ago, but it did not improve her symptoms. Which of the following is the most likely diagnosis?

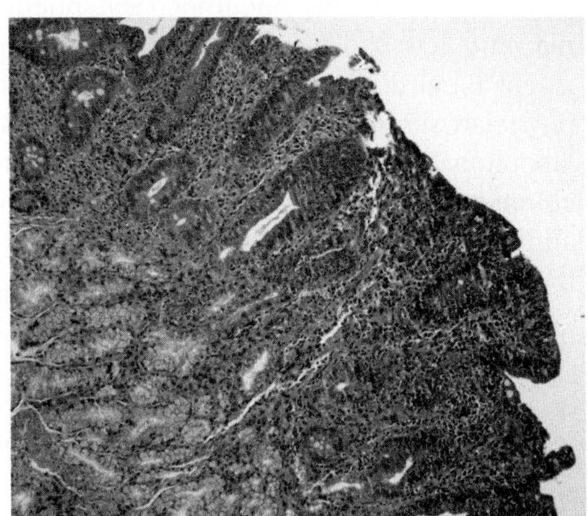

Reproduced, with permission, from USMLERx.com.

(A) Abetalipoproteinemia
(B) Celiac sprue
(C) Lactase deficiency
(D) Viral enteritis
(E) Whipple disease

20. A pediatrician becomes concerned after learning about the family and the medical history of an 18-month-old child who is currently suffering from pneumonia, with a presumed diagnosis of *Streptococcus pneumoniae* infection. Over the past year, the patient has suffered from erysipelas as well as a previous bout of pneumococcal pneumonia; both were treated successfully with antibiotics. The patient's mother says that her son's maternal uncle also suffered from repeated bacterial infections and was successfully treated with antibiotics. On physical examination, it appears that the patient does not have tonsils. His mother denies a previous tonsillectomy. Analysis of the boy's serum would most likely yield which of the following results?

(A) $< 200/mm^3$ CD4 T lymphocytes
(B) Absence of T lymphocytes
(C) IgA, IgG, and IgM levels normal
(D) IgG and IgM levels markedly decreased, no IgA
(E) IgG and IgM levels normal, IgA markedly decreased

21. A 26-year-old woman presents to the clinic with joint pain in her hands and wrists, difficulty breathing, and redness over her cheeks and nose. She also notes that her fingertips change color from white to blue to red when she is cold. Which of the following describes the renal pathology commonly associated with this patient's condition?

(A) Histopathology reveals glomerulonephritis with subendothelial immune deposits evident on immunofluorescence electron microscopy
(B) It has a "railroad track" or "tram track" appearance on light microscopy
(C) It is a homogeneous renal disease
(D) It is associated with elevated serum complement levels
(E) It is immune mediated by anti-mitochondrial antibodies

22. A clinician is concerned that an Rh-negative mother may be pregnant with an Rh-positive fetus. The potential pathology that the clinician is concerned about is classified as which of the following immune reactions?

(A) Graft-versus-host disease
(B) Type I hypersensitivity
(C) Type II hypersensitivity
(D) Type III hypersensitivity
(E) Type IV hypersensitivity

23. A 14-year-old boy presents to the physician with recurrent pyogenic infections. Physical examination shows that the boy has pruritic papulovesicular dermatitis. Laboratory tests show low serum IgM level and a normal serum

IgG level. Which of the following laboratory abnormalities is most likely to also be present?

(A) Hypocalcemia
(B) Low IgA level
(C) Low IgE level
(D) Lymphopenia
(E) Thrombocytopenia

24. A 30-year-old woman presents to the emergency department with a right-sided facial droop and bilateral swelling on the face near the angles of the mandible. She reports that these signs occurred suddenly while she was at home. On further questioning she says that for the past few weeks she has been feeling short of breath and tired, and has had a dry cough. She denies any recent exposure to wooded areas. Her temperature is 38.4°C (101.2°F), heart rate is 93/min, blood pressure is 110/85 mm Hg, respiratory rate is 22/min, and oxygen saturation is 93% on room air. Physical examination reveals red, tearing eyes; smooth, nontender bulging of both cheeks; a right-sided drooping of the mouth; cervical nodes; and bilateral dry râles. Results of a purified protein derivative test are negative. X-ray of the chest is shown in the image. What process is most likely to be causing this patient's symptoms?

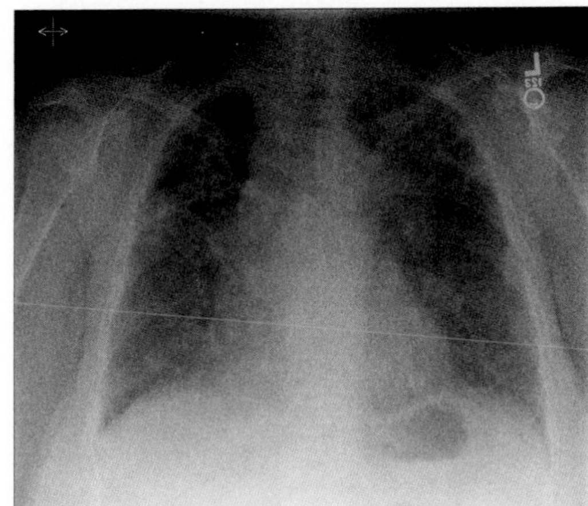

Reproduced, with permission, from USMLERx.com.

(A) Lyme disease
(B) Pneumonia
(C) Sarcoidosis
(D) Systemic lupus erythematosus
(E) Tuberculosis

25. A 58-year-old man presents to his physician because of fatigue, edema, and worsening kidney function. After extensive laboratory work-up, his physician decides to perform a kidney biopsy. The pathologist notes numerous green-colored, proteinaceous deposits when he uses polarized light microscopy to view the sample. Which of the following is most likely abnormal in this patient?

(A) C2
(B) CD8
(C) Fab fragment
(D) Ig light chain
(E) Major histocompatibility complex II

26. A 7-year-old boy is brought to the physician by his parents because of recurrent sinus infections. The parents state that the boy also has had multiple lung infections and intermittent diarrheal infections since birth. Which of the following results would most likely be found on further testing?

(A) A high IgE level
(B) A low IgA level
(C) A low IgM level, with increased IgA
(D) A negative nitroblue tetrazolium dye test
(E) A normal immunoglobulin level for all isotypes

27. A patient is administered a tuberculin test. Which of the following types of hypersensitivity reaction is being tested, and which cells would be expected to mediate a positive test result?

(A) Type I hypersensitivity, mast cells
(B) Type II hypersensitivity, cytotoxic T lymphocytes
(C) Type IV hypersensitivity, mast cells
(D) Type IV hypersensitivity, T-helper 1 cells
(E) Type IV hypersensitivity, T-helper 2 cells

28. A 24-year-old, previously healthy woman presents to the outpatient clinic with a two-week history of drooping eyelids and difficulty rising from a chair. Stimulation with a reversible acetylcholinesterase inhibitor leads to the resolution of her symptoms. Which of the following is most responsible for the three-dimensional structure of the key mediator in this woman's condition?

(A) Disulfide bonds
(B) Hydrogen bonds
(C) Ionic bonds
(D) Triple covalent bonds
(E) Van der Waals forces

29. A 3-year-old boy is brought to his pediatrician because of worsening cough and rhinorrhea. His parents state that he has had multiple similar episodes over the past year with two brief hospitalizations for pneumonia. Physical examination of the skin reveals the lesion seen in the image. Laboratory tests show very low serum levels of IgA. Which of the following is most likely to also be seen in this child?

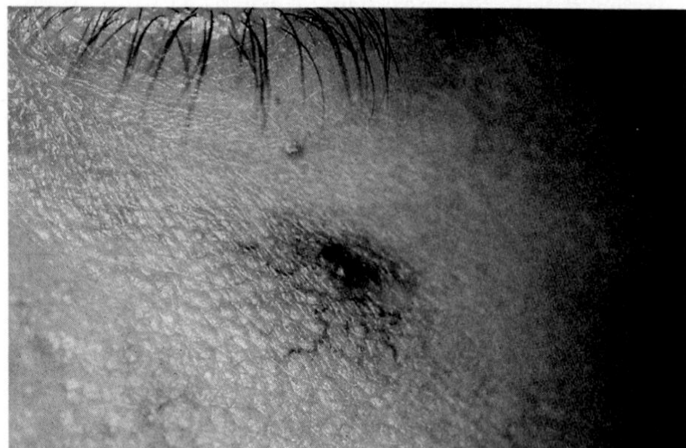

Reproduced, with permission, from Wolff K, et al, *Fitzpatrick's Color Atlas & Synopsis of Clinical Dermatology*, 6th edition. New York: McGraw-Hill, 2009.

(A) A noninflamed skin abscess
(B) A repaired cleft palate
(C) Frequent falls
(D) Skin granulomas
(E) Visual hallucinations

30. A 50-year-old man comes to the physician with hemoptysis and diffuse joint pain. He states that both his father and cousin had similar symptoms and were diagnosed with microscopic polyangiitis, a disease affecting medium- to small-sized arteries that is believed to have an autoimmune component to its pathogenesis. Antibody levels were measured to confirm the diagnosis. What other disease is most closely correlated with the same type of autoantibodies as present in this patient?

(A) Churg-Strauss syndrome
(B) CREST variant of scleroderma
(C) Sjögren syndrome
(D) Systemic lupus erythematosus
(E) Wegener granulomatosis

ANSWERS

1. **The correct answer is E.** This patient suffers from rejection of his recently transplanted organ. There are three types of rejection: hyperacute, acute, and chronic. A hyperacute rejection is mediated by pre-formed antibodies to the transplanted organ. In most cases, it can be observed while still in the operating theater. Acute rejection can occur at any time but is most likely in the first three months after transplantation. It is due to human leukocyte antigen discrepancies between host and graft, and is more common in highly vascular organs such as the liver or kidney. Finally, chronic rejection is a slow process that leads to fibrosis of the transplanted tissue due to increased fibroblast activity. This patient experienced acute rejection, which is mediated by cytotoxic T cells (CD8).

   Answer A is incorrect. CD20 is a B-cell marker. Because they are a precursor to plasma cells, they would only be indirectly involved in hyperacute rejection.

   Answer B is incorrect. CD27 is a marker of plasma cells. Plasma cells are responsible for antibody production and therefore would be the culprit in hyperacute rejections.

   Answer C is incorrect. CD34 is a fibrocyte marker. Fibrocytes leave the bloodstream and differentiate into fibroblasts in the transplanted organ. They are the cell type that leads to chronic rejection of the graft.

   Answer D is incorrect. CD4 is the marker of T-helper cells. They do not attack pathogens or tissues and are not implicated in the pathology of acute rejection and negative selection.

2. **The correct answer is A.** Severe combined immunodeficiency can be caused by multiple factors: failure to synthesize major histocompatibility complex II antigens, defective interleukin-2 receptors, or adenosine deaminase deficiency. This defect in early stem cell differentiation results in a lack of T and B lymphocytes. Without T and B lymphocytes, patients are at significantly increased risk of bacterial, viral, and fungal infections. Treatment includes bone marrow transplantation.

   Answer B is incorrect. Failure of the third and fourth pharyngeal pouches to descend is known as DiGeorge syndrome, and results in no thymus or parathyroid glands. Chromosome 22q11 deletions are associated with DiGeorge syndrome. Tetany from hypocalcemia and viral and fungal infections are common due to the lack of T lymphocytes, while normal B lymphocytes are present.

   Answer C is incorrect. A CD40 ligand defect causes hyper-IgM syndrome, because the CD4 T-helper cells are unable to switch classes from IgM. Although these patients present with multiple infections such as pneumonia, sinusitis, infectious diarrhea, and central nervous system (CNS) infections, the most common laboratory finding is neutropenia, not low levels of lymphocytes.

   Answer D is incorrect. The lack of reduced NADPH oxidase activity results in chronic granulomatous disease. *Staphylococcus aureus*, *Escherichia coli*, and *Aspergillus* are common pathogens. The nitroblue tetrazolium dye reduction test shows no activity in these patients. Because the question stem says that the nitroblue tetrazolium dye test turned blue, this patient must have normal NADPH oxidase activity, and thus cannot have chronic granulomatous disease.

   Answer E is incorrect. An X-linked tyrosine kinase defect causes Bruton agammaglobulinemia, resulting in decreased levels of all immunoglobulin molecules. Infections begin to occur after the maternal IgG antibodies decline, typically after six months of life.

3. **The correct answer is C.** This patient has signs and symptoms of rheumatoid arthritis, a disorder of immune dysregulation. Many parallel and sequential events occur within the synovium to cause joint destruction, including activation of T lymphocytes and release of many proinflammatory cytokines such as

interleukin (IL) 1. Transforming growth factor-β plays a role in dampening the immune response, and in the case of rheumatoid arthritis works as a reparative agent by inhibiting T lymphocyte activation and proliferation, inhibiting biosynthesis of metalloproteinases, protecting cartilage from degradation by IL-1, and inhibiting tumor necrosis factor secretion by macrophages.

Answer A is incorrect. Interferon-γ is secreted by helper T lymphocytes and helps stimulate macrophages.

Answer B is incorrect. IL-7 is secreted by macrophages and is one of the main cytokines involved in mounting an acute phase response. IL-7 has been shown to stimulate bone erosion in rheumatoid arthritis.

Answer D is incorrect. Tumor necrosis factor-α is one of the main cytokines involved in mounting an acute-phase response; it is secreted by macrophages.

Answer E is incorrect. Tumor necrosis factor-β has functions similar to tumor necrosis factor-α in that it helps mount an acute-phase response. However, it is secreted by activated T lymphocytes instead of macrophages.

4. **The correct answer is C.** Dendritic cells arise from both myeloid and lymphoid bone marrow precursors and then establish sites of residence within the peripheral tissues. Immature dendritic cells located within the epidermis are named Langerhans cells, and they are highly phagocytic. The exact function of Birbeck granules is unknown, but they are present only with Langerhans cells. Upon antigen encounter, Langerhans cells upregulate costimulatory molecules (such as major histocompatibility complex class II) and then migrate to the draining lymph node, where they play an integral part in the activation of T lymphocytes and the subsequent induction of an adaptive immune response.

   Answer A is incorrect. Kupffer cells are tissue-resident macrophages within the liver.

   Answer B is incorrect. Kupffer cells are tissue-resident macrophages; the image depicts a Langerhans cell.

   Answer D is incorrect. Langerhans cells are specialized, tissue-resident dendritic cells, not macrophages.

   Answer E is incorrect. Microglia are tissue-resident macrophages within the CNS.

5. **The correct answer is D.** When an Rh-negative mother gives birth to an Rh-positive fetus, fetal RBCs may enter the mother's circulation, and the body may recognize the Rh antigen as foreign and produce antibodies against it. As maternal IgG freely crosses the placenta, any subsequent Rh-positive fetus is at risk for hemolytic disease. Thus, the indirect Coombs test is an important laboratory tool to monitor for Rh incompatibilities that may complicate fetal health. The test result given in this question indicates that the patient possesses anti-Rh antibodies in her serum. Therefore, it would be logical for the clinician to suspect previous pregnancy with an Rh-positive fetus.

   Answer A is incorrect. The laboratory protocol described in the question stem is correct. Rh-positive RBCs must be added because the test is assaying for the presence anti-Rh antibodies, which will bind the Rh antigen on the RBCs.

   Answer B is incorrect. The presence of anti-Rh antibodies within the patient's serum suggests that she has been exposed to the blood of at least one Rh-positive fetus.

   Answer C is incorrect. The results of the test cannot be used to determine the Rh status of a current fetus; only direct typing of fetal blood can determine its Rh status.

   Answer E is incorrect. The test yielded a positive result. Agglutination occurs when the anti-IgG antibody binds to the anti-Rh antibodies that are already bound to the Rh-positive RBCs.

6. **The correct answer is E.** Vancomycin can cause two types of hypersensitivity reactions: **anaphylaxis,** which is a type I hypersensitivity reaction, and the **"red man" syndrome**

(RMS), which is an anaphylactic reaction. This patient most likely has RMS due to rapid infusion of vancomycin. Although her symptoms also may be consistent with anaphylaxis, the patient has never been exposed to vancomycin; therefore, she would not have preformed IgE antibodies against the drug. By contrast, a vancomycin-induced anaphylactic reaction involves histamine release from mast cells and basophils **without** binding of preformed IgE antibodies to Fc receptors. RMS can be prevented by slow infusion of vancomycin, which is preferable to discontinuing the drug. Another method of prevention is pretreatment with antihistamine.

Answer A is incorrect. Type II hypersensitivity reactions are characterized by IgM or IgG molecules binding to an antigen on a cell, which leads to destruction of the cell via activation of the complement cascade. Examples include autoimmune hemolytic anemia, Goodpasture syndrome, rheumatic fever, and Graves disease.

Answer B is incorrect. Type I hypersensitivity reactions are mediated by pre-formed IgE antibodies that bind a particular antigen to which the patient has already been exposed. Binding of the antigen-IgE complexes to Fc receptors on mast cells results in degranulation and release of vasoactive substances such as histamine. The reaction occurs rapidly after antigen exposure. Examples include anaphylaxis, asthma, hives, wheals, and flare.

Answer C is incorrect. Type III hypersensitivity reactions involve antibodies binding to antigen in plasma, leading to antibody-antigen immune complexes. Examples include polyarteritis nodosa, immune complex glomerulonephritis, lupus, rheumatoid arthritis, serum sickness, and the Arthus reaction (local complex deposition).

Answer D is incorrect. Type IV hypersensitivity reactions involve sensitized T lymphocytes that encounter the antigen and release lymphokines. Examples include a tuberculosis (TB) skin test, transplant rejection, and contact dermatitis (poison oak, poison ivy).

7. **The correct answer is D.** This child is suffering from acute epiglottitis, caused by *Haemophilus influenzae* type B (HiB). The incidence of this illness has decreased drastically in recent years because of immunization efforts. The HiB vaccine consists of two parts: the bacterial capsule antigen and diphtheria toxoid protein. Because the bacterial capsule is a polysaccharide, it alone will not generate a sufficient immune response. Therefore, a protein (the toxoid) is added to the vaccine in order to generate an antibody response.

   Answer A is incorrect. Whereas attachment pili are an important virulence factor of *H influenzae*, they are not the reason why the vaccine must contain a toxoid protein.

   Answer B is incorrect. Whereas *H influenzae* is a gram-negative rod, its Gram stain characteristics do not play a role in the body's ability to generate antibodies against it.

   Answer C is incorrect. IgA protease is an important virulence factor in *H influenzae*. It functions to cleave IgA, which allows the bacteria to colonize the mucosa. It does not, however, play a role in vaccination.

   Answer E is incorrect. *H influenzae* does not generate protein A. This is a virulence factor found in *Staphylococcus aureus* that binds the Fc portion of IgG and thus helps prevent opsonization.

8. **The correct answer is A.** This clinical scenario would result in hyperacute rejection (within minutes of transplantation; clinical presentation within minutes to hours) mediated by pre-formed anti-donor antibodies in the recipient. The recipient would possess anti-type A antibodies, which react to the A antigen present not only on RBCs but on most other cell types. Hyperacute rejection occurs almost immediately, as the anti-donor antibodies bind directly to vascular endothelial cells, initiating complement and clotting cascades and resulting in hemorrhage and necrosis of the transplanted kidney. It should be noted that it is not only ABO blood group mismatches but any anti-donor antibodies possessed by the recipient that can lead to hyperacute rejection; thus,

it is important to carefully cross-match donor and recipient.

Answer B is incorrect. Macrophages provide a secondary immune response in this situation but are not initially involved in acute or hyperacute reactions.

Answer C is incorrect. Hyperacute rejection is typically mediated by pre-formed anti-donor antibodies that are possessed by the recipient.

Answer D is incorrect. Graft-versus-host disease (GVHD) is a serious adverse effect of bone marrow transplantation mediated by donor-derived T lymphocytes. Acute GVHD usually occurs within the first three months after an allogeneic bone marrow transplantation, whereas chronic GVHD usually develops after the third month post-transplant.

Answer E is incorrect. Acute rejection is cell-mediated and occurs within weeks after transplantation of an organ that is major histocompatibility (MHC)-mismatched; rejection is the result of cytotoxic T lymphocytes reacting to foreign MHC molecules. In this scenario, hyperacute rejection would be expected to occur first (within the first few hours after transplant).

9. **The correct answer is B.** This patient's recurrent viral and fungal infections and hypocalcemia are consistent with DiGeorge syndrome. This condition is caused by the failure of development of the third and fourth pharyngeal pouches, and thus the thymus and parathyroid glands. The recurrent viral and fungal infections are caused by a T-lymphocyte deficiency. In lymph nodes, T lymphocytes are found in the paracortical region, thus this region is often underdeveloped in patients with DiGeorge syndrome.

   Answer A is incorrect. Follicles are areas of mostly B-lymphocyte aggregation, and are not usually affected in DiGeorge syndrome.

   Answer C is incorrect. The medullary sinuses contain macrophages and communicate with lymphatics.

   Answer D is incorrect. This pattern is characteristic of follicular lymphoma, not DiGeorge syndrome.

   Answer E is incorrect. The medullary cords contain lymphocytes and plasma cells, and are not usually affected in DiGeorge syndrome.

10. **The correct answer is D.** The smear would have a hypersegmented neutrophil, classically associated with vitamin B_{12} deficiency or folate deficiency. In this patient's case, symptoms and laboratory findings suggest a deficiency in vitamin B_{12}, most likely resulting in pernicious anemia, given the patient's age. Autoimmune gastritis/pernicious anemia is associated with two forms of autoantibodies: (1) antibodies directed against the transmembrane proton pumps of parietal cells (the cells that secrete gastric acid and intrinsic factor [IF]) and (2) antibodies directed against IF itself. Parietal cell autoantibodies lead to their destruction, thereby decreasing IF and acid production (which then hinders vitamin B_{12} release from food). IF autoantibodies, on the other hand, prevent either the binding of vitamin B_{12} to IF, or the binding of the vitamin B_{12}-IF complex to its receptor in the distal ileum. Symptoms of vitamin B_{12} deficiency include fatigue, pallor, mild to moderated jaundice, glossitis (a painful, beefy tongue), and neuropathies (particularly of the lower extremities due to atrophy of the posterior and lateral columns in the spinal cord). Serum levels of homocysteine and methylmalonic acid can be elevated, and a complete blood cell count can show thrombocytopenia. Vitamin B_{12} deficiency also causes a megaloblastic anemia with hypersegmented neutrophils on peripheral blood smear. Folate deficiency also results in a similar megaloblastic anemia, although is not accompanied by neurologic symptoms.

    Answer A is incorrect. Acute blood loss would result in a normocytic normochromic anemia. However, this patient shows signs of vitamin B_{12} deficiency, which would result in a macrocytic anemia with polysegmented neutrophils on peripheral blood smear.

Answer B is incorrect. Anemia of chronic disease results in a microcytic, hypochromic anemia (late manifestation) on peripheral blood smear with decreased serum iron levels and decreased total iron-binding capacity. This patient shows signs of vitamin B_{12} deficiency, which would result in a macrocytic anemia with polysegmented neutrophils.

Answer C is incorrect. Iron deficiency anemia can result in hypersegmented neutrophils but also results in a microcytic, hypochromic anemia (late manifestation) on peripheral blood smear with decreased serum iron and increased total iron-binding capacity. This patient shows signs of vitamin B_{12} deficiency, which would result in a macrocytic anemia with polysegmented neutrophils.

Answer E is incorrect. Pyridoxine deficiency (vitamin B_6), often caused by isoniazid therapy, results in an acquired sideroblastic anemia (often macrocytic, anisocytosis). However, this patient shows signs of vitamin B_{12} deficiency, which would result in a macrocytic anemia with polysegmented neutrophils on peripheral blood smear.

11. **The correct answer is A.** The cell on the left is a macrophage and the cell on the right is a helper T cell. The image depicts a macrophage secreting interleukin-12 (IL-12), which causes the naïve helper T cell to differentiate into a Th1 cell. In turn, the T cell secretes interferon-γ (IFN-γ), stimulating the macrophage to increase antigen presentation and lysosome production. This series of events is an important mechanism for increasing killing of intracellular pathogens such as mycobacteria.

    Answer B is incorrect. Eosinophils do not present antigens to Th1 cells and are not clasically thought to secrete IL-12. Plasma levels of eosinophils increase in hypersensitivity diseases such as asthma and in parasitic infection.

    Answer C is incorrect. Basophils and mast cells are the primary mediators of the immediate allergic, or type I, hypersensitivity reaction. These cells are activated by attached IgE and produce histamine and other inflammatory chemicals. IL-12 and IFNγ are not directly involved.

    Answer D is incorrect. IFN-γ, IL-8, and C5a are major chemotactic factors for neutrophils. Neutrophils are not antigen-presenting cells and would not secrete IL-12.

12. **The correct answer is B.** This patient is likely suffering from one of the two major types of scleroderma, known as CREST syndrome. The **CREST** acronym indicates the major symptoms: **C**alcinosis, **R**aynaud phenomenon, **E**sophageal dysmotility, **S**clerodactyly, and **T**elangiectasia. Often, CREST syndrome patients test positive for anticentromere antibodies. The answer describes Raynaud phenomenon, which may be triggered by cold weather or even emotional stimuli.

    Answer A is incorrect. These symptoms are not usually associated with CREST syndrome.

    Answer C is incorrect. These symptoms are suggestive of Sjögren syndrome, not CREST syndrome.

    Answer D is incorrect. This is not a symptom usually associated with CREST syndrome. Note that urethritis, conjunctivitis/anterior uveitis, and arthritis make up the classic triad in Reiter syndrome.

    Answer E is incorrect. This is not usually a hallmark of CREST syndrome but rather of diffuse scleroderma. Note that diffuse scleroderma is associated with anti-Scl-70 antibody.

13. **The correct answer is C.** This patient most likely has hyper-IgM syndrome, which is caused by a defect in the CD40 ligand on CD4 T helper cells. This defect leads to an inability to class switch between the different immunoglobulin isotypes. Since IgM is initially created and subsequently switched to the other isotypes, an inability to do so leads to elevated IgM levels and low levels of all other isotypes. Two prominent clinical problems are *Pneumocystis jiroveci* and neutropenia.

    Answer A is incorrect. Ataxia-telangiectasia is caused by a defect in DNA repair enzymes. The disease is associated with an IgA deficiency. The typical presentation of the disease is given away by the name, as symptoms include cerebellar problems (ataxia) and spider angiomas (telangiectasia).

Answer B is incorrect. Leukocyte adhesion deficiency syndrome is caused by a defect in the LFA-1 adhesion protein on the surface of neutrophils. The disease usually presents with marked leukocytosis and localized bacterial infections that are difficult to detect until they have progressed to an extensive life-threatening level. Since neutrophils are unable to adhere to the endothelium and transmigrate into tissues, infections in patients with leukocyte adhesion deficiency syndrome act similarly to those observed in neutropenic patients.

Answer D is incorrect. Job syndrome involves the failure of helper T lymphocytes to produce interferon-γ (IFN-γ). Because IFN-γ is a potent activator of phagocytic cells, a decrease in its production leads to a failure of neutrophils to respond to chemotactic stimuli. Job syndrome presents with recurrent staphylococcal abscesses, eczema, and high levels of IgE.

Answer E is incorrect. In thymic aplasia (DiGeorge syndrome), the third and fourth pharyngeal pouches, and thus the thymus and parathyroid glands, fail to develop. The disease often presents with many congenital defects, such as cardiac abnormalities, cleft palate, and abnormal facies. Thymic aplasia can also present with tetany due to hypocalcemia.

14. **The correct answer is B.** Patients suffering from microscopic polyangiitis often have autoantibodies against the enzyme myeloperoxidase, which stains in a perinuclear pattern and is therefore commonly called P-ANCA (perinuclear anti-neutrophil cytoplasmic antibody). Wegener granulomatosis is a vasculitis characterized by necrotizing granuloma formation in the lungs and kidneys. These patients often have autoantibodies specific for proteinase-3, which stains in a cytoplasmic distribution and is therefore commonly called C-ANCA (cytoplasmic anti-neutrophil cytoplasmic antibody). In both of these diseases, the patient's autoantibody titer is usually a good indicator of disease severity, particularly in Wegener granulomatosis, for which specificity and sensitivity of antibody testing are both >90%.

Answer A is incorrect. Kawasaki disease is not associated with serum P-ANCA, and Buerger disease is not associated with serum C-ANCA.

Answer C is incorrect. "Classic" polyarteritis nodosa is not associated with P-ANCA, and Buerger disease is not associated with C-ANCA.

Answer D is incorrect. Takayasu arteritis is not associated with serum P-ANCA.

Answer E is incorrect. Takayasu arteritis is not associated with serum P-ANCA, and Buerger disease is not associated with serum C-ANCA.

Answer F is incorrect. Temporal arteritis is not associated with serum P-ANCA.

15. **The correct answer is A.** The image reveals Reed-Sternberg cells, which are found in Hodgkin lymphoma and can be identified by their distinctive "owl's eye" bilobular nuclei. Most studies support a B-lymphocyte origin for Reed-Sternberg cells. Evidence supporting this includes rearrangements at immunoglobulin gene loci and the expression of MHC class II and B7 molecules. Additionally, they are CD 30+ and CD 15+, but CD45-.

Answer B is incorrect. Fibroblasts are elevated in chronic inflammation and in granulation tissue. Tumors that are derived from fibroblasts are called fibrosarcomas.

Answer C is incorrect. Activated macrophages tend to form granulomas, which are groups of epithelial-like macrophages that are surrounded by a collar of mononuclear lymphocytes and plasma cells. They lack the "owl's-eyes" nuclei that characterize Reed-Sternberg cells.

Answer D is incorrect. Neutrophil levels are elevated in acute infection and inflammation. Their appearance is characterized by a three- to four-lobed nucleus and basophilic granules.

Answer E is incorrect. T lymphocytes are elevated in T-lymphocyte leukemias such as T-cell acute lymphocytic leukemia and T-cell chronic lymphocytic leukemia.

16. **The correct answer is E.** Juvenile rheumatoid arthritis (JRA) may appear with a different presentation than adult-onset rheumatoid arthritis (RA). By definition, JRA begins before age 16 years and must include arthritis in at least one joint for at least six weeks. Additionally, the morphologic joint pathology is similar to that of adult-onset RA. However, there are several signs and symptoms that occur more commonly in JRA than in adult-onset RA, including an increased likelihood of systemic onset (with symptoms including high fevers, lymphadenopathy, and hepatomegaly), large-joint involvement, and anti-nuclear antibody seropositivity. Furthermore, JRA patients are less likely to have rheumatoid nodules and rheumatoid factor.

    Answer A is incorrect. There are several signs and symptoms that occur more commonly in JRA than in adult-onset RA, including increased likelihood of systemic onset, increased likelihood of large-joint involvement, and increased likelihood of anti-nuclear antibody seropositivity. Age at onset is <16 years.

    Answer B is incorrect. Systemic symptoms are more likely, but high levels of serum rheumatoid factor are less likely, in patients with JRA.

    Answer C is incorrect. Both systemic symptoms and large-joint involvement are more likely in patients with JRA.

    Answer D is incorrect. Systemic symptoms are more likely, but high levels of serum rheumatoid factor are less likely, in patients with JRA.

17. **The correct answer is D.** This patient has already had several bacterial infections, most notably an infection with *Streptococcus pneumoniae*. Complement, part of the innate immune system, is a group of serum proteins that work with antibody activity to eliminate pathogens. Specifically, the protein C3b is responsible for the opsonization of bacteria, and is likely the protein that is missing in this child's immune system. Opsonins adhere to microorganisms and promote leukocyte chemoattraction, antigen binding and phagocytosis, and activation of macrophage and neutrophil killing mechanisms. The antibody IgG is also an opsonin, and C3b and IgG are the two primary opsonins responsible for defense against bacteria.

    Answer A is incorrect. IgA patrols mucosal barriers and prevents attachment of bacteria and viruses. It does not fix complement, nor is it an opsonin.

    Answer B is incorrect. IgD is found on the surface of many B lymphocytes and in the serum, but its function is unclear.

    Answer C is incorrect. IgE mediates immediate (type I) hypersensitivity and immunity to helminths by facilitating the activation of eosinophils.

    Answer E is incorrect. IgM fixes (activates) complement but does not function by opsonization. It exists as a monomer on the surface of B lymphocytes, or as a pentamer in the serum.

18. **The correct answer is A.** This patient has become susceptible to opportunistic disease due to infection with HIV. Risk factors for contracting HIV include high-risk sexual behavior and intravenous drug use. HIV preferentially infects T-helper cells, which stain positive for CD3 and CD4. However, CD3 stains all T lymphocytes, while CD4 is specific for T-helper cells. At this point in time, the patient can be diagnosed with AIDS based on the presence of AIDS-defining opportunistic infections or by a CD4+ cell count <200/mm^3. This patient should be started on highly active antiretroviral therapy, which commonly includes the nucleoside reverse transcriptase inhibitor zidovudine.

    Answer B is incorrect. CD8 is specific for cytotoxic T lymphocytes. HIV affects only T-helper cells and does not affect cytotoxic T lymphocytes.

    Answer C is incorrect. CD20 is a marker that is specific for B lymphocytes, which are activated by T-helper cells. A person with HIV infection will not be deficient in B lymphocytes. In fact, individuals with HIV may produce a large amount of antibodies from B lymphocytes.

Answer D is incorrect. CD40 is found on B lymphocytes. Costimulation with T lymphocytes occurs via the CD40 ligand and is required for activation of B lymphocytes. CD40 is not found on T lymphocytes

Answer E is incorrect. CD56 is a marker that is specific for natural killer cells, which are unaffected in HIV infection. It should be noted that natural killer cells are an important part of the body's defense against tumors.

19. **The correct answer is B.** Celiac sprue is also known as gluten-sensitive enteropathy, nontropical sprue, and celiac disease. It is due to a sensitivity to gluten, which is found in wheat, grains, and many cereals. Biopsy shows marked atrophy, total loss, or flattening of the villi of the small bowel.

Answer A is incorrect. Abetalipoproteinemia is an autosomal recessive disease that causes a defect in the synthesis and export of lipids by mucosal cells because of the inability to synthesize apolipoprotein B. These patients usually have acanthocytes (or spur cells, RBCs that have spiny projections) and do not have any characteristic features of the intestine found in celiac disease.

Answer C is incorrect. Lactase deficiency causes osmotic diarrhea from the inability to break down lactose into glucose and galactose.

Answer D is incorrect. Viral enteritis, usually caused by a rotavirus, is common in children and can cause diarrhea. However, the clinical time course, suggested gluten sensitivity, and findings on biopsy make viral enteritis unlikely.

Answer E is incorrect. Whipple disease usually presents in middle-aged men who have malabsorptive diarrhea, and the hallmark is the presence of periodic acid-Schiff-positive macrophages in the intestinal mucosa. Rod-shaped bacilli of the causal agent, *Tropheryma whippelii*, are found on electron microscopy.

20. **The correct answer is D.** The infant's family history is suggestive of a trait with X-linked inheritance, and the preponderance of bacterial infections suggests a defect in the humoral (antibody-mediated) immune response. These two clues are most suggestive of a diagnosis of Bruton X-linked agammaglobulinemia. The molecular defect occurs in a signaling molecule named *BTK* (Bruton tyrosine kinase), leading to maturing arrest of developing B cells at the pre-B-cell stage. Arrest at the pre-B-cell stage would result in an inability to produce immunoglobulins; thus, the patient would have very low levels of all immunoglobulins in his serum. In the first several months of life, the infant can get by without problems because of the mother's IgG (still present). Indeed, it should be noted that these patients are particularly susceptible to extracellular pyogenic bacterial infections with organisms such as *Haemophilus influenzae*, *Streptococcus pyogenes*, *Staphylococcus aureus*, and *Streptococcus pneumoniae*. The only physical finding for Bruton patients is the absence, or near absence, of tonsils and adenoids, which are B-cell-rich tissues. Patients diagnosed with Bruton will need to be treated with replacement immunoglobulin.

Answer A is incorrect. A CD4 T-lymphocyte count $<200/mm^3$ suggests a diagnosis of AIDS, not an inherited genetic defect. Without any indication that his mother has HIV, there would be no reason to suspect HIV for the boy. AIDS patients have a defect in cell-mediated immunity, but the repeated bacterial infections in this case indicate the patient has a defect in humoral immunity.

Answer B is incorrect. Absence of T lymphocytes would result in a defect in cell-mediated immunity, and the patient would be more highly susceptible to viral and intracellular bacterial pathogens. Decreased T cells are seen in DiGeorge syndrome because of absence of thymus.

Answer C is incorrect. The physical examination and family and patient history are all highly suggestive of an immunoglobulin deficiency.

Answer E is incorrect. Low serum IgA levels are suggestive of selective IgA deficiency, the most common inherited immunodeficiency in the European population and, interestingly enough, one that appears to have no striking disease associations. These patients may produce autoantibodies to IgA that make them susceptible to anaphylactic reactions when transfused with normal blood products containing IgA.

21. **The correct answer is A.** Systemic lupus erythematosus (SLE) is a chronic autoimmune disease that affects multiple organ systems, including the kidney. It presents with a variety of symptoms including arthropathy, malar rash, Raynaud phenomenon, and pleural and pericardial effusions. SLE affects young adults (women almost three times more than men) and usually presents with a combined nephritic and nephrotic picture. Lupus nephropathy is a heterogeneous renal disease that is a consequence of immune complexes deposited in the glomerulus. Anti-dsDNA antibodies and low serum complement levels are markers for renal involvement in lupus. Histologic sections of biopsies from an SLE-affected kidney have a peculiar wire-loop appearance with subendothelial basement membrane deposits. In general, immunosuppressants are used to minimize the inflammatory effects of lupus on the kidney.

    Answer B is incorrect. A "tram track" appearance is typically seen in membranoproliferative glomerulonephritis.

    Answer C is incorrect. Lupus nephritis is considered a heterogeneous renal disease that can have a variety of presentations including active or inactive diffuse, segmental, or global glomerulonephritis.

    Answer D is incorrect. Immune complex deposition causes complement activation and leads to low serum complement levels.

    Answer E is incorrect. SLE is associated with anti-dsDNA and anti-Smith antibodies, not antimitochondrial antibodies.

22. **The correct answer is C.** This clinician is concerned that the fetus may have erythroblastosis fetalis (hemolytic disease of the newborn). This disease is mediated by maternally derived IgG anti-Rh antibodies developed in Rh-negative mothers that are directed at the Rh antigen present on the fetal RBCs of a Rh+ fetus in a previous pregnancy. If the mother possesses the antibodies developed from a previous exposure to an Rh+ fetus, they may cross the placenta (antibodies of the IgG isotype readily cross the placenta) and coat the fetal RBCs of a Rh+ fetus if the mother is now pregnant with another Rh+ child. Antibody coating of the RBCs leads to phagocytosis of RBCs (via Fc receptors) and/or destruction of the RBCs by the complement system and potentially fatal anemia. This antibody-mediated cytotoxic reaction is an example of a type II hypersensitivity reaction.

    Answer A is incorrect. Graft-versus-host disease is a potentially lethal side effect of bone marrow transplantation.

    Answer B is incorrect. Type I hypersensitivity reactions are antibody-mediated but require antigen binding to IgE, which is prebound to the surface of mast cells. Mast cell degranulation then ensues. Examples include anaphylaxis, asthma, hives, and local wheal and flare.

    Answer D is incorrect. Type III hypersensitivity reactions are immune complex-mediated. Examples include polyarteritis nodosa, glomerulonephritis, rheumatoid arthritis, and SLE.

    Answer E is incorrect. Type IV hypersensitivity reactions are a group of T-cell-mediated pathologies. Examples include the tuberculin skin test, transplant rejection, and contact dermatitis.

23. **The correct answer is E.** This patient has Wiskott-Aldrich syndrome, an X-linked disorder resulting in the body's inability to mount an IgM response to bacteria. Recurrent pyogenic infections, eczema, and thrombocytopenia are the typical triad of symptoms. Wiscott-Aldrich syndrome does not present with any specific enzyme abnormality.

Answer A is incorrect. Hypocalcemia is characteristic of thymic aplasia (DiGeorge syndrome), in which the third and fourth pharyngeal pouches, and thus the thymus and parathyroid glands, fail to develop. As a result patients may experience tetany. Thymic aplasia often presents with congenital defects such as cardiac abnormalities, cleft palate, and abnormal facies.

Answer B is incorrect. IgA levels are elevated in Wiskott-Aldrich syndrome. They are low in hyper-IgM syndrome, ataxia-telangiectasia, and in selective IgA deficiency.

Answer C is incorrect. IgE levels are elevated in Wiskott-Aldrich syndrome. They are low in hyper-IgM syndrome, in which B cells are unable to class switch because of a defect in helper T cells; these patients have high levels of IgM and low IgG, IgA and IgE levels.

Answer D is incorrect. Wiskott-Aldrich syndrome is characterized by thrombocytopenia and small platelets, rather than lymphopenia. Lymphopenia is typical of patients with severe combined immunodeficiency, who also have reduced levels of all immunoglobulin isotypes and are infected early in life by opportunistic pathogens.

24. **The correct answer is C.** Sarcoidosis is a systemic inflammatory process that involves an exaggerated Th_1 immune response of unknown etiology. It generally causes respiratory symptoms, with the appearance of hilar lymphadenopathy and noncaseating granulomas in the lungs, but can affect any organ system. Acute sarcoidosis can develop suddenly over a period of weeks, with both constitutional and respiratory symptoms. The Heerfordt-Waldenström syndrome of acute sarcoidosis includes the development of fever, parotid enlargement, anterior uveitis, and facial nerve palsy, as seen in this patient. Of the neurologic symptoms seen in sarcoidosis, seventh nerve involvement is the most common.

Answer A is incorrect. Lyme disease is a multisystem infection caused by the spirochete *Borrelia burgdorferi*, carried by the *Ixodes scapularis* tick. Within the first few weeks after an infected bite, patients may develop erythema migrans at the site of the bite and additional annular lesions. They may also display symptoms of cardiac and neurologic involvement, including first-degree heart block, myopericarditis, meningitis, cerebellar ataxia, and seventh nerve facial palsy. In addition, patients often experience a migratory musculoskeletal pain. They do not, however, experience respiratory or ocular symptoms.

Answer B is incorrect. Pneumonia is an infection of the lung involving the alveoli, interstitia, and distal airways whereupon the alveoli become consolidated with WBCs, RBCs, and fibrin. The patient with pneumonia may have fever, cough, and an increased respiratory rate, as this patient does. However, physical exam would display findings of dullness to percussion in a lobar distribution in addition to other breath sounds such as wheezes or râles, and findings would be unlikely to be bilateral. Coughing often produces sputum.

Answer D is incorrect. SLE is an autoimmune disease in which circulating antibodies and immune complexes cause systemic damage to the body. SLE is most prevalent in women and African-American people. Symptoms can affect all organ systems and cause polyarthritis, malar rash, nephritis, vascular occlusions, and pericarditis. Neurologic symptoms include headache, cognitive dysfunction, seizures, and myelopathy, but seventh nerve involvement is not particularly common. Pulmonary symptoms usually manifest as a pleuritis with or without pleural effusion, but one would not see granulomas on radiography.

Answer E is incorrect. TB is caused by the acid-fast bacterium *Mycobacterium tuberculosis*, which produces a primary infection of the lungs. Symptoms include fever, night sweats, malaise, weakness, and dry cough. Radiography may reveal paratracheal or hilar lymphadenopathy, as in this patient. However, while it is possible that her nonpulmonary symptoms may occur with extrapulmonary TB, her purified protein derivative test is negative, making it less likely that she has been exposed to the bacterium.

25. **The correct answer is D.** This patient is likely presenting with renal amyloidosis. (Remember, amyloid deposits show apple-green birefringence in polarized light). Clonal plasma cells express abnormal amounts of light chain protein. The organs most affected are the kidneys and the heart. Symptoms include neuropathy, proteinuria, edema, hepatosplenomegaly, and congestive heart failure.

    Answer A is incorrect. C2 is a complement protein; complement is a system of proteins that aid in humoral immunity and inflammation. It is not involved in amyloidosis pathogenesis.

    Answer B is incorrect. CD8 is a protein found on cytotoxic T lymphocytes and is involved in immune response. It is not involved in amyloidosis.

    Answer C is incorrect. The Fab fragment is the part of the antibody that binds to the antigen and includes both light and heavy chains. Amyloidosis is associated only with abnormal light chain protein.

    Answer E is incorrect. Major histocompatibility complex II is a protein complex that is involved in presenting antigens to immune cells. It is not involved in amyloid protein deposition.

26. **The correct answer is B.** Selective immunoglobulin deficiency is a deficit in a specific class of immunoglobulins. IgA deficiency is the most common of these. Because IgA is the most prominent immunoglobulin found in mucous membranes, patients suffering from a deficiency of it can present with sinus and lung infections.

    Answer A is incorrect. A very high IgE level and normal levels of all other immunoglobulins are characteristic of Job syndrome. Job syndrome is a disorder of the immune system that involves the failure of helper T cells to produce interferon-γ. It presents with multiple "cold" (or noninflamed) skin lesions and high IgE levels.

    Answer C is incorrect. A low IgM level in conjunction with an elevated IgA level and a normal IgG level is characteristic of Wiskott-Aldrich syndrome. Wiskott-Aldrich syndrome is an X-linked disorder that results in a reduced IgM response to encapsulated bacteria. The triad of symptoms consists of recurrent pyogenic infections, eczema, and thrombocytopenia.

    Answer D is incorrect. Normal immunoglobulin levels and a negative nitroblue tetrazolium dye reduction test are characteristic of chronic granulomatous disease. Chronic granulomatous disease results from an NADPH oxidase deficiency that reduces the ability of phagocytes to kill catalase-positive bacteria. It does not present with low levels of immunoglobulins. The definitive test for this disorder is a negative nitroblue tetrazolium dye reduction test.

    Answer E is incorrect. Normal immunoglobulin levels can be seen in thymic aplasia (DiGeorge syndrome). Thymic aplasia, in which the thymus and parathyroids fail to develop, results from the failure of the third and fourth pharyngeal pouches to develop. Consequently, T cells are completely absent. Patients with thymic aplasia typically present with recurrent viral and fungal infections. They may also have disorders of the great vessels and heart and may experience tetany due to hypocalcemia.

27. **The correct answer is D.** Type IV hypersensitivity reactions (also known as delayed-type hypersensitivity) are mediated by previously activated T-helper 1 (Th_1) cells. These cells recognize the TB-derived peptide and carbohydrate mixture that is administered during the tuberculin test. These Th_1 cells become activated to secrete interferon-γ and tumor necrosis factor-b, which mediate a local inflammatory response within 24-48 hours after administration of the injection. These Th_1 effector cells are present only in individuals who have previously been exposed to *Mycobacterium tuberculosis* or those who were vaccinated with bacille Calmette-Guérin. It is important to note that other type IV hypersensitivity reactions include celiac disease and contact hypersensitivities such as poison ivy.

Answer A is incorrect. While mast cells are involved in the pathogenesis of type I hypersensitivity reactions, the tuberculin test is an example of a type IV reaction.

Answer B is incorrect. While cytotoxic T lymphocytes are involved in the pathogenesis of type II hypersensitivity reactions, the tuberculin test is an example of a type IV reaction.

Answer C is incorrect. Mast cells are not directly involved in the pathogenesis of type IV hypersensitivity reactions.

Answer E is incorrect. While a positive tuberculin test is an example of a type IV hypersensitivity reaction, it is mediated by T-helper 1 (Th_1) cells, not Th_2 cells. Th_2 cells are those that help the humoral (antibody-mediated) arm of the immune response.

28. **The correct answer is A.** The patient in this scenario has myasthenia gravis. This condition is characterized by ptosis, limb weakness, and difficulty breathing. The key mediator is an autoantibody to the acetylcholine receptor on the postsynaptic membrane. All antibody molecules consist of two identical heavy chains and two identical light chains that are held together by disulfide bonds.

    Answer B is incorrect. Hydrogen bonds are weaker than disulfide bonds and do not connect the antibody chains.

    Answer C is incorrect. Ionic bonds are found in chemicals such as sodium chloride but are not responsible for holding antibody chains together.

    Answer D is incorrect. Triple covalent bonds are seen between some atoms, such as nitrogen, but are not responsible for holding the chains of antibody molecules together.

    Answer E is incorrect. Van der Waals forces are weak attraction forces and do not play a significant role in holding antibody chains together.

29. **The correct answer is C.** The image shows spider angiomas, which are common on the ears and cheeks of patients with ataxia-telangiectasia. Ataxia-telangiectasia is an autosomal recessive disorder caused by a mutation on chromosome 11q22-23 that results in a defect in DNA repair enzymes. It manifests as a variable combination of progressive neurologic impairment, cerebellar ataxia, variable immunodeficiency (usually IgA deficiency) with susceptibility to sinopulmonary infections, impaired organ maturation, x-ray hypersensitivity, ocular and cutaneous telangiectasia, and a predisposition to malignancy.

    Answer A is incorrect. A noninflamed or "cold" abscess is characteristic of Job syndrome which results from a failure of interferon-γ production by helper T cells. The lack of interferon-γ leads to the failure of the neutrophil response to chemotactic stimuli. Patients with Job syndrome present with eczema, coarse facies, retained primary teeth, and high levels of IgE.

    Answer B is incorrect. Cleft palate is a common feature of thymic aplasia (DiGeorge syndrome). Thymic aplasia results from failure of the third and fourth pharyngeal pouches (and thus the thymus and parathyroid glands) to develop. The disease often presents with congenital defects such as cardiac abnormalities, cleft palate, and abnormal facies. Thymic aplasia can also present with tetany due to hypocalcemia.

    Answer D is incorrect. Granulomas are collections of cells seen in (among other things) chronic granulomatous disease. This disease is caused by an inability of neutrophils to kill bacteria once they have phagocytosed them.

    Answer E is incorrect. Visual hallucinations are not a symptom of any of the known immune deficiencies.

30. **The correct answer is A.** Microscopic polyangiitis is one of the trio of diseases (with Wegener granulomatosis and Churg-Strauss syndrome) that are referred to as the ANCA (antineutrophil cytoplasmic antibody)-associated vasculitides. Over 80% of patients with this disease have ANCA, namely the perinuclear pattern of staining (P-ANCA) type. Inflammation of the pulmonary capillaries,

which can lead to hemoptysis, is common in these patients, and 90% of patients have necrotizing glomerulonephritis (leading to hematuria). Other common symptoms include intestinal pain/bleeding, muscle pain, and weakness. Churg-Strauss syndrome also involves the pulmonary vasculature and is associated with eosinophilia as well as elevated P-ANCA levels.

Answer B is incorrect. The CREST variant of scleroderma is associated with anti-centromere antibodies, which are not particularly associated with microscopic polyangiitis.

Answer C is incorrect. Sjögren syndrome is associated with antiribonucleoprotein (anti-RNP) antibody SS-A (Ro), which is present in 70%-95% of patients, and SS-B (La), which is present in 60-90% of patients. Neither antibody is associated with microscopic polyangiitis.

Answer D is incorrect. SLE is associated with anti-nuclear, anti-dsDNA, anti-Smith antibodies. None of these are particularly associated with microscopic polyangiitis.

Answer E is incorrect. While the clinical presentation is similar, Wegener granulomatosis is associated with cytoplasmic (not perinuclear) ANCA, which is not very common in patients with microscopic polyangiitis.

CHAPTER 6

Pathology

QUESTIONS

1. A 19-year-old college student is admitted to the hospital for bacterial meningitis. The patient initially recovers and responds to treatment. However, later in her hospital stay she begins to experience headache and blurred vision. Her physicians note cognitive decline and a gait disturbance that was not evident during her brief recovery phase. CT of the head shows enlarged ventricles. Which of the following mechanisms is most likely responsible for the patient's deterioration?

   (A) Destruction of brain parenchyma
   (B) Excessive cerebrospinal fluid production
   (C) Fusion of the cranial sutures
   (D) Impaired cerebrospinal fluid resorption
   (E) Obstruction of the cerebral aqueduct

2. A 41-year-old man visits his physician because of increasingly painful headaches. CT of the head reveals an abnormality and an MRI of the brain with contrast (shown below) is performed for further evaluation. If a biopsy of this tumor were obtained, what would the pathologist likely see under the microscope?

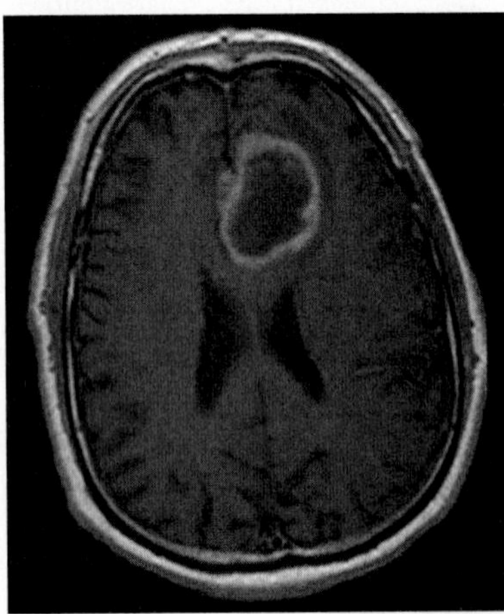

Courtesy of Dr. Per-Lennart Westesson, University of Rochester Medical Center.

   (A) Densely packed cells with halos of cytoplasm surrounding large round nuclei
   (B) Perivascular pseudorosettes with tumor cells surrounding vessels
   (C) Pseudopalisading tumor cells surrounding necrotic regions
   (D) Sharply demarcated areas of tumor cells located at the grey-white matter junction
   (E) Whorled pattern of concentrically arranged spindle cells with psammoma bodies

3. A 43-year-old woman presents to her primary care physician for a regular check-up. A neurologic examination shows that when the patient looks to the left, the right eye stops at the midline and the left eye shows monocular horizontal nystagmus. When the patient looks to the right, both eyes seem to move appropriately. Convergence is normal. What is the most likely cause of this patient's findings?

   (A) Lesion of the left medial longitudinal fasciculus
   (B) Lesion of the left sixth cranial nerve
   (C) Lesion of the right medial longitudinal fasciculus
   (D) Lesion of the right oculomotor nerve
   (E) Pupillary light-near dissociation
   (F) Relative afferent pupillary defect

4. A 22-year-old man presents to his primary care physician with complaints of weakness and a rash. Physical examination shows slight oral mucosal bleeding and diffuse petechiae. He has a history of generalized tonic-clonic seizures that are well controlled with medication but is otherwise healthy. Results of a bone marrow aspirate are shown in the image. Which of the following is the most likely cause of his symptoms?

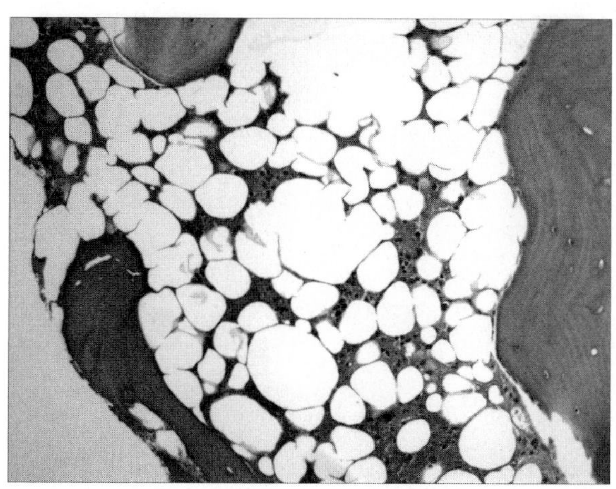

Reproduced, with permission, from USMLERx.com.

(A) Adverse drug reaction
(B) Alcoholism
(C) Idiopathic thrombocytopenic purpura
(D) Pernicious anemia
(E) Vitamin C deficiency

5. A 57-year-old man presents with a cough and progressively increasing shortness of breath. The patient has been a plumber for 20 years, and before that job he worked on ships. High-resolution CT reveals areas of pleural thickening with calcified plaques. A specially stained specimen from a patient with a similar condition is shown in the image. Which of the following best describes the patient's condition?

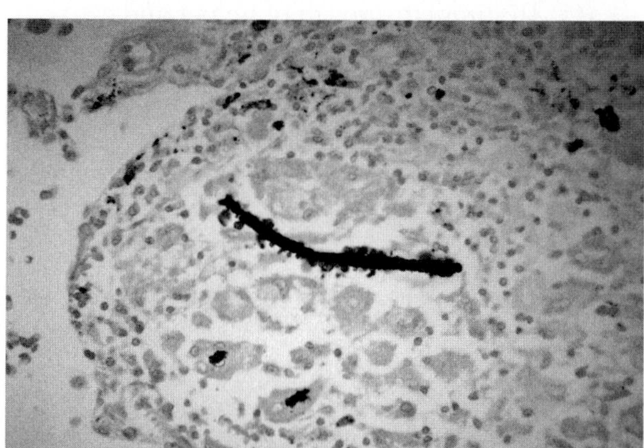

Courtesy of Dr. Edwin P. Ewing Jr, Centers for Disease Control and Prevention.

(A) Compared to the general population, smoking would present an increased risk of bronchogenic cancer in this patient
(B) Lungs in this patient will have silicotic nodules
(C) The findings are associated with exposure to air pollution
(D) The patient does not have an increased risk of mesothelioma
(E) The patient has a condition associated with increased tuberculosis susceptibility
(F) The patient will have localized intra-alveolar fibrosis

6. A 7-year-old African-American boy is brought to the pediatrician's office by his mother after he begins crying inconsolably and complaining that his fingers hurt. His mother reports that he had been playing in the sun all day long. A peripheral blood smear is shown in the image. Which of the following complications is associated with this patient's disease?

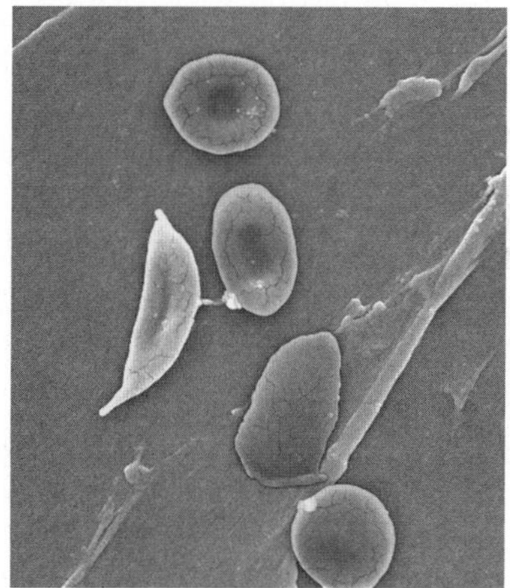

Courtesy of the Sickle Cell Foundation of Georgia: Jackie George, Beverly Sinclair.

(A) Myelofibrosis
(B) Cyclical fevers
(C) Eosinophilia
(D) Microangiopathic hemolytic anemia
(E) Acute chest syndrome

7. A mother takes her previously healthy 7-year-old son to the doctor because he appears "puffy." Physical examination reveals pitting edema bilaterally in his lower limbs and swelling of his eyelids. Urinalysis reveals a pH of 5 with 4+ proteinuria; glucose and ketones are absent. What is most likely the cause of the patient's edema?

   (A) Congestive heart failure
   (B) A thickening of the glomerular basement membrane
   (C) A loss of the negative charge in the glomerular filtration barrier
   (D) Inadequate dietary protein
   (E) Split glomerular basement membrane secondary to a mutation in type IV collagen

8. A 26-year-old woman visits her physician with complaints of vaginal bleeding after sexual intercourse. She started menses at age 14 years and has 32-day cycles. She acknowledges having unprotected sex with multiple partners. Cytologic specimens are taken from the cervix and vagina. On microscopy, cervical cells have large nuclei with open chromatin; several cells have mitotic figures. What additional findings would most likely be present in the specimens that account for these findings?

   (A) Double-stranded DNA virus
   (B) Gram-negative diplococci
   (C) Gram-positive cocci
   (D) Single-stranded RNA
   (E) Squamous cells covered with bacteria

9. A 67-year-old man is admitted to the hospital after fracturing the neck of his right femur. A pathologic fracture is suspected. Serum protein electrophoresis shows an abnormal monoclonal paraprotein spike. Subsequent bone marrow biopsy demonstrates an abnormal proliferation of the cells shown in the image. Which of the following describes the function of the secretory product these cells normally produce?

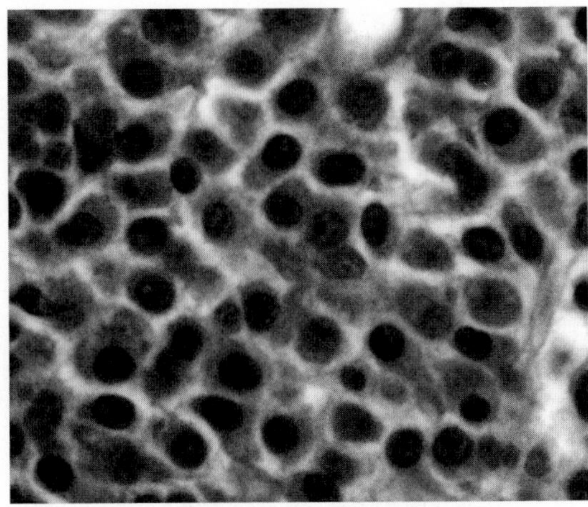

Reproduced, with permission, from USMLERx.com.

   (A) To block attachment of bacteria and viruses to mucous membranes
   (B) To fix complement and serve as an antigen receptor on the surface of B lymphocytes in the primary immune response
   (C) To increase interleukin-2 receptor synthesis by helper T-lymphocyte and B-lymphocyte proliferation
   (D) To mediate a type I hypersensitivity reaction by causing the release of secretory products from basophils or mast cells
   (E) To opsonize bacteria, neutralize toxins and viruses, and fix complement in the secondary immune response
   (F) To promote vasodilation and leukocyte extravasation
   (G) To stimulate growth of helper and cytotoxic T lymphocytes

10. Autopsy of a patient shows bilaterally enlarged, cystic kidneys and a vascular lesion at the base of the brain, as seen in the image. Which chromosome was most likely mutated in the patient?

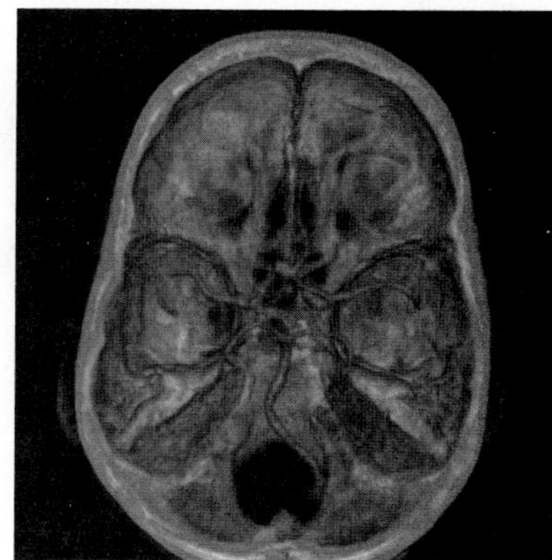

Reproduced, with permission, from USMLERx.com.

(A) 4
(B) 15
(C) 16
(D) 22
(E) X

11. A 3-year-old developmentally delayed girl presents to the pediatric neurologist for evaluation of new onset seizures. The parents are also concerned because the child frequently exhibits inappropriate outbursts of laughter. Physical examination is significant for abnormal facies marked by microcephaly, deep-set eyes, and a large mouth with a protruding tongue. The child's gait is unstable. The most likely diagnosis is an example of which of the following genetic phenomena?

(A) Anticipation
(B) Heteroplasmy
(C) Imprinting
(D) Locus heterozygosity
(E) Mosaicism

12. A 51-year-old man complains lately of recurrent vomiting. He cannot remember when it began, but he says he is concerned because sometimes he throws up blood. On physical examination, there is some lower extremity edema, and some tortuous veins on the surface of his abdomen. He admits to having several recent sexual partners, and has never been tested for sexually transmitted diseases. He also reports drinking a "few" drinks a night. Results of a liver biopsy are shown in the image. Which of the following best describes the pathologic process occurring in this patient's liver?

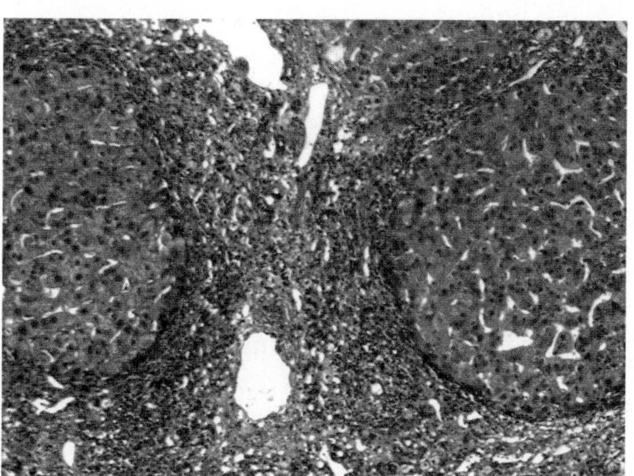

Reproduced, with permission, from USMLERx.com.

(A) At this stage in disease, hepatocytes fail to regenerate
(B) Lipid deposition is taking place
(C) Mallory bodies are commonly seen in this condition
(D) The architectural changes that are occurring are irreversible
(E) The liver will be enlarged

13. A 55-year-old recent immigrant from Taiwan presents to the clinic with a three-month history of worsening nasal congestion, epistaxis, and recurrent ear infections. Physical examination reveals painless firm lymph node enlargement in the neck. CT of the head reveals a large mass situated in the upper nasopharynx. Biopsy of the lesion shows large epithelioid cells intermixed with numerous infiltrating lymphocytes. The infectious agent directly associated with this patient's pathology is best described by which category?

(A) DNA virus
(B) Eubacterium
(C) Fungus
(D) Mycobacterium
(E) RNA virus

14. A 56-year-old man is admitted to the emergency department with a chief complaint of severe abdominal and flank pain. The physician orders x-ray of the abdomen, as shown in the image. The patient's condition necessarily implies which of the following?

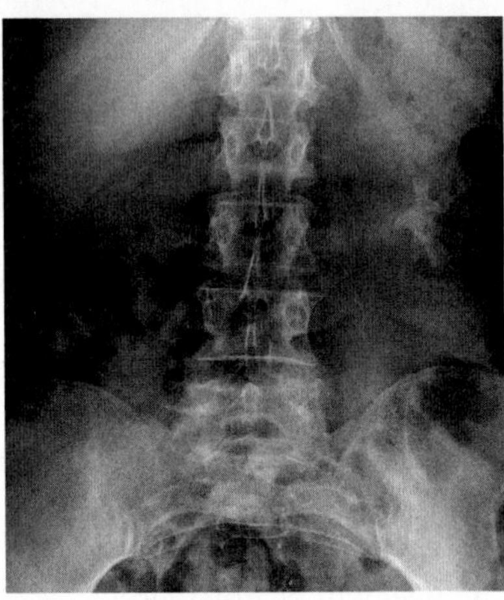

Reproduced, with permission, from USMLERx.com.

(A) Acidic urine, pH <7.2
(B) Alkaline urine, pH >7.2
(C) Ammonium in the urinary tract
(D) Sodium chloride in the collecting ducts
(E) Uric acid in the renal pelvis

15. A patient with AIDS and a CD4+ cell count $<50/\text{mm}^3$ is suffering from an infection that affects his lungs, eyes, gastrointestinal tract, and central nervous system. Results of a biopsy are shown in the image. With what is the patient most likely infected?

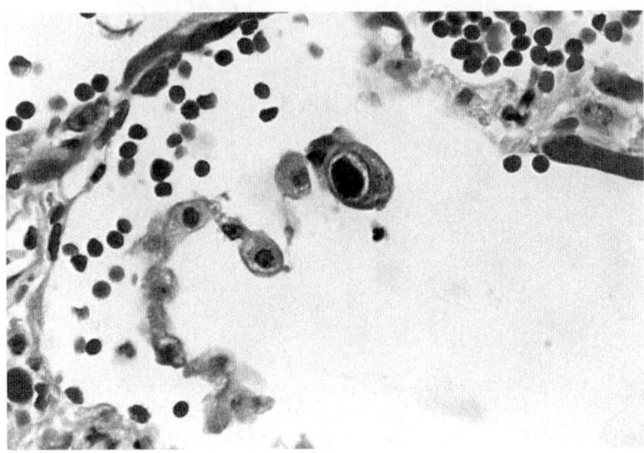

Courtesy of Dr. Edwin P. Ewing Jr, Centers for Disease Control and Prevention.

(A) *Candida albicans*
(B) *Cryptococcus neoformans*
(C) Cytomegalovirus
(D) Herpes simplex virus
(E) *Mycobacterium avium*
(F) *Pneumocystis jiroveci*

16. The attending pathologist reviews a hematoxylin-eosin-stained slide from the liver biopsy of a 50-year-old man suffering from dyspnea on exertion, lower extremity edema, and orthopnea. In addition, the patient has recent onset diabetes mellitus and testicular atrophy. One of the patient's four brothers also has the same set of medical problems. The pathologist performs one more study, which confirms the suspected diagnosis (see image). Which of the following is the most likely diagnosis?

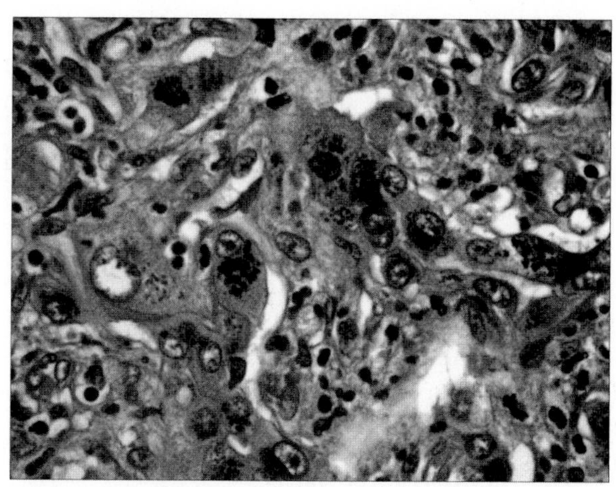

Reproduced, with permission, from USMLERx.com.

(A) α_1-Antitrypsin deficiency
(B) Alcoholic hepatitis
(C) Cystic fibrosis
(D) Hereditary hemochromatosis
(E) Wilson disease

17. A 37-year-old HIV-positive man presents for evaluation of anogenital lesions. He states that the lesions have been present for years, but have recently grown in size and become pruritic and tender. On examination he is circumcised and has multiple hyperkeratotic papules on his penis shaft, perineum, and anal area. He also has a palpable rectal mass with guaiac-positive stool and conjunctival pallor. On further questioning, he admits to recent unintentional weight loss, constipation, and bloating. His CD4+ cell count is 150/mm^3 and his hematocrit is 26%. CT of the abdomen shows a 3 × 4-cm rectal mass with multiple metastatic lesions in his liver. What tumor-suppressor protein is targeted by the virus causing this patient's rectal cancer?

(A) APC
(B) BRCA1
(C) MSH2
(D) NF1
(E) p53

18. A 5-year-old boy presents with an unsteady gait and severe vertigo and nausea. A brain lesion is seen on CT scan. A biopsy of the lesion is shown in the image. Where in the brain is the patient's lesion?

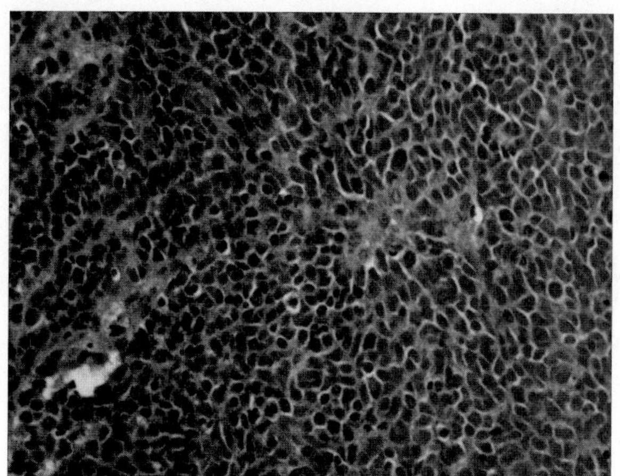

Reproduced, with permission, from USMLERx.com.

(A) Cerebellar vermis
(B) Intermediate section of the cerebellar hemisphere
(C) Lateral section of the cerebellar hemisphere
(D) Occipital cortex
(E) Postcentral gyrus of the parietal lobe

19. A 64-year-old retired shipyard worker has been experiencing shortness of breath, a cough, and chest pain for five months. In that time he has lost 14.5 kg (32 lb). He develops progressive ascites, and ultimately dies due to a pulmonary embolus. Autopsy results are shown in the image. Exposure to which substance is a risk factor for this patient's disorder?

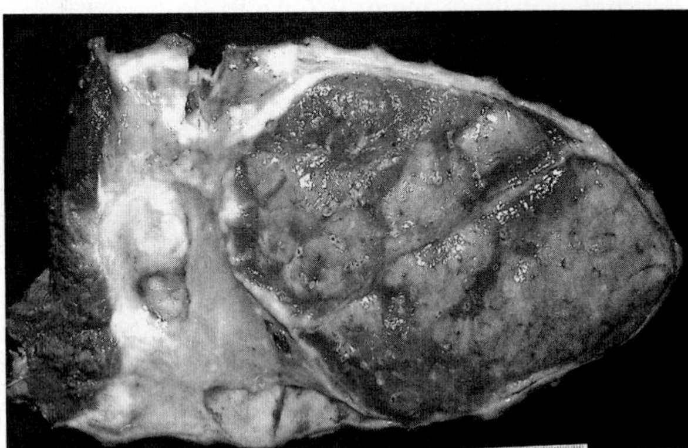

Reproduced, with permission, from USMLERx.com.

(A) Aflatoxin B
(B) Asbestos
(C) Benzene
(D) Cadmium
(E) Silica

20. A 12-year-old boy is brought to the doctor for progressive fatigue and shortness of breath on exertion. He was born full term and has been generally healthy until a few months ago, when his parents noticed that he became tired after only five minutes of playing with his siblings. Physical examination reveals a loud, holosystolic murmur and mild cyanosis of his lips. Examination of his hands reveals clubbing of the fingers. Which of the following cardiac defects is most likely to be found on echocardiogram?

(A) Bicuspid aortic valve
(B) Left-to-right shunt
(C) Mitral regurgitation
(D) Right-to-left shunt
(E) Valvular vegetations

ANSWERS

1. **The correct answer is D.** The arachnoid granulations are outgrowths of the arachnoid mater through the dura mater and into the superior sagittal sinus. They are responsible for returning fluid from the cerebrospinal fluid (CSF) into general circulation. Following irritation of the meninges secondary to meningitis or subarachnoid hemorrhage, the arachnoid granulations may become scarred and fail to resorb adequate CSF. This causes CSF to build up in both the subarachnoid space and the ventricles, producing communicating hydrocephalus.

   Answer A is incorrect. Enlarged ventricles are commonly seen in advanced neurodegenerative diseases such as Alzheimer's. As brain mass is progressively lost, CSF accumulates to fill the void, a phenomenon known as hydrocephalus ex vacuo. Substantial loss of brain parenchyma is not generally seen in meningitis and thus is an unlikely mechanism for the development of hydrocephalus in this setting.

   Answer B is incorrect. Overproduction of CSF by the choroid plexus is an uncommon cause of hydrocephalus. It may occur in the setting of a choroid plexus papilloma but would not be a consequence of meningitis.

   Answer C is incorrect. Closure of the cranial sutures is a normal phenomenon that occurs as infants grow and is not responsible for the development of hydrocephalus. In young infants, the flexibility of the cranium prior to suture fusion allows the head to enlarge noticeably in the setting of hydrocephalus.

   Answer E is incorrect. Obstruction of the flow of CSF within the ventricular system leads to noncommunicating hydrocephalus, in which pressure builds up within the ventricles, but not in the subarachnoid space. Such obstruction is commonly the result of brain tumors (particularly neoplasms of the ependymal cells lining the ventricles), or congenital malformations.

2. **The correct answer is C.** This patient has a lesion consistent with glioblastoma multiforme (GBM), which is the most common primary brain tumor. The MRI shows an irregular mass lesion with avid peripheral contrast enhancement and central hypoenhancement, which is due to central necrosis suggestive of high-grade malignancy. Note the "butterfly" shape of the lesion due to fact that it narrows as it passes through the corpus collosum while crossing the midline—this is a classic imaging finding in GBM. On histopathology, the lesion consists of highly malignant astrocyte tumor cells that surround areas of necrosis; this is known as pseudopalisading. GBM has been associated with genetic alterations, including loss of *p53* function, increased activity of the epidermal growth factor receptor gene (*EGFR*), and loss of heterozygosity on chromosome arm 10q. GBM has a poor prognosis, with a mean survival of 8-10 months after diagnosis; most patients die within two years.

   Answer A is incorrect. Densely packed cells with halos of cytoplasm surrounding large round nuclei are characteristic of oligodendrogliomas, which are slow-growing tumors originating in the cerebral hemispheres. These lesions have a better prognosis than astrocytomas, with a mean patient survival of 5-10 years.

   Answer B is incorrect. Perivascular pseudorosettes with tumor cells surrounding vessels are characteristic of ependymomas, which are tumors located in the periventricular space or in the spinal cord that may obstruct the flow of CSF.

   Answer D is incorrect. Sharply demarcated areas of tumor cells located at the grey-white matter junction are characteristic of secondary metastatic lesions from a primary tumor elsewhere in the body, most commonly the breast, lung, thyroid, skin, kidney, and gastrointestinal (GI) tract.

   Answer E is incorrect. A whorled pattern of concentrically arranged spindle cells with calcified psammoma bodies is characteristic of meningiomas, which are the second most common primary intracranial neoplasm. Meningiomas are benign, slow-growing tumors of the meninges.

3. **The correct answer is C.** The description is consistent with internuclear ophthalmoplegia, which consists of ipsilateral medial rectus palsy on attempted lateral conjugate gaze away from the lesion with associated monocular horizontal nystagmus in the contralateral abducting eye with preserved convergence. It results from damage to the ipsilateral medial longitudinal fasciculus (MLF), which is the connection between the abducent and oculomotor nuclei, so that the two nerves' actions become unlinked. The third nerve and medial rectus muscle function normally in convergence but not during actions that require conjugate eye movements. In young patients, it is most commonly the result of central nervous system infection or multiple sclerosis, whereas in older patients it is more commonly the result of vascular disease.

   Answer A is incorrect. A lesion of the left medial longitudinal fasciculus (MLF) would produce an internuclear opthalmoplegia, as in this case. However, the findings of a left MLF lesion would include impaired left (ipsilateral) eye adduction with rightward gaze as well as right (contralateral) eye horizontal nystagmus. The clinical description in the vignette is the mirror image, consistent with a lesion of the right MLF.

   Answer B is incorrect. A pure sixth-nerve palsy would have almost the opposite effect of this scenario and would cause a lateral rectus palsy as opposed to a medial rectus palsy seen here.

   Answer D is incorrect. Recall that cranial nerve (CN) III, or the oculomotor nerve, innervates all the extraocular muscles with the exception of the lateral rectus (innervated by CN VI) and the superior oblique (innervated by CN IV). In a lesion of CN III the affected eye looks "down and out" while at rest, or abducted and depressed.

   Answer E is incorrect. Pupillary light-near dissociation is also known as Argyll Robertson pupil and is an absent miotic reaction to light with preserved accommodation. This condition can occur in neurosyphilis, diabetes, and systemic lupus erythematosus.

   Answer F is incorrect. A relative afferent pupillary defect is also known as a Marcus Gunn pupil. It results from a lesion in the afferent limb of the pupillary light reflex and can be seen in the retrobulbar neuritis of multiple sclerosis. It would not result in medial rectus palsy on attempted lateral conjugate gaze.

4. **The correct answer is A.** The bone marrow aspirate is hypocellular without any abnormal cells, suggestive of aplastic anemia. Given the clinical history, this patient's seizures were likely treated with carbamazepine, which can cause aplastic anemia. Other causes of aplastic anemia include viruses (Epstein-Barr virus, hepatitis C, and parvovirus B19), toxins (benzene and insecticides), and other drugs (cancer chemotherapeutics). Aplastic anemia can also be idiopathic.

   Answer B is incorrect. Alcoholism has many metabolic and clinical sequelae, including decreases in all cell lines due to marrow suppression. Therefore, this patient's clinical picture could be explained by alcoholic cirrhosis. However, the hypoplastic bone marrow and known antiepileptic drug use make the diagnosis of aplastic anemia most likely.

   Answer C is incorrect. This patient does have symptoms of thrombocytopenia, but the bone marrow aspirate should appear normal in idiopathic thrombocytopenic purpura.

   Answer D is incorrect. Pernicious anemia, the leading cause of megaloblastic anemia, does uncommonly occur in this age group. However, the bone marrow aspirate is not consistent with pernicious anemia, as this disease does not affect neutrophils, platelets, or any myeloid cell line other than erythrocytes.

Answer E is incorrect. Although vitamin C deficiency can cause gingival bleeding, it does not cause anemia or a hypoplastic bone marrow.

5. **The correct answer is A.** The image shows the classic "barbell" ferruginous bodies seen in asbestosis. These bodies can only be seen when the slide is stained with Prussian blue. Asbestosis is most common in plumbers, construction workers, and shipbuilders. Pleural plaques are suggestive of asbestos exposure. Patients with asbestosis have an increased risk of bronchogenic carcinoma. This risk is compounded greatly by smoking, making smoking an even riskier habit in someone with asbestosis.

   Answer B is incorrect. Silicotic nodules are seen in the lungs of patients with silicosis, while ferruginous bodies and ivory-white pleural plaques are seen in lungs of patients with asbestosis. The ferruginous bodies can be detected on biopsy by Prussian blue staining.

   Answer C is incorrect. Anthracosis (carbon deposits) is seen in patients exposed to pollution (usually seen in city-dwellers). This would grossly look like black spots on the lung, and is not considered to be pathologic.

   Answer D is incorrect. The patient has an increased risk of both mesothelioma and bronchogenic carcinoma.

   Answer E is incorrect. Silicosis, a disease caused by exposure to free silica dust, is associated with increased tuberculosis susceptibility. Asbestosis is not associated with this increased susceptibility.

   Answer F is incorrect. Lungs with asbestosis have diffuse pulmonary interstitial fibrosis caused by inhaled asbestos fibers. The distribution is not localized or intra-alveolar.

6. **The correct answer is E.** This patient's blood smear is strongly suggestive of sickle cell anemia, an autosomal recessive disorder caused by defective hemoglobin S (HbS). Hypoxic conditions result in the polymerization and "sickling" of HbS, leading to vulnerable RBCs and hemolytic anemia. This patient's history likely is explained by a vasoocclusive crisis, a situation in which sickled cells clog the microvasculature and produce painful tissue ischemia. Sickle cell anemia also is characterized by splenic sequestration (with eventual functional asplenia and an increased risk for sepsis and osteomyelitis), cerebrovascular accidents, and acute chest syndrome. Acute chest syndrome is a severe complication of vasoocclusive disease and presents with chest pain, hypoxemia, and chest infiltrates. Because hypoxemia can instigate further sickling and pulmonary vasoocclusion, acute chest syndrome is an indication for emergent exchange transfusion.

   Answer A is incorrect. Myelofibrosis (agnogenic myeloid metaplasia) is associated with teardrop cells and nucleated RBCs on peripheral blood smear. In this disorder, dysplastic megakaryocytes produce increased fibroblast growth factors, leading to marrow fibrosis and marrow failure.

   Answer B is incorrect. Cyclical fevers are characteristic of malaria. Intracorpuscular parasites would be anticipated on peripheral blood smear.

   Answer C is incorrect. Eosinophilia is associated with parasite infection and would not explain the sickled cells seen in the image. In addition parasite infections are associated more often with iron deficiency anemia and fatigue, rather than with acute painful episodes.

   Answer D is incorrect. Microangiopathic hemolytic anemia is found in both disseminated intravascular coagulation and thrombotic thrombocytopenic purpura. Schistocytes (fragmented RBCs) are found on the blood smear.

7. **The correct answer is C.** The presentation described is typical of nephrotic syndrome. Minimal change disease is the most common cause of nephrotic syndrome in children. It is characterized by a lack of abnormalities visible by light microscopy, and it usually does not involve any abnormalities that can be seen using immunofluorescence. Only when examined with electron microscopy does the tissue show effacement of the foot processes of visceral epithelial cells (podocytes). It is thought that the

selective proteinuria that is present in minimal change disease is caused by a loss of the fixed negative charge in the glomerular filtration barrier. The disease usually responds to treatment with steroids.

Answer A is incorrect. Edema is most often caused by cirrhosis, nephrotic syndrome, or congestive heart failure (CHF). CHF in a child is uncommon. If the patient were to have CHF, a different set of symptoms would be seen, including exertional dyspnea and paroxysmal nocturnal dyspnea.

Answer B is incorrect. Thickening of the glomerular basement membrane (GBM) is seen in patients with membranous glomerulopathy, which is a leading cause of nephrotic syndrome in adults. It has characteristic findings on light microscopy (thickening of the GBM), and this is in contrast with the lack of light microscope changes for minimal change disease.

Answer D is incorrect. Urinalysis shows that the patient is losing protein in the urine, and his physical appearance is not that of protein-calorie malnutrition.

Answer E is incorrect. The answer choice describes Alport syndrome, which often causes a nephritic syndrome with gross hematuria, but less significant protein loss. This child has significant edema, suggesting that a nephrotic syndrome may be the culprit.

8. **The correct answer is A.** The findings on microscopy indicate a malignant transformation of normal cells. Increased nuclear-to-cytoplasm ratio, open chromatin, and mitotic figures indicate that cells are actively dividing. Given the patient's history of multiple sexual partners and postcoital bleeding, these cells likely indicate the presence of cervical cancer. Cervical cancer is commonly linked to human papillomavirus infection. The virus can be isolated during cytology through various methods. It is a double-stranded DNA virus.

   Answer B is incorrect. Gram-negative diplococci are not associated with cervical cancer. However, they can be found in gonorrhea cervicitis.

   Answer C is incorrect. There are no gram-positive cocci associated with cervical cancer.

   Answer D is incorrect. There is no single-stranded virus associated with cervical cancer.

   Answer E is incorrect. Squamous cells covered with bacteria can be found in bacterial vaginosis, which causes foul-smelling discharge. There is no known association between bacterial vaginosis and cervical cancer.

9. **The correct answer is E.** This patient most likely has multiple myeloma, a hematologic cancer in which the primary pathologic process is a neoplastic, monoclonal proliferation of plasma cells within the bone marrow. Common manifestations of the disease include bone pain, lytic bone lesions (which can lead to pathologic fractures), renal insufficiency, susceptibility to infection, and hypercalcemia. The primary secretory product of the plasma cells in multiple myeloma is IgG (55% of cases). IgG functions to opsonize bacteria, neutralize toxins and viruses, and fix complement in the immune response.

   Answer A is incorrect. This choice describes the function of IgA, which blocks attachment of bacteria and viruses to mucous membranes. Although IgA also is produced by plasma cells, IgA-producing multiple myelomas comprise only 25% of all cases of multiple myeloma.

   Answer B is incorrect. This choice describes the function of IgM. Although IgM also is produced by plasma cells, IgM-producing multiple myelomas are rare. Waldenström macroglobulinemia is an uncommon form of lymphoma that secretes monoclonal IgM paraprotein. This condition, however, typically is not associated with bone lesions.

   Answer C is incorrect. This answer describes the function of tumor necrosis factor-α, a critical inflammatory cytokine produced by macrophages.

   Answer D is incorrect. This choice describes the function of IgE, which mediates type I hypersensitivity reactions. Multiple myelomas producing IgE are rare.

Answer F is incorrect. This answer describes the function of histamine, which is stored in granules in mast cells and basophils. It is released in response to the cross-linking of IgE molecules on the surfaces of these cells.

Answer G is incorrect. This choice describes the function of interleukin-2, a cytokine that is important in triggering the secondary immune response. It is produced by helper T lymphocytes rather than plasma cells.

10. **The correct answer is C.** The patient most likely had adult polycystic kidney disease (APKD). Eighty-five percent of patients with this disease have a mutation in the *PKD1* gene, which is located on the short arm of chromosome 16. Patients with APKD suffer from renal failure due to multiple, large cysts in the kidney. These patients can also develop intracranial berry aneurysms (as seen in the image).

    Answer A is incorrect. Huntington disease is caused by a nucleotide repeat expansion in the Huntington gene on the short arm of chromosome 4.

    Answer B is incorrect. Marfan syndrome is caused by a mutation in the fibrillin-1 gene on the long arm of chromosome 15.

    Answer D is incorrect. Neurofibromatosis type 2 is caused by a mutation in the merlin tumor suppressor gene on the long arm of chromosome 22.

    Answer E is incorrect. Many diseases are due to mutations of the X chromosome. One example is fragile X syndrome, which is due to a nucleotide repeat expansion in the FMR1 RNA-binding protein gene on the X chromosome.

11. **The correct answer is C.** This child most likely has Angelman syndrome. Individuals with this phenotype have a characteristic facies with microcephaly, maxillary hypoplasia, deep-set eyes, and a large mouth with tongue protrusion. Their gait is jerky and "puppet-like," and their behavior is marked by frequent paroxysms of inappropriate laughter. Severe mental retardation and speech impairment are usually present, and 80%-90% of patients have epilepsy. Angelman syndrome, along with Prader-Willi syndrome, is a classic example of imprinting, which occurs when the phenotype differs depending on whether the mutation is of paternal or maternal origin. Deletions in Prader-Willi syndrome, a phenotypically distinct disorder, occur exclusively on the paternal chromosome 15, whereas deletions at the same site of chromosome 15 on the maternal chromosome result in Angelman syndrome.

    Answer A is incorrect. Anticipation is the phenomenon in which the severity of a disease worsens in succeeding generations. This occurs, for example, in triplet repeat diseases such as Huntington disease, wherein the triplet repeat tends to lengthen, age of onset decreases, and disease severity increases with successive generations. This does not occur in Angelman syndrome.

    Answer B is incorrect. Heteroplasmy describes the presence of both normal and mutated mitochondrial DNA. This phenomenon is responsible for the variable expression of mitochondrial inherited diseases.

    Answer D is incorrect. Locus heterozygosity describes the phenomenon by which mutations at different loci can result in the same phenotype. An example of this is albinism, which can be caused by a number of different mutations.

    Answer E is incorrect. Mosaicism occurs when cells in the body have different genetic makeup. This sometimes occurs, for example, in Turner syndrome. This does not occur in Angelman syndrome.

12. **The correct answer is D.** The image demonstrates micronodular cirrhosis, typically seen with regenerative nodules with thick collagenous septa. Some proliferation of bile ducts is also seen. This microscopic view of the liver is most consistent with cirrhosis. In end-stage disease, it is often difficult to determine the primary etiology, but the most common cause in the Western World is alcoholic liver disease (60-70% of cases), followed by viral

hepatitis. An important feature of cirrhosis is that the normal architecture is disrupted. This can lead to impedance of blood and bile flow, causing portal hypertension and/or cholestasis with jaundice. The early stages of alcoholic liver disease, such as steatosis (build-up of lipid droplets within cells) and alcoholic hepatitis, are reversible if alcohol use is discontinued. However, once the process of fibrosis begins, it is irreversible.

Answer A is incorrect. In cirrhosis, hepatocyte regeneration continues between the fibrous septae, forming uniform "micronodules." Thus, although the liver ultimately loses its function and normal architecture, regeneration of hepatocytes still occurs.

Answer B is incorrect. Steatosis is characterized by accumulation of lipid droplets within hepatocytes. This is a common characteristic in many disease states such as alcoholic and nonalcoholic steatohepatitis, the latter of which is strongly associated with obesity and hyperlipidemia. It is important to remember that these disease states are often reversible when the offending agent (eg, alcohol use or high serum lipid levels) is removed. However, if untreated, these conditions can eventually progress to cirrhosis. Regenerative nodules and fibrotic bands are not seen in steatosis.

Answer C is incorrect. Mallory bodies, degenerating hepatocytes full of eosinophilic cytoplasmic inclusions, are common in alcoholic hepatitis. Alcoholic hepatitis is also characterized by neutrophilic infiltrates, ballooning of hepatocytes, and cytokeratin intermediate filaments. However, the characteristic nodular regeneration with scarring seen in cirrhosis is not a feature of alcoholic hepatitis. If alcohol use continues over years, alcoholic hepatitis progresses to cirrhosis. However, Mallory bodies are rare in the cirrhotic liver.

Answer E is incorrect. In alcoholic hepatitis, the fatty and inflamed liver will be larger than normal and usually weighs >2 kg. However, as cirrhosis develops over years of continued alcohol use, the liver becomes fibrotic and shrinks. It can sometimes weigh as little as 1 kg.

13. **The correct answer is A.** This patient has developed nasopharyngeal carcinoma, a condition common in certain parts of the world, including Asia and Africa. Development of this tumor is always associated with infection by Epstein-Barr virus (EBV), a DNA virus in the herpesvirus family. Development of this tumor is believed to be related to a synergistic interaction between EBV and a diet high in carcinogenic nitrosamines (common in foods that has been smoked or preserved). Common symptoms include nasal congestion, epistaxis, ear infections (due to tumor-induced blockage of the eustachian tubes), and headache.

    Answer B is incorrect. Many bacteria are capable of infecting the nasopharynx; however, none are directly associated with malignancy.

    Answer C is incorrect. Nasopharyngeal zygomycosis is a condition that could present with these symptoms in an immunocompromised patient. However, biopsy would show filamentous nonseptate hyphae and a granulomatous response.

    Answer D is incorrect. Although a tuberculoma in the nasopharynx can be confused with a nasopharyngeal tumor, biopsy would show caseating granulomas with multinucleated giant cells.

    Answer E is incorrect. Although a retrovirus such as HIV can create an immunocompromised state favoring the development of a malignancy, it is not the direct cause of tumor formation. Lymphomas can be associated with the retrovirus human T-cell lymphoma virus; however, biopsy would show sheets of malignant T lymphocytes typical of this lymphoma. Other RNA viruses are not associated with malignancy.

14. **The correct answer is B.** The abdominal radiograph shows staghorn renal calculus in the left kidney. A stone that involves the renal medulla and extends into at least two calyces is considered a staghorn calculus. Approximately three quarters of all staghorn calculi are caused by struvite stones. Struvite stones are made up of a phosphate mineral that requires an alkaline urine to precipitate.

Answer A is incorrect. Acidic urine would hinder formation of staghorn calculi.

Answer C is incorrect. Presence of ammonia (not ammonium) in urine is a requirement for formation of staghorn calculi, which allows for crystallization of magnesium ammonium phosphate and carbonate apatite.

Answer D is incorrect. Sodium chloride is not usually a component of renal calculi and is not required for their formation.

Answer E is incorrect. Uric acid is a component of some renal calculi but is not radiopaque and is not part of staghorn calculi.

15. **The correct answer is C.** The image shows the typical large, round, intranuclear inclusion with perinuclear halo that is seen in cells affected by cytomegalovirus (CMV) infection. These structures are called "owl's eyes" due to their microscopic appearance. In immunocompromised patients, CMV infection can present as retinitis, pneumonitis, inflammation along the GI tract, polyradiculopathy, transverse myelitis, and focal encephalitis. In patients with HIV/AIDS, these sequelae occur most prominently when the CD4+ cell count is $<100/mm^3$ or when the HIV viral load is $>10,000$ copies/mm^3. CMV can cause further immunosuppression, leading to other opportunistic infections such as *Pneumocystis* and *Aspergillus* pneumonia.

Answer A is incorrect. *Candida* is a fungus that produces a wide spectrum of diseases, ranging from superficial mucocutaneous disease in immunocompetent hosts to invasive illnesses in immunocompromised hosts. Histology reveals round or ovoid yeast cells, hyphae, or pseudohyphae.

Answer B is incorrect. *Cryptococcus neoformans* causes meningitis and meningoencephalitis in patients with AIDS. This fungus is difficult to observe with routine hematoxylin and eosin stains, so methenamine silver or periodic acid-Schiff stains are used to identify the characteristic narrow-based buds and round-to-oval yeast, surrounded by a polysaccharide capsule.

Answer D is incorrect. Herpes simplex virus in HIV-infected individuals can cause recurrent orolabial, genital, and perianal lesions. A Tzanck smear is positive for multinucleated epithelial giant cells. It does not cause the large intranuclear inclusion body shown.

Answer E is incorrect. *Mycobacterium avium* causes lung disease in immunocompromised hosts and is subsequently spread via the blood to the liver, spleen, bone marrow, and other sites. Histology of mycobacterium is not consistent with this image. Rather, acid-fast staining would show organisms in foamy macrophages, granulomas, giant cells, and cells with eosinophilic necrosis.

Answer F is incorrect. *Pneumocystis jiroveci* (formerly *carinii*) causes pneumonia in immunocompromised individuals.

16. **The correct answer is D.** Hereditary hemochromatosis is an iron-overload disease caused by mutations in the *HFE* gene. Patients classically present with the triad of diabetes, cirrhosis, and bronze skin pigmentation. This patient has many of the signs of advanced hereditary hemochromatosis: diabetes due to pancreatic iron deposition, heart failure as a result of cardiac iron deposition, cirrhosis from hepatic iron deposition, and testicular atrophy as a result of dysfunction of the hypothalamic-pituitary system from iron deposition. In addition, one of his siblings is also affected, indicating the autosomal recessive nature of the disease. The brown granular pigment in hepatocytes seen in the image suggests hemosiderosis, but an iron stain (Prussian blue) is also necessary because the brown pigment resembles lipofuscin in hematoxylin and eosin stains.

Answer A is incorrect. α_1-Antitrypsin deficiency is due to mutations in the protease inhibitor gene on chromosome 14. α_1-Antitrypsin is a protein produced in the liver and has a number of functions, the most common being protection of the lungs from elastase, an enzyme produced by neutrophils. Patients with a deficiency in this protein may present with respiratory complaints and can develop emphysema. In some patients, cirrhosis may occur due to accumulation of α_1-antitrypsin in the liver. Histopathologic examination would not show brown granular pigment in hepatocytes. Rather, microscopic examination of a liver biopsy would show periodic acid Schiff-positive, diastase-resistant globules in hepatocytes.

Answer B is incorrect. Intracytoplasmic hyaline inclusions derived from cytokeratin intermediate filaments called Mallory bodies and microvesicular steatosis are common findings in alcoholic hepatitis. Accumulation of iron is not associated with this condition.

Answer C is incorrect. Cystic fibrosis is an autosomal recessive disease caused by mutations in the *CFTR* gene on chromosome 7. This gene encodes for a chloride ion channel. Patients typically present early in life with meconium ileus, multiple respiratory tract infections, or failure to thrive. Patients typically have a number of upper and lower pulmonary manifestations, especially recurrent respiratory infections. Patients also have GI symptoms due to insufficient release of pancreatic enzymes for digestion. This causes protein and fat malabsorption, leading to steatorrhea and fat-soluble vitamin deficiencies.

Answer E is incorrect. Wilson disease is an autosomal recessive disease of copper accumulation in various tissues. It is due to mutations in the *ATP7B* gene, which encodes a copper-transporting ATPase. Patients may have a variety of hepatic manifestations, ranging from asymptomatic hepatomegaly to acute fulminant hepatitis. They also have neurologic manifestations such as tremor, dysarthria, or gait abnormalities. Psychiatric manifestations, such as mood or personality changes, are also common, and Kayser-Fleischer rings are evident on ophthalmic exam in almost all patients. This patient's liver biopsy does not show any changes specific to Wilson disease.

17. **The correct answer is E.** This HIV-positive patient has multiple anogenital warts, or condylomata acuminata, which are caused by human papillomavirus (HPV) types 6 and 11. A feared complication of condylomata acuminata is anorectal cancer, as seen here. Immunodeficiency predisposes to the development of HPV-induced transformation. The mechanism of HPV-induced transformation involves the production of a viral protein, E6, which binds to a cellular ubiquitin ligase E6AP. On binding to E6, E6AP polyubiquitinates the tumor suppressor p53, leading to dysregulated cell proliferation and, eventually, oncogenesis.

    Answer A is incorrect. *APC* is a tumor suppressor gene mutated in certain hereditary forms of colon cancer. The APC protein normally degrades the transcription factor β-catenin, which is involved in colonic epithelial cell proliferation. In the absence of APC, increased levels of β-catenin accumulate, eventually leading to oncogenesis.

    Answer B is incorrect. *BRCA1* is a tumor suppressor gene commonly mutated in hereditary forms of breast and ovarian cancers. The BRCA1 protein functions in DNA repair processes, and inherited mutations in BRCA1 interfere with DNA repair, leading to the accumulation of mutations and, eventually, oncogenesis.

    Answer C is incorrect. The *MSH2* gene regulates a mismatch repair enzyme and is mutated in certain hereditary forms of colon cancer. In the absence of MSH2, increased levels of DNA mutations accumulate, leading to eventual cellular transformation.

    Answer D is incorrect. *NF1* is a tumor suppressor gene mutated in neurofibromatosis type 1. The NF1 protein functions as a GTPase activating protein for the small G protein Ras. Because Ras is only active when it is GTP-bound, NF1-mediated GTP hydrolysis leads to inactivation of Ras. In the absence of NF1, Ras is hyperactive, leading to enhanced growth factor signal transduction and, eventually, oncogenesis.

18. **The correct answer is A.** The boy's brain biopsy demonstrates medulloblastoma. This is a poorly differentiated neuroectodermal tumor that occurs predominantly in children and exclusively in the cerebellum. The cerebellar vermis is the medial section of the cerebellum and is responsible for proximal muscle coordi-

nation, balance, and vestibulo-ocular reflexes. As seen in this patient, lesions of the vermis lead to vertigo, nausea, and difficulties in coordinating movement of trunk and proximal limb muscles. The presence of medulloblastoma commonly leads to obstruction of the outflow of CSF and the potential for hydrocephalus, a life-threatening condition.

Answer B is incorrect. Medulloblastomas arise in the midline of the cerebellum in children. The intermediate section of the cerebellar hemisphere is more lateral than the vermis. Lesions in the intermediate section would cause deficits in coordinating movements of the ipsilateral distal extremities, not the vertigo and proximal limb problems seen in this patient.

Answer C is incorrect. Medulloblastomas arise in the midline of the cerebellum in children. Lesions of the lateral hemisphere would likely cause deficits in planning movements of the ipsilateral distal extremities, not the vertigo and proximal limb problems seen in this patient.

Answer D is incorrect. Medulloblastomas arise in the midline of the cerebellum in children, not in the occipital cortex. Occipital cortex lesions could lead to defects in vision, not the vertigo and proximal limb problems seen in this patient.

Answer E is incorrect. Medulloblastomas arise in the midline of the cerebellum in children, not in the parietal cortex. The postcentral gyrus of the parietal lobe is the primary somatosensory cortex. Lesions of this area would cause sensory deficits, not the vertigo and proximal limb problems seen in this patient.

19. **The correct answer is B.** This image demonstrates an advanced case of mesothelioma, diffusely involving the pleura and encasing lung parenchyma. The clinical history supports this diagnosis. Asbestos is present in certain building materials and fire-resistant materials, and exposure to asbestos is a risk factor for the development of mesothelioma.

Answer A is incorrect. Aflatoxin B is produced by *Aspergillus* and is a common contaminant of cereals, spices, and nuts. It has been associated with carcinoma of the liver.

Answer C is incorrect. Long-term exposure to high levels of benzene can lead to leukemia and Hodgkin lymphoma. Benzene is the main component of light oil, and is found in gasoline and other fuels.

Answer D is incorrect. Cadmium is a carcinogen associated with the development of prostate cancer. It can be found in batteries and in metal coatings.

Answer E is incorrect. Exposure to silica may occur in the manufacturing of several materials, such as glass, ceramics, and electronics. Silicosis is characterized by bilateral, fine nodularity in the upper lung lobes. It is slowly progressive. Its role as a carcinogen is controversial.

20. **The correct answer is D.** This boy most likely suffers from Eisenmenger syndrome, which is demonstrated by the cyanosis and digital clubbing. In Eisenmenger syndrome a ventricular septal defect (VSD), atrial septal defect (ASD), or patent ductus arteriosus causes a left-to-right shunt and thus an acyanotic lesion, which is why he has been asymptomatic for much of his life. Over time the uncorrected shunt reverses as the right ventricle hypertrophies in response to increased pulmonary vascular resistance, and becomes a right-to-left shunt and thus acyanotic heart disease. The resultant low blood oxygen levels can lead to the development of exercise intolerance, cyanosis, and clubbing of the fingers as seen in this patient.

Answer A is incorrect. Patients with bicuspid aortic valves often have no symptoms, but later in life the valve can become calcified, leading to premature aortic stenosis in the fifth and sixth decades. However, bicuspid aortic valve is an unlikely cause of symptoms such as cyanosis and clubbing in a 12-year-old child.

Answer B is incorrect. Before the development of Eisenmenger syndrome, congenital defects such as VSD, ASD, and patent ductus arteriosus produced a left-to-right shunt. However, this boy's symptoms indicate that the direction of the shunt has reversed.

Answer C is incorrect. Mitral regurgitation classically produces a holosystolic murmur that radiates to the axilla. Although chronic mitral regurgitation can lead to CHF, it is an unlikely cause of symptoms such as cyanosis and clubbing in a 12-year-old child.

Answer E is incorrect. A holosystolic murmur may be heard in the setting of endocarditis, and valvular vegetations would be seen on echocardiogram. However, this would not explain the boy's other symptoms.

CHAPTER 7

Pharmacology

QUESTIONS

1. AIDS is currently managed with highly active anti-retroviral therapy, combining a series of medications to overwhelm the virus and minimize its ability to form resistance to any one of the medications. Currently, protease inhibitors, nucleoside reverse transcriptase inhibitors, and non-nucleoside reverse transcriptase inhibitors are three types of medications that can be used in combination. Which of the following is a non-competitive reverse transcriptase inhibitor?

   (A) Didanosine
   (B) Lamivudine
   (C) Nevirapine
   (D) Saquinavir
   (E) Zidovudine

2. A patient is being treated with β-blockers for hypertension. Which of the following describes the effects of β-blockers on end-diastolic volume (EDV), blood pressure (BP), contractility, heart rate (HR), and ejection time?

Choice	EDV	BP	Contractility	HR	Ejection time
A	no effect or ↓	↓	little/no effect	↓	little/no effect
B	↓	↓	↓	↑	↓
C	↓	↓	↓	↓	↓
D	↑	↓	↓	↓	↑
E	↓	↓	↑	↑	↓

   (A) A
   (B) B
   (C) C
   (D) D
   (E) E

3. A 68-year-old woman with type 2 diabetes mellitus and a 30-pound weight loss over the past two months presents to the physician with a history of nausea and bloating. Symptoms are most prominent following a meal. An outpatient gastric emptying study shows esophageal dysmotility. The best treatment option for this patient is which of the following?

   (A) Esophageal resection
   (B) Metoclopramide
   (C) Omeprazole
   (D) Ondansetron
   (E) Vagotomy

4. Patients with hyperthyroidism have several options to treat their disease, including subtotal thyroidectomy and radioactive ablation. When a patient is unwilling or unable to undergo these procedures, pharmacological therapy is often pursued. One particular medication inhibits the conversion of iodide to iodine and inhibits the organification of iodine with tyrosine. Which of the following is an additional mechanism of action of this drug?

   (A) Permanently reducing thyroid activity
   (B) Binding to and blocking the iodide transport mechanism of thyroid follicular cells
   (C) Binding to intracellular nuclear receptors of peripheral tissue and activating genes
   (D) Blocking the peripheral conversion of thyroxine to triiodothyronine
   (E) Inhibiting the binding of thyroxine to thyroid-binding globulin

5. A 36-year-old man who works at an explosives factory comes to the clinic for an annual check-up. He is concerned about long-term exposure to industrial chemicals. He reports that although he is in excellent health otherwise, he experiences headaches, dizziness, and palpitations every Monday. Laboratory studies show:

   WBC count: 8000/mm^3
   Hematocrit: 46%
   Hemoglobin: 15 g/dL
   Platelet count: 310,000/mm^3
   Na^+: 137 mEq/L
   K^+: 3.5 mEq/L
   Cl^-: 102 mEq/L

HCO_3^-: 24 mEq/L
Blood urea nitrogen: 12 mg/dL
Creatinine: 1.0 mg/dL

An ECG shows normal sinus rhythm with no Q wave changes. Which of the following is the most likely serious complication that can occur as a result of his exposure?

(A) Anemia
(B) Atherosclerosis
(C) Cardiac arrest
(D) Congestive heart failure
(E) Dementia

6. A 30-year-old woman presents to her physician with a two-month history of menorrhagia. She has also noticed significant fatigue over the past five weeks and some blood on her toothbrush every day during this time. Laboratory tests show a WBC count of 80,000/mm^3, hemoglobin of 8.6 g/dL, hematocrit of 25%, and platelet count of 80,000/mm^3. Bone marrow smear reveals the following image. Which of the following is the best choice for therapy?

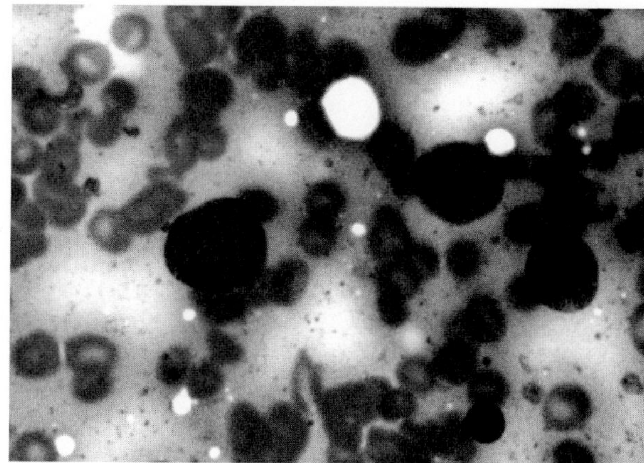

Reproduced, with permission, from USMLERx.com.

(A) All-*trans* retinoic acid
(B) Cytarabine
(C) Daunorubicin
(D) Fludarabine
(E) Irinotecan

7. A 70-year-old man presents to his cardiologist with shortness of breath, crackles along both lung bases, and 1+ pitting edema in his lower extremities. His cardiologist diagnoses him with mild congestive heart failure and places him on a thiazide diuretic. Two days later, the patient comes to the emergency department obtunded and oliguric, with a highly elevated creatinine level of 8.3 mg/dL. His wife reports that the only medication that he took besides his diuretic was "some ibuprofen for his headache." Which of the following is the most likely reason for this patient's sudden renal failure?

(A) Decrease of prostaglandin E_2 production in both arterioles of the kidney
(B) Decrease of prostaglandin E_2 production in the afferent arterioles of the kidney
(C) Decrease of prostaglandin E_2 production in the efferent arterioles of the kidney
(D) Increase of prostaglandin E_2 production in the afferent arterioles of the kidney
(E) Increase of prostaglandin E_2 production in the efferent arterioles of the kidney

8. A 42-year-old woman comes to a follow-up appointment complaining of weight gain two weeks after beginning a new medication for her refractory schizophrenia. Laboratory studies show a low WBC count and low absolute neutrophil count. Peripheral blood smear shows a total absence of neutrophils and bands. The rest of the laboratory results are within normal limits. Which of the following drug therapies did this patient most likely begin two weeks ago?

(A) Chloramphenicol
(B) Clozapine
(C) Metronidazole
(D) Penicillin
(E) Polymyxin B

9. A 64-year-old man develops chronic renal failure. He has an extensive medical history, and also complains of increasingly poor vision in his right eye. After a kidney biopsy is taken (see image), his physician immediately starts him on a new medication. What pharmacologic treatment has been shown to most effectively delay the progression of the pathology shown in this photomicrograph?

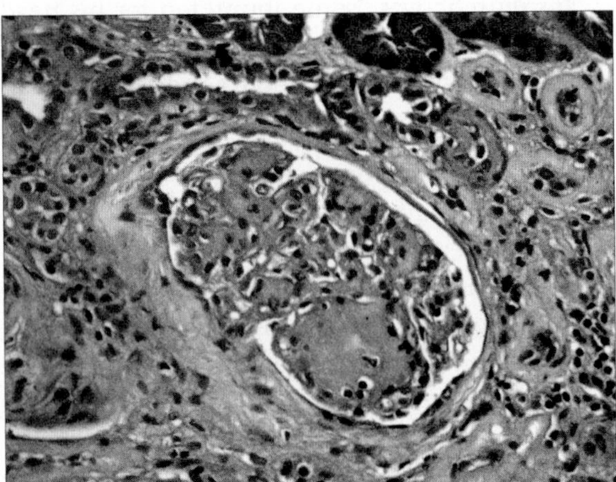

Reproduced, with permission, from USMLERx.com.

(A) Angiotensin-converting enzyme inhibitors
(B) β-Blockers
(C) Cyclophosphamide
(D) Prednisone
(E) Thiazides

10. A 74-year-old man comes to the physician complaining of increased urinary frequency along with difficulty starting and stopping urination. His wife states that he wakes her up multiple times throughout the night when he hurries to the bathroom, yet is unable to urinate. Diagnostic work-up reveals a benign condition. Which of the following is the mechanism of action of a common medication used to treat this condition?

(A) Formation of superoxide radicals that attack DNA bonds
(B) Gonadotropin-releasing hormone analog
(C) Inhibition of 5-α-reductase
(D) Inhibition of cGMP-specific phosphodiesterase type 5
(E) Inhibition of cytochrome P450 enzymes
(F) Inhibition of testosterone's negative feedback on gonadotropin secretion

11. Following the discovery of a suspicious abandoned package on the subway, a number of passengers present to the emergency department with abdominal cramps, vomiting, shortness of breath, and generalized weakness. Physical examination of these patients reveals excessive perspiration, bilateral wheezes, bradycardia, and miosis. Which of the following is the most appropriate treatment for these patients?

(A) Echothiophate
(B) Hexamethonium
(C) Pancuronium
(D) Pralidoxime
(E) Pyridostigmine

12. The targets of multiple lipid-lowering agents are labeled in the image. Which of the targets corresponds to the therapy associated with the most significant decrease in triglyceride levels?

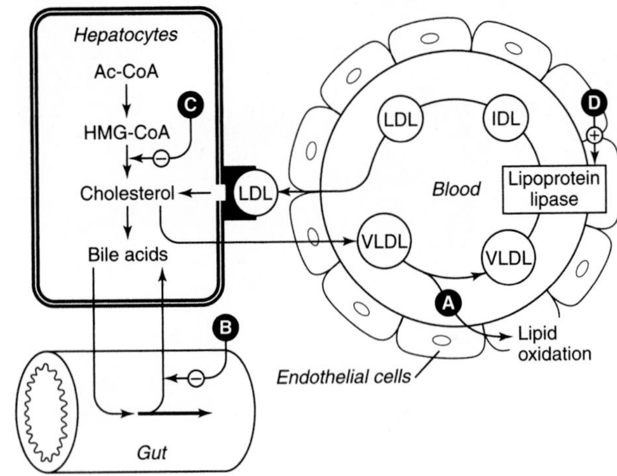

Reproduced, with permission, from USMLERx.com.

(A) A
(B) B
(C) C
(D) D

13. A 67-year-old man previously diagnosed with Hodgkin lymphoma complains of severe shortness of breath when he walks or climbs stairs. Examination reveals regular venous pressure of 18 cm H_2O, bi-basilar rales, an S_3 gallop, and 2+ lower-extremity edema. His physician suspects an adverse effect of treatment is causing this patient's symptoms. The pharmacologic agent most likely responsible for the symptoms in this patient has the same mechanism of action as which of the following cancer drugs?

(A) Cisplatin
(B) Cyclophosphamide
(C) Dactinomycin
(D) Methotrexate
(E) Paclitaxel

14. A 68-year-old man with a history of stroke and hypertension comes to the emergency department because of a five-hour history of palpitations and light-headedness. He states that he has experienced shorter episodes of palpitations before, but nothing as severe as this. Physical examination reveals an irregular heart rhythm that eventually improves with various atrioventricular node blocking agents. The patient is prescribed a regimen of daily medications including a drug to prevent a potential complication of his condition. Which of the following drugs is most likely prescribed long-term to prevent such complications?

(A) Aspirin
(B) Protamine sulfate
(C) Streptokinase
(D) Unfractionated heparin
(E) Warfarin

15. Drug X has a half-life of 50 hours and a volume of distribution of 5 L. Which of the following is the clearance of drug X?

(A) 0.07 L/h
(B) 0.1 L/h
(C) 70 L/h
(D) 175 L/h
(E) 250 L/h

16. A 33-year-old immigrant from Peru comes to a women's health clinic because she has missed her period for the past two months. When her pregnancy test comes back positive, she becomes distraught, saying that she has been taking oral contraceptive pills for the past year and has not missed a single dose. As she starts to cry, her tears are noted to have an orange tint. The physician tells her that the most likely reason her oral contraceptives were ineffective is an interaction with one of her other medications. What is the mechanism of action of the drug that the patient is taking?

(A) Formation of toxic metabolites that has a bactericidal effect
(B) Blocks sodium channels, which prevents the release of the excitatory neurotransmitter glutamate from the presynaptic neurons
(C) Cationic and basic proteins bind to the cell membrane and disrupt the osmotic properties
(D) Blocks RNA synthesis by inhibiting DNA-dependent RNA polymerase
(E) Prolongs action potential phases I and III via blockage of sodium and potassium channels

17. A patient presents to his primary care physician. On his last visit, he was diagnosed with hypertension and started on hydrochlorothiazide. What electrolyte changes would you now expect to see in this patient with diuretic use?

Choice	Urine sodium	Urine potassium	Blood pH
A	↓	↑	↑
B	↑	↓	↓
C	↑	↑	↓
D	↑	↑	↑

Reproduced, with permission, from USMLERx.com.

(A) A
(B) B
(C) C
(D) D

18. A 35-year-old African-American woman presents to her gynecologist because of lower abdominal pain. She is diagnosed with an eight-week gestational age, ectopic pregnancy and treated medically. A few months later she returns complaining of vaginal bleeding and is diagnosed with a gestational choriocarcinoma. Her physician chooses the same drug to treat this cancer that he used to treat her ectopic pregnancy. Which of the following drugs is indicated in the treatment of both ectopic pregnancy and gestational choriocarcinoma?

    (A) Methotrexate
    (B) Mifepristone
    (C) Misoprostol
    (D) Rifampin
    (E) Tamoxifen

19. A 24-year-old law student has been experiencing frequent headaches over the course of the last several months, for which he has been taking increasing doses of aspirin. After a long night of studies, he takes a particularly large dose of aspirin; he later becomes disoriented, confused, and then experiences a seizure. He is brought to the emergency department by his roommate, where his serum salicylate level is 130 mg/dL. Which of the following is the most appropriate treatment?

    (A) Protamine
    (B) Glucagon
    (C) N-acetylcysteine
    (D) Bicarbonate
    (E) Vitamin K

20. A 59-year-old man who is receiving immunosuppressive therapy develops the tender red vesicles seen in this image. His lesions respond to acyclovir. Which of the following best describes the infection shown in this image?

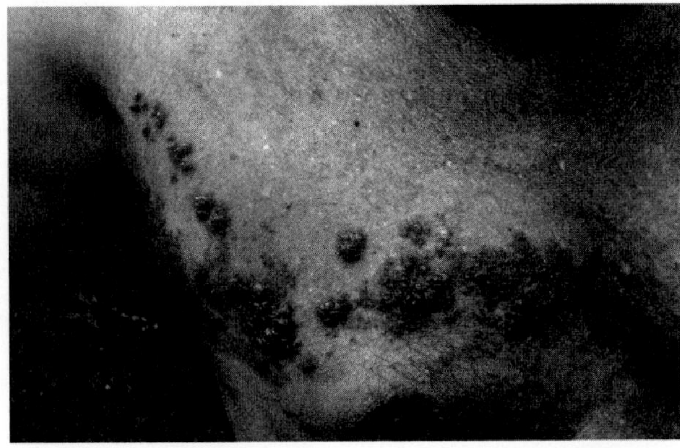

Courtesy of Wikipedia.

    (A) The current symptoms are only manifest once the virus has developed a novel RNA polymerase
    (B) The infective virions contain viral thymidine kinase
    (C) The viral reverse transcriptase may be inhibited by acyclovir
    (D) The virus incorporates host cell proteases into its genome in order to cleave and activate the viral polyprotein
    (E) Treatment with acyclovir is preventing the virus from synthesizing its own guanine nucleotides

21. A 4-year-old girl is brought by her mother to the emergency department complaining of severe abdominal pain. Her mother reports that the girl has ingested 10-15 chocolate-coated iron tablets she had found in her grandmother's purse, presumably thinking they were candy. Soon after arriving the patient begins to vomit bright red blood. Physical examination shows hypotension and tachycardia. Which of the following is the best initial treatment for this patient?

    (A) Aminocaproic acid
    (B) Deferoxamine
    (C) Dimercaprol
    (D) Oral bicarbonate
    (E) Penicillamine

22. A 43-year-old woman presents to the emergency department following a motor vehicle collision. She did not sustain any serious physical injuries, but she appears drowsy and states that she is feeling very sleepy. Emergency medical staff collected several open medication bottles from the floor of her automobile. Although the contents of two of the bottles could not be determined, the patient's recently filled bottle of diazepam was almost empty. The patient quickly becomes unresponsive and stops breathing. Administration of which of the following agents will reverse these symptoms?

(A) Flumazenil
(B) Glucagon
(C) Midazolam
(D) Naloxone
(E) Physostigmine

23. The image shows the dose-response curves for the agonist drug X administered alone, and several possible curves representing drug X administered with other agents. Which of the following curves, A through E, represents the activity of drug X when it is administered with a noncompetitive antagonist?

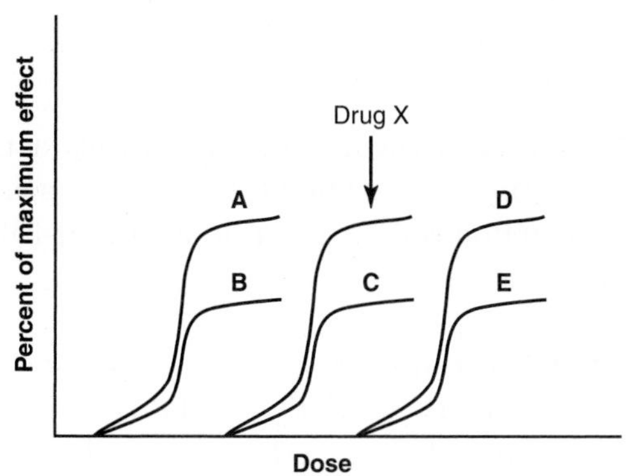

Reproduced, with permission, from USMLERx.com.

(A) Curve A
(B) Curve B
(C) Curve C
(D) Curve D
(E) Curve E

24. Class I antiarrhythmics are sodium channel blockers that slow or block cardiac conduction, especially in depolarized cells. Which of the following antiarrhythmics will increase both the action potential and the effective refractory period?

(A) Encainide
(B) Mexiletine
(C) Procainamide
(D) Propafenone
(E) Tocainide

25. A 68-year-old man complains of gradually progressive fatigue, shortness of breath, and a 5.9-kg (13-lb) unintentional weight gain. He denies chest pain, fevers, chills, and night sweats. Physical examination reveals 3+ bilateral pitting edema in the lower extremities. X-ray of the chest shows cardiomegaly and pulmonary venous congestion. Echocardiography shows severe left ventricular dilatation and global hypokinesis, with an ejection fraction of 25%. He is placed on a pharmacologic regimen including digoxin. At which point in the image is digoxin a direct inhibitor?

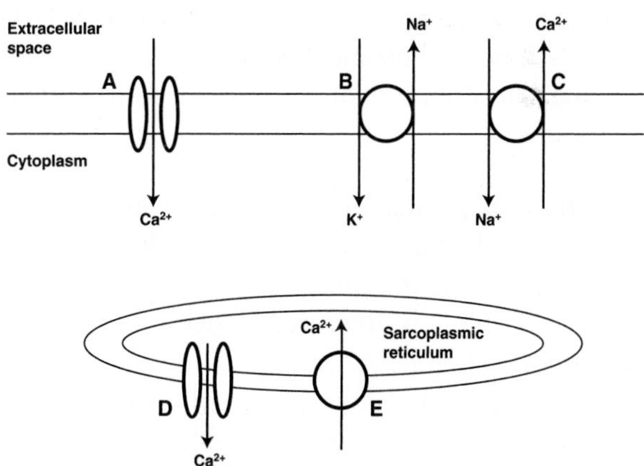

Reproduced, with permission, from USMLERx.com.

(A) A
(B) B
(C) C
(D) D
(E) E

ANSWERS

1. **The correct answer is C.** Nevirapine is a non-nucleoside reverse transcriptase inhibitor (NNRTI). NNRTIs function by binding to the reverse transcriptase enzyme and acting as a noncompetitive inhibitor. Noncompetitive inhibitors bind to a site on the enzyme other than the active site.

   Answer A is incorrect. Didanosine is a nucleoside reverse transcriptase inhibitor. It can cause pancreatitis in some individuals.

   Answer B is incorrect. Lamivudine is a nucleoside reverse transcriptase inhibitor. It functions by binding to the active site of the reverse transcriptase enzyme to inactivate it. It has very few adverse effects and can also be used to treat hepatitis B.

   Answer D is incorrect. Saquinavir is a protease inhibitor that blocks the enzyme necessary for the creation of new viral proteins.

   Answer E is incorrect. Zidovudine, or AZT, is a nucleoside reverse transcriptase inhibitor. It functions by binding to the active site of the reverse transcriptase enzyme to inactivate it. HIV will quickly become resistant to AZT if not taken in conjunction with other antiretroviral drugs.

2. **The correct answer is D.** β-Blockers decrease contractility and heart rate (resulting in decreased oxygen consumption) by inhibiting β-1 receptors in the heart. A decrease in heart rate will then allow more time for diastolic filling (increasing EDV) and systolic ejection (increasing ejection time). In addition, β-blockers will decrease the secretion of renin, which will decrease aldosterone by extension and further reduce blood pressure.

   Answer A is incorrect. Answer A does not reflect the effects of β-blockers.

   Answer B is incorrect. Answer B does not reflect the effects of β-blockers.

   Answer C is incorrect. Answer C does not reflect the effects of β-blockers.

   Answer E is incorrect. Answer E is compatible with the effects of nitrates. These drugs serve to decrease the afterload on the heart by vasodilation. However, vasodilation produces a reflex increase in both contractility and heart rate. An increase in heart rate causes a decrease in EDV and ejection time.

3. **The correct answer is B.** This patient presents with gastroparesis, specifically esophageal dysmotility, secondary to her diabetes. Other causes of esophageal dysmotility include diabetic gastroparesis, Chagas disease, lupus, and other collagen vascular diseases. Initial treatment consists of promotility agents, with metoclopramide being first-line therapy.

   Answer A is incorrect. Esophageal resection is the treatment for squamous cell carcinoma or adenocarcinoma of the esophagus or for high-grade Barrett esophagus.

   Answer C is incorrect. Omeprazole is a proton pump inhibitor used to treat gastroesophageal reflux disease, peptic ulcer disease, and acid hypersecretion.

   Answer D is incorrect. Ondansetron is a 5-HT_3 receptor antagonist used to treat refractory or severe nausea and vomiting.

   Answer E is incorrect. Vagotomy is a treatment option for peptic ulcer disease or acid hypersecretion states such as in Zollinger-Ellison syndrome.

4. **The correct answer is D.** The drug described is propylthiouracil (PTU), a standard agent in the treatment of hyperthyroidism. This agent inhibits both the conversion of iodide to elemental iodine and the organification of iodine with tyrosine, therefore blocking the production of mono- and diiodotyrosine within thyroid follicular cells. In addition, PTU inhibits the peripheral conversion of thyroxine (T_4) to triiodothyronine (T_3), the most active biological form of thyroid hormone; T_3 is approximately 10 times more potent than T_4. The majority of T_3 is converted in the periph-

eral tissue, liver, and kidneys. Two important adverse effects of PTU are exfoliative skin rash (most common) and agranulocytosis (most severe, but fortunately quite rare).

Answer A is incorrect. Propylthiouracil has no effect on the binding of T_3 to the thyroid hormone receptor.

Answer B is incorrect. Perchlorate and thiocyanate are two ionic inhibitors that block the thyroid's ability to sequester iodide. These drugs are rarely used today but have been used to treat Graves disease and amiodarone-induced thyrotoxicosis.

Answer C is incorrect. This describes the mechanism of levothyroxine, the drug most commonly used in to treat hypothyroidism. It is an analog of endogenous T_4. Also used in neonates with thyroid deficiency, this medication can prevent mental retardation if administered within two weeks of delivery.

Answer E is incorrect. This describes radioactive iodine, which is used patients >21 years old who have hyperthyroidism. It is the preferred drug to treat Graves disease that it is refractory to antithyroid drugs or when surgery fails.

5. **The correct answer is C.** This patient's symptoms suggest that he is experiencing nitroglycerin withdrawal. Nitroglycerine is a vasodilator. Chronic industrial exposure leads to tolerance for vasodilatation on work days and a compensatory vasoconstriction on weekends when the exposure is removed, thus resulting in the "Monday disease." The most severe consequence is when the compensatory vasoconstriction is unopposed in critical areas such as the coronary vessels, leading ischemia due to decreased blood flow.

   Answer A is incorrect. Anemia can be a result of lead or other heavy metal poisoning, but not nitroglycerin.

   Answer B is incorrect. Atherosclerosis is formed by fatty streak deposition, which along with endothelial damage results in plaque formation over time. It is not linked to nitroglycerin exposure.

   Answer D is incorrect. Congestive heart failure (CHF) can be a complication of long-term coronary artery disease or a myocardial infarction (MI), but not of nitroglycerin exposure.

   Answer E is incorrect. Dementia can be a result of neurotoxin exposures (eg, mercury). Nitroglycerin exposure does not cause dementia.

6. **The correct answer is A.** This patient is presenting with acute promyelocytic leukemia (APL), the cancer most frequently associated with disseminated intravascular coagulation and bleeding diatheses. Typically these patients present with anemia, fatigue, and bleeding. The age of this patient points to acute myelogenous leukemia (AML), and the image confirms that this patient has the promyelocytic type by showing abundant promyelocytes with azurophilic granules. APL can often be treated by differentiating the malignant cells into mature neutrophils, which have a life span of approximately seven days. The cells harbor a t(15;17) translocation, making the retinoic acid receptor responsible for their transformation, and the cells can be differentiated using high-dose all-*trans* retinoic acid.

   Answer B is incorrect. Cytarabine is a nucleotide analog that is incorporated into DNA, subsequently inhibiting DNA polymerase and RNA polymerase. It is used to treat AML, but is not as specific or effective in APL therapy.

   Answer C is incorrect. Daunorubicin is an anthracycline that inhibits topoisomerase II and intercalates into DNA, preventing relegation during mitosis and, in turn, introducing double-strand breaks. It is used in acute lymphocytic leukemia and AML, but is not as specific or helpful in treating APL.

   Answer D is incorrect. Fludarabine is an ATP analog that inhibits DNA polymerase, DNA primase, and RNA reductase, blocking DNA synthesis. It is often used to treat chronic lymphocytic leukemia. It can also be used to treat AML, but is not specific to APL.

   Answer E is incorrect. Irinotecan is a topoisomerase I inhibitor, preventing ligation of single-strand breaks when it forms a complex with DNA and this enzyme. As the cell attempts to replicate its DNA, much damage is done when DNA polymerase encounters the complex, leading to cell death. Again, this drug is not specific to APL.

7. **The correct answer is A.** The photomicrograph shows Kimmelstiel-Wilson nodules, which are pathognomonic for diabetic nephropathy. Even without recognizing this specific histopathology, however, one should be reminded of diabetes due to the combination of renal and visual findings (diabetic nephropathy and retinopathy). Angiotensin-converting enzyme (ACE) inhibitors are the drugs of choice in the control of diabetes-induced renal disease because they reduce systemic blood pressure, reduce the effects of angiotensin II (AT II) on efferent arterioles, and attenuate the stimulatory effect of AT II on glomerular cell growth and matrix production. ACE inhibitors have been conclusively shown to delay the time to end-stage renal disease by 50% in type 1 diabetics and to significantly delay progression of renal disease in type 2 diabetics. All diabetics should begin ACE inhibitor therapy at the onset of microalbuminuria, even in the absence of hypertension. In addition, one should consider starting patients with diabetes on statins and low-dose aspirin as they are at a higher risk of coronary artery disease.

   Answer B is incorrect. β-Blockers are used to control essential hypertension, not diabetic nephropathy. These drugs have been shown to reduce mortality in patients with CHF.

   Answer C is incorrect. Cyclophosphamide is often used in conjunction with prednisone to treat immunologically mediated kidney disease.

   Answer D is incorrect. Prednisone is used to treat immune-mediated nephropathy, not diabetic nephropathy.

   Answer E is incorrect. Thiazides are often used in the initial treatment of hypertension, which could ultimately lead to renal failure. However, they have not specifically been shown to reduce the progression of diabetic nephropathy.

8. **The correct answer is B.** Clozapine is an atypical antipsychotic used primarily to treat schizophrenia. The patient here is exhibiting agranulocytosis, which is the most serious risk associated with clozapine use. Consequently, clozapine is reserved for schizophrenia that is otherwise refractory to treatment. Patients must be regularly monitored for neutropenia for the first six months of treatment. Other adverse effects include weight gain, hypotension, mild sedation, and, in some cases, extrapyramidal effects.

   Answer A is incorrect. Chloramphenicol is associated with aplastic anemia, which is characterized by neutropenia, thrombocytopenia, and decreased RBCs. It would not be used to treat schizophrenia.

   Answer C is incorrect. Metronidazole is associated with disulfiramlike reactions and not agranulocytosis.

   Answer D is incorrect. Penicillin is associated with gastrointestinal (GI) distress, urticaria, and anaphylaxis, not agranulocytosis.

   Answer E is incorrect. Polymyxins are associated with neurotoxicity and renal tubular acidosis, not agranulocytosis.

9. **The correct answer is B.** Renal failure is a very dangerous adverse event associated with nonsteroidal anti-inflammatory drugs (NSAIDs). The patient was in CHF when he first presented. His cardiologist consequently treated him with a diuretic, intending to reduce his total body fluids. When the amount of fluids in the body contracts, the body attempts to compensate by releasing angiotensin II, a potent vasoconstrictor. In order to protect the kidney from losing its perfusion due to this vasoconstriction, the kidney simultaneously releases prostaglandins at both the afferent and efferent arterioles, where they act as vasodilators. By taking an NSAID like ibuprofen and inhibiting the cyclooxygenase (COX)-1 and COX-2 enzymes, this patient blocked the pathway producing the prostaglandins that were keeping

the afferent arterioles dilated and thus keeping his kidneys perfused. His renal failure is prerenal in origin, resulting from the constriction of these arterioles.

Answer A is incorrect. NSAIDs will block the production of prostaglandin E_2 at both arterioles, but the constriction of the afferent arteriole is the primary cause of this man's renal failure.

Answer C is incorrect. While NSAIDs would also have blocked the production of prostaglandin E_2 at the efferent arteriole, this would not cause renal failure, it would actually increase glomerular filtration rate (blocking the outflow without blocking the inflow will increase filtration). This would not cause the patient to present with oliguria or a rising creatinine level.

Answer D is incorrect. Ibuprofen blocks the synthesis of prostaglandins, and thus a decrease in the prostaglandin level would be seen, not an increase.

Answer E is incorrect. Ibuprofen blocks the synthesis of prostaglandins, and thus a decrease in the prostaglandin level would be seen, not an increase.

10. **The correct answer is C.** This man presents with classic symptoms of benign prostatic hypertrophy (BPH), which include difficulty starting and maintaining a urine stream, feeling as though the bladder is never emptied, having the urge to urinate again soon after voiding, and pain on urination or dysuria. Finasteride is most commonly used to treat this condition. Finasteride acts by inhibiting the conversion of testosterone to dihydrotestosterone (DHT) by inhibiting 5α-reductase. Normally DHT binds to the nuclear androgen receptors and stimulating mitogenic growth factors that cause stromal and epithelial hyperplasia along with promoting secondary sexual characteristics (in men and women). DHT, not testosterone, is the culprit behind prostatic hyperplasia because of DHT's slow dissociation from the prostatic nuclear androgen receptor. Inhibiting 5α-reductase and thus DHT formation leads to a reduction in the size of the prostate, providing symptomatic relief.

Answer A is incorrect. Bleomycin acts by chelating mechanisms to attack the phosphodiester bonds of DNA. It is used to treat testicular tumors and lymphomas (especially Hodgkin), not benign prostatic hypertrophy.

Answer B is incorrect. Leuprolide is a gonadotropin-releasing hormone analog that binds the luteinizing hormone-releasing hormone receptor in the pituitary. This leads to desensitization of the receptor and, subsequently, to reduced release of luteinizing hormone (LH). Leuprolide is used to treat metastatic carcinoma of the prostate, not BPH, and also plays a role in in vitro fertilization.

Answer D is incorrect. Sildenafil inhibits cGMP-specific phosphodiesterase type 5, resulting in increased concentrations of cGMP, which increases vasodilation leading to increased blood flow to the corpus cavernosum. Sildenafil is used primarily to treat erectile dysfunction.

Answer E is incorrect. Ketoconazole is an antifungal with antiandrogenic properties that acts by inhibiting cytochrome P450 enzymes (CYP450). It is not used to treat BPH, but is used commonly to treat fungal infection such as athlete's foot and ringworm.

Answer F is incorrect. Flutamide is a potent androgen receptor antagonist that has limited efficacy when used alone because the increased LH secretion stimulates higher serum testosterone levels. Thus the increase in serum testosterone can overcome the androgen receptor antagonism. This drug is used primarily in conjunction with a gonadotropin-releasing hormone analog in the treatment of metastatic prostate cancer.

11. **The correct answer is D.** This scenario is commonly observed in cases of organophosphate poisoning. Organophosphates lead to phosphorylation and deactivation of acetylcholinesterase, causing an increase in acetylcholine levels and their associated cholinergic effects and subsequent symptoms described in the

vignette. Pralidoxime dephosphorylates the acetylcholinesterase and reactivates it, primarily in the neuromuscular junction. It thus reverses the toxic process triggered by organophosphates. Atropine, a muscarinic receptor antagonist, is commonly added for symptomatic relief of salivation, cramping, sweating, and wheezing.

Answer A is incorrect. Echothiophate is an acetylcholinesterase inhibitor; it would further increase acetylcholine levels in the neuromuscular junction and worsen the symptoms.

Answer B is incorrect. Hexamethonium is a nicotinic receptor antagonist and would be inappropriate, as it does not interact with muscarinic receptors.

Answer C is incorrect. Pancuronium is a long-lasting nicotinic receptor antagonist. It does not act at the muscarinic receptors responsible for the patient's sweating, salivation, cramping, and wheezing.

Answer E is incorrect. Pyridostigmine is an acetylcholinesterase inhibitor; it would further increase acetylcholine levels in the neuromuscular junction and worsen the symptoms.

12. **The correct answer is D.** Fibrates like gemfibrozil act at point D. They are ligands for the peroxisome proliferator-activated receptor-α (PPAR-α) protein, a receptor that regulates the transcription of genes involved in lipid metabolism. Increased expression of the PPAR-α protein results in increased expression of lipoprotein lipase on endothelial cells and thus increased clearance of triglyceride-rich lipoproteins. Fibrates have been shown to decrease triglyceride levels by as much as 35%-50%.

    Answer A is incorrect. There are no lipid-lowering drugs that act at point A.

    Answer B is incorrect. Bile acid sequestrants such as cholestyramine act at point B by blocking the reabsorption of bile acids. The liver must then metabolize more cholesterol to replace the bile acids, thereby primarily lowering LDL-cholesterol levels.

    Answer C is incorrect. 3-Hydroxy-3-methylglutaryl coenzyme A (HMG CoA) reductase inhibitors act at point C by competitively inhibiting the synthesis of mevalonate by HMG CoA reductase, an essential step in the production of cholesterol in the liver. Serum LDL cholesterol levels are, in turn, decreased as the liver upregulates LDL receptor expression to compensate for diminished capacity to endogenously synthesize cholesterol.

13. **The correct answer is C.** This patient has dyspnea on exertion but normal pulmonary function tests, and most likely has dilated cardiomyopathy due to the toxic effects of doxorubicin, a DNA intercalating agent that is used as a part of the **ABVD** (**A**driamycin [doxorubicin], **B**leomycin, **V**inblastine, and **D**acarbazine) treatment regimen for Hodgkin lymphoma. Doxorubicin also is used to treat myelomas, sarcomas, and some solid-tissue tumors (breast, lung, and ovary). Dactinomycin has a mechanism of action similar to that of doxorubicin, as it also acts via DNA intercalation. Dactinomycin is used to treat Wilm tumor, germ cell tumors, rhabdomyosarcoma, and various other sarcomas.

    Answer A is incorrect. Cisplatin is an alkylating-like agent that cross-links DNA, thus causing apoptosis. It is used to treat testicular, bladder, ovarian, and lung carcinomas. Nephrotoxicity and acoustic nerve damage are prominent adverse effects of cisplatin treatment.

    Answer B is incorrect. Cyclophosphamide is an alkylating agent that acts by attaching alkyl groups to DNA bases, ultimately causing DNA damage. It is used to treat non-Hodgkin lymphomas, and breast and ovarian carcinomas. Hemorrhagic cystitis is an adverse effect of cyclophosphamide treatment.

    Answer D is incorrect. Methotrexate inhibits the metabolism of folic acid by inhibiting dihydrofolate reductase, thereby preventing the conversion of dihydrofolate to tetrahydrofolate. Because tetrahydrofolate is essential for thymidine synthesis, methotrexate has a toxic effect on replicating cells. Methotrexate is used to treat many cancers including choriocarcinoma, leukemia in the spinal fluid, osteosarcoma, breast cancer, lung cancer, non-Hodgkin lymphoma, and head and neck cancers.

Answer E is incorrect. Paclitaxel inhibits microtubule disassembly by binding to the β subunit of tubulin, which ultimately disrupts cellular function and leads to apoptosis. Paclitaxel is used to treat ovarian, breast, and lung cancer in addition to Kaposi sarcoma.

14. **The correct answer is E.** This patient has chronic atrial fibrillation, which is a risk factor for clot formation and systemic embolization. Given his age, history of hypertension, and previous stroke, he needs ongoing anticoagulation to prevent possible complications, such as cerebrovascular accidents or mesenteric infarction. Warfarin inhibits gamma-carboxylation of vitamin K-dependent clotting factors and is used for chronic anticoagulation. It is taken orally and has a long half-life. The degree of anticoagulation must be followed by measuring the International Normalized Ratio (INR).

Answer A is incorrect. Aspirin is an antiplatelet agent used to prevent MI. It also has antipyretic, analgesic, and anti-inflammatory effects.

Answer B is incorrect. Protamine sulfate is used for rapid reversal of heparinization in the setting of overzealous anticoagulation.

Answer C is incorrect. Streptokinase is used to break down existing clots.

Answer D is incorrect. Heparin is used for acute, not long-term, anticoagulation.

15. **The correct answer is A.** The formula for half-life ($t_{1/2}$) is: (0.7 × volume of distribution) / (clearance). Rearranging the formula yields: Clearance = (0.7 × volume of distribution) / ($t_{1/2}$) = (0.7 × 5 L) / (50 h) = 0.07 L/h.

Answer B is incorrect. Calculation error.

Answer C is incorrect. Calculation error.

Answer D is incorrect. Calculation error.

Answer E is incorrect. Calculation error.

16. **The correct answer is D.** Rifampin suppresses RNA synthesis by inhibiting DNA-dependent RNA polymerase and is an antibiotic used to treat tuberculosis. One major adverse effect of rifampin is that it is metabolized by and also induces the CYP450 isoenzyme system; thus drugs such as oral contraceptives, warfarin, and ketoconazole may need to be given in higher doses in order to be therapeutic. This is probably the reason why this woman's oral contraceptive pills failed. Another well-known adverse effect that can be frightening to patients is that rifampin turns all bodily fluids (tears, sweat, and urine) orange. Other uses of rifampin include treatment of leprosy, for meningococcal prophylaxis, and for *Haemophilus influenzae* type b chemoprophylaxis.

Answer A is incorrect. Metronidazole forms toxic metabolites that have a bactericidal effect. It is an effective antibiotic against amoebae and anaerobes. It is also used in *Giardia* infection. One of metronidazole's best known adverse effects is a disulfiram-like reaction when taken with ethanol. Metronidazole is also highly teratogenic and should not be taken by pregnant women.

Answer B is incorrect. Phenytoin acts by blocking sodium channels, which inhibits glutamate release from excitatory presynaptic neurons. It is used to treat epilepsy, particularly tonic-clonic and partial seizures. It has many adverse effects, including induction of the CYP450 isoenzyme system, and thus would interact with oral contraceptive pills. However, phenytoin does not cause red-orange bodily fluids. Some other adverse effects of phenytoin include gingival hyperplasia, megaloblastic anemia secondary to folate deficiency, and central nervous system depression. Phenytoin is also teratogenic and causes fetal hydantoin syndrome (prenatal growth deficiency, mental retardation, and congenital malformations).

Answer C is incorrect. Polymyxins B and E are cationic basic proteins that act as detergents that bind to cell membranes and disrupt the osmotic and cell membrane integrity of the bacteria. They are used in resistant gram-negative infections. Adverse effects include neurotoxicity and acute renal tubular necrosis.

Answer E is incorrect. Amiodarone prolongs the action potential in cardiac phases I and III via blockage of sodium and potassium channels. It is an antiarrhythmic drug that has properties of both class I and class III antiarrhythmics, and is most often used to treat refractory atrial fibrillation and ventricular tachyarrhythmias. Amiodarone is infamous for its many adverse effects, including interstitial pulmonary fibrosis, thyroid dysfunction (both hyper- and hypothyroidism), and hepatocellular necrosis. Amiodarone and other antiarrhythmic drugs do not cause orange bodily fluids, though it does turn the skin bluish with chronic use.

17. **The correct answer is A.** Hydrochlorothiazide decreases blood, not urine, sodium by blocking reuptake of NaCl in the distal convoluted tubule.

Answer B is incorrect. Hydrochlorothiazide causes decreased blood potassium and increased urine potassium through loss of potassium in the distal nephron.

Answer C is incorrect. Hydrochlorothiazide will cause a metabolic alkalosis, not acidosis, through volume contraction, loss of hydrogen ion into cells in exchange for potassium, and loss of hydrogen ion in the urine.

Answer D is incorrect. Patients taking any type of diuretic, with the exception of potassium-sparing diuretics such as spironolactone, will have increased loss of potassium into the urine. All diuretics also increase urine sodium, as they inhibit reuptake of sodium at various points along the nephron. Thiazide diuretics inhibit sodium reuptake in the distal tubule. Finally, thiazide diuretics cause a metabolic alkalosis through several mechanisms: volume contraction, low potassium leading to loss of hydrogen ion in principle cells, and potassium exiting cells into the blood in exchange for hydrogen ion going into cells.

18. **The correct answer is A.** Methotrexate, a folic acid analog, can be used as an immunosuppressant, an abortifacient, or an antineoplastic agent. It is used to terminate an ectopic pregnancy, or in combination with misoprostol to terminate an intrauterine first-trimester pregnancy. It also can be used alone or in combination with other agents to treat malignant gestational trophoblastic disease (GTD) such as choriocarcinoma. Most patients with choriocarcinoma have metastatic disease at the time of diagnosis, with spread to the lungs, liver, vagina, or central nervous system. Of note, malignant GTD after an ectopic pregnancy is rare; it is much more likely to develop after a molar pregnancy.

Answer B is incorrect. Mifepristone is a partial progesterone agonist that can be used alone or in combination with misoprostol to induce a first-trimester medical abortion. It has been studied as an agent to treat ectopic pregnancy, but it is not used to treat GTD.

Answer C is incorrect. Misoprostol is a synthetic analog of prostaglandin$_1$. It promotes uterine contractions and so is used in combination with mifepristone to induce a first-trimester medical abortion. It is not used to treat either ectopic pregnancy or GTD.

Answer D is incorrect. Rifampin inhibits DNA-dependent RNA polymerase. It is used to treat *Mycobacterium tuberculosis* infection, to delay resistance to dapsone in patients with leprosy, and for chemoprophylaxis in patients exposed to *Neisseria meningitides* and unimmunized children exposed to *Haemophilus influenzae* type B. It is not used to treat ectopic pregnancy or GTD.

Answer E is incorrect. Tamoxifen is a partial estrogen agonist that is used to treat estrogen-dependent cancers of the breast. It is not indicated in the treatment of ectopic pregnancy or GTD.

19. **The correct answer is D.** Administration of bicarbonate alkalinizes the urine, thereby promoting the excretion of acidic drugs such as aspirin and not allowing them to be reabsorbed. Highly basic urine deprotonates acids such as salicylates within the renal tubules, resulting in an ionic charge. In general, charged molecules are cleared, while uncharged molecules

are easily reabsorbed from the tubules. Thus bicarbonate administration is indicated because it promotes "trapping" of salicylates in the urine and their subsequent excretion.

Answer A is incorrect. Protamine is used to treat heparin toxicity.

Answer B is incorrect. Glucagon is used to treat β-blocker toxicity.

Answer C is incorrect. N-acetylcysteine is used to treat acetaminophen toxicity.

Answer E is incorrect. Vitamin K is used to treat warfarin toxicity.

20. **The correct answer is B.** Herpes zoster is characterized by reactivation of a latent varicella-zoster infection. Original infection is characterized by chickenpox, after which the virus lives in the ganglia of spinal nerve roots. When the infection is reactivated, as often happens in immunosuppressed patients, eruptive vesicles develop in a dermatomal pattern and do not cross the midline. Acyclovir is the primary treatment of zoster infection. Acyclovir is an inactive precursor that is activated by viral thymidine kinase when absorbed by infected cells. When activated, it forms a guanine analog that results in chain termination when read by viral DNA polymerase.

Answer A is incorrect. Reactivation of the patient's latent varicella zoster virus infection is most likely secondary to his immunosuppression. While herpesviruses can develop resistance to acyclovir by modifications to the viral DNA polymerase, mutations in the viral RNA polymerase do not lead to an increased incidence of reactivation.

Answer C is incorrect. Reverse transcriptase is not present in varicella-zoster virus.

Answer D is incorrect. Herpes zoster virus encodes its own proteases. Host cell proteases are not incorporated into the zoster DNA, nor do they cleave the viral polyprotein.

Answer E is incorrect. The action of acyclovir does not affect the production of the virion's native nucleotides. Chain termination occurs as long as the virus contains thymidine kinase.

21. **The correct answer is B.** Symptoms of iron overdose include onset of nausea, vomiting (including hemorrhagic gastroenteritis), and abdominal pain within four hours of ingestion. Other symptoms may include hyperglycemia, leukocytosis, shock, and coma. Deferoxamine is an iron-specific chelating agent that binds to both ferric and ferrous ions to form ferrioxamine. Deferoxamine can capture iron from ferritin and hemosiderin outside the bone marrow, but leaves iron in hemoglobin, cytochromes, and myoglobin untouched. Although deferoxamine can effectively and rapidly reduce effective blood iron levels, adverse effects include hypotensive shock secondary to histamine release, allergic reaction, and rare cases of neural and renal toxicity.

Answer A is incorrect. Aminocaproic acid is used in the treatment of tissue plasminogen activator or streptokinase overdose.

Answer C is incorrect. Dimercaprol is used to treat poisoning by arsenic, mercury, and gold.

Answer D is incorrect. Bicarbonate can be used to inactivate iron in the GI tract. Although this treatment may prevent iron from being absorbed in the GI tract, it would do nothing to remove excess iron already in the bloodstream.

Answer E is incorrect. Penicillamine is used to treat lead and arsenic toxicity, not iron poisoning.

22. **The correct answer is A.** The patient has overdosed on diazepam, a benzodiazepine. Flumazenil is a competitive antagonist at the benzodiazepam GABAergic receptor. Its use can prevent or reverse the central nervous system effects of benzodiazepine overdose.

Answer B is incorrect. Glucagon can be used to counter β-blocker overdose. It would not be used to treat diazepam overdose.

Answer C is incorrect. Midazolam is a shorter-acting benzodiazepine and would exacerbate this patient's symptoms.

Answer D is incorrect. Naloxone is used to reverse the effects of opiates such as heroin or morphine.

Answer E is incorrect. Physostigmine is used to reverse the effects of anticholinergic agents.

23. **The correct answer is C.** Graphs of this nature display two important characteristics about a drug in a given reaction—its potency and its efficacy. Potency is used to describe the amount of drug needed to produce a given effect. A drug with high potency will be given at a lower dose to produce the same effect as a drug with low potency. On the graph, more potent drugs are located toward the left (indicating lower doses). Efficacy is a property intrinsic to a drug that reflects how well it generates a response on binding to its receptor. A drug that is highly efficacious will better generate a response than the comparable quantity of a less efficacious drug. On the graph, more efficacious drugs are located toward the top (indicating higher maximal effects). Using this framework, we can now understand the definition of a noncompetitive antagonist. Antagonist indicates that it will decrease the efficacy of the drug in question. The fact that it is noncompetitive means that it cannot be overcome (or "out-competed") simply by adding more of the agonist drug. Molecularly, a competitive antagonist is one that resembles the agonist and thus can fill up receptor sites that the agonist would normally bind. A noncompetitive antagonist does not bind to the same receptor as the agonist. Instead, it binds to the receptor to change its conformation, so that when the agonist binds, it is less able to do its job (decreased efficacy). This phenomenon is displayed by curve C in the graph, which will never reach the same height (efficacy) as the agonist administered alone.

Answer A is incorrect. Curve A represents a dose-response curve with the same efficacy but increased potency. In order to be a noncompetitive antagonist, by definition, it must lower the drug's efficacy.

Answer B is incorrect. Curve B represents a drug with a lower efficacy but a greater potency than drug X. This could occur with a type of drug known as a partial agonist, which binds to the receptor as well as (or better than) the original agonist, but when bound, exerts only a fraction of the effect that could be produced by the original agonist.

Answer D is incorrect. Curve D represents a drug with a decreased potency but the same efficacy. This could occur with the addition of a competitive antagonist. Remember that this antagonist would bind to the same receptor site as the agonist and take up its binding spots, effectively making it appear as though there is less of the agonist around to bind the receptor.

Answer E is incorrect. Curve E represents a drug with lower efficacy and potency. This could occur with the addition of a partial antagonist, which operates with logic similar to that of a partial agonist.

24. **The correct answer is C.** Class IA antiarrhythmics, such as procainamide, affect both atrial and ventricular arrhythmias. They block sodium channels and thus slow conduction velocity in the atria, ventricles, and Purkinje fibers. This decreased conduction velocity slows phase 0 of the action potential (AP) and is manifested as an increased QRS duration on ECG. In addition to blocking sodium channels, class IA antiarrhythmics also block potassium channels and thus increase the AP duration by prolonging the effective refractory period (ERP).

Answer A is incorrect. Encainide is a class IC antiarrhythmic.

Answer B is incorrect. Mexiletine is a class IB antiarrhythmic.

Answer D is incorrect. Class IC antiarrhythmics, such as propafenone, slow phase 0 of the AP, but have no effect on the AP duration. These antiarrhythmics have no affect on the ERP.

Answer E is incorrect. Class IB antiarrhythmics, such as tocainide, slow phase 0 of the AP, but decrease the AP duration. These antiarrhythmics affect ischemic or depolarized Purkinje and ventricular tissues. These antiarrhythmics have no affect on the ERP.

25. **The correct answer is B.** Digoxin is a direct inhibitor of Na^+/K^+-ATPase (point B on the image). The increased levels of intracellular Na^+ indirectly inhibit the function of the Na^+/Ca^{2+} exchanger (point C on the image), resulting in increased intracellular Ca^{2+} concentration. This in turn results in the inotropic properties of digoxin.

Answer A is incorrect. A is the voltage-gated calcium channel, which is not inhibited by digoxin.

Answer C is incorrect. C is the Na^+/Ca^{2+} exchanger, which is not the direct site of action for digoxin.

Answer D is incorrect. D is the ryanodine calcium channel, which releases calcium from the sarcoplasmic reticulum. It is not the site of action for digoxin.

Answer E is incorrect. E is the ATP-dependent calcium pump, which pumps calcium back into the sarcoplasmic reticulum.

SECTION II

Organ Systems

- Cardiovascular
- Endocrine
- Gastrointestinal
- Hematology-Oncology
- Musculoskeletal
- Neurology
- Psychiatry
- Renal
- Reproductive
- Respiratory

CHAPTER 8

Cardiovascular

QUESTIONS

1. A 36-year-old man presents with sudden-onset dizziness and chest palpitations. He had been healthy previously. An ECG is shown in the image. Laboratory work-up reveals normal levels of RBCs and WBCs and a normal cardiac panel. The drug commonly used to treat this condition inhibits which of the following?

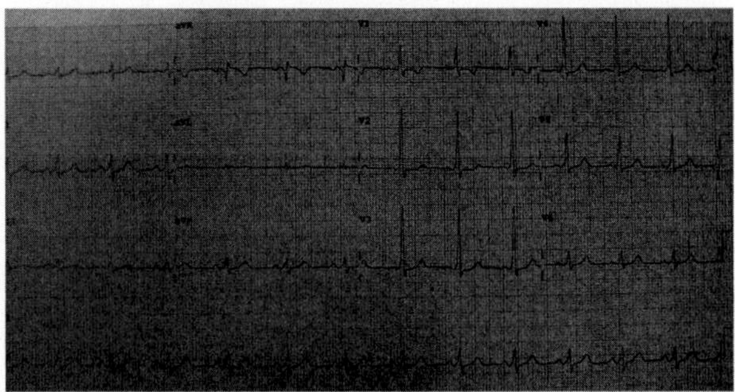

Courtesy of Dr. James Heilman.

   (A) β-Adrenergic receptor
   (B) Acetylcholine receptor
   (C) Calcium channel
   (D) Potassium channel
   (E) Sodium-potassium ATPase enzyme

2. A 64-year-old woman with a history of diabetes, hypertension, and congestive heart failure was brought to the emergency department after she complained of a headache and blurred vision and was found to have a blood pressure of 220/95 mm Hg. The intern who saw her wanted to treat her with drug X, but the attending physician rejected this choice because of its tendency to cause compensatory tachycardia and exacerbate fluid retention, as well as its potential to cause a lupus-like syndrome with long-term use. What is the mechanism of action of drug X?

   (A) Block calcium channels
   (B) Decreased production of cGMP
   (C) Increased production of cGMP
   (D) Inhibit angiotensin-converting enzyme
   (E) Inhibit carbonic anhydrase
   (F) Inhibit sodium chloride reabsorption

3. 3-Hydroxy-3-methylglutaryl coenzyme A (HMG CoA) reductase inhibitors, commonly known as the statins, are the most effective drugs available for reducing LDL cholesterol levels. Statins cause several downstream effects by inhibiting the rate-limiting step in hepatic cholesterol synthesis. What is the primary effect of statins on hepatocytes?

   (A) Decreased hepatic production of LDL cholesterol
   (B) Decreased production of triglycerides
   (C) Downregulation of cell surface LDL cholesterol receptors
   (D) Increased production of HDL cholesterol
   (E) Upregulation of cell surface LDL cholesterol receptors

4. A 45-year-old man who takes spironolactone and digoxin for his congestive heart failure is admitted to the hospital because he is experiencing an altered mental status. The ECG changes shown in the image are noted on testing. Urinalysis would most likely reveal which of the following?

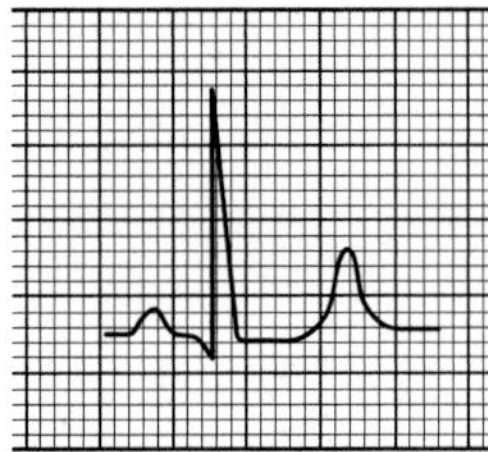

Reproduced, with permission, from USMLERx.com.

   (A) High K^+, high Na^+, high-normal urine volume
   (B) High K^+, low Na^+, low urine volume
   (C) High K^+, low Na^+, normal urine volume
   (D) Low K^+, high Na^+, high-normal urine volume
   (E) Low K^+, low Na^+, normal urine volume

5. A 2-year-old boy is brought to the clinic by his parents because he suffers from sudden cyanotic attacks that can be improved only by squatting. He is referred to a cardiologist, who informs the parents that their son's right ventricle is abnormally large. Which of the following is most likely the root cause of this boy's heart defect?

(A) Anterosuperior displacement of the infundibular septum
(B) Overriding aorta
(C) Patent ductus arteriosus
(D) Pulmonary stenosis
(E) Ventricular septal defect

6. A 55-year-old man with hypertension is prescribed an antiarrhythmic agent that alters the flow of cations in myocardial tissue. The image is a trace of a myocardial action potential. Each phase is associated with the opening and/or closing of various ion channels. Which of the following would be affected by an agent that affects phase 0 of the myocardial action potential?

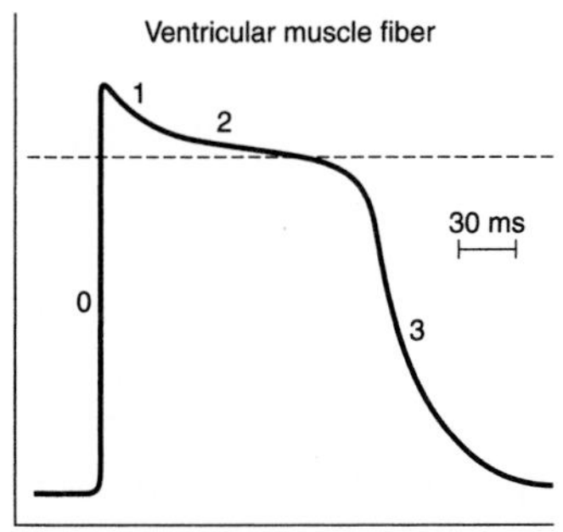

Reproduced, with permission, from USMLERx.com.

(A) Ligand-gated calcium channels opening
(B) Ligand-gated potassium channels closing
(C) Ligand-gated sodium channels opening
(D) Voltage-gated calcium channels opening
(E) Voltage-gated potassium channels closing
(F) Voltage-gated sodium channels closing
(G) Voltage-gated sodium channels opening

7. A 50-year-old man presents to the emergency department because of substernal chest pain that started four hours ago and is becoming severe. After a thorough work-up he is diagnosed with an acute myocardial infarction (MI). Which of the following laboratory test elevations is most specific for MI?

(A) Alanine aminotransferase
(B) Aspartate aminotransferase
(C) Creatine kinase-MB fraction
(D) Lactate dehydrogenase
(E) Troponin I

8. Following the administration of drug X, there is an increase in systolic, diastolic, and mean arterial pressures. After the effect of drug X has worn off completely, drug Y is then added, resulting in little or no change to the baseline blood pressure. When drug X is re-administered, there is a net decrease in blood pressure (see image). Which of the following drug combinations represents drug X and drug Y, respectively?

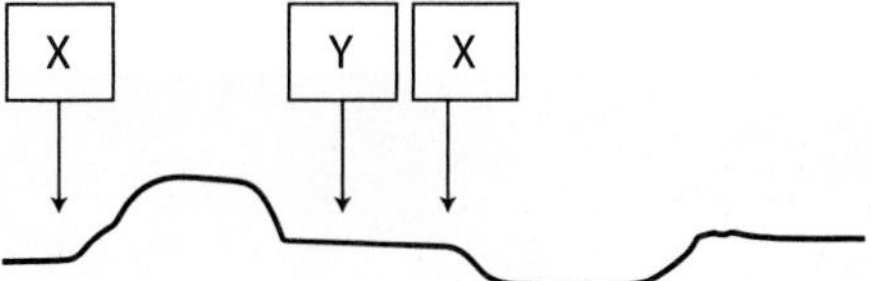

Reproduced, with permission, from USMLERx.com.

(A) Epinephrine, phentolamine
(B) Isoproterenol, clonidine
(C) Norepinephrine, propranolol
(D) Phenylephrine, metoprolol
(E) Phenylephrine, phentolamine

9. A 56-year-old woman arrives in the emergency department complaining of dizziness and headache. Her blood pressure is 210/140 mm Hg. She is currently not taking any medications and has not seen a doctor for several years. The physician decides to address her hypertension urgently. Which of the following drugs is contraindicated in this patient?

(A) Intravenous diltiazem
(B) Intravenous labetalol
(C) Intravenous metoprolol
(D) Oral captopril
(E) Sublingual nifedipine

10. A 64-year-old man is brought to the emergency department for chest pain. An electrocardiogram demonstrates an ST-elevation myocardial infarction in the posterior leads. After the initial management, he is admitted to the critical care unit for monitoring. On the fifth hospital day, he experiences a sudden onset of dyspnea and hypotension. An echocardiogram shows severe mitral regurgitation. An occlusion in which vessel is responsible for these findings?

    (A) Left anterior descending artery
    (B) Left circumflex artery
    (C) Left marginal artery
    (D) Posterior descending artery
    (E) Right marginal artery

11. A 17-year-old boy dies suddenly while playing basketball for his high school team. His heart is examined at autopsy. According to the image, which of the following is the most likely cause of this person's death?

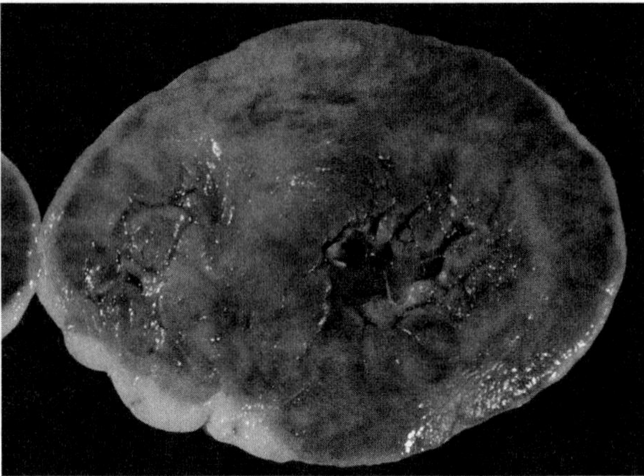

Reproduced, with permission, from USMLERx.com.

    (A) *Enterovirus* infection
    (B) Immune-mediated destruction of cardiomyocytes
    (C) Mutation in a sarcomere gene such as myosin-binding protein C
    (D) Protein deposits such as transthyretin
    (E) Trypanosome transmitted by insect bite

12. A 72-year-old African-American man undergoes hip surgery. On his third hospital day, he develops chest pain, tachycardia, dyspnea, and a low-grade fever. The man goes into cardiac arrest and efforts to resuscitate him are unsuccessful. On autopsy a massive pulmonary embolus is discovered. Which of the following would most likely predispose the patient to this event?

    (A) Factor VIII deficiency
    (B) Low serum homocysteine levels
    (C) Mutation in the factor V gene
    (D) Overproduction of protein C
    (E) Von Willebrand factor deficiency

13. A 16-year-old Asian girl sees her physician because she has been experiencing fever, night sweats, and arthralgias. The physician diagnoses her with a disorder that is characterized by thickening of the great vessels. Which of the following signs and symptoms most likely will be detected on history and physical examination?

    (A) Abdominal pain and melena
    (B) Intermittent jaw claudication
    (C) Pneumonitis
    (D) Strawberry tongue
    (E) Weak pulses in the upper extremities

14. A 67-year-old woman presents to the emergency department complaining of dizziness. During the interview, she experiences two episodes of near-syncope. Physical examination reveals palpitations and slight bradycardia. Her daughter, who accompanies her, states that the patient is taking a medication for "heart troubles," but she cannot remember its name. Results of ECG are shown in the image. Which of the following medications is this patient likely taking that could both explain her symptoms and produce the abnormalities shown in this ECG?

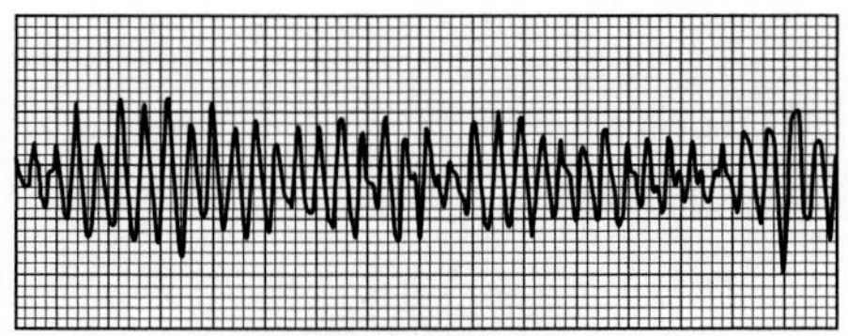

Reproduced, with permission, from USMLERx.com.

(A) Adenosine
(B) Bretylium
(C) Propranolol
(D) Quinidine
(E) Verapamil

15. A 65-year-old African-American man is admitted to the hospital for severe shortness of breath. He states that he has been having increased difficulty breathing when performing physical activity. Lung auscultation reveals bilateral crackles. His blood pressure is 125/85 mm Hg, and his heart rate is 85/min. Cardiac auscultation detects no rubs or murmurs. Blood tests are not suggestive of infection. Coronary artery angiography is performed and shows no significant vascular disease. What is the most likely cause of this patient's disease manifestations?

(A) Aortic stricture
(B) Fibrosis of the endocardium
(C) Fibrotic debris within the pericardial membrane
(D) Ischemia of the myocardium
(E) Ventricular dysfunction

16. A 25-year-old pregnant woman goes to her gynecologist for her 36-week checkup. She complains of light-headedness when she lies down in bed at night. In the office her blood pressure is 120/70 mm Hg while sitting upright and 90/50 mm Hg while lying supine. Which of the following is the most likely cause of this hypotension?

(A) Anemia
(B) Cardiogenic shock
(C) Inferior vena cava compression
(D) Third spacing of fluid
(E) Vasodilation

17. Atherosclerosis is associated with numerous well-known risk factors, such as age, smoking, diabetes, hyperlipidemia, and a family history of atherosclerosis. LDL cholesterol is believed to be a key factor in the pathway through which hyperlipidemia causes atherosclerosis. What is most likely the first step in the pathogenesis of atherosclerosis caused by hyperlipidemia?

(A) Endothelial dysfunction
(B) Foam cell formation
(C) LDL cholesterol oxidation
(D) Monocyte activation
(E) Plaque formation

18. Jugular venous pressure (JVP) curves are designed to show the pressure changes that normally take place in the right atrium throughout the cardiac cycle. A JVP curve consists of two, or sometimes three, positive waves and two negative troughs. A normal JVP curve is shown in the image. Which of the following points on the normal jugular venous tracing below would be most prominently affected in tricuspid regurgitation?

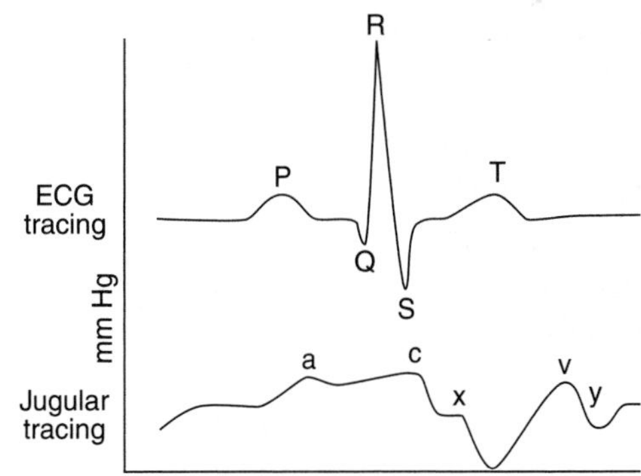

Reproduced, with permission, from USMLERx.com.

(A) C and X
(B) A and Y
(C) A and C
(D) V and Y

19. A 56-year-old Asian man with hypertension, hypercholesterolemia, and type 2 diabetes mellitus comes to a physician for a check-up. It has been several years since he has been to the doctor. His past medical history is significant for an acute illness at the age of nine, which involved a high fever, pleuritic chest pain, migrating joint pain, and a pink, nonpruritic rash on his torso. His blood pressure is 155/100 mm Hg and heart rate is 70/min. Auscultation of the heart reveals a low-pitched diastolic rumble heard best at the apex. What is the most likely pressure change that would be seen in this patient's heart?

(A) Decreased left atrial pressure
(B) Decreased left ventricular pressure
(C) Increased left atrial pressure
(D) Increased left ventricular pressure
(E) Increased right atrial pressure

20. A common location for an abdominal aortic aneurysm is inferior to the renal arteries and extending to the bifurcation of the common iliac arteries. Repair involves resecting the diseased portion of the aorta and replacing it with a synthetic graft. Based on anatomic considerations, which structure is most at risk of ischemia during repair of an aneurysm at this specific location?

(A) Ascending colon
(B) Sigmoid colon
(C) Small intestine
(D) Spleen
(E) Stomach

21. A 52-year-old African-American man is brought to the emergency department unresponsive. Efforts to resuscitate him are unsuccessful. On autopsy, they discover that he suffered from a ruptured aneurysm of the aortic root. A picture of his dilated aorta is shown below. In addition, inspection of the man's skin reveals several nodular lesions that are present throughout his trunk and extremities. Which of the following is most likely associated with the underlying etiology of this patient's aneurysm?

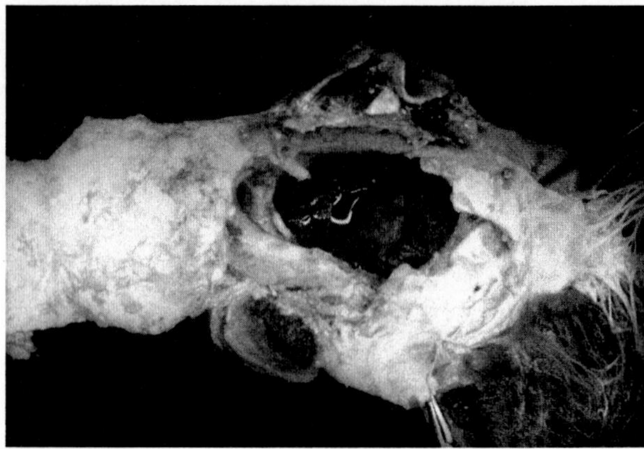

Courtesy of Dr. Susan Lindsley, Centers for Disease Control and Prevention.

(A) Atherosclerosis
(B) Congenital medial weakness
(C) Cystic medial necrosis
(D) Disruption of the vasa vasorum
(E) Hypertension

22. A baby is born to a mother who was not immunized as a child. On gross physical examination, the infant appears normal, but on cardiac examination is found to have a continuous murmur in both systole and diastole. The physician prescribes a particular drug for the infant, and on follow-up the murmur has disappeared. What is the mechanism of action of the drug most likely prescribed?

(A) Increases thromboxane A_2
(B) Inhibits prostaglandin E_2 formation
(C) Stimulates M_2-receptors
(D) Stimulates prostaglandin E_2-receptors
(E) Stimulates prostaglandin $F_2\alpha$-receptors

23. A 25-year-old white woman with no past medical history presents to the emergency department for "a racing heartbeat." It is determined that she has paroxysmal supraventricular tachycardia. Which of the following is the drug of choice used for diagnosing and abolishing atrioventricular nodal arrhythmias by virtue of its effectiveness and its low toxicity?

(A) Adenosine
(B) Bretylium

(C) Encainide
(D) Lidocaine
(E) Sotalol

24. Gemfibrozil has been proven to modestly decrease LDL cholesterol levels, modestly increase HDL cholesterol levels, and significantly decrease triglyceride levels. The mechanism of gemfibrozil is best described by which of the following?

(A) Slows the conversion of VLDL to LDL cholesterol
(B) Increases expression of triglyceride receptors
(C) Inhibits peroxisome proliferator-activated receptor α nuclear transcription (PPAR-α) regulator
(D) Promotes hepatocyte lipolysis
(E) Activates lipoprotein lipase

25. A 48-year-old executive presents to the emergency department because of chest tightness and shortness of breath. ECG shows ST-segment elevations in leads V4, V5, and V6. He has a history of high blood pressure, and his father died of heart problems at a young age. Assuming no other cardiac history, which of the following myocardial abnormalities would most likely be seen via light microscopy eight hours after his symptoms began?

(A) Contraction bands
(B) Granulation tissue
(C) Monocytic infiltrate
(D) Neutrophilic infiltrate
(E) No change can be detected with light microscopy at this time

26. A 58-year-old man with a past medical history of hypertension goes to his physician for a routine visit. On physical examination the physician is able to detect an S_4 heart sound, and refers the patient to a cardiologist. After a thorough work-up, he is found to have left ventricular hypertrophy. The image below plots left ventricular pressure versus left ventricular volume for a single cardiac cycle. This patient's S_4 heart sound heard on auscultation would best correspond to which of the following points?

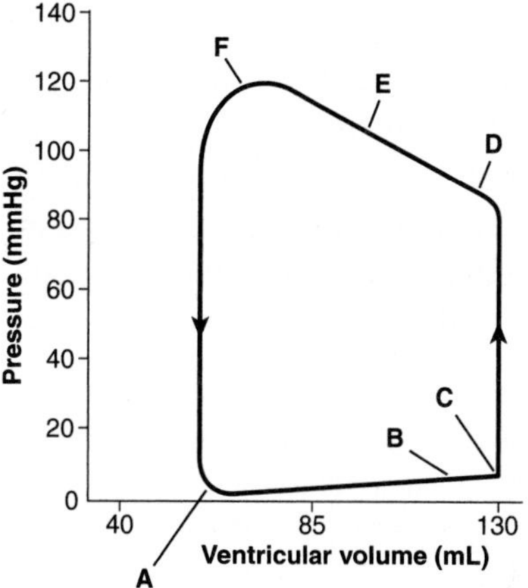

Reproduced, with permission, from USMLERx.com.

(A) A
(B) B
(C) C
(D) D
(E) E
(F) F

27. A 67-year-old woman with a long history of poorly controlled diabetes mellitus and chronic renal failure is admitted to the hospital for treatment of cellulitis. Two days into her hospital stay she complains of chest pain that is relieved when she leans forward. An ECG shows diffuse ST segment elevations with PR depressions; her echocardiogram is normal. Which of the following is the most appropriate treatment at this time?

(A) Cardiac catheterization
(B) Dialysis
(C) Nonsteroidal anti-inflammatory drugs
(D) Pericardiocentesis
(E) Switch her to another antibiotic regimen

28. An 87-year-old man suffered an acute ST-elevation myocardial infarction a few minutes ago. He was subsequently treated with aspirin, metoprolol, and heparin. Immediately before being taken to the catheterization laboratory, the patient becomes unresponsive. He is placed on telemetry and his rhythm strip is shown in the image. Although the patient receives a series of emergent defibrillations, he does not convert to sinus rhythm. Due to failure to respond, the patient is given an agent associated with which of the following potential adverse effects?

Reproduced, with permission, from USMLERx.com.

(A) Bleeding
(B) Increased post-myocardial infarction mortality
(C) Malar rash
(D) Pulmonary fibrosis
(E) Yellow-green vision

29. A 24-year-old man presents to the emergency department with fever, chills, night sweats, malaise, and fatigue that started three days ago. In the past 24 hours, he has become short of breath. He admits to using intravenous drugs regularly. At presentation the patient is shaking and appears pale. Physical examination is remarkable for a temperature of 39.4°C (103°F), hypoxia to 88% on room air, jugular venous distention, bilaterally decreased breath sounds at the bases of the lungs, and a grade III/VI systolic murmur heard best at the lower left sternal border. Which pathogen is most likely responsible for this patient's condition?

(A) *Enterococcus faecalis*
(B) *Haemophilus aphrophilus*
(C) *Staphylococcus aureus*
(D) *Streptococcus bovis*
(E) *Streptococcus viridans*

30. A 65-year-old woman with type 2 diabetes mellitus is prescribed a drug by her physician to treat her hypertension. She returns complaining of facial swelling and a cough. Her physician promptly switches her to a new drug, which has the same desired effect but fewer adverse effects. What is the mechanism of action of the replacement drug?

(A) Blockade of β1 receptors
(B) Inhibition of angiotensin II receptors
(C) Inhibition of angiotensin-converting enzyme
(D) Inhibition of calcium channels
(E) Inhibition of NaCl reabsorption in the early distal tubule

31. A 75-year-old man with a history of small cell lung cancer diagnosed six weeks ago presents to the emergency department in shock. He is found to have a heart rate of 137/min, respiratory rate of 25/min, and blood pressure of 85/45 mm Hg that decreases to 70/40 mm Hg with inspiration. On examination the patient has jugular venous distension and distant heart sounds but clear lungs. ECG shows sinus tachycardia with electrical alternans. Which of the following is the best next step in management?

(A) Administer diltiazem
(B) Administer metoprolol
(C) Diuresis
(D) Intravenous fluids
(E) Surgery

32. A 25-year-old college student presents to his primary care physician. He said he first started to notice problems a few months ago after returning from a hike in the woods at a park in upstate New York. He originally had an expanding rash starting on his calf and flu-like symptoms that resolved spontaneously. Recently, he started having symptoms of dizziness, syncope, dyspnea, chest pain, and palpitations for several weeks' duration. His physician obtains an ECG, as shown in the image. The vector that carries the organism responsible for the student's symptoms is also responsible for transmitting which of the following diseases?

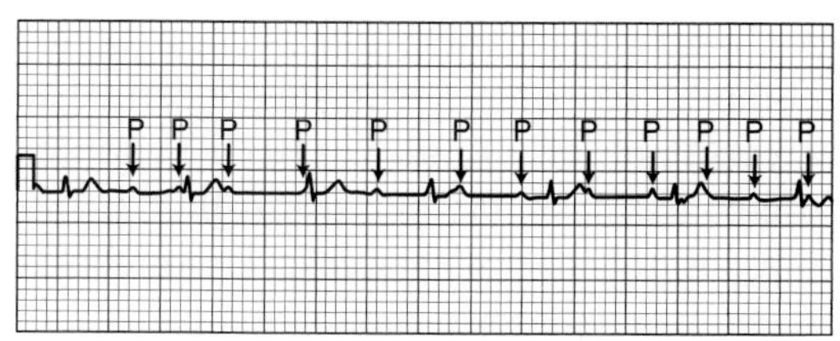

Reproduced, with permission, from USMLERx.com.

(A) Babesiosis
(B) Epidemic typhus
(C) Malaria
(D) Plague
(E) Rocky Mountain spotted fever

33. A 55-year-old woman with a history of myocardial infarction (MI) in the area of distribution of the left anterior descending artery (LAD) presents to her cardiologist because of fatigue, orthopnea, nocturnal dyspnea, weight gain, and "swollen ankles." Echocardiography reveals normal timing of the cardiac cycle and normal cardiac valves. Which of the following would most likely be heard in this patient on auscultation?

(A) Holosystolic, harsh-sounding murmur, loudest at tricuspid area
(B) Paradoxically split S_2
(C) Pulmonary flow murmur
(D) S_3
(E) S_4
(F) Widened splitting of S_2

34. Elevations in cardiac enzymes are used to diagnose a myocardial infarction (MI). The diagram below shows the duration of elevation of several of these enzymes following an MI. Which cardiac enzyme becomes elevated approximately four hours after an MI and remains elevated 7-10 days afterward?

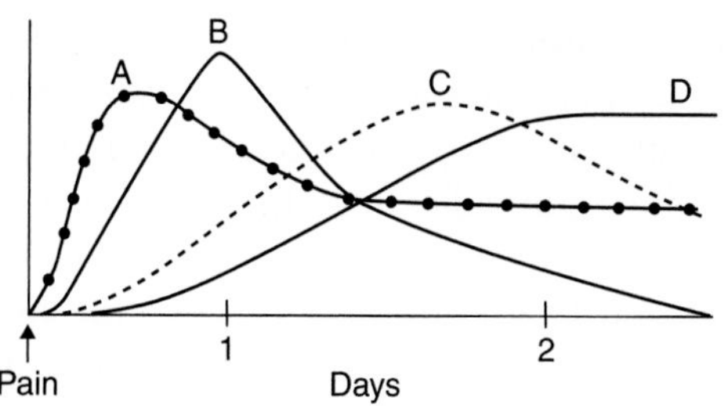

Reproduced, with permission, from USMLERx.com.

(A) Aspartate aminotransferase
(B) Brain natriuretic peptide
(C) C-reactive protein
(D) Creatine kinase-MB fraction
(E) Lactate dehydrogenase
(F) Myoglobin
(G) Troponin

35. A girl is born prematurely at 26 weeks' gestation. She is placed in an incubator and appears to be in stable condition. During a cardiac examination on her second day of life, the physician hears a machine-like murmur in the second intercostal space at the left sternal border. He prescribes indomethacin to eliminate the condition before complications arise. What is the embryonic origin of the structure targeted by this drug?

(A) First aortic arch
(B) Fourth aortic arch
(C) Second aortic arch
(D) Sixth aortic arch
(E) Third aortic arch

36. A 61-year-old man is rushed to the emergency department after losing consciousness for a few minutes at a shopping mall. His wife explained to the paramedics that he was walking up a flight of stairs when he became short of breath and fell to the ground. Once at the hospital, the patient reports to the physician that over the past three months, he has been feeling dizzy frequently, in addition to becoming short of breath after walking five blocks. He reports that two years ago he was able to walk a mile with no difficulty. On physical examination, the physician notes some crackles in the lung bases bilaterally and carotid pulses that seem somewhat weak and delayed in comparison to the patient's heart sounds. Which other physical finding is likely to be found in this patient?

    (A) Blowing holosystolic murmur that radiates to the axilla
    (B) Crescendo-decrescendo systolic murmur that radiates to the axilla
    (C) Crescendo-decrescendo systolic murmur that radiates to the carotids
    (D) Diastolic decrescendo murmur that radiates to the apex
    (E) Diastolic decrescendo murmur that radiates to the axilla
    (F) Opening snap followed by a mid-diastolic rumble that radiates to the axilla

37. A 65-year-old man presents to the emergency department because of chest pain. He is found to have a large inferior wall myocardial infarction with 2-mm ST-segment elevations in leads II, III, and aVF. ECG also demonstrates gradual lengthening of the PR interval until one QRS complex is dropped. He is sent to the cardiac catheterization laboratory, where a stent is placed in one of his major coronary arteries. In which coronary artery was the stent most likely placed?

    (A) Diagonal branch of the LAD
    (B) Left anterior descending artery
    (C) Left circumflex artery
    (D) Left marginal artery
    (E) Right coronary artery

38. A 2-year-old Japanese girl is brought to the clinic by her parents, who are concerned about a persistent fever of 40°C (104°F) and an erythematous rash on her trunk that has been present for the past week. Laboratory tests show an erythrocyte sedimentation rate of 80 mm/hr, a C-reactive protein level of 15 mg/L, and a platelet count of 700,000/mm³. The doctors decide to treat her with intravenous immunoglobulin and aspirin to avoid a life-threatening complication. What other signs might this patient's doctors have seen that led them to initiate this therapy?

    (A) Hypothermia
    (B) Optic neuritis
    (C) Proteinuria
    (D) Pulmonary edema
    (E) Strawberry tongue

39. A 54-year-old woman comes to the physician three months after a undergoing a root canal, with primary complaints of persistent general malaise and fever. The symptoms developed slowly over the weeks following her root canal, but have not abated. The patient has a temperature of 38.3°C (100.1°F). Ophthalmic examination reveals retinal hemorrhages with clear central regions. Examination of the extremities reveals painful red nodules on her digits and dark macules on her palms and soles. On cardiac examination, a click and a systolic murmur are auscultated over the mitral valve. She tells the physician that the click is due to a mechanical valve replacement done four years ago because she had rheumatic fever as a child. Which of the following is the most appropriate treatment?

    (A) Acyclovir
    (B) Caspofungin
    (C) Clindamycin
    (D) Mebendazole
    (E) Metronidazole
    (F) Penicillin
    (G) Pentamidine

40. A 60-year-old diabetic man is brought to the emergency department by ambulance. His wife told paramedics that he had been progressively drowsy over the previous two-three hours. Forty-five minutes earlier he had announced that he was going to the bedroom to administer his nightly dose of insulin. When he didn't return to the living room, she went to check on him, and found him lying face down on the bed with an empty insulin needle beside him and an open bottle of propranolol on the nightstand. Upon arrival in the emergency department the patient is unresponsive. Heart rate is 45/min and his serum glucose level is 80 mg/dL. Which of the following is the most appropriate treatment to reverse the most likely cause of this patient's condition?

(A) Albuterol
(B) Cocaine
(C) Digitalis
(D) Glucagon
(E) Phenylephrine

41. Nitrates often are given as part of the management of angina. What is the primary mechanism by which nitrates work in the treatment of this condition?

(A) Decrease atrioventricular node conduction velocity
(B) Decrease heart rate and contractility
(C) Increase oxygen delivery to myocytes
(D) Stimulate dilation of coronary arterioles
(E) Stimulate venodilation

42. The image depicts the relationship of left ventricular pressure and volume in the cardiac cycle. The various phases of the cardiac cycle are labeled I through IV. During which phase are the pressures in the left atrium and left ventricle most equal?

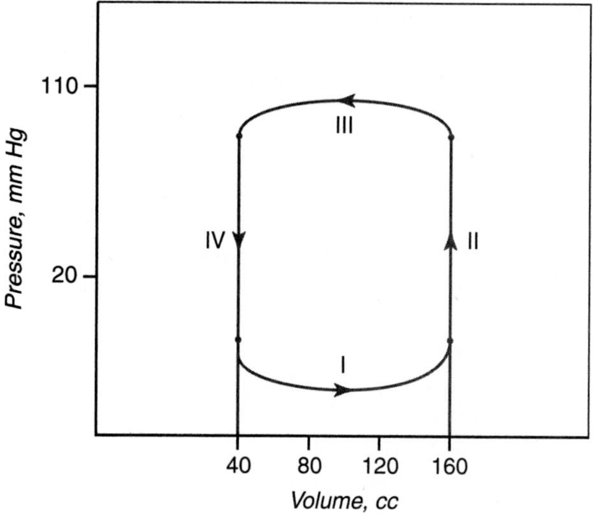

Reproduced, with permission, from USMLERx.com.

(A) Phase I
(B) Phase II
(C) Phase III
(D) Phase IV

43. A 32-year-old man with diabetes presents to his physician with orthostatic hypotension. A deficiency in the normal physiologic response carried out by arterial baroreceptors located in the aortic arch and the carotid sinus is suspected. What is the mechanism of the normal physiologic response to hypotension?

(A) Decreased baroreceptor afferent firing in the aortic arch leads to increased sympathetic efferent firing
(B) Decreased baroreceptor afferent firing in the carotid sinus leads to increased parasympathetic efferent firing
(C) Decreased baroreceptor afferent firing in the carotid sinus leads to increased sympathetic efferent firing
(D) Increased baroreceptor afferent firing in the aortic arch leads to increased parasympathetic efferent firing
(E) Increased baroreceptor afferent firing in the carotid sinus leads to increased sympathetic efferent firing

44. A 56-year-old woman presents to her physician due to recent onset of chest pain and dyspnea. Six weeks prior, the patient suffered a myocardial infarction. Her physical examination is remarkable for a friction rub over the fifth intercostal space in the midclavicular line, along with an elevated jugular venous pressure. What is the most likely cause of this patient's presentation?

    (A) Cardiac arrhythmia
    (B) Dressler syndrome
    (C) Left ventricular failure
    (D) Thromboembolism
    (E) Ventricular rupture

45. A 45-year-old African-American man is brought to the emergency department because of sudden chest pain radiating to the back. The pain started while the patient was taking his morning jog. X-ray of the chest is immediately done and shows a widened mediastinum. The patient has a history of anaphylaxis related to the type of iodinated contrast agent used in CT. Therefore, an MRI is performed to confirm the expected diagnosis. Findings on a sagittal bright blood MRI are shown in the image. Which of the following co-morbidities is most directly responsible for the patient's potentially fatal condition?

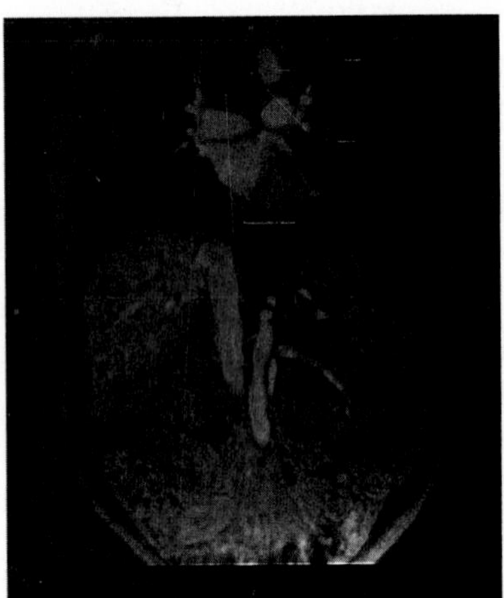

Reproduced, with permission, from USMLERx.com.

    (A) Cocaine abuse
    (B) Diabetes
    (C) Hypercholesterolemia
    (D) Hypertension
    (E) Sickle cell disease

46. A 76-year-old man receives a pacemaker to treat a dangerous form of heart block. His condition is characterized by an ECG with a constant PR interval, with the random absence of QRS complexes. Which of the following abnormalities is the most likely cause of this type of heart block?

    (A) Atrioventricular node abnormality
    (B) Defect in the His-Purkinje system
    (C) Independently contracting atria and ventricles
    (D) Retrograde conduction
    (E) Sinoatrial node abnormality

47. A 56-year-old white man is rushed to the emergency department after complaining of crushing substernal chest pain. He is morbidly obese, diaphoretic, tachypneic, and clutching his chest. Initial ECG reveals ST-segment elevations in the anterior leads. The patient is stabilized and seems to be doing well, but then he suddenly experiences cardiac arrest and dies. Which of the following is the most likely cause of death in this patient?

    (A) Arrhythmia
    (B) Formation of ventricular septal defect
    (C) Mural thrombosis
    (D) Myocardial pump failure
    (E) Rupture of ventricular free wall
    (F) Ruptured papillary muscle

48. The image is a representation of the pressure-volume (P-V) relationship in the left ventricle during a typical cardiac cycle. The phases of the cardiac cycle are labeled I through IV. Which of the following occurrences alone would increase the width of the P-V loop?

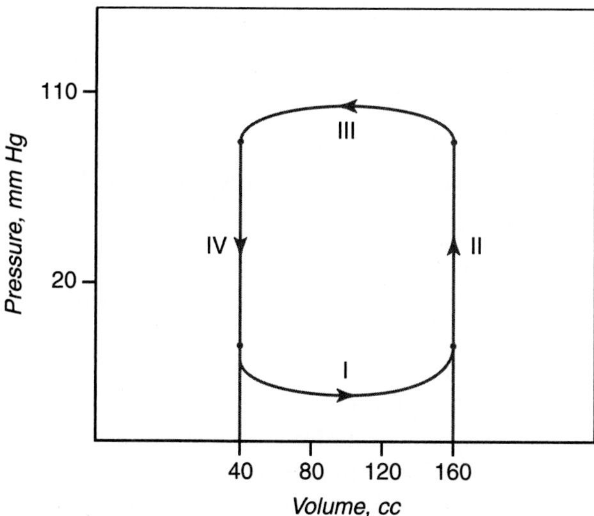

Reproduced, with permission, from USMLERx.com.

(A) Decreased afterload
(B) Decreased contractility
(C) Decreased preload
(D) Increased arterial pressure
(E) Increased end-systolic volume

49. Cardiac output is a function of stroke volume and heart rate. Stroke volume increases when contractility increases, preload increases, or afterload decreases. There are a number of factors that affect each of these components and ultimately cardiac output. Which of the following variations would increase cardiac output in an otherwise normal patient?

(A) β-Blocker treatment
(B) Cardiac glycoside administration
(C) Increasing extracellular sodium concentration
(D) Lowering intracellular calcium concentration
(E) Metabolic acidosis

50. A 54-year-old woman presents to her physician with swelling in her extremities. Palpation produces significant pitting. Which of the following conditions represents the most likely physiologic basis for this physical finding?

(A) Decreased capillary permeability
(B) Decreased capillary pressure
(C) Increased interstitial fluid pressure
(D) Increased interstitial oncotic pressure
(E) Increased plasma protein levels

ANSWERS

1. **The correct answer is D.** This patient has Wolff-Parkinson-White (WPW) syndrome, a condition whereby the heart is abnormally stimulated by an accessory electrical pathway (often known as the bundle of Kent). The presence of Δ-wave (a sloping upstroke of the QRS complex) is diagnostic. Amiodarone is an effective pharmacologic agent for this condition. This is a potassium channel blocker (class III antiarrhythmic). Procainamide also can be used; however, it is a sodium channel blocker (class Ia), which is not one of the answer choices.

   Answer A is incorrect. An example of a β-adrenergic receptor blocker is metoprolol. It is used to treat hypertension and atrial fibrillation (to slow down the ventricular rate) but is contraindicated WPW sndrome. This is a class II antiarrhythmic agent.

   Answer B is incorrect. Acetylcholine receptor is blocked by atropine, among other anticholinergic agents. Atropine has a wide variety of clinical uses such as increasing sinoatrial node firing (to treat bradycardia) and decreasing bronchiole secretion (such as during anesthesia).

   Answer C is incorrect. An example of a calcium channel blocker is verapamil (class IV antiarrhythmic). It is used to treat hypertension and atrial fibrillation (to slow down the ventricular rate) but is contraindicated in WPW syndrome.

   Answer E is incorrect. The sodium-potassium ATPase enzyme is inhibited by digoxin, which is used to increase myocardial contraction in the symptomatic treatment of congestive heart failure (CHF).

2. **The correct answer is C.** Drug X is hydralazine, a vasodilator used to treat essential hypertension and CHF (although rarely used today). It works by increasing cGMP levels, which causes smooth muscle relaxation. The effect is greater on arterioles than veins, causing a reduction in afterload.

   Answer A is incorrect. This is the mechanism of calcium channel blockers such as nifedipine, not of hydralazine.

   Answer B is incorrect. Hydralazine works by increasing cGMP, not decreasing it.

   Answer D is incorrect. This is the mechanism of angiotensin-converting enzyme (ACE) inhibitors, not of hydralazine.

   Answer E is incorrect. This is the mechanism of acetazolamide, not hydralazine.

   Answer F is incorrect. Hydrochlorothiazide acts on the early distal tubule in the kidney.

3. **The correct answer is E.** The inhibition of de novo cholesterol synthesis results in reduced intrahepatic cholesterol concentrations, which then stimulates hepatocytes to upregulate surface LDL cholesterol receptors. This facilitates the clearance of LDL cholesterol from the circulation. In addition, circulated LDL cholesterol precursors, including VLDL cholesterol remnants, are cleared more rapidly from circulation because of their cross-recognition with hepatic LDL cholesterol receptors.

   Answer A is incorrect. Although statins decrease hepatic synthesis of cholesterol, they have no direct effect on LDL cholesterol production.

   Answer B is incorrect. Statins only mildly reduce the plasma concentrations of triglycerides.

   Answer C is incorrect. Statins cause upregulation, not downregulation, of surface LDL cholesterol receptors.

   Answer D is incorrect. Statins do not directly increase HDL cholesterol production. They can have a mild beneficial effect on HDL cholesterol in some patients, but it is not a consistent result.

4. **The correct answer is D.** The key is to realize that the question is asking for results of urinalysis (not serum electrolyte values). The

ECG shows peak T waves and a widened QRS interval, which are classic changes seen in hyperkalemia. Spironolactone is the most likely medication to affect urinary electrolytes. As an inhibitor of aldosterone receptors in the collecting tubule and an inhibitor of Na^+ channels, spironolactone greatly decreases the excretion of K^+ and mildly increases the excretion of Na^+. Urine volume will be high-normal because the diuretic will increase saltwater wasting.

Answer A is incorrect. Spironolactone decreases K^+ excretion, so there will be decreased levels of K^+ in the urine sample.

Answer B is incorrect. Na^+ excretion will be increased with the use of spironolactone; also, diuretics will increase the amount of urine volume excreted.

Answer C is incorrect. Spironolactone will increase Na^+ excretion and decrease K^+ excretion so that K^+ concentrations will be decreased in the urine and Na^+ concentrations will be increased. Treatment involves cystidine or uridine to bypass this step in pyrimidine synthesis and also to negatively downregulate orotic acid production.

Answer E is incorrect. Spironolactone decreases K^+ excretion but increases Na^+ excretion; therefore, Na^+ concentrations will be elevated in the urine.

5. **The correct answer is A.** This patient has tetralogy of Fallot, which is defined by the combined symptoms of ventricular septal defect (VSD), overriding aorta, pulmonary stenosis, and right ventricular hypertrophy. The cause of these abnormalities, however, is an anterosuperior displacement of the infundibular septum during heart development in utero. Patients with tetralogy of Fallot learn to squat during cyanotic spells, which causes compression of the femoral arteries, thereby decreases their right-to-left shunt.

   Answer B is incorrect. An overriding aorta is one of the four manifestations of tetralogy of Fallot, not the cause.

   Answer C is incorrect. Patent ductus arteriosus is not the cause of tetralogy of Fallot. In fact, a patent ductus arteriosus is protective in patients with tetralogy of Fallot because it causes some of the unoxygenated blood from the overriding aorta to return to the pulmonary artery to be oxygenated.

   Answer D is incorrect. Pulmonary stenosis is one of the four manifestations of tetralogy of Fallot, not the cause.

   Answer E is incorrect. VSD is one of the four manifestations of tetralogy of Fallot, not the cause.

6. **The correct answer is G.** Voltage-gated Ca^+ channels (L type) open slowly in response to the sodium upstroke (approximately around -40 mV), allowing calcium to flow down its concentration gradient and into the cell. Concurrently, there is an outward potassium current via voltage-gated channels that leads to the plateau. The result is a slow conduction velocity that prolongs the transmission from the atria to the ventricles.

   Answer A is incorrect. Ion channels in the myocardium are voltage gated.

   Answer B is incorrect. During phase 2, voltage-gated potassium cells open to allow potassium efflux.

   Answer C is incorrect. Ion channels in the myocardium are voltage gated.

   Answer D is incorrect. Voltage-gated sodium channels are responsible for the upstroke in ventricular cells (phase 0).

   Answer E is incorrect. During phase 2, voltage-gated potassium cells open to allow potassium efflux.

   Answer F is incorrect. Closing voltage-gated sodium channels would hyperpolarize the cell. Voltage-gated sodium channels are responsible for the upstroke in ventricular cells (phase 0). These open in response to depolarization to the -55mV threshold value, allowing sodium to rapidly flow down its concentration gradient into the cell. These channels are then inactivated and cannot be opened again until the cell is repolarized.

7. **The correct answer is E.** Troponin is a protein found along the sarcomeres that assist in muscle contraction. With muscle injury, troponin is leaked into the serum. Different fractions show different specificities for different tissues. In cardiac tissue, troponin I has been shown to be more specific and equally if not more sensitive than cardiac enzymes, CK-MB in particular.

   Answer A is incorrect. Alanine aminotransferase (ALT) is found mostly in the liver and is therefore a specific marker of damage to hepatocytes. Elevations of ALT are not associated with myocardial infarction (MI).

   Answer B is incorrect. Aspartate aminotransferase (AST) is an enzyme found in the heart, liver, and skeletal muscle, and an elevation in it is nonspecific for damage to those tissues. Although commonly elevated in the setting of liver disease, AST levels peak around day two post-MI.

   Answer C is incorrect. Creatinine kinase (CK) is located on the inner mitochondrial membrane, on myofibrils, and in the muscle cytoplasm and catalyzes the production of ATP. It is released during skeletal muscle injury (MM), cardiac injury (MB), and brain injury (BB). In this case, there is an infiltration of neutrophils and the cardiac muscle strand is lysing and losing its striations. These findings are consistent with an acute MI one-three days earlier. During an acute MI, the most specific serum elevations are seen in CK-MB and troponin I. Between the two, however, troponin I has been proven to be more specific, and equally if not more sensitive than CK-MB.

   Answer D is incorrect. Lactate dehydrogenase (LDH) is an enzyme found in many tissues throughout the body. It is a useful marker for liver disease, MI, and hemolysis but is not specific for any one tissue. Before CK-MB (cardiac injury) and troponin I detection, it was the test of choice in diagnosing MI.

8. **The correct answer is A.** Epinephrine is a nonselective agonist of α- and β-adrenergic receptors. Administering a large dose of epinephrine causes an increase in blood pressure via an increased heart rate and in contractility through stimulation of β_1 receptors; and net a increase in systemic vascular resistance through α_1-mediated vasoconstriction (the β_2-mediated vasodilation is negligible compared to the α_1 effects). Adding phentolamine, a selective α_1 antagonist, blocks the α effects of epinephrine. Therefore re-administration leaves only the β_1-receptor actions (increased contractility and heart rate) and the β_2-mediated increase in vasodilation, causing a net decrease in blood pressure.

   Answer B is incorrect. Isoproterenol is an agonist of β- and α-adrenergic receptors, although its primary action is at the β receptor. Hence, adding isoproterenol actually would cause a decrease in pressure through β_2-mediated vasodilation. Clonidine is an α agonist, and would lead to decreased sympathetic outflow and possibly cause an additional decrease in pressure. Adding isoproterenol after clonidine administration would lead to a further decrease in blood pressure.

   Answer C is incorrect. Norepinephrine is an agonist at mainly α-adrenergic receptors but also some β_1 activity. This leads to an increase in vasoconstriction. Propranolol is a nonspecific β blocker, which would not block the effects of norepinephrine, so readministration would cause an increase in blood pressure.

   Answer D is incorrect. Phenylephrine is an α_1 agonist that would cause an increase in pressure through α_1-stimulated vasoconstriction. Metoprolol is a β_1 blocker, which would not inhibit the effects of phenylephrine. Therefore re-administration of phenylephrine would cause another increase in blood pressure.

   Answer E is incorrect. Phenylephrine is an α_1 agonist that would cause an increase in pressure through α_1-stimulated vasoconstriction. Phentolamine is a nonselective α blocker, which would block the increase in pressure caused by phenylephrine and cause no change in pressure after repeat phenylephrine administration.

9. **The correct answer is E.** Nifedipine is a dihydropyridine class calcium channel blocker that could be used in the long-term control of hypertension. However, in the case of a hypertensive emergency, nifedipine used sublingually can cause dangerous fluctuations in blood pressure that are difficult to control and can lead to more harm than good.

   Answer A is incorrect. Diltiazem is a benzothiazepine class calcium channel blocker that reduces myocardial demand and also causes vasodilation. It is not contraindicated in this patient.

   Answer B is incorrect. Labetalol is a combined α/β-blocker that has effects on both receptors. It can be used in a hypertensive situation as an emergent option for treatment. It is not contraindicated in this patient.

   Answer C is incorrect. Metoprolol is a β-blocker used to treat angina by reducing heart rate and contractility. It also reduces the metabolic demand of the myocardium. It is often used to control hypertension, but is not contraindicated in this patient.

   Answer D is incorrect. Captopril is an ACE inhibitor used in the control of chronic hypertension. It is especially useful for patients who have signs of renal disease and can slow the progression of damage to the kidneys. It is not contraindicated in this patient.

10. **The correct answer is D.** This patient most likely suffered from acute mitral regurgitation secondary to rupture of the posterior papillary muscle. The anterior and posterior papillary muscles anchor the chordae tendineae, which prevent the cusps of the mitral valve from being forced into the left atrium. An occlusion of the posterior descending artery can lead to an infarction of the posterior papillary muscle and subsequent rupture of the muscle several days later. Patients will present with a sudden onset of pulmonary edema and frequently cardiogenic shock.

    Answer A is incorrect. The anterior papillary muscle is supplied by both the left anterior descending artery and the left circumflex artery. Because of its dual blood supply, the anterior papillary muscle is less likely to rupture after a MI. Furthermore, the patient's initial MI involved the posterior aspect of the myocardium.

    Answer B is incorrect. The anterior papillary muscle is supplied by both the left anterior descending artery and the left circumflex artery. Because of its dual blood supply, the anterior papillary muscle is less likely to rupture after a MI. Furthermore, the patient's initial MI involved the posterior aspect of the myocardium.

    Answer C is incorrect. The left (or obtuse) marginal artery, which is a branch of the left circumflex artery, follows the left border of the heart to supply the left ventricle.

    Answer E is incorrect. The right marginal artery follows the inferior border of the heart to supply the right ventricle.

11. **The correct answer is C.** The key finding is hypertrophy with asymmetric septal enlargement without free ventricular wall enlargement. This is seen in patients with hypertrophic obstructive cardiomyopathy (HOCM). Mutation in a sarcomere gene such as myosin-binding protein C is one of the most common genetic causes of HOCM. This type of cardiomyopathy is inherited in an autosomal dominant fashion. The anatomic distortion can lead to a dynamic ventricular outflow obstruction during systolic ejection, which leads to a systolic murmur, dyspnea, lightheadedness, syncope, and in many cases sudden death. On histologic examination, HOCM would show disoriented, tangled, hypertrophied myocardial fibers.

    Answer A is incorrect. Infection with an *Enterovirus*, namely coxsackie B virus, initially causes a subacute myocarditis but can eventually lead to dilated cardiomyopathy (DCM). Pathologically, DCM produces a grossly enlarged heart with dilation of all four chambers and normal ventricular wall thickness. Other etiologies for DCM include alcohol abuse, wet beriberi, cocaine use, Chagas disease, doxorubicin toxicity, hemochromatosis, and peripartum cardiomyopathy.

Answer B is incorrect. Immune-mediated destruction of cardiomyocytes is the cause of cardiac damage in rheumatic fever. This disease is a consequence of pharyngeal infection with group A β-hemolytic streptococci. Early deaths from rheumatic heart disease are due to myocarditis, whereas late sequelae include damage to the heart valves. Histologically, this disease is associated with Aschoff bodies, which are granulomas with giant cells. The heart muscle itself, however, would appear grossly normal.

Answer D is incorrect. Deposits of protein such as light chains, heavy chains, or transthyretin are associated with amyloidosis. Amyloidosis produces a restrictive cardiomyopathy, in which the ventricular wall and chamber size grossly appear normal, which is not consistent with the reduced chamber size seen in this specimen. In addition, amyloidosis is generally a disease of the elderly, and is thus not as likely in this 17-year-old patient.

Answer E is incorrect. Chagas disease is caused by a trypanosome that is primarily endemic to South America. Eighty percent of those infected will develop myocarditis, and 10% will suffer acute cardiac death later. Grossly, the myocardium can appear normal or slightly dilated, with minute hemorrhagic lesions.

12. **The correct answer is C.** A mutation in the factor V gene, also known as factor V Leiden, causes resistance to deactivation of factor V by protein C. Uninhibited factor V activity leads to a hypercoagulable state, which predisposes to deep vein thrombosis (DVT) and subsequent pulmonary embolism (PE).

Answer A is incorrect. Factor VIII deficiency (hemophilia A) would predispose an individual to bleeding. Factor VIII is an integral part of the intrinsic coagulation cascade.

Answer B is incorrect. High, rather than low, homocysteine levels lead to a hypercoagulable state.

Answer D is incorrect. Proteins C and S act as negative regulators of the coagulation cascade. Therefore a deficiency, rather than overproduction, will lead to a hypercoagulable state.

Answer E is incorrect. Von Willebrand factor allows platelets to adhere to a defect where collagen is exposed and binds inactive factor VIII in circulation. A deficiency (von Willebrand disease) leads to bleeding complications such as epistaxis, menorrhagia, and gastrointestinal (GI) bleeds.

13. **The correct answer is E.** This girl has Takayasu arteritis, a large-vessel vasculitis usually found in women <40 years of age of Asian descent. It is characterized by a thickening of the aortic arch and/or the proximal great vessels. The most prominent feature is weak pulses in the upper extremities. Complications of untreated late-stage Takayasu include aortic aneurysms and typically involve the aortic arch. This leads to narrowing, or possible obliteration, of the major arteries associated with the aortic arch. Treatment involves high doses of oral prednisone that are tapered over many months as the clinician and patient agree to minimize the adverse effects of corticosteroids.

Answer A is incorrect. Abdominal pain and melena can be present in patients with polyarteritis nodosa, a vasculitis of small- or medium-sized arteries. These symptoms are due to ischemia and infarction of the intestines. Classically, Takayasu disease affects the aortic arch, although the aortic root (dilation with subsequent valvular insufficiency) and coronary arteries (narrowing and potential infarction) may be involved in the later stages of the disease.

Answer B is incorrect. Intermittent jaw claudication is indicative of temporal (giant-cell) arteritis. Giant-cell arteritis is a medium/large vessel vasculitis that typically affects arteries on the head. It usually is seen in women >70 years, and common symptoms include fever, headache (temporal area), jaw claudication, reduced visual acuity, and sudden vision loss. The diagnosis is achieved via a tissue biopsy of the temporal artery and treatment is with corticosteroids. Giant-cell arteritis may present as sudden monocular blindness, and emergent corticosteroids are needed to save that eye.

Answer C is incorrect. Pneumonitis is a classic symptom of Wegener granulomatosis, a necrotizing small-vessel vasculitis primarily affecting the kidneys and the lungs. The classic clinical vignette for Wegener will describe a patient who presents with hemoptysis and hematuria and who has classical antineutrophil cytoplasmic antibodies on serologic evaluation.

Answer D is incorrect. Strawberry tongue is seen in children with Kawasaki disease, an arteritis that often involves the coronary arteries, but can affect vessels of any size. In children, the symptoms of Kawasaki's can relent without treatment and the major complications are coronary artery aneurysms and MIs. The diagnostic criteria for this disease are five days of fever plus four of five of the following: (1) erythema of the lips or oral cavity or cracking of the lips; (2) rash on the trunk; (3) swelling or erythema of the hands or feet; (4) red eyes (conjunctival injection); and (5) a swollen lymph node in the neck >15 mm.

14. **The correct answer is D.** The ECG demonstrates a pattern characteristic of torsades de pointes. Quinidine, a class IA antiarrhythmic agent, is used to treat supraventricular arrhythmias by slowing conduction. A simultaneous increase of the QT interval caused by quinidine risks torsades de pointes.

Answer A is incorrect. Adenosine is used both to diagnose and to treat supraventricular tachyarrhythmias. However, it is not associated with torsades des pointes.

Answer B is incorrect. Although the class III antiarrhythmics tend to be associated with torsades des pointes, bretylium is an exception to this rule and has no association with this condition.

Answer C is incorrect. Propranolol is a class II antiarrhythmic, but it is not associated with torsades de pointes. β Blockers such as propranolol are used to suppress abnormal pacemakers by decreasing the slope of phase 4 of the cardiac cycle; in other words, it slows the diastolic depolarization of pacemaker cells.

Answer E is incorrect. Bepridil, not verapamil, is a calcium channel blocker and class IV antiarrhythmic known to be associated with torsades de pointes. Verapamil and diltiazem are two calcium channel blockers used in the prevention of nodal arrhythmias (eg, supraventricular tachycardia).

15. **The correct answer is E.** This patient presents with shortness of breath and dyspnea on exertion. The bilateral crackles detected on physical examination indicate pulmonary edema. This spectrum of signs and symptoms are suggestive of left ventricular dysfunction leading to CHF. CHF itself has many causes, but the lack of other clinical findings (no rubs or murmurs) indicates either hypertensive heart disease or cardiomyopathy as likely etiologies. Cardiomyopathy can be divided into dilated, hypertrophic, or restrictive. Alcoholism and coxsackie virus B have been strongly associated with dilated cardiomyopathy.

Answer A is incorrect. Aortic strictures are typically associated with the congenital defect known as coarctation of the aorta. Twice as common in men as in women, coarctation is fairly common in patients with Turner syndrome. While pumping against a permanently elevated afterload may cause left ventricular hypertrophy and eventually failure, this condition would result in a slightly different clinical picture. The patient would have higher blood pressure in the upper extremities than in the lower extremities, causing additional symptoms of claudication and coldness in the feet. Also, coarctations often produce a detectable systolic murmur.

Answer B is incorrect. Fibrosis of the endocardium is associated with the effects of a carcinoid tumor on the heart. Signs that are usually detected on auscultation are pulmonic stenosis or tricuspid regurgitation. Classic symptoms of carcinoid syndrome include flushing, diarrhea, and bronchospasm.

Answer C is incorrect. Fibrotic debris within the pericardial membrane occurs in constrictive pericarditis. A pericardial friction rub would be detectable on auscultation.

Answer D is incorrect. Ischemia of the myocardium is usually the result of coronary artery disease and typically presents with complaints of chest pain. An active coronary artery disease process has been ruled out by angiography.

16. **The correct answer is C.** Inferior vena cava (IVC) compression is common in women during the third trimester of pregnancy. The large uterus compresses the IVC, decreasing venous return to the heart. This reduction in preload reduces stroke volume, thus reducing cardiac output. Recall that mean arterial pressure = cardiac output × total peripheral resistance; an acute decrease in either of these parameters will reduce blood pressure. Pregnant women can avoid this problem by placing a pillow under their right side or by lying on their left side to remove the weight of the gravid uterus from the IVC.

    Answer A is incorrect. During pregnancy the total plasma volume increases to 30%-50% greater than normal at term. RBC mass increases during pregnancy as well due to increased circulating erythropoietin levels. The expansion of intravascular volume is relatively greater than the increase in RBC mass, resulting in a physiologic anemia. However, this generally does not cause adverse symptoms for the mother, and would not cause hypotension in a supine position.

    Answer B is incorrect. Cardiogenic shock can cause hypotension by decreasing the stroke volume and cardiac output, but it would not occur only in the supine position.

    Answer D is incorrect. When fluid leaves the intravascular space and enters the interstitial space, it is referred to as third spacing. In pregnancy, there is a physiologic amount of third spacing, which causes dependent edema in the hands and feet. Some women may even experience pulmonary edema, which can be dangerous. Third spacing does cause hypotension if the intravascular volume is not replaced, but it would not cause isolated hypotension in the supine position.

    Answer E is incorrect. Vasodilation will reduce blood pressure, and pregnant women do have a constant amount of vasodilation that is greater than that in nonpregnant women. Blood pressure decreases by about 10 mm Hg during pregnancy, particularly during the first and second trimesters. However, this vasodilation should remain relatively constant when transferring from an upright to a supine position, and would not account for the sudden hypotension seen in this case.

17. **The correct answer is C.** Hyperlipidemia is a recognized risk factor for atherosclerosis. Current concepts describing the pathogenesis of this process suggest that the first step is the oxidation of LDL cholesterol. This then causes endothelial damage that leads to monocyte activation, formation of foam cells, smooth muscle proliferation, and subsequent arterial plaques. The oxidation of LDL cholesterol increases monocyte receptor affinity for the molecule and stimulates the monocytes to migrate into the subendothelial space of the artery. Macrophages that phagocytose these molecules become foam cells, which then lead to other downstream effects of atherosclerosis such as calcification and occlusion of the vessel lumen. This in turn can lead to ischemia of various tissues, most notably the heart.

    Answer A is incorrect. Endothelial dysfunction is one of the primary steps in the pathogenesis of atherosclerosis. Endothelial dysfunction can be caused by numerous factors, such as the toxins found in cigarette smoke, and is not necessarily caused by oxidized LDL cholesterol. However, when looking specifically at the relationship between hyperlipidemia and atherosclerosis, LDL oxidation generally occurs before endothelial dysfunction.

    Answer B is incorrect. Foam cells are formed from macrophages that phagocytosed oxidized LDL cholesterol. In fact, they only uptake LDL cholesterol once it has undergone oxidation, which then causes changes in the LDL cholesterol that signal activation of macrophage "scavenger" receptors (CD36). Foam cells play an important role in the pathogenesis of atherosclerosis, but they are not the first step in the pathway between hyperlipidemia and atherosclerosis.

Answer D is incorrect. Monocyte activation plays a role in the pathogenesis of atherosclerosis, but it is not the first step in the pathway between hyperlipidemia and atherosclerosis.

Answer E is incorrect. Plaque formation is the result of many of these steps, and it contributes to the pathogenesis of atherosclerosis. However, it is not the first step in the pathway between hyperlipidemia and atherosclerosis.

18. **The correct answer is A.** In tricuspid regurgitation, blood flows backward into the atria during ventricular systole. This would affect the C and X waves, replacing them with a large positive deflection. This positive deflection effectively joins the C wave and the V wave, creating the "CV wave." The C wave is thought to be due to pressure on the tricuspid valve during ventricular systole. If the valve allows backflow during ventricular systole, the increased ventricular pressures would be transmitted back into the right atrium and the jugular vein. The downward movement of the ventricle causes the x descent during ventricular systole. This would also be replaced by a positive deflection from blood regurgitating into the atria during ventricular systole.

    Answer B is incorrect. These points are not the most likely to be affected in tricuspid regurgitation.

    Answer C is incorrect. These points are not the most likely to be affected in tricuspid regurgitation.

    Answer D is incorrect. These points are not the most likely to be affected in tricuspid regurgitation. The V wave is increased pressure because of right atrial filling against a closed tricuspid valve. With tricuspid regurgitation, there is little effect on the V wave itself, but rather it becomes the end point for the new CV-wave change.

19. **The correct answer is C.** The patient's history of a prior illness with features of fever, pleuritic chest pain, joint pain, and rash (probably erythema marginatum) is indicative of rheumatic fever. If left untreated, rheumatic fever can evolve into rheumatic heart disease, which typically presents with mitral valve stenosis. This can be heard on auscultation as a high-pitched opening snap that follows S_2, and a low-frequency decrescendo diastolic murmur heard best over the apex of the heart. The increased resistance to flow from the left atrium to the left ventricle leads to an increase in left atrial pressure.

    Answer A is incorrect. Left atrial pressure would increase, not decrease, with mitral stenosis.

    Answer B is incorrect. Mitral stenosis would not result in an overall decrease in left ventricular pressure; pressure will only be decreased relative to the left atrium.

    Answer D is incorrect. Left ventricular pressure would increase with aortic stenosis. Rheumatic heart disease most typically presents as mitral stenosis, although aortic stenosis is the next most common presentation.

    Answer E is incorrect. Right atrial pressure would increase in response to pulmonic valve stenosis or tricuspid valve stenosis. The tricuspid valve is sometimes affected in rheumatic heart disease and would also cause a diastolic murmur. However, this is far less common than mitral stenosis in the setting of rheumatic heart disease. In fact, the pulmonic valve is the least likely to be affected in rheumatic heart disease.

20. **The correct answer is B.** The inferior mesenteric artery (IMA) originates from the aorta inferior to the renal arteries and superior to the bifurcation of the aorta into the common iliac arteries. The IMA supplies blood to the distal one-third of the transverse colon, descending and sigmoid colons, and the upper portion of the rectum. The IMA may sometimes be sacrificed during an infrarenal aortic aneurysm repair rather than being reattached to a healthy segment of aorta. Usually there is enough collateral flow to the hindgut from the superior mesenteric artery and the hypogastric arteries that the loss of the IMA does not result in co-

lonic ischemia. However, ischemia of the sigmoid colon occurs in 1%-7% of repairs, and should be considered if bloody diarrhea or an increased WBC count occurs postoperatively.

Answer A is incorrect. The ascending colon receives its blood supply from the superior mesenteric artery. This vessel is located superior to the renal arteries and thus would not be disrupted during resection of the infrarenal aorta.

Answer C is incorrect. The small intestine, as well as the distal duodenum and proximal two-thirds of the transverse colon, receive blood supply from the superior mesenteric artery, which branches off the aorta above the level of the renal arteries. Thus blood flow to these structures would not be affected.

Answer D is incorrect. The spleen receives its blood supply from the splenic artery. This vessel is a branch of the celiac trunk that emerges from the aorta superior to the renal arteries. Thus blood flow to the spleen would not be affected.

Answer E is incorrect. The stomach receives its blood supply from various branches of the celiac trunk, which emerges from the aorta above the level of the renal arteries, and would thus not be affected.

21. **The correct answer is D.** Syphilitic aortitis is characterized by obliterative endarteritis of the vasa vasorum of the tunica media. This disruption of the vasa vasorum can lead to an aneurysm, typically involving the ascending aorta, and is a manifestation of the tertiary stage of the disease. Syphilitic aneurysms are often complicated by atherosclerosis. The patient's skin lesions are likely "gummas" of tertiary syphilis, which appear as fibrous nodules on the skin surface. Less commonly, these lesions can be ulcerative.

    Answer A is incorrect. Atherosclerosis is most frequently associated with a descending aortic aneurysm, especially one involving the abdominal aorta, and is rarely associated with ascending aortic aneurysms in the absence of underlying pathology, such as that of tertiary syphilis.

    Answer B is incorrect. Congenital medial weakness is actually associated with the development of berry aneurysms, which typically occur along the circle of Willis. They are the most frequent cause of subarachnoid hemorrhage and are also associated with adult polycystic kidney disease.

    Answer C is incorrect. Cystic medial necrosis (cystic degeneration of the tunica media of the aorta) is the most frequent pre-existing histologic lesion in aortic dissection. It is associated with dilation of the ascending aorta, particularly in relation to Marfan syndrome. Although this answer choice is possible, the skin lesions point to tertiary syphilis as the most likely cause of the cardiac pathology.

    Answer E is incorrect. Hypertension is often implicated in the etiology of dissecting aneurysms due to a longitudinal intraluminal tear. Dissection is usually not associated with aortic dilation.

22. **The correct answer is B.** This infant is presenting with a patent ductus arteriosus (PDA), a left-to-right shunt that rarely causes cyanosis. PDA is associated with maternal rubella infection during pregnancy. During fetal development, the ductus arteriosus remains patent through the action of prostaglandin E_2 (PGE_2). PDA at birth is closed with indomethacin, a nonsteroidal anti-inflammatory drug (NSAID) that inhibits PGE_2 formation. Remember, there are, in general, three congenital heart lesions that cause late cyanosis as a result of left-to-right shunt: VSD, atrial septal defect (ASD), and PDA. The classic murmur heard with PDA is a continuous, machine-like murmur.

    Answer A is incorrect. Thromboxane A_2 causes platelet aggregation and vasoconstriction. Indomethacin would decrease thromboxane formation by inhibiting cyclooxygenase-1 and -2 enzymes.

    Answer C is incorrect. M_2-receptors are G-protein-linked and are responsible for lowering both heart rate and heart contractility.

Answer D is incorrect. Prostaglandin E_2-receptor activation increases body temperature.

Answer E is incorrect. Prostaglandin $F_2\alpha$-receptor activation causes uterine contractions and bronchoconstriction.

23. **The correct answer is A.** Adenosine is extremely useful in abolishing atrioventricular (AV) nodal arrhythmias when given in high-dose intravenous (IV) boluses. Adenosine works by hyperpolarizing AV node tissue by increasing the conductance of potassium and by reducing calcium current. As a result, the conduction through the AV node is markedly reduced. In addition to this, adenosine's extremely short duration of action (15 seconds) limits the occurrence of its toxicities (ie, hypotension, flushing, chest pain, and dyspnea).

 Answer B is incorrect. Bretylium, a potassium channel blocker (class III), is used when other antiarrhythmics fail.

 Answer C is incorrect. Encainide is used when ventricular tachycardia progresses to ventricular fibrillation; it is also used in intractable supraventricular tachycardia.

 Answer D is incorrect. Lidocaine, a class Ib antiarrhythmic, is used in the treatment of acute ventricular arrhythmias such as post-MI arrhythmias.

 Answer E is incorrect. Sotalol, which is both a β-adrenergic-receptor blocker (class II) and a potassium channel blocker (class III), is used when other antiarrhythmics fail.

24. **The correct answer is E.** Gemfibrozil is a fibrate that stimulates lipoprotein lipase by activation of the PPARα protein. In so doing, it has beneficial effects on the serum lipid profile. Adverse effects of fibrates include elevation of liver enzymes and myositis.

 Answer A is incorrect. Gemfibrozil speeds the conversion of VLDL to LDL cholesterol.

 Answer B is incorrect. Gemfibrozil has no effect on triglyceride receptors.

 Answer C is incorrect. Gemfibrozil promotes PPAR-α activation.

 Answer D is incorrect. Gemfibrozil inhibits lipolysis.

25. **The correct answer is A.** This man has suffered a MI. He demonstrates two of the five important risk factors for developing heart disease, which include hypertension, hyperlipidemia, tobacco use, diabetes, and a family history of heart disease. The changes that occur in the affected cardiac tissue can be helpful in assessing when the infarct occurred. During the first day after an MI, the affected tissue begins to undergo coagulative necrosis and releases enzymes such as troponin I and CK-MB from the dying cells. Coagulative necrosis is marked in the early stages by preservation of general tissue architecture, with myocytes becoming increasingly eosinophilic. Contraction bands will also be seen, causing myocytes to take on a wavy appearance.

 Answer B is incorrect. The presence of granulation tissue indicates that remodeling of damaged tissue is occurring. It is characterized by the presence of fibroblasts and vascular proliferation. This would first be seen, along with a mixed inflammatory picture, beginning 5-10 days after a MI.

 Answer C is incorrect. Macrophages are seen in the development of chronic inflammation. Five to ten days after an MI, macrophages come to the scene to aid in cleaning up areas of dead tissue. It is important to remember that it usually takes time for macrophages and other signs of chronic inflammation to appear in any setting.

 Answer D is incorrect. Neutrophils are the hallmark of an acute inflammatory process. A massive influx of neutrophils, along with extensive coagulative necrosis, begins at 12-24 hours and continues until about four days after an MI. Although neutrophils are generally considered the first responders in any inflammatory process, they appear after the start of coagulative necrosis in the evolution of an MI.

 Answer E is incorrect. In the first 2-4 hours following an MI, no change can be detected using light microscopy. However, by eight hours changes associated with coagulative necrosis would certainly be visible.

26. **The correct answer is B.** Point A corresponds to the opening of the mitral valve at the beginning of diastole, and the line from A to C shows the increase in ventricular volume during diastole. Point C marks the beginning of systole as left ventricular pressure becomes greater than left atrial pressure, causing the mitral valve to close. This closure (in conjunction with the closure of the tricuspid valve) represents S_1. The line from point C to D corresponds to isovolumetric contraction, during which both the mitral and aortic valves remain closed as the left ventricular pressure increases. At point D the left ventricular pressure becomes greater than the aortic pressure and the aortic valve opens. Between points D and F the left ventricular pressure continues to increase as the ventricle continues to contract and blood is ejected from the left ventricle into the aorta. At point F the aortic valve closes when the left ventricle begins to relax and the left ventricular pressure becomes less than aortic pressure. This closure (in conjunction with the closure of the pulmonic valve) represents S_2. The line from point F to point A represents the isovolumetric relaxation at the end of ventricular systole. When the left ventricular pressure becomes less than the pressure in the left atrium, the mitral valve opens, thus beginning a new loop of the cardiac cycle (diastole plus systole). Point B corresponds to the point near the end of diastole when S_4 may be heard. An S_4, commonly called the "atrial kick," is not normally present in adults. Its presence suggests a decrease in ventricular compliance, such as occurs in ventricular hypertrophy resulting from chronic hypertension. S_4 is thought to result from vibration of a stiff, noncompliant ventricular wall as blood is rapidly ejected into the ventricle from the atrium.

    Answer A is incorrect. Point A represents the opening of the mitral valve at the beginning of diastole, not an S_4 heart sound. Normally no sound is heard when the mitral valve opens. However, in cases of mitral stenosis, an opening click may be audible if the valve leaflets are stiff. In addition, in some cases a third heart sound (S_3) may be heard shortly after point A at the beginning of diastole. S_3 is due to the vibration of the distended ventricular wall during rapid filling and is usually soft and low in frequency. While the presence of an S_3 is normal in children, in adults it usually suggests volume overload, such as occurs in CHF.

    Answer C is incorrect. Point C corresponds to S_1, which is heard normally when the mitral and tricuspid valves close at the end of diastole. The S_4 sound would be heard just before this at point B.

    Answer D is incorrect. Point D represents the opening of the aortic valve. While this normally creates no audible sound on auscultation, there may be an ejection click at this point in some cases of aortic stenosis.

    Answer E is incorrect. Point E may correspond to an audible ejection murmur in cases of aortic stenosis. However, this is not the point in the cardiac cycle when one expects to hear an S_4 heart sound.

    Answer F is incorrect. Point F represents the sound of the aortic valve closing when the left ventricle begins to relax and the left ventricular pressure becomes less than aortic pressure. The closure of the aortic valve (in conjunction with the closure of the pulmonic valve) can be heard on auscultation as the second heart sound (S_2).

27. **The correct answer is B.** The patient is experiencing pericarditis due to uremia secondary to chronic kidney disease in the setting of long-standing diabetes mellitus (DM). Pericarditis presents with pleuritic, positional chest pain that is often relieved by sitting forward and with a pericardial friction rub on physical examination. Diffuse ST segment elevations may be found on ECG, while an echocardiogram may be normal unless an effusion is also present. Pericarditis has multiple etiologies, including viral (coxsackie virus, echovirus, adenovirus, and HIV), bacterial (tuberculosis or *Streptococcus pneumoniae* or *Staphylococcus aureus* in the setting of endocarditis, pneumonia, or post-cardiac surgery), neoplastic, auto-

immune, uremic, cardiovascular, or idiopathic. Treatment of pericarditis secondary to uremia is dialysis.

Answer A is incorrect. Cardiac catheterization is indicated in patients who are experiencing acute coronary syndrome. While this patient is certainly at risk for ischemic heart disease given her age and history of diabetes, her symptoms and ECG findings of diffuse ST segment elevations are more indicative of pericarditis. In contrast, acute myocardial ischemia is more likely to present with chest pain that is not relieved by changes in position and ECG findings that show ST segment elevations in contiguous leads only.

Answer C is incorrect. NSAIDs are the appropriate treatment for viral or idiopathic pericarditis. However, this patient is experiencing pericarditis due to uremia secondary to chronic kidney disease in the setting of longstanding DM, and therefore the most effective treatment for her is dialysis.

Answer D is incorrect. Pericardiocentesis would be indicated if this patient had evidence of a pericardial effusion, such as distant heart sounds on physical examination, electrical alternans on ECG, cardiomegaly on x-ray of the chest, or fluid in the pericardial space on echocardiogram. However, this patient does not have any of these findings, and therefore pericardiocentesis is not indicated.

Answer E is incorrect. Changing the patient's antibiotic regimen is indicated if she is suspected of having an allergic reaction (such as the development of a rash or anaphylaxis) to a particular medication. However, in this case her symptoms are not consistent with an allergic reaction, and therefore her antibiotic regimen does not need to be changed.

28. **The correct answer is D.** Ventricular fibrillation is an irregular ventricular rhythm without any distinct QRS complexes, ST segments, or T waves. This is an important cause of sudden cardiac death, as well as mortality within the first 24 hours of an acute MI. If defibrillation fails to convert to sinus rhythm, the next treatment choice is the use of antiarrhythmics. There are four general classes of antiarrhythmics: class I blocks sodium channels, class II blocks β-adrenergic receptors, class III blocks potassium channels, and class IV blocks calcium channels. Epinephrine, amiodarone (class IA and class III properties), or lidocaine (class IB) are the agents indicated after a round of unsuccessful defibrillation. Of these agents, only amiodarone may produce the adverse effect of pulmonary fibrosis. Amiodarone is also associated with hypotension, thyroid dysfunction (both hypo- and hyperthyroidism), hepatotoxicity, ocular changes, and other arrhythmias (namely, bradyarrhythmias and torsades de pointes). In patients taking amiodarone, remember to check pulmonary function tests, liver function tests, and thyroid function tests.

Answer A is incorrect. There is no increased risk of bleeding associated with any of the antiarrhythmic drugs. Warfarin and heparin are commonly used drugs that can cause bleeding. However, they would not be used during ventricular fibrillation.

Answer B is incorrect. Class IC agents (ie, flecainide and encainide) are contraindicated in the post-MI population, due to their association with increased post-MI mortality. These drugs work at phase 3 of the action potential and have no effect on action potential duration. They are most often used in cases of ventricular tachycardia that progress to ventricular fibrillation, or intractable supraventricular tachycardia.

Answer C is incorrect. Procainamide, a type 1A antiarrhythmic drug, is a common cause of drug-induced lupus, but it is not used to treat a patient in ventricular fibrillation. It acts by increasing action potential duration and increasing QT interval. It is most often used for treatment of re-entrant and ectopic supraventricular and ventricular tachycardia. Other drugs in this class include quinidine (which has the adverse effect of cinchonism), amiodarone (which is also a class III antiarrhythmic), and disopyramide.

Answer E is incorrect. Digoxin toxicity can lead to disturbances in color vision, including yellow-green vision, as well as nausea, vomiting, diarrhea, and arrhythmias. Digoxin directly inhibits Na^+/K^+-ATPase, leading to indirect inhibition of the Na^+/Ca^{2+} exchanger. Therefore there is an increase in intracellular calcium, leading to positive inotropy. This drug is most often used for chronic heart failure and control of atrial fibrillation, not for ventricular fibrillation.

29. **The correct answer is C.** This is a classic case of acute bacterial endocarditis (ABE). Endocarditis often is characterized by constitutional symptoms (fever, malaise, chills), new-onset cardiac murmur, and a combination of other signs and symptoms (eg, Janeway lesions, Osler's nodes, Roth's spots). Acute and subacute endocarditis can be differentiated based on history, because the acute case will have the most severe and sudden onset, as in this patient. ABE also is seen most often in cases of IV drug use and indwelling catheters, and *Staphylococcus aureus* is the most common bacterial pathogen isolated in these cases, because it is part of the skin flora and enters the blood at needle sites. This patient's history of IV drug abuse, as well as auscultation of a murmur consistent with tricuspid regurgitation, point to a right-sided ABE infection. In right-sided endocarditis, one more often sees septic emboli to the lungs, leading to bilateral infiltrates. This patient is manifesting signs of bilateral infiltrates with hypoxia, decreased breath sounds, and dullness to percussion. It is important to note that many of the classic signs of endocarditis, such as Janeway lesions, Osler's nodes, and Roth's spots, are seen mostly as a complication of left-sided endocarditis, in which septic emboli leave the heart and enter the systemic circulation.

    Answer A is incorrect. *Enterococcus faecalis* also causes subacute endocarditis. The classic picture is a slow onset of constitutional symptoms with low-grade fever. *Enterococcus* infection is not seen as frequently as *Streptococcus viridans*, but it is known to colonize damaged heart valves, especially in patients with a history of rheumatic fever.

    Answer B is incorrect. *Haemophilus aphrophilus* is part of the **HACEK** group of fastidious gram-negative bacilli (***H**aemophilus aphrophilus*, ***A**ctinobacillus actinomycetemcomitans*, ***C**ardiobacterium hominis*, ***E**ikenella corrodens*, and ***K**ingella kingae*) that cause 5%-10% of cases of bacterial endocarditis that are not related to IV drug use. These organisms are slow growing and difficult to culture from blood samples, making diagnosis more complex.

    Answer D is incorrect. *Streptococcus bovis* also causes subacute bacterial endocarditis, which presents with low-grade fever and insidious onset. It normally inhabits the lower GI tract, and lesions in the colon, such as those that occur in colon cancer, allow the bacteria access to the bloodstream. It most commonly affects the aortic valve.

    Answer E is incorrect. *Streptococcus viridans* is the most common cause of bacterial endocarditis overall. This group of bacteria is seen most often in subacute cases in which the onset of symptoms usually is chronic and low-grade fevers are common. *Streptococcus viridans* commonly colonizes heart valves previously damaged by rheumatic fever, thus causing left-sided infective endocarditis as opposed to the right-sided version seen more commonly with *Staphylococcus aureus*. One common source of infection is dental procedures during which normal flora of the oropharynx can enter the bloodstream.

30. **The correct answer is B.** Angiotensin II receptor blockers such as losartan have similar blood pressure-lowering properties as ACE inhibitors, but have fewer adverse effects. Adverse effects of angiotensin II receptors include hyperkalemia and fetal renal toxicity.

    Answer A is incorrect. Blockade of β_1 receptors is the mechanism of action of acebutolol, betaxolol, esmolol, atenolol, and metoprolol. These drugs are used to treat hypertension, in addition to angina, supraventricular tachycardia, CHF, and glaucoma. These drugs also decrease post-MI mortality. Common toxicities include impotence, exacerbation of asthma, sedation, bradycardia, and atrioventricular block.

Answer C is incorrect. ACE inhibitors, such as captopril and enalapril, are antihypertensive drugs commonly prescribed to diabetics due to their possible renal-sparing properties. However, these drugs have common adverse effects such as hyperkalemia, cough, angioedema, taste changes, hypotension, and rash. In addition, ACE inhibitors are teratogenic, causing fetal renal problems. This patient was taking an ACE inhibitor before. The adverse effects of cough and angioedema prompted her physician to switch her to an angiotensin II receptor blocker.

Answer D is incorrect. Nifedipine, verapamil, and diltiazem are drugs that act through inhibition of calcium channels in cardiac and smooth muscle. They are commonly used in the treatment of hypertension, angina, Prinzmetal's angina, and Raynaud syndrome. Verapamil and diltiazem are also used as antiarrhythmics.

Answer E is incorrect. This is the mechanism of action of thiazide diuretics such as hydrochlorothiazide, which are commonly used antihypertensive agents. Adverse effects include hypokalemic metabolic alkalosis, hyponatremia, hyperglycemia, hyperlipidemia, hyperuricemia, hypercalcemia, and allergic reactions.

31. **The correct answer is D.** This patient is suffering from cardiogenic shock due to pericardial tamponade secondary to his small cell lung cancer. Cardiac tamponade can occur secondary to trauma, hypothyroidism, myocardial rupture, or as a complication of pericarditis (especially in the setting of malignancy or uremia). Specifically, cardiac tamponade results when the pericardial space fills with enough fluid to cause increased intrapericardial pressure, compression of the heart throughout its cycle, and subsequent decreased diastolic filling of the heart. As a result of the decreased preload, stroke volume falls and cardiogenic shock (in the absence of pulmonary edema) results. Classic physical examination findings in cardiac tamponade include Beck's triad of distant heart sounds, increased jugular venous pressure, and hypotension. Pulsus paradoxus may also be seen, which occurs when the systolic blood pressure drops by >10 mm Hg on inspiration. ECG is often low voltage and may reveal electrical alternans. Because patients in cardiac tamponade are in a low-output state, they are preload dependent and require immediate volume resuscitation to maintain cardiac output. Positive inotropes such as dobutamine and pericardiocentesis would also be indicated in this patient after he has begun receiving IV hydration.

Answer A is incorrect. Diltiazem is a calcium channel blocker that has a negative inotropic effect on the heart. In the setting of cardiac tamponade, a negative inotrope like diltiazem is contraindicated because it would decrease his already low cardiac output and therefore worsen his hypotension and shock.

Answer B is incorrect. Metoprolol is a selective β_1-blocker that has negative inotropic effects on the heart. In the setting of cardiac tamponade, a negative inotrope like metoprolol is contraindicated because it would decrease his already low cardiac output and therefore worsen his hypotension and shock.

Answer C is incorrect. Because patients in cardiac tamponade are in a low-output state due to the compression of the heart by the surrounding fluid within the pericardial sac, their cardiac output is preload dependent. Any intervention that decreases his preload would be contraindicated in this setting because it would lead to decreased cardiac output and worsening hypotension and shock; therefore, diuresis is not indicated in this patient.

Answer E is incorrect. In the setting of cardiac tamponade, surgery is indicated only if fluid has reaccumulated after catheter drainage, the effusion is loculated, there is a special need for biopsy material, or the patient has a coagulopathy. Moreover, general anesthesia is usually required, and may be unsafe if needle drainage is not performed first to reduce the severity of the tamponade. Therefore, surgery is not the most appropriate next step in the management of this patient.

32. **The correct answer is A.** This patient presents with symptoms consistent with Lyme disease.

He had a characteristic expanding rash (erythema migrans) and resolving flu-like symptoms. Lyme disease can often lead to cardiac symptoms such as those described, as well as heart block that can require cardiac pacing. Lyme disease is carried by the *Ixodes* tick. *I scapularis* is also the vector of disease for babesiosis, a malaria-like parasitic disease common in the northeastern corner of the United States.

Answer B is incorrect. Epidemic typhus is known as "louse-borne typhus." The vector for transmission is *Pediculus corporis*. Epidemic typhus is unusual because the vector for disease feeds only on humans and not other animals. The bacterium responsible is *Rickettsia prowazekii*.

Answer C is incorrect. Malaria is a protozoan parasitic disease responsible for one-three million deaths per year worldwide. Its vector of transmission (and target for disease control) is the female *Anopheles* mosquito.

Answer D is incorrect. Plague is an infectious disease caused by the bacterium *Yersinia pestis*. It is mainly transmitted by fleas that live on infected rodents such as the oriental rat flea, *Xenopsylla cheopis*.

Answer E is incorrect. Rocky Mountain spotted fever is caused by *Rickettsia rickettsii*, a species of bacteria spread to humans by the ticks of the *Dermacentor* family such as *D variabilis*.

33. **The correct answer is D.** This woman has CHF, which is causing pulmonary and systemic edema due to elevated venous pressures ("backward failure") and fatigue due to an insufficient cardiac output to meet the metabolic demands of the body ("forward failure"). In an attempt to compensate for the decreased cardiac output, the heart operates at higher end-diastolic and end-systolic volumes, which often produces a third heart sound (S_3), most likely due to the increased tension of the chordae tendinae during the rapid filling phase of early ventricular diastole. While the presence of an S_3 is normal in children, in adults it is often a sign of volume overload, as in CHF.

Answer A is incorrect. VSD causes a harsh holosystolic murmur heard best over the tricuspid area. VSD is a relatively common congenital cardiac anomaly; however, this murmur would not be heard in heart failure, which is the most likely disease process occurring in this case.

Answer B is incorrect. In the absence of disease, the sounds made by the closing of the aortic and pulmonic valves (S_2) occur simultaneously during expiration, but are split during inspiration as the decrease in intrathoracic pressure causes a delay in the closing of the pulmonic valve. Paradoxical splitting occurs in cases of aortic stenosis or left bundle branch block, when the closing of the aortic valve is delayed and thus the pulmonic valve closes before the aortic valve on expiration, but the delayed closure of the pulmonic valve on inspiration causes the sounds to be simultaneous on inspiration. This patient does not have any signs or symptoms of aortic stenosis or a left bundle branch block, but she does have signs of volume overload due to CHF. Thus she would likely have an abnormal S_3, not a paradoxically split S_2.

Answer C is incorrect. A pulmonary flow murmur is a systolic murmur heard best over the pulmonic area, associated with increased flow across the pulmonary valve. This occurs in conditions such as an ASD, in which blood from the left heart flows to the right heart, thus increasing the volume of blood that flows through the pulmonic valve. ASD can also cause a diastolic rumble due to increased flow over the tricuspid valve. However, an ASD murmur would not be heard in this clear case of heart failure.

Answer E is incorrect. The fourth heart sound (S_4) occurs in late diastole and coincides with atrial contraction in cases in which the atrium contracts against a stiffened ventricle. An S_4 is not present in normal children or adults, and suggests a decrease in ventricular compliance, as is seen in the ventricular hypertrophy that develops in chronic hypertension. This patient has signs of volume overload and would be more likely to present with an S_3 due to systolic dysfunction than an S_4 due to diastolic dysfunction.

Answer F is incorrect. In the absence of disease, the sounds made by the closing of the aortic and pulmonic valves (S_2) occur simultaneously during expiration, but are split during inspiration, as the decrease in intrathoracic pressure causes a delay in the closing of the pulmonic valve. In cases of pulmonic valve stenosis or right bundle branch block, there may be an increased delay in the closure of the pulmonic valve, causing an accentuation of the normal splitting of S_2 during inspiration. S_2 may be audibly split during expiration as well, as the pulmonic valve closes after the aortic valve, regardless of respiratory cycle.

34. **The correct answer is G.** Cardiac troponin I levels (line A) become elevated in the first four hours after an MI and remain elevated for 7-10 days. It is the most specific protein marker for MI. However, creatine kinase (CK)-MB is the enzyme of choice for the detection of reinfarction within the first week. If re-infarction occurs, CK-MB levels would again increase, whereas troponin levels remain elevated from the previous event.

    Answer A is incorrect. AST (line C) is the third enzyme to become elevated, as it gradually increases over the first two days, then slowly declines. The serum level of this enzyme is not specific for cardiac cell damage.

    Answer B is incorrect. Brain natriuretic peptide becomes elevated as the atria are stretched chronically as a result of volume overload, as occurs in CHF. It is not represented in the image, as it is not acutely elevated in MI.

    Answer C is incorrect. C-reactive protein is a marker of inflammation. It has recently been shown in the JUPITER trial as possibly valuable as beginning statin use to lower cardiac risk in a person with a normal LDL cholesterol level. It is not represented in the image, as it is not used to diagnose MI.

    Answer D is incorrect. CK-MB (line B) levels peak in the first 24 hours and then decrease.

    Answer E is incorrect. Lactate dehydrogenase (line D) is the last cardiac enzyme to become significantly elevated, on approximately day two post-MI, and it remains elevated for up to seven days.

    Answer F is incorrect. Myoglobin typically rises and falls within 6 hours post-MI. It, like AST, is nonspecific, as it is also found in skeletal muscle throughout the body. It is not typically used clinically in the diagnosis of MI and is also not represented in the image.

35. **The correct answer is D.** This infant has a patent ductus arteriosus (PDA). The sixth aortic arch gives rise to the proximal pulmonary arteries and, on the left side, to the ductus arteriosus. In the fetus the ductus arteriosus connects the pulmonary trunk to the aorta and allows blood from the right ventricle to bypass the lungs (which do not function at this time), enter the aorta, and return to the umbilical arteries. At birth, the increase in oxygen with the infant's first breath results in decreased prostaglandin levels, which allows the ductus arteriosus to close. Closure is assisted by increased oxygen stimulating the opening of the pulmonary vessels, which decreases vascular resistance, thus leading to increased blood flow to the lungs. Failure of the ductus arteriosus to close completely results in a PDA. This condition is almost always present in premature infants with low surfactant production and low oxygen levels. Indomethacin, a NSAID, inhibits prostaglandins and is frequently used to close a PDA in neonates.

    Answer A is incorrect. The first aortic arch contributes part of the maxillary artery.

    Answer B is incorrect. The fourth aortic arch gives rise to the aortic arch on the left and the proximal right subclavian artery on the right.

    Answer C is incorrect. The second aortic arch produces the stapedial artery and the hyoid artery.

    Answer E is incorrect. The third aortic arch gives rise to the common carotid artery and the proximal part of the internal carotid artery.

36. **The correct answer is C.** This patient is most likely presenting with symptomatic aortic stenosis. One of the most common presentations of this condition is new-onset syncope in an older adult during an episode of exertion. This results from the inability to increase cardiac output during exertion due to a stenotic (usually calcified) valve. In addition, the stenotic valve also causes a pressure build-up on the left side of the heart, resulting in pulmonary congestion, as suggested by the bilateral crackles in this patient. The classic heart murmur of aortic stenosis is a harsh crescendo-decrescendo systolic murmur usually heard best along the right upper sternal border, which radiates to the carotids or the apex. Other findings on cardiovascular examination that suggest aortic stenosis include a weak and delayed carotid pulse (pulsus parvus et tardus), soft or absent A_2 component of S_2, displaced point of maximal impulse (PMI) with left ventricular hypertrophy, and later left ventricular dysfunction (which results in a wide and displaced PMI).

    Answer A is incorrect. Mitral regurgitation is associated with a blowing holosystolic murmur best heard along the apex. When moderate to severe, this condition can result in dyspnea, but it generally is not associated with syncope, unless there is associated severe left ventricular dysfunction. This condition generally is not associated with a weak and delayed carotid pulse. Mitral regurgitation is often caused by myxomatous degeneration of the valve, ischemic heart disease, infective endocarditis, or collagen vascular disease.

    Answer B is incorrect. While a crescendo-decrescendo systolic murmur certainly fits with this patient's likely aortic stenosis, the murmur would not radiate to the axilla. Cardiac murmurs radiate in the direction of flow that is being affected. Flow through the aortic valve goes from the apex of the heart (the left ventricle) up through the aortic valve into the aortic arch and carotid arteries. Thus on auscultation you would expect to hear the murmur radiating through the carotids and to the apex of the heart. Murmurs associated with radiation to the axilla usually involve pathology of the mitral valve.

    Answer D is incorrect. An early diastolic decrescendo murmur radiating to the apex would be associated with aortic insufficiency (also known as aortic regurgitation). This condition can result in dyspnea, but generally is not associated with syncope unless there is associated severe left ventricular dysfunction. Aortic regurgitation will also present with a widened pulse pressure.

    Answer E is incorrect. An early diastolic decrescendo murmur could be associated with aortic insufficiency; however, the murmur of aortic insufficiency would not radiate to the axilla. A murmur of this nature in the axilla may be suggestive of mitral regurgitation; however, this patient's symptoms do not match with this condition.

    Answer F is incorrect. Mitral stenosis is associated with an opening snap followed by a mid-diastolic rumble. Mitral stenosis most commonly presents with dyspnea, but is generally not associated with syncope, and does not produce a weak and delayed carotid pulse. Mitral valve stenosis is often associated with a history of rheumatic fever.

37. **The correct answer is E.** The ECG findings are consistent with MI and a second-degree Mobitz type 1 atrioventricular (AV) block or Wenckebach block. AV block occurs in 12%-25% of patients with acute MI; first-degree AV block occurs in 2%-12%, second-degree AV block occurs in 3%-10%, and third-degree AV block occurs in 3%-7%. Second-degree type I AV block occurs more commonly in inferior than anterior MIs. The right coronary artery (RCA) supplies the inferior wall of the heart. It also supplies the sinoatrial and AV nodes. The sinus node receives blood supply from the right coronary artery in 59% of patients, from the left circumflex artery in 38%, and from both arteries with a dual blood supply in 3%. The AV node is supplied by the RCA in 90% of patients. Thus the AV block is likely due to injury to the AV node as a result of an occlusion in the RCA causing ischemia to the right

posterior atrium, where the AV nodal cells are located.

Answer A is incorrect. The diagonal branches of the LAD are one or two large branches of the LAD that descend anteriorly across the surface of the left ventricle. A lesion here will not cause an inferior wall infarct of the heart.

Answer B is incorrect. The left anterior descending (LAD) branch of the left coronary artery supplies the anterior two-thirds of the interventricular septum and the entire anterior wall of the left ventricle, as it travels along the anterior interventricular groove toward the apex of the heart. A lesion in the LAD would result in an anterior wall MI. It does not supply the inferior wall of the heart, as described in the vignette. A large proximal LAD infarction may also affect the conduction system, but it typically affects the area below the AV node that courses through the interventricular septum. This can sometimes result in bundle-branch blocks, higher-degree AV blocks, and even complete heart block.

Answer C is incorrect. The left circumflex artery is a branch of the LAD that travels toward the left side of the heart. A lesion here will not cause an infarct on the inferior wall of the heart.

Answer D is incorrect. The left marginal artery is a large branch of the left circumflex artery. It continues on the left side of the heart across its rounded obtuse margin. A lesion here does not cause an AV block or an inferior wall infarct.

38. **The correct answer is E.** The child in this question likely has Kawasaki disease, a vasculitis of unknown etiology that is hypothesized to be an infectious or autoimmune response (ie, molecular mimicry). The major symptoms include a high fever of more than five days' duration, bilateral conjunctivitis, lip fissures, strawberry tongue, palmar and plantar desquamation, and cervical lymphadenopathy. Minor criteria may include elevated acute phase reactants, leukocytosis, thrombocytosis, and mild elevation of liver function test results. The most important complication of Kawasaki disease is the development of coronary artery aneurysms, which can result in MI. IV immunoglobulin and aspirin is the appropriate therapy.

Answer A is incorrect. Kawasaki disease is associated with a high fever rather than with hypothermia.

Answer B is incorrect. Kawasaki disease is not associated with optic neuritis. This finding is more commonly associated with multiple sclerosis.

Answer C is incorrect. Kawasaki disease typically does not involve the kidney, which is in contrast to Henoch-Schönlein purpura, a vasculitic disease affecting mostly children.

Answer D is incorrect. Kawasaki disease often occurs after an upper respiratory infection, but it is not usually associated with pulmonary symptoms.

39. **The correct answer is F.** This woman is likely suffering from prosthetic valve endocarditis. She may not have taken appropriate prophylactic antibiotics before her root canal procedure, and her susceptible mitral valve after rheumatic fever has been exposed to transient bacteremia. Her symptoms, including low-grade persistent fever, new-onset murmur, and insidious onset, suggest subacute bacterial endocarditis. This is further supported by her physical examination, which reveals the presence of Roth spots (retinal hemorrhages), Osler's nodes (painful red nodules on digits), and Janeway lesions (dark macules on palms and soles). Given her clinical history and symptoms, the bacterium most likely to have caused this episode is *Streptococcus sanguis*, part of the viridans group. The most appropriate treatment for such an infection is penicillin G.

Answer A is incorrect. Acyclovir is a guanosine analogue antiviral drug used to treat herpes simplex and herpes zoster. This is a bacterial endocarditis and not a viral infection.

Answer B is incorrect. Caspofungin is an antifungal used to treat aspergillosis. It would not treat a gram-positive cocci infection.

Answer C is incorrect. Clindamycin, the treatment for several important anaerobic infections, works by blocking peptide bond formation at the 50S ribosomal subunit. This is not an anaerobic infection.

Answer D is incorrect. Mebendazole is an antiparasitic drug used to treat roundworm infections such as pinworm and whipworm. Mebendazole is not used to treat bacterial endocarditis.

Answer E is incorrect. Metronidazole is a bactericidal agent used to treat protozoal infections, specifically *Giardia*, *Entamoeba*, and *Trichomonas* species, as well as anaerobes, specifically *Bacteroides* and *Clostridium* species. Gram-positive cocci are not within metronidazole's spectrum.

Answer G is incorrect. Pentamidine is an antiparasitic drug used for prophylaxis against *Pneumocystis jiroveci* pneumonia. Pentamidien is not used to treat bacterial endocarditis.

40. **The correct answer is D.** This patient is experiencing a propranolol overdose. Propranolol, a β-adrenergic receptor blocker, reduces heart rate and contractility due to antagonism of β_1-receptors in the sinoatrial node. This lowers cardiac output. The goal of therapy should be restoring myocardial contractility and increasing cardiac output. Glucagon acts as a positive inotropic agent. It increases intracellular cAMP levels independently of adrenergic receptor signaling. Because its mechanism is unaffected by adrenergic blockade, glucagon is the drug of choice in β-blocker toxicity.

    Answer A is incorrect. Albuterol is primarily a β_2 agonist and has little positive inotropic effect.

    Answer B is incorrect. Cocaine causes vasoconstriction and may lead to arrhythmia. It is not indicated as treatment for β-blocker overdose.

    Answer C is incorrect. Although digitalis is also a positive inotropic agent, it commonly leads to atrioventricular block in the setting of bradycardia due to its strong parasympathomimetic actions. It would thus not be indicated in this clinical scenario.

    Answer E is incorrect. Phenylephrine is an α-adrenergic receptor agonist that causes vasoconstriction and rapid increases in total peripheral resistance. This dramatic increase in afterload would be very dangerous for this patient.

41. **The correct answer is E.** Nitrates are first-line treatment in the management of angina. They act by stimulating the release of nitric oxide in smooth muscle, causing an increase in cGMP levels and subsequent smooth muscle relaxation, primarily in the venous system. Such venodilation causes a decrease in preload, which reduces left ventricular wall stress and in turn minimizes myocardial oxygen consumption.

    Answer A is incorrect. Many antiarrhythmic medications, including calcium channel blockers and adenosine, act by decreasing the conduction velocity across the atrioventricular node. However, this is not the mechanism by which nitrates work in the treatment of angina.

    Answer B is incorrect. β-Blockers are also used to treat angina. They act by decreasing heart rate and contractility to effectively reduce myocardial oxygen consumption. However, this is not the mechanism by which nitrates work in the treatment of angina.

    Answer C is incorrect. Nitrates act primarily by stimulating venodilation to decrease preload and thereby reduce myocardial oxygen consumption. They do not act by increasing the oxygen supply to the myocardium.

    Answer D is incorrect. Angina is caused by atherosclerotic stenosis within coronary arteries that limit blood flow through those vessels. Coronary arterioles in patients with flow-limiting coronary stenosis are already dilated to maintain resting blood flow. Therefore, any vasodilating effects nitrates have on coronary arteries are negligible in the setting of already maximally dilated coronary arteries. Thus, stimulating the vasodilation of coronary arterioles is not the primary mechanism of nitrates in the treatment of angina.

42. **The correct answer is B.** Isovolumetric contraction (phase II in the image) is the period between mitral valve closing and aortic valve opening. The cardiac musculature contracts against the closed aortic valve to drastically elevate ventricular pressure.

    Answer A is incorrect. Ventricular filling (phase I in the image) is the period between mitral valve opening and closing. Ventricular pressure remains roughly equal to atrial pressure, as they are in direct communication while the mitral valve is open.

    Answer C is incorrect. Ventricular ejection (phase III in the image) is the period between aortic valve opening and closing. Volume falls precipitously as blood rushes into the aorta.

    Answer D is incorrect. Isovolumetric relaxation (phase IV in the image) is the period in which both the aortic and mitral valves are closed, thus keeping ventricular volume constant. This phase ends when the ventricular pressure falls below the level of the atrial pressure, and the mitral valve opens to allow filling.

43. **The correct answer is C.** The carotid sinus baroreceptor sends an afferent signal via the glossopharyngeal nerve to the medulla, which in turn responds by increasing sympathetic outflow. This results in systemic vasoconstriction, increased heart rate, increased contractility, and increased blood pressure.

    Answer A is incorrect. The baroreceptor located in the aortic arch responds only to an increase in blood pressure.

    Answer B is incorrect. The correct efferent response to a decreased baroreceptor afferent firing rate would be increased sympathetic activity and decreased parasympathetic activity.

    Answer D is incorrect. The baroreceptor located in the aortic arch responds only to an increase in blood pressure. The parasympathetic nervous system is not activated to correct hypotension.

    Answer E is incorrect. The afferent firing rate would decrease, not increase, with hypotension.

44. **The correct answer is B.** Dressler syndrome is an autoimmune phenomenon that results in fibrinous pericarditis. This delayed pericarditis typically develops 2-10 weeks post-MI and presents clinically as chest pain and a pericardial friction rub. It is generally treated with nonsteroidal anti-inflammatory agents or corticosteroids.

    Answer A is incorrect. Cardiac arrhythmia is a common cause of post-MI death, typically occurring the first few days following the event. It is not associated with a friction rub.

    Answer C is incorrect. Left ventricular failure occurs in 60% of people who suffer an MI and can present as CHF, which can cause chest pain, dyspnea, and an elevated jugular venous pressure. No friction rub is typically present.

    Answer D is incorrect. Because ischemic/scarred myocardial tissue lacks normal contractility, there is increased blood stasis and formation of large mural thrombi. Smaller thromboemboli can break off these large mural thrombi and lead to cerebrovascular accidents, transient ischemic attacks, and renal artery thrombosis. Post-MI arrhythmias are also a promoter of blood stasis and subsequent thromboembolic events. However, a friction rub does not indicate thromboembolism.

    Answer E is incorrect. Ventricular rupture is a serious cause of post-MI death that typically occurs 4-10 days after the initial event. It can present with persistent chest pain, syncope, and distended jugular veins, but most often it presents with sudden death. A friction rub would not be observed.

45. **The correct answer is D.** This patient experienced an aortic dissection, characterized by a transverse tear through the intima and internal media of the aortic wall. A blood-filled channel subsequently forms within the wall and is at great risk of rupture, resulting in massive hemorrhage (the "pseudolumen" is the darker of the two lumens in the image). Hyperten-

sion is the major risk factor contributing to the damage of the blood vessel. Other risk factors include connective tissue diseases (eg, Ehlers-Danlos and Marfan syndromes), pregnancy, trauma, and aortic coarctation.

Answer A is incorrect. Cocaine abuse can lead to hypertension, which can later contribute to aortic dissection. Cocaine abuse would not be the direct cause of the aortic dissection, however.

Answer B is incorrect. Diabetes is a risk factor for MI but not for aortic dissection.

Answer C is incorrect. Hypercholesterolemia contributes more significantly to atherosclerosis and subsequent MI than aortic dissection.

Answer E is incorrect. Sickle cell disease is not a direct cause of aortic dissection.

46. **The correct answer is B.** The ECG findings describe Mobitz type II second-degree heart block. A defect in the His-Purkinje system transmitting impulses from the atrioventricular (AV) node to the myocardium is usually, but not always, responsible for this type of heart block.

Answer A is incorrect. In contrast to this patient's findings, AV node abnormalities lengthen the PR interval and are responsible for first-degree heart block and Mobitz type I second-degree heart block. While AV nodal abnormalities can occasionally cause Mobitz type II second-degree heart block, defects in the His-Purkinje system are more commonly the culprit.

Answer C is incorrect. Independently contracting atria and ventricles occur in the complete absence or ablation of the His-Purkinje system. There is no consistency in the length of the PR interval.

Answer D is incorrect. Retrograde conduction would result in an increase in the number of P waves and a decrease in the PR interval. P waves would also show flipping or other abnormalities.

Answer E is incorrect. Sinoatrial node abnormalities are responsible for problems in overall automaticity of the conduction system and would not result in randomly dropped QRS complexes.

47. **The correct answer is A.** The patient died suddenly a few hours after an acute MI. Fatal arrhythmias are the most common cause of death (also known as sudden cardiac death) in the first few hours of an infarction. Arrhythmias are due to disruption of the vascular supply to the conduction system, combined with myocardial irritability after injury. The patient likely suffered from polymorphic ventricular tachycardia or ventricular fibrillation. Also, ventricular tachyarrhythmias and intraventricular conduction abnormalities (such as a left bundle branch block) are common long-term complications of an MI after the myocardium becomes scar tissue and loses its intrinsic conducting abilities.

Answer B is incorrect. Although less likely than a ventricular free-wall rupture, the interventricular septum also may rupture three-seven days after infarction, leading to a VSD, a left-to-right intracardiac shunt, and a low cardiac output.

Answer C is incorrect. After MI, there is a risk of thrombus formation over the infarcted area of endocardium due to turbulence in the blood flow. Clot formation can lead to a left-sided embolism; however, this is not the most common cause death in the acute post-MI setting. Additionally, left ventricular emboli more likely would lead to ischemic strokes, not sudden cardiac death.

Answer D is incorrect. MI can lead to further complications such as CHF and cardiogenic shock. However, these complications rarely cause sudden cardiac death in a stabilized patient in the acute setting. Myocardial failure leading to CHF and poor cardiac output may take weeks to months to occur, and is the result of ventricular remodeling. Hence β-blockers and ACE inhibitors are used widely in the post-MI period to alter the neurohormonal milieu imposed by the renin-angiotensin-aldosterone system, and to counteract deleterious ventricular remodeling.

Answer E is incorrect. Ventricular free-wall rupture is a complication that usually occurs three-seven days after infarction because of the weakened wall of the damaged area during the inflammatory cellular reorganization process. The left ventricular free wall is the most likely site of rupture. Rupture, should it occur, leads to bleeding into the pericardial space and fatal cardiac tamponade.

Answer F is incorrect. A ruptured papillary muscle is a possible complication of MI, but it most commonly occurs three-seven days after the ischemic event. Papillary muscle rupture is not typically the underlying etiology of death in the acute setting. Rather, it could cause a low cardiac output and acute pulmonary edema, likely requiring intubation until surgery can be performed to repair the valve.

48. **The correct answer is A.** The width of the P-V loop represents the stroke volume. Afterload refers to the aortic pressure against which the left ventricle pumps. Decreases in afterload decrease the resistance against which the left ventricle must pump and, therefore, increase the stroke volume of the cardiac cycle. Other physiologic changes that increase the stroke volume include increased preload and increased contractility.

Answer B is incorrect. Contractility describes the intrinsic ability of the myocardium to pump against a given resistance. Decreased contractility in effect weakens the heart, reducing stroke volume.

Answer C is incorrect. Decreased preload is a reduction in the volume of blood that fills the ventricle during diastole. Based on the Starling relationship, in which force of contraction is proportional to the initial length of cardiac muscle fibers, this decreased ventricular filling results in a reduction of stroke volume.

Answer D is incorrect. Increased arterial pressure is synonymous with increased afterload. Increased afterload results in decreased stroke volume based on an increase in pressure against which the left ventricle must pump.

Answer E is incorrect. Increased end-systolic volume in the ventricle without a corresponding increase in preload would represent a decreased ejection fraction and therefore a decreased stroke volume.

49. **The correct answer is B.** Cardiac glycosides such as digoxin inhibit the Na^+-K^+-ATPase transport system to increase intracellular sodium concentration, which in turn increases intracellular calcium concentration via the sodium-calcium exchange carrier mechanism. This increased intracellular calcium level allows greater amounts of calcium to be released to the myofilaments during excitation, resulting in a positive inotropic effect. Increased contractility of the heart increases stroke volume, which in turn increases cardiac output. Glycosides are largely not used today because of the advent of newer drugs that have fewer adverse effects. The outstanding exception is digoxin, which is still widely used to treat heart failure and atrial fibrillation.

Answer A is incorrect. β-Blockers inhibit sympathetic cardiac activation by blocking the activity of catecholamines on the heart, decreasing heart rate and thus cardiac output. These agents are specifically used in CHF in order to decrease myocardial energy use and cardiac oxygen demand.

Answer C is incorrect. Increased extracellular sodium levels in isolation would not increase cardiac output. Increasing cardiac output would require an increase in intracellular calcium levels, which is released from the sarcoplasmic reticulum. This may be achieved by the calcium influx triggered by sodium-calcium exchange channels. Thus increasing intracellular sodium concentrations would increase contractility, but increased extracellular sodium would not.

Answer D is incorrect. A decreased intracellular calcium level would decrease the contractility of the heart, resulting in decreased stroke volume and thus decreased cardiac output.

Answer E is incorrect. Metabolic acidosis decreases contractility and stroke volume; thus this would decrease cardiac output.

50. **The correct answer is D.** Net fluid movement is governed by the equation $J_V = K_f[(P_c - P_i) -(p_c - p_i)]$, where K_f is the filtration coefficient (factoring in membrane permeability), P_c is capillary pressure, P_i is interstitial fluid pressure, p_c is capillary oncotic pressure, and p_i is interstitial oncotic pressure. Increasing P_c, p_i, or the permeability of the capillaries will lead to a net flow of fluid from the capillaries into the interstitium, leading to the edema that is seen in this patient. Likewise, decreasing p_c and P_i will also lead to net outward flow and edema.

Answer A is incorrect. Decreasing capillary permeability would result in fluid being trapped in the vascular space.

Answer B is incorrect. Decreased capillary pressure would decrease the pressure differential driving fluid into the interstitial space.

Answer C is incorrect. Increased interstitial fluid pressure would lead to greater resistance to net fluid flow from the capillaries.

Answer E is incorrect. Increased plasma protein levels would cause an increase in capillary oncotic pressure, leading to fluid retention in the vascular space.

CHAPTER 9

Endocrine

QUESTIONS

1. A 42-year-old woman with a history of pernicious anemia presents to her physician complaining of anxiety and occasional palpitations. She has unexplained weight loss of 10 lb (4.5 kg) and multiple daily bowel movements. She has not had a menstrual period in four months. She has a thyroid bruit and a 10 × 4 cm oval, nontender soft-tissue mass anterior to the thyroid cartilage. Which of the following is the most likely etiology of this patient's disease?

   (A) Autoantibody stimulation of thyroid-stimulating hormone receptors
   (B) Idiopathic replacement of thyroid tissue with fibrous tissue
   (C) Papillary thyroid cancer
   (D) Thyroid adenoma
   (E) Viral infection leading to destruction of thyroid tissue

2. A 57-year-old man with hypertension and coronary artery disease presents to the clinic for his annual check-up. His physical examination is notable for a solitary thyroid nodule. The patient denies any symptoms such as cough, difficulty swallowing, or hoarseness. The physician refers him to an ear, nose, and throat specialist for further evaluation. Results of a fine-needle aspiration biopsy are shown in the image. Which of the following thyroid tumors does this patient have?

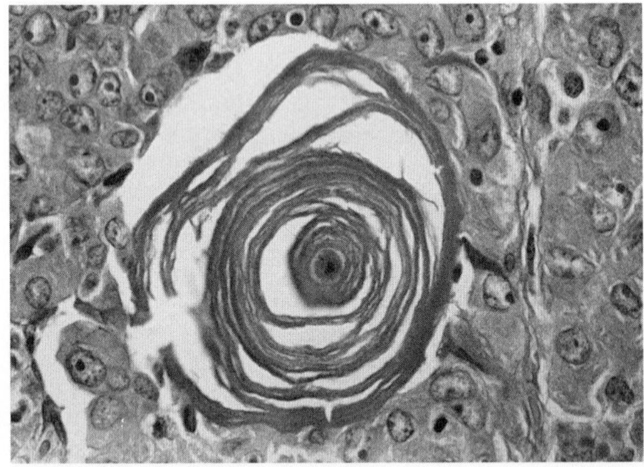

Courtesy of Armed Forces Institute of Pathology.

   (A) Anaplastic
   (B) Follicular
   (C) Hürthle cell
   (D) Medullary
   (E) Papillary

3. A 21-year-old woman presents to the emergency department complaining of diarrhea, heart palpitations, anxiety, and diffuse abdominal pain. Vital signs show tachycardia. The patient wanted to lose weight and started taking her mother's medication to do so; she does not know for which condition the medication was prescribed. Her friend had similar symptoms not long ago and was treated for her condition. Which of the following most likely accounts for this patient's presentation?

   (A) Dobutamine
   (B) Iodide
   (C) Levothyroxine
   (D) Methimazole
   (E) Propylthiouracil

4. The parents of an 18-month-old girl bring her to the pediatrician because she has been having frequent fevers, has developed dark circles around her eyes, and has seemed paler than usual. On physical examination the physician notices an abdominal mass that is palpable in the right upper and left upper quadrants. Imaging studies show involvement of the left adrenal gland and the liver. Which the following would be consistent with this patient's likely diagnosis?

   (A) Bilateral underdevelopment of the iris
   (B) Elevated urine free cortisol
   (C) Elevated urine vanillylmandelic acid
   (D) Symptoms of hypotensive shock
   (E) WBC count >60,000/mm^3

5. A 60-year-old patient from an underserved, impoverished family complains of being "really thirsty, really hungry, and always having to urinate." The patient also reports worsening fatigue and weight loss. Urinalysis reveals severe proteinuria, which prompted a renal biopsy; the histologic section is shown in the image. Which of the following histologic findings is apparent in the renal tissue?

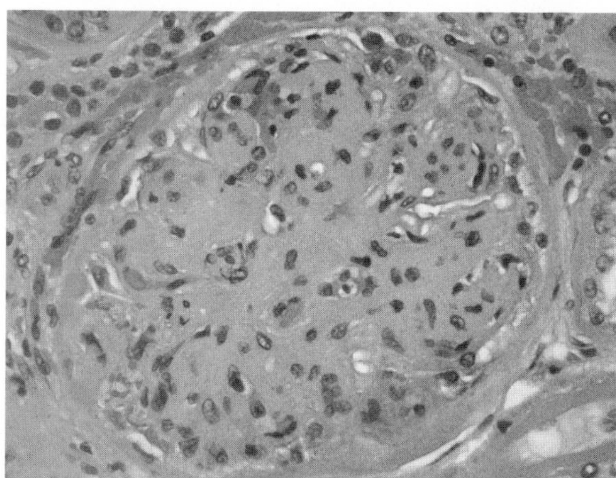

Reproduced, with permission, from USMLERx.com.

(A) Crescent formation
(B) Hyaline arteriolosclerosis
(C) Leukocytic infiltration
(D) Nodular glomerulosclerosis
(E) Wire-loop abnormality

6. A 35-year-old man presents to his physician complaining of increased urinary frequency, polyuria, and an insatiable thirst. He was recently started on a new medication after visiting his psychiatrist. Laboratory studies show that the patient is hypernatremic and has decreased urine osmolarity. Which of the following drugs is most likely contributing to this patient's current condition?

(A) Carbamazepine
(B) Lithium
(C) Fluoxetine
(D) Clomipramine
(E) Phenobarbital

7. A 45-year-old man with type 2 diabetes mellitus presents to his physician for regular follow-up. On neurologic examination, the patient demonstrates the most common initial sensory impairment in patients with diabetes mellitus. Which of the following receptors is most likely affected in this patient?

(A) Krause end bulbs
(B) Meissner corpuscle
(C) Merkel nerve endings
(D) Pacinian corpuscle
(E) Ruffini corpuscle

8. A certain tumor-associated syndrome may manifest as diarrhea, cutaneous flushing, asthmatic wheezing, and right-sided valvular heart disease. These symptoms are attributable to high circulating levels of particular tumor-secreted substance. Which of the following acts primarily by blocking the reuptake of this same substance?

(A) Buspirone
(B) Fluphenazine
(C) Isocarboxazide
(D) Maprotiline
(E) Quetiapine
(F) Trazodone

9. A 45-year-old woman presents to her doctor with feelings of fatigue, increased appetite, increased sweating, and palpitations. Her doctor also notes that her eyes appear unusual (see image). She receives pharmacologic treatment for her condition, but soon develops a fever and multiple infections in her throat and gastrointestinal tract. Her doctor quickly discontinues the medication. Which medication was she most likely prescribed?

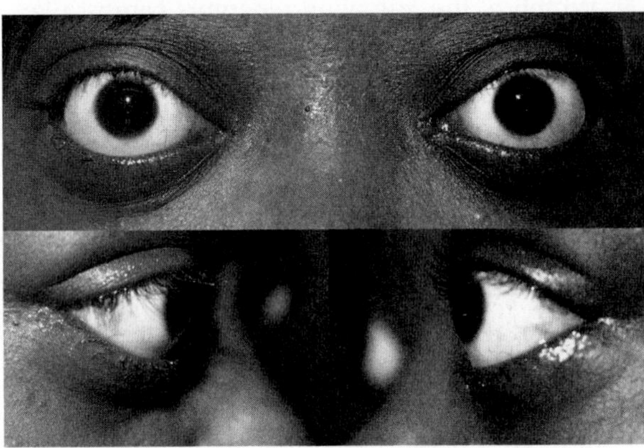

Reproduced, with permission, from USMLERx.com.

(A) Folic acid
(B) Levothyroxine
(C) Propranolol
(D) Propylthiouracil
(E) Radioactive iodine

10. A 40-year-old man with AIDS and chronic adrenocortical insufficiency presents to the emergency department with acute-onset nausea, vomiting, and abdominal pain. He is febrile and hypotensive. He was started recently on a new drug for a fungal infection. Laboratory tests reveal a potassium level of 5.2 mEq/L. Which of the following agents is most likely to have caused this patient's symptoms?

(A) Amphotericin B
(B) Caspofungin
(C) Flucytosine
(D) Ketoconazole
(E) Trimethoprim-sulfamethoxazole

11. A normal-appearing, 23-year-old man sees a physician, because he was awakened on several occasions by severe headaches, anxiety, and heart palpitations. Vital signs are within normal limits. On physical examination, he has pectus excavatum, a high arched palate, bilateral pes cavus, and scoliosis. Which of the following laboratory measures would likely be elevated in this patient?

(A) Calcitonin
(B) Calcium
(C) Insulin
(D) Phosphate
(E) Thyroglobulin

12. A 23-year-old woman visits her primary care physician because of fatigue. Laboratory studies show:

WBC count: 5000/mm^3
Hematocrit: 28.0%
Hemoglobin: 9.8 g/dL
Mean corpuscular volume: 105 fL
Glucose: 98 mg/dL
Platelet count: 322,000/mm^3
Na^+: 139 mEq/L
K^+: 4.3 mEq/L
Cl^-: 101 mEq/L
Blood urea nitrogen: 15 mg/dL
Creatinine: 0.9 mg/dL

A Schilling test is performed: A dose of radiolabeled vitamin B_{12} is administered orally, and shortly thereafter a nonradiolabeled dose is given via injection. A 24-hour urine collection reveals no vitamin B_{12} excretion. One week later, another dose of radiolabeled vitamin B_{12} is administered, along with intrinsic factor. This time, vitamin B_{12} excretion in the urine is normal. The secretion of what substance is likely altered?

(A) Bicarbonate
(B) Gastrin
(C) Hydrochloric acid
(D) Insulin
(E) Trypsin

13. Overactivity of the smaller, pale cells with round nuclei shown in the image can lead to fibrous tissue with hemorrhagic foci and cyst formation in bone marrow. What are these cells called?

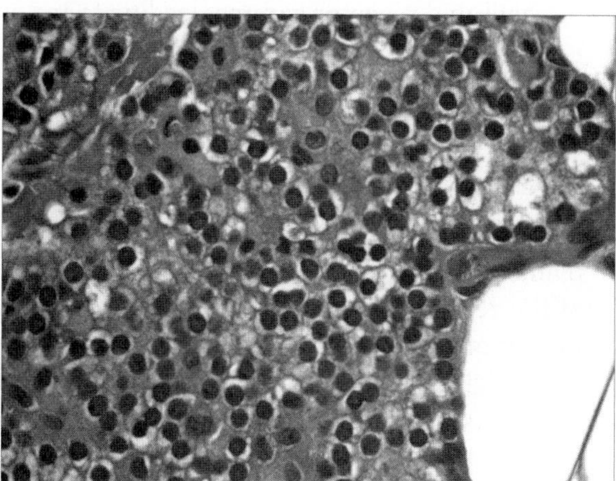

Reproduced, with permission, from USMLERx.com.

(A) Adipocytes
(B) Parathyroid oxyphil cells
(C) Parathyroid chief cells
(D) Thyroid follicle cells
(E) Thyroid C cells

14. A 66-year-old man with a 50-pack-year history of cigarette smoking comes to the clinic complaining of chronic cough, dyspnea, and blood in his sputum. He says he has been feeling lethargic and has lost 18 kg (40 lb) over the past three months with no changes in diet or exercise. While awaiting x-ray of the chest, the patient suffers a seizure and is rushed to the emergency department of the nearest hospital. Laboratory studies show a serum sodium level of 120 mEq/dL. Which of the following is most likely to be elevated in this patient?

(A) ACTH
(B) ADH
(C) Parathyroid hormone
(D) Renin
(E) Tumor necrosis factor-α

15. A 65-year-old woman comes to her primary care physician complaining of progressive weakness and fatigue. On further questioning she notes recent weight gain and constipation, and states that she often feels cold. Physical examination shows a moderate-sized, non-tender goiter. Histologic examination of the goiter shows a lymphocytic infiltrate. Which of the following best describes this patient's thyroid-stimulating hormone and thyroid hormone levels relative to normal baseline values?

Choice	Thyroid-stimulating hormone	Total thyroxine	Free thyroxine
A	↑	↑	↑
B	↑	↓	↑
C	↑	↓	↓
D	↓	↓	↑
E	↓	↓	↓

Reproduced, with permission, from USMLERx.com.

(A) A
(B) B
(C) C
(D) D
(E) E

16. A 25-year-old woman is brought to the hospital by her parents because she told them she constantly hears voices that insult her and tell her to perform various actions. After a brief stay on the psychiatric floor she was discharged with a prescription for haloperidol. Which of the following is an adverse effect of this medication?

(A) Ataxia
(B) Diarrhea
(C) Galactorrhea
(D) Hypertension
(E) Insomnia

17. A 43 year-old woman presents with fatigue, a 4.5-kg (9.9-lb) weight gain over the past three months, cold intolerance, hair loss, and concentration problems. Physical examination is significant for dry, coarse skin and bradycardia. She states that she had some slight swelling of her lower neck several months ago, which resolved without treatment. Results of antithyroglobulin antibody and antinuclear antibody tests are negative, but a thyroid peroxidase antibody test is positive. For which other autoimmune diseases does this patient have an increased risk?

(A) Graves disease and pernicious anemia
(B) Osteoarthritis and Addison disease
(C) Rheumatoid arthritis and vitiligo
(D) Type 1 diabetes mellitus and celiac disease
(E) Whipple disease and type 1 diabetes mellitus

18. A 26-year-old man presents to a clinic complaining of intermittent muscle cramping for the past three months. On physical examination, his blood pressure is found to be 190/105 mm Hg. Blood is drawn, and this reveals his sodium level to be 155 mEq/L, potassium level 3.2 mEq/L, and bicarbonate level 33 mEq/L. Otherwise, his extended metabolic panel and complete blood count are normal. What is the most likely cause of this patient's findings?

(A) Addison disease
(B) Conn syndrome
(C) Cushing syndrome
(D) Hyperparathyroidism
(E) Pheochromocytoma

19. A 44-year-old woman presents to her physician with a one month history of fatigue, polyuria, and polydipsia. Laboratory studies show a glucose level of 350 mg/dL. The physician decides to prescribe a medication to treat diabetes mellitus. He warns the patient that an adverse effect of the medication is lactic acidosis. Which of the following is the most likely mechanism of action of the medication?

(A) Binding to the insulin receptor, increasing glycogen storage in the liver and glycogen and protein synthesis in muscle
(B) Inhibition of intestinal brush border α-glucosidase and delayed sugar hydrolysis
(C) Stimulation of glycolysis in peripheral tissues and decrease in hepatic gluconeogenesis
(D) Stimulation of peroxisome proliferator-activated receptor-gamma, leading to increased glucose uptake in muscle and adipose tissue
(E) Stimulation of the release of endogenous insulin stores

20. A 42-year-old white man presents with a complaint of a "sugar problem." He brings a copy of the report that was obtained on his routine insurance screening test. The report shows his fasting glucose level was 136 mg/dL, and a follow-up fasting glucose level was 142 mg/dL. During a review of systems the patient complains of weight gain, trouble speaking, and vision problems over the past several months. He specifically comments that his favorite hat is now too small on him. During examination of the patient's cranial nerves, which of the following visual field cuts would be expected?

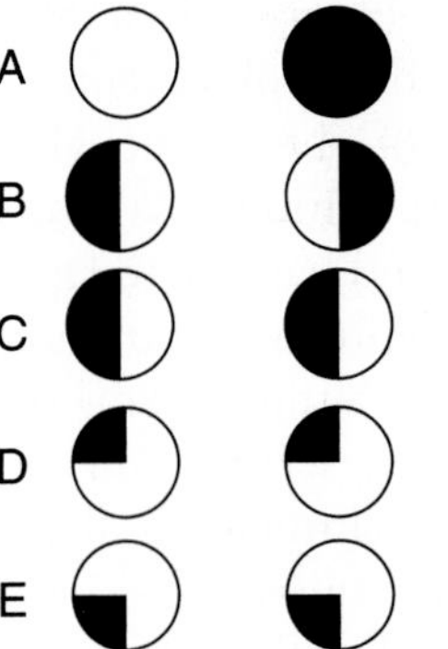

Reproduced, with permission, from USMLERx.com.

(A) A
(B) B
(C) C
(D) D
(E) E

21. A 34-year-old woman gives birth to a child with ambiguous genitalia. The child is hypotensive. A geneticist tells the mother that her child is genotypically a female, although the child seems to have partially virilized external genitalia. Which of the following enzymes is most likely deficient in this infant?

(A) 5α-Reductase
(B) 17α-Hydroxylase
(C) 11β-Hydroxylase
(D) 21-Hydroxylase

22. Glucocorticoids are important in the treatment of inflammatory diseases; however, their use is associated with many adverse effects on multiple systems. The utility of glucocorticoids has to be weighed against the patient's ability to withstand the problems that are likely to arise. High-dosage glucocorticoid treatment can result in which ECG changes?

(A) Appearance of delta wave
(B) Appearance of U wave
(C) Peaked T wave
(D) PR segment elongation
(E) ST segment elevation

23. A 30-year-old woman with no prior medical history is diagnosed with diastolic hypertension. The patient reports symptoms of weakness, fatigue, polyuria, polydipsia, and headache. Laboratory results indicate she is hypokalemic and hypernatremic, has decreased renin levels, and has a metabolic alkalosis. CT of the abdomen shows a 4-cm mass located on the right side of the body. In order to immediately relieve the patient's condition surgically, the surgeon must first ligate the primary venous drainage of the mass. Into which of the following structures does the primary venous drainage flow?

(A) Abdominal aorta
(B) Inferior vena cava
(C) Portal vein
(D) Right gonadal vein
(E) Right renal vein

24. A 42-year-old woman with a history of breast cancer presents to the emergency department with hématuria and costovertebral tenderness. She rates her pain as 8 out of 10 in severity, but says that it seems to "come and go," fluctuating in intensity. She also complains of mild fatigue, along with nausea and constipation for the past few months. Physical examination reveals tenderness of the joints and muscle weakness. Radionuclide imaging demonstrates one area of increased uptake corresponding to her superior left parathyroid gland. Which laboratory values are most likely to be seen in this patient?

Choice	Parathyroid hormone	1,25-Dihydroxy-cholecalciferol	Serum calcium	Serum phosphate
A	↓	↓	↓	↑
B	↓	↑	↑	↓
C	↑	↓	↓	↑
D	↑	normal to ↓	↓	↑
E	↑	↑	↑	↓

Reproduced, with permission, from USMLERx.com.

(A) A
(B) B
(C) C
(D) D
(E) E

25. A 27-year-old white woman comes to the physician because of a six-month history of progressive weakness and fatigue, and occasional mild abdominal pain. She also has noticed that her skin has become more tan, especially at the elbows, knees, and knuckles, despite the fact that she is not usually in the sun. Laboratory tests show decreased serum levels of sodium, bicarbonate, chloride, and glucose and increased levels of potassium. Which of the following is the most likely diagnosis?

(A) Addison disease
(B) Conn syndrome
(C) Cushing syndrome
(D) Pheochromocytoma
(E) Waterhouse-Friderichsen syndrome

26. A 34-year-old woman goes to her primary care physician complaining of visual changes and a recent feeling that "her heart was racing." During the interview, the physician notices that the patient is clearly anxious. During the review of systems, the patient reveals a recent unintentional 4-kg (8.8-lb) weight loss. On physical examination, the physician notes that the patient is tachycardic and has 2+ nonpitting edema in her lower extremities. Which of the following is the most likely etiology of this disease?

(A) Autoantibodies to the thyroid-stimulating hormone receptor
(B) Circulating antibodies to thyroid peroxidase and thyroglobulin
(C) Hyperfunctioning thyroid nodule
(D) Iodine deficiency
(E) Reaction to radiation

27. An 18-year-old woman is referred to a specialist, because she never began menstruating. She reports generalized weakness and occasional bouts of nausea and vomiting. Her blood pressure is 160/99 mm Hg. Laboratory studies show a serum potassium level of 2.2 mEq/L. She is diagnosed with a condition that affects the production of two of the three major adrenal hormones, leaving only one functioning hormone. In which area of the adrenal gland is this one functioning hormone produced?

(A) Capsule
(B) Medulla
(C) Zona fasciculata
(D) Zona glomerulosa
(E) Zona reticularis

28. A 7-year-old girl with a viral upper respiratory infection is brought to the emergency department because of severe confusion, abdominal pain, and vomiting. Her respirations are deep and rapid, and her breath has a fruity odor. The child's mother notes that she has been drinking large quantities of water and has had an increased appetite. Despite her increased appetite, she has been losing weight. An arterial blood gas analysis shows:

pH: 7.25
Partial oxygen pressure: 90 mm Hg
Partial carbon dioxide pressure: 30 mm Hg
Bicarbonate: 18 mEq/L

Based on the probable diagnosis, which of the following is the child's most likely human leukocyte antigen type?

(A) HLA-A3
(B) HLA-B27
(C) HLA-DQ2 and -DQ8
(D) HLA-DR2 and -DR3
(E) HLA-DR3 and -DR4

29. The image below depicts the arterial network of the brain. Infarction of which artery would lead to contralateral deficits of the leg and foot?

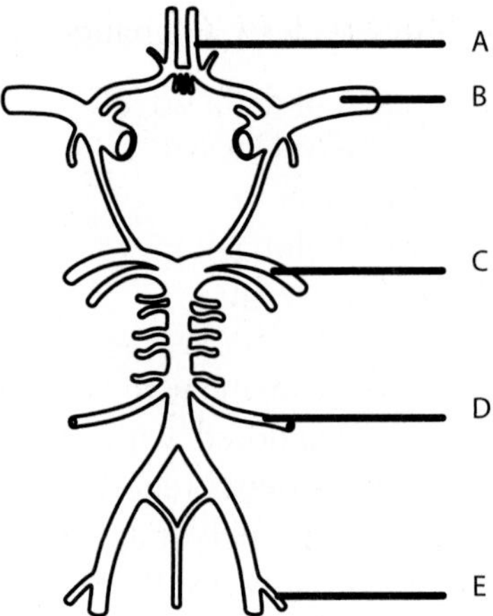

Reproduced, with permission, from USMLERx.com.

(A) A
(B) B
(C) C
(D) D
(E) E

30. A researcher is investigating hormones that act via nuclear hormone receptors. She has developed an assay to analyze the activity of these hormones by assessing mRNA levels of known downstream products in various tissues. What hormone can be studied by this technique?

(A) Glucagon
(B) Histamine
(C) Insulin
(D) Norepinephrine
(E) Thyroid hormone

31. A 6-year-old girl is brought to the clinic by her parents, because they thought she looked like she was "growing breasts." On physical examination, she indeed is developing breasts, but she also has pubic hair. The diagnosis is precocious puberty, and leuprolide is prescribed. The parents are told that leuprolide will suppress their daughter's increased expression of sex hormones. The vasculature of the hypothalamus and pituitary gland is uniquely designed and functionally resembles the design of the gastrointestinal vasculature in that it includes a portal system. Which of the following is the functional significance of this specialized vascular system?

(A) Delivery of hormones for processing
(B) Delivery of hormones for storage
(C) Delivery of hormones in high concentrations
(D) Delivery of hormones to the hypothalamus
(E) Delivery of pre-formed trophic hormones systemically

32. A 24-year-old nulliparous woman presents to her physician with galactorrhea and bilateral hemianopsia. Medical history is significant for hypercalcemia and recurrent duodenal ulcers. Which of the following shares the genetic inheritance pattern of this patient's disorder?

(A) Fabry disease
(B) Familial dysautonomia
(C) Hypokalemic periodic paralysis
(D) Mitochondrial myopathy, encephalopathy, lactic acidosis, and stroke-like (MELAS) episodes
(E) X-linked hypophosphatemic rickets

33. A 59-year-old man with no prior medical history presents to his physician with marked hyperglycemia, diarrhea, and weight loss. CT scan of the abdomen reveals a pancreatic mass. A trial period on an oral hypoglycemic agent has not succeeded in reducing his glucose levels. Physical examination is significant for the painful rash shown in the image. Which of the following is the most likely diagnosis?

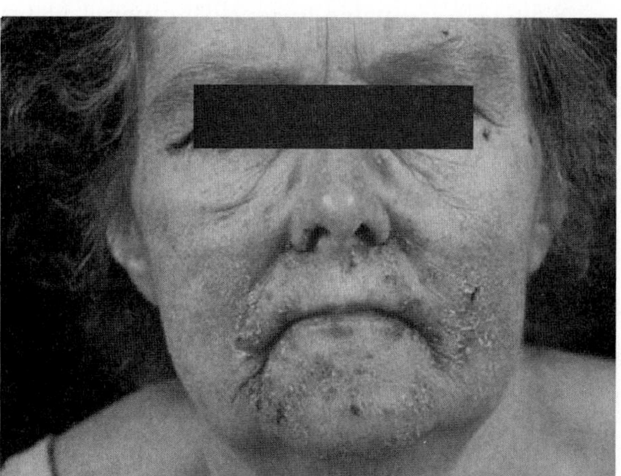

Reproduced, with permission, from Wolff K, Johnson RA, Suurmond D. *Fitzpatrick's Color Atlas & Synopsis of Clinical Dermatolgy*, 5th edition. New York: McGraw-Hill, 2005; Fig. 17-12.

(A) Glucagonoma
(B) Insulinoma
(C) Pancreatic adenocarcinoma
(D) Type 1 diabetes mellitus
(E) VIPoma

34. A particular hormone stimulates the enzyme that converts testosterone to 17β-estradiol in granulosa cells. What is a second function of this hormone?

(A) Causes endometrial proliferation
(B) Induces inhibin secretion
(C) Stimulates desmolase
(D) Stimulates secretion of luteinizing hormone and follicle-stimulating hormone
(E) Triggers ovulation

35. A 44-year-old man is brought to the emergency department after collapsing at his office. The patient has diabetes mellitus and was recently diagnosed with hypertension. He is complaining of blurry vision, fatigue, and dizziness. His coworkers report that he was confused and agitated before he collapsed. He denies chest pain, palpitations, tremor, fever, or chills. His diabetes has been poorly controlled with glyburide, and his most recent HbA_{1c} level was 8.5%. He is unable to recall the name of his antihypertensive drug. Which of the following agents is most likely responsible for this patient's condition?

(A) Enalapril
(B) Hydrochlorothiazide
(C) Metoprolol
(D) Propranolol
(E) Triamterene

36. A 10-year-old girl with no prior medical history presents to the clinic because she's not feeling well. Her mother says the girl has been very thirsty lately and urinating more frequently; she has also lost 4.5 kg (10 lb) over the past year. Laboratory studies show a markedly elevated blood glucose level and a decreased insulin level; levels of a specific antibody are also elevated. Antibodies against which of the following organs are most likely present in this girl?

(A) Adrenal gland
(B) Kidney
(C) Liver
(D) Pancreas
(E) Spleen

37. A tumor biopsy reveals cells with numerous large vacuolar spaces within the cytoplasm (see image). The patient is later prescribed phenoxybenzamine. From what cells is this tumor derived?

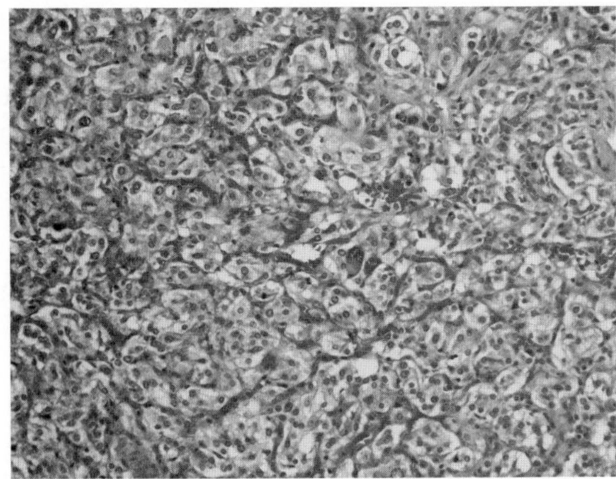

Reproduced, with permission, from USMLERx.com.

(A) C cells
(B) Chromaffin cells
(C) Islet beta cells
(D) Plasma cells
(E) Somatotrophs

38. A 25-year-old woman who was recently diagnosed with hypothyroidism comes to the clinic for a follow-up examination. In addition to levothyroxine, she has been taking a number of daily supplements to help accelerate her recovery. Although she initially reported an improvement in her symptoms, the patient now complains of constipation, brittle hair, and fatigue. Which of the following supplements best accounts for the decline in the patient's clinical course?

(A) Iodine
(B) Magnesium
(C) Vitamin C
(D) Vitamin E
(E) Zinc

39. A 65-year-old man presents to his physician complaining of nocturia. He reports awakening five to six times per night to urinate and difficulty starting a stream. Biopsy of the prostate shows enlargement and dilation of the prostatic glands but no dysplasia. Which of the following is the most appropriate pharmacological treatment for this patient?

(A) Finasteride
(B) Flutamide
(C) Ketoconazole
(D) Spironolactone
(E) Yohimbine

40. A mother brings her 2-year-old daughter to the pediatrician because she has noticed that her daughter's ribs appear knobby on either side of her midline. The mother says that she and her daughter live in an inner-city apartment and rarely go outside. She also notes that she is still breast-feeding her daughter. Which laboratory result would the pediatrician expect to see in this patient?

Choice	Calcium	Phosphate	Parathyroid hormone
A	↓	↓	↓
B	↓	↓	↑
C	↓	↑	↑
D	↑	↓	↑
E	↑	↑	↓

Reproduced, with permission, from USMLERx.com.

(A) A
(B) B
(C) C
(D) D
(E) E

41. A 12-year-old girl presents with her mother to her pediatrician complaining of a lump in her neck. She states that the lump has been there as long as she can remember, but within the past three days has become red, swollen, and very painful. On physical examination, the pediatrician notes a warm, fluctuant mass in the anterior midline of the neck that is exquisitely sensitive to touch and moves with swallowing. During embryologic development, this patient's lesion most likely originated from which of the following structures?

(A) Esophagus
(B) First branchial arch
(C) First branchial pouch
(D) Pharynx
(E) Second branchial arch
(F) Second branchial pouch
(G) Trachea

42. A 25-year-old woman with a history of obesity presents for her annual physical examination. She is seeking advice on how to lose weight. She has been on a diet and exercise program for the past year without much success and wants to try pharmaceutical intervention. The mechanism of action of which of the following drugs is most similar to that of sibutramine?

(A) Methylphenidate
(B) Orlistat
(C) Selegiline
(D) Tranylcypromine

43. A 19-year-old female college student presents with rapid onset of malaise, myalgias, vomiting, photophobia, and a temperature of 39.8°C (103.6°F). Because she quickly develops leg pains along with a purpuric rash, she is transferred from university health services to a local hospital, where she is found to have a blood pressure of 82/49 mm Hg after receiving 2 L intravenous normal saline. Physical examination reveals positive Kernig and Brudzinski signs, a petechial rash on her lower extremity, and diffuse abdominal tenderness. Her arterial oxygen pressure is 58 mm Hg, platelet count is 81,000/mm^3, International Normalized Ratio is 2.1, and D-dimer levels are elevated at 41,000 ng/mL. Cerebrospinal fluid shows 1300 WBCs/mm^3 and 10. RBCs/mm^3. Gram stain shows multiple gram-negative diplococci. Which aspect of this disease process most likely contributes to her hypotension, vomiting, and diffuse abdominal tenderness?

(A) Bilateral adrenal hemorrhage
(B) Disseminated intravascular coagulation
(C) Hypoxemia
(D) Meningitis
(E) Viral gastroenteritis

44. A 65-year-old man is diagnosed with the syndrome of inappropriate ADH secretion (SIADH) in the setting of small cell lung cancer. To treat his SIADH, the patient is started on drug X. He soon begins producing large quantities of dilute urine and drinking copious amounts of water. Despite fluid restriction, the patient continues to produce dilute urine. Laboratory tests reveal an increased serum ADH level, serum hyperosmolarity, and hypernatremia. Drug X might also be used to treat which of the following?

(A) Acute gouty arthritis
(B) Conn syndrome
(C) Enuresis
(D) Lyme disease
(E) Pheochromocytoma

45. A neonate with a cleft palate undergoes a full evaluation. Abnormalities on physical examination include low-set ears and ocular hypertelorism. Echocardiogram reveals a ventricular septal defect, and x-ray of the chest reveals absence of a thymic shadow. Complete blood cell count with differential reveals lymphopenia. What would be the expected serum calcium, parathyroid hormone, and phosphorus levels for this infant relative to normal?

Choice	Calcium	Parathyroid hormone	Phosphorus
A	↓	↓	↓
B	↓	↓	↑
C	↑	↓	↑
D	↑	↑	↑

Reproduced, with permission, from USMLERx.com.

(A) A
(B) B
(C) C
(D) D

46. A 25-year-old man with no significant medical history comes to the emergency department after experiencing tremors. On questioning he admits to a recent history of sweating, nausea, vomiting, and lightheadedness. On physical examination he is visibly anxious. Laboratory studies show a blood glucose level of 50 mg/dL. CT of the abdomen shows a 1.5-cm mass in the head of an organ. Surgical resection of this mass will necessitate ligation of branches from which of the following vascular structures?

(A) The gastroduodenal and inferior mesenteric arteries
(B) The gastroduodenal and superior mesenteric arteries
(C) The proper hepatic and inferior mesenteric arteries
(D) The proper hepatic and superior mesenteric arteries
(E) The left gastric and inferior mesenteric arteries
(F) The left gastric and superior mesenteric arteries

47. A 54-year-old woman presents to the physician with diabetes mellitus, osteoporosis, and hypertension. She has noted a recent weight gain and abdominal striae. Laboratory studies show a decreased ACTH level. A single mass is noted adjacent to the right kidney on abdominal CT scan. Neither low- nor high-dose dexamethasone suppresses the patient's cortisol production. Which of the following is the most likely explanation for these findings?

(A) Adrenal adenoma
(B) Bilateral adrenal hyperplasia
(C) Ectopic ACTH secretion
(D) Exogenous corticosteroid administration
(E) Pituitary adenoma

48. A 60-year-old woman with a 55-pack-year smoking history presents to the emergency department complaining of nausea and vomiting, headache, malaise, and diffuse bone pain. CT shows a solitary nodule in the upper lobe of the right lung. Laboratory studies are significant for a serum calcium level of 14.2 mg/dL, serum phosphate of 1.5 mg/dL, and serum alkaline phosphatase activity of 81 U/L. The factor that accounts for this patient's laboratory findings acts primarily at which of the following locations?

(A) Adrenal cortex and intestines
(B) Adrenal cortex and renal tubules
(C) Intestine and bones
(D) Renal tubules and bones
(E) Renal tubules and pancreas

49. A researcher studying type 2 diabetes mellitus is attempting to induce insulin resistance in normal mice. Inhibition of which of the following would produce this effect?

(A) Adenylate cyclase
(B) Guanylate cyclase
(C) Serine kinases
(D) Threonine kinases
(E) Tyrosine kinases

50. A 48-year-old man with a history of thyroid carcinoma for which he underwent thyroidectomy five years ago presents to his primary care physician complaining of a six-week history of intermittent palpitations, diaphoresis, headaches, and anxiousness. His blood pressure is 180/90 mm Hg and heart rate is 135/min. After a complete work-up, the patient is diagnosed with a pheochromocytoma, and his physician recommends surgery. Which of the following is the most appropriate preoperative management for this patient?

(A) α-Blockade followed by β-blockade
(B) β-Blockade followed by α-blockade
(C) Levothyroxine
(D) Prednisone
(E) Propylthiouracil

ANSWERS

1. **The correct answer is A.** This patient presents with Graves disease. In Graves disease, thyroid-stimulating IgG antibodies bind to thyroid-stimulating hormone (TSH) receptors on the thyroid, leading to excess thyroid hormone production. This causes glandular hyperplasia and enlargement, resulting in a characteristic goiter (the 10 × 4 cm nontender soft-tissue mass is the goiter, which has obliterated the normal thyroid anatomy.) Graves disease is the most common cause of thyrotoxicosis. Patients with Graves disease are at higher risk of other autoimmune diseases, such as pernicious anemia or type 1 diabetes mellitus (DM), than are patients without Graves disease. Presenting symptoms of Graves disease include anxiety, irritability, tremor, heat intolerance with sweaty skin, tachycardia and cardiac palpitations, weight loss, increased appetite, fine hair, diarrhea, and amenorrhea or oligomenorrhea. Signs include diffuse goiter, exophthalmos, periorbital edema, and hyperreflexia. Laboratory values reveal increased thyroid hormone levels and decreased TSH levels.

   Answer B is incorrect. Idiopathic replacement of thyroid and surrounding tissue with fibrous tissue is seen in Riedel thyroiditis; patients may present with dysphagia, stridor, dyspnea, and hypothyroidism, although more than 50% of patients are euthyroid. The disease can mimic thyroid carcinoma, which is high on the list of differential diagnoses for a patient with Riedel thyroiditis.

   Answer C is incorrect. A large, nontender mass in the region where one usually would expect to palpate the thyroid could be concerning for a locally advanced thyroid malignancy; however, the symptoms of hyperthyroidism that this patient is experiencing make this much less likely, because the vast majority of thyroid malignancies do not produce thyroid hormones. Furthermore, the exam is more consistent with a diffuse goiter than a focal nodule, which tends to be more discrete and firm.

   Answer D is incorrect. Most thyroid adenomas present as solitary nodules and usually are nonfunctional.

   Answer E is incorrect. Viral infections such as mumps or coxsackievirus can lead to destruction of thyroid tissue and granulomatous inflammation, as seen in subacute granulomatous thyroiditis. Patients typically present with flu-like symptoms and thyroid tenderness. The disease is typically self-limited and can include a transient hyperthyroid state.

2. **The correct answer is E.** As shown in the image, psammoma bodies, which are calcified remnants belonging to the tumor that likely infarcted, are present in about one-half of patients with papillary carcinoma. Papillary thyroid cancer is the most common type of thyroid cancer and has the best prognosis. Papillary carcinoma is the most common thyroid tumor, and results from neck irradiation, a common therapy between 1920 and 1960. Patients often present as the man in our scenario: asymptomatic with an incidental finding on palpation of the thyroid gland.

   Answer A is incorrect. Anaplastic thyroid cancer is rare, undifferentiated, and tends to have a worse prognosis. It is the most aggressive type of thyroid gland carcinoma. Patients often present with a rapidly-growing nodule or mass and a complaint of dysphagia, dyspnea, neck pain, and/or cough. Histologically, this tumor shows infiltration of adjacent structures with regions of necrosis and hemorrhage. Treatment for this disease is mostly palliative, as this cancer is very aggressive and has often metastasized by the time of diagnosis.

   Answer B is incorrect. Follicular thyroid cancer tends to have a good prognosis, but there is the risk of early metastasis. It is a well-differentiated tumor, but has the potential to become invasive. The most common presentation is subclinical, with a thyroid mass or nodule felt upon palpation of the neck. Histologically, this tumor appears encapsulated and is often found in necrotic or hemorrhagic areas. It can also have well-defined follicles.

Answer C is incorrect. Hürthle cell is a rare variant of follicular cell carcinoma with the following differences: (1) it tends to be bilateral and multifocal, and (2) it is more likely to metastasize to lymph nodes than follicular carcinoma. Patients often present with a palpable mass in the neck, and complaints of pressure on the throat resulting in pain, coughing, dyspnea, dysphagia, or hoarseness.

Answer D is incorrect. Medullary thyroid cancer arises from the parafollicular cells (unlike papillary, follicular, and anaplastic, which arise from the epithelial cells). Since the parafollicular cells (C cells) produce calcitonin, this can serve as a marker by which the tumor can be monitored. Carcinoembyronic antigen can also serve as a marker for medullary thyroid cancer, but it is not as sensitive. This tumor can be seen alone or as a part of multiple endocrine neoplasia (MEN) types II and III.

3. **The correct answer is C.** This patient's symptoms are caused most likely by surreptitious use of levothyroxine. This medication can cause weight loss but also thyrotoxicosis. Levothyroxine is a synthetic form of thyroxine (T_4) that is used to treat hypothyroidism. Excessively high serum levels of levothyroxine result in symptoms of thyrotoxicosis, including those described in the vignette in addition to heat intolerance, unexplained weight loss, agitation, and confusion. Her friend also had these symptoms because of her thyrotoxicosis caused by Graves disease, in which TSH receptor antibodies are produced. Graves disease also causes exophthalmos; this autoimmune disease affects the periorbital region, resulting in proptosis and extraocular muscle swelling.

   Answer A is incorrect. Dobutamine is an α-adrenergic agonist that is useful in the acute treatment of congestive heart failure (CHF). Whereas the effects of this drug can mimic the symptoms and signs of thyrotoxicosis, this agent cannot account for the gastrointestinal (GI) symptoms, weight loss, and heat intolerance that are characteristic of thyrotoxicosis.

   Answer B is incorrect. Pharmacologic doses of iodide are used to treat hyperthyroidism. They inhibit the synthesis of thyroid hormone and the release of pre-formed thyroid hormone. Iodide is administered orally, and adverse effects include sore mouth and throat, rashes, ulcerations of mucous membranes, and a metallic taste in the mouth.

   Answer D is incorrect. Methimazole is used to treat hyperthyroidism by inhibiting the addition of iodine to thyroglobulin by the enzyme thyroperoxidase. Adverse effects include agranulocytosis, which should be suspected if the patient develops a fever or sore throat while on this medication. In the event of an overdose, iatrogenic hypothyroidism would result.

   Answer E is incorrect. Propylthiouracil, which inhibits the synthesis of T_4 and the peripheral conversion of T_4 to tri-iodothyronine, is used to treat hyperthyroidism. Rare toxicities caused by this agent include agranulocytosis, rash, and edema.

4. **The correct answer is C.** Neuroblastoma is a tumor that often affects the adrenal medulla, although it can involve any site along the sympathetic chain. It is most commonly seen in children, with a median age of presentation of 17 months. The condition may present with constitutional symptoms as well as periorbital ecchymosis, proptosis, limp, bone pain, hypertension, and/or involvement of the skin (bluish, nontender subcutaneous nodules). Urine vanillylmandelic acid and homomandelic acid levels are typically elevated in these patients. Therapy involves resection, radiation, and/or chemotherapy.

   Answer A is incorrect. Bilateral underdevelopment of the iris, also known as aniridia, would be consistent with symptoms of WAGR, in which the W stands for Wilms tumor (**WAGR** means **W**ilms tumor, **A**niridia, **G**enitourinary malformations, and mental **R**etardation). Wilms tumor is the most common primary renal tumor, commonly presenting with an asymptomatic flank mass that classically does not cross the midline, while this patient's mass does cross the midline on physical examination. Mean age at presentation is 42 months.

Answer B is incorrect. Adrenal adenocarcinoma may cause Cushing syndrome, resulting in findings such as truncal obesity, moon facies, buffalo hump, purple striae, muscle wasting, osteoporosis, and psychiatric disturbances. However, this patient's age and symptoms are far more consistent with neuroblastoma.

Answer D is incorrect. Symptoms of hypotensive shock without hypovolemia in this young child would be consistent with adrenal insufficiency due to adrenocortical atrophy. Other symptoms may include nausea and vomiting, which this patient does not have. Adrenocortical atrophy would not present with a mass on physical examination or imaging.

Answer E is incorrect. A WBC count >60,000/mm^3 in this patient would be consistent with an acute leukemia. However, while acute leukemias can present with systemic symptoms, they do not involve the presence of abdominal masses.

5. **The correct answer is D.** This is a classic case of a patient with type 2 DM: polydipsia, polyuria, and polyphagia in an individual >40 years of age. This condition is due to increased resistance to insulin. The image shows nodular glomerulosclerosis, also known as Kimmelstiel-Wilson glomerulosclerosis. This represents the accumulation of nodules in the mesangial matrix, which is pathognomonic for DM. Kidneys of diabetic patients also show increased basement membrane thickness and diffuse mesangial matrix proliferation.

   Answer A is incorrect. Crescent formation results from a proliferation of Bowman capsule epithelial cells, which appear to "crowd out" the glomerular tufts. It is classically seen in nephritic syndromes and suggests a poor prognosis.

   Answer B is incorrect. Hyaline arteriolosclerosis is a homogeneous, eosinophilic thickening of arteriolar walls that results in a narrowed vessel lumen. It is a feature of benign nephrosclerosis often seen in long-standing hypertension, a common cause of chronic renal failure. The image shown is of a glomerulus, not a renal arteriole.

   Answer C is incorrect. Leukocytic infiltration is characteristic of inflammatory diseases of the glomerulus; it is observed most often in poststreptococcal glomerulonephritis, but also can be seen in membranoproliferative glomerulonephritis and rapidly progressive glomerulonephritis.

   Answer E is incorrect. The wire-loop abnormality is characteristic of type IV lupus nephropathy. This condition is caused by thickening of the glomerular basement membrane associated with immune complex deposition.

6. **The correct answer is B.** This patient is presenting with nephrogenic diabetes insipidus (DI), which is a rare toxicity of lithium. Patients with DI either lack the ability to produce ADH (central DI), or cannot produce an appropriate renal response to ADH (nephrogenic DI). Patients present with symptoms of insatiable thirst, polyuria, and an inability to concentrate urine. Lithium, which is used as a mood stabilizer for bipolar affective disorder, is an iatrogenic cause of nephrogenic diabetes insipidus.

   Answer A is incorrect. Carbamazepine is an antiepileptic drug that can cause diplopia, ataxia, and liver toxicity.

   Answer C is incorrect. Fluoxetine is a selective serotonin reuptake inhibitor that can cause symptoms of central nervous system (CNS) stimulation such as anxiety, tremor, and nausea.

   Answer D is incorrect. Clomipramine is a tricyclic antidepressant that can cause convulsions, coma, and arrhythmias.

   Answer E is incorrect. Phenobarbital is a barbiturate that can cause symptoms of CNS depression and induce the cytochrome P450 (CYP450) enzyme system.

7. **The correct answer is D.** The most common initial sensory impairment in patients with

diabetes is a loss of vibrational sensation. This finding is most clearly demonstrated on physical examination by placing a vibrating tuning fork on the big toe. The sensory receptors responsible for transducing the sensation of vibration, pressure, and tension are the large, encapsulated pacinian corpuscles, which are located in the deeper layers of the skin, ligaments, and joint capsules. They can be distinguished histologically by their onion-like appearance on cross section. This patient is presenting with one of the complications of diabetes, neuropathy, and because pacinian corpuscles are responsible for transducing vibratory stimuli, it is these receptors that are involved in this patient's presentation.

Answer A is incorrect. Krause end bulbs are sensory receptors found in the oropharynx and conjunctiva of the eye.

Answer B is incorrect. Meissner corpuscles, which are responsible for conveying the sensation of light touch, are small and encapsulated sensory receptors found just beneath the dermis of hairless skin, most prominently in the fingertips, soles of the feet, and lips. Meissner corpuscles are involved in the reception of light discriminatory touch, not vibratory sensation, as is being tested in this case.

Answer C is incorrect. Merkel nerve endings are non-encapsulated and found in all skin types (both hairy and hairless) and, along with Meissner corpuscles, are believed to be responsible for discriminatory touch.

Answer E is incorrect. Ruffini corpuscles are spindle-shaped, encapsulated mechanoreceptors that are found in the soles of the feet and are responsible for transducing pressure.

8. **The correct answer is F.** Carcinoid syndrome is an uncommon syndrome caused by tumors of neuroendocrine origin. When these tumors metastasize to the liver, the high levels of serotonin (the substance referenced in the question stem) secreted by the tumor are no longer metabolized by first-pass hepatic metabolism, leading to characteristic symptoms of diarrhea, cutaneous flushing, asthmatic wheezing, and right-sided heart disease. Serotonin levels are increased in these patients. Trazodone is an antidepressant whose primary mechanism of action is inhibiting serotonin reuptake in the CNS.

Answer A is incorrect. Buspirone is a 5-HT_{1A} agonist used to treat generalized anxiety disorder.

Answer B is incorrect. Fluphenazine is a typical antipsychotic that acts by blocking dopamine D_2 receptors. It does not significantly inhibit serotonin reuptake.

Answer C is incorrect. Isocarboxazide is an antidepressant whose mechanism of action consists of inhibiting an enzyme called monoamine oxidase. While this results in elevated serotonin levels, isocarboxazide itself does not inhibit serotonin reuptake.

Answer D is incorrect. Maprotiline is an antidepressant that acts by blocking the reuptake of norepinephrine.

Answer E is incorrect. Quetiapine is an atypical antipsychotic. These agents act by blocking 5-HT_2 and dopamine receptors.

9. **The correct answer is D.** The patient most likely has Graves disease-induced hyperthyroidism, the most prominent feature being the exophthalmos seen in the image. In addition, her fatigue, sweating, palpitations, and increased appetite are also symptoms of hyperthyroidism. She could be treated with an agent such as propylthiouracil at this point, which would help with the symptoms, although it will not reverse the eye changes. Unfortunately, it can have the adverse effect of agranulocytosis, and thus blood work needs to be done when first prescribing this agent to a patient. Agranulocytosis can lead to infection and may be life threatening.

Answer A is incorrect. Folic acid is not used in the treatment of hyperthyroidism. It also does not cause agranulocytosis. It is often given to patients who are anemic. It is important that pregnant women receive adequate amounts of folic acid to reduce the incidence of neural tube defects.

Answer B is incorrect. Levothyroxine is used to treat hypothyroidism and would be contraindicated in this patient as it would worsen her current symptoms.

Answer C is incorrect. Propranolol is also used to treat hyperthyroidism. However, it is not associated with agranulocytosis. Its most common adverse effect is fatigue.

Answer E is incorrect. Radioactive iodine is used to treat hyperthyroidism. The treatment is permanent and often results in hypothyroidism. It does not cause agranulocytosis.

10. **The correct answer is D.** HIV-infected patients commonly have endocrine dysfunction caused by HIV itself, other infections, or medications. In this patient, who has baseline chronic adrenal insufficiency, ketoconazole can precipitate acute adrenal crisis, which often presents with nonspecific symptoms such as nausea, vomiting, abdominal pain, fever, weakness, and fatigue. Ketoconazole is an imidazole whose mechanism of action is primarily inhibition of ergosterol synthesis. As ergosterol is a major component of the fungal cell membrane, ketoconazole is an effective antifungal agent. Unfortunately, CYP450 activity and steroid synthesis are also inhibited by this agent, as seen in this patient.

    Answer A is incorrect. Amphotericin B is an antifungal medication that can cause fevers and chills, hypotension, nephrotoxicity, and arrhythmias.

    Answer B is incorrect. Caspofungin is an antifungal medication that can cause GI upset and flushing.

    Answer C is incorrect. Flucytosine is an antifungal medication that can cause nausea, vomiting, diarrhea, and bone marrow suppression.

    Answer E is incorrect. Trimethoprim-sulfamethoxazole is used as treatment and prophylaxis against *Pneumocystis jiroveci* pneumonia in patients with AIDS. It may cause adverse effects such as hypersensitivity reactions, nephrotoxicity, and leukopenia.

11. **The correct answer is A.** This patient has a presentation suspicious of MEN type 2B. These patients have a classic triad of pheochromocytoma, marfanoid body habitus, and medullary thyroid carcinoma. This patient's paroxysms of severe headaches, anxiety, and heart palpitations suggest a possible excess of catecholamines, the hallmark of pheochromocytoma. The physical examination findings suggest a marfanoid body habitus. Because the patient has two of the three signs of MEN-2B, one must have a high level of suspicion for the third, medullary thyroid carcinoma. This is a neoplasm of the medullary C cells, which produce calcitonin. Hence, the patient's laboratory findings would be significant for an elevated serum calcitonin level.

    Answer B is incorrect. An elevated serum calcium is seen in patients with MEN type 1 or type 2A. These patients present with hypercalcemia in the setting of a parathyroid adenoma. However, neither of these two syndromes presents with a marfanoid body habitus. Thus, the patient's physical exam findings should lead to a diagnosis of MEN-2B, in which serum calcium levels would be normal.

    Answer C is incorrect. An insulinoma is a pancreatic islet cell tumor that could be seen in a patient with MEN type 1 and would secrete large amounts of insulin, causing hypoglycemia with symptoms of nervousness, sweating, trembling, and weakness. MEN-1 consists of pancreatic islet cell tumors (eg, gastrinomas, vasoactive intestinal peptide tumors [VIPomas], and insulinomas), parathyroid adenomas, and pituitary adenomas. This patient has a history suggestive of MEN-2B, so an insulinoma is unlikely and thus serum insulin levels would be normal.

    Answer D is incorrect. An elevated serum phosphate is not present in any of the MEN syndromes. In patients with MEN-1 or MEN-2A who have parathyroid adenomas, the serum phosphate will actually be low. This is because these patients produce excess amounts of parathyroid hormone (PTH), which acts on the kidneys to cause secretion of phosphate. The patient in the vignette has MEN-2B, a syndrome that does not produce any pathophysiology in phosphate balance. Thus, this patient's serum phosphate levels would be normal.

Answer E is incorrect. Although patients with MEN-2B have medullary thyroid carcinoma, laboratory values of thyroglobulin will not be elevated. This is because the neoplasm consists of the medullary C cells, which produce calcitonin. Serum thyroglobulin is a useful post-operative tumor marker in papillary thyroid carcinoma, but it would not be elevated in this patient.

12. **The correct answer is C.** The patient suffers from a megaloblastic anemia secondary to pernicious anemia, as evidenced from the mean corpuscular volume >100 fL and the hematocrit <35%. The Schilling test is performed to determine whether the body is absorbing vitamin B_{12}, and to identify why if it is not. During part 1 of the test, nonradiolabeled vitamin B_{12} is given to saturate tissue stores and to prevent the binding of radioactive vitamin B_{12} in body tissues. The absence of vitamin B_{12} excretion indicates that the intestines are not absorbing the vitamin normally. Results of part 2 of the Schilling test indicate a problem with the secretion of intrinsic factor (IF). Because IF is secreted by the parietal cells, which are destroyed by an autoimmune process, other substances secreted by these cells, such as hydrochloric acid, are also likely altered.

    Answer A is incorrect. Bicarbonate is secreted to buffer the hydrochloric acid from the parietal cells; however, bicarbonate is not secreted by the parietal cells themselves.

    Answer B is incorrect. Gastrin is secreted by G cells, not by parietal cells.

    Answer D is incorrect. Insulin is secreted by the pancreatic β cells in the islets of Langerhans, not by parietal cells of the stomach.

    Answer E is incorrect. Trypsin is secreted in the pancreas by acinar cells, not by the parietal cells.

13. **The correct answer is C.** Parathyroid chief cells are small, pale cells with round central nuclei. These cells secrete PTH, which raises serum calcium levels in three ways: (1) it acts directly on bone to increase osteoclastic resorption; (2) it acts directly on the kidney to increase resorption of calcium and inhibit resorption of phosphate; and (3) it promotes GI absorption of calcium via increased levels of activated vitamin D. Hyperparathyroidism can lead to osteitis fibrosa cystica, which consists of fibrous tissue with cysts and hemorrhagic foci in the bone marrow with a very thin cortex.

    Answer A is incorrect. Adipose tissue in the parathyroid gland increases with age but does not secrete hormones related to calcium regulation. The cells contain large vacuoles that appear white on hematoxylin and eosin stain.

    Answer B is incorrect. Parathyroid oxyphil cells tend to occur in nodules and have abundant eosinophilic cytoplasm. They are larger than chief cells and do not secrete PTH.

    Answer D is incorrect. Thyroid follicular cells are simple cuboidal cells that line colloid follicles. They are responsible for the synthesis and secretion of triiodothyronine (T_3) and T_4.

    Answer E is incorrect. Thyroid C cells secrete calcitonin, which decreases bone resorption of calcium, leading to a decrease in serum calcium levels. C cells are distinguished by their extensive clear cytoplasm. Think "C" for "Clear Cytoplasm."

14. **The correct answer is B.** This vignette is most consistent with the syndrome of inappropriate ADH secretion (SIADH) due to a lung neoplasm. ADH is normally secreted by the posterior pituitary and stimulates the expression of aquaporins in the renal collecting ducts. This results in transport of water into the renal medulla from the ductal lumen, thus increasing water reabsorption by the kidneys. When levels of this hormone are inappropriately elevated, excessive water retention results in hyponatremia, which can lead to seizures. ADH can be produced ectopically in the setting of malignancy such as small cell lung cancer.

    Answer A is incorrect. ACTH can be produced ectopically in the setting of small cell lung cancer. However, excessive levels of ACTH would result in Cushing syndrome, with symptoms of hypertension, weight gain, moon facies, truncal obesity, buffalo hump, insulin resistance, skin thinning/striae, osteoporosis, and amenorrhea. The vignette provides no signs or symptoms that would be consistent with Cushing syndrome.

Answer C is incorrect. PTH-related peptides can be produced ectopically in the setting of malignancy and are associated with a variety of neoplasms, including squamous cell lung cancer, breast cancer, renal cell carcinoma, and multiple myeloma. However, excessive levels of PTH would result in hypercalcemia, and the vignette does not provide any indication that would be consistent with this condition.

Answer D is incorrect. Hyperreninemia does not typically occur as a paraneoplastic syndrome and is most commonly caused by renal artery stenosis. Renin is normally released by the kidneys upon sensing decreased blood pressure. Renin plays a role in the conversion of angiotensinogen to angiotensin I, which is then converted by angiotensin-converting enzyme (ACE) into angiotensin II. Angiotensin II stimulates the release of aldosterone from the adrenal glands. Therefore, hyperreninemia leads to increased levels of angiotensin II and aldosterone, resulting in hypertension and hypokalemia. The vignette does not mention any signs or symptoms of hypokalemia, such as nausea, vomiting, muscle weakness, and cardiac arrhythmias.

Answer E is incorrect. Tumor necrosis factor-α (TNF-α) can be produced ectopically in the setting of malignancy. Increased TNF-α secretion can be caused by the same cancers that produce PTH-related peptide, including squamous cell lung cancer, breast cancer, renal cell carcinoma, and multiple myeloma. TNF-α is associated with fever and cachexia, among many other findings.

15. **The correct answer is C.** The vignette describes a classic history for primary hypothyroidism caused by Hashimoto thyroiditis. Hashimoto thyroiditis is caused by circulating antibodies against one or more thyroid antigens, leading to autoimmune-mediated destruction of the thyroid gland (as reflected by the lymphocytic infiltrate). It is characterized by reduced secretion of both free and total T_4. This leads to an increase in TSH levels due to a decrease in negative feedback by T_4 and T_3 on the anterior pituitary.

Answer A is incorrect. In the setting of primary hypothyroidism, both total and free T_4 levels should be decreased rather than increased. An elevated TSH level in the setting of high total and free T_4 levels could be seen in a TSH-secreting pituitary adenoma or, less commonly, in patients with thyroid hormone resistance syndrome. A TSH-secreting adenoma, however, would result in symptoms of hyperthyroidism, such as weight loss, hyperactivity, heat intolerance, and palpitations.

Answer B is incorrect. Both total and free T_4 levels should be decreased in the setting of primary hypothyroidism. An elevated T_4 level is usually associated with hyperthyroidism, not hypothyroidism. Free and total T_4 levels should vary in opposite directions only when there is a change in the amount of thyroxine-binding globulin (TBG), which binds thyroid hormone in the blood. A good example is in pregnancy, where TBG levels increase in response to estrogen, thus decreasing the amount of free T_4. However, TSH levels are high due to decreased negative feedback to the pituitary, and therefore the total T_4 level will be high.

Answer D is incorrect. In Hashimoto thyroiditis, both total and free T_4 levels should be decreased and TSH levels should be increased due to a decrease in negative feedback on the pituitary gland.

Answer E is incorrect. There are three types of hypothyroidism: primary, secondary, and tertiary. In primary hypothyroidism, such as Hashimoto thyroiditis, the cause is malfunctioning of the thyroid gland which leads to reduced free and total T_4 levels and increased TSH levels. In secondary hypothyroidism (much less prevalent than the primary form), the pituitary gland does not produce sufficient

TSH, leading to decreased TSH levels in addition to low total and free T_4 levels. Tertiary hypothyroidism (also rare) presents with low levels of TSH and thyroid hormones, but is caused by a hypothalamic abnormality leading to decreased thyrotrophin-releasing hormone production in the hypothalamus.

16. **The correct answer is C.** The patient presents with auditory hallucinations, which are suggestive of schizophrenia. Schizophrenia is a psychiatric disorder characterized by positive symptoms such as delusions, hallucinations (mainly auditory), disorganized thought, and disorganized behavior, and negative symptoms that include flat or blunted affect, apathy, and anhedonia. Although not fully understood, it is believed that schizophrenia is related to increased dopamine activity in certain neural pathways. Consequently, typical antipsychotics, such as haloperidol, that block dopamine D_2 receptors, have been used. Unfortunately, dopamine antagonism has adverse effects, such as interfering with the normal feedback inhibition of dopamine in the hypothalamic-pituitary axis. Since dopamine inhibits prolactin secretion from the anterior pituitary, the blockade of dopamine receptors may cause hyperprolactinemia and galactorrhea. Although the cause is unknown, neuroleptic malignant syndrome (NMS) is another important adverse event, and is believed to be due to dopamine antagonism. NMS is a neurologic emergency, characterized by mental status change, rigidity, fever, and dysautonomia.

    Answer A is incorrect. Antipsychotics may cause an imbalance in dopamine and muscarinic receptor antagonism, which results in extrapyramidal adverse effects, such as dystonia, akinesia, akathisia, and tardive dyskinesia. Dystonia is characterized by sustained and prolonged contraction of agonist and antagonist muscles producing abnormal postures. Akinesia is the absence of movement, while akathisia refers to the feeling of restlessness that is relieved by movement. Tardive dyskinesia commonly presents as involuntary choreiform movements of the lower face, characterized by rhythmic protrusion of the tongue, lip smacking, and chewing. Ataxia, or poor coordination, is a known adverse effect of lithium but not neuroleptics.

    Answer B is incorrect. Typical antipsychotics have an antimuscarinic effect that can cause constipation, not diarrhea.

    Answer D is incorrect. Typical antipsychotics have anti-α-receptor effects that can cause hypotension, not hypertension.

    Answer E is incorrect. Typical antipsychotics have an antihistamine effect that causes sedation, not insomnia.

17. **The correct answer is D.** This patient has Hashimoto thyroiditis, an autoimmune disorder in which patients have antibodies attacking thyroglobulin, thyroid peroxidase, or another part of the thyroid gland or thyroid hormone synthesis pathway. Patients with Hashimoto thyroiditis have a 20 times greater prevalence of celiac disease and type 1 DM than the general population.

    Answer A is incorrect. This patient has Hashimoto thyroiditis. She would not have Graves disease as well.

    Answer B is incorrect. Addison disease does have a high prevalence in patients with Hashimoto thyroiditis. However, osteoarthritis is not an autoimmune disease.

    Answer C is incorrect. Rheumatoid arthritis and vitiligo are both autoimmune diseases, but they do not have as high of an association with Hashimoto thyroiditis as do type 1 DM and celiac disease.

    Answer E is incorrect. Whipple disease is caused by *Tropheryma whippelii.*

18. **The correct answer is B.** Conn syndrome, which is also known as primary hyperaldosteronism, usually results from a solitary aldosterone-secreting adenoma of the adrenal cortex. In patients with Conn syndrome, the high levels of aldosterone cause sodium retention; this leads to hypertension and excess potassium excretion, which likely caused the patient's muscle cramping. Metabolic alkalosis

is another finding of Conn syndrome. The plasma renin level is decreased in patients with this condition.

Answer A is incorrect. Addison disease, unlike Conn syndrome, results from a deficiency of aldosterone. Signs of this condition include hypotension, skin hyperpigmentation, hyponatremia, and hyperkalemia. Addison disease does not explain the clinical scenario described.

Answer C is incorrect. Cushing syndrome occurs from excess secretion of cortisol. The clinical picture is marked by hypertension, weight gain, moon facies, truncal obesity, hyperglycemia, striae, and osteoporosis. Cushing syndrome does not explain the clinical scenario described.

Answer D is incorrect. Hyperparathyroidism results in elevated calcium levels. Depression, constipation, and fractures are symptoms that are associated with hyperparathyroidism. Other commonly associated symptoms include kidney stones, chronic renal insufficiency, gallstones, pancreatitis, weakness, fatigue, and valvular calcifications. Hyperparathyroidism does not explain the clinical scenario described.

Answer E is incorrect. Pheochromocytoma usually results from neoplasms of the adrenal medulla that secrete catecholamines. Classic symptoms of Pheochromocytoma include the "5 Ps": elevated blood **P**ressure, **P**ain (headache), **P**erspiration, **P**alpitations, and **P**allor with diaphoresis. Pheochromocytoma does not explain the above patient presentation.

19. **The correct answer is C.** Though its mechanism of action is poorly understood, metformin, a biguanide, is thought to decrease serum glucose levels by stimulating glycolysis in peripheral tissues and decreasing hepatic gluconeogenesis. Biguanides may cause lactic acidosis.

    Answer A is incorrect. Insulin and insulin analogs bind the insulin receptor on cell membranes, subsequently activating a tyrosine kinase that leads to the absorption of glucose into the cell. Insulin binding leads to increased glycogen storage in the liver and glycogen and protein synthesis in muscle.

    Answer B is incorrect. α-Glucoside inhibitors such as acarbose and miglitol are carbohydrate analogs. They inhibit intestinal brush border α-glucosidase and decrease sugar hydrolysis.

    Answer D is incorrect. Glitazones such as rosiglitazone and pioglitazone are thiazolidinediones used to increase sensitivity to insulin. They stimulate peroxisome proliferator-activated receptor-gamma, leading to increased glucose uptake in muscle and adipose tissue.

    Answer E is incorrect. Sulfonylureas such as glyburide and glipizide stimulate the release of endogenous insulin stores. They close potassium channels in β cells, leading to an influx of calcium, cell depolarization, and insulin release.

20. **The correct answer is B.** This patient has symptoms of acromegaly, which is caused by increased release of growth hormone (GH), most likely due to a pituitary adenoma. The pituitary sits immediately behind the optic chiasm, and increases in its size may lead to impingement on the nasal tracts that cross in the midline of the chiasm, causing bi-temporal hemianopia.

    Answer A is incorrect. Loss of vision only in the right eye is caused by lesions of the right eye or right optic nerve that are distal to the optic chiasm.

    Answer C is incorrect. Left homonymous hemianopia is caused by a lesion of the right optic tract that is just proximal to the optic chiasm.

    Answer D is incorrect. Left-upper-quadrant anopia is caused by a lesion in Meyer loop in the temporal lobe on the right.

    Answer E is incorrect. Left-lower-quadrant anopia is caused by a lesion in the dorsal optic radiation that goes through the parietal lobe.

21. **The correct answer is D.** This patient has symptoms consistent with congenital adrenal hyperplasia, a group of syndromes involving

deficiency of enzymes produced in the adrenal glands involved in aldosterone production for salt retention (zona glomerulosa), cortisol production (zona fasciculata), and androgen production for sexual development (zona reticularis). 21-Hydroxylase is part of the mineralocorticoid- and glucocorticoid-producing pathways. Deficiency of this enzyme decreases aldosterone and cortisol levels, causing decreased blood pressure. Additionally, the block in the production of these hormones shunts additional intermediary products toward sex hormone production, resulting in overproduction of sex hormones, especially testosterone; this results in masculinization of the fetus' phenotypic characteristics.

Answer A is incorrect. 5α-Reductase converts testosterone into dihydrotestosterone and is responsible for secondary sexual development in males (ie, external genitalia). A deficiency in this enzyme would not affect mineralocorticoid, glucocorticoid, or testosterone production, but infants born XY would have female genitalia at birth. At puberty, genitalia would become masculinized as a result of the surge of testosterone that occurs during this time. This deficiency cannot account for hypotension and virilization.

Answer B is incorrect. 17α-Hydroxylase deficiency is a rare disorder that blocks glucocorticoid and sex hormone production, resulting in excess production of mineralocorticoid, namely aldosterone. This syndrome would present with sodium retention and hypertension, as well as a default genotypic female gender (lack of müllerian inhibiting factor) with an immature female phenotype caused by a lack of sex hormone production.

Answer C is incorrect. 11β-Hydroxylase deficiency also affects the mineralocorticoid- and glucocorticoid-producing pathways (similar to 21-hydroxylase deficiency). The effects of 11β-hydroxylase deficiency occur later in the adrenal pathways, and the result is the buildup of a precursor (11-deoxycorticosterone) that can act as a weak mineralocorticoid, producing masculinization, hypertension, and salt retention.

22. **The correct answer is B.** Acute high-dosage glucocorticoid treatment can cause a change in electrolyte levels by their cross-reactivity to the mineralocorticoid receptors, thus causing sodium retention and potassium depletion. Hypokalemia is manifested on ECG as a U wave, which is a small wave that follows the T wave.

    Answer A is incorrect. Delta waves are the result of accessory conduction pathways, not hypokalemia. They are often seen in Wolff-Parkinson-White syndrome and look like slurred upstrokes in the QRS complex.

    Answer C is incorrect. Peaked T waves on ECG are suggestive of hyperkalemia. In this case, the more likely result is hypokalemia instead of hyperkalemia; thus, T waves would not be expected to be peaked.

    Answer D is incorrect. PR segment elongation is indicative of increased time for conduction between the atria and the ventricles. This is typically seen with first-degree heart block, which is not caused by glucocorticoid treatment.

    Answer E is incorrect. ST segment elevation suggests transmural myocardial ischemia, which is not an adverse effect of glucocorticoids.

23. **The correct answer is B.** This is a case of primary hyperaldosteronism, or Conn syndrome. It is caused by increased aldosterone secretion, and an adrenal adenoma is the most common cause, as in this case. In addition to the symptoms seen in this patient, Conn syndrome is associated with failure to suppress aldosterone with salt loading. Pathologic examination would reveal a single, well-circumscribed adenoma with lipid-laden clear cells. In terms of primary venous drainage, the right adrenal gland is drained via the right adrenal vein, which flows directly into the inferior vena cava (IVC). Thus a right-sided hyperfunctioning adrenal adenoma is drained via the right adrenal vein into the IVC. In contrast, the left adrenal gland is drained via the left adrenal vein into the left renal vein, which then flows into the IVC.

Answer A is incorrect. The abdominal aorta plays no role in the vascular drainage of any organ but rather provides arterial supply to the abdominal organs, including the kidneys and adrenals glands.

Answer C is incorrect. The portal vein is superior and anterior to the adrenal and renal vasculature and is not involved in the drainage of either of the adrenal glands. Instead, it drains most of the GI tract down to the rectum into the liver.

Answer D is incorrect. The right gonadal vein drains the testes or ovaries directly into the inferior vena cava but does not drain the right adrenal gland in either sex.

Answer E is incorrect. Drainage of the right adrenal gland and hence a right-sided adrenal adenoma does not flow through the right renal vein, but instead the adrenal vein flows directly into the inferior vena cava.

24. **The correct answer is E.** This patient has symptoms of nephrolithiasis or kidney stones, a common symptom of hyperparathyroidism. The hypercalcemia and imaging findings suggest a parathyroid adenoma, which is a benign growth of the parathyroid gland. Parathyroid adenomas are three times more often in women than men and generally presenting during middle age. They are the most common cause of primary hyperparathyroidism. Parathyroid adenomas are often asymptomatic, but may present with the classic tetrad of "stones, bones, abdominal groans, and psychic moans," including nephrolithiasis (stones); osteoporosis or osteitis fibrosa cystica (bones); constipation, nausea, vomiting, ulcers, pancreatitis, or gallstones (abdominal groans); and depression, lethargy, and eventually seizures (psychic moans). Imaging studies are often used for diagnosis. Treatment is surgical. Preoperative scintigraphy is useful in distinguishing adenomas from parathyroid hyperplasia, in which more than one gland would demonstrate increased uptake. High levels of PTH increase calcium levels by increasing renal calcium absorption in the distal tubule and by stimulating the production of 1,25-dihydroxycholecalciferol in the kidney, leading to hypercalcemia. Hypophosphatemia is caused by PTH inhibition of renal phosphate reabsorption in the proximal tubule.

Answer A is incorrect. These laboratory values are consistent with hypoparathyroidism, commonly caused by surgical removal of the thyroid or congenital absence, such as in a patient with DiGeorge syndrome. The low PTH level leads to decreased 1,25-dihydroxycholecalciferol production, decreased serum calcium (both through decreased uptake and decreased reabsorption), and increased phosphate retention. Patients with hypoparathyroidism generally present with increased neuromuscular excitability and tetany, symptoms of severe hypocalcemia.

Answer B is incorrect. These laboratory values are consistent with humoral hypercalcemia of malignancy, caused by a PTH-related peptide (PTHrP) secreted by some types of malignant tumors, such as breast or bronchogenic squamous cell carcinoma. PTHrP has all the same physiologic functions of PTH, including increased bone resorption, increased renal calcium reabsorption, and increased phosphate excretion. Laboratory findings are similar to those of primary hyperparathyroidism, except that in this case the increased calcium is caused by PTHrP, not PTH. Thus PTH levels are low due to the hypercalcemia, but all other laboratory values are the same.

Answer C is incorrect. These laboratory values are associated with secondary hyperparathyroidism, commonly associated with chronic renal failure. This is referred to as "secondary" because other changes in body chemistry precede the increase in PTH. In the case of chronic renal failure, a decreased glomerular filtration rate leads to decreased phosphate excretion and, ultimately, hyperphosphatemia. Hyperphosphatemia in turn decreases α-hydroxylase activity, lowering 1,25-dihydroxycholecalciferol production and decreasing serum calcium. In addition, 1-25-dihydroxycholecalciferol is already lowered due to poor renal function. Serum phosphate complexes with calcium in the blood, which further decreases the serum calcium level. This low calcium level stimulates an increase in PTH production. Individuals with renal failure are generally older than this patient and have other metabolic imbalances, such as acidosis, hyperkalemia, and hypertension.

Answer D is incorrect. These laboratory values are consistent with pseudohypoparathyroidism, also known as type Ia Albright's hereditary osteodystrophy. This is an autosomal dominant disease caused by a defective G_s protein in kidney and bone, leading to resistance to PTH. The inability to respond to PTH results in hypocalcemia and hyperphosphatemia, and the low calcium levels stimulate release of more PTH. Patients with this disease tend to have short stature, a round face, and shortened fourth and fifth digits (brachydactyly), along with symptoms of hypocalcemia such as tetany and positive Chvostek and Trousseau signs. Impaired mentation is also found in about half of patients with pseudohypoparathyroidism. This patient's presentation is not consistent with this disease. In addition, this condition generally presents before age 42 years, and hypocalcemia, not hypercalcemia, would be found.

25. **The correct answer is A.** This patient has Addison disease (also known as primary adrenocortical deficiency), which is adrenal insufficiency (remember the "**GFR**" of the adrenal gland: **G**lomerulosa is the outer layer, which makes mineralocorticoids, namely aldosterone; **F**asciculata is the middle layer, which makes glucocorticoids such as cortisol; and **R**eticularis is the inner layer, which makes sex steroids such as estrogens and androgens). Decreased levels of aldosterone lead to hypotension, increased levels of potassium, and decreased levels of sodium, chloride, and bicarbonate. Decreased levels of cortisol lead to decreased glucose levels. Decreased cortisol also leads to increased levels of ACTH (as the pituitary attempts to increase stimulation of the adrenal gland), causing hyperpigmentation (from a precursor hormone to ACTH that stimulates melanocytes), especially at physical pressure points such as the elbows, knees, and knuckles.

    Answer B is incorrect. Conn syndrome is defined as a chronic excess of aldosterone secretion from an aldosterone-secreting adenoma in one adrenal gland. Unlike patients with Addison disease, people with Conn syndrome would have, among other findings, hypertension, increased serum sodium, decreased serum potassium, low serum renin, and increased serum aldosterone.

    Answer C is incorrect. Cushing syndrome is a name for any condition that causes an excess of glucocorticoids, such as cortisol. Early signs include hypertension and weight gain, which progress to truncal obesity, moon facies, and a "buffalo hump" from accumulation of fat in the posterior neck and back.

    Answer D is incorrect. A pheochromocytoma is neoplasm of the chromaffin cells (neural crest derivatives that synthesize and release mostly catecholamines). Most cases present with hypertension, headache, tremor, sweating, and a sense of apprehension. The hypertension may occur in isolated bursts or chronically and may be associated with palpitations,

    Answer E is incorrect. Waterhouse-Friderichsen syndrome is characterized by rapidly developing adrenocortical insufficiency (days to weeks) accompanied by an overwhelming bacterial infection (classically *Neisseria meningitidis*), rapidly progressive hypotension, shock, disseminated intravascular coagulation (DIC), and widespread purpura.

26. **The correct answer is A.** This patient has Graves disease, an autoimmune disorder resulting from IgG-type autoantibodies to the TSH receptor. The three classic findings associated with Graves disease are hyperthyroidism, ophthalmopathy, and dermopathy/pretibial myxedema.

    Answer B is incorrect. Hashimoto thyroiditis is an autoimmune disorder characterized by antibodies attacking thyroglobulin or thyroid peroxidase (the two most common autoantibodies in these patients) or antibodies against another part of the thyroid or thyroid hormone synthesis pathway. Although some cases of Hashimoto thyroiditis may present as a transient hyperthyroidism (with symptoms including palpitations and increased metabolic rate) from an initial disruption of thyroid follicles, the majority of cases present with signs and symptoms of hypothyroidism, such as intolerance to cold weather, weight gain, and mental and physical slowness.

Answer C is incorrect. Plummer disease is characterized by a nodular goiter that has a hyperfunctioning nodule, causing hyperthyroidism. As opposed to Graves disease, Plummer disease is not accompanied by ophthalmopathy or dermopathy/pretibial myxedema.

Answer D is incorrect. Iodine deficiency causes hypothyroidism, manifested with signs and symptoms that include intolerance to cold weather, weight gain, and mental and physical slowness.

Answer E is incorrect. Papillary carcinoma of the thyroid, the most common form of thyroid cancer, usually presents as an asymptomatic thyroid nodule with signs of obstruction from the tumor such as hoarseness, cough, dysphagia, or dyspnea or a cervical lymph node mass (as opposed to symptoms of hyper- or hypothyroidism). Radiation is a common cause of thyroid cancer.

27. **The correct answer is D.** 17α-Hydroxylase deficiency, a form of congenital adrenal hyperplasia, is characterized by deficits in glucocorticoid and sex steroid synthesis. This is coupled with increased mineralocorticoid (aldosterone) production due to the shunting of precursors, such as pregnenolone and progesterone, through mineralocorticoid pathways. The increased levels of aldosterone lead to increased sodium retention and potassium excretion (hence, the patient's hypertension and hypokalemia). The low sex steroid levels manifest clinically as a female phenotype with no sexual maturation. Aldosterone is produced in the zona glomerulosa. Aldosterone synthesis requires 21β-hydroxylase but not 17α-hydroxylase. Remember the mnemonic "Salt, Sugar, and Sex" for the layers of the adrenal cortex and their respective products, with "salt" corresponding to the outer zona glomerulosa, "sugar" corresponding to the middle zona fasciculata, and "sex" corresponding to the inner zona reticularis. 11β-Hydroxylase deficiency is another form of congenital adrenal hyperplasia and causes decreased cortisol, aldosterone, and corticosterone production and excess production of sex hormones and 11-deoxycorticosterone. The symptoms are similar to those of 17α-hydroxylase deficiency, manifesting as hypertension and hypokalemia; however, virilization would also be present.

Answer A is incorrect. The capsule does not produce any hormones.

Answer B is incorrect. The medulla produces catecholamines (epinephrine and norepinephrine); neither 17α-hydroxylase nor 21β-hydroxylase is required for the synthesis of catecholamines.

Answer C is incorrect. Cortisol is produced in the zona fasciculata of the adrenal cortex. Cortisol synthesis requires 21β-hydroxylase and 17α-hydroxylase and is therefore deficient in this patient.

Answer E is incorrect. Sex hormones are produced in the zona reticularis. Synthesis of the sex hormones requires 17α-hydroxylase, but not 21β-hydroxylase, and is therefore deficient in this patient, leading to her primary amenorrhea. 11β-Hydroxylase deficiency is another form of congenital adrenal hyperplasia, and causes decreased cortisol, aldosterone, and corticosterone production and excess production of sex hormones and 11-deoxycorticosterone. The symptoms are similar to those of 17α-hydroxylase deficiency, manifesting as hypertension and hypokalemia; however, virilization would also be present.

28. **The correct answer is E.** This patient has ketoacidosis due to uncontrolled type 1 DM. The stress caused by the viral upper respiratory infection likely increased her insulin requirements, precipitating fat breakdown and ketogenesis. These are often the presenting events of previously undiagnosed type 1 DM:

The patient has a subclinical disease that becomes a clinical disease in the setting of an acute comorbid illness. Signs and symptoms of ketoacidosis include rapid deep breathing (Kussmaul's respirations), nausea/vomiting, abdominal pain, hyperthermia, psychosis/dementia, and dehydration. A fruity odor to the breath from the ketone bodies is commonly present. Labs demonstrate hyperglycemia, increased ketone levels, leukocytosis, and a metabolic acidosis. Type 1 DM is associated with HLA-DR3 and -DR4.

Answer A is incorrect. HLA-A3 is associated with hemochromatosis.

Answer B is incorrect. HLA-B27 is associated with a number of inflammatory conditions, including psoriasis, ankylosing spondylitis, Reiter syndrome, and inflammatory bowel disease.

Answer C is incorrect. HLA-DQ2 and -DQ8 are associated with celiac disease.

Answer D is incorrect. HLA-DR2 and -DR3 are associated with lupus fibrillation.

29. **The correct answer is A.** The image depicts the circle of Willis. The artery labeled A is the anterior cerebral artery (ACA), which supplies the medial surface of the brain, the area responsible for the contralateral leg and foot areas of the motor and sensory cortices. Thus, a lesion in the artery would lead to deficits in contralateral motor function of the leg and foot.

    Answer B is incorrect. Label B points to the middle cerebral artery (MCA). A deficit in the MCA would cause contralateral face and arm paralysis and sensory loss.

    Answer C is incorrect. Label C points to the posterior cerebral artery (PCA). A deficit in the PCA would cause contralateral hemianopia with macular sparing.

    Answer D is incorrect. Label D points to the anterior inferior cerebellar artery (AICA). A deficit in the AICA would lead to lateral inferior pontine syndrome.

    Answer E is incorrect. Label E points to the posterior inferior cerebellar artery (PICA). A deficit in the PICA would lead to lateral medullary syndrome.

30. **The correct answer is E.** Thyroid hormones act via nuclear hormone receptors. On binding with its ligand, the receptor translocates from the cytoplasm into the cell nucleus, and the ligand-receptor complex acts as a transcription factor. This results in gene transcription and new protein synthesis. Other hormones that act through nuclear steroid hormone receptors include cortisol, aldosterone, vitamin D, testosterone, estrogen, and progesterone.

    Answer A is incorrect. Glucagon acts via G-protein receptors located in the plasma membrane. G proteins are activated, and the α subunit activates adenylate cyclase. Glucagon does not act via nuclear hormone receptors.

    Answer B is incorrect. Histamine and vasopressin activate phospholipase C, resulting in the cleavage of phosphatidylinositol diphosphate into inositol triphosphate and diacylglycerol. It does not act via nuclear hormone receptors.

    Answer C is incorrect. Intracellular insulin acts via a tyrosine kinase cascade and not via nuclear hormone receptors.

    Answer D is incorrect. Norepinephrine acts by binding to and activating adrenergic receptors. It does not bind to nuclear hormone receptors.

31. **The correct answer is C.** The hypophyseal portal system allows delivery of releasing hormones (GH-releasing hormone, corticotropin-releasing hormone, thyrotropin-releasing hormone, and gonadotropin-releasing hormone) and inhibiting hormones (somatostatin and dopamine) from the neuroendocrine cells in the hypothalamus directly to the anterior pituitary gland, where they control the production and release of tropic hormones into the systemic circulation. Portal systems consist of two capillary beds directly connected by veins; these keep hormones from being diluted before reaching the pituitary. Hormones are de-

livered to the pituitary gland in high concentrations and are not needed elsewhere in the body.

Answer A is incorrect. The cells of the pituitary gland do not carry out any processing of hypothalamic hormones. The posterior pituitary serves as a storage site for ADH and oxytocin, which are synthesized in the hypothalamic supraoptic and paraventricular nuclei and then transported to the posterior pituitary via the supraopticohypophyseal tract.

Answer B is incorrect. The supraopticohypophyseal tract is the conduit through which ADH and oxytocin, both produced in the hypothalamus, are delivered to the posterior pituitary for storage and later release. Note that this circuit does not involve any vascular structures.

Answer D is incorrect. Hormones are delivered from the anterior pituitary to the hypothalamus via the systemic circulation, just as they are delivered to other tissues. This process does not involve the hypophyseal portal system.

Answer E is incorrect. Tropic hormones of the hypothalamic-pituitary axis (GH, ACTH, TSH, luteinizing hormone (LH), and follicle-stimulating hormone) are synthesized and secreted by the anterior pituitary gland in response to hormonal stimulation by the hypothalamus, but they are not produced in the hypothalamus. These hormones are secreted from the pituitary into the systemic circulation.

32. **The correct answer is C.** The patient has tumors involving the "3 Ps" of MEN type 1, also known as Wermer syndrome. Her galactorrhea and bilateral hemianopsia likely are due to a **P**rolactin-secreting pituitary tumor encroaching on her optic chiasm, and her hypercalcemia likely is due to a **P**arathyroid adenoma. Her recurrent duodenal ulcers are a manifestation of a gastrin-secreting tumor that frequently is located in the **P**ancreas, as seen in Zollinger-Ellison syndrome. The genetic inheritance of MEN-1 is autosomal dominant, as is the inheritance of hypokalemic periodic paralysis, a disorder characterized by episodes of paralysis/weakness accompanied by hypokalemia. Although not necessary as a part of the question stem, as are all three characteristic tumors, the USMLE often will mention that multiple family members have been affected by similar or a variety of tumors. This is a clear indication that the disorder is most likely autosomal dominant in inheritance pattern.

Answer A is incorrect. Fabry disease is an X-linked recessive disorder characterized by peripheral neuropathy, cardiovascular disease, and angiokeratomas. It results from a deficiency in the enzyme α-galactosidase A.

Answer B is incorrect. Familial dysautonomia is an autosomal recessive disorder in which individuals have a poorly developed autonomic nervous system, resulting in such manifestations as labile blood pressure, reduced production of tears, and an inappropriate response to stress.

Answer D is incorrect. MELAS (**M**itochondrial myopathy, **E**ncephalopathy, **L**actic **A**cidosis, and **S**troke-like episodes) is a disorder characterized by mitochondrial inheritance. Mitochondrial inheritance is characterized by transmission of a trait to the offspring of an affected mother but never to the offspring of an affected father, because mitochondria are inherited from only the egg and not the sperm.

Answer E is incorrect. Hypophosphatemic rickets is inherited in an X-linked dominant fashion.

33. **The correct answer is A.** This patient has symptoms of a glucagonoma, a rare glucagon-secreting tumor that can cause hyperglycemia, diarrhea, and weight loss. The hyperglycemia seen in these patients will not respond to oral hypoglycemic agents because of the uncontrolled excess glucagon production that continues despite increased insulin levels. Glucagonomas also are associated with necrolytic migratory erythema, a skin rash consisting of painful, pruritic erythematous papules that blister, erode, and crust over.

Answer B is incorrect. An insulinoma would be expected to cause hypoglycemia rather than hyperglycemia.

Answer C is incorrect. Pancreatic adenocarcinoma could explain this patient's weight loss and abdominal mass. Adenocarcinoma of the pancreatic tail also could account for his hyperglycemia, as these lesions sometimes infiltrate and compromise the pancreatic islets, resulting in insulin deficiency. However, this patient's painful skin rash would not be consistent with pancreatic adenocarcinoma. Rather, these patients may manifest migratory thrombophlebitis (Trousseau syndrome), a condition in which the extremities become red and tender.

Answer D is incorrect. The patient's age makes less likely, though does not exclude, an initial presentation of type 1 DM. However, the pancreatic mass and rash cannot be explained by the diagnosis of type 1 DM.

Answer E is incorrect. VIPomas are rare endocrine tumors that arise in the pancreatic islets. Although VIPomas can cause diarrhea, hyperglycemia, and a pancreatic mass on CT, they are not associated with the rash observed in this patient.

34. **The correct answer is B.** Testosterone is produced in the theca cells. From the theca cells, it diffuses into the granulosa cells. There, follicle-stimulating hormone (FSH) stimulates the enzyme aromatase within the cells to convert testosterone to 17β-estradiol. In males, FSH is also responsible for inducing Sertoli's cells to secrete inhibin, which works in a negative-feedback fashion to inhibit FSH formation.

Answer A is incorrect. Estrogen causes the endometrium to proliferate. It does not stimulate the granulosa cells to convert testosterone to estradiol.

Answer C is incorrect. ACTH stimulates the enzyme desmolase. Desmolase is responsible for converting cholesterol to pregnenolone, a key step in the synthesis of adrenocortical steroids. ACTH does not stimulate the granulosa cells to convert testosterone to estradiol.

Answer D is incorrect. Gonadotropin-releasing hormone stimulates the production of LH and FSH in the anterior pituitary. It does not directly affect the conversion of testosterone to estradiol.

Answer E is incorrect. LH acts on the theca cells to produce testosterone. LH surges also trigger ovulation.

35. **The correct answer is D.** This patient is most likely suffering from hypoglycemia due to his sulfonylurea medication, glyburide. Symptoms of hypoglycemia can be categorized as neuroglycopenic (resulting from the lack of glucose to the CNS) or neurogenic (adrenergic symptoms resulting from the catecholamine response to hypoglycemia). Neuroglycopenic symptoms include weakness, confusion, drowsiness, dizziness, syncope, difficulty speaking and blurry vision. Neurogenic symptoms include diaphoresis, hunger, tingling, tremor, palpitations, chest pain, and anxiety. Nonselective β-blockers, such as propranolol, can block the sympathetic surge that triggers the body's response to insulin-induced hypoglycemia. This can cause "hypoglycemia unawareness" and is especially seen in patients with diabetes. This is mainly a β_2-mediated effect, as noncardiac β_2-receptors are the trigger for catecholamine-induced glycogenolysis. Selective β_1 blockers, such as metoprolol, are therefore less likely to cause this effect.

Answer A is incorrect. Enalapril is an ACE inhibitor. Its most common adverse effects are cough, hypotension, and edema. Dizziness and syncope have been associated with ACE inhibitors, but agitation and confusion have not been reported. Propranolol is therefore the better answer.

Answer B is incorrect. Hydrochlorothiazide is a thiazide diuretic. Its adverse effects include hyperglycemia, hyperlipidemia, hyperuricemia, and hypercalcemia. It is not associated with hypoglycemia unawareness.

Answer C is incorrect. Metoprolol is a β_1-selective blocker and is therefore less likely to cause hypoglycemia unawareness.

Answer E is incorrect. Triamterene is a potassium-sparing diuretic. Its most common adverse effect is hyperkalemia. It is not associated with hypoglycemia unawareness.

36. **The correct answer is D.** This patient has type 1 DM. The pancreas contains the islets of Langerhans, which secrete insulin (β cells), glucagons (α cells), and somatostatin (δ-cells) and comprise the endocrine component of the pancreas. This patient has marked, absolute insulin deficiency, resulting from diminished β cell mass; the pathophysiology often involves islet antibodies. Insulin acts on the liver, muscle, and adipose, and ultimately decreases blood glucose levels. An acute metabolic complication seen primarily in type 1 diabetes is diabetic ketoacidosis, which results from accumulation of ketones. Even though the blood glucose level is elevated, the body is unable to utilize it due to the lack of insulin. The high blood glucose causes dehydration via an osmotic diuresis. Patients are treated with insulin to normalize the metabolism of carbohydrates, proteins, and fats and with fluids to correct the dehydration.

Answer A is incorrect. The adrenal gland had several important synthetic functions, including production of aldosterone, cortisol, sex steroids, and epinephrine, but it does not play a role in insulin production.

Answer B is incorrect. The kidney produces renin, the first component of the renin-angiotensin-aldosterone system.

Answer C is incorrect. The liver has numerous important synthetic functions, including production of insulin-like growth factors/somatomedins in response to GH stimulation, but is not involved in insulin synthesis or secretion. It is, however, one of the targets of insulin. Insulin acts on the liver to increase glucose uptake via an enzymatic effect, triglyceride synthesis, protein synthesis, and glycogen synthesis and to decrease gluconeogenesis, glycogenolysis, lipolysis, protein catabolism, ureagenesis, ketogenesis, and blood glucose levels.

Answer E is incorrect. The spleen is an important component of the reticuloendothelial system; however, it has no significant synthetic or endocrine function.

37. **The correct answer is B.** The biopsy reveals a pheochromocytoma, a tumor derived from chromaffin cells of the adrenal medulla. The punctate blue-black granules seen in the image are dense-core neurosecretory granules containing catecholamines, and episodic release of these granules produces classic hyperadrenergic symptoms (the "**5 Ps**": elevated blood **P**ressure, **P**ain [headache], **P**erspiration, **P**alpitations, and **P**allor/diaphoresis) as well as increased urinary vanillylmandelic acid levels (metabolites from catecholamine breakdown). Initial treatment is with phenoxybenzamine, a nonspecific, irreversible α-blocker that can help manage symptoms related to pheochromocytoma, such as hypertension and excessive sweating. Pheochromocytomas also should be remembered by the "**rule of 10s**": **10%** are malignant, **10%** are bilateral, **10%** are extra-adrenal, **10%** are calcified, **10%** are in children, and **10%** are familial.

Answer A is incorrect. Parafollicular C cells of the thyroid produce calcitonin and can lead to medullary carcinoma, which appears histologically as sheets of cells in an amyloid stroma.

Answer C is incorrect. Malignancy of the pancreatic islet beta cells can lead to insulin-secreting insulinomas. Patients present with severe intractable hypoglycemia.

Answer D is incorrect. Plasma cells produce antibodies as part of the humoral immune response and can become malignant in multiple myeloma. Monoclonal plasma cells can take on a "fried-egg" appearance in the marrow.

Answer E is incorrect. Somatotrophs release GH from the anterior pituitary, and somatotroph adenomas can lead to acromegaly or gigantism (in adolescents).

38. **The correct answer is A.** Iodine is essential for the normal synthesis and secretion of T_4; however, at excess levels iodine can actually inhibit this process by blocking its own transport into the thyroid follicular cells. This occurs because of an escape mechanism by the thyroid: A shutdown in the presence of excessive iodine protects the body from excessive production of T_3, which can cause thyrotoxicosis.

This inhibition can actually result in clinical hypothyroidism, manifesting in this patient as constipation, brittle hair, and fatigue. In her case, overzealous supplementation of iodine resulted in hypothyroidism secondary to iodine excess.

Answer B is incorrect. Magnesium is important in the maintenance of normal cardiac rhythms and in the generation and transduction of action potentials. Hypermagnesemia is associated with dysrhythmias, neurologic symptoms, neuromuscular deficits, and pulmonary symptoms, but it is not associated with hypothyroidism.

Answer C is incorrect. Vitamin C (ascorbic acid) is a necessary cofactor for collagen synthesis and the conversion of dopamine to norepinephrine, and it facilitates iron absorption by keeping iron in a reduced oxidation state. Deficiency of vitamin C causes scurvy, which involves skin and gum breakdown due to collagen fragility. Excess vitamin C is not associated with hypothyroidism.

Answer D is incorrect. Vitamin E is an antioxidant that protects RBCs from hemolysis. Deficiency of this vitamin is associated with increased RBC fragility and hemolysis but not hypothyroidism. Excessive vitamin E can actually lead to an increased risk of bleeding, and can consequently cause hemorrhagic stroke.

Answer E is incorrect. Zinc is important for normal wound healing and immune function, and deficiency results in symptoms of hypogonadism, decreased skeletal muscle maturation, and cataracts. However, zinc intake is not associated with hypothyroidism.

39. **The correct answer is A.** Benign prostatic hyperplasia (BPH) is a common entity in men >50 years old and increases in prevalence with increasing age. Pathophysiologically, estradiol levels increase with age and they are thought to sensitize the prostate to the effects of dihydrotestosterone (DHT), causing the prostatic cells to grow. Common symptoms of BPH include increased frequency of urination, nocturia, problems with initiating and stopping urination, and pain on urination. Finasteride is a 5-α-reductase inhibitor that inhibits the conversion of testosterone to DHT, therefore preventing further growth of the prostate. Finasteride also promotes hair growth.

    Answer B is incorrect. Flutamide is a competitive inhibitor of testosterone and its receptor and is used to treat prostatic carcinoma, not BPH. The biopsy did not show dysplasia, so treatment of carcinoma is not appropriate.

    Answer C is incorrect. Ketoconazole is a commonly used antifungal that also has antiandrogen effects. In the latter capacity, it is used in the treatment of polycystic ovarian syndrome to prevent hirsutism.

    Answer D is incorrect. Spironolactone is a K^+-sparing diuretic that also has antiandrogenic effects. In addition to use in the treatment of hyperaldosteronism, hypokalemia, and CHF, it can be used in preventing hirsutism in polycystic ovarian syndrome.

    Answer E is incorrect. Yohimbine is an α_2-selective inhibitor with questionable usage in the treatment of impotence. While this patient has multiple genitourinary complaints, impotence is not one of them.

40. **The correct answer is B.** To answer this question, one must first arrive at the diagnosis of rickets. The knobbiness of the patient's ribs suggests the rachitic rosary often seen with rickets. The next step is to realize that in this case, rickets is secondary to vitamin D deficiency, as evidenced by the risk factors listed: living in an inner-city apartment, rarely going outside, and continuing to be breast-fed (breast milk has little or no vitamin D, unlike vitamin D-supplemented cow's milk). In vitamin D deficiency one expects to see a decrease in calcium and phosphate levels because vitamin D has a key role in increasing their uptake from the GI tract. The decrease in calcium levels would result in an increase in PTH levels, making this the correct answer.

    Answer A is incorrect. This combination of laboratory values would rarely be seen.

    Answer C is incorrect. This combination of laboratory values could be seen with renal insufficiency. In such a case, the poor kidney function would result in decreased excretion of phosphate. The increased serum phosphate could then complex with serum calcium, causing a decrease in calcium levels. This decrease in calcium would in turn stimulate an increase in PTH. This chronic stimulation of PTH levels can result in secondary hyperparathyroidism.

Answer D is incorrect. This combination of laboratory values could be seen with hyperparathyroidism because the increased PTH level would cause an increase in calcium levels and a decrease in phosphate levels. This occurs because PTH stimulates calcium absorption from the GI tract, calcium reabsorption from the kidney, and calcium release from bone. At the same time, PTH inhibits reabsorption of phosphate from the kidney.

Answer E is incorrect. This combination of laboratory values could be seen with vitamin D intoxication. High levels of vitamin D would result in high levels of calcium and phosphate. The high calcium levels would suppress secretion of PTH.

41. **The correct answer is D.** This is a case of a thyroglossal duct cyst, resulting from a failure of the thyroglossal duct to involute during development. It usually remains asymptomatic unless it becomes infected, which often occurs during childhood. These cysts are differentiated from other conditions such as branchial cleft cysts by their midline location. Embryologic development of the thyroid begins in the pharynx.

Answer A is incorrect. Thyroid development does not originate in the esophagus. It originates in the pharynx, above the beginning of the esophagus.

Answer B is incorrect. The first branchial arch gives rise to the malleus and incus, the muscles of mastication, and other structures innervated by cranial nerve V. It is not involved in thyroid development.

Answer C is incorrect. The first branchial pouch gives rise to the auditory tube and tympanic cavity. It is not involved in thyroid development.

Answer E is incorrect. The second branchial arch gives rise to the stapes, styloid process, hyoid bone, the muscles of facial expression, and other structures innervated by the facial nerve. It does not give rise to the thyroid.

Answer F is incorrect. The second branchial pouch gives rise to the lining of the palatine tonsils. It is not involved in thyroid development.

Answer G is incorrect. Thyroid development begins in the pharynx, and the thyroid eventually moves to its final anatomic position anterior to the trachea. Thyroid development does not involve the trachea.

42. **The correct answer is A.** Both methylphenidate and sibutramine are stimulants that function by inhibiting neurotransmitter reuptake. Sibutramine is a drug used to treat obesity that inhibits the reuptake of serotonin, norepinephrine, and dopamine; methylphenidate treats attention deficit/hyperactivity disorder by inhibiting the reuptake of norepinephrine and dopamine.

Answer B is incorrect. Orlistat is a diet drug that inhibits pancreatic lipase. It is also used in the treatment of obesity with the idea that reducing the activity of the lipase will reduce absorption of dietary fats. Its function is not similar to that of sibutramine.

Answer C is incorrect. Selegiline is a selective monoamine oxidase inhibitor used to treat Parkinson disease. Its main function is to increase the amount of dopamine available in these patients.

Answer D is incorrect. Tranylcypromine is a monoamine oxidase inhibitor used as an antidepressant. Although it also increases the amount of neurotransmitters at the neuronal synapse, it does so by preventing the breakdown as opposed to the reuptake.

43. **The correct answer is A.** This patient has disseminated meningococcal infection, characterized by meningitis (cerebrospinal fluid [CSF]

pleocytosis and positive examination findings), hypoxemia, DIC, and acute onset adrenal insufficiency. Acute onset adrenal insufficiency in the context of disseminated meningococcemia is termed Waterhouse-Friderichsen syndrome and is caused by bilateral adrenal hemorrhage. It is important to recognize that the clinical presentation of adrenal insufficiency is often nonspecific, and may include fever, nausea, vomiting, diffuse abdominal tenderness, and hypotension that is mainly refractory to large amounts of intravenous hydration.

Answer B is incorrect. Although this patient indeed has DIC (thrombocytopenia, coagulopathy, elevated D-dimer, and a petechial rash), these findings are not likely contributing to her abdominal tenderness.

Answer C is incorrect. This patient's hypoxemia is likely due to sepsis secondary to meningococcal bacteremia. Hypoxemia may cause cyanosis and dyspnea, but it does not cause hypotension and diffuse abdominal tenderness.

Answer D is incorrect. This patient also has meningitis, characterized by photophobia, fevers, positive Kernig and Brudzinski signs, and CSF pleocytosis with positive Gram stains. However, meningitis alone does not cause diffuse abdominal tenderness.

Answer E is incorrect. Viral gastroenteritis is a common cause of hypotension, vomiting, and diffuse abdominal tenderness. However, in this case of Waterhouse-Friderichsen syndrome (which is due to disseminated meningococcemia), a concomitant viral gastroenteritis is unlikely.

44. **The correct answer is D.** Treatments for SIADH include demeclocycline (drug X in this vignette) and water restriction. This patient appears to have developed a complication of demeclocycline therapy: nephrogenic diabetes insipidus (DI). In nephrogenic DI the kidney is unable to resorb sufficient water in response to ADH, resulting in the production of large quantities of relatively dilute urine. Symptoms of nephrogenic DI include polydipsia, polyuria, hypotonic urine, serum hyperosmolarity, and hypernatremia. In addition, serum ADH levels tend to be elevated; this represents the body's effort to compensate for a diminished renal response to ADH. Demeclocycline is just one cause of nephrogenic DI; others include lithium toxicity and hypercalcemia. Demeclocycline is a tetracycline analog (an antibiotic) that might also be used to treat Lyme disease.

    Answer A is incorrect. Acute gouty arthritis is often treated with nonsteroidal anti-inflammatory drugs, including indomethacin. The patient in this vignette has developed nephrogenic DI. Indomethacin is actually used to treat nephrogenic DI, and it does not have a role in the treatment of SIADH.

    Answer B is incorrect. Conn syndrome (primary hyperaldosteronism) is a disorder characterized by excessive aldosterone secretion. Medical treatment includes spironolactone, a potassium-sparing diuretic that acts as an aldosterone antagonist. Spironolactone is not a conventional treatment for SIADH, nor would it explain the development of nephrogenic DI in this patient.

    Answer C is incorrect. Medical treatment options for enuresis (bedwetting) include desmopressin (a synthetic form of ADH) and tricyclic antidepressants. Neither of these agents would be used in the therapy of SIADH, nor would they be expected to cause nephrogenic DI. The offending agent in this vignette (drug X) is demeclocycline.

    Answer E is incorrect. Medical treatment for pheochromocytoma includes α-blocking agents such as phenoxybenzamine and phentolamine. This patient appears to have developed nephrogenic DI in response to demeclocycline therapy for SIADH. Demeclocycline is an antibiotic and is not commonly used to treat pheochromocytomas.

45. **The correct answer is A.** Parathyroid hypoplasia results in a decreased PTH level, which leads to elevated, not low, serum phosphorus levels.

    Answer B is incorrect. This patient most likely has DiGeorge syndrome, a collection of signs and symptoms associated with defective development of the pharyngeal pouch system (usually caused by a deletion on chromosome 22q11.2). The classic presentation for DiGeorge syndrome is the triad of conotruncal cardiac anomalies, hypoplastic thymus, and hypocalcemia. Cleft palate and abnormal facies are also common. The thymus may be hypoplastic or completely absent, resulting in T-lymphocyte deficiency. Hypocalcemia results from parathyroid hypoplasia and is thus accompanied by low PTH and elevated serum phosphorus levels.

Answer C is incorrect. Parathyroid hypoplasia results in a decreased PTH level, which in turn leads to decreased, not elevated, serum calcium levels.

Answer D is incorrect. Parathyroid hypoplasia results in a decreased rather than elevated PTH level, which in turn leads to decreased, not elevated, serum calcium levels.

46. **The correct answer is B.** This patient has a mass in the head of the pancreas, an organ that is both an exocrine and endocrine gland, and is both secondarily retroperitoneal and peritoneal. As an exocrine gland it produces bicarbonates and digestive enzymes, and as an endocrine gland it produces glucagons, insulin, somatostatin, and pancreatic polypeptide. This patient's symptoms and low blood glucose level suggest that there is an abundance of insulin production, such as in a tumor. The CT findings support a mass, which likely is the source. Treatment involves resection of the mass, and ligation of its blood supply in the case of a possible tumor. The head of the pancreas and the duodenum share a dual blood supply from the gastroduodenal artery, a branch of the celiac trunk. This artery supplies the anterior and posterior superior pancreaticoduodenal arteries as well as the superior mesenteric artery, which supplies the anterior and posterior inferior pancreaticoduodenal arteries. Therefore, to resect any portion of the duodenum or the head of the pancreas, branches from both the gastroduodenal and superior mesenteric arteries must be ligated.

Answer A is incorrect. While the gastroduodenal artery is an important source of vascular supply to the head of the pancreas, the inferior mesenteric artery does not provide any vascular supply to this structure and thus provides no branches that would need to be ligated to remove the mass described in the question stem.

Answer C is incorrect. Neither the proper hepatic nor the inferior mesenteric arteries provide any significant arterial supply to the head of the pancreas; thus no branches from either of these vessels would need to be ligated to complete the resection.

Answer D is incorrect. While the superior mesenteric artery is an important source of vascular supply to the head of the pancreas, the proper hepatic artery does not provide any vascular supply to this structure and therefore provides no branches that would need to be ligated to remove the mass.

Answer E is incorrect. Neither the left gastric nor the inferior mesenteric arteries provide any significant arterial supply to the head of the pancreas; thus no branches from either of these vessels would need to be ligated to complete the resection.

Answer F is incorrect. While the superior mesenteric artery is an important source of vascular supply to the head of the pancreas, the left gastric artery does not provide any vascular supply to this structure and thus provides no branches that would need to be ligated to remove the mass.

47. **The correct answer is A.** The patient has signs and symptoms suggestive of hypercortisolism, also known as Cushing syndrome. Etiologies of hypercortisolism include a cortisol-producing adrenal adenoma, an ACTH-producing pituitary adenoma, paraneoplastic ectopic production of ACTH, and exogenous cortisol or ACTH administration. The dexamethasone suppression test can help distinguish between possible etiologies of hypercorticism. In normal individuals, low doses of dexamethasone suppress cortisol production. In patients with ACTH-producing pituitary adenomas, high

doses of dexamethasone are needed to suppress cortisol production. In patients with adrenal adenomas or ectopic sources of ACTH, both low and high doses of dexamethasone fail to suppress cortisol production. Unlike patients with ectopic ACTH production, patients with an adrenal adenoma are expected to have low levels of ACTH due to negative feedback inhibition from the increased cortisol levels, as noted in this patient.

Answer B is incorrect. Bilateral adrenal hyperplasia suggests increased stimulation of the adrenal glands due to increased ACTH production from either a pituitary adenoma or an ectopic ACTH source.

Answer C is incorrect. Ectopic ACTH production is seen in paraneoplastic syndromes associated with bronchogenic cancer, pancreatic cancer, and thymomas. Bilateral adrenal hyperplasia and failed dexamethasone suppression are characteristics of ectopic ACTH production. A single mass noted on abdominal CT scan adjacent to a kidney is more suggestive of an adrenal adenoma than bilateral adrenal hyperplasia.

Answer D is incorrect. Although exogenous corticosteroid administration, like adrenal adenomas, results in decreased levels of ACTH, a mass on abdominal CT scan would be unlikely in a patient with exogenous corticosteroid administration.

Answer E is incorrect. An ACTH-secreting pituitary adenoma would cause bilateral adrenal hyperplasia and elevated ACTH levels, which are usually suppressed with high-dose dexamethasone.

48. **The correct answer is D.** The patient's hypercalcemia and hypophosphatemia in the setting of increased serum alkaline phosphatase activity are consistent with elevated PTH levels. This is likely caused by ectopic production of PTH-related peptide (PTHrP), which produces physiologic effects that mimic those of PTH: increased bone resorption (causing elevated alkaline phosphatase activity), increased renal reabsorption of calcium (resulting in elevated serum calcium levels), decreased renal reabsorption of phosphate (resulting in decreased serum phosphate levels), and increased vitamin D activation. Squamous cell lung cancer is known to be associated with ectopic PTHrP production.

Answer A is incorrect. PTH and PTHrP do not act at the adrenal cortex or the intestine. The adrenal cortex is the primary site of action for ACTH and ACTH-like peptide; the intestine is the primary site of action for 1,25-dihydroxycholecalciferol. Additionally, the adrenal glands are not normally involved in regulating serum calcium and phosphate levels.

Answer B is incorrect. PTH and PTHrP have no action at the adrenal cortex. ACTH and ACTH-like peptide (both of which can be secreted by neoplastic cells, resulting in Cushing syndrome) act primarily at the adrenal cortex. Additionally, the adrenal glands are not normally involved in regulating serum calcium and phosphate levels.

Answer C is incorrect. The intestine and bones are primary sites of action for 1,25-dihydroxycholecalciferol (activated vitamin D), which causes increased calcium and phosphate absorption in the intestines and increased bone resorption of calcium and phosphate. While PTH and PTHrP stimulate the production of 1,25-dihydroxycholecalciferol, producing secondary effects at the intestine, these hormones do not act primarily on the intestine.

Answer E is incorrect. PTH and PTHrP act primarily at the renal tubules and bones to increase serum calcium levels and decrease phosphate levels. These hormones do not influence the pancreas, although pancreatic tumors have been shown to occasionally secrete PTHrP. Additionally, the pancreas is not normally involved in regulating serum calcium and phosphate levels.

49. **The correct answer is E.** The actions of insulin are mediated at the cellular level by binding of the insulin to its receptor followed by autophosphorylation of tyrosine residues on the insulin receptor; this generates a tyrosine kinase that participates in an intracellular sig-

naling cascade. Inhibition of tyrosine kinase function would preclude downstream signaling and block the physiologic changes associated with insulin action, regardless of the amount of insulin present in the blood.

Answer A is incorrect. Adenylate cyclase and its product, cAMP, are involved in numerous important intracellular signaling systems, including the systems that mediate autonomic sympathetic nervous stimulation, ADH action, renal calcium and phosphate transport, and glucagon action. However, adenylate cyclase and cAMP are not involved in the system that mediates insulin action.

Answer B is incorrect. Guanylate cyclase and its product, cGMP, are involved in many intracellular signaling systems, including those that mediate the transduction of visual stimuli into electrical signals in the nervous system, and the relaxation of vascular smooth muscle throughout the body. However, guanylate cyclase and cGMP are not known to be involved in the system that mediates insulin action.

Answer C is incorrect. Serine kinases are involved in a number of intracellular signaling cascades, but they are not known to be involved in the signaling cascade that mediates insulin action.

Answer D is incorrect. Threonine kinases are involved in a number of intracellular signaling cascades, but they are not known to be involved in the signaling cascade that mediates insulin action.

50. **The correct answer is A.** This patient has a pheochromocytoma, a chromaffin cell tumor of the adrenal medulla that secretes excess epinephrine and norepinephrine. Signs and symptoms of pheochromocytoma include episodic hypertension, headache, sweating, tachycardia, palpitations, and pallor. Pheochromocytomas may occur sporadically or as part of the MEN syndromes, which are a group of autosomal dominant syndromes in which more than one endocrine organ is dysfunctional. Given his history of thyroid carcinoma requiring a thryoidectomy, this patient most likely has MEN type II, which is characterized by the combination of medullary carcinoma of the thyroid, pheochromocytoma, and parathyroid hyperplasia. Pheochromocytomas are treated surgically, but must first be managed preoperatively with both a nonselective α-antagonist (usually phenoxybenzamine) to normalize blood pressure, followed by a β-blocker (eg, propranolol) to control tachycardia. The β-blocker should never be started prior to α-blockade because it would result in unopposed α-receptor stimulation, leading to a further elevation in blood pressure.

Answer B is incorrect. Pheochromocytomas are treated surgically, but must first be managed preoperatively with both a nonselective α-antagonist (usually phenoxybenzamine) to normalize blood pressure, followed by a β-blocker (eg, propranolol) to control tachycardia. The β-blocker should never be started prior to α-blockade because it would result in unopposed α-receptor stimulation, leading to a further elevation in blood pressure.

Answer C is incorrect. Levothyroxine is thyroid hormone replacement that is used to treat hypothyroidism and myxedema. It is not indicated in the treatment of pheochromocytoma.

Answer D is incorrect. Prednisone is a glucocorticoid that is used to treat many inflammatory, allergic, and immunologic disorders, but is not indicated in the treatment of pheochromocytoma.

Answer E is incorrect. Propylthiouracil is used to treat hyperthyroidism. It acts by inhibiting the organification and coupling of thyroid hormone synthesis, and by decreasing the peripheral conversion of T_4 to T_3. It is not indicated in the treatment of pheochromocytoma.

CHAPTER 10

Gastrointestinal

QUESTIONS

1. A 35-year-old woman who is HIV positive presents to the physician because of jaundice and right upper quadrant abdominal pain. She reports having had multiple episodes of jaundice over the past 10 years. Physical examination is remarkable for scleral icterus, marked ascites, and splenomegaly. A hepatitis panel is positive for HBsAg and anti-HBc IgM, but negative for HBsAb and anti-HAV IgM. Which of the following would most likely be lower than the normal reference range in this patient?

    (A) Alkaline phosphatase
    (B) Bilirubin
    (C) Platelet count
    (D) Prothrombin time
    (E) Transaminases

2. An 85-year-old woman presents to the emergency department because of sudden onset of abdominal pain, maroon-colored stools, and abdominal distention. She denies any past abdominal surgery. An upper gastrointestinal fluoroscopy study is performed with the results shown below. Which of the following is the most likely cause of this patient's symptoms?

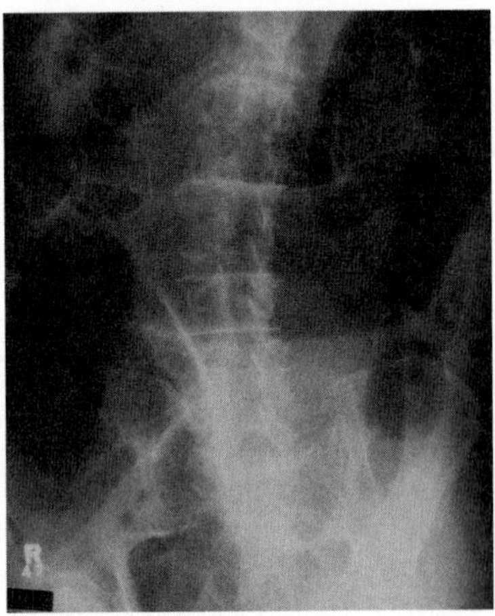

Reproduced, with permission, from USMLERx.com.

    (A) Duodenal hematoma
    (B) Esophageal stricture
    (C) Intussusception
    (D) Perforated esophagus
    (E) Volvulus

3. A 22-year-old woman with no significant medical history complains of diffuse abdominal pain. Physical examination reveals rebound tenderness in the right lower quadrant. The patient denies being sexually active and has not traveled recently. However, she does mention eating "funny tasting" potato salad at an outdoor party three days ago. Which of the following is the most appropriate next step in management?

    (A) Emergency appendectomy
    (B) Initiation of metronidazole, bismuth, and amoxicillin therapy
    (C) Measurement of serum β-human chorionic gonadotropin level
    (D) Measurement of serum lipase level
    (E) Stool culture

4. A 43-year-old overweight woman presents to her doctor's office because of right upper quadrant abdominal pain. She has experienced similar episodes of this type of pain in the past and admits that it is worse after meals. Increased secretion of which of the following is responsible for this patient's postprandial pain?

    (A) Cholecystokinin
    (B) Decreasing the secretion of gastrin
    (C) Pepsin
    (D) Somatostatin
    (E) Vasoactive intestinal peptide

5. A 25-year-old man presents to his physician with a complaint of "yellow eyes" for the past day. For the past five days, he has been ill with a low-grade fever, rhinorrhea, myalgias, and generalized malaise. The physical examination confirms scleral icterus, but is otherwise unremarkable. Electrolytes and complete blood cell count are all within normal limits. Laboratory tests show:

    Aspartate aminotransferase: 31 IU/L
    Alanine aminotransferase: 25 IU/L
    Alkaline phosphatase: 45 IU/L

Total bilirubin: 3 mg/dL
Lactate dehydrogenase: 40 IU/L
Haptoglobin: 76 mg/dL (normal: 46-316 mg/dL)

His urinalysis demonstrates a normal bilirubin level. What is the most appropriate treatment for this patient's condition?

(A) Corticosteroids
(B) No treatment is required
(C) Pegylated interferon
(D) Phenobarbital
(E) Ursodeoxycholic acid

6. A 39-year-old white woman who suffers from polycythemia vera presents to the clinic complaining of severe and constant right upper quadrant pain over the past two days. Physical examination reveals an enlarged liver. What other finding would most likely be seen at presentation?

(A) Ascites
(B) Asterixis
(C) Esophageal varices
(D) Hyperpigmented skin
(E) Spider angiomata

7. A 29-year-old woman presents to her primary care physician complaining of "trouble eating." She says she has had pain when swallowing both solids and liquids for the past nine months. She states that it has been difficult to maintain an appetite over this time and reports a weight loss of 2.3 kg (5 lb). Symptoms have remained constant since they appeared nine months ago. The patient does not exhibit tightening of the facial skin, claw-like hands, or any other systemic symptoms. Which of the following drug mechanisms of action is most likely to improve the patient's symptoms?

(A) Decreasing calcium availability in smooth muscle cells
(B) Decreasing proton secretion into the stomach lumen
(C) Enhancing the phosphorylation of myosin light chains
(D) Inhibiting the degradation of acetylcholine

8. A 57-year-old white man is brought to the emergency department by ambulance because of sudden-onset, bright red emesis. His blood pressure is 80/40 mm Hg and heart rate is 124/min. Physical examination is notable for jaundice and an enlarged abdomen that is dull to percussion and positive for a fluid wave. Which of the following vessel anastomoses is responsible for the patient's bleeding?

(A) Left gastric artery and left gastric vein
(B) Left gastric vein and azygos vein
(C) Paraumbilical vein and inferior epigastric vein
(D) Portal vein and inferior vena cava
(E) Splenic vein and left renal vein

9. An 18-year-old man with no significant medical history presents to the clinic with pain in the right lower quadrant, mild diarrhea, and fever. This has happened twice within the past 12 months, but he has been asymptomatic between episodes. The patient denies recent travel or camping. Physical examination reveals a perianal fistula. The gross appearance of the terminal ileum from a similar patient is shown in the image. Which of the following screening measures would be least useful in this patient?

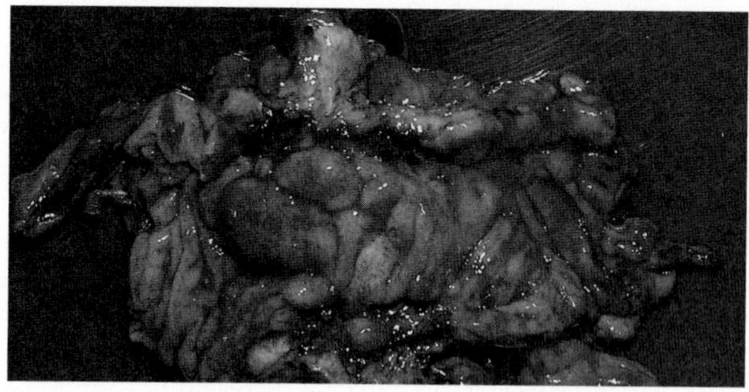

Reproduced, with permission, from USMLERx.com.

(A) Fundoscopic examination
(B) Yearly alkaline phosphatase level
(C) Intermittent hemoglobin levels
(D) Intermittent blood urea nitrogen and creatinine levels
(E) Yearly colonoscopy

10. A 16-year-old boy presents to the clinic with "skin boils." The lesions are erythematous and tender, concerning for skin abscesses due to methicillin-resistant *Staphylococcus aureus*. The patient is promptly given an oral medication to treat the infection. The abscesses eventually resolve. Three days later, the boy develops fever and watery, foul-smelling diarrhea. What is the mechanism of action of the antibiotic the patient is taking?

    (A) Blocking the 30S ribosomal subunit
    (B) Blocking the 50S ribosomal subunit
    (C) Forming toxic metabolite
    (D) Inhibiting cell-wall synthesis
    (E) Inhibiting the translocation step of protein synthesis

11. A 65-year-old woman presents to the emergency department with persistent right upper quadrant pain with nausea and vomiting. CT of the abdomen reveals a polypoid mass of the gallbladder protruding into the lumen, diffuse thickening of the gallbladder wall, and enlarged lymph nodes. This patient most likely has a history of which of the following?

    (A) *Ascaris lumbricoides*
    (B) Cigarette smoking
    (C) Gallstones
    (D) *Schistosoma haematobium*
    (E) Tuberculosis

12. A 35-year-old woman presents to the emergency department because of abdominal pain and diarrhea mixed with mucus and blood. She also has ulcerated lesions with violaceous borders on her legs. Gross blood is present on rectal examination. A biopsy of her colon reveals inflammation confined to the mucosa and submucosa, as shown in the image. Which of the following would most likely be used to treat this patient?

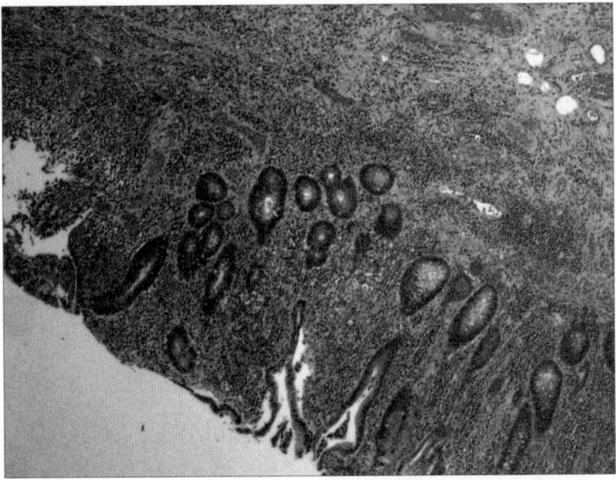

Reproduced, with permission, from USMLERx.com.

    (A) Infliximab
    (B) Nizatidine
    (C) Omeprazole
    (D) Ondansetron
    (E) Sucralfate
    (F) Sulfasalazine

13. A fourth-year medical student is working in a medical relief group in Haiti for several months. Several parents bring their children to the clinic and explain that the children have had profuse, watery stool along with watery vomiting. All of the children are afebrile, slightly hypotensive, and tachycardic but have a normal respiratory rate. Urine output is reduced. What would be the best immediate management of this diarrhea?

    (A) Antibiotics
    (B) Diphenoxylate
    (C) Intravenous normal saline with 5% dextrose
    (D) Loperamide
    (E) Oral rehydration solutions

14. A 79-year-old woman presents with 5.4-kg (12-lb) weight loss over the past two months, associated with progressively worsening dull, constant abdominal pain, early satiety, and nausea. Her examination is notable for a palpable periumblicial node as well as left supraclavicular adenopathy. Which of the following is the most likely diagnosis?

(A) Adenocarcinoma of the pancreas
(B) Adenocarcinoma of the stomach
(C) Ductal carcinoma in situ of the breast
(D) Esophageal carcinoma
(E) Krukenberg tumor

15. A medical student presents to an infectious disease specialist complaining of abdominal distention and tenderness. The patient reports no recent changes in normal bowel habits. Physical examination shows hepatosplenomegaly. Bowel sounds are normal. On questioning, the patient reports that he traveled to Brazil several months ago to study tribal medical practices. He frequently went swimming in the Amazon River to wash himself. Several weeks after returning from his trip, he recalls having fever, diarrhea, weight loss, and "funny looking" stools. Which of the following conditions is most likely responsible for this patient's present symptoms?

(A) Appendicitis
(B) Bowel obstruction
(C) Enterocolitis
(D) Portal hypertension
(E) Ruptured viscus

16. A 34-year-old man is brought to the emergency department after being involved in a high-speed collision with an oncoming car. He has multiple fractures and contusions. Results of fundoscopy are shown in the image. The patient is stabilized and transferred to the intensive care unit. Two days later, there is evidence of gastrointestinal (GI) hemorrhage. What is the most likely mechanism of the GI bleeding?

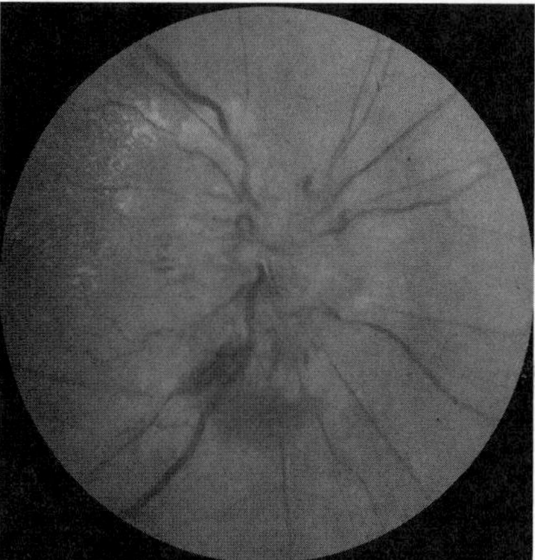

Reproduced, with permission, from USMLERx.com.

(A) Chronic irritation of the gastroesophageal junction by caustic acid secretions
(B) Dilated submucosal veins in the esophagus due to portal hypertension
(C) Increased vagal stimulation secondary to elevated intracranial pressure
(D) Inhibited gastric secretion of mucus secondary to bacterial infection in the stomach
(E) Overuse of oral analgesics leading to superficial gastric erosions

HIGH-YIELD SYSTEMS

Gastrointestinal

17. A 20-year-old man has Crohn disease that is refractory to treatment with high-dose methylprednisolone. He is started on therapy with infliximab, a chimeric monoclonal antibody with anti-inflammatory effects. This drug is administered intravenously every two months and produces substantial improvement in the patient's symptoms between doses. Which of the following best describes infliximab's mechanism of action?

(A) Binds to a growth factor receptor to target a cell for killing
(B) Binds to and neutralizes soluble tumor necrosis factor-α
(C) Binds to and neutralizes tumor necrosis factor-α receptors on T cells
(D) Inhibits a fusion protein with tyrosine kinase activity
(E) Inhibits macrophage production of tumor necrosis factor-α

18. A 2-month-old boy is brought to his pediatrician for a regular check-up. His parents report that he has a poor appetite and is very constipated. He has small bowel movements once a week, which his parents say appear to be very painful. Although he was at the 75th percentile for both height and weight at birth, he is currently at the 25th percentile for height and is below the fifth percentile for weight. His abdomen is distended, but his bowel sounds are normal and his abdomen does not appear to be tender. Barium enema shows a narrow rectosigmoid with a dilation of the segment above the narrowing, and a rectosigmoid biopsy shows a conspicuous absence of ganglion cells. Which of the following genetic conditions is most commonly associated with this patient's disease?

(A) Cystic fibrosis
(B) Down syndrome
(C) Sickle cell disease
(D) Tay-Sachs disease
(E) Turner syndrome

19. An 8-year-old boy presents to the emergency department because of 18 hours of severe vomiting. Arterial blood gas analysis reveals a pH of 7.48, a bicarbonate level of 35 mEq/L, and a partial carbon dioxide pressure of 48 mm Hg. Which of the following best describes the acid-base disturbance occurring in this patient?

(A) Metabolic acidosis
(B) Metabolic acidosis with respiratory compensation
(C) Metabolic alkalosis and metabolic acidosis
(D) Metabolic alkalosis and respiratory acidosis
(E) Metabolic alkalosis and respiratory alkalosis
(F) Metabolic alkalosis with respiratory compensation

20. A 43-year-old multiparous woman with no other medical history presents to her physician because of crampy abdominal pain, fever, and jaundice. Laboratory studies show:

Total bilirubin: 4.8 mg/dL
Direct bilirubin: 4.2 mg/dL
Amylase: 50 U/L
Lipase: 70 U/L
Aspartate aminotransferase: 75 U/L
Alanine aminotransferase: 70 U/L

The patient subsequently is sent for endoscopic retrograde cholangiopancreatography; results are shown in the image. What is the most likely cause of the obstruction seen in the image?

HIGH-YIELD SYSTEMS
Gastrointestinal

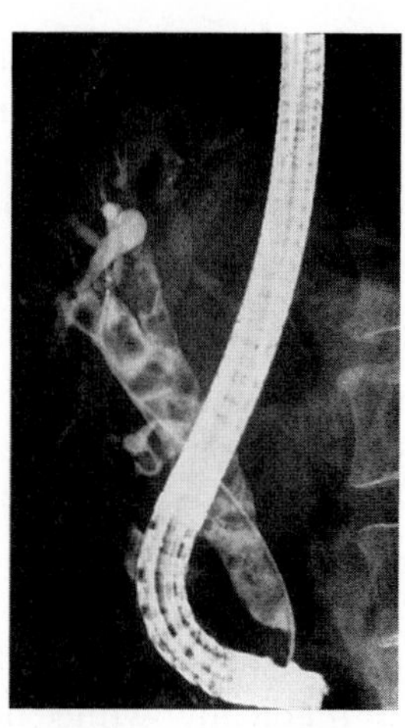

Fauci AS, et al, eds. *Harrison's Principles of Internal Medicine,* 17th ed. New York: McGraw-Hill, 2008; Fig. 305-2C.

(A) Choledocholithiasis
(B) High-fiber diet
(C) Malignancy
(D) Primary biliary cirrhosis
(E) Primary sclerosing cholangitis

21. A 75-year-old woman is taken to the hospital by her son after two bouts of bilious vomiting. Although she normally has a healthy appetite, over the past three days she has had little interest in eating. Furthermore, her belly has become rigid and diffusely tender. X-ray of the abdomen reveals dilated loops of small intestines. Which of the following predisposes this patient to this condition?

(A) Celiac sprue
(B) Chronic *Helicobacter pylori* infection
(C) History of abdominal surgery
(D) Smoking
(E) Ulcerative colitis

22. A 27-year-old man presents to his family physician for an annual physical examination. On rectal examination, masses are palpated. The patient is referred for a colonoscopy, which reveals adenomatous polyps located diffusely throughout the colon. When asked about his family history, the patient states that his father passed away from colon cancer. Which of the following inheritance patterns is characteristic of this condition?

(A) Autosomal dominant
(B) Autosomal recessive
(C) Autosomal trisomy
(D) Sex chromosome abnormality
(E) X-linked recessive

23. A 10-year-old girl living in Grand Haven, Michigan, is brought to the physician because she has had a fever and headache accompanied by vomiting and bloody diarrhea over the last few days. She has no history of recent travel or sick contacts but has a pet puppy, which the mother says has also had diarrhea for the past week. A stool culture incubated at 42°C in a microaerophilic environment shows many gram-negative, comma-shaped organisms, each with a single polar flagellum. The organism responsible for this patient's sickness is associated with the possible development of which of the following symptoms?

(A) Acute renal failure and thrombocytopenia with hemolytic anemia
(B) Fever, migratory polyarthritis, and carditis
(C) Fever, new murmur, small erythematous lesions on the palms, and splinter hemorrhages on the nail bed
(D) Petechial rash and bilateral hemorrhage into the adrenal glands
(E) Symmetric ascending muscle weakness beginning in the distal lower extremities

24. A 2-year-old girl who has recently been adopted from Southeast Asia is brought to the clinic by her adopted parents. They are concerned because the child seems to be having trouble with her vision in low-light conditions. The nutrient most likely deficient in this child is absorbed by the gastrointestinal system using what mechanism?

(A) Apoferritin-mediated transport
(B) Intrinsic factor-mediated transport
(C) Micelle-mediated transport
(D) Sodium-dependent cotransport
(E) Vitamin D-dependent binding protein-mediated transport

25. A 34-year-old man visits his physician because he has experienced increasing "itchiness" and fatigue over the past three months. Medical history is significant for a total colon resection; pathologic findings at resection are shown in the image. Physical examination reveals scleral icterus. Given his past medical history, ultrasound studies are performed, which reveal obliteration of the intrahepatic bile ducts. What is this man's most likely underlying condition?

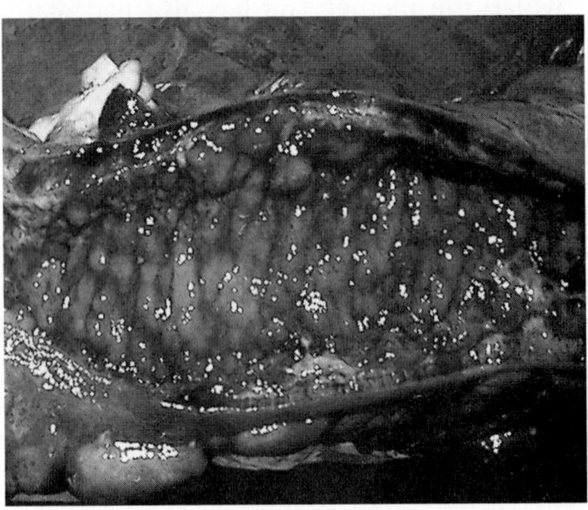

Reproduced, with permission, from USMLERx.com.

(A) Hepatitis C infection
(B) Primary biliary cirrhosis
(C) Systemic lupus erythematosus
(D) Ulcerative colitis
(E) Wilson disease

26. A 29-year-old man complains to his physician of chronic diarrhea. On further questioning he reveals that the diarrhea is watery and intermittent, and that he also suffers from flatulence and weight loss of 3.6 kg (8 lb) over the past year. He denies fever, nausea, vomiting, abdominal pain, and recent travel. Stool examinations for ova and parasites and for occult blood are negative, and stool culture does not grow any pathogens. Endoscopy is performed and biopsy of the upper part of the small intestine demonstrates diffuse blunting of villi and a chronic inflammatory infiltrate in the lamina propria. Which therapeutic option will most likely benefit this patient?

(A) Gluten-free diet
(B) Corticosteroid therapy
(C) Antibiotic therapy
(D) Thiamine and vitamin B_{12}
(E) Vitamins A, D, E, and K

27. A 26-year-old man with hepatitis C is being treated medically while he awaits liver transplantation. One of the drugs he is taking causes him to have periodic fevers and chills and a sense of depression that he did not have prior to treatment. Which of the following drugs most likely is responsible for this patient's adverse effects?

(A) Intravenous immunoglobulin
(B) Lamivudine
(C) Pegylated interferon
(D) Ribavirin
(E) Tumor necrosis factor-α

28. A 10-year-old boy is brought to the emergency department by his parents with a low-grade fever, anorexia, nausea, vomiting, and abdominal pain. The parents report that the pain initially began periumbilically and developed into severe right lower quadrant pain after several hours. On physical examination the child is diaphoretic and lies still; involuntary guarding and rebound are present. Pain is elicited when the child is placed on his left side and the right leg is hyperextended against resistance. Which of the following provides innervation to the muscle involved in this maneuver?

(A) Inferior gluteal nerve
(B) Lumbar plexus and femoral nerve
(C) Obturator nerve
(D) Sciatic nerve
(E) Superior gluteal nerve

29. A 4-year-old child is brought to the pediatrician because of abdominal pain, vomiting, and diarrhea containing mucus and blood. The child has a fever of 39.4°C (103°F). On stool culture, the causative organism is shown to be a non-lactose-fermenting, non-hydrogen sulfide-producing bacterium that is extremely virulent. Which of the following is/are most likely to result from continued infection by this organism?

(A) Ascending muscle weakness
(B) Headache and rose spots on abdomen
(C) Pulmonary hemorrhage, mediastinitis, and shock
(D) Renal failure, microangiopathic hemolytic anemia, and thrombocytopenia
(E) Subcutaneous nodules, polyarthritis, chorea, and a heart murmur

30. A 62-year-old man with a long history of alcoholism presents to the emergency department with steatorrhea and abdominal pain. CT of the abdomen is shown in the image. The intern on duty recalls learning about a drug indicated for acromegaly that may also reduce the secretion of pancreatic fluids and possibly decrease the patient's pain. The drug works by mimicking the levels of which hormone?

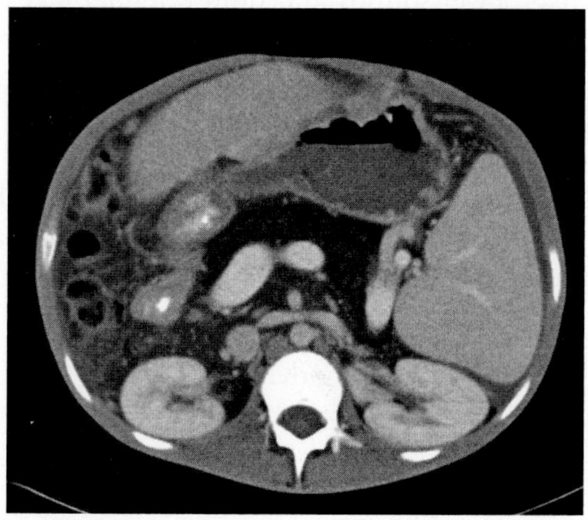

Reproduced, with permission, from USMLERx.com.

(A) Cholecystokinin
(B) Gastrin
(C) Secretin
(D) Somatostatin
(E) Vasoactive intestinal peptide

31. A 27-year-old woman with no significant medical history complains of a month of sharp, nonradiating, epigastric pain. Her pain is relieved after eating food, and she has experienced weight gain. What is the most likely primary treatment for this patient?

(A) Amoxicillin, clarithromycin, and omeprazole
(B) Avoidance of nonsteroidal anti-inflammatory drugs
(C) Gastrinoma resection
(D) Metoclopramide
(E) Ranitidine

32. A 34-year-old woman presents with three weeks of abdominal pain and diarrhea. She says the diarrhea appears to be greasy. She also admits to a lot of flatulence since the gastrointestinal symptoms began. A stain of the stool is shown in the image. What drug(s) should be used to treat the organism causing her symptoms?

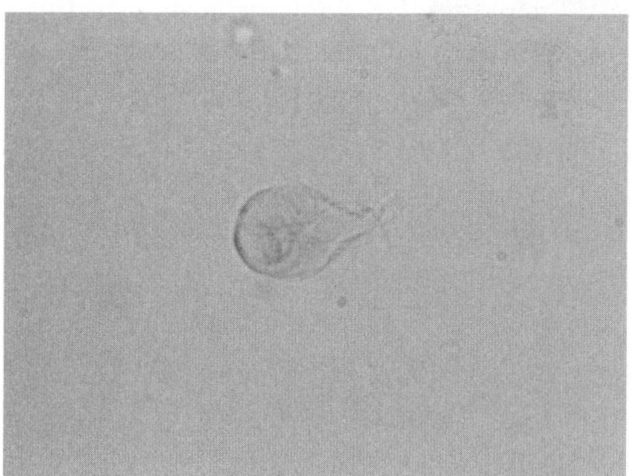

Courtesy of Dr. Mae Melvin, Centers for Disease Control and Prevention.

(A) Chloroquine
(B) Dapsone
(C) Melarsoprol
(D) Metronidazole
(E) Nifurtimox
(F) Sulfadiazine and pyrimethamine

33. A 40-year-old man with no significant past medical history presents to the emergency department because of a two day history of fever, vomiting, and diarrhea. His blood pressure is 90/65 mm Hg and pulse is110/min. An intravenous line is started and he is given 3 L of fluid and then admitted for monitoring. On admission, laboratory studies are unremarkable except for a serum albumin level of 3.0 g/dL. Which of the following is the most likely cause of this patient's laboratory abnormality?

    (A) Hemodilution
    (B) Liver disease
    (C) Malabsorption
    (D) Nephrotic syndrome
    (E) Poor nutritional status

34. A 33-year-old man with gastroesophageal reflux disease returns to his physician for the second time in two weeks complaining of worsening soreness in his throat. Two weeks earlier he was diagnosed with penicillin-sensitive *Streptococcus pyogenes* on throat culture and was prescribed ciprofloxacin (since he is allergic to penicillin). Review of the patient's medication history reveals a possible drug interaction. Which of the following medications is this patient most likely taking that would reduce the effectiveness of his antibiotic?

    (A) Aspirin
    (B) Calcium carbonate
    (C) Cimetidine
    (D) Misoprostol
    (E) Omeprazole

35. A 46-year-old man presents to the emergency department complaining of severe abdominal pain following a weekend of tailgating during which he consumed "a ton" of beer. On physical examination the patient has a temperature of 38.2°C (100.8°F), with pain located in the epigastric region that periodically radiates to his back. Laboratory tests show a serum amylase level of 400 U/L and WBC count of 16,000/mm³. What is the most likely complication of this disease?

    (A) Cholecystitis
    (B) Chronic gastritis
    (C) Pancreatic carcinoma
    (D) Pancreatic pseudocyst
    (E) Small bowel obstruction

36. A 51-year-old man with a lengthy history of medication-dependent reflux esophagitis sees his physician for an annual physical examination. Laboratory tests reveal a blood gastrin level three times the upper limit of normal. His physician expresses concern that the patient is at risk of developing atrophic gastritis. Which of the following medications is this patient most likely taking?

    (A) Aluminum hydroxide
    (B) Bismuth
    (C) Cimetidine
    (D) Misoprostol
    (E) Omeprazole

37. A 25-year-old man presents to his primary care physician after several episodes of severe crampy abdominal pain relieved by the passage of loose stool mixed with blood and mucus. He says he has been feeling fatigued for the past three months and has lost 6.8 kg (15 lb). He has a fever of 37.3°C (99.1°F); abdominal examination is notable for hypoactive bowel sounds and diffuse tenderness with guarding. Colonoscopy reveals diffuse, continuous ulcerations of the intestinal mucosa extending proximally from the rectum to the splenic flexure. A diagnosis is made and genetic testing reveals the patient carries an HLA subtype commonly associated with the disease. Which other disease is associated with the same human leukocyte antigen subtype?

    (A) Ankylosing spondylitis
    (B) Diabetes mellitus type 1
    (C) Graves disease
    (D) Multiple sclerosis
    (E) Rheumatoid arthritis

38. A 67-year-old Chinese immigrant with a history of alcohol abuse and chronic hepatitis B virus infection has been experiencing fatigue, weight loss, and vague abdominal pain for several months. Physical examination reveals a palpable mass in the liver. Before the mass can be surgically resected, the patient dies of respiratory failure. The appearance of his liver at autopsy is shown in the image. How does this lesion migrate to other organs in the body?

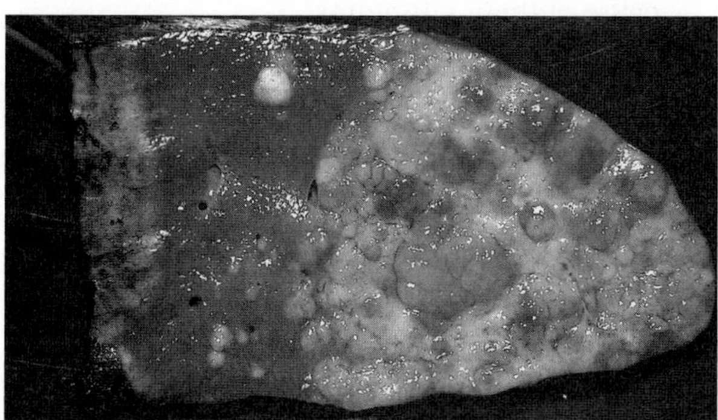

Reproduced, with permission, from USMLERx.com.

(A) Contiguous spread
(B) Direct dissemination into the peritoneal cavity
(C) Hematogenous dissemination
(D) Lymphatic drainage
(E) Secretion into bile

39. A 35-year-old man with a history of drinking one-two bottles of vodka per day for the past 15 years presents to the emergency department because of massive hematemesis and severe epigastric pain. He takes antacids to manage mild acid reflux but has no other known medical problems or medications. His temperature is 36.7°C (98.1°F), pulse is 110/min, respiratory rate is 23/min, and blood pressure is 80/40 mm Hg. Physical examination reveals a regular rate and rhythm with no murmurs and his lungs are clear to auscultation. No jaundice is present. There is no abdominal tenderness or distension, no hepatosplenomegaly, and bowel sounds are present. His stool is negative for blood. Which of the following is the most likely diagnosis?

(A) Esophageal laceration
(B) Esophageal metaplasia
(C) Esophageal squamous cell carcinoma
(D) Esophageal stricture
(E) Esophageal varices

40. A 32-year-old woman complains of alternating bouts of diarrhea and constipation and reports chronic abdominal pain relieved by frequent bowel movements. Her symptoms are exacerbated by stress. The patient denies fever or weight loss. She has a negative fecal occult blood test. Colonoscopy and endoscopy reveal no abnormalities. The most likely diagnosis in this patient is commonly associated with which of the following findings?

(A) Leukocytosis
(B) Normal biopsy
(C) Primary sclerosing cholangitis
(D) Strictures in the small bowel
(E) Villous flattening in the small intestine

41. An obese 40-year-old multiparous woman comes to the physician because she has been experiencing right upper quadrant pain with nausea and vomiting precipitated by fatty foods. Results of a right upper quadrant ultrasound are shown in the image. Laboratory studies show:

Total cholesterol: 280 mg/dL
LDL cholesterol: 170 mg/dL
HDL cholesterol: 33 mg/dL
Triglycerides: 420 mg/dL

Which of the following drugs is relatively contraindicated in this patient's treatment?

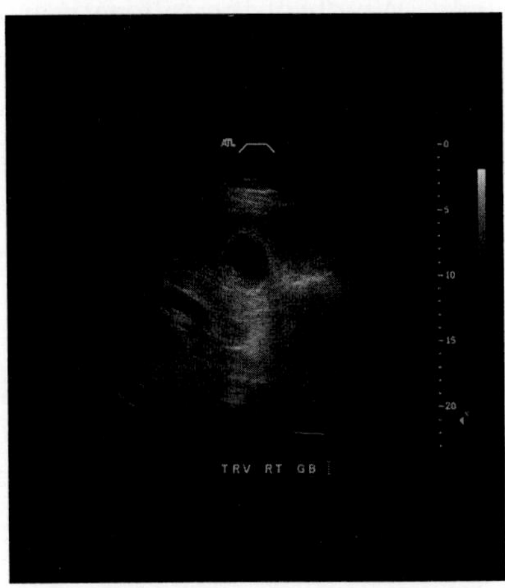

Reproduced, with permission, from USMLERx.com.

(A) Ezetimibe
(B) Gemfibrozil
(C) Niacin
(D) Pravastatin
(E) Simvastatin

42. A healthy 55-year-old woman presents to the physician with a one-year history of an unchanging, non-painful palpable mass in her left cheek. A parotid gland biopsy reveals groups of well-differentiated epithelial cells in a chondromyxoid stroma surrounded by a fibrous capsule; multiple cell types are visible on light microscopy. The pathologic description of the mass is most consistent with which of the following conditions?

(A) Adenoid cystic carcinoma
(B) Mucoepidermoid carcinoma
(C) Pleomorphic adenoma
(D) Sialic duct stone
(E) Warthin tumor

43. A 45-year-old woman who was diagnosed with scleroderma five years ago presents to her physician with increasing difficulty swallowing. Which of the following abnormalities of esophageal muscle function is the most likely cause of these symptoms?

(A) Atrophy of smooth muscle in the lower half of the esophagus
(B) Atrophy of smooth muscle in the lower two thirds of the esophagus
(C) Atrophy of smooth muscle in the upper two thirds of the esophagus
(D) Atrophy of striated muscle in the lower half of the esophagus
(E) Atrophy of striated muscle in the lower two-thirds of the esophagus
(F) Atrophy of striated muscle in the upper two-thirds of the esophagus

44. A 78-year-old man is brought to the hospital because of fever and acute onset of left lower quadrant abdominal pain. About a week ago, he was seen by his family physician for painless rectal bleeding. Laboratory tests show:

RBC count: 5 million/mm^3
Hematocrit: 36%
Hemoglobin: 12 g/dL
WBC count: 93,000/mm^3
Mean corpuscular volume (MCV): 75 fL

Which of the following is the most appropriate follow-up test after the patient is discharged?

(A) Abdominal ultrasound
(B) Colonoscopy
(C) CT of the abdomen
(D) MRI of the abdomen
(E) Upright abdominal X-ray

45. A 26-year-old man presents to the clinic with bradykinesia, rigidity, and resting tremor. Serum aminotransferase levels are mildly elevated. A liver biopsy is shown in the image. What is the chance that this patient's sister will have the same condition?

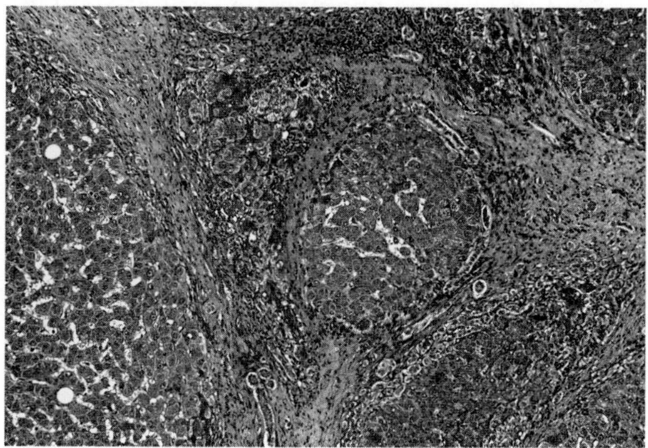

Courtesy of Wikipedia.

(A) 0%
(B) 25%
(C) 50%
(D) 66.6%
(E) 100%

46. A woman comes to the physician because of profuse vomiting and watery, non-bloody diarrhea that developed five hours after she had eaten tuna salad. She is diagnosed with food poisoning. Which of the following is the most likely cause of her symptoms?

(A) A β-hemolytic, gram-positive rod
(B) A gram-positive, catalase-positive, coagulase-positive coccus
(C) A pre-formed enterotoxin
(D) A pre-formed superantigen
(E) An invasive gram-negative rod

47. A newborn develops marked jaundice and kernicterus within weeks of birth. Blood tests reveal alanine aminotransferase = 16 U/L, aspartate aminotransferase = 14 U/L, and total bilirubin = 3.8 mg/dL. Urine tests are negative for bilirubin. Treatment attempts with phenobarbital, plasmapheresis, and phototherapy are unsuccessful. The infant's condition deteriorates over the next two months and he dies. What is the underlying cause of the infant's death?

(A) Elevated antimitochondrial antibodies
(B) Problem with bilirubin conjugation
(C) Problem with bilirubin uptake
(D) Problem with excretion of conjugated bilirubin
(E) Problem with hepatic copper excretion

48. A 45-year-old man presents to the emergency department complaining of a high fever, malaise, and confusion since waking up earlier in the morning. He underwent abdominal surgery two weeks ago and was discharged two days postoperatively without complication. On examination, his temperature is 39.0°C (102.2°F), heart rate is 110/min, blood pressure is 80/50 mm Hg, and respiratory rate is 18/min. His abdomen is warm and erythematous, there is purulent discharge draining from the surgical incision site, and a rash is evident on his chest and abdomen. The patient receives appropriate therapy. Days later, a blood culture reveals high levels of gram-positive bacteria, and molecular studies reveal high levels of interleukin (IL)-1, IL-6, and tumor necrosis factor-α. What cellular process initiated this patient's presentation?

(A) Antigen binding to normal cellular receptors and interfering with proper function
(B) Binding to the macrophage CD14 receptor
(C) Free antigen cross-linking of mast cell IgE
(D) Protein A binding of the IgG Fc receptor
(E) Simultaneous antigen binding of the T-cell receptor and major histocompatibility complex class II

49. A 40-year-old white man presents to the emergency department complaining of burning retrosternal chest pain after meals. The pain is relieved by antacids. The patient's ECG is normal, and x-ray of the chest is remarkable for an 8-cm hiatal hernia. This patient is at risk for developing which of the following types of cancer?

(A) Adenocarcinoma of the esophagus
(B) Gastric adenocarcinoma
(C) Krukenberg tumor
(D) Non-small cell adenocarcinoma of the lung
(E) Squamous cell carcinoma of the esophagus

50. A 50-year-old man presents to his physician because of a 6.8-kg (15-lb) weight loss over the past month, epigastric pain radiating to the back, and jaundice. He also complains of redness, swelling, and tenderness of his left lower extremity. Laboratory studies show an amylase level of 500 U/L, a lipase level of 300 U/L, and an alkaline phosphatase level of 500 U/L. Which tumor markers are most likely to be elevated in this patient?

(A) α-Fetoprotein and β-human chorionic gonadotropin
(B) α-Fetoprotein and CA 19-9
(C) α-Fetoprotein and carcinoembryonic antigen
(D) β-Human chorionic gonadotropin and carcinoembryonic antigen
(E) CA 19-9 and carcinoembryonic antigen

ANSWERS

1. **The correct answer is C.** This patient has a flare-up of her chronic hepatitis B virus (HBV) infection, as evidenced by the presence of HBsAg and anti-HBc IgM and lack of HBsAb. HBV typically presents with jaundice and right upper quadrant pain and can be transmitted via parenteral, sexual, and maternal-fetal routes. About 5% of adults with acute HBV infection will develop chronic hepatitis, and 12%-20% of these will go on to develop cirrhosis. Chronic HBV infection is marked by the presence of HBsAg for >6 months. While most patients will develop HBsAb and eliminate HBsAg from the blood, chronically infected patients do not. A patient with HIV may have a history of risky sexual behavior and would be at increased risk for HBV infection; in fact, chronic HBV infection affects about 10% of HIV-infected patients worldwide. This patient's signs of scleral icterus, ascites, and splenomegaly indicate that her chronic liver disease may have progressed to cirrhosis. The fibrotic liver can induce portal hypertension, causing engorgement of the spleen due to increased pressures within the portal circulation. This enlarged spleen sequesters increased numbers of platelets within it. Thus in this patient we might expect a low platelet count.

   Answer A is incorrect. An elevation in alkaline phosphatase activity occurs most commonly in obstructive liver disease due to a blockage in the biliary tree caused by acute cholecystitis, primary biliary cirrhosis, and other causes. Because viral hepatitis is not an obstructive disease, alkaline phosphatase level would not likely be abnormal.

   Answer B is incorrect. A patient with chronic liver disease would have an elevated serum bilirubin level, because damage to hepatocytes would lead to difficulty releasing bilirubin into the bile, causing it to leak out into the blood.

   Answer D is incorrect. A patient with chronic liver disease would have an increase in prothrombin time due to a decrease in coagulation factors, as the liver is the site of production of all major coagulation factors except factor VIII.

   Answer E is incorrect. A patient with chronic liver disease would be more likely to have an elevation of transaminase levels, as these indicate hepatocellular damage. If the patient's liver disease has progressed to cirrhosis, one might expect the transaminase levels to be normal since the liver would be small and fibrotic, thus no longer capable of releasing large amounts of these enzymes. However, an abnormally low value would not be the most likely finding.

2. **The correct answer is E.** This is an example of volvulus, a twisting of the large intestine in a closed-loop obstruction. The elderly and debilitated are at a particular risk for volvulus. This patient has the common symptoms of colonic obstruction, with abdominal pain, abdominal distention, and bloody stools. The image shows the nonspecific "double-bubble," which is a sign of proximal small-bowel obstruction. Colonoscopy frequently is both diagnostic and therapeutic, as insufflations of air and passing the colonoscope through the point of volvulus frequently results in reduction of the volvulus. The condition frequently recurs, and definitive surgical treatment is a sigmoid colectomy, though a sigmoidopexy (fixing of the sigmoid colon to anterior abdominal) can be performed in those patients who are too sick to tolerate an intestinal resection.

   Answer A is incorrect. Duodenal hematoma is a potential consequence of abdominal trauma. Signs and symptoms include pain, gastric distention, and anorexia. Radiologic findings can resemble an obstruction in the upper or middle gastrointestinal (GI) tract, and hence are not congruent with the image shown. The treatment for duodenal hematomas usually is nonoperative, as these hematomas often resolve on their own, except in the case of penetrating abdominal trauma, when the abdomen must be explored to the examine the duodenal hematoma as well as search for other sites of injury).

Answer B is incorrect. Esophageal strictures can cause an obstruction in the upper GI tract, leading to impaired passage of both food and liquid. The consequences include vomiting, anorexia, and aspiration. On x-ray of the chest the esophagus is greatly distended, and stomach often is collapsed. Because the obstruction is proximal to the stomach, the vomitus usually does not include bile, and the ingested food usually is not digested.

Answer C is incorrect. Intussusception occurs when one segment of the intestine (frequently small intestine, or distal ileum into cecum) telescopes into the immediately distal segment of the bowel. Intussusception is a common cause of small-bowel obstruction in children, but not in the adult or elderly populations. Furthermore, the radiologic findings make volvulus, and not intussusceptions (the classic radiographic finding of intussusceptions is the "target sign"), the better answer.

Answer D is incorrect. A perforated esophagus, also known as Boerhaave syndrome, is a medical emergency, because gastric contents and air are released into the mediastinum. The patient usually experiences excruciating chest pain, dyspnea, dysphagia, and hemodynamic instability. Radiography would reveal air within the mediastinum. There would be no bilious vomiting or hematochezia. Furthermore, the patient usually has a history of trauma or violent retching (most commonly secondary to alcohol consumption).

3. **The correct answer is C.** The possibility of ectopic pregnancy should always be considered in a woman of reproductive age who presents with abdominal pain, regardless of the patient's history. The history of eating potato salad is a distracter, and should not change the clinician's decision to measure the β-human chorionic gonadotropin (β-hCG). The symptoms of ectopic pregnancy may closely mimic those of acute appendicitis, making measurement of the β-hCG level especially critical in cases of suspected appendicitis. Furthermore, an undiagnosed ectopic pregnancy can result in morbidity and even death.

   Answer A is incorrect. Surgery to remove the appendix would be indicated once appendicitis had been confirmed by CT or upon ruling out other significant diagnostic possibilities. Proceeding with appendectomy prior to ruling out ectopic pregnancy would be inappropriate in a young woman.

   Answer B is incorrect. The triple therapy listed is indicated for the eradication of *Helicobacter pylori*, the causative agent of most gastric and duodenal ulcers. This patient's severe, acute-onset pain in the right lower quadrant is not suggestive of an ulcer.

   Answer D is incorrect. Acute pancreatitis classically presents with epigastric pain radiating to the back, often preceded by nausea and vomiting. Elevated serum lipase levels are often present. This patient's pain is not demonstrative of that typically seen in acute pancreatitis.

   Answer E is incorrect. A stool culture would be performed if the physician were suspicious of an infectious diarrhea. Although the "funky tasting" potato salad might suggest infectious causes, this patient denies diarrhea, and thus the clinical suspicion remains low. Furthermore, a stool culture is certainly not the first test to be performed, as more pressing tests such as measuring the β-hCG level would need to be done first.

4. **The correct answer is A.** This is a classic presentation of cholelithiasis, or gallstones. Patients with cholelithiasis experience pain after meals as a result of the duodenal release of cholecystokinin (CCK), which causes the gallbladder to contract while the stone obstruct the cystic duct. CCK is stimulated by fatty acids and amino acids.

   Answer B is incorrect. Gastrin is released by the G cells of the stomach in response to proteins or peptides in the stomach. Gastrin leads to increased secretion of gastric acid and low pH inhibits its secretion, leading to a negative feedback loop. Gastrin does not have an effect on gallbladder contraction.

Answer C is incorrect. Pepsin is a digestive protease released by chief cells in the stomach. Pepsinogen, which is the precursor protein, autocleaves in the acidic environment of the stomach. It is released under the influence gastrin and the influence of the vagus nerve. It does not cause gallbladder contraction.

Answer D is incorrect. Somatostatin is release by the D cells of the duodenum. It reduces smooth muscle contractions and inhibits the release of both insulin and glucagon from the pancreas. It does not cause gallbladder contraction.

Answer E is incorrect. Vasoactive intestinal peptide induces smooth muscle relaxation in the lower esophageal sphincter, stomach, gallbladder and stimulate secretion of water into pancreatic juice and bile. It also inhibits gastric acid secretion and absorption from the intestinal lumen. It causes relaxation rather than contraction of the gallbladder.

5. **The correct answer is B.** This patient has Gilbert syndrome, the most common inherited disorder of bilirubin conjugation. It is due to a gene mutation that results in a decreased level of uridine diphosphate glucuronyl transferase (UDPGT). The disease is autosomal recessive; in the Western world, approximately 9% of people are homozygous for the mutation, and 30% are heterozygous (heterozygotes are asymptomatic). The disease commonly first manifests in young adults after an inciting event, such as a febrile illness, physical exertion, stress, or fasting. Laboratory tests will demonstrate unconjugated hyperbilirubinemia, but will be otherwise normal. The disease is benign and requires no treatment. This patient has a mild unconjugated hyperbilirubinemia and is otherwise healthy besides a mild flu-like illness, so Gilbert is the most likely diagnosis.

Answer A is incorrect. Corticosteroids would be useful for treatment of autoimmune hemolytic anemia. In hemolytic anemia, lactate dehydrogenase is commonly elevated, haptoglobin is decreased, and hemoglobin is low. All of these levels are normal in this patient, so autoimmune hemolytic anemia is unlikely.

Answer C is incorrect. Pegylated interferon is useful in treating chronic hepatitis C infection (HCV). HCV would present with increased aspartate aminotransferase and alanine aminotransferase, and if advanced, signs of cirrhosis. This patient has an isolated hyperbilirubinemia, so HCV is unlikely. An acute HCV infection can present in a variety of ways, including hyperbilirubinemia, but interferon is not used for acute HCV, so this is not the best answer.

Answer D is incorrect. Crigler-Najjar syndrome is similar to Gilbert syndrome in that it is caused by a mutation in the gene coding for UDPGT. However, in Crigler-Najjar syndrome the enzyme is severely lacking or completely absent. Type I is most severe, causing death early in life from kernicterus. Type II is milder and more responsive to treatment. Phenobarbital is useful in lowering the bilirubin concentration in type II but not type I disease. This patient is asymptomatic and is presenting later in life; thus this cannot be Crigler-Najjar syndrome.

Answer E is incorrect. Ursodeoxycholic acid (ursodiol) is used for gallstone dissolution in patients who cannot tolerate surgery. This patient has normal alkaline phosphatase levels, which would be elevated in cholelithiasis. Furthermore, if this patient did have gallstones, he would likely be treated with surgery, which is much more effective than ursodiol.

6. **The correct answer is A.** This is an acute presentation of Budd-Chiari syndrome, or thrombosis of two or more hepatic veins. This condition is associated with hypercoagulable states such as myeloproliferative disorders, inherited coagulation disorders, intra-abdominal cancers, oral contraceptive use, and pregnancy. The increased intrahepatic pressure leading to ascites is present in 90% of patients with Budd-Chiari syndrome. The disease can also present in a subacute manner or in a chronic manner, and diagnosing this condition may then be more challenging because the classic triad

of abdominal pain, hepatomegaly, and ascites may not be present.

Answer B is incorrect. Asterixis is associated with hepatic encephalopathy in the setting of liver failure. The underlying mechanisms linking liver failure to asterixis are not completely understood.

Answer C is incorrect. Esophageal varices are associated with portal hypertension, in which portosystemic shunts occur to bypass the hepatic circulation and return blood to the heart.

Answer D is incorrect. Skin hyperpigmentation can occur in several settings, such as hemochromatosis or Addison disease (adrenal atrophy), but none of these diseases fit the present clinical picture.

Answer E is incorrect. Spider angiomata are usually associated with cirrhosis; their pathogenesis is not completely understood but they are believed to occur in the setting of defects in the metabolism of sex hormones. They can also be present in pregnant women and malnourished patients.

7. **The correct answer is A.** The patient's dysphagia for both solids and liquids suggest a motility problem. Due to loss of the myenteric (Auerbach's) plexus, the lower esophageal sphincter (LES) fails to relax. The majority of patients with achalasia have difficulty swallowing both solids and liquids for >6 months, as well as an increased risk of esophageal cancer. Esophageal manometry is the gold standard of diagnosing achalasia by documenting loss of coordinated peristalsis along the esophagus and abnormally high lower esophageal sphincter tone. Upper endoscopy is also performed to rule out cancer. Surgical corrections include pneumatic dilation and esophageal myotomy. Medical approaches to treating achalasia include using a calcium channel blocker, nitroglycerin, or botulinum toxin. Calcium channel blockers such as nifedipine decrease the availability of calcium to the myosin-actin complex, leading to smooth muscle relaxation. Nitroglycerin works through a cGMP-mediated mechanism to dephosphorylate and inactivate myosin light chains. Botulinum toxin causes muscle paralysis by inhibiting the exocytosis of acetylcholine from presynpatic neurons.

   Answer B is incorrect. Decreasing proton secretion into the stomach lumen is the mechanism of action of proton pump inhibitors (eg, omeprazole), which are used to treat gastroesophageal reflux disease and dyspepsia as well as peptic ulcer disease. This patient has achalasia, which is unrelated to acid secretion. This mechanism would not relieve the patient's symptoms.

   Answer C is incorrect. Enhancing phosphorylation of myosin light chains would enhance muscle contraction, which is the opposite of the mechanism of action of nitroglycerin, and would worsen this patient's symptoms.

   Answer D is incorrect. Inhibiting the degradation of acetylcholine is the mechanism of action of acetylcholinesterase inhibitors (eg, physostigmine), which are used to treat organophosphate poisoning and to reverse the effects of neuromuscular junction blockers (eg, pancuronium). This mechanism would lead to increased availability of acetylcholine at the neuromuscular junction, leading to more active muscle contraction, and would actually worsen this patient's symptoms.

8. **The correct answer is B.** The patient's presentation is consistent with ruptured esophageal varices, a dangerous complication of portal hypertension. When the liver becomes extremely fibrotic, as it does with years of exposure to alcohol (note the jaundice and ascites in this patient), there is an increase in resistance in blood flow through the liver, causing portal hypertension. When the pressure in the portal system is greater than the systemic venous pressure, blood will find alternate routes to return to the heart. One of those alternate routes is from the left gastric vein into the azygos vein, which leads to esophageal varices.

   Answer A is incorrect. The portal system is a system of veins that drain the GI tract and deliver the blood to the liver. The left gastric artery is upstream of the portal system, and an anastomosis between the left gastric artery and vein would bypass the portal system altogether and therefore would not contribute to the formation of esophageal varices.

Answer C is incorrect. Anastomoses between the paraumbilical vein and the inferior epigastric vein lead to the formation of caput medusae, the spokes-of-a-wheel veins that radiate from the umbilicus in patients with portal hypertension.

Answer D is incorrect. There is no natural route for blood to flow from the portal vein to the inferior vena cava. Creating a portacaval shunt, which is a current treatment option for portal hypertension, can relieve the pressure in the portal system and reduce the risk of bleeding from varices.

Answer E is incorrect. Anastomoses between the splenic vein and the left renal vein are retroperitoneal vessels that are not near the esophagus.

9. **The correct answer is D.** The picture of intermittent abdominal pain, fever, and diarrhea should lead you to a diagnosis of irritable bowel disease. The presence of an anal fistula strongly suggests Crohn disease rather than ulcerative colitis, given that it causes transmural inflammation. There are no renal disorders associated with Crohn disease, so blood urea nitrogen and creatinine would not be reasonable screening tests.

   Answer A is incorrect. A much-feared extraintestinal manifestation of Crohn disease is anterior uveitis. If untreated, it can lead to blindness. Migratory polyarthritis may also travel with this condition and can develop either before or soon after intestinal symptoms develop.

   Answer B is incorrect. Primary sclerosing cholangitis can occasionally occur with Crohn disease, but the association is much stronger in ulcerative colitis. Testing for elevated alkaline phosphatase would prompt investigation and further testing for primary sclerosing cholangitis.

   Answer C is incorrect. Iron deficiency anemia may develop as a result of blood loss secondary to GI tract inflammation.

   Answer E is incorrect. There is a fivefold increased incidence of GI tract cancer in patients with long-standing progressive Crohn disease compared to age-matched patients. Screening with yearly colonoscopy is usually started approximately eight years after diagnosis of Crohn disease.

10. **The correct answer is B.** Methicillin-resistant *Staphylococcus aureus* (MRSA) is an organism that is resistant to traditional penicillin family of antibiotics. Therefore, MRSA must be treated with clindamycin, trimethoprim-sulfamethoxazole, or vancomycin. Watery, foul-smelling stool in the presence of fever following antibiotic treatment usually is caused by *Clostridium difficile* superinfection. Of these various therapies for MRSA, clindamycin is the only one that is known to cause a *C difficile* colitis from antibiotic-induced bacterial overgrowth. Clindamycin disrupts bacterial protein synthesis by blocking the 50S subunit of the ribosome. It is used frequently to treat anaerobic infections and has proven efficacy against MRSA infections. In this patient, clindamycin would have been a good choice for treatment of a community acquired MRSA infection.

    Answer A is incorrect. Blocking the 30S ribosomal subunit is the main mechanism of the aminoglycosides (for example, gentamicin) and tetracycline. Gentamicin is an aminoglycoside that works by binding to bacterial ribosomes and preventing protein synthesis. It is used to treat infections with gram-negative rods. Adverse effects include nephrotoxicity and ototoxicity. It is not a common treatment for MRSA, nor a well-documented cause of *C difficile*. Tetracyclines such as doxycycline may be used to treat MRSA but do not cause *C difficile* colitis.

    Answer C is incorrect. Forming toxic metabolite is the main mechanism of metronidazole. Metronidazole is the treatment of choice for *C difficile* superinfection, yeast infections, and bacterial vaginosis. It destroys bacteria through the production of toxic free radicals and is used commonly to treat anaerobic and protozoan infections. Metronidazole is not used to treat MRSA infections. Adverse effects of metronidazole include a disulfiram-like reaction to alcohol, GI upset, and headache.

Answer D is incorrect. Many antibiotics work by inhibiting cell-wall synthesis. A classic example is penicillin, which inhibits peptidoglycan crosslinking. Another class of cell-wall synthesis blocker is vancomycin, which binds to the D-ala-D-ala portion of cell-wall precursors. Vancomycin, although a good treatment option for MRSA, rarely causes C *difficile* superinfection. It can be administered orally to treat C *difficile* superinfection, but is generally a second-line agent because of concern about the spread of vancomycin-resistant enterococci. Adverse effects of vancomycin include nephrotoxicity, ototoxicity, and red man syndrome.

Answer E is incorrect. Inhibiting the translocation step of protein synthesis is the mechanism of macrolides (azithromycin, erythromycin). Macrolides are good choices for treating community acquired pneumonia (particularly azithromycin), but not MRSA-related infections. Moreover, macrolides are not commonly associated with pseudomembranous colitis.

11. **The correct answer is C.** The patient's clinical presentation is consistent with adenocarcinoma of the gallbladder. Gallbladder adenocarcinoma is associated with chronic gallbladder inflammation, typically from a history of gallstones, which can be seen with the thickening of the gallbladder wall on CT. Gallbladder polyps, the polypoid lesion, are also associated with an increased risk of gallbladder adenocarcinoma. The enlarged lymph nodes point to local invasion and spread, which is unfortunately common on initial presentation. Gallbladder cancer is a disease of the elderly and is more common in women than men. Most (90%) patients with gallbladder cancer have concomitant stones. In general, the treatment for adenocarcinoma of the gallbladder is surgical excision but prognosis is generally poor if not found incidentally.

Answer A is incorrect. *Ascaris lumbricoides* is associated with GI irritation, cough, and eosinophilia.

Answer B is incorrect. Cigarette smoking is associated with many malignancies, particularly of the lung, pancreas, and esophagus; it has not been linked to adenocarcinoma of the gallbladder.

Answer D is incorrect. *Schistosoma haematobium* infection is associated with the development of squamous cell carcinoma of the bladder.

Answer E is incorrect. Tuberculosis is associated with hemoptysis, cough, and weight loss.

12. **The correct answer is F.** The patient has ulcerative colitis. The leg lesions represent pyoderma gangrenosum and are the first clue of an extra-intestinal manifestation of ulcerative colitis. The diagnosis is confirmed with the biopsy showing that the inflammation is contained to the mucosal and the submucosal layers (remember that in Crohn disease the inflammation is transmural, leading to fistula formation). Sulfasalazine is a combination of sulfapyridine, which is an antibacterial drug, and mesalamine, which is an anti-inflammatory drug. Its adverse effects include malaise, nausea, sulfonamide toxicity, and reversible oligospermia. Immunosuppressive drugs such as 6-mercatopurine and methotrexate can be used to treat ulcerative colitis and Crohn disease.

Answer A is incorrect. Infliximab is a monoclonal antibody to tumor necrosis factor-α. It is used to treat patients with Crohn disease, especially when anal fistulas are present, but it is second-line therapy for ulcerative colitis, after the aminosalicylates (eg, sulfasalazine).

Answer B is incorrect. Nizatidine is a reversible histamine-2 blocker. It is used to treat patients with peptic ulcer, gastritis, and mild esophageal reflux. It has no role in the treatment of ulcerative colitis.

Answer C is incorrect. Omeprazole is a proton pump inhibitor that irreversibly inhibits sodium-potassium-ATPase in stomach parietal cells. It is used in cases of peptic ulcer, gastritis, esophageal reflux, and Zollinger-Ellison syndrome. It has no role in the treatment of ulcerative colitis.

Answer D is incorrect. Ondansetron is a 5-hydroxytryptamine-3 antagonist that serves as a powerful central-acting anti-emetic. It can be used to treat patients symptomatically for nausea and vomiting, but it has no role in the treatment of ulcerative colitis.

Answer E is incorrect. Sucralfate binds to an ulcer base to provide physical protection. It improves ulcer healing, and it also is used to treat traveler's diarrhea. It has no role in the treatment of ulcerative colitis.

13. **The correct answer is E.** The presentation and history suggest cholera. Cholera is caused by *Vibrio cholerae*, a gram-negative comma-shaped bacterium. It can cause profuse secretory diarrhea with watery vomiting in some patients. It has been a problem in many parts of the world, especially after natural disasters, as mortality in untreated patients exceeds 50%. Initial management in the setting of moderate or mild dehydration secondary to diarrhea is oral rehydration therapy (ORT). The presentation of these patients suggests moderate dehydration. ORT consists of administering glucose-containing sodium solution in a ratio not exceeding two glucose molecules per one sodium molecule. Dehydration is prevented by shifting fluid from the intestinal lumen into the circulation, secondary to glucose-coupled sodium transport in the mucosal cells.

    Answer A is incorrect. Although antibiotics might be helpful in treating a bacterial diarrhea, the first-line treatment for dehydration of any etiology is to correct the volume loss. This is achieved by ORT. Although one could make a case for using antibiotics concomitantly with ORT, almost all cases of cholera subside if the patient is well hydrated. Furthermore, antibiotics are not recommended in certain bacterial diarrheas such as with *Salmonella* infection in which antibiotics can, in fact, lengthen the course and severity of the disease.

    Answer B is incorrect. Diphenoxylate is an antidiarrheal opiate that is used in the management of diarrhea. However, it would not be the treatment of choice, as this is likely a secretory diarrhea and not due to increased peristalsis. Anti-peristaltic medications also exacerbate infections and would be undesirable in this case of possible viral/bacterial infection.

    Answer C is incorrect. A bolus of normal saline could be given immediately to a child presenting with dehydration. However, intravenous (IV) normal saline with dextrose is considered maintenance IV fluid and usually would not be given immediately. In addition, IV fluids would be less desirable than ORT because of the potential risk of developing iatrogenic electrolyte imbalances such as hypernatremia. When patients present with severe dehydration (hypotensive, anuric, sunken eyes, cool skin with acrocyanosis, mental status changes, tachypneic, >10% volume loss), then rapid IV infusion of isotonic saline is indicated.

    Answer D is incorrect. Loperamide is an antidiarrheal opiate that inhibits peristalsis by interfering with calcium channels. Although this medication is used in diarrhea management, it would not be the treatment of choice, as this is likely a secretory diarrhea and not due to increased peristalsis. Anti-peristaltic medications also exacerbate infections and would be undesirable in this case of possible viral/bacterial infection.

14. **The correct answer is B.** Patients with gastric cancer tend to present with abdominal pain, anorexia, early satiety, nausea, and/or dysphagia. Weight loss tends to be secondary to insufficient food intake, but may also be due to gastric stasis or outlet obstruction. The abdominal pain progressively worsens as the disease spreads. Lymphatic spread is common and resulting examination findings may show a periumbilical nodule (Sister Mary Joseph's node) as well as left supraclavicular adenopathy (Virchow node).

    Answer A is incorrect. Cancer of the body or tail of the pancreas typically presents with pain and weight loss, while cancer in the head of the pancreas tends to present earlier, with steatorrhea, weight loss, and jaundice. Other presenting symptoms include recent onset of atypical diabetes mellitus (DM), unexplained thrombophlebitis, and unexplained pancreatitis.

Answer C is incorrect. Nonmetastatic breast cancer does not present with abdominal pain.

Answer D is incorrect. Esophageal cancer tends to present with dysphagia associated with weight loss as well as regurgitation of food. Hoarseness may be a symptom if the tumor has invaded the recurrent laryngeal nerve.

Answer E is incorrect. Krukenberg tumor is secondary to peritoneal spread of gastric cancer and tends to present with an enlarged ovary.

15. **The correct answer is D.** Schistosomiasis is a parasitic disease with hepatic involvement. *Schistosoma mansoni* larva, which are commonly found in fresh waters of South America, penetrate the host's skin, invade the peripheral vasculature, and eventually settle in the portal or pelvic venous vasculature. Several weeks following infection, patients may develop symptoms similar to the ones described, such as fever, diarrhea, and weight loss; the "funny looking" stools likely represent *S mansoni* eggs. Chronic infection may eventually lead to portal hypertension and hepatosplenomegaly, leading in turn to ascites and eventually cirrhosis. In addition, the hepatosplenomegaly leads to esophageal varices, producing bleeding that can often be the first clinical sign.

Answer A is incorrect. Appendicitis commonly presents with right lower quadrant abdominal pain, fever, nausea, vomiting, and leukocytosis. The ascites seen in this patient is not a typical finding with appendicitis.

Answer B is incorrect. Bowel obstruction generally presents with nausea, vomiting, and decreased or absent bowel sounds. This patient has none of these signs or symptoms. The patient does not have risk factors for bowel obstructions, which include hernias, previous abdominal surgeries, or colon cancer. It should also be noted that this patient reports no changes in his normal bowel habits. If a bowel obstruction were producing his symptoms, he would not be passing gas or having bowel movements.

Answer C is incorrect. Enterocolitis would not present with signs and symptoms of ascites. It usually manifests with diarrhea; however, this patient's current symptoms do not include changes in bowel habits. It is not a chronic disease and cannot cause portal hypertension.

Answer E is incorrect. Ruptured viscera may present with signs of peritonitis such as rebound tenderness. Rupture may result from ischemic bowel disease or obstruction. This patient's history, physical examination, and imaging studies are inconsistent with this etiology. A ruptured viscus is often fatal within several days because of infection and subsequent sepsis.

16. **The correct answer is C.** Cushing ulcer is a type of acute stress ulcer that is associated with elevated intracranial pressure in trauma or severe illness. Increased intracranial pressure stimulates the vagus nucleus, causing increased acid secretion in the stomach. A Curling's ulcer tends to occur in the fundus of the stomach and results in superficial capillary bleeding, but may also involve heavier bleeding if the submucosa is eroded. In this case, the elevated intracranial pressure from the high-speed collision is markedly demonstrated as papilledema in the image.

Answer A is incorrect. This answer choice describes the mechanism behind gastroesophageal reflux disease (GERD). Esophageal irritation by acid reflux is generally associated with intestinal metaplasia of the esophagus and Barrett esophagus with predisposition to esophageal cancer. GERD is unlikely to be the cause for bleeding ulcers.

Answer B is incorrect. Esophageal varices are commonly caused by portal hypertension, which is frequently seen in chronic alcoholics or in patients with cirrhosis. Elevated hepatic portal pressure can cause the development of lower esophageal varices, which can be a source of massive bleeding. This patient does not have a history of alcohol use or cirrhosis.

Answer D is incorrect. Duodenal ulcers are a type of peptic ulcer that is highly associated with *Helicobacter pylori*. The patient such an ulcer often complains of abdominal pain that is ameliorated by eating. The peptic ulcers are characteristically more insidious and often linked to *H pylori*, not to the acute stress associated with trauma or severe illness.

Answer E is incorrect. Oral analgesics such as nonsteroidal anti-inflammatory drugs (NSAIDs), when used **long-term**, are associated with gastric ulcerations and superficial erosions. Given that the patient was just injured two days ago, not only is there insufficient exposure to oral NSAIDs, but he is likely still on IV analgesia. Also, NSAID use is not associated with the papilledema shown in the image.

17. **The correct answer is B.** Recent studies have demonstrated the benefit of infliximab (Remicade) in the treatment of Crohn disease that is refractory to steroid treatment. It also is approved for use in a variety of other autoimmune diseases such as ulcerative colitis, ankylosing spondilitis, psoriasis, and psoriatic arthritis. Infliximab is a monoclonal chimeric antibody that binds soluble tumor necrosis factor-α (TNF-α), and as a result blocks its effects. TNF-α is a pro-inflammatory cytokine secreted by macrophages that is found in high concentrations in the stool of Crohn patients. The chimeric antibody is 75% human and 25% murine. A single infusion produces a clinical response in 65% of patients. Common adverse effects are increased susceptibility to upper respiratory infections, headache, and GI distress.

Answer A is incorrect. The drug trastuzumab (Herceptin) is a monoclonal antibody specific for c-erbB2 (HER-2/neu), the epidermal growth factor receptor. Over-expression of this cell marker is a poor prognostic factor for carcinoma of the breast.

Answer C is incorrect. Infliximab remains in the serum, and binds soluble TNF-α molecules and inhibits binding to the TNF-α receptor, thereby preventing receptor activation and its subsequent effects. Infliximab does not bind to cell surface receptors.

Answer D is incorrect. Imatinib (Gleevec) is a tyrosine kinase receptor inhibitor. The tyrosine kinase receptor is mutated in the *bcr-abl* protein that results from the 9;22 translocation (Philadelphia chromosome). This mutation has been linked with chronic myelogenous leukemia and some GI stromal tumors. It results in an overly active *abl* tyrosine kinase that has oncogenic effects.

Answer E is incorrect. Infliximab binds soluble TNF-α but does not affect the total amount of TNF-α produced by macrophages.

18. **The correct answer is B.** This patient suffers from Hirschsprung disease, which manifests when neural crest cells fail to migrate to the distal colon. Consequently, enteric neurons do not form in a segment of the rectosigmoid; these neurons are normally responsible for relaxation of the rectum to allow defecation. If this condition is left untreated, these infants run the risk of developing enterocolitis or a bowel perforation. Ten percent of cases of Hirschsprung disease occur in children with Down syndrome, caused by trisomy 21. Children with Down syndrome also have an increased risk of duodenal atresia, congenital heart disease, and acute lymphoblastic leukemia.

Answer A is incorrect. Cystic fibrosis (CF) is caused by recessive mutations in the *CFTR* gene on chromosome 7. Infants with CF have an increased risk of meconium ileus, and also show a variable spectrum of pancreatic insufficiency. Later in life, patients with CF develop characteristic bronchiectasis with chronic lung infections with *Pseudomonas* species. There is, however, no association between CF and Hirschsprung disease.

Answer C is incorrect. Sickle cell disease is caused by homozygous mutations in the β-globin gene. Neonates with sickle cell disease are often asymptomatic as long as fetal hemoglobin persists. There is no known association between sickle cell disease and Hirschsprung disease.

Answer D is incorrect. Tay-Sachs disease is caused by a deficiency in the hexosaminidase A enzyme, leading to accumulation of GM2 ganglioside. Infants with Tay-Sachs disease show progressive neurodegeneration, cherry red spots on the retina, and developmental delay. There is, however, no known association between Tay-Sachs disease and Hirschsprung disease.

Answer E is incorrect. Infants with Turner syndrome (XO) commonly show coarctation of the aorta, but there is no association between Turner syndrome and Hirschsprung disease.

19. **The correct answer is F.** This patient is presenting with only slight alkalemia (normal arterial pH is 7.35-7.45). However, the bicarbonate level is substantially elevated, about 11 mEq/L above normal. This implies that a metabolic alkalosis is occurring, which can be explained by the patient's recent history of severe protracted vomiting. Vomiting causes a loss of hydrochloric acid from the GI tract; this acid must be replaced, which is done by drawing hydrogen from body stores and leaving bicarbonate behind. Normally with this level of bicarbonate elevation alone, a higher pH would be expected. However, this patient's partial carbon dioxide pressure (PCO_2) is elevated to 48 mm Hg. This implies that a normal respiratory compensation has occurred in order to normalize the pH by retaining acid by the formation of carbonic acid from carbon dioxide. The expected compensation is an increase of 0.7 mm Hg of carbon dioxide for every 1-mEq/L increase in bicarbonate. This patient's bicarbonate level has increased by about 11 mEq/L, and the PCO_2 has increased by about 8 mm Hg, an appropriate compensation.

Answer A is incorrect. Because this patient's pH is greater than normal, an alkalosis must be present.

Answer B is incorrect. Metabolic acidosis with respiratory compensation would result in a low pH, a low bicarbonate level, and a decreased PCO_2.

Answer C is incorrect. Vomiting typically induces a metabolic alkalosis due to a loss of hydrogen ions from the stomach, leading to an increase in pH. This leaves an increased bicarbonate concentration (generally >24 mEq/L) in the bloodstream; therefore this patient does indeed have a metabolic alkalosis. However, some patients present with more than one condition causing an acid-base imbalance, which is known as a complicated or mixed condition. If a metabolic acidosis were occurring simultaneously (such as in ketoacidosis or diarrhea), the bicarbonate level would be closer to normal because the two processes would have opposing effects on bicarbonate levels and effectively cancel each other out.

Answer D is incorrect. This patient has a metabolic alkalosis, as evidenced by the increased pH with increased bicarbonate level. PCO_2 is elevated as well, indicating that appropriate respiratory compensation is occurring. If a simultaneous respiratory acidosis were occurring, the PCO_2 would be even higher than anticipated based on normal compensatory mechanisms. Generally, PCO_2 should rise by 0.7 mm Hg for every 1-mEq/L increase in bicarbonate level. So if carbon dioxide levels increase by more than that, a coexistent respiratory acidosis should be suspected.

Answer E is incorrect. This patient has an alkalosis, as evidenced by the elevated pH with increased bicarbonate. PCO_2 is elevated as well, indicating that there is appropriate respiratory compensation occurring. If a simultaneous respiratory alkalosis were occurring, the PCO_2 would be normal (meaning there is a failure of respiratory compensatory mechanisms) or it would be decreased. In an isolated metabolic alkalosis, respiratory compensation should occur. If it does not or if PCO_2 is low, a concurrent respiratory alkalosis should be suspected.

20. **The correct answer is A.** The elevated direct bilirubin level and the imaging findings are consistent with a common duct obstruction, most likely secondary to a gallstone (consider this woman's risk factors: female, fertile, and >40 years). An obstruction in the common

duct (choledocholithiasis) does not allow drainage of bile from the liver or gallbladder, and can lead to cholangitis, which is characterized by Charcot's triad of jaundice, fever, and right upper quadrant pain. About 80% of gallstones are made of cholesterol; these occur when solubilizing bile acids and lecithin are overwhelmed by excess cholesterol. The remaining 20% are pigment stones containing mainly calcium bilirubinate; these can occur during periods of increased hemolysis.

Answer B is incorrect. No clear relationship has been established between gallstone formation and diet, but it has been suggested that low-fiber and high-cholesterol diets are contributing factors.

Answer C is incorrect. A tumor at the head of the pancreas could cause this patient's signs and symptoms, but the patient would likely be older and present with other associated symptoms such as weight loss and back pain.

Answer D is incorrect. Although the patient's age and sex are consistent with a diagnosis of primary biliary cirrhosis, endoscopic retrograde cholangiopancreatography would demonstrate the small intrahepatic bile duct destruction associated with this autoimmune disease. Additionally, the patient's lab work-up would reveal increased serum mitochondrial antibodies.

Answer E is incorrect. Primary sclerosing cholangitis also may cause Charcot's triad. However, endoscopic retrograde cholangiopancreatography would reveal "beading," or alternating strictures and dilation of the biliary tree due to intra- and extrahepatic inflammation and fibrosis of the bile ducts. This disease frequently is associated with ulcerative colitis.

21. **The correct answer is C.** This patient has a small bowel obstruction. Dilated loops of small intestines on x-ray of the abdomen and a clinical history of anorexia, vomiting, and abdominal pain are usually sufficient to make the diagnosis. In the United States, the leading cause of small bowel obstructions is adhesion formation, which obstructs the lumen of the small bowel. These adhesions are formed during the healing process secondary to abdominal surgery. Other conditions that predispose patients to small bowel obstructions are hernias and intraluminal cancers of the small intestine.

Answer A is incorrect. Celiac sprue can present with GI upset, diarrhea, and flatulence, but does not have a correlation with small bowel obstruction. Dermatitis herpetiformis is a dermatologic manifestation of gluten insensitivity that presents with erythematous, grouped, pruritic papules.

Answer B is incorrect. Infection with *Helicobacter pylori* is limited to gastric and duodenal mucosa and is not known to cause strictures or adhesions. Therefore even chronic infections have no potential to cause small bowel obstructions. Long-standing *H pylori* infection can cause MALT lymphoma and peptic ulcers.

Answer D is incorrect. Although smoking has multiple detrimental effects on health, it has no correlation to the progression of small bowel obstructions.

Answer E is incorrect. Ulcerative colitis does not predispose patients to small bowel obstruction because this inflammatory disease process is limited to mucosa and submucosa. Crohn disease, on the other hand, can lead to small bowel obstruction, as it can cause transmural inflammatory and bowel strictures.

22. **The correct answer is A.** Familial adenomatous polyposis (FAP) is an autosomal dominant condition characterized by a germline mutation on chromosome 5, specifically at the adenomatous polyposis coli (APC) locus. The *APC* gene is thought to have tumor-suppressive effects, and its loss is associated with more than colonic cancers. In addition to duodenal neoplasms for which these patients with FAP must undergo lifelong upper endoscopic surveillance, increased risk exists in these patients for developing gastric, liver, thyroid, and central nervous system neoplasms.

Answer B is incorrect. Examples of autosomal recessive conditions include cystic fibrosis, sickle cell anemia, and hemochromatosis.

Answer C is incorrect. Examples of autosomal trisomy conditions include Down syndrome (trisomy 21), Edwards syndrome (trisomy 18), and Patau syndrome (trisomy 13).

Answer D is incorrect. Examples of conditions related to sex chromosome abnormalities include Klinefelter syndrome (XXY), Turner syndrome (XO), and double-Y males (XYY).

Answer E is incorrect. Examples of X-linked recessive conditions include hemophilia A and B, glucose-6-phosphate dehydrogenase deficiency, and Lesch-Nyhan syndrome.

23. **The correct answer is E.** Guillain-Barré syndrome is characterized by rapidly progressing ascending paralysis. It is an autoimmune-mediated illness that can occur following a variety of infectious diseases, but is particularly associated with prior infection by *Campylobacter jejuni*. *C jejuni* gastroenteritis is characterized in this patient by her vomiting and bloody diarrhea together with the finding of comma-shaped organisms with a single polar flagellum when cultured at 42°C in a microaerophilic environment. Other enteric pathogens with this morphology include bacteria of the *Vibrio* genus (*V cholera* and *V parahaemolyticus*). These species, however, are not endemic to the United States and would not be expected in a patient without a recent travel history, nor do the symptoms match. *C jejuni* is transmitted to humans via the fecal-oral route from either domestic animals or eating undercooked poultry.

Answer A is incorrect. Hemolytic-uremic syndrome (HUS) is characterized by acute renal failure and thrombocytopenia with hemolytic anemia. HUS can be a complication of infection caused by *Escherichia coli* O157:H7, not *Campylobacter jejuni*. Like *C jejuni*, *E coli* O157:H7 is a gram-negative rod that can cause enteritis. *E coli*, however, is characterized by numerous flagella and aerobic metabolism.

Answer B is incorrect. Rheumatic fever is characterized by fever, migratory polyarthritis, and carditis. It is known to occur after Group A streptococcal pharyngitis. There is no evidence of *Streptococcus pyogenes* infection in this patient, as she does not have symptoms of pharyngitis or culture findings of gram-positive cocci in chains.

Answer C is incorrect. Fever, a new murmur, Janeway lesions, and nail bed hemorrhages are signs of bacterial endocarditis. Acute endocarditis is most often caused by *Staphylococcus aureus*, and subacute infection are often caused by viridans group streptococci. Endocarditis is not a known sequelae of *C jejuni* infection.

Answer D is incorrect. Waterhouse-Friderichsen syndrome is characterized by high fever, shock, purpura, and adrenal insufficiency. It is classically associated with *Neisseria meningitides* septicemia. This patient's symptoms do not resemble meningitis nor does the culture match the gram-negative diplococci of *Neisseria*.

24. **The correct answer is C.** This patient most likely has vitamin A deficiency, which is characterized by early symptoms of night blindness, dry conjunctivae, and gray plaques, or late symptoms of corneal ulceration and necrosis leading to perforation and blindness. This deficiency is typically seen in children and pregnant women whose diets are deficient in vitamin A. It can also be seen in alcoholics, after intestinal surgery (especially when the ileum is involved), and in patients with fat malabsorption, cholestasis, or inflammatory bowel disease. Vitamins A, D, E, and K (fat-soluble vitamins) are absorbed in the small intestine and absorption requires micelles formed with bile salts.

Answer A is incorrect. Ferrous iron is absorbed in the small intestine and absorption requires apoferritin binding. Iron deficiency may be caused by chronic bleeding, inadequate intake of iron, or malabsorption syndromes. Symptoms include fatigue, pallor, or weakness. Iron deficiency may affect many other processes because iron is needed for the normal functioning of many enzymes.

Answer B is incorrect. Vitamin B_{12} is a water-soluble vitamin that is absorbed in the terminal ileum. Its absorption requires binding to intrinsic factor, which is secreted by gastric parietal cells. Thus, in pernicious anemia, where there is damage to gastric parietal cells, vitamin B_{12} deficiency may develop and may lead to megaloblastic anemia.

Answer D is incorrect. Water-soluble vitamins are absorbed in the small intestine and absorption requires sodium cotransport. Vitamin A is a fat-soluble vitamin.

Answer E is incorrect. Calcium is absorbed in the small intestine and absorption is facilitated by a vitamin D-dependent calcium binding protein. Hypocalcemia may result in numerous situations, including parathyroid hormone deficiency, eating disorders, and following parathyroidectomy. Symptoms include perioral tingling, ECG changes, tetany, and Chvostek sign (tapping the facial nerve will produce facial spasms on the same side).

25. **The correct answer is D.** The image shows inflammatory pseudopolyps in a patient with ulcerative colitis. Primary sclerosing cholangitis (PSC) is an extraintestinal complication of ulcerative colitis. About 70% of patients with PSC also have ulcerative colitis; however, only about 4% of patients with ulcerative colitis will develop PSC. PSC leads to obliterative fibrosis of intrahepatic and extrahepatic bile ducts, and can over time lead to cirrhosis. Patients with PSC also have an increased risk of developing cholangiocarcinoma.

Answer A is incorrect. HCV infection can cause cirrhosis, and subsequent hepatic adenocarcinoma, but it is not associated with PSC.

Answer B is incorrect. Primary biliary cirrhosis is a disease commonly found in middle-aged women that affects smaller bile ducts and, as the name suggests, can lead to cirrhosis over time. The etiology is likely autoimmune, and 90% of patients have antimitochondrial antibodies. This disease can manifest with destruction of intrahepatic ducts. However, this would not explain this patient's prior colon resection nor his colon pathology.

Answer C is incorrect. While systemic lupus erythematosus (SLE) is associated with a constellation of immunologically related conditions, PSC is not one of them.

Answer E is incorrect. Wilson disease does cause hepatic manifestations such as chronic hepatitis, which may lead to jaundice and cirrhosis. However, the obliteration of intrahepatic ducts seen on imaging studies is consistent with PSC, rather than hepatitis. Furthermore, hepatitis would not explain the purpose of his total colectomy nor his colon pathology shown in image.

26. **The correct answer is A.** The patient's clinical, laboratory, and histologic features are indicative of celiac sprue. The classical presentation of this disease is during infancy, but it may also present any time between the ages of 10 and 40. Classic signs include diarrhea, foul-smelling, bulky, floating stools, weight loss, growth failure, and vitamin deficiencies. These symptoms follow exposure to the protein gliadin, which results in intestinal inflammation. A gluten-free diet usually relieves symptoms and restores mucosal histology, and therefore it is the most appropriate therapeutic measure.

Answer B is incorrect. Corticosteroids may be employed in the treatment of refractory sprue, but a gluten-free diet is the most appropriate step at this time.

Answer C is incorrect. Antibiotic therapy does not have a place in the treatment of celiac sprue.

Answer D is incorrect. While patients with celiac sprue are often deficient in B vitamins, treating the underlying pathology is the best course.

Answer E is incorrect. While patients with celiac sprue are often deficient in fat-soluble vitamins, treating the underlying pathology is the best course.

27. **The correct answer is C.** Pegylated interferon is a cytokine derivative that improves the body's antiviral response. It is used in the treatment of HBV and HCV. Adverse effects of interferon therapy include a flu-like reaction that manifests as episodic fevers and chills,

as well as occasional profound depression. As a result, interferon is contraindicated in severely depressed or suicidal patients. Although interferon is not a cure for hepatitis, it is recommended to slow the progression of cirrhotic liver disease in some patients. Pegylated interferon is a longer-acting form of interferon.

Answer A is incorrect. IV immunoglobulin is an engineered antibody that is used to clear the serum of protein products. It often is used in treatment of autoimmune diseases such as Guillain-Barré syndrome. Adverse effects include flu-like reaction and anaphylactic reaction.

Answer B is incorrect. Lamivudine is a nucleotide reverse transcriptase inhibitor used in the treatment of HIV and HBV. Its principal adverse effect is hepatotoxicity.

Answer D is incorrect. Ribavirin is an antiviral drug used in the treatment of HCV, respiratory syncytial virus, and, occasionally, other viral illnesses. It is not associated with depression or a flu-like reaction.

Answer E is incorrect. Tumor necrosis factor-α is a cytokine involved in the antiviral and antitumor response. It is not used currently as a treatment for HCV.

28. **The correct answer is B.** This patient presents with the classic signs and symptoms of appendicitis. When the right leg is hyperextended, the iliopsoas muscle group pushes against the appendix and causes significant pain and irritation. Pain with hyperextension will also be present in pancreatic cancers and inflammation of the cecum and the sigmoid colon. The psoas muscle is innervated by the lumbar plexus, and the iliacus muscle is innervated by the femoral nerve.

    Answer A is incorrect. The inferior gluteal nerve innervates the gluteus maximus. This muscle is not utilized in the psoas sign maneuver.

    Answer C is incorrect. The obturator nerve originates from the lumbar plexus and innervates the medial thigh muscles. These muscles are not utilized in the psoas sign maneuver.

    Answer D is incorrect. The sciatic nerve innervates the hip joint, the muscular knee flexors in the thigh, and all the leg and foot muscles. These muscles are not utilized in the psoas sign maneuver.

    Answer E is incorrect. The superior gluteal nerve innervates the gluteus medius and gluteus minimus muscles. These muscles are not utilized in the psoas sign maneuver.

29. **The correct answer is D.** *Shigella* species produce gastroenteritis characterized by abdominal pain, bloody diarrhea, and nausea and/or vomiting. Additionally, because *Shigella* species invade intestinal epithelial cells, the illness is accompanied by fever. *Shigella* is a nonlactose fermenter, and it does not produce gas or hydrogen sulfide. Infection usually affects preschool-age children and populations in nursing homes. Transmission occurs by the fecal-to-oral route via fecally contaminated water and hand-to-hand contact. It's an extremely virulent organism requiring only 10 organisms for infection. *Shigella* also produces Shiga toxin, which can cleave host rRNA and enhance cytokine release, resulting in hemolytic uremic syndrome. This syndrome develops after the endothelium is damaged in the kidney and results in renal failure, thrombocytopenia, and microangiopathic hemolytic anemia.

    Answer A is incorrect. This describes Guillain-Barré syndrome, which is often associated with *Campylobacter jejuni* infection. While *C jejuni* is a common cause of dysentery, it does not fit this lab description (it's a gram-negative, curved rod).

    Answer B is incorrect. These two symptoms, along with diarrhea and fever, are characteristic of typhoid fever caused by *Salmonella typhi*. However, unlike *S enteritidis*, *S typhi* does not cause dysentery. Furthermore, *Salmonella* produce hydrogen sulfide, which *Shigella* does not. *Salmonella* infection results from fecal-oral transmission and the pathogen lives in the GI tract of animals. It infects humans when there is contamination of food or water by animal feces.

Answer C is incorrect. This describes an inhaled infection by *Bacillus anthracis*, which is not connected to any of the other symptoms this child has.

Answer E is incorrect. These symptoms describe rheumatic fever, which is caused by an infection by *Streptococcus pyogenes*. *S pyogenes* does not cause dysentery, nor does it fit the laboratory description of the causative organism in this case.

30. **The correct answer is D.** This patient's symptoms and pancreatic calcifications on the CT scan are consistent with chronic pancreatitis. The intern is thinking about octreotide, a somatostatin analog used to treat acromegaly. Among its various actions, somatostatin is a potent inhibitor of growth hormone secretion; it also suppresses the release of a number of digestive hormones, such as gastrin, cholecystokinin, secretin, and vasoactive intestinal peptide (VIP). It also decreases the secretion of pancreatic fluids. By inhibiting the secretion of pancreatic fluids, octreotide may be able to alleviate this patient's chronic abdominal pain.

    Answer A is incorrect. Cholecystokinin (CCK) is a hormone synthesized by duodenal I cells. Once chyme enters the duodenum, CCK is secreted to decrease gastric acid secretion and to slow the release of chyme into the duodenum. CCK stimulates the release of pancreatic digestive enzymes and induces gallbladder contraction. CCK is not indicated for the treatment of acromegaly, and no analogs have been created.

    Answer B is incorrect. Gastrin is a hormone released by stomach G cells in response to stomach distention, vagal stimulation, and proteins. Through the actions of gastrin on parietal cells, the end result of gastrin release is increased acid secretion. Gastrin also causes chief cells to release pepsinogen for breakdown of proteins. Gastrin is not indicated for the treatment of acromegaly and does not have a role in exocrine pancreas function.

    Answer C is incorrect. Secretin is a hormone produced by duodenal S cells and secreted in response to increased duodenal fatty acids and acidity. It maintains duodenal pH by stimulating bicarbonate secretion by the pancreas, thus neutralizing gastric acid. It is not indicated for the treatment of acromegaly and does not control pancreatic enzyme secretion.

    Answer E is incorrect. VIP is a hormone produced in the intestines and pancreas. In the intestines VIP induces smooth muscle relaxation, whereas in the pancreas it stimulates pancreatic bicarbonate secretion. VIP is not indicated for the treatment of acromegaly.

31. **The correct answer is A.** This patient is likely suffering from a duodenal ulcer. *Helicobacter pylori* is the most common cause of duodenal and gastric ulcers (involved in 100% and 70% of lesions, respectively). It can be diagnosed with esophagogastroduodenoscopy or a urease breath test. A key distinction between these two ulcers is that eating food often relieves duodenal ulcer pain and patients tend to report resulting weight gain. Duodenal ulcer symptoms are exacerbated when acid is secreted without any food to act as a buffer, causing pain on an empty stomach. The standard first-line therapy is one-week triple therapy consisting of the antibiotics amoxicillin and clarithromycin, and a proton pump inhibitor such as omeprazole.

    Answer B is incorrect. NSAIDs are the second leading cause of both gastric and duodenal ulcers, but are more commonly associated with gastric ulcers. Unlike duodenal ulcers, gastric ulcers are worsened by food; patients usually complain of resulting early satiety and weight loss. Although NSAIDs should be avoided, this would not be a primary part of the treatment plan for this patient with confirmed *Helicobacter pylori* infection.

    Answer C is incorrect. Patients with Zollinger-Ellison syndrome have gastrin-secreting tumors of the pancreas and duodenum. They will have findings indicative of acid hypersecretion, such as several refractory ulcers. It is associated with multiple endocrine neoplasia type 1 (MEN-1). Although this syndrome can result in a duodenal ulcer, the question stem makes no mention of other tumors associated with MEN-1 (pituitary adenoma, parathyroid adenoma), and does not indicate that the patient has an elevated serum gastrin. Thus, the patient's pathology is more likely due to *Helicobacter pylori* infection.

Answer D is incorrect. Metoclopramide is used primarily as an anti-emetic and a prokinetic agent. It would not be first-line therapy for a patient with a duodenal ulcer.

Answer E is incorrect. Ranitidine is a histamine$_2$-receptor antagonist. It is frequently used as a treatment for gastroesophageal reflux disease to reduce the amount of acid in the stomach. It would not target *Helicobacter pylori*.

32. **The correct answer is D.** The organism causing the patient's symptoms is the protozoan *Giardia lamblia*. *G lamblia* trophozoites commonly cause chronic diarrhea. This parasite is treated with metronidazole. It spreads via oral-fecal transmission in its cyst form and then colonizes the GI tract in its trophozoite form. *G lamblia* is found primarily in the duodenum and jejunum, and causes a combination of malabsorption with diarrhea through a still incompletely understood mechanism. The patient's complaints of greasy stool and flatulence are classic signs of this type of infection. Diagnosis is made via direct examination of stool for cysts as well as duodenal fluid sampling and small-bowel biopsy.

Answer A is incorrect. Chloroquine is used to treat *Plasmodium*, the organism that causes malaria.

Answer B is incorrect. Dapsone is used to treat *Pneumocystis jiroveci*, a common cause of pneumonia in HIV.

Answer C is incorrect. Melarsoprol is used to treat *Trypanosoma brucei gambiense* and *Trypanosoma brucei rhodesiense*, the causes of African sleeping sickness. Specifically, it is used in cases of central nervous system penetration.

Answer E is incorrect. Nifurtimox is the primary treatment for *Trypanosoma cruzi*, the cause of Chagas disease.

Answer F is incorrect. Sulfadiazine plus pyrimethamine is the primary treatment for *Toxoplasma*, which causes brain abscesses in HIV and birth defects.

33. **The correct answer is A.** This patient is most likely suffering from acute gastroenteritis, probably of viral origin. While there are several causes of hypoalbuminemia, the most likely cause in this otherwise healthy man is simply a dilutional effect due to the large amounts of fluid he was given. This type of hypoalbuminemia is also seen in congestive heart failure.

Answer B is incorrect. Chronic liver disease causes hypoalbuminemia as albumin is produced in the liver. However, this loss of synthetic liver function typically does not occur until the final stage of liver disease, cirrhosis. It is unlikely that this young and healthy individual has severe enough liver disease to cause a dysfunction in albumin synthesis.

Answer C is incorrect. Malabsorptive states, such as short bowel syndrome and celiac sprue, can lead to decreased ability to absorb protein. Over time this leads to hypoalbuminemia. This patient's two day illness would not cause a protein deficiency severe enough to cause hypoalbuminemia.

Answer D is incorrect. Nephrotic syndrome causes hypoalbuminemia due to excessive protein loss. This syndrome would also be classically accompanied by massive proteinuria, peripheral and periorbital edema, and hyperlipidemia. However, the vignette does not describe any of these findings, and the recent large fluid load is the most likely culprit for the hypoalbuminemia.

Answer E is incorrect. Poor nutritional status causes hypoalbuminemia due to insufficient protein intake. However, this patient's two-day history of vomiting would not cause a severe enough nutritional deficit to induce hypoalbuminemia, which is generally seen only after long-term protein deficiency.

34. **The correct answer is B.** The oral absorption of ciprofloxacin is impaired by divalent cations,

including those in common antacids such as calcium carbonate, which this patient is likely taking to treat GERD. Ciprofloxacin belongs to the family of fluroquinolones, which block bacterial DNA synthesis by inhibiting bacterial DNA gyrase. Inhibition of DNA gyrase prevents the relaxation of positively supercoiled DNA that is required for normal transcription and replication.

Answer A is incorrect. Unlike the other drugs listed, aspirin is not used as a pharmacotherapeutic agent for treating GERD. In fact, it is known to cause gastric ulcers. Although many patients take aspirin for its antiplatelet effect, this patient has no reason to be using aspirin. Furthermore, no drug interactions would be expected between aspirin and ciprofloxacin.

Answer C is incorrect. Cimetidine, an H_2-receptor antagonist, is associated with gynecomastia, thrombocytopenia, and inhibition of the cytochrome P450 (CYP450) system. However, it does not significantly affect the metabolism or pharmacokinetics of ciprofloxacin.

Answer D is incorrect. Misoprostol is a prostaglandin E_1 analog that can be used to prevent NSAID-induced peptic ulcers. It is also used as a medical abortifacient in many countries and is therefore strictly contraindicated in pregnant women. Misoprostol would not decrease the absorption nor increase the metabolism of ciprofloxacin.

Answer E is incorrect. Omeprazole is a proton pump inhibitor considered first-line therapy for GERD. Omeprazole decreases intragastric acidity, but does not affect the intestinal absorption, metabolism, or excretion of ciprofloxacin.

35. **The correct answer is D.** This patient's presentation is classic for acute pancreatitis. This process often occurs in young patients after consuming large amounts of alcohol. Other causes include gallstone obstruction, medications, infection, hypertriglyceridemia, and trauma. Pseudocysts often arise after a bout of acute pancreatitis and consist of necrotic, hemorrhagic debris with pancreatic enzymes. These cysts lack a true epithelial lining.

Answer A is incorrect. Cholecystitis is not a common complication of acute pancreatitis.

Answer B is incorrect. Chronic gastritis is not a common complication of acute pancreatitis.

Answer C is incorrect. Pancreatic carcinoma does not arise from a bout of acute pancreatitis, although evidence exists to suggest that chronic pancreatitis may be a risk factor for pancreatic carcinoma.

Answer E is incorrect. Small bowel obstruction is not a common complication of acute pancreatitis.

36. **The correct answer is E.** Omeprazole is a proton pump inhibitor (PPI) that works by covalently binding, and irreversibly inactivating the H^+/K^+/ATPase on the luminal surface of the gastric parietal cell. Gastrin levels are regulated by a feedback loop. Intragastric acidity stimulates D-cells in the gastric antrum to release somatostatin, which works in a paracrine fashion, binding to G-cells in the gastric antrum and inhibiting gastrin release. PPIs will effectively raise the intragastric pH so that gastrin levels rise two- to four-fold. Omeprazole is associated with atrophic gastritis due to hypergastrinemia. It may also be associated with carcinoid tumors, headaches, and GI disturbances.

Answer A is incorrect. Aluminum hydroxide is an antacid that is not absorbed and thus does not cause systemic adverse effects. It is associated with constipation and hypophosphatemia.

Answer B is incorrect. Bismuth binds to ulcers, providing a physical protective barrier. It has no known adverse effects.

Answer C is incorrect. Cimetidine is an H_2-antagonist and is associated with headache, confusion, thrombocytopenia, and inhibition of the CYP450 system. Inhibition of the proton pumps by PPIs such as omeprazole has a greater effect on the intragastric acidity that regulates the gastrin feedback loop than antagonizing the H_2-receptors by drugs such as cimetidine.

Answer D is incorrect. Misoprostol is a prostaglandin E_1 analog that can be used to prevent NSAID-induced peptic ulcers. It is also used as a medical abortifacient in many countries and is therefore strictly contraindicated in pregnant women.

37. **The correct answer is A.** This patient suffers from ulcerative colitis (UC), an inflammatory bowel disease of unknown etiology that affects rectum and may extend proximally to the colon; disease is rarely found in the small intestine. UC is characterized by mucosal and submucosal inflammation. Friable mucosal pseudopolyps may be evident on colonoscopy. Patients typically present with crampy abdominal pain and bloody diarrhea. UC is associated with the HLA B27 subtype. Diseases associated with the HLA B27 subtype can be remembered with the mnemonic **PAIR**, and include **P**soriasis, **A**nkylosing spondylitis, **I**nflammatory bowel disease, and **R**eiter syndrome.

Answer B is incorrect. DM is associated with the HLA-DR3 and -DR4 subtypes.

Answer C is incorrect. Graves disease and celiac sprue are associated with the HLA-B8 subtype.

Answer D is incorrect. Multiple sclerosis, hay fever, SLE, and Goodpasture syndrome are associated with the HLA-DR2 subtype.

Answer E is incorrect. Rheumatoid arthritis is associated with the HLA-DR4 subtype.

38. **The correct answer is C.** This is a case of hepatocellular carcinoma (HCC). As are renal cell carcinoma and follicular thyroid carcinoma, HCC is spread commonly via hematogenous dissemination. Accordingly, metastases often develop in the lung, portal vein, periportal nodes, brain, or bones. The patient's chronic HBV infection and alcohol abuse likely led to the development of cirrhosis and then HCC.

Answer A is incorrect. Hodgkin lymphoma, many benign neoplasms, and some sarcomas spread in a contiguous manner without metastasizing to distant sites.

Answer B is incorrect. Ovarian cancer and appendiceal cancers can disseminate directly throughout the peritoneal cavity. This often happens well before the diagnosis of ovarian cancer is made. This process is known as pseudomyxoma peritonei, and is characterized by a diffuse collection of gelatinous materials in the abdomen, peritoneal surfaces, and pelvis. HCC does not spread in this manner.

Answer D is incorrect. Many cancers, including breast cancer, colon cancer, papillary thyroid carcinoma, and melanoma, metastasize via lymphatic drainage. HCC, however, is notable for hematogenous dissemination.

Answer E is incorrect. There is no evidence that HCC or any other cancer metastasizes in this manner.

39. **The correct answer is A.** This patient has Mallory-Weiss syndrome. Repeated bouts of prolonged vomiting (such as after an alcohol binge or in eating disorders) can cause longitudinal lacerations in the distal esophagus, normally at the gastroesophageal junction or in the proximal gastric mucosa, with extension to submucosal arteries that can bleed massively. Left untreated, this bleeding can be fatal. Mallory-Weiss syndrome generally presents with hematemesis after a bout of retching or vomiting; however, new research suggests that this classic history may be obtained in only about 50% of patients. Bleeding from esophageal varices might also be expected if the patient has chronic liver disease. However, this patient is relatively young and shows no other signs of liver disease. Furthermore, variceal bleeding is usually painless, while Mallory-Weiss tears are more commonly associated with pain. Thus of the two choices, Mallory-Weiss syndrome is the better answer.

Answer B is incorrect. Metaplasia of esophageal mucosa, called Barrett esophagus, is associated with chronic reflux causing inflammation and possibly ulceration. This can lead to bleeding, but it is usually not massive as in this patient. Barrett esophagus is of concern primarily because of its strong association with adenocarcinoma.

Answer C is incorrect. Esophageal squamous cell carcinoma might cause ulceration of the esophageal mucosa, but massive bleeding is uncommon.

Answer D is incorrect. Esophageal stricture is typically caused by scarring from reflux, ingestion of toxic or caustic substances, or scleroderma. It most commonly manifests as chronic dysphagia, not hematemesis.

Answer E is incorrect. Esophageal varices are seen in chronic liver disease that has resulted in portal hypertension. The increased pressure in the portal circulation causes dilation of submucosal veins in the lower esophagus. Bleeding from varices can be massive and even fatal, but it is generally not painful. Furthermore, this patient is rather young and shows no symptoms of liver disease.

40. **The correct answer is B.** Any biopsy would likely show normal structures. Irritable bowel syndrome is a functional GI disorder characterized by abdominal pain and altered bowel habits in the absence of demonstrable organic pathology. It is a diagnosis of exclusion based on clinical features such as the ones presented. Most commonly, patients have alternating diarrhea and constipation, chronic abdominal pain that improves with stools, a change in stool frequency and consistency, and onset after emotional and/or stressful life events. These symptoms occur in the absence of fevers, lower GI bleeding, leukocytosis, and weight loss.

Answer A is incorrect. Pseudomembranous colitis usually follows antibiotic therapy and is characterized by bloody diarrhea, fever, and leukocytosis. Absence of these manifestations in this patient argues against this diagnosis.

Answer C is incorrect. Primary sclerosing cholangitis is an extra-intestinal manifestation of ulcerative colitis. On colonoscopy, the mucosa demonstrates continuous superficial ulcerations with resultant inflammatory pseudopolyps.

Answer D is incorrect. Crohn disease has a highly variable presentation; however, skip lesions, fissures, and strictures are generally evident on colonoscopy, endoscopy, and radiography.

Answer E is incorrect. Celiac sprue is a disease of malabsorption characterized by bulky, fatty stools following meals. Endoscopy reveals villous flattening in the small intestine.

41. **The correct answer is B.** The patient has gallstones, as evidenced by her symptoms and ultrasound findings of multiple gallstones. She fits the demographics of the classic patient with cholesterol gallstones: **F**at, **F**emale, **F**ertile, and **F**orty (the "4 F's"). Gemfibrozil, a fibrate, is contraindicated in the treatment of hypertriglyceridemia in the presence of gallstones. Fibrates can increase the development of gallstones, thus increasing the risk of cholecystitis.

Answer A is incorrect. Ezetimibe, in combination with a statin, is an appropriate choice for treatment of this patient.

Answer C is incorrect. Niacin would not be the first line of treatment for this patient, but it is not contraindicated.

Answer D is incorrect. Pravastatin is an appropriate choice for treatment of her metabolic profile.

Answer E is incorrect. Simvastatin is an appropriate choice for treatment of this patient.

42. **The correct answer is C.** The most common tumor of the parotid gland is the pleomorphic adenoma or the mixed tumor, accounting for 50% of salivary tumors. The pleomorphic adenoma is a benign, well-differentiated, well-circumscribed mass that grows slowly over the course of months to years. On histopathology, it is characterized by the presence of multiple cell types, classically epithelial cells in a chondromyxoid stroma.

Answer A is incorrect. Adenoid cystic carcinoma (ACC) is an invasive, poorly differentiated cancer characterized by gland-forming tissue and a cystic, fluid-filled cavity. It tends to infiltrate perineurial spaces and cause pain. ACC constitutes 5% of salivary tumors and is malignant.

Answer B is incorrect. Mucoepidermoid carcinoma is an invasive, poorly differentiated cancer composed of mucosal and epidermal cell types. This type constitutes 15% of salivary gland tumors and is malignant. The fact that this patient's tumor has not changed over the course of one year suggests that the mass is not an invasive, malignant carcinoma.

Answer D is incorrect. A sialic duct stone is an inorganic precipitate mechanically obstructing the opening of the sialic duct, resulting in an erythematous and inflamed oral mass. Sialic duct stones typically present with pain while eating due to the stone obstructing saliva from exiting the gland through the salivary duct.

Answer E is incorrect. Warthin tumor is a benign mass of lymphoid cells. A well-circumscribed mass of lymphoid cells in a salivary gland is virtually pathognomonic for a Warthin tumor, which make up 5-10% of salivary tumors. Although this patient's tumor is well-circumscribed (surrounded by a fibrous capsule), it is composed of tissues of mixed origin—not lymphocytes.

43. **The correct answer is B.** The upper third of the esophagus is made up of striated muscle (allows some voluntary control). The middle third of the esophagus is made up of both striated and smooth muscle. The lower third of the esophagus is made up of smooth muscle (entirely involuntary). Patients with scleroderma develop dysphagia (usually to solids) secondary to atrophy of smooth muscle of the lower two-thirds of the esophagus and incompetence of the lower esophageal sphincter (LES). The wall of the esophagus becomes thin and atrophic and can have regions of fibrosis.

    Answer A is incorrect. Patients with scleroderma develop dysphagia secondary to atrophy of smooth muscle in the lower two-thirds (not the lower half) of the esophagus and incompetence of the LES.

    Answer C is incorrect. Patients with scleroderma develop dysphagia secondary to atrophy of smooth muscle in the lower (not upper) two-thirds of the esophagus and incompetence of the LES.

    Answer D is incorrect. Patients with scleroderma develop dysphagia secondary to atrophy of smooth (not striated) muscle in the lower two-thirds (not the lower half) of the esophagus and incompetence of the LES.

    Answer E is incorrect. Patients with scleroderma develop dysphagia secondary to atrophy of smooth (not striated) muscle in the lower two-thirds of the esophagus and incompetence of the LES.

    Answer F is incorrect. Patients with scleroderma develop dysphagia secondary to atrophy of smooth (not striated) muscle in the lower (not upper) two-thirds of the esophagus and incompetence of the LES.

44. **The correct answer is B.** Painless rectal bleeding in an elderly individual (especially with a history of constipation or poor fiber intake) suggests diverticulosis, a condition in which the mucosa and submucosa herniate through the muscular layer of the GI tract (frequently along the sigmoid colon), forming pockets called diverticula. This patient's lower left quadrant abdominal pain indicates that he is now suffering from acute diverticulitis, which is inflammation of one or more diverticula. The laboratory values show marked leukocytosis, which is actually a common finding in acute diverticulitis. More notably, the patient appears to have iron-deficient, microcytic anemia (low hemoglobin and low MCV) This could result from his past bleeding episodes; however, it could also be a sign of chronic occult bleeding from an undiagnosed carcinoma. After the patient is stabilized and the acute diverticulitis has resolved, the patient should undergo colonoscopy to rule out malignancy. Colonoscopy is contraindicated during an acute episode of diverticulitis due to increased risk of bowel perforation.

    Answer A is incorrect. An abdominal ultrasound can be quickly carried out in the emergency setting. It is helpful in the diagnosis of some genitourinary, gynecologic, and biliary pathologies as well as appendicitis. Its usefulness in diagnosing diverticulitis is limited. It has no role in screening for colon cancer.

Answer C is incorrect. CT of the abdomen with infusion is useful in the diagnosis of acute diverticulitis. It may show the presence of diverticula and signs of adjacent inflammatory changes such as edema and fat stranding. Once the patient's symptoms resolve, there is no need for a follow-up CT scan. This imaging modality has no role in screening for colon cancer.

Answer D is incorrect. MRI of the abdomen is not useful in the diagnosis or management of diverticulitis. It has no role in screening for colon cancer.

Answer E is incorrect. An upright abdominal x-ray is cheap and easily obtained. However, it is not used to diagnose diverticulitis nor is it used to rule out colon cancer.

45. **The correct answer is B.** This is a presentation of Wilson disease. The patient has parkinsonian symptoms due to the death of neurons in the basal ganglia (particularly in the putamen and globus pallidus). In addition, the liver biopsy shows evidence of cirrhosis (although this is a trichrome stain and not a copper stain, so the histopathology findings alone in this case are not specific). Wilson disease is an autosomal recessive disease in which there is a mutation in *ATP7B*, a gene in chromosome 13 that encodes for a copper-transporting ATPase. Copper accumulates in the liver, basal ganglia, bones, joints, kidneys, and Descemet membrane in the cornea (Kayser-Fleischer rings). Because Wilson disease follows an autosomal recessive pattern of inheritance, the patient's sister has a 25% chance of also having the disease.

 Answer A is incorrect. The patient's sister would have nearly 0% chance of getting the disease if this condition followed an X-linked pattern of inheritance. Examples of X-linked disorders include Duchenne muscular dystrophy and Lesch-Nyhan syndrome.

 Answer C is incorrect. Fifty percent would be the answer in the case of an autosomal dominant disorder such as hereditary spherocytosis, familial adenomatous polyposis, and adult polycystic kidney disease.

 Answer D is incorrect. If the sister were healthy, she would have a 66.6% chance of being a carrier of the mutated gene.

 Answer E is incorrect. A 100% chance of getting a disease is not common, unless one is referring to the likelihood a child has of inheriting a disease with a mitochondrial pattern of inheritance from a mother with the condition. Examples of diseases with this inheritance pattern include mitochondrial myopathies and Leber hereditary optic neuropathy.

46. **The correct answer is C.** The rapid onset of vomiting and diarrhea associated with *Staphylococcus aureus* food poisoning is not due to the bacterium itself but rather to ingestion of pre-formed enterotoxin. Mayonnaise and egg products are common sources.

 Answer A is incorrect. *Bacillus cereus* is a gram-positive, β-hemolytic rod that is often associated with food poisoning from reheated rice. Much like *S aureus*, it can produce a pre-formed toxin that can result in food poisoning.

 Answer B is incorrect. Gram-positive, catalase-positive, coagulase-positive bacteria include *S aureus*, which is likely the source of the pre-formed enterotoxin. However, the pre-formed enterotoxin is responsible for this patient's symptoms of food poisoning.

 Answer D is incorrect. *S aureus* can also produce the superantigen TSST-1, which mediates toxic shock syndrome. This patient is not exhibiting symptoms of toxic shock syndrome, which include fever, rash, and shock.

 Answer E is incorrect. Raw or undercooked seafood is a common cause of *Vibrio parahaemolyticus* or *V vulnificus* infection. These pathogens cause disease by direct invasion of the intestinal mucosa. The incubation period from ingestion to illness is about three days;

S aureus toxin causes illness within hours of ingestion.

47. **The correct answer is B.** The patient has Crigler-Najjar syndrome type 1. Patients with this condition lack uridine diphosphate glucuronyl transferase, leading to an inability to conjugate bilirubin. This leads to increased unconjugated bilirubin, which causes jaundice, kernicterus, and bilirubin deposition in the brain. Crigler-Najjar syndrome type 1 presents early in life and it is fatal. Type 2 of the syndrome is less severe and responds to phenobarbital.

Answer A is incorrect. Elevated antimitochondrial antibodies are found in the serum of patients with primary biliary cirrhosis, an intrahepatic autoimmune disorder often associated with scleroderma and CREST syndrome (CREST = **C**alcinosis and anti-**c**entromere antibodies, **R**aynaud phenomenon, **E**sophageal dysmotility, **S**clerodactyly, and **T**elangiectasias). Patients present with severe obstructive jaundice, steatorrhea, pruritus, and hypercholesterolemia.

Answer C is incorrect. A problem with bilirubin uptake describes Gilbert syndrome. Gilbert syndrome is a benign unconjugated hyperbilirubinemia that is caused directly by decreased bilirubin uptake or by mildly decreased uridine diphosphate glucuronyl transferase. It is asymptomatic except for jaundice during periods of psychological or physiologic stress and has no clinical consequences.

Answer D is incorrect. A problem with excretion of conjugated bilirubin is the etiology of both Dubin-Johnson syndrome and Rotor syndrome. Dubin-Johnson syndrome is a conjugated hyperbilirubinemia that is the result of defective liver excretion. This patient has unconjugated hyperbilirubinemia, evident in the absence of bilirubin in the urine (unconjugated bilirubin is not water soluble). Gross examination would reveal a black liver. Rotor syndrome is a rare idiopathic form of hyperbilirubinemia that affects both sexes, with onset occurring shortly after birth or during childhood. Rotor syndrome, like Dubin-Johnson syndrome, has a relatively benign course.

Answer E is incorrect. Inadequate hepatic copper excretion is the cause of Wilson disease, an autosomal recessive disease associated with asterixis, parkinsonian symptoms, choreiform movements, dementia, and characteristic corneal deposits known as Kayser-Fleischer rings.

48. **The correct answer is E.** The clinical presentation (fever, rash, hypotension) is characteristic of toxic shock syndrome (TSS) produced by *Staphylococcus aureus*. The *S aureus* TSST-1 superantigen simultaneously binds the β region of the T-cell receptor and the major histocompatibility complex class II of antigen-presenting cells, leading to the release of interferon-γ from T helper cells type 1 and IL-1, IL-6, and tumor necrosis factor-α from macrophages. Prolonged use of a single tampon is a common cause of TSS in women, but other causes in either sex include staphylococcal infection of surgical wounds, burns, and catheters.

Answer A is incorrect. This answer choice describes one type of antibody-mediated (type II) hypersensitivity, such as that of myasthenia gravis.

Answer B is incorrect. Binding of the macrophage CD14 receptor is characteristic of endotoxin/lipopolysaccharide of gram-negative bacteria. This process is capable of initiating a clinical presentation similar to that described here, but it is specific to gram-negative bacteria, thus contradicting other information contained in the stem.

Answer C is incorrect. Antigen cross-linking of IgE on mast cells and basophils describes the initiating event of anaphylaxis, a type I hypersensitivity reaction that results in histamine-induced vasodilation. Although anaphylaxis can result in some of the signs and symptoms seen in this patient, the specific molecular cascade described is indicative of *S aureus* superantigen infection.

Answer D is incorrect. Protein A binding of IgG Fc receptors is a virulence mechanism utilized by *S aureus* that leads to the inhibition of complement fixation and phagocytosis. Although protein A is seen with the organism implied in the stem, it does not initiate the signs and symptoms of TSS. Instead, it inhibits immune function.

49. **The correct answer is A.** The quality and location of this patient's pain, combined with its alleviation with medication and the radiographic findings, are suggestive of GERD. GERD increases the risk of developing esophageal mucosal metaplasia (squamous is replaced by columnar), called Barrett esophagus. In turn, patients with Barrett esophagus are at increased risk for developing adenocarcinoma of the distal esophagus. Barrett esophagus is diagnosed by endoscopy, and must be followed with annual endoscopy and biopsy to monitor for adenocarcinoma.

    Answer B is incorrect. Stomach cell adenocarcinoma is not associated with GERD. Risk factors for gastric adenocarcinoma include *Helicobacter pylori* infection, nitrosamine exposure, excessive salt intake, and low intake of fresh fruits and vegetables. This type of carcinoma is predisposed by achlorhydria and chronic gastritis. Alarming signs and symptoms of gastric adenocarcinoma include unexplained weight loss, persistent vomiting, dysphagia, family history of upper GI tract cancer, left supraclavicular adenopathy, and hematemesis. Current treatment of gastric adenocarcinoma consists of different multidrug therapies with agents such as 5-fluorouracil, doxorubicin, cisplatin, etoposide, and/or irinotecan.

    Answer C is incorrect. Krukenberg tumor is involvement of the ovaries (typically bilateral) by metastatic carcinoma of the stomach, intestines, or breasts. This neoplasm bears no relation to GERD nor is it possible for this male patient to have ovarian metastases assuming normal reproductive development. Patients with Krukenberg tumor might present with disproportionate abdominal pain, left supraclavicular adenopathy, bloody stools, iron deficiency anemia, palpable pelvic masses, and/or cystic masses on ultrasound. Current treatment includes obtaining a tissue diagnosis of the ovarian mass to differentiate primary from metastatic lesions. There is no agreed-upon medical treatment, but survival can be improved with bilateral oophrectomy if the metastasis is limited to the ovaries. This would accompany treatment of the underlying primary tumor.

    Answer D is incorrect. Non-small cell adenocarcinoma of the lung (NSCLC) is commonly caused by cigarette smoking but is not associated with GERD. A patient with NSCLC might present with hemoptysis, cough, chronic lung infections, history of smoking, chest wall pain, shortness of breath, and/or hoarseness. The only current treatment regimens for NSCLC that have proven to improve survival are the cisplatin-based regimens, which combine cisplatin with various other antineoplastic agents (eg, paclitaxel, docetaxel, gemcitabine, and vinorelbine).

    Answer E is incorrect. Squamous cell carcinoma is not known to correlate with GERD. Squamous cell carcinoma is thought to be associated with tobacco and alcohol use. It tends to involve the proximal and mid-sections of the esophagus rather than the distal esophagus. Combination therapy with 5-fluorouracil and cisplatin is currently the mainstay of treatment in esophageal squamous cell carcinoma.

50. **The correct answer is E.** This patient has signs and symptoms characteristic of pancreatic adenocarcinoma. This malignancy often presents with jaundice, epigastric pain radiating to the back, and weight loss. The red, swollen, tender lower extremity indicates a possible deep vein thrombosis. Patients with pancreatic adenocarcinoma may present with migratory thrombophlebitis, which is called Trousseau sign. Laboratory studies show increased amylase, lipase, and alkaline phosphatase levels. Tumor markers such as CA 19-9 and carcinoembryonic antigen (CEA) are often elevated in pancreatic cancer. These markers are generally not sensitive or specific enough to be used for diagnosis, but they do have use in monitoring the course of the disease and response to therapy. CEA is also a marker for colorectal cancer. Pancreatic cancers are more common in patients with a history of smoking, DM, and

chronic pancreatitis. Treatment for pancreatic adenocarcinoma is surgical removal, yet for most patients this is impossible, as the cancer has already metastasized prior to its discovery. If possible, pancreaticoduodenectomy or distal pancreatectomy is preferred to a total pancreatectomy in order to preserve some of the pancreatic function.

Answer A is incorrect. This patient clearly shows signs of pancreatic adenocarcinoma, and neither α-fetoprotein nor β-hCG elevations are associated with this neoplasm.

Answer B is incorrect. The CA 19-9 level is indeed elevated in many cases of pancreatic adenocarcinoma. However, an α-fetoprotein level is not found in pancreatic malignancies; rather, it is elevated in hepatocellular carcinomas and nonseminomatous germ cell tumors of the testis. While hepatocellular carcinomas can occasionally present with jaundice and derangements in liver function tests, they are unlikely to cause elevations in amylase and lipase levels. Furthermore, the characteristic signs of migratory thrombophlebitis (Trousseau sign) should lead you to think of pancreatic adenocarcinoma as the most likely diagnosis.

Answer C is incorrect. The CEA level is elevated in both pancreatic adenocarcinoma and colorectal cancer. However, the α-fetoprotein level is elevated in hepatocellular carcinomas and nonseminomatous germ cell tumors of the testis. Neither of these is likely in this patient, so this is not the best answer.

Answer D is incorrect. The CEA level is elevated in both pancreatic adenocarcinoma and colorectal cancer. However, β-hCG is a tumor marker for gynecologic neoplasms such as gestational trophoblastic tumors, choriocarcinomas, and hydatidiform moles. It is also elevated in the setting of several types of testicular germ cell tumors, such as seminomas and choriocarcinomas. Given the clinical presentation, none of these is the best diagnosis for this patient, so this is not the best answer.

CHAPTER 11

Hematology-Oncology

QUESTIONS

1. The image shows a section of biopsied tissue from a skin lesion on the forehead of a 60-year-old farmer. Which of the following is the most likely gross description of the skin lesion?

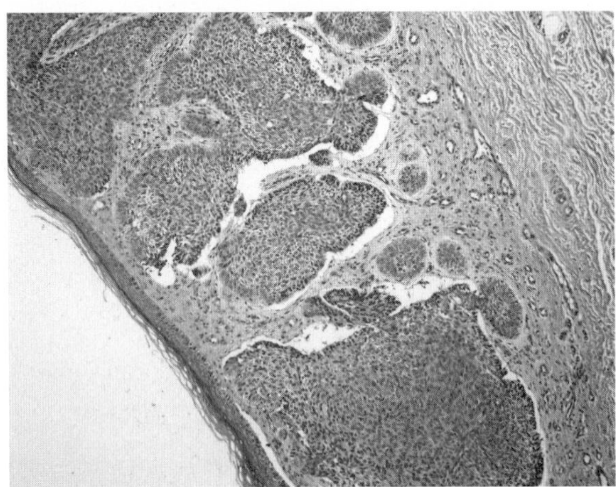

Reproduced, with permission, from USMLERx.com.

(A) 5- to 10-mm oval, tan-brown patches that do not darken with sunlight
(B) Raised, pearly borders surrounded by fine telangiectasias
(C) Sharply defined red, scaling plaques
(D) Tan-brown, rough lesion <1 cm in diameter
(E) Thickened, hyperpigmented skin with velvet-like texture

2. A 55-year-old man comes to his physician for a routine health maintenance examination. He has never smoked and does not drink alcohol. Toward the end of the visit, he tells his physician that he has worked in the textiles industry for 30 years. He knows that he has been exposed to aniline dyes and is concerned about how this may affect his health. This patient's occupational exposure increases his risk for which of the following neoplasms?

(A) Esophageal adenocarcinoma
(B) Hepatocellular carcinoma
(C) Mesothelioma
(D) Nasopharyngeal carcinoma
(E) Transitional cell carcinoma of the bladder

3. A 43-year-old man comes to the physician complaining of heartburn and black, tarry stools. He states that he has been eating much less than usual, although he still manages to drink at least one beer per day, which he reports having done for the past 20 years. On physical examination the patient exhibits diffuse tenderness and guarding over the entire epigastric area. Serum levels of which of the following substances are likely to be elevated in this patient?

(A) Cholecystokinin
(B) Gastrin
(C) Intrinsic factor
(D) Secretin
(E) Somatostatin

4. A 65-year-old man presents with a two-month history of cough, severe left-sided shoulder pain, and hoarseness. Most concerning to him, however, is the droop of his left eyelid, which developed over the previous few weeks. The patient worked as a technician in a nuclear power plant before retiring last year and has a 40-year history of smoking. Physical examination reveals that his left pupil is smaller than his right, and the skin on the left side of his face is extremely dry. CT of the chest reveals a 3-cm nodule in one lung. Which type and in which part of the lung is this man's tumor most likely located?

(A) Adenocarcinoma located in the apex of left lung
(B) Adenocarcinoma located in the apex of the right lung
(C) Squamous cell carcinoma located in the apex of left lung
(D) Squamous cell carcinoma located in the apex of the right lung
(E) Squamous cell carcinoma located in the hilum of the left lung

5. A 58-year-old man presents to his primary care physician complaining of years of heartburn that has not resolved with over-the-counter drugs. His physician refers him to have an esophagoduodenostomy (EGD) performed. The image was taken during the patient's EGD. Following the EGD, what medication should this patient start taking?

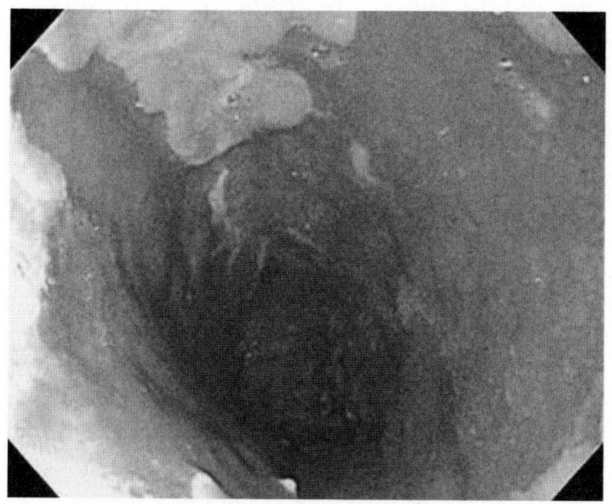

Reproduced, with permission, from Greenberger NJ, et al. *Current Diagnosis & Treatment: Gastroenterology, Hepatology, & Endoscopy*, New York: McGraw-Hill, 2009; Plate15.

(A) Bismuth subsalicylate
(B) Calcium carbonate
(C) Omeprazole
(D) Ranitidine
(E) Sucralfate

6. A 38-year-old woman returning to the US from a trip to Japan complains of sudden chest pain and shortness of breath. She is taking no medication other than an oral contraceptive pill. She is tachycardic and tachypneic, and her right calf is swollen and tender. She is admitted for appropriate therapy. Which of the following laboratory tests is important in monitoring her initial therapy?

(A) Bleeding time
(B) International Normalized Ratio
(C) No monitoring is needed
(D) Partial thromboplastin time
(E) Prothrombin time

7. A 4-year-old girl is brought to the emergency department with an eight-hour history of projectile vomiting and headache. Her parents say that the patient was well until two months ago, when they noted that she was becoming increasingly clumsy. Physical examination shows nystagmus in all directions of gaze, as well as truncal ataxia. Laboratory blood studies show a WBC count of $7200/mm^3$, a hemoglobin level of 12.3 g/dL, and a platelet count of $225{,}000/mm^3$. Which of the following is most likely to be evident on histopathologic examination of the lesion?

(A) Deeply staining nuclei with scant cytoplasm arranged in pseudorosettes
(B) Pleomorphic, anaplastic cells with foci of necrosis in a palisading pattern
(C) Regular round cells featuring spherical nuclei with finely granular chromatin surrounded by clear cytoplasm
(D) Stratified squamous epithelial cells embedded in spongy reticular stroma with prominent peripheral gliosis
(E) Whorls of meningothelial cells with oval-shaped nuclei with indistinct cytoplasm and psammoma bodies

8. A 17-year-old boy presents to the emergency department with severe abdominal pain. Laboratory tests show a deficit in uroporphyrinogen I synthetase and excess δ-aminolevulinate and porphobilinogen in the urine. Which of the following symptoms would most likely also be present in this patient?

(A) Chest pain
(B) Hypotension
(C) Neuropsychiatric disturbances
(D) Polyphagia
(E) Stiff neck

9. A 7-year-old child from Africa presents with a neck mass and painless cervical lymphadenopathy. On nasopharyngoscopy, a mass arising in the nasopharynx is visible. The mass is biopsied. Under light microscopy, the cells are arranged in a syncytial pattern with vesiculated nuclei and prominent nucleoli. Immunohistochemistry is consistent with nonkeratinizing nasopharyngeal carcinoma, undifferentiated. The virus associated with this carcinoma is also associated with what other malignancy, as shown in the image?

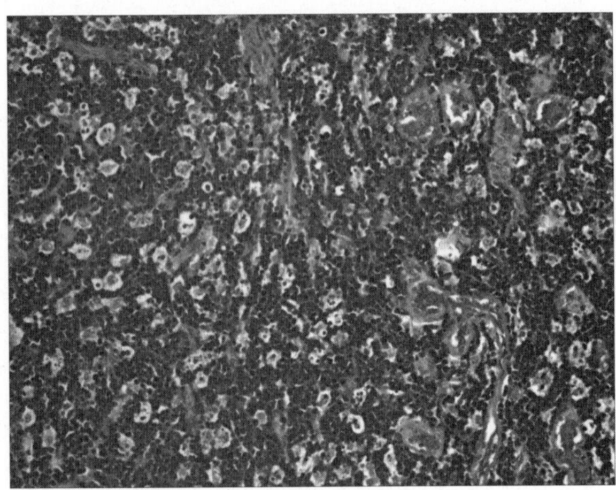

Reproduced, with permission, from USMLERx.com.

(A) Adult T-lymphocyte leukemia
(B) Burkitt lymphoma
(C) Cervical carcinoma
(D) Hepatocellular carcinoma
(E) Kaposi sarcoma

10. A 22-year-old man presents to the emergency department with mucosal bleeding and epistaxis. Laboratory tests show an increased bleeding time and an increased partial thromboplastin time. His mother was anemic throughout her life and required several blood transfusions after a minor operation. Which of the following is the most likely diagnosis?

(A) Bernard-Soulier syndrome
(B) Glanzmann thrombocytopenia
(C) Hemophilia A
(D) Vitamin K deficiency
(E) Von Willebrand disease

11. A 9-year-old African-American boy is brought to the emergency department with sudden onset of chest pain and dyspnea. Initial examination reveals tachycardia and hypoxemia. A chest x-ray demonstrates bilateral patchy infiltrates. Last year, the patient was diagnosed with cholecystitis with multiple radiopaque stones. There is a history of a "blood problem" that runs in the family. Which of the following peripheral blood smear findings is most consistent with his clinical condition?

(A) Heinz bodies
(B) Howell-Jolly bodies
(C) Microcytes
(D) Ringed sideroblasts
(E) Spherocytes

12. A 55-year-old man presents to his physician because of easy bruising, splenomegaly, and fatigue. Results of peripheral blood smear are shown in the image. Rapid treatment of this patient's condition could lead to release of the contents of the pictured cells and the development of a serious hematologic complication. If this complication were to develop, which of the following would most likely be seen on a peripheral blood smear?

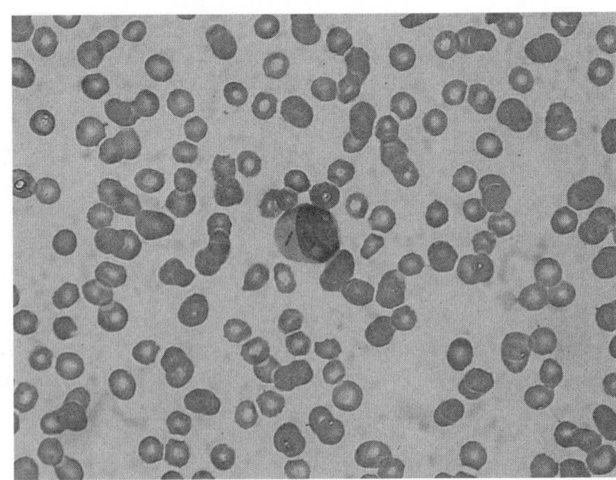

Courtesy of Wikipedia.

(A) Acanthocytes
(B) Burr cells
(C) Schistocytes

(D) Target cells
(E) Teardrop cells

13. An autopsy is performed on a 65-year-old woman. On examination of the liver, the pathologist finds multiple tumors of various sizes throughout both lobes. Without direct pathologic correlation, which of the following is most likely the location of the primary tumor?

(A) Breast
(B) Colon
(C) Kidney
(D) Liver
(E) Lung

14. A child is brought to the pediatrician because her parents are concerned about lead poisoning since their house is known to contain lead-based paint. A complete blood count reveals anemia. Lead poisoning causes anemia because it does which of the following?

(A) Disrupts heme synthesis by causing decreased iron absorption from the gut
(B) Disrupts heme synthesis by increasing the activity of aminolevulinate dehydratase
(C) Disrupts heme synthesis by inhibiting ferrochelatase
(D) Disrupts hemoglobin function by binding to hemoglobin with high affinity, preventing oxygen binding
(E) Disrupts RBC DNA synthesis, causing megaloblastic changes in RBCs

15. A 59-year-old woman is admitted to the hospital because of a brief episode of right-sided hemiparesis. Medical history is significant for an eight-week history of bleeding from the gums, nosebleeds, throbbing and burning sensations in the hands and feet, and mild left upper quadrant pain. A blood panel shows a hemoglobin level of 15 g/dL, hematocrit of 45%, and platelet count of 900,000/mm^3. Erythrocyte sedimentation rate, C-reactive protein, and WBC count are within normal range. Based on the patient's symptoms and abnormal laboratory results, the patient begins treatment with hydroxyurea. Which of the following is the most likely diagnosis?

(A) Essential thrombocytosis
(B) Immune thrombocytopenic purpura
(C) Polycythemia vera
(D) Sickle cell disease
(E) Thrombotic thrombocytopenic purpura

16. Physical examination of a 60-year-old woman reveals gait instability and decreased proprioception in her lower extremities. Blood tests show a normal hematocrit level and near-normal mean cell volume. Her physician orders additional tests. Which of the following laboratory results supports a diagnosis of cobalamin deficiency?

(A) Decreased homocysteine levels
(B) Decreased level of lactate dehydrogenase
(C) Elevated methylmalonic acid
(D) Elevated WBC count
(E) Negative anti-intrinsic factor antibody
(F) Negative result of Schilling's test

17. A 28-year-old previously healthy woman who is six months pregnant comes to the physician complaining of excessive fatigue for the past several months. Physical examination reveals pallor of her mucous membranes. A peripheral blood smear shows small RBCs containing a narrow rim of hemoglobin at the periphery. Which of the following laboratory values are most likely to be found in this patient?

Choice	Ferritin	Iron-binding capacity	Mean corpuscular volume
A	↓	↓	normal
B	↓	↓	↑
C	↓	↑	↓
D	↓	↑	↑
E	↑	↑	↓

Reproduced, with permission, from USMLERx.com.

(A) A
(B) B
(C) C
(D) D
(E) E

18. A 40-year-old woman is diagnosed with metastatic breast cancer. Analysis of her biopsy specimen shows tumor cells that overexpress *HER2*, a member of the epidermal growth factor receptor family. She begins chemotherapy that will specifically target the extracellular domain of the HER2 receptor on the cancer cells. Which of the following drugs has most likely been prescribed for this patient?

    (A) All-*trans* retinoic acid
    (B) Imatinib mesylate
    (C) Methotrexate
    (D) Rituximab
    (E) Trastuzumab

19. A 47-year-old woman from the Middle East presents to the clinic with fever, general malaise, and weight loss. Physical examination reveals hepatomegaly and massive splenomegaly, along with edema. Laboratory tests show moderate anemia and a peripheral WBC count <4000/mm^3. Macrophages containing amastigotes are seen on histologic analysis. From which of the following hosts did this woman most likely acquire the parasite that she now harbors?

    (A) *Aedes* mosquito
    (B) *Anopheles* mosquito
    (C) *Ixodes* tick
    (D) Reduviid bug
    (E) Sandfly

20. A type of lymphoma is characterized by onset in middle age and by neoplastic cells that resemble normal germinal center B lymphocytes. What characteristic chromosomal translocation and protein are produced by this translocation?

    (A) t(8;14), *c-Myc*
    (B) t(9;22), *Bcr-Abl*
    (C) t(11;22), *EWS-Fli-*1
    (D) t(14;18), *Bcl-*2
    (E) t(15;17), *PML/RARα*

21. A 52-year-old heart transplant patient receiving chronic immunosuppressive therapy develops bacterial sinusitis. His list of medications includes cyclosporine. The patient's physician decides to start him on antibiotic therapy but is having difficulty choosing between amoxicillin and erythromycin to treat the infection. Compared to using each agent alone, concurrent use of erythromycin and cyclosporine would most likely lead to which of the following?

    (A) Decreased risk of renal failure
    (B) Increased cyclophilin concentration
    (C) Increased cyclosporine serum concentrations
    (D) Increased risk of infection with *Clostridium difficile*
    (E) Increased risk of QTc prolongation

22. A 34-year-old man presents to his primary care physician complaining of a low-grade fever, drenching sweats at night, and an unintentional 5-kg (12-lb) weight loss over the past three months. CT of the chest reveals mediastinal lymphadenopathy. Subsequent biopsy of an involved node is remarkable for the cell shown in the image. Which of the following is part of the multidrug regimen that would be used to manage this patient's disease?

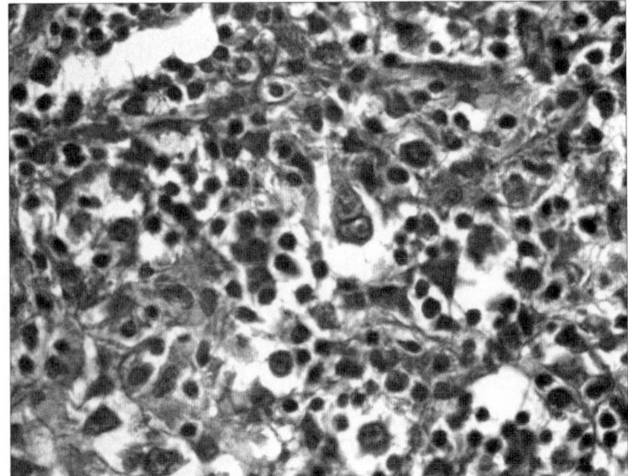

Reproduced, with permission, from USMLERx.com.

(A) Cyclosporine
(B) Hydroxyurea
(C) Imatinib
(D) Isoniazid
(E) Vinblastine

23. A 30-year-old woman comes to the physician because of bruising easily. She is currently taking no medications and has no significant past medical history. Laboratory studies are significant for a platelet count of 25,000/mm^3 and the presence of high levels of antiplatelet antibodies. Which of the following features is most likely to be seen on peripheral blood smear?

(A) Bite cells
(B) Drepanocytes
(C) Enlarged platelets
(D) Howell-Jolly bodies
(E) Pappenheimer bodies

24. A 2-year-old boy is brought to a clinic because of a large, unilateral, painless abdominal mass his mother noticed while bathing him. While performing an ultrasound-guided biopsy, the technician notes that the kidney calyces are highly distorted by the mass. Which of the following is most likely the origin of this lesion?

(A) A mutation of the *APKD1* gene on chromosome 16
(B) Embryonic renal cells from the embryonic kidney
(C) Malignant transformation of renal tubular cells
(D) Malignant transformation of uroepithelial cells
(E) Primitive neural crest cells

25. A 44-year-old woman comes to the physician because of a four-month history of fatigue, joint pain, malaise, and morning stiffness that sometimes persist for more than an hour after waking. Laboratory tests show:

WBC count: 15,100/mm^3
Hemoglobin: 8.8 g/dL
Hematocrit: 26.7%
Platelet count: 267,000/mm^3
Mean corpuscular volume: 87 fL
Total iron binding capacity: 200 µg/dL
Haptoglobin: 100 mg/dL
LDH cholesterol: 85 mg/dL

Peripheral blood smear shows a normochromic, normocytic anemia. Which of the following is the most likely cause of her fatigue?

(A) Anemia of chronic disease
(B) Autoimmune hemolytic anemia
(C) Iron deficiency anemia
(D) Megaloblastic anemia
(E) Sideroblastic anemia

26. A 32-year-old man is diagnosed with Hodgkin lymphoma and begins chemotherapy. Shortly after completing treatment, the patient complains of a chronic cough and difficulty catching his breath after climbing stairs. He also says he thinks his skin is "getting darker." Throughout chemotherapy his complete blood cell counts revealed minimal myelosuppression. Which of the following drugs is most likely responsible for these adverse effects?

(A) Bleomycin
(B) Busulfan
(C) Dactinomycin
(D) Doxorubicin
(E) Vinblastine

27. A 61-year-old woman complains of a tingling sensation in her feet that has become progressively worse over the past several months. On physical examination she appears mildly jaundiced and her tongue has a glazed appearance. Neurologic findings include decreased vibrational sense in her lower extremities. A peripheral blood smear is shown in the image. Which of the following is the most common cause of the disorder seen in this patient?

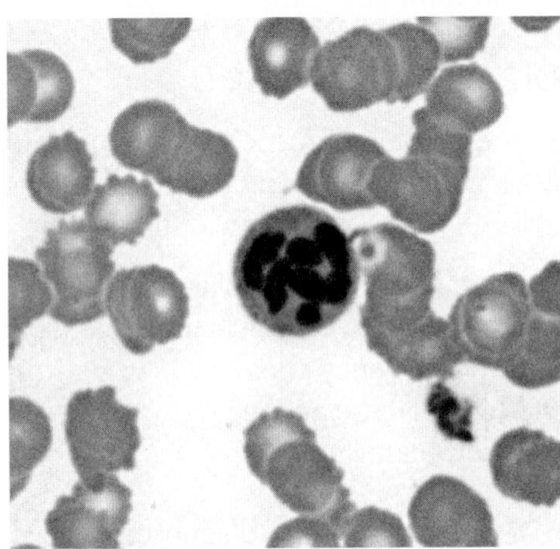

Reproduced, with permission, from USMLERx.com.

(A) Bacterial overgrowth
(B) Gastrectomy
(C) Infection with *Diphyllobothrium latum*
(D) Nutritional deficiency
(E) Pancreatic insufficiency
(F) Pernicious anemia

28. A 57-year-old woman is diagnosed with small-cell lung carcinoma. She has gained weight, and she says that her face has recently "ballooned." Which of the following symptoms is this patient likely to be experiencing in addition to the ones mentioned?

(A) Cold intolerance and constipation
(B) Increased bone density
(C) Insatiable thirst and polyuria
(D) Poor wound healing and facial plethora
(E) Proximal muscle weakness and palpitations

29. A 45-year-old woman arrives at the emergency department complaining of intense pain in her upper abdomen for the past four hours. She had a similar episode many months ago, but the pain resolved within an hour without treatment. Physical examination reveals scleral icterus, jaundice, and splenomegaly. Ultrasound demonstrates radiopaque gallstones. Results of a Coombs test are negative. A peripheral blood smear shows small RBCs, several of which have no central pallor. Which of the following is the most likely cause of this patient's condition?

(A) A mechanical heart valve
(B) A mutation in the gene encoding ankyrin
(C) A mutation in the gene encoding glucose-6-phosphate dehydrogenase
(D) Circulating antibodies targeted against RBCs
(E) Iron deficiency

30. A 19-year-old man is referred to an oncologist after his primary care physician detects a soft tissue mass along the distal femur. The oncologist diagnoses the patient with osteosarcoma and places him on a chemotherapeutic regimen that includes a dihydrofolate reductase inhibitor. A week later, he returns to the clinic with nausea, vomiting, and diarrhea. Which of the following is the best course of intervention?

(A) Administer erythropoietin
(B) Administer filgrastim
(C) Folic acid supplementation
(D) Iron supplementation
(E) Vitamin B_{12} supplementation

31. A 72-year-old man with a chronic cough comes to a local clinic complaining of a sharp pain in his ribs that started this morning after he had an episode of severe coughing. He notes that he has also been feeling very fatigued lately and has lost 10 lb (4.5 kg) in the past three months. The physician orders a chest x-ray, which reveals a rib fracture on the lateral view. Suspicious, the physician then orders a bone marrow biopsy. The results are shown in the image. Which of the following additional pathologic findings is this patient most likely to have?

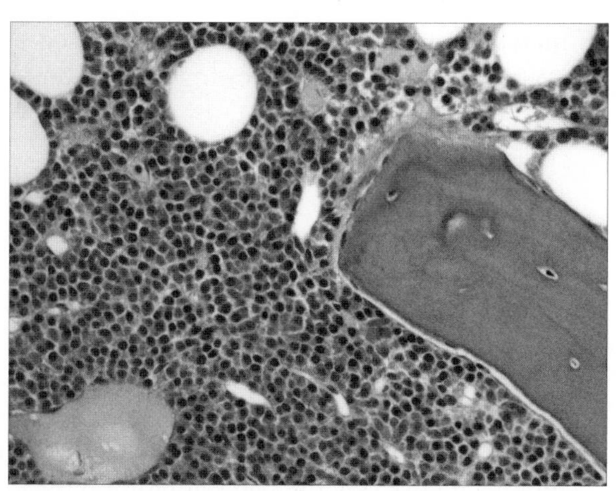

Reproduced, with permission, from USMLERx.com.

(A) Aplastic anemia
(B) Hypercalcemia
(C) Hypocalcemia
(D) Reed-Sternberg cells
(E) Severely elevated prostate-specific antigen level

32. A 62-year-old man with a history of hyperlipidemia and multiple transient ischemic attacks presents to the emergency department after two hours of left-sided weakness in his upper extremity and face. After a CT of the head shows no evidence of intracranial hemorrhage, a fibrinolytic enzyme is administered. Two hours later the man develops bleeding from his gums as well as several large subcutaneous ecchymoses. Which of the following drugs could stop this man's bleeding?

(A) Aminocaproic acid
(B) Protamine sulfate
(C) Recombinant factor VIII
(D) Tissue plasminogen activator
(E) Vitamin K

33. A 60-year-old woman presents with weight loss, fatigue, and new-onset ascites. Ascitic fluid cytology shows atypical glandular cells with dysplastic nuclei, blood, and increased protein content. The patient has a palpable left clavicular mass, a hard mass beneath her umbilicus, and diffuse abdominal and pelvic pain. Results of biopsy of the stomach are shown in the image. Which of the following factors most likely contributed to the development of this patient's pathology?

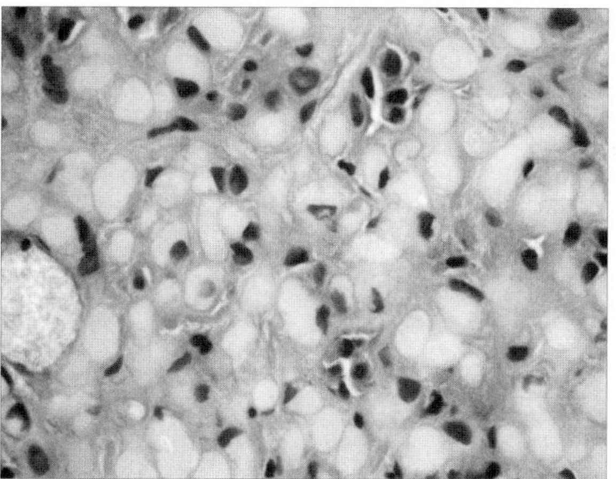

Reproduced, with permission, from USMLERx.com.

(A) Dietary nitrosamines
(B) History of oral contraceptive use
(C) Low dietary folate
(D) Polyvinyl chloride exposure
(E) Prior tuberculosis

34. A patient with relapsing Hodgkin disease presents with weight gain, foot ulcers, vision problems, elevated blood sugar, oral candidiasis, and new onset of wildly swinging mood changes. What is the most likely etiology of this patient's psychiatric symptoms?

(A) Adverse effects of bleomycin
(B) Adverse effects of prednisone
(C) Adverse effects of vincristine
(D) Normal psychiatric response to having cancer
(E) Progression of disease

35. A 41-year-old pregnant woman sees her obstetrician because of new-onset vaginal bleeding. Although she is only four months pregnant, her doctor notes that her uterus is the size usually seen at six months of gestation. Maternal blood works shows a β-human chorionic gonadotropin level >5 times the upper limit of normal. If left untreated, what is a possible consequence of the patient's condition?

(A) Choriocarcinoma
(B) Coma
(C) Fetal neural tube defects
(D) Ovarian cancer
(E) Uterine bleeding and exsanguination

36. A 9-month-old girl is found to be anemic. Her mother and several great aunts have a similar history. Results of a peripheral blood smear suggest thalassemia major. What laboratory values are most likely to be seen in this patient?

Choice	Hemoglobin (g/dL)	Reticulocyte count (%)	Mean corpuscular hemoglobin (pg/cell)	Mean corpuscular volume (fL)	Serum iron (μg/dL)
A	5.5	6%	18	60	100
B	7.5	3%	26	65	65
C	8.0	1%	27	100	75
D	9.0	2%	31	92	225
E	10.5	2%	30	91	85

Reproduced, with permission, from USMLERx.com.

(A) A
(B) B
(C) C
(D) D
(E) E

37. A 56-year-old man who is a health care worker presents to his physician with vague abdominal discomfort. A physical examination reveals a tender liver, palpable to 6 cm below the costal margin and scleral icterus. His laboratory studies are significant for an aspartate aminotransferase activity of 200 U/L and an alanine aminotransferase activity of 450 U/L. CT of the abdomen shows a dominant solid nodule in the liver. The tumor marker most likely to be increased in this patient is also likely to be elevated in which of the following malignancies?

(A) Choriocarcinoma
(B) Colorectal carcinoma
(C) Melanoma
(D) Neuroblastoma
(E) Prostatic carcinoma
(F) Yolk sac carcinoma

38. A 57-year-old man presents to his internist because of abnormal bleeding following a routine dental cleaning. Over the past several months he has experienced symptoms of headache, dizziness, fatigue, decreased vision, and occasional epistaxis. He has also begun noticing "lumps" on his armpits and groin region. The spleen tip is palpable on physical examination. Laboratory tests show a hemoglobin level of 11 g/dL, blood urea nitrogen of 25 mg/dL, calcium of 9.1, and total protein of 15 g/dL. Immunofixation shows high levels of IgM. Results of bone marrow biopsy are shown in the image. Which of the following is the most likely explanation for the patient's symptoms?

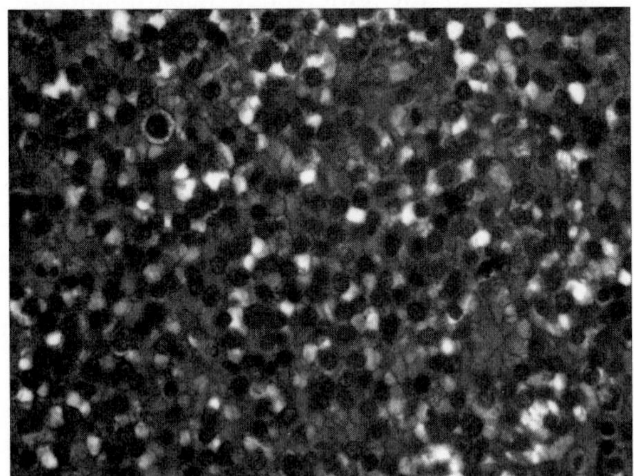

Reproduced, with permission, from USMLERx.com.

(A) Heavy-chain disease
(B) Monoclonal gammopathy of undetermined significance
(C) Multiple myeloma
(D) Primary amyloidosis
(E) Waldenström macroglobulinemia

39. A 29-year-old man presents to his primary care physician with a painless testicular mass. Which of the following lymph nodes are most likely involved?

(A) Deep inguinal
(B) External iliac
(C) Gluteal
(D) Para-aortic
(E) Superficial inguinal

40. A 20-year-old woman comes to her family physician for a routine check-up. She exhibits mild mental retardation. Physical examination shows an oval-shaped, slightly pigmented nevus on the lower back and an angiofibroma on the forehead that the patient reports having had since birth. The patient has a history of a cardiac rhabdomyoma that spontaneously regressed in childhood. A previous MRI showed multiple nodules of glial proliferation in the basal ganglia, ventricles, and cortex. This patient most likely also has which of the following conditions?

(A) Bilateral hearing loss
(B) Central scotoma
(C) Epilepsy
(D) Retinal detachment
(E) Severe sun sensitivity

41. A 29-year-old woman, who is 32 weeks pregnant and has been in the hospital for 3 days because of pyelonephritis, starts oozing blood from her intravenous lines and bleeding from her gums. Petechiae are also noted in her skin. Laboratory tests show:

Platelet count: 98,000/mm³
Hematocrit: 38%
WBC count: 8000/mm³
Prothrombin time: prolonged

What other laboratory anomaly would also be expected?

(A) Elevated D-dimer levels
(B) Elevated factor VII levels
(C) Elevated fibrinogen levels
(D) Elevated protein C levels
(E) Elevated protein S levels

42. A 62-year-old woman presents to the clinic complaining of frequent bleeding while brushing her teeth and easy bruising. She reports she recently had pneumonia and was treated with a broad-spectrum antibiotic. Laboratory tests show:

Prothrombin time: 18 seconds
Partial thromboplastin time: 37 seconds
Platelet count: 231,000/mm³
Hematocrit: 37%
WBC count: 4800/mm³

The cofactor that is deficient in this patient is needed for the carboxylation of glutamate residues of which of the following?

(A) Factors II, VII, VIII, and X
(B) Factors VII, VIII, IX, and XII
(C) Proteins C and S and factors IX, X, XI, and XII
(D) Proteins C and S and factors XII, IX, and X
(E) Proteins C and S, prothrombin, and factors VII, IX, and X

43. A 50-year-old man comes to the physician's office with weight loss, fatigue, night sweats, easy bruising, and nosebleeds. He also complains of pain near his first metatarsophalangeal joint in his left foot. Physical examination is remarkable for hepatosplenomegaly. Laboratory studies show a preponderance of WBCs (>50,000/mm³) and a full spectrum of myeloid cells in the peripheral blood smear. On genetic analysis, a translocation of chromosomes 9 and 22 is found. Which of the following is the first-line treatment for this condition?

(A) Allopurinol
(B) Busulfan
(C) Hydroxyurea
(D) Imatinib
(E) Interferon-α

44. Several drugs are used to prevent myocardial infarction in patients with acute coronary syndrome. One class of drugs binds to the glycoprotein receptor IIb/IIIa on activated platelets, thereby interfering with platelet aggregation. This prevents renewed formation of clots that could block the lumen of the cardiac vessels. Which of the following is an example of this class of drug?

(A) Abciximab
(B) Clopidogrel
(C) Leuprolide
(D) Selegiline
(E) Ticlopidine

45. A 36-year-old white woman with a history of uncomplicated systemic lupus erythematosus presents to her physician with edema and pain in her right foot that began two days ago. Physical examination reveals a positive Homan sign (pain on dorsiflexion of the foot), and an ultrasound reveals a non-occlusive thrombus in the right popliteal vein. Laboratory studies show a platelet count of 175,000/mm³, a prothrombin time of 26 seconds, and partial thromboplastin time of 89 seconds. What is the most likely cause of this patient's condition?

(A) Antibodies directed against factor VIII
(B) Antibodies directed against heparin
(C) Antibodies directed against platelet glycoprotein IIb/IIIa
(D) Antibodies directed against platelet phospholipids
(E) Antibodies directed against RBCs

46. A 58-year-old hospitalized woman who has been complaining of dysuria develops a high fever and a sudden drop in blood pressure. The patient has petechiae and purpura, bleeding from her intravenous sites, and epistaxis. Laboratory tests show an elevated white blood cell count, low platelet count, elevated creatinine, increased prothrombin time and partial thromboplastin time, and elevated of D-dimers. A peripheral blood smear is shown in the image. Which of the following is the most likely underlying cause of this woman's acute symptoms?

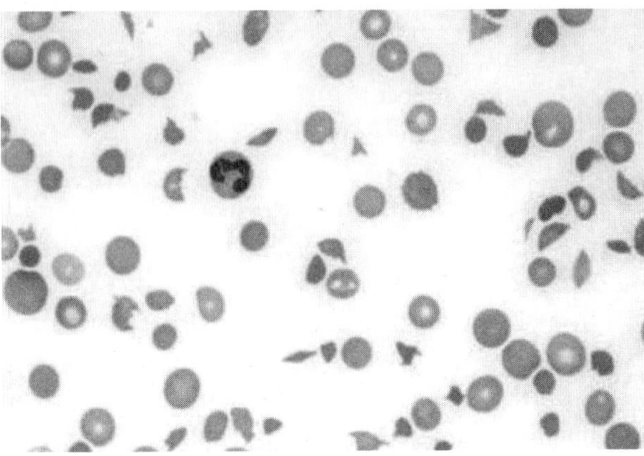

Reproduced, with permission, from USMLERx.com.

(A) Absence of glycoprotein Ib
(B) Absence of protease responsible for cleaving von Willebrand factor
(C) Activation of the coagulation cascade
(D) Deficiency of factor VIII
(E) An invasive gram-negative rod

47. A 70-year-old African-American man presents to his physician for a routine physical examination. The patient denies any current or past medical problems, and results of physical examination are normal. Routine laboratory tests show an abnormal monoclonal serum immunoglobulin level. Additional studies including a bone scan, CT of the abdomen, and a 24-hour urine collection reveal no abnormalities. Which of the following is the best next step in management?

(A) Prescribe a bisphosphonate
(B) Prescribe high-dose steroids
(C) Prescribe vinca alkaloids
(D) Recommend daily anticoagulation with aspirin
(E) Repeat laboratory tests in six months

48. An 8-year-old boy has a history of chronic and severe hemolytic anemia, hepatosplenomegaly, and maxillary overgrowth. He has received blood transfusions since early infancy but has not received a transfusion in >4 months. Hemoglobin (Hb) electrophoresis shows marked elevation of HbF, increased HbA_2, and absence of HbA_1. Which of the following diagnoses is most consistent with this patient's electrophoresis?

(A) α-Thalassemia minor
(B) β-Thalassemia major
(C) β-Thalassemia minor
(D) Glucose 6-phosphate dehydrogenase deficiency
(E) HbH disease histocompatibility complex class II
(F) RBCs containing Hb Bart

49. A 69-year-old man has a tumor removed from the cerebellopontine angle because a CT scan shows a 2-cm, sharply circumscribed mass adjacent to the right pons and extending into the right cerebellar hemisphere. The patient reports a three-month history of dizziness. The tumor specimen appears as a single irregular fragment of tan-pink soft tissue that measures slightly less than two cm. A microscopic pathology report indicates that the specimen consists of compact areas of spindle cells with pink cytoplasm that form whorls and palisades. Which of the following types of tumors would most likely result in these findings?

(A) Medulloblastoma
(B) Meningioma
(C) Neurofibroma
(D) Oligodendroglioma
(E) Schwannoma

50. A 22-year-old man is diagnosed with medullary thyroid carcinoma, and a comprehensive metabolic panel is significant for hypercalcemia. He notes that he has episodes of dizziness accompanied by sweating and feeling lightheaded. He says he remembers his mother having her thyroid gland removed when he was a young child but cannot remember the exact reason. These findings suggest a possible mutation in which of the following genes?

(A) *braf*
(B) *erb*-B2
(C) *MEN1*
(D) *ras*
(E) *ret*

ANSWERS

1. **The correct answer is B.** The classic gross signs of pearly borders and fine telangiectasias lead one to suspect basal cell carcinoma. The photomicrograph confirms this, as the nuclei are arranged in palisades, and there are islands of tumor cells. These histologic characteristics are hallmarks of basal cell carcinoma. Also note that the lesion is on the face of a farmer, someone who presumably has extensive sun exposure.

   Answer A is incorrect. This description is that of lentigo, which is characterized histologically by linear basal hyperpigmentation from melanocyte hyperplasia. This skin lesion most often occurs in childhood and is benign.

   Answer C is incorrect. Squamous cell carcinoma of the skin may also be seen in a patient such as this farmer, who has had frequent sun exposure over many years. However, it is frequently preceded by actinic keratosis, can occur on mucous areas (such as lips, unlike basal cell carcinoma), and is characterized histologically by keratin pearls. Keratin pearls appear as pink, extracellular concretions on hematoxylin and eosin staining, and these are not evident on the image shown here.

   Answer D is incorrect. Actinic keratosis, which can progress to squamous cell carcinoma, is the most common precancerous dermatosis. The histologic description is characterized by cytologic atypia in the lower-most layers of the epidermis, and a thickened stratum corneum in which nuclei are often retained. In contrast to basal cell carcinoma, intercellular bridges are also present.

   Answer E is incorrect. Acanthosis nigricans involves thickened hyperpigmented zones. These lesions can be associated with benign or malignant conditions elsewhere in the body, such as endocrine disorders or adenocarcinomas. Histologically, there is hyperkeratosis with prominent rete ridges and basal hyperpigmentation without melanocyte hyperplasia.

2. **The correct answer is E.** Aniline dyes such as naphthalene increase the risk of transitional cell carcinoma of the bladder. Other general risk factors include advanced age (typically a patient's sixth or seventh decade), tobacco use, and exposure to nitrosamines. Clinical symptoms of bladder cancer include hematuria, dysuria, and incontinence.

   Answer A is incorrect. Exposure to nitrosamines (compounds often found in smoked foods) increases one's risk of esophageal and gastric cancer.

   Answer B is incorrect. Infection with hepatitis B (HBV) and hepatitis C (HCV) viruses, as well as exposure to carbon tetrachloride, aflatoxins, and vinyl chloride, increase one's risk of hepatocellular carcinoma.

   Answer C is incorrect. Asbestos exposure increases the risk of mesothelioma and lung cancer.

   Answer D is incorrect. Infection with Epstein-Barr virus increases the risk of nasopharyngeal carcinoma.

3. **The correct answer is B.** The question describes a case of Zollinger-Ellison syndrome. Although gastrin-secreting tumors (called gastrinomas) are just as likely to arise in the duodenum and peripancreatic soft tissue as in the pancreas itself, the patient's long history of alcohol consumption makes a gastrinoma of pancreatic origin most likely secondary to malignant pancreatic islet cell tumors. Zollinger-Ellison syndrome arises from hypergastrinemia. Gastrin, which is normally produced by the G cells of the stomach antrum and duodenum, stimulates acid secretion by parietal cells in the stomach. Excess gastrin typically leads to excess acid production. Laboratory values commonly seen in this condition include increased basal and maximal acid output and serum gastrin levels >1000 pg/mL. Multiple peptic ulcerations are often the result. Excess gastrin secretion also promotes hypertrophy of the stomach mucosa. Increased stomach acid

leads to symptoms of gastroesophageal reflux disease, and to ulceration and gastric bleeding, as evidenced by this patient's melena. An elevated serum gastrin level would be diagnostic of gastrinoma.

Answer A is incorrect. Cholecystokinin (CCK) is produced by the I cells of the duodenum and jejunum. CCK stimulates gallbladder contraction and pancreatic enzyme secretion. CCK inhibits gastric acid secretion.

Answer C is incorrect. Intrinsic factor is released by the parietal cells of the stomach. Its principle function is to bind vitamin B_{12} to promote its absorption.

Answer D is incorrect. Secretin is produced normally by the S cells of the duodenum and promotes pancreatic bicarbonate secretion. It inhibits gastric acid secretion.

Answer E is incorrect. Somatostatin is produced by the pancreatic islets and gastrointestinal (GI) mucosa. Somatostatin inhibits gastric acid and pepsinogen secretion and also counteracts cholecystokinin and secretin activity. Somatostatin also inhibits the release of insulin and glucagons.

4. **The correct answer is C.** The vignette describes a superior sulcus tumor, otherwise known as Pancoast tumor. Although Pancoast tumors may be lung neoplasms of any type, primary squamous cell carcinomas are the most commonly seen. Located in the apex of the affected lung, the tumor compresses the cervical sympathetic plexus as it grows, resulting in shoulder pain, Horner syndrome (ipsilateral ptosis, miosis, and anhidrosis), and sometimes neurologic deficits such as ipsilateral hand weakness and hoarseness. Because the patient's symptoms are ipsilateral to the damaged plexus, the tumor must be located in the apex of the left lung.

   Answer A is incorrect. Pancoast tumor is a squamous cell carcinoma.

   Answer B is incorrect. Pancoast tumor is a squamous cell carcinoma. A tumor in the right apex would not result in left-sided symptoms, as described in this patient.

   Answer D is incorrect. A tumor in the right apex would not result in left-sided symptoms.

   Answer E is incorrect. Although squamous cell carcinoma of the lung usually appears centrally about the hilum, a tumor in this location would not cause Horner syndrome.

5. **The correct answer is C.** The lighter epithelium well above the gastroesophageal junction in the image is the characteristic appearance of Barrett esophagus. It may also be described as velvety Barrett esophagus, which is a precursor lesion to esophageal adenocarcinoma in which intestinal epithelium replaces normal squamous epithelium of the distal esophagus. If not already taking a proton-pump inhibitor, the patient should be started on one to prevent and reverse dysplasia.

   Answer A is incorrect. Bismuth can be used to acutely treat reflux and is part of "triple therapy" to eradicate *Helicobacter pylori*; however, it is not used to treat Barrett esophagus.

   Answer B is incorrect. Calcium carbonate is an over-the-counter treatment for the acute relief of gastroesophageal reflux disease. It has no role in preventing reflux or treating Barrett esophagus.

   Answer D is incorrect. Ranitidine is an H_2-blocker that can be used to treat mild reflux. This patient has a precancerous lesion (Barrett esophagus) as a result of his long-standing gastroesophageal reflux disease; thus, treatment with an H_2-blocker alone is inappropriate.

   Answer E is incorrect. Sucralfate works by coating the gastric mucosa. It is not indicated to treat Barett's esophagus.

6. **The correct answer is D.** This patient likely has a deep vein thrombosis (DVT) complicated by a pulmonary embolus. She is predisposed to DVT by long hours of inactivity and use of oral contraception. Unfractionated heparin is the most appropriate initial therapy. It works by catalyzing the activation of antithrombin III, decreasing the level of available thrombin, and inhibiting factor Xa. The

degree of heparinization can be monitored by measuring the partial thromboplastin time (PTT), which is a measure of the intrinsic coagulation pathway.

Answer A is incorrect. Bleeding time is a measure of platelet function. Any disorder of platelet function or one that affects platelet function, such as von Willebrand disease, would result in an increase in bleeding time.

Answer B is incorrect. The International Normalized Ratio (INR) is a means of standardizing prothrombin time (PT) measurements from laboratory to laboratory. INR must be monitored in patients who are treated with warfarin. Therapeutic INR is between 2 and 3.

Answer C is incorrect. A patient who is treated with low-molecular-weight heparin (LMWH) needs no laboratory monitoring. However, this patient is unlikely to be treated with LMWH, which is more expensive and more difficult to reverse in the case of supratherapeutic anticoagulation. The initial therapy of choice for inpatient anticoagulation (absent specific contraindications) is still heparin.

Answer E is incorrect. PT is a measure of the extrinsic coagulation pathway. This value must be monitored when warfarin is used as an anticoagulant.

7. **The correct answer is A.** Symptoms of increased intracranial pressure (nausea and vomiting), in conjunction with cerebellar signs of nystagmus and truncal ataxia in a young child are highly suspicious for a diagnosis of medulloblastoma, which arises in the cerebellum. This lesion is the most common malignant brain tumor in children. Histologically, tumor cells are small, with reduced cytoplasm and crescent-shaped, deeply-staining nuclei (due to high mitotic activity) arranged in pseudorosettes that form sheets of anaplastic cells. These tumors often respond to radiotherapy.

   Answer B is incorrect. This description is characteristic of glioblastoma multiforme, the most common primary adult brain tumor. It is generally localized to the cerebral cortex, and typically presents with severe headache and symptoms consistent with increased intracranial pressure. The prognosis is poor, with most mortality occurring within the first year, and a five-year survival rate of near zero. Glioblastoma multiforme is rarely found in children.

   Answer C is incorrect. This description is consistent with a diagnosis of oligodendroglioma, a relatively rare, slow-growing, benign tumor that is most often found in the frontal lobes. General symptoms include headaches, seizures, and changes in cognition, while focal lesions can present with localized weakness, sensory loss, or aphasia. The tumor consists of cells that have round nuclei with clear cytoplasm (an appearance resembling a fried egg), and are often associated with areas of calcification.

   Answer D is incorrect. This describes a craniopharyngioma, the most common supratentorial tumor in children, which is derived from embryological remnants of Rathke pouch. The clinical presentation typically involves severe headaches, visual changes, and growth failure secondary to pituitary dysfunction. Incidence peaks in children and in the fifth decade of life.

   Answer E is incorrect. This is a description of a meningioma, a benign primary intracranial neoplasm localized to the meninges. Clinically, these tumors often present with seizures or a neurologic deficit that gradually worsens over time secondary to mass effect. Focal symptoms can vary by location; however, a meningeally-derived neoplasm is unlikely to result in radiologic findings localized to the cerebellar vermis, as in this case.

8. **The correct answer is C.** This patient suffers from acute intermittent porphyria (AIP), an autosomal-dominant disorder caused by a lack of uroporphyrinogen I synthetase. The buildup of toxic levels of δ-aminolevulinate (ALA) and porphobilinogen lead to the associated symptoms of abdominal pain (more than 90% of cases), neuropathy, high sympathetic tone, and neuropsychiatric disturbances, including anxiety, depression, seizures, and paranoia. AIP almost never presents before puberty, and

it can be hard to diagnose because of its acute nature. Untreated, it can lead to paralysis and death.

Answer A is incorrect. The differential diagnosis for chest pain is long and includes cardiac, pulmonary, GI, and musculoskeletal etiologies. However, attacks of acute intermittent porphyria are not associated with chest pain.

Answer B is incorrect. Due to the high sympathetic tone caused by the pain of the crisis, hypertension may be associated with acute intermittent porphyria, but not hypotension.

Answer D is incorrect. Polyphagia, or greatly increased hunger, is one of the cardinal symptoms associated with diabetes mellitus, not acute intermittent porphyria.

Answer E is incorrect. A stiff neck may be associated with meningeal irritation and can be found in meningitis or with musculoskeletal problems, but it is not found in acute intermittent porphyria.

9. **The correct answer is B.** Epstein-Barr virus is closely associated with the African and AIDS cases of Burkitt lymphoma. By light microscopy, Burkitt lymphoma has a classic "starry-sky" appearance, made up of monomorphic medium-size cells with deep basophilic cytoplasm and numerous tingible body macrophages. Immunohistochemistry stains demonstrate that the tumor cells are made up of CD10-positive monoclonal B lymphocytes. Ninety percent of Burkitt lymphoma cases contain a *c-myc* translocation.

Answer A is incorrect. Adult T-lymphocyte leukemia is most commonly associated with human T-cell lymphotropic virus-1 (HTLV-1). HTLV-1 is endemic to southwest Japan, South America, central Africa, and the Caribbean, and is transmitted through blood products, breast milk, and sexual secretions. Adult T-lymphocyte leukemia arises in 1%-5% of HTLV-1-positive patients. In adult T-lymphocyte leukemia, the neoplastic cells have multilobated nuclei (in a clover leaf pattern), and will often invade the dermis and subcutaneous tissue layers.

Answer C is incorrect. Epidemiologic studies indicate human papilloma virus (HPV) infections as the most important risk factor for the development of cervical cancer. The majority of anal, perianal, vulvar, and penile cancers, as well as some oropharyngeal squamous cell cancers, also appear to be linked to HPV infection. There are high- and low-risk strains of HPV, the major difference being that the low-risk strains are maintained as extrachromosomal DNA episomes in infected cells, whereas the high-risk HPV genome becomes integrated into the host cellular DNA. This recombination event often leaves the viral oncogenes E6 and E7 coupled to the viral promoter and enhancer sequences, allowing their continued expression after integration. E7 inactivates the *Rb* protein, whereas E6 causes destruction of p53. This leads to resistance to apoptosis and allows cells with DNA damage to survive and proliferate. Ultimately, there may be progression to malignancy. Histologically, 90%-95% of invasive cervical cancers are squamous cell carcinomas (<5% are adenocarcinoma). On light microscopy, early invasive cancers appear as a tiny bud of invasive cells penetrating through the basement membrane and pushing into the underlying stroma. Lymphocytic collections in the stroma represent a reaction to invasion.

Answer D is incorrect. Both HBV and HCV infections are associated with the development of hepatocellular carcinoma (HCC). HBV causes HCC through a combination of chronic hepatic inflammation and integration of the viral genome into the host DNA. Histopathology of HCC from HBV or HCV varies, depending on the degree of differentiation of the tumor, but most commonly has a trabecular pattern and is closely associated to cirrhosis.

Answer E is incorrect. Human herpesvirus 8 genome segments have been identified in >90% of patients with Kaposi sarcomas, suggesting a causative role. Kaposi sarcoma is caused by a proliferation of spindle cells from a single clone of endothelial cell origin. Histologic findings include proliferation of spindle cells, prominent slit-like vascular spaces, and extravasated RBCs.

10. **The correct answer is E.** This patient suffers from von Willebrand disease (vWD), the most common inherited bleeding disorder. This disorder is a result of functional problems with vWD factor. This factor serves as the ligand for platelet adhesion to a damaged vessel wall. It also is the plasma carrier for factor VIII. The disease may be acquired (via malignancy, autoimmunity, or drug therapy) through antibodies directed against the factor, or it may be inherited (typically in an autosomal dominant pattern). The unique lab findings in vWD (platelet dysfunction and lack of a carrier for factor VIII) result in increased bleeding time and an increased PTT.

    Answer A is incorrect. Bernard-Soulier disease is an inherited defect in platelet adhesion due to decreased surface expression of glycoprotein Ib. Laboratory tests would reveal an increased bleeding time, normal platelet count, normal PT, and normal PTT.

    Answer B is incorrect. Glanzmann thrombocytopenia is an autosomal recessive disorder in which platelets do not have the glycoprotein IIb/IIIa receptor, which normally binds fibrinogen. This defect results in abnormal platelet aggregation. However, PTT is normal.

    Answer C is incorrect. Hemophilia A is an X-linked disorder that causes factor VIII deficiency. Bleeding frequently occurs in joints and the retroperitoneal space. Laboratory tests would reveal an increased PTT and normal bleeding time (because there is no inherent platelet disorder).

    Answer D is incorrect. Vitamin K deficiency impairs coagulation factors II, VII, IX, and X, the function of which depends on vitamin K-mediated γ-carboxylation. Laboratory tests would reveal an elevated PT, elevated PTT, and a deficiency in factors II, VII, IX, and X.

11. **The correct answer is B.** This patient has sickle cell disease, an autosomal recessive disorder common in African-Americans. It arises from a missense mutation on the β-globin chain (valine to glutamic acid substitution). Under certain conditions such as dehydration, acidosis, and hypoxemia, sickle cell patients are at risk for RBC sickling, leading to microvascular occlusions and tissue ischemia. Vasoocclusion of the pulmonary capillaries causes acute chest syndrome. In addition, other complications include aseptic necrosis of the femoral head, aplastic crisis, sequestration crisis in the spleen, autosplenectomy, and increased susceptibility to infection by encapsulated bacteria. Chronic intravascular hemolysis predisposes these patients to calcium bilirubinate gallstones, which are radiopaque more often than cholesterol stones (10%-15% of cholesterol stones and ~50% of pigment stones contain enough calcium to be radiopaque). On the peripheral blood smear, one would detect normocytic RBCs admixed with sickle-shaped RBCs, increased reticulocytes, and Howell-Jolly bodies. Howell-Jolly bodies are nuclear remnants in RBCs that are a result of splenic dysfunction.

    Answer A is incorrect. Heinz bodies are precipitated hemoglobin, often associated with glucose-6-phosphate dehydrogenase (G6PD) deficiency. Heinz bodies can cause membrane damage, which the spleen recognizes and removes, producing the so-called "bite cells." Patients with G6PD deficiency do not present with acute chest syndrome.

    Answer C is incorrect. Microcytic RBCs are seen in iron deficiency anemia, not in sickle cell patients. In fact, peripheral smears from sickle cell patients show normocytic RBCs with increased reticulocytes.

    Answer D is incorrect. Ringed sideroblasts result from iron accumulation in the mitochondria secondary to defective heme synthesis. This is seen in patients with chronic alcoholism, vitamin B_6 deficiency, and lead poisoning. Clinical symptoms depend largely on the specific cause. However, ringed sideroblastic anemia does not produce vasoocclusive symptoms.

    Answer E is incorrect. Spherocytes are RBCs that appear round and lack the central indentation found normally in mature RBCs. Spherocytes may be acquired or congenital. Congenital or hereditary spherocytosis is an autosomal dominant disorder involving mutations in the ankyrin or spectrin proteins; these proteins provide RBC membrane with its structural integrity. A portion of this unstable membrane is removed by the spleen during the RBCs' life cycle, resulting in the characteristic spherical shape of this disease. These patients may present with splenomegaly and aplastic crisis but not vasoocclusive symptoms.

12. **The correct answer is C.** This patient has symptoms, physical findings, and a peripheral blood smear suggestive of acute myelogenous leukemia (AML). The image has a classic "Auer rod" in the cytoplasm. Auer rods are are fused lysosomal granules. A sudden release of Auer's rods may cause acute disseminated intravascular coagulation (DIC) and fatal hemorrhage. DIC is a disorder in which activation of the coagulation cascade leads to the development of microthrombi and the consumption of platelets, fibrin, and coagulation factors. Lab findings in DIC include increased PT and PTT, an elevation in fibrin split products, and thrombocytopenia. A peripheral blood smear of a patient with DIC would reveal helmet-shaped cells and schistocytes. Schistocytes are irregularly shaped or fragmented RBC forms that are generated when RBCs attempt to squeeze through the fibrin meshwork associated with small vessel thrombi.

    Answer A is incorrect. Acanthocytes (sometimes called spur cells) are spiny RBCs that are associated with abetalipoproteinemia as well as severe liver disease.

    Answer B is incorrect. Burr cells (also known as echinocytes) are abnormal RBCs with short, blunt projections around the periphery. These cells can be seen in hemolytic-uremic syndrome, pyruvate kinase deficiency, uremia, and other disorders.

    Answer D is incorrect. Target cells are abnormal RBCs with a "bull's-eye" appearance. They are seen in a variety of conditions including asplenia, liver disease, and thalassemia.

    Answer E is incorrect. Teardrop cells are abnormal RBCs seen in the setting of myeloid metaplasia with myelofibrosis. Some have posited that the teardrop morphology results from the RBCs trying to squeeze out of fibrotic bone marrow.

13. **The correct answer is B.** The liver and lung are the most common sites of metastasis (after lymph nodes) because of the high blood flow through these organs. Therefore, primary tumors in any of the locations listed as possible answers may metastasize to the liver. However, given that the blood vessels from the GI tract drain into the hepatic circulation, the most likely primary tumor that metastasizes to the liver would be from a GI source such as the colon.

    Answer A is incorrect. Breast tumors may also metastasize to the liver, but with less frequency than GI cancers. Breast metastases are found more often in brain and bone.

    Answer C is incorrect. Tumors of the kidney, such as renal cell carcinoma, metastasize to the brain and bone, and less so to the liver.

    Answer D is incorrect. Metastatic involvement of the liver is far more common than primary neoplasia. Multiple tumors in the liver suggests that the primary tumor exists in another organ.

    Answer E is incorrect. Lung tumors often metastasize to brain and bone, and less often to the liver.

14. **The correct answer is C.** Lead inhibits ALA dehydratase and ferrochelatase, preventing both porphobilinogen formation and the incorporation of iron into protoporphyrin IX, the final step in heme synthesis. Inhibition of both of these steps results in ineffective heme synthesis and subsequent microcytic (hemoglobin-poor) anemia.

    Answer A is incorrect. Lead poisoning does not affect iron absorption from the gut.

    Answer B is incorrect. Lead inhibits ALA dehydratase, preventing porphyrin synthesis beyond the formation of ALA; it does not increase its actions. This causes ALA to accumulate in the urine.

Answer D is incorrect. Lead does not have a high affinity for hemoglobin. This type of pathology is seen in carbon monoxide (CO) poisoning. CO binds to hemoglobin with much higher affinity than oxygen, resulting in decreased oxygen-carrying capacity.

Answer E is incorrect. Lead does not interrupt RBC DNA synthesis. Folate and/or vitamin B_{12} deficiencies disrupt DNA synthesis, specifically thiamine synthesis, resulting in megaloblastic changes in RBCs.

15. **The correct answer is A.** Based on the patient's symptoms and blood count, the physician suspects essential thrombocytosis and begins the patient on hydroxyurea. Essential thrombocytosis is a myeloproliferative disorder characterized by platelet overproduction by megakaryocytes; its cause is unknown. Patients exhibit epistaxis, thrombosis, bruising, bleeding, and mild splenomegaly. Patients also complain of erythromelalgia, which is burning and redness of the hands and feet caused by platelets obstructing blood flow in capillaries and arterioles. Older patients also may experience transient ischemic attacks. Hydroxyurea interferes with DNA synthesis by inhibiting ribonucleotide reductase, preventing conversion of ribonucleotides to deoxyribonucleotides. Hydroxyurea would thus decrease platelet production in this patient.

Answer B is incorrect. Immune thrombocytopenic purpura (ITP) is characterized by a low platelet count due to antibodies against platelets. The antibodies opsonize the platelets for phagocytosis by macrophages, causing platelet levels to fall. Patients usually are asymptomatic, but once the platelet level falls below 20,000/mm^3, they may have bleeding, manifested as bruising, petechiae, nosebleeds, or intracerebral hemorrhage. ITP usually is treated with steroids. This patient has thrombocytosis, not thrombocytopenia, so ITP is not a correct choice.

Answer C is incorrect. Polycythemia vera is a chronic myeloproliferative disorder characterized by increases in all three hematopoietic lineages, leading to excess RBC production (erythrocytosis), WBC production (leukocytosis), and platelet production (thrombocytosis). Patients can have constitutional findings such as headache or weakness; neurologic symptoms such as dizziness, tinnitus, or changes in vision; or abdominal pain from massive hepatosplenomegaly. The thrombocytosis associated with polycythemia vera is milder than that seen in essential thrombocytosis. In addition, this patient has no leukocytosis or changes in hemoglobin or hematocrit (Hct), making polycythemia vera an unlikely diagnosis.

Answer D is incorrect. Sickle cell disease is caused by hemoglobin S, a mutated variant of hemoglobin that leads to RBC "sickling" in deoxygenated blood. The sickled RBCs occlude blood vessels, depriving tissue of oxygen and leading to ischemia and vasoocclusive crises. Patients with sickle cell disease are anemic and functionally asplenic; this patient has neither condition. In addition, platelet levels are normal in sickle cell disease. Hydroxyurea is approved for use in sickle cell disease, because it increases expression of fetal globin chains, thereby providing a pool of functional hemoglobin.

Answer E is incorrect. Thrombotic thrombocytopenic purpura (TTP) is characterized by the formation of many blood clots, leading to a variety of symptoms. The classical findings are hemolytic anemia, thrombocytopenia, neurologic findings, impaired kidney function, and fever. TTP is a result of aggregation of platelets, setting off the coagulation cascade in blood vessels. When these microthrombi form, they circulate. Treatment is with plasmapheresis. This patient has none of these signs or symptoms; in fact, the patient has increased platelet levels.

16. **The correct answer is C.** In a minority of patients with cobalamin (vitamin B_{12}) deficiency, the Hct and mean corpuscular volume are normal. In these cases, laboratory testing for elevated methylmalonic acid can be used to make the diagnosis.

Answer A is incorrect. In patients with cobalamin deficiency, homocysteine levels typically are elevated. Homocysteine levels can be used to diagnose cobalamin deficiency in symptomatic patients in whom the Hct and mean corpuscular volume are normal.

Answer B is incorrect. Lactate dehydrogenase is increased in cobalamin deficiency because of failed hematopoiesis.

Answer D is incorrect. Because cobalamin deficiency impairs DNA synthesis in all cell lines, neutropenia with hypersegmented neutrophils typically is seen in cobalamin-deficient patients.

Answer E is incorrect. A positive anti-intrinsic factor antibody test suggests inhibition of the binding between intrinsic factor and cobalamin. Because this decreases absorption of the vitamin, antibodies against intrinsic factor can result in cobalamin deficiency and pernicious anemia.

Answer F is incorrect. The Schilling test localizes the cause of cobalamin deficiency, once a diagnosis has been made. Patients suspected of cobalamin deficiency are administered combinations of radioactive cobalamin, antibiotics, intrinsic factor, and pancreatic extracts, after which radioactivity in the urine is measured. A positive Schilling test implies a defect in cobalamin absorption.

17. **The correct answer is C.** This woman most likely suffers from iron deficiency anemia, as supported by her fatigue and signs of mucous membrane pallor. Furthermore, the peripheral blood smear showing small RBCs is consistent with the microcytic, hypochromic anemia of iron deficiency. In premenopausal women, pregnancy is a common cause of iron deficiency anemia due to increased iron demands. Other causes of iron deficiency anemia include blood loss, menorrhagia or GI bleeding, hookworm, poor diet, and malabsorption. Other causes of microcytic anemia include thalassemia, lead poisoning, and sideroblastic anemia. These are less likely causes of anemia than iron deficiency in a previously healthy pregnant woman. Iron deficiency anemia is characterized by a low ferritin level, high iron-binding capacity, and low mean corpuscular volume (MCV).

    Answer A is incorrect. A blood smear showing small RBCs is suggestive of a microcytic anemia with a low mean corpuscular volume (MCV), not a normocytic anemia with a normal MCV. Normocytic anemia can be caused by acute hemorrhage, enzyme defects (eg, glucose-6-phosphate dehydrogenase deficiency), RBC membrane defects, bone marrow disorders, hemoglobinopathies, autoimmune hemolytic anemia, and anemia of chronic disease.

    Answer B is incorrect. Iron deficiency anemia is a microcytic anemia and thus is accompanied by low, not high, MCV. High MCV indicates a macrocytic anemia, such as folate deficiency or vitamin B_{12} deficiency. Furthermore, iron deficiency anemia is associated with a high, not low, iron-binding capacity.

    Answer D is incorrect. Iron deficiency anemia is a microcytic anemia and thus is accompanied by low, not high, MCV. High MCV indicates a macrocytic anemia, which can be caused by a folate or vitamin B_{12} deficiency.

    Answer E is incorrect. Iron deficiency anemia is accompanied by a low, not high, ferritin level.

18. **The correct answer is E.** Trastuzumab is a recombinant human monoclonal antibody to human epidermal growth factor receptor 2 (*HER*-2). Trastuzumab is used to treat women with metastatic breast cancer that overexpresses the *HER*-2 oncogene. It acts by binding to the extracellular domain of the *HER*-2 receptor on cancer cells, preventing receptor stimulation and inhibiting cell growth.

    Answer A is incorrect. All-*trans* retinoic acid (ATRA) is a vitamin A derivative used to induce remission in patients with acute promyelocytic leukemia. ATRA is thought to bind to nuclear receptors and induce terminal cell division and differentiation of the neoplastic promyelocytes into mature WBCs.

    Answer B is incorrect. Imatinib mesylate is used to treat chronic myeloid leukemia. It works by blocking the ATP-binding site in the *bcr-abl* tyrosine kinase domain, thereby preventing autophosphorylation, and repressing signals for cell proliferation.

Answer C is incorrect. Methotrexate is an antimetabolite that acts as a folic acid analog. Methotrexate is used to treat trophoblastic neoplasms, leukemias, and cancers of the breast, head and neck, and lung. Given that this patient's cancer is known to overexpress *HER*-2, trastuzumab is the best answer.

Answer D is incorrect. Rituximab is a monoclonal antibody that interacts with the surface protein found on non-Hodgkin lymphoma cells. It is not used to treat breast cancer.

19. **The correct answer is E.** This patient is infected with *Leishmania donovani*, which is transmitted by the sandfly. Infection presents with hepatosplenomegaly, malaise, anemia, leukopenia, and weight loss. Microscopically, macrophages containing amastigotes are observed. Sodium stibogluconate is used to treat *L donovani* infection.

Answer A is incorrect. The *Aedes* mosquito spreads the flaviviruses responsible for dengue fever and yellow fever. Dengue fever is characterized by headache, myalgais, arthralgias, and a petechial rash; laboratory tests show thrombocytompenia and a relative leukopenia. Treatment is supportive. Yellow fever presents with fever, headache, back pain, and jaundice; the best treatment is prevention via vaccination.

Answer B is incorrect. The *Anopheles* mosquito transmits the *Plasmodium* species of protozoa that are responsible for malaria. Malaria presents with fevers accompanied by headaches, sweats, malaise, and anemia (due to lysed RBCs), but not leukopenia. Diagnosis is made by examining the patient's RBCs on blood films. Treatment is tailored to the geographic area of infection and the *Plasmodium* species involved; agents include chloroquine, hydroxychloroquine, and atovaquone-proguanil.

Answer C is incorrect. The *Ixodes* tick transmits the pathogens that cause babesiosis (*Babesia microti*, a protozoan), Lyme disease (*Borrelia burgdorferi*, a spirochete bacterium) and erlichiosis (*Ehrlichia chaffeensis*, a rickettsial bacterium). Infection with *Babesia* species presents with a malaria-like syndrome. On microscopic examination one observes the Maltese cross-appearing parasite but no RBC pigment. Quinine is used to treat babesiosis. Lyme disease classically presents with a circular, expanding rash that takes on the appearance of a bull's eye; it can proceed to involve many organs, notably the central and peripheral nervous systems, the joints, the eyes, and the heart. Lyme disease is diagnosed by exam findings and exposure history, with corroboration from serological testing. Treatment in adults is usually with doxycycline. Erlichiosis presents with a high fever, fatigue, and myalgias, and can cause leukopenia, thryombocytopenia and renal insufficiency. Diagnosis is again by exam and exposure history, with corroboration by serological testing. Treatment is with doxycycline.

Answer D is incorrect. The reduviid bug spreads the protozoan *Trypanosoma cruzi*. Chronic infection with *T cruzi* causes Chagas disease, a condition characterized by cardiomegaly and, often, dilation of the intestinal tract. Microscopic examination reveals flagellated trypomastigotes in the blood and nonmotile amastigotes in tissue culture. Nifurtimox is used to treat *T cruzi*.

20. **The correct answer is D.** This answer describes follicular lymphoma, the most common type of non-Hodgkin lymphoma in the US. The characteristic chromosomal translocation is t(14;18), which juxtaposes the immunoglobulin heavy-chain (IgH) locus on chromosome 14 next to the *BCL2* locus on chromosome 18. This causes overproduction of the *Bcl*-2 protein, an anti-apoptotic factor, facilitating the survival of the cancer. An important simplifying fact to help remember the different chromosomal translocations is that those involving the immunoglobulin loci on chromosome 14 tend to be cells that normally produce antibodies (eg, B lymphocytes). Thus these translocations are common in B-lymphocyte lymphomas.

Answer A is incorrect. The t(8;14) rearrangement is found most commonly in Burkitt lymphoma as well as in some cases of acute lymphocytic leukemia (ALL). Translocation of the *c-myc* gene next to the immunoglobulin heavy-chain (IgH) locus results in constitutive overproduction of the *c-myc* oncogene, promoting neoplastic proliferation.

Answer B is incorrect. The t(9;22) translocation results in the Philadelphia chromosome, which is found most commonly in chronic myelogenous leukemia (CML) as well as in other chronic myeloproliferative disorders and ALL, where it confers a poor prognosis. The translocation results in a *Bcr-Abl* fusion protein that functions as a constitutively active tyrosine kinase to promote leukemia growth. This fusion has allowed not only easier diagnosis and monitoring of disease, but the recent development of imatinib mesylate (Gleevec) for the treatment of CML. Imatinib is a competitive inhibitor of *Bcr-Abl*, platelet-derived growth factor, and *c-kit* tyrosine receptor kinases.

Answer C is incorrect. The t(11;22) chromosomal translocation is associated with Ewing sarcoma. (Note that it does not involve the immunoglobulin locus.) It overproduces a chimeric transcription factor that activates the *c-myc* promoter and produces excessive amounts of the *EWS-Fli*-1 protein. Ewing sarcoma is a small, round cell tumor of the bone usually found in the long bones of teenagers. X-ray will show a lytic tumor with reactive bone deposited around it in an onion-skin fashion.

Answer E is incorrect. The t(15;17) translocation denotes the acute pro-myelocytic leukemia (APL) subtype of AML. The characteristic fusion of the pro-myelocytic leukemia gene with the retinoic acid receptor-α(*RAR*α) gene blocks differentiation of immature myeloid blasts, most likely by blocking activity of other retinoic acid receptors. Treatment with all-*trans* retinoic acid (termed differentiation therapy) overwhelms the blockade of the other retinoic acid receptors, restores differentiation, and can induce temporary remission. Combination differentiation treatment together with conventional chemotherapy can result in long-term survival rates of 70%-80%, unique among the acute leukemias. APL patients typically also present with dysfunctional coagulopathies, predisposing them to excess bleeding, a major source of mortality.

21. **The correct answer is C.** Cyclosporine is an immunosuppressant that binds to cyclophilins. This complex inhibits calcineurin, triggering the inhibition of the production of interleukin-2 (IL-2) and blocking the differentiation and activation of T lymphocytes. Cyclosporine is metabolized by the cytochrome P450 system in the liver. Erythromycin is an inhibitor of P450 and causes increased concentrations of drugs processed via the system. Other inhibitors include isoniazid, sulfonamides, cimetidine, ketoconazole, and grapefruit juice.

Answer A is incorrect. Cyclosporine is notorious for causing nephrotoxicity. Erythromycin alone does not cause renal failure. However, by increasing the serum levels of cyclosporine, erythromycin treatment will increase the likelihood of renal failure.

Answer B is incorrect. Cyclophilin concentration is decreased as cyclosporine is increased and binds cyclophilin. Because erythromycin increases cyclosporine, cyclophilin levels fall.

Answer D is incorrect. Erythromycin and other macrolide antibiotics are known to cause *C difficile* colitis. *C difficile* infection is not opportunistic but is instead caused by overgrowth of *C difficile* in the colon when normal gut flora are killed by antibiotic treatment. Although the combination of erythromycin and cyclosporine therapy increases the serum concentration of cyclosporine, it has no effect on the concentration of erythromycin. There is therefore no increased risk of *C difficile* infection.

Answer E is incorrect. One rare complication of erythromycin treatment is prolongation of the QT_c interval and the risk for cardiac arrhythmia. Although the combination of erythromycin and cyclosporine therapy increases the serum concentration of cyclosporine, it has no effect on the concentration of erythromycin. There is therefore no increased risk of

QT_c prolongation with this drug combination compared with the use of erythromycin alone.

22. **The correct answer is E.** This patient presents with the classic signs and "symptoms" (night sweats, fever, and weight loss) of Hodgkin lymphoma. The diagnosis is confirmed by the presence of a Reed-Sternberg cell, which is shown in the image and is diagnostic for Hodgkin lymphoma. These cells are large, with lobed nuclei that look like "owl eyes." Vinblastine is part of the **ABVD** regimen (**A**driamycin [doxorubicin], **B**leomycin, **V**inblastine, and **D**acarbazine) used to treat Hodgkin lymphoma. It inhibits microtubular formation of the mitotic spindle, so affected cells cannot pass through metaphase. Vinblastine is used to treat both Hodgkin and non-Hodgkin lymphomas as well as many solid tumors. Adverse effects include alopecia, constipation, myelosuppression, and, rarely, neurotoxicity.

    Answer A is incorrect. Cyclosporine is an immunosuppressant used in transplant patients and patients with autoimmune disorders. It works by inhibiting the production and release of IL-2, a cytokine involved in the activation of cytotoxic T lymphocytes. Adverse effects of cyclosporine include GI upset, headache, and tremor. Notably, myelosuppression is not a common adverse effect.

    Answer B is incorrect. Hydroxyurea is used to treat sickle cell anemia, and to decrease the burden of high WBC counts in acute leukemia and CML. Hydroxyurea is an antimetabolite, and although its exact mechanism is unknown, it is believed to affect the synthesis (S) phase of the cell cycle. Its major adverse effect is myelosuppression.

    Answer C is incorrect. Imatinib is used to treat CML and GI stromal tumors, and would not be helpful in a patient with Hodgkin lymphoma. Patients with CML present with increased neutrophils and metamyelocytes. Imatinib is a tyrosine kinase inhibitor that specifically targets the continuously active *Bcr-Abl* receptor in CML, promoting apoptosis in these cells. Adverse effects include weight gain, GI distress, musculoskeletal pain, and myelosuppression.

    Answer D is incorrect. Isoniazid is one of the drugs used to treat tuberculosis (TB), along with rifampin, pyrazinamide, streptomycin, and ethambutol. Night sweats, fever, and weight loss are common in patients with TB; however, the presence of Reed-Sternberg cells in this patient strongly suggests Hodgkin lymphoma. Isoniazid inhibits mycolic acid synthesis, thereby disrupting the *Mycoplasma* cell wall. Adverse effects include hepatotoxicity, neuropathy, and potentially psychiatric symptoms.

23. **The correct answer is C.** This patient most likely has immune thrombocytopenic purpura, an autoimmune disease characterized by a low platelet count and easy bruising or bleeding through skin or mucous membranes. On blood smear platelets may be abnormally large, because of increased platelet production; there also tend to be more megakaryocytes in the marrow.

    Answer A is incorrect. Bite cells are RBCs with portions removed by splenic macrophages. They are often found in patients with hemolysis related to an enzyme deficiency.

    Answer B is incorrect. Drepanocytes, or sickled RBCs, are found in patients with sickle cell disease.

    Answer D is incorrect. Howell-Jolly bodies are retained chromosomes found in the RBCs of patients who have undergone splenectomy.

    Answer E is incorrect. Pappenheimer bodies are siderosomes, or iron bodies, seen on Wright stain of RBCs in patients with excess iron.

24. **The correct answer is B.** Wilms tumor arises from neoplastic embryonic renal cells of the metanephros. Wilms tumor is the most common solid tumor of childhood (most commonly occurring between the ages of two and four years) and is rarely seen in adults. It commonly presents with a large palpable flank mass and hemihypertrophy (abnormal enlarge-

ment of one side of the body). It is associated with the deletion of tumor suppressor gene *WT1* on chromosome 11. Because it arises from the kidney parenchyma, it distorts the kidney calyces as it grows

Answer A is incorrect. Adult polycystic kidney disease is an autosomal dominant disorder that presents with bilateral cystic enlargement of the kidneys. Individuals with this disorder also suffer from cystic enlargement of the liver, berry aneurysms, and mitral valve prolapse.

Answer C is incorrect. Clear cell carcinoma of the kidney is a malignancy derived from the renal tubular cells. It is common for patients to present with an abdominal mass, but patients with clear cell carcinoma are commonly men around 50-70 years of age, with an increased incidence found in smokers. Patients with renal cell carcinoma present with a range of symptoms, such as hematuria, a palpable mass, polycythemia, flank pain, and fever.

Answer D is incorrect. Transitional cell carcinoma (TCC) is a malignant tumor that arises from the uroepithelial cells of the urinary tract. TCC is the most common tumor of the urinary tract, and can occur in the renal calyx, renal pelvis, ureters, and bladder. Painless hematuria and urinary outflow obstruction are the most common presenting signs of TCC.

Answer E is incorrect. Neuroblastoma results from primitive neural crest cells and presents as an abdominal mass in young children. The tumor does not arise in the kidney; instead, it forms from the adrenal medulla and paraspinal sympathetic ganglia. Therefore it does not distort the kidney architecture.

25. **The correct answer is A.** This patient's history and physical exam, including prolonged morning stiffness and symmetrical joint involvement, are consistent with rheumatoid arthritis (RA). RA is often associated with anemia of chronic disease (ACD). ACD typically presents as a normocytic anemia as evidenced by a normal mean corpuscular volume (MCV). ACD occurs in patients with chronic inflammatory, infectious, malignant, or autoimmune diseases and is caused by ineffective iron incorporation into developing RBCs. ACD is associated with low total iron binding capacity as well as elevated ferritin levels. Other causes of normocytic anemia include acute hemorrhage, enzyme defects, RBC membrane defects, bone marrow disorders, hemoglobinopathies, and autoimmune hemolytic anemia.

Answer B is incorrect. Autoimmune hemolytic anemia (AIHA) is a normocytic anemia caused by antibody-mediated RBC destruction. There is no association between AIHA and RA. Significant laboratory findings include a positive direct antiglobulin test (also known as the Coombs test), low haptoglobin level, and elevated LDH cholesterol level. AIHA can be further categorized as warm or cold depending on whether the antibody causes a stronger reaction at 37°C or 4°C. Blood smears show numerous microspherocytes (warm) or marked RBC agglutination (cold).

Answer C is incorrect. Iron deficiency anemia is a common cause of anemia that is often due to occult blood loss in adults and dietary deficiency in young children. This type of anemia has no direct association with RA or most other chronic diseases. Blood smear should show a microcytic, hypochromic anemia, instead of a normocytic anemia. Other significant laboratory values include a decreased serum iron level, decreased serum ferritin level, decreased MCV, and increased total iron binding capacity.

Answer D is incorrect. Megaloblastic anemia is usually due to lack of either vitamin B_{12} or folate. Common causes include pernicious anemia, gastrectomy, disease of the terminal ileum, and dietary deficiency. This patient has a normocytic picture, not a macrocytic one, which makes megaloblastic anemia unlikely.

Answer E is incorrect. Sideroblastic anemia is a condition in which a defect exists in heme synthesis such that iron is deposited in a ring around the nucleus of the erythroblast. Blood smear should show the presence of these distinctive ring sideroblasts. Furthermore, sideroblastic anemia is a microcytic, microchromic anemia, not a normocytic anemia. This type of anemia can be found congenitally through gene defects such as a mutation in the alanine synthase gene or can be seen as a part of acquired diseases such as the myelodysplastic syndromes.

26. **The correct answer is A.** This patient is experiencing bleomycin toxicity, which causes pulmonary fibrosis, interstitial pneumonitis, and skin changes, especially hyperpigmentation. The pulmonary complications of bleomycin are dose dependent and therefore occur late in the treatment course when the cumulative dose becomes high. The incidence of pulmonary toxicity is approximately 10%. Bleomycin is notable for causing minimal myelosuppression compared to other chemotherapeutic agents.

    Answer B is incorrect. Busulfan, an alkylating agent, is also known for causing pulmonary fibrosis and hyperpigmentation. Unlike bleomycin, however, busulfan causes myelosuppression in almost 100% of patients.

    Answer C is incorrect. Dactinomycin is an antineoplastic agent that intercalates in DNA, inhibiting DNA and RNA synthesis. Its adverse effects include cardiotoxicity, nausea, vomiting, and myelosuppression.

    Answer D is incorrect. The toxic effects of doxorubicin include cardiotoxicity, myelosuppression, and alopecia. Toxic injury to the myocardium is dose dependent, and cardiotoxicity results from doses >500 mg/m^2. Congestive heart failure could present with a nonproductive cough and exertional dyspnea, but this patient is also suffering from hyperpigmentation and minimal myelosuppression, making bleomycin the best answer.

    Answer E is incorrect. The toxic effects of vinblastine include neurotoxicity (areflexia, peripheral neuropathy, paralytic ileus) and bone marrow suppression. Remember the mnemonic, "Vin**blast**ine **blasts** bone marrow."

27. **The correct answer is F.** This patient has signs and symptoms of cobalamin (vitamin B_{12}) deficiency. Cobalamin deficiency can present with pallor and mild jaundice because of increased RBC breakdown stemming from ineffective erythropoiesis. Other physical findings include angular stomatitis (fissuring at the corners of the mouth) and painful glossitis (a shiny, "beefy" tongue). Patients with cobalamin deficiency also experience symmetric neuropathy, especially of the lower extremities. The peripheral blood smear demonstrates macrocytosis and hypersegmented neutrophils. The most common cause of cobalamin deficiency is pernicious anemia, a disorder in which dietary cobalamin is not absorbed as a result of gastric parietal cell atrophy and the subsequent absence of intrinsic factor.

    Answer A is incorrect. Bacterial overgrowth in an intestinal blind loop can lead to competition for dietary cobalamin. Provided cobalamin intake is adequate, floral overgrowth is a less common cause of cobalamin deficiency.

    Answer B is incorrect. Gastrectomy can result in insufficient intrinsic factor secretion and subsequent cobalamin deficiency. However, it is not the most common cause of this megaloblastic anemia.

    Answer C is incorrect. Infection with the fish tapeworm *Diphyllobothrium latum* can also result in competition for dietary cobalamin.

    Answer D is incorrect. Nutritional deficiency is a rare cause of cobalamin deficiency and is seen in patients who have adhered to strict vegan diets over several years. Bodily stores of cobalamin are large (on the order of years) and must be depleted before a deficiency can develop.

    Answer E is incorrect. Pancreatic insufficiency results in decreased or absent levels of pancreatic proteases, which free cobalamin from carrier proteins and allow it to bind intrinsic factor. Pancreatic insufficiency is a less common cause of cobalamin deficiency.

28. **The correct answer is D.** Although her symptoms may be somewhat nonspecific, the fact that this patient has small-cell lung carcinoma (SCLC) hints that her symptoms may be part of a paraneoplastic syndrome. SCLC is notorious for production of ACTH and ADH. In this case, excessive ACTH production has led

to increased glucocorticoids. Weight gain and redistribution of body fat (in contrast to the cachexia typical of cancers alone) and moon facies are classic signs of Cushing syndrome. Poor wound healing (due to inhibition of collagen synthesis by glucocorticoids) and facial plethora are also part of Cushing syndrome.

Answer A is incorrect. Cold intolerance and constipation are symptoms of hypothyroidism.

Answer B is incorrect. This patient is likely suffering from decreased bone density secondary to increased glucocorticoid activity. Patients with Cushing syndrome often develop osteoporosis.

Answer C is incorrect. Insatiable thirst and polyuria are symptoms of ADH deficiency or diabetes insipidus.

Answer E is incorrect. Proximal muscle weakness and palpitations are symptoms of hyperthyroidism. Although Cushing syndrome can also cause proximal limb weakness from selective atrophy of fast-twitch (type 2) myofibers, it does not have the cardiac effects of hyperthyroidism.

29. **The correct answer is B.** This woman suffers from hereditary spherocytosis (HS), typically caused by mutations in the genes that code for either ankyrin or spectrin; these are proteins that contribute to the RBC cytoskeleton. Instability in the RBC cytoskeleton results in the formation of spherocytes, which are small RBCs with a characteristic lack of central pallor. HS is a type of hemolytic anemia often associated with splenomegaly, jaundice, and pigmented gallstones. An osmotic fragility test is used to confirm the diagnosis. Coombs test is negative in patients with HS.

Answer A is incorrect. A mechanical heart valve can cause a hemolytic anemia due to mechanical trauma to the RBCs as they flow across the foreign surface. This results in schistocytes in the peripheral blood smear, not spherocytes. Furthermore, it would not account for this patient's symptoms.

Answer C is incorrect. A mutation in the gene encoding glucose 6-phosphate dehydrogenase (G6PD) can cause G6PD deficiency. This is an X-linked mutation and therefore typically occurs only in male patients. Heinz bodies may be found in the peripheral blood smear.

Answer D is incorrect. Circulating antibodies targeted against RBCs can cause autoimmune hemolytic anemia. This will result in a positive Coombs test.

Answer E is incorrect. Iron deficiency can cause a nonhemolytic, microcytic anemia that can result in microcytic RBCs with increased central pallor in the peripheral blood smear, not spherocytes.

30. **The correct answer is C.** This patient's cancer was treated with methotrexate, a folic acid analog that inhibits dihydrofolate reductase, halting DNA synthesis. It is specific for the S-phase of the cell cycle, so rapidly dividing cancer cells are targeted. Myelosuppression may occur, because the production of blood cell progenitors in the bone marrow is also inhibited. Myelosuppression can be reversed with leucovorin, an analog of folate, which counters the effects of methotrexate.

Answer A is incorrect. Epoetin can be used to ameliorate bone marrow toxicity through stimulation of erythroid proliferation. However, this will not correct the pancytopenia caused by methotrexate.

Answer B is incorrect. Administration of a granulocyte colony stimulating factor drug such as filgrastim is useful in correcting neutropenia post-chemotherapy, but it does not correct pancytopenia as seen in this patient.

Answer D is incorrect. Iron supplementation is useful to correct for iron deficiency anemia, which is a microcytic, hypochromic anemia, and usually results from blood loss due to menstruation or GI bleeding. This patient has pancytopenia due to methotrexate therapy, which is reversed with leucovorin.

Answer E is incorrect. A vitamin B_{12} replacement is often administered via intramuscular injection. This vitamin reverses megaloblastic anemia due to autoimmune-mediated deficiency of intrinsic factor produced by the parietal cells of the stomach. This patient has pancytopenia due to methotrexate therapy, which is reversed with leucovorin.

31. **The correct answer is B.** Multiple myeloma (MM) must be on the differential diagnosis in any elderly patient with pathologic fractures. MM is a bone marrow neoplasm, specifically the plasma cell. The bone marrow biopsy findings are consistent with MM. Plasma cells can be seen throughout this image, recognized by their off-center nuclei and clock-face chromatin distribution. Also commonly seen on a blood smear are stacked RBCs, in what is known as a rouleaux formation. Because MM is a tumor arising from bone, it causes destructive bone lesions, which causes hypercalcemia.

    Answer A is incorrect. Aplastic anemia is a pancytopenia that manifests as anemia, thrombocytopenia, and neutropenia. Biopsies show a hypocellular marrow with fatty infiltration. This slide (image) has too many cells to represent aplastic anemia.

    Answer C is incorrect. Because MM is a tumor arising from within bone, it causes destructive bone lesions that result in elevated (not reduced) serum calcium levels.

    Answer D is incorrect. Lymphoma is a neoplastic disorder of the lymphoid tissue. There are many different types of lymphoma, two of the most distinctive histologic types being Burkitt lymphoma and Hodgkin lymphoma. Burkitt lymphoma shows a "starry sky" pattern on histology. This pattern is created by macrophage ingestion of tumor cells. Hodgkin lymphoma is distinguished by its Reed-Sternberg cells. The Reed-Sternberg cells are binucleate and display prominent nucleoli. There are no Reed-Sternberg cells in this image, and the clinical picture is more consistent with MM than lymphoma.

    Answer E is incorrect. While a slight increase in prostate-specific antigen is normal with aging, severely elevated levels indicate prostate cancer. It commonly metastasizes to the axial skeleton and can cause back pain and spinal cord compression. It causes osteoblastic lesions in bone, although the rib would be an unusual location. However, bone marrow biopsies should be normal.

32. **The correct answer is A.** This man appears to be suffering from an acute stroke (cerebrovascular accident or CVA). After confirming that it is not a hemorrhagic stroke with a CT scan, the next step in treatment is administration of tissue plasminogen activator (tPA) if the duration of stroke has been <3 hours. The major adverse effect of tPA is bleeding. Excess bleeding must be reversed with aminocaproic acid, which blocks the conversion of plasminogen to plasmin.

    Answer B is incorrect. Protamine sulfate is used to reverse the effects of heparin. It is a positively-charged molecule that binds to negatively charged heparin molecules, thereby neutralizing the molecule and rendering it ineffective. Protamine sulfate would not reverse bleeding associated with tPA.

    Answer C is incorrect. Recombinant factor VIII is used to treat hemophilia A. These patients do not make factor VIII so it must be replaced. It would not reverse bleeding associated with tPA.

    Answer D is incorrect. tPA is an enzyme that normally cleaves plasminogen to plasmin. Plasmin then facilitates the breakdown of fibrin clots. It is the cause of the bleeding in this individual, not the antidote.

    Answer E is incorrect. Vitamin K is cofactor for epoxide reductase, which is responsible for making clotting factors II, VII, IX, and X. It is used to treat warfarin overdose along with fresh frozen plasma. Vitamin K would not reverse bleeding associated with tPA.

33. **The correct answer is A.** This patient presents with metastatic gastric adenocarcinoma and peritoneal carcinomatosis. The image shows a diffusely infiltrating signet ring cell carcinoma of the stomach, with large vacuoles of mucin displacing the nuclei of cells. Physical findings may include Virchow node (left clavicular node), Sister Mary Joseph node (umbilical nodes), Blumer's shelf node (superior rectum), and new-onset ascites. Gastric cancer is associ-

ated with dietary nitrosamines, Japanese ethnicity, *Helicobacter pylori* infection, and pernicious anemia.

Answer B is incorrect. Oral contraceptives are associated with hepatic adenomas.

Answer C is incorrect. Low dietary folate is associated with neural tube defects in pregnancy.

Answer D is incorrect. Polyvinyl chloride is associated with hepatic angiosarcomas.

Answer E is incorrect. Prior TB is associated with disseminated, miliary, or reactivation TB, with classic lesions in vertebral bodies (Pott disease) and the psoas muscle.

34. **The correct answer is B.** This patient presents with some of the classic adverse effects of steroid therapy, which is often part of treatment for Hodgkin disease via the **MOPP** cancer chemotherapy regimen: **M**echlorethamine, vincristine (**O**ncovin), **P**rocarbazine, and **P**rednisone. These include the physical signs of Cushing syndrome (weight gain, moon facies, thin skin, muscle weakness, and brittle bones), along with cataracts, hypertension, increased appetite, elevated blood sugar level, indigestion, insomnia, nervousness, restlessness, and immunosuppression. Prednisone is known to produce profound mood changes known as glucocorticoid psychosis.

Answer A is incorrect. The typical adverse effects of bleomycin are pulmonary fibrosis, skin changes, and myelosuppression. Bleomycin is part of the **ABVD** cancer chemotherapy regimen against Hodgkin: **A**driamycin (doxorubicin), **B**leomycin, **V**inblastine, and **D**acarbazine.

Answer C is incorrect. Common adverse effects of vincristine are areflexia and peripheral neuritis. Vincristine is part of the **MOPP** cancer chemotherapy regimen used against Hodgkin disease: **M**echlorethamine, vincristine (**O**ncovin), **P**rocarbazine, and **P**rednisone.

Answer D is incorrect. Wildly swinging mood is suggestive of cyclothymic disorders, which are common in patients with chronic medical illness. Cyclothymic disorders cannot be diagnosed until the patient has experienced two years of mood symptoms.

Answer E is incorrect. The progression of Hodgkin disease typically does not involve profound psychiatric symptoms.

35. **The correct answer is A.** The patient has a hydatidiform mole. Hydatidiform moles are cystic swellings of the chorionic villi. They usually present in the fourth and fifth months of pregnancy with vaginal bleeding. On examination, the uterus is larger than expected for gestational age, and the serum β-human chorionic gonadotropin (β-hCG) level is much higher than normal. Moles can be either partial or complete and are caused by either fertilization of an egg that has lost its chromosomes or fertilization of a normal egg with two sperm. Partial moles may contain some fetal tissue but no viable fetus, and a complete mole contains no fetal tissue. Hydatidiform moles must be surgically removed, because the chorionic villi may embolize to distant sites and because hydatidiform moles may lead to choriocarcinoma, an aggressive neoplasm that metastasizes early but is very responsive to chemotherapy.

Answer B is incorrect. Coma is a possible outcome of eclampsia, not an outcome of a hydatidiform mole. Preeclampsia is the triad of hypertension, proteinuria, and edema seen in pregnancy. Eclampsia occurs when seizures accompany the symptoms of preeclampsia. This patient has none of these symptoms.

Answer C is incorrect. Neural tube defects are usually detected in utero by increased α-fetoprotein levels in amniotic fluid and maternal serum; β-hCG levels are normal in these patients.

Answer D is incorrect. Ovarian cancers are often accompanied by an increase in blood cancer antigen 125 levels, not β-hCG levels. This patient has a hydatidiform mole, not ovarian cancer. Hydatidiform moles do not predispose patients to ovarian cancer.

Answer E is incorrect. If undetected, tubal pregnancies may rupture, causing unilateral lower quadrant pain and uterine bleeding. Because the patient may exsanguinate, ruptured ectopic pregnancy is a surgical emergency. This patient does not have the symptoms of a tubal pregnancy. Also, because of the small size of the fallopian tubes, tubal pregnancies present long before four months of gestation.

36. **The correct answer is A.** In thalassemia major, hypochromic, microcytic anemia is seen, and the reticulocyte count is elevated due to increased production of RBCs by the bone marrow.

Answer B is incorrect. These indices are consistent with iron-deficiency anemia.

Answer C is incorrect. A mean corpuscular volume $\geq$100 suggests megalobastic anemia, which is not consistent with the patient's thalassemia major observed on the peripheral blood smear. Classically, megaloblastic anemia is caused by either vitamin B_{12} or folate deficiency.

Answer D is incorrect. The mean corpuscular volume suggests a normocytic, normochromic anemia, which includes the hemolytic anemias. However, because the serum iron level is increased, sideroblastic anemia should be suspected if these lab values are found.

Answer E is incorrect. These RBC parameters (Hct, hemoglobin) are consistent with anemia, and the mean corpuscular volume suggests a normocytic, normochromic anemia. The anemia is most likely due to chronic disease.

37. **The correct answer is F.** This vignette suggests a hepatoma (hepatocellular carcinoma), which is associated with an elevated α-fetoprotein level. Hepatomas are highly associated with chronic HBV and HCV infections. Other risk factors include Wilson disease, hemochromatosis, alcoholic cirrhosis, α_1-antitrypsin deficiency, and exposure to toxins and carcinogens such as aflatoxin. α-Fetoprotein is a marker for hepatomas, but levels can also be elevated in patients with germ cell tumors, such as yolk sac tumors. Yolk sac tumors (also known as endodermal sinus tumors) arise from the germ cells that eventually become the adult gonads. Yolk sac tumors are the most common malignant testicular and ovarian tumors in children. Remember, tumor markers should not be used to make the primary diagnosis, but for confirmation and to monitor the response to therapy.

Answer A is incorrect. The marker for choriocarcinoma is β-hCG. This marker is also elevated with hydatidiform moles and gestational trophoblastic tumors. Hepatomas are not known to elevate β-hCG levels.

Answer B is incorrect. The marker for colorectal carcinoma is carcinoembryonic antigen (CEA). This marker is nonspecific and is also produced by pancreatic, gastric, and breast carcinomas. Most tumors of endoderm origin can release CEA excluding hepatomas. However, secondary tumors in the liver from malignant colon cancer may also present with increased CEA levels.

Answer C is incorrect. The marker for melanoma is S-100. This marker also is elevated with neuroendocrine tumors such as astrocytomas and even carcinoid tumors. Hepatomas are not known to elevate S-100 levels.

Answer D is incorrect. The marker for neuroblastoma is bombesin. This marker also is elevated with lung and gastric cancers. Hepatomas are not known to elevate bombesin levels.

Answer E is incorrect. The marker for prostatic carcinoma is prostate-specific antigen. Hepatomas are not known to elevate prostate-specific antigen levels.

38. **The correct answer is E.** High levels of IgM on immunofixation, coupled with the predominance of plasma cells in the bone marrow biopsy, are consistent of Waldenström macroglobulinemia. Waldenström macroglobulinemia is a B-lymphocyte lymphoproliferative disorder that often results in a syndrome of blood hyperviscosity secondary to increased levels of IgM (both heavy and light chains), which are secreted by neoplastic plasma cells. It is most commonly seen in adults who have lymphoplasmacytic lymphoma. Bone marrow biopsy reveals diffuse infiltrates of lymphocytes, plasma cells, and intermediate

plasmacytoid lymphocytes; there is often reactive hyperplasia of mast cells. Patients with Waldenström macroglobulinemia often present with similar abnormalities to those listed (mild anemia, blood urea nitrogen on the upper limit of normal, and increased total protein). They experience a variety of signs and symptoms such as constitutional symptoms, episodic bleeding, lymphadenopathy, and hepatosplenomegaly. Visual changes, dementia, ataxia, and vertigo are symptoms of hyperviscosity.

Answer A is incorrect. Heavy-chain disease encompasses a number of disorders including chronic lymphocytic leukemia/small lymphocytic lymphoma, lymphoplasmacytic lymphoma, and Mediterranean lymphoma. The common feature of these disorders is that they secrete free heavy-chain fragments. Bone marrow biopsy reflects the underlying disorder. Although the image depicts lymphoplasmacytic lymphoma, the findings of increased IgM, rather than only increased free heavy chains, makes this diagnosis less likely.

Answer B is incorrect. Monoclonal gammopathy of undetermined significance (MGUS) is common in elderly asymptomatic patients with high M components in the blood. One percent of cases progress to a symptomatic monoclonal gammopathy (eg, multiple myeloma). Bone marrow biopsy is normal with <10% abnormal plasma cells. MGUS is distinguished from myeloma by the lack of lytic lesions and little to no plasmacytosis.

Answer C is incorrect. Multiple myeloma is also a monoclonal plasma cell neoplasm characterized by lytic bone lesions at multiple sites. It can also spread to lymph nodes and other extranodal sites. Bone marrow biopsy reveals the replacement of normal marrow cells with abnormal plasma cells featuring multiple nuclei, prominent nucleoli, and cytoplasmic droplets containing Ig molecules. Although multiple myeloma can also demonstrate similar bone marrow biopsy findings as Waldenström macroglobulinemia, multiple myeloma is not associated with hyperviscosity syndrome. Additionally, multiple myeloma typically presents with hypercalcemia due to osteoclast activation. The patient in this vignette, on the other hand, has normal calcium levels. High levels of monoclonal Ig chain, usually IgG or IgA, are secreted into the serum. Ig light chains, known as Bence-Jones proteins, are often secreted in the urine, leading to renal failure. In this patient, immunofixation shows high levels of IgM, which is consistent with Waldenström macroglobulinemia.

Answer D is incorrect. Primary amyloidosis results from a monoclonal proliferation of plasma cells that secrete abnormal immunoglobulins containing light chains (usually λ) that deposit in various tissues. Bone marrow biopsy may show normal bone marrow or a modest increase in the number of plasma cells with pale pink amorphous deposits and increased histiocytes. Diagnosis is made by positive Congo red staining and apple green birefringence by polarizing microscopy.

39. **The correct answer is D.** A painless testicular mass is the classic presentation of testicular cancer. Young and middle-aged men are most commonly affected. In development, the testes begin high in the abdomen and descend to their final resting place in the scrotum. The lymphatic drainage from the testes, therefore, is to the para-aortic lymph nodes in the lumbar region just inferior to the renal arteries.

Answer A is incorrect. The deep inguinal nodes drain the vessels in the spongy urethra and may become enlarged in some sexually transmitted diseases or other causes of urethritis, or in anal cancer.

Answer B is incorrect. External iliac nodes drain the bladder.

Answer C is incorrect. Gluteal lymph nodes drain the deep tissue of the buttocks.

Answer E is incorrect. Tumors of the scrotum itself, but not of the testes, may spread to the superficial inguinal lymph nodes. The scrotum is an outpouching of abdominal skin, and drainage of this skin is to the superficial inguinal nodes. The testes, however, which lie inside the scrotum, begin life in the abdomen, and lymph drainage follows embryologic origins.

40. **The correct answer is C.** This patient has tuberous sclerosis, an autosomal dominant disorder affecting tuberin and hamartin proteins, which regulate cellular growth and differentiation. Two gene loci for tuberous sclerosis have been identified on chromosomes 9 and 16. Tuberous sclerosis has a strong association with tumors such as cortical tubers, renal angiomyolipomas, cardiac rhabdomyomas, astrocytomas, and pulmonary lymphangioleiomyomatosis. Typical skin findings include the ash-leaf spot, Shagreen patch, and facial angiofibromas. Patients with tuberous sclerosis typically present with mental retardation and epilepsy.

    Answer A is incorrect. Neurofibromatosis is an autosomal dominant disorder caused by mutations in either the *NF1* gene on chromosome 17 (neurofibromatosis type 1) or the *NF2* gene on chromosome 22 (neurofibromatosis type 2). Patients with neurofibromatosis type 1 have characteristic café-au-lait spots, cutaneous neurofibromas, and Lisch nodules in the iris, along with central nervous system tumors such as optic gliomas and astrocytomas. Patients with neurofibromatosis type 2 have bilateral acoustic neuromas as a characteristic finding, and may present with bilateral tinnitus and hearing loss.

    Answer B is incorrect. Leber hereditary optic neuropathy is due to a mitochondrial mutation that causes degeneration of the optic nerve with rapid loss of central vision, leading to a central scotoma that is permanent. More males than females are affected, with symptoms usually starting in the third decade.

    Answer D is incorrect. Von Hippel-Lindau syndrome is an autosomal dominant disorder characterized by abnormal blood vessel growth. The overgrowth of blood vessels leads to angiomas and hemangioblastomas in the retina, brain, and spinal cord as well as in other regions of the body. Patients also show cystic growths in the kidneys and pancreas, pheochromocytomas (resulting in apparently essential hypertension), islet cell tumors, and clear cell renal carcinoma. The disease is due to deletion of the *VHL* tumor suppressor gene on the short arm of chromosome 3. Untreated retinal hemangiomas can rupture, leading to retinal detachment.

    Answer E is incorrect. Sun sensitivity would be associated with xeroderma pigmentosum, an autosomal recessive disease caused by a deficiency in DNA repair of thymine dimers. Patients are very sensitive to UV radiation-induced thymine dimers, which can cause keratoses, skin cancers, and premature aging. These patients have an increased tendency to develop basal cell and squamous cell carcinomas of the skin. Lesions are often seen around the eyes and eyelids.

41. **The correct answer is A.** DIC can occur in the setting of obstetric complications, sepsis, malignancy, and other conditions. It is described as a thrombohemorrhagic process because there are microthrombi throughout the body, and coagulation factors and platelets are consumed actively. The active conversion of fibrinogen to fibrin as part of the convergence of both clotting cascades leads to decreased levels of fibrinogen. At the same time, anticoagulation factors such as plasmin and protein C are being activated, leading to fibrinolysis and increased levels of D-dimers in the circulation.

    Answer B is incorrect. DIC leads to consumption of coagulation factors; therefore, a drop in factor VII levels would be expected.

    Answer C is incorrect. Fibrinogen is actively converted to fibrin in the setting of DIC; therefore, a decrease in the levels of fibrinogen would be expected.

    Answer D is incorrect. Because the anticoagulation factors are also being activated and consumed during DIC, protein C levels would decrease.

    Answer E is incorrect. The patient has a prolonged PT, likely indicating a deficiency in one of the factors involved with the extrinsic pathway. Vitamin K is a fat-soluble vitamin that is a cofactor for the γ-carboxylation of glutamate residues of prothrombin; factors VII,

IX, and X; and proteins C and S. Vitamin K deficiency is uncommon; however, it can occur in the setting of oral broad-spectrum antibiotics, which suppress the flora of the bowel and interfere with the absorption and synthesis of this vitamin. It can also be associated with other conditions related to fat malabsorption and diffuse liver disease, or in the neonatal period when the intestinal flora have not developed and the liver reserves of vitamin K are small. Vitamin K deficiency usually presents with bleeding diathesis, hematuria, melena, bleeding gums, and ecchymoses.

42. **The correct answer is E.** The most common tumor of the parotid gland is the pleomorphic adenoma or the mixed tumor, accounting for 50% of salivary tumors. The pleomorphic adenoma is a benign, well-differentiated, well-circumscribed mass that grows slowly over the course of months to years. On histopathology, it is characterized by the presence of multiple cell types, classically epithelial cells in a chondromyxoid stroma.

Answer A is incorrect. The activity of factor VIII does not depend on vitamin K.

Answer B is incorrect. The activities of factors VIII and XII do not depend on vitamin K.

Answer C is incorrect. The activities of factors IX and XII do not depend on vitamin K.

Answer D is incorrect. The activity of factor XII does not depend on vitamin K.

43. **The correct answer is D.** This patient is suffering from CML caused by the t(9;22) chromosomal translocation, creating the Philadelphia chromosome. This translocation generates a fusion protein, *Bcr-Abl*, that functions as a constitutively active tyrosine kinase, promoting dysregulated cell growth and division. Imatinib (Gleevec or STI571) is a specific inhibitor of tyrosine kinase. It acts by binding to the ATP-binding pocket of tyrosine kinase, thus inhibiting its ability to phosphorylate.

Answer A is incorrect. Allopurinol is often used with other chemotherapeutic agents in the initial treatment of CML to prevent attacks of gout due to release of nucleic acids into the plasma from dying WBCs. It does not treat the underlying CML.

Answer B is incorrect. Busulfan used to be a treatment in patients intolerant of hydroxyurea. Like the others, it has now been supplanted by imatinib.

Answer C is incorrect. Hydroxyurea is moderately effective in bringing the disease under control and maintaining a normal white count, but its use has been superseded by imatinib.

Answer E is incorrect. Interferon-α was once the treatment of choice for this condition but has been superseded by imatinib.

44. **The correct answer is A.** Abciximab functions by binding to the glycoprotein receptor IIb/IIIa on activated platelets, preventing fibrinogen from binding and interfering with platelet aggregation. It is used in acute coronary syndrome and angioplasty.

Answer B is incorrect. Both clopidogrel and ticlopidine function by inhibiting the ADP pathway involved in the binding of fibrinogen to platelets during platelet aggregation.

Answer C is incorrect. Leuprolide is a gonadotropin-releasing hormone analog that acts as an agonist when administered in a pulsatile fashion and as an antagonist when administered in a continuous fashion. It is used to treat infertility (when administered as an agonist), prostate cancer (when administered as an antagonist), and uterine fibroids.

Answer D is incorrect. Selegiline is a selective monoamine oxidase B inhibitor that causes an increase in the availability of dopamine. It is used with levodopa in the treatment of Parkinson disease.

Answer E is incorrect. Both clopidogrel and ticlopidine function by inhibiting the ADP pathway involved in the binding of fibrinogen to platelets during platelet aggregation.

45. **The correct answer is D.** This patient has developed a lupus anticoagulant, which is an-

other name for acquired antiphospholipid antibody syndrome. Platelet phospholipids are required for both the intrinsic and extrinsic clotting pathways. Antiphospholipid antibodies bind to platelet phospholipids, thereby making them accessible to clotting factors and leading to recurrent venous and arterial thrombosis. Because both the PT and PTT assays use exogenous phospholipids, the antibodies inhibit their function and paradoxically show an increase in coagulation time.

Answer A is incorrect. Factor VIII antibodies are a rare cause of acquired hemophilia in the elderly. Their presence would cause bleeding rather than thrombus formation. They would also elevate the PTT but not the PT.

Answer B is incorrect. Heparin-induced thrombocytopenia is a hypercoagulable state caused by an immune reaction to exogenous heparin. This patient has no history of heparin exposure.

Answer C is incorrect. Antibodies directed against platelet glycoproteins, especially IIb/IIIa, lead to idiopathic thrombocytopenic purpura. This is characterized by extremely low platelet levels but normal PT and PTTs.

Answer E is incorrect. Antibodies directed against RBC antigens lead to hemolytic anemia. They are unrelated to clotting disorders.

46. **The correct answer is C.** This woman is suffering from DIC secondary to gram-negative sepsis that resulted from a hospital-acquired urinary tract infection. Common causes of DIC are gram-negative sepsis, malignancy, acute pancreatitis, trauma, transfusion reactions, and obstetric complications. The underlying mechanism of DIC is activation of the coagulation cascade, which leads to microthrombi and global consumption of platelets, fibrin, and coagulation factors. Thrombus formation in the microvasculature results in microangiopathy with schistocytes and helmet-shaped cells, which are shown in the image. Complications include bleeding, thrombosis, and organ failure. Laboratory findings include elevated PT, elevated PTT, elevated D-dimer level, and decreased platelet count.

Answer A is incorrect. This abnormality underlies Bernard-Soulier disease, an inherited disorder in platelet adhesion due to the absence of the glycoprotein Ib receptor. Peripheral blood smear may show increased platelet size (macrothrombocythemia) but no schistocytes. Laboratory findings include a normal PT, normal PTT, and decreased platelet count.

Answer B is incorrect. This abnormality underlies thrombotic thrombocytopenic purpura, which is characterized by the classic pentad of fever, thrombocytopenia, microangiopathic hemolysis, neurologic symptoms, and renal insufficiency. Schistocytes may be present on the peripheral blood smear. However, laboratory findings include a decreased platelet count with normal PT and PTT.

Answer D is incorrect. Hemophilia A is an X-linked disorder leading to deficiency of factor VIII that may manifest as excessive or spontaneous bleeding. Laboratory findings include a normal PT, elevated PTT, and normal platelet count. Schistocytes would not be present on the peripheral blood smear.

Answer E is incorrect. This answer describes the abnormality underlying von Willebrand disease, an inherited bleeding disorder that affects both platelet adhesion and factor VIII half-life. Schistocytes would not be present on the peripheral blood smear. Laboratory findings include a normal PT, elevated PTT, and normal platelet count.

47. **The correct answer is E.** This patient likely has MGUS, a premalignant dysproteinemia affecting nearly 1%-3% of asymptomatic individuals >50 years old. MGUS is defined by the presence of <3 g/dL of monoclonal immunoglobulin (M protein) in the serum in the absence of evidence for malignancy. This rule-out includes performing a metastatic bone survey, CT of the abdomen, 24-hour urine collection, serum protein electrophoresis, and potentially bone marrow aspiration. There is no treatment for MGUS, and approximately 1% of patients per year with MGUS will progress to an overt plasma cell dyscrasia. It is essential

to monitor M protein levels, as well as Bence Jones proteinuria, in these patients at periodic intervals for the remainder of their lives.

Answer A is incorrect. Bisphosphonates such as alendronate and risedronate are used to treat multiple myeloma, which is known to cause bone destruction as a result of increased osteoclast activity. Bisphosphonates have been shown to decrease pain and fractures in multiple myeloma by reducing the number and activity of osteoclasts.

Answer B is incorrect. High-dose steroids are not a treatment modality for MGUS, as there is no treatment for MGUS.

Answer C is incorrect. Vinca alkaloids such as vincristine and vinblastine are microtubule inhibitors used to treat some cancers, including leukemias and lymphomas.

Answer D is incorrect. A patient with an abnormal monoclonal serum immunoglobulin level but no other signs of malignancy (MGUS) should be monitored at regular intervals for progression of disease, but no treatment is indicated.

48. **The correct answer is B.** Thalassemias are inherited diseases involving decreased synthesis or complete absence of either the α-globin chain or the β-globin chain of Hb. This patient has classic symptoms of severe β-thalassemia (Cooley anemia): hemolytic anemia, hepatosplenomegaly, and "chipmunk facies" (reflecting the extramedullary hematopoiesis in the bones of the face). The requirement for blood transfusions since birth should raise the suspicion for β-thalassemia major, but the Hb electrophoresis results alone can be used to arrive at this conclusion. This patient shows increased HbF ($\alpha 2\gamma 2$) and HbA_2 ($\alpha 2\delta 2$); thus synthesis of the α-chain is intact. Absence of HbA_1 ($\alpha 2\beta 2$) supports an absence of β-chain synthesis and, therefore, a diagnosis of β-thalassemia major. Death in these individuals often is caused by cardiac failure secondary to hemochromatosis.

Answer A is incorrect. α-Thalassemia minor is associated with a two-gene deletion of α-globin (two gene regions out of four are intact). A mild anemia will be present, but the electrophoresis results will be normal, because the two remaining α-globin genes produce sufficient α-globin chains for normal HbA_1 levels. Deletion of only a single α-gene results in an asymptomatic carrier with no hematologic manifestations.

Answer C is incorrect. β-Thalassemia minor (the heterozygous defect) would show decreased but not absent HbA_1. This is a less severe form of the disease. β-Thalassemia minor confers a mild protective effect against *Plasmodium falciparum* malaria because of the shortened lifespan of the RBCs.

Answer D is incorrect. Glucose-6-phosphate dehydrogenase deficiency does not present with an abnormal Hb electrophoresis.

Answer E is incorrect. HbH is associated with three-gene deletion of α-globin. The abnormal Hb molecule (HbH) contains four β-chains, and is detected by electrophoresis. The β-thalassemias are more prevalent in Mediterranean people, whereas the α-thalassemias are more prevalent in Asian and African populations.

Answer F is incorrect. Hb Bart is the most severe of the hemoglobinopathies, involving deletion of all four α-globin genes. This results in the absence of all hemoglobins that require this chain and the sole production of Hb Bart, a tetramer of the γ-chain (normally a component of HbF). This condition leads to hydrops fetalis and intrauterine fetal death. Hb Bart is detected by electrophoresis.

49. **The correct answer is E.** This patient had an acoustic schwannoma removed from the cerebellopontine angle. Schwann cell tumors are the third most common primary intracranial tumor, are often localized to cranial nerve VIII (acoustic neuroma), and are commonly seen at the cerebellopontine angle. The most common signs and symptoms of schwannomas include hearing loss, tinnitus, vertigo, hydrocephalus, and increased intracranial pressure. Most are benign, slow-growing tumors that can be resected. Histologically, two patterns are found: (1) Antoni A, or spindle cells palisad-

ing and forming a whorl appearance; and (2) Antoni B, or loosely arranged tissue after degeneration in the tumor. The histopathologic description of this patient's tumor is consistent with Antoni A.

Answer A is incorrect. Medulloblastomas are highly malignant radiosensitive tumors that are typically found in the posterior fossa. These tumors are of neuroectodermal origin, and histopathologic examination shows a rosette or perivascular pseudorosette pattern. Peak incidence occurs in childhood.

Answer B is incorrect. Meningiomas are slow-growing tumors that occur most often in the hemispheric convexities and parasagittal regions. They rarely appear in the cerebellopontine angle. However, the histology would classically show psammoma bodies, or areas of calcification.

Answer C is incorrect. Neurofibromas are tumors of peripheral origin. This patient's tumor is intra-axial, as shown on the CT scan. Histologically, these cells appear as loosely arranged spindle cells with intervening collagen.

Answer D is incorrect. Oligodendrogliomas are relatively uncommon, slow-growing tumors that occur most often in the frontal lobes. The tumor is composed of homogeneous sheets of cells with uniformly rounded nuclei and an associated network of finely branching blood vessels.

50. **The correct answer is E.** The characteristics described in the question are found in patients with multiple endocrine neoplasia (MEN) type 2, also known as Sipple's syndrome. MEN-2 is associated with parathyroid hyperplasia or tumor leading to hypercalcemia, medullary carcinoma of the thyroid, and pheochromocytoma (which commonly causes elevated plasma catecholamine levels). The patient's episodes of lightheadedness and sweating may be attributed to the elevated catecholamine level found in pheochromocytoma. The MEN syndromes follow an autosomal dominant pattern of inheritance, and MEN-2A and MEN-2B are both linked to distinct mutations in the *ret* proto-oncogene.

Answer A is incorrect. Mutations in *braf* have been associated with papillary carcinoma of the thyroid. This is the most common thyroid malignancy, and it has been associated with a remote history of radiation exposure. It is not associated with any of the MENs.

Answer B is incorrect. The *erb*-B2 oncogene is associated with breast, ovarian, and gastric carcinomas.

Answer C is incorrect. Mutations in the *MEN1* tumor suppressor gene are found in patients with MEN type 1, also known as Wermer syndrome. This disease is characterized by hyperplasia or tumor of the "**3 Ps**": **P**ituitary, **P**arathyroid, and **P**ancreas. It may manifest its pancreatic component by the Zollinger-Ellison syndrome, hyperinsulinemia, or pancreatic cholera. Although this patient does have hypercalcemia that may be attributed to hyperplasia or tumor of the parathyroid gland, he does not have any pancreatic symptoms. MEN-1 syndrome is not associated with medullary thyroid carcinoma.

Answer D is incorrect. The *ras* oncogene mutation is associated with follicular thyroid carcinoma, not medullary thyroid carcinoma.

CHAPTER 12

Musculoskeletal

QUESTIONS

1. A 68-year-old man presents to his physician's office with diffuse pelvic pain. X-ray of the abdomen is shown in the image. Which of the following would help diagnose the primary tumor most commonly responsible for these radiologic findings?

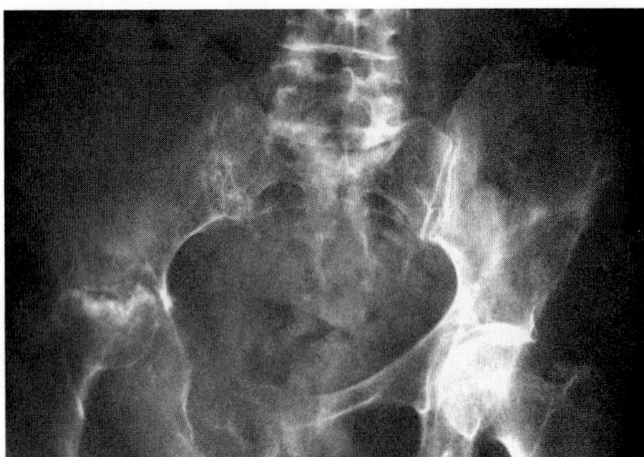

Reproduced, with permission, from Skinner HB. *Current Diagnosis & Treatment in Orthopedics*, 4th ed. New York: McGraw-Hill, 2006; Fig. 6-78A.

(A) Digital rectal examination
(B) Palpation of the abdomen
(C) Palpation of the costovertebral angle
(D) Palpation of the neck
(E) Thorough skin examination

2. A 17-year-old boy presents to his pediatrician with pain in his right leg. Biopsy reveals a malignancy in the distal femur. He has a family history of "eye cancer" in a younger sister. Which of the following is the most likely diagnosis?

(A) Chondrosarcoma
(B) Enchondroma
(C) Ewing sarcoma
(D) Osteochondroma
(E) Osteosarcoma

3. A 76-year-old man is scheduled to undergo elective repair of an abdominal hernia that is easily reducible. During the repair, the surgeon sees that the sac protrudes directly through the external inguinal ring without coursing through the inguinal canal. Which of the following types of hernia does this patient most likely have?

(A) Diaphragmatic hernia
(B) Direct inguinal hernia
(C) Femoral hernia
(D) Hiatal hernia
(E) Indirect inguinal hernia

4. A 22-year-old college student presents to the school health service complaining of worsening weakness in his arms and legs. He says that over the past day he has also begun to feel weakness in his chest and back. He mentions that he thinks he had food poisoning earlier in the week, which caused stomach pain and bloody diarrhea. Physical examination reveals that the deep tendon reflexes in his lower extremities are absent. His physician sends his stool to be cultured. The results show infection with *Campylobacter jejuni*. Which one of the following statements is most consistent with the disease process connecting the patient's gastrointestinal infection and his neurological symptoms?

(A) An excessive immune response to a gastrointestinal *Campylobacter jejuni* infection led to an autoimmune inflammation of peripheral nerves
(B) Dissemination of *Campylobacter jejuni* gastrointestinal infection led to infiltration of peripheral muscle cells with *C jejuni*
(C) Dissemination of *Campylobacter jejuni* gastrointestinal infection led to infiltration of peripheral nerves with *C jejuni*
(D) Toxins secreted by *Campylobacter jejuni* infiltrated into peripheral muscle cells
(E) Toxins secreted by *Campylobacter jejuni* infiltrated into peripheral nerves, causing their destruction

5. A 37-year-old man presents to his physician with a rash. Physical examination reveals the lesions shown in the image; the man says the lesions do not itch. Which family of viruses is responsible for causing this rash?

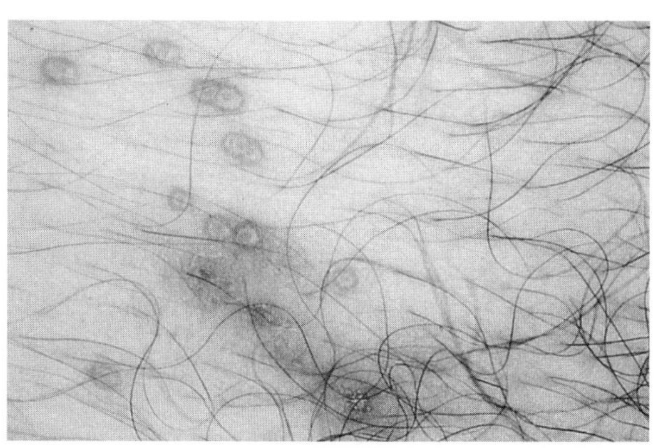

Reproduced, with permission, from Fauci AS, et al, eds. *Harrison's Principles of Internal Medicine*, 17th ed. New York: McGraw-Hill, 2008; Fig. 176-1.

(A) Adenovirus
(B) Hepadnavirus
(C) Herpes simplex virus
(D) Papillomavirus
(E) Polyomavirus
(F) Poxvirus

6. A 17-year-old girl complains of a painful, swollen left elbow and fever. In the previous few days her right knee was also swollen and slightly painful. The physician notices several oral ulcers and an edematous and tender left elbow. Laboratory tests are notable for weakly positive antinuclear antibodies and anemia, and the results of Venereal Disease Research Laboratory testing are positive. The patient is shocked when informed of her positive result for syphilis, stating that she has no sexual history. Which of the following is the most specific antibody for the patient's condition?

(A) Anti-IgG
(B) Anti-Jo-1
(C) Anti-Smith
(D) Anticentromere
(E) Antimicrosomal

7. A 32-year-old man recently underwent a liver transplant and was prescribed cyclosporine to reduce the chance of immune rejection. After a few weeks of taking the drug, he started experiencing acute pain, tenderness, warmth, and swelling of his right great toe. His physician takes a fluid sample from the affected area. Examination of the contents reveals the presence of intracellular crystals. Which of the following medications would prevent this problem from recurring?

(A) Allopurinol
(B) Calcitonin
(C) Collagenase
(D) Furosemide
(E) Warfarin

8. A 16-year-old gymnast presents to the emergency department after landing awkwardly on her ankle subsequent to dismounting from the parallel bars. She reports that she felt her ankle "roll inward," essentially inverting her ankle as a result of a misaligned axial load. On physical examination of the injured ankle, there appears to be a forward displacement of the talus. Which of the following ligaments has she most likely injured?

(A) Anterior talofibular ligament
(B) Calcaneofibular ligament
(C) Talonavicular ligament
(D) Tibiocalcaneal ligament
(E) Tibiotalar ligament

9. A 3-year-old boy is brought to the pediatrician by his mother, who notes that, despite no history of trauma, her son has been crying, rubbing his forearm, and guarding this area. This child's medical history is significant for normal, full-term birth and satisfactory achievement of developmental milestones, but poor dentition and two previous instances of skeletal fracture. The posterior area of the forearm is tender and erythematous. There is a bluish discoloration to the sclera and diminished auditory acuity. Which of the following is the most likely diagnosis?

(A) A defect in dystrophin
(B) A defect in fibrillin
(C) A defect in type I collagen
(D) A defect in type III collagen
(E) Child abuse
(F) Hemophilia A

10. A 32-year-old man is brought into the emergency department by ambulance after falling from a ladder while cleaning his roof gutters. His vital signs are stable, he is fully alert and oriented, and he reports having no past medical problems. He is in excruciating pain, which he states is located in his left arm. An x-ray of the left upper extremity is shown in the image. If left untreated, which of the following muscles is at risk of losing function due to this injury?

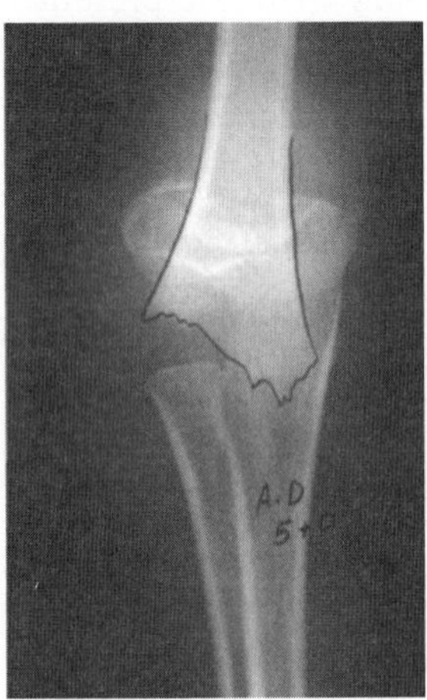

Reproduced, with permission, from Skinner HB. *Current Diagnosis & Treatment in Orthopedics*, 4th ed. New York: McGraw-Hill, 2006; Fig. 11-44.

(A) First and second lumbricals
(B) Brachioradialis
(C) Flexor carpi ulnaris
(D) Opponens pollicis
(E) Palmaris longus
(F) Pronator teres

11. A 52-year-old woman presents to her physician with three weeks of skin blisters. She says when these blisters rupture they leave painful ulcerations. On examination, tender ulcerations are found on her back and trunk. Biopsy is performed and direct immunofluorescence of the lesion reveals a net-like deposit of immunoglobulin surrounding keratinocytes. What aspect of epithelial cell junctions is targeted by autoantibodies in this condition?

(A) Gap junctions
(B) Hemidesmosomes
(C) Macula adherens
(D) Zona adherens
(E) Zona occludens

12. A 27-year-old man presents to his dermatologist with several red, tender nodules on his lower legs. On histopathology, there is inflammation of the subcutaneous fat, tissue septal widening, neutrophilia, and fibrin exudation. Which of the following diseases often goes along with these skin findings?

(A) Acne vulgaris
(B) Crohn disease
(C) Eczema
(D) Pancreatitis
(E) Psoriasis

13. A previously healthy 30-year-old woman who performs as a contortionist in the circus is found unconscious in her dressing room. By the time she receives medical attention, she cannot be revived. An autopsy is performed and an abnormality is discovered in the circle of Willis, as shown in the image. The patient was also reported to have a history of easy bruising and bleeding. Which of the following proteins was most likely defective in this patient?

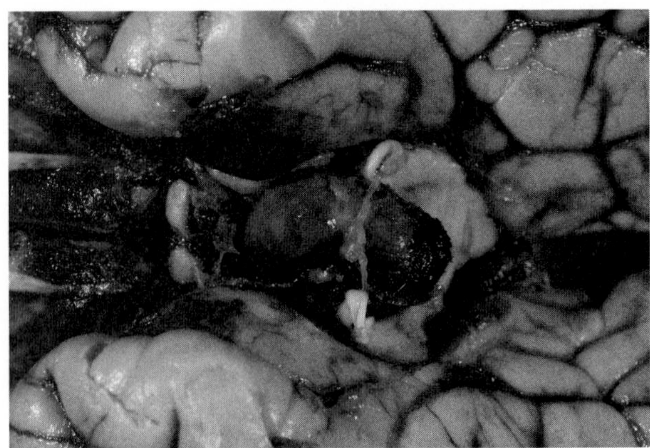

Reproduced, with permission, from USMLERx.com.

(A) Fibrillin-1
(B) Keratin 14
(C) Type I procollagen

(D) Type III procollagen
(E) Type IV collagen

14. A couple brings their 3-year-old son to the emergency department, reporting that he fell down the stairs and broke his arm. The boy has a tearful face and gingerly holds his right arm by the elbow, but refuses to look the physician in the eye or to answer any questions. An x-ray of the boy's arm is performed. Which of the following types of fracture is most likely to suggest an etiology of child abuse?

(A) Bowing fracture
(B) Buckle fracture
(C) Greenstick fracture
(D) Spiral fracture

15. A 31-year-old man comes to the clinic complaining of red and itchy eyes for the past eight hours. The patient has had pain on urination and diffuse joint pain for 1 month, but tested negative for gonorrhea and chlamydial infection on a previous visit three weeks ago. He has also tested negative for rheumatoid factor, and his human leukocyte antigen (HLA) status is HLA-B27. When asked about any recent illnesses, the patient recalls going to the emergency department two months ago for a bad case of diarrhea. Which of the following is the most likely diagnosis?

(A) Anklyosing spondylitis
(B) Lyme arthritis
(C) Psoriatic arthritis
(D) Reactive arthritis
(E) Systemic lupus erythematosus

16. A 70-year-old man complains of a long history of pain in his ankles, toes, and fingers. He has experienced intermittent acute attacks of exquisite pain every few months, followed by completely asymptomatic periods. In recent years, he has had near-constant discomfort at baseline, and now has permanent "swelling" in many of the joints of his fingers and toes. Joint fluid is aspirated, and the fluid is examined under polarized light (shown in the image). Treatment is initiated, and the patient's uric acid levels gradually fall. What is the mechanism of action of the best treatment?

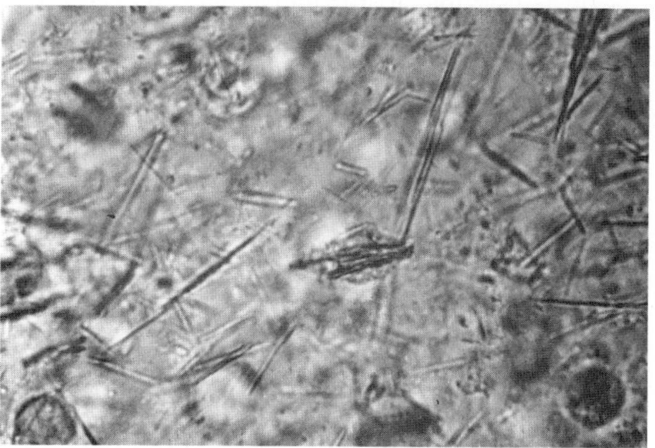

Reproduced, with permission, from Fauci AS, et al, eds. *Harrison's Principles of Internal Medicine*, 17th edition. New York: McGraw-Hill, 2008; Figure 327-1.

(A) Binds tubulin
(B) Blocks formation of prostaglandins and thromboxane from arachidonic acid
(C) Inhibits release of phospholipase A2
(D) Inhibits xanthine oxidase
(E) Selective, competitive angiotensin II receptor inhibition

17. A 57-year-old automotive factory worker with no significant past medical history reports to the clinic complaining of weakness and pain in his right shoulder with any movement. He says that for the past two weeks he has had trouble lifting his right arm above his head. He reports using his left arm to lift his right arm slightly, and then he can lift his right arm the rest of the way without help. Which of the following muscles is most likely injured in this patient?

(A) Deltoid
(B) Infraspinatus
(C) Subscapularis
(D) Supraspinatus
(E) Teres minor

18. A 49-year-old man is lifting a heavy box above his head when he experiences a sudden tearing sensation and pain that travels along his left arm. When he attempts to move his arm he is not able to medially rotate it. Which of the following muscles is most likely injured?

    (A) Deltoid muscle
    (B) Infraspinatus muscle
    (C) Subscapularis muscle
    (D) Supraspinatus muscle
    (E) Teres minor

19. A 22-year-old emergency room nurse has a positive purified protein derivative test. Results of radiography of the chest are unremarkable. She begins a nine-month prophylaxis regimen, but two months into treatment she complains of the sudden onset of fever, rash, and swelling of her joints. What is the mechanism of the medication that caused these adverse effects?

    (A) Decreases synthesis of folate
    (B) Decreases synthesis of messenger RNA
    (C) Decreases synthesis of mycolic acids
    (D) Decreases synthesis of peptidoglycan
    (E) Increases synthesis of cGMP

20. A young man complains of difficulty eating. His neurologic examination reveals a symmetric smile, symmetric palate elevation, midline tongue, as well as good shoulder shrug and head turning strength. However, he has difficulty opening his mouth and biting down firmly. Damage to what cranial nerve could explain his condition?

    (A) V_2
    (B) V_3
    (C) VII
    (D) X
    (E) XII

21. A 32-year-old woman is incidentally found to have a mediastinal mass (see image) while having a plain film x-ray of the chest performed. She subsequently reports that lately she has been "feeling more fatigued, especially at the end of the day." In the office, she has difficulty rising from her chair to move to the examination table. On physical examination the patient has asymmetric left-sided ptosis, a subjective feeling of "blurred vision" when reading the eye chart on the wall, and a facial droop bilaterally. What test would confirm the most likely diagnosis in this patient?

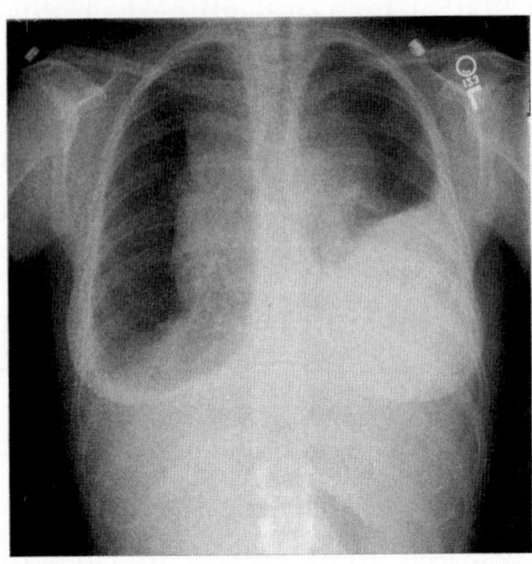

Reproduced, with permission, from USMLERx.com.

    (A) Acetylcholine receptor antibody assay
    (B) Complete blood cell count
    (C) Parathyroid hormone level
    (D) Thyroid stimulating hormone level
    (E) Urine catecholamine levels

22. A 12-year-old African-American girl is brought to the physician with complaints of fever, malaise, and pain in her left forearm for the past four days. Her mother reports no history of trauma or fracture, but recounts an upper respiratory infection a few days ago. The patient has been hospitalized three times for abdominal pain, for which she takes hydroxyurea. Her temperature is 39.8°C (103.6°F) and the rest of her vital signs are stable. On examination the left forearm is erythematous, warm, and tender to palpation. Blood samples for culture are drawn. Which of the following organisms is most likely to be isolated from this patient's blood?

    (A) *Escherichia coli*
    (B) *Pseudomonas aeruginosa*
    (C) *Salmonella* species
    (D) *Staphylococcus aureus*
    (E) *Streptococcus pyogenes*

23. A 9-month-old girl presents to her pediatrician because of abnormal stature and growth. The child displays short stature, shortening of the proximal limbs, short fingers, and frontal bossing. Which of the following is the most likely etiology of this infant's condition?

(A) Bone resorption
(B) Collagen formation
(C) Endochondral ossification
(D) Mucopolysaccharide degradation

24. A 64-year-old woman with no prior medical history has had increasing back pain and right hip pain for the past decade. The pain is worse at the end of the day. On physical examination, she has bony enlargement of the distal interphalangeal joints (see image). Which of the following diseases is most likely the cause of this patient's symptoms?

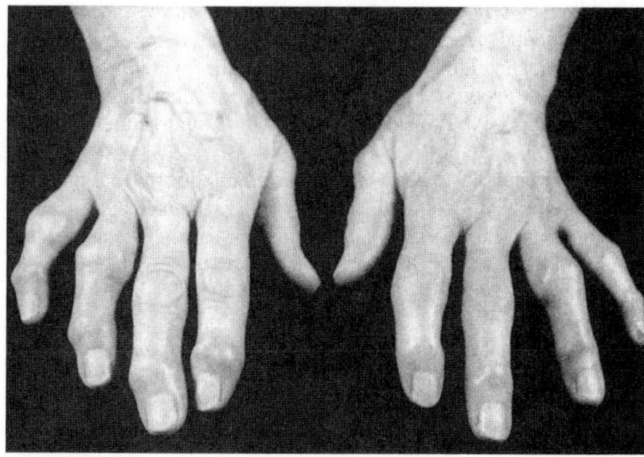

Reproduced, with permission, from Fauci AS, et al, eds. *Harrison's Principles of Internal Medicine*, 17th edition. New York: McGraw-Hill, 2008; Figure 326-2.

(A) Gout
(B) Osteoarthritis
(C) Osteomyelitis
(D) Pseudogout
(E) Rheumatoid arthritis

25. A 42-year-old woman comes to the clinic complaining of blurry vision. She states that for the past three weeks her eyes have been very dry and itchy, and she is unable to make tears. She also states that she has had a very dry mouth despite drinking adequate fluids. Physical examination reveals bilateral dry, ulcerated corneas and fissures on the sides of her lips. In addition, both of her knees are erythematous and swollen. When asked about her knees, she says, "Yes, my knees and wrists tend to be swollen and stiff in the morning, but my mom had arthritis." Testing for several autoantibodies reveals she is rheumatoid factor-positive and antibody-SS-B (La)-positive. Which of the following is the most likely diagnosis?

(A) CREST syndrome
(B) Cystic fibrosis
(C) Sicca syndrome
(D) Sjögren syndrome
(E) Sjögren-Larsson syndrome

26. An 18-year-old man is injured during a soccer game when the goalie dives for the ball but tackles the player on the lateral aspect of his leg. He is helped off the field and brought to the emergency department, where he tells the physician that he heard a pop when he was tackled. Physical examination reveals an anterior drawer sign and MRI reveals a torn anterior cruciate ligament and medial collateral ligament. Which one of the following structures is also likely to be injured?

(A) Lateral collateral ligament
(B) Lateral meniscus
(C) Medial meniscus
(D) Patellar ligament
(E) Posterior cruciate ligament

27. A mother brings her 12-year-old son to the pediatrician's office because he is complaining of leg pain. The pain is located at the distal right tibia and has persisted over the past two weeks. The mother also notes that the child has had intermittent fevers during this time. On examination, the site is erythematous and swollen. A plain film x-ray is taken, the results of which are shown in the image. Biopsy of the site shows sheets of many uniform cells with scant, clear cytoplasm and no evidence of normal bony matrix. Which of the following is the most likely diagnosis?

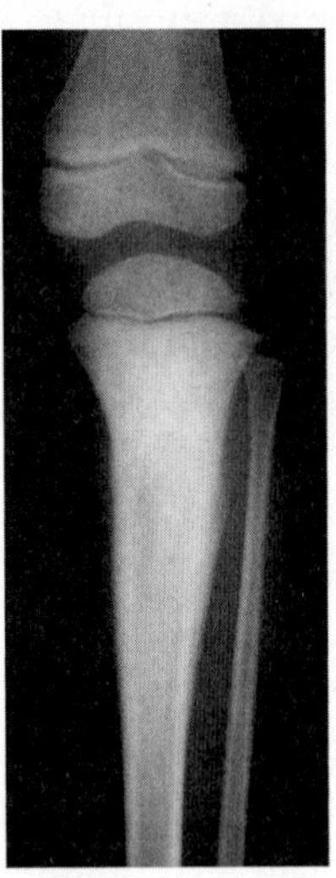

Courtesy of Dr. Jeevak Almast, University of Rochester Medical Center.

(A) Ewing sarcoma
(B) Giant cell tumor
(C) Osteochondroma
(D) Osteomyelitis
(E) Osteosarcoma

28. A 1-year-old adopted, darkly pigmented boy is brought to the pediatrician for his first well-child check-up. The adoptive parents do not know any of the infant's past medical history or family history. Physical examination reveals an unusual widening of the child's wrists and ankles and marked enlargement of the child's costochondral junctions. What is a characteristic laboratory finding used to support the most likely diagnosis?

(A) Increased intact parathyroid hormone level
(B) Increased serum 1,25-dihydroxycholecalciferol level
(C) Increased serum 25-hydroxycholecalciferol level
(D) Increased serum calcium level
(E) Increased serum phosphorus level

29. A 45-year-old woman who recently underwent a left mastectomy and axillary dissection for breast cancer now presents to her physician with a chief complaint that she feels like her shoulder blade sticks out sometimes. She denies any pain. This patient's injured nerve originates at which spinal levels?

(A) C3, C4, and C5
(B) C5 and C6
(C) C5, C6, and C7
(D) C7 and C8
(E) C7, C8, and T1

30. A 42-year-old woman has had increasing pain and swelling of the joints of her hands and feet for several months. It is becoming very difficult for her to perform common household tasks. A microscopic image of the synovium of a proximal interphalangeal joint in her hand is shown in the image. Which of the following laboratory serologic findings would most likely be positive in this patient?

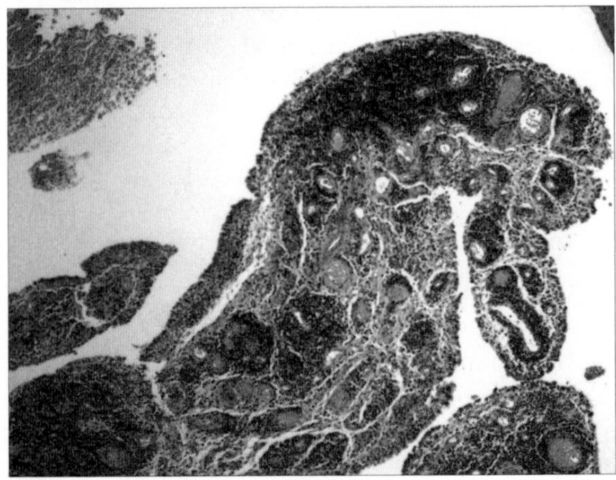

Reproduced, with permission, from USMLERx.com.

(A) Anti-centromere antibody
(B) Anti-nuclear antibody
(C) *Borrelia burgdorferi* antibody
(D) HLA-B27
(E) IgM anti-IgG

31. A 6-year-old child is brought to the emergency department by his parents after they all returned from a trip to East Africa. His parents report that approximately two weeks ago he had a fever and diarrhea that resolved. However, he now has a fever and weakness of his left leg. On further questioning, his parents state that he is home-schooled and that he has never received vaccinations. Which of the following sequelae is most likely to result in this patient?

(A) Neuron loss in the posterior horns
(B) Reflex preservation in affected limbs
(C) Respiratory muscle paralysis
(D) Sensory loss in affected limbs
(E) Short-term memory loss

32. A 15-year-old boy presents to the emergency department after falling off his skateboard. On physical examination he is unable to dorsiflex or evert at the ankle. In addition, the patient reports pain and numbness in the lateral leg and dorsum of the foot. When asked to walk, he raises his affected leg high off the ground and his foot slaps the ground when walking. He is diagnosed with a fracture. Which of the following structures is most likely to be compromised by this fracture?

(A) Common peroneal nerve
(B) Femoral nerve
(C) L4 nerve root
(D) Obturator nerve
(E) Tibial nerve

33. A 27-year-old homeless man presents to the clinic because of a five-day history of pain and swelling in his right upper arm. MRI of the area reveals diffuse soft tissue and bone inflammation. Results of bone biopsy are shown in the image. Blood cultures grow *Pseudomonas*. Which of the following would a complete history of this patient most likely reveal?

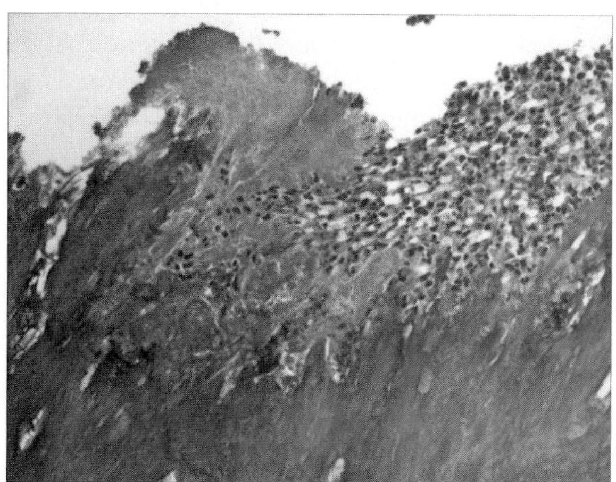

Reproduced, with permission, from USMLERx.com.

(A) Corticosteroid use
(B) Intravenous drug use
(C) Miliary tuberculosis
(D) Multiple sexual partners
(E) Sickle cell anemia

34. A 22-year-old woman who is a professional tennis player presents to her physician because of pain on the lateral aspect of her elbow radiating down her forearm. She describes the pain as shooting and constant. Repetitive use of which of the following muscles most likely led to this patient's condition?

(A) Biceps
(B) Extensor carpi radialis
(C) Extensor carpi ulnaris
(D) Flexor carpi ulnaris
(E) Pronator teres

35. A 50-year-old man who recently returned from visiting family in northern New Mexico comes to the physician with exquisitely tender and enlarged lymph nodes. He also complains of fever, chills, and general weakness. On physical examination, the physician notes a painful ulcer surrounded by dark, hemorrhagic purpura on the right arm in the area where, according to the patient, a flea had bitten him five days ago. After being admitted to the hospital, the patient soon develops abnormal coagulation times and is quickly started on a regimen of streptomycin and tetracycline. Which of the following organisms is most likely responsible for this patient's symptoms?

(A) *Babesia microti*
(B) *Bacillus anthracis*
(C) *Leishmania donovani*
(D) *Trichinella spiralis*
(E) *Yersinia pestis*

36. A 63-year-old man and known alcoholic has been unable to afford alcohol. He now presents with hypertension and profuse sweating, and is agitated because he believes that insects are crawling all over his skin. During the examination, he loses consciousness and begins to seize on the stretcher. The seizure-induced muscle contractions result in which of the following changes in length within each sarcomere?

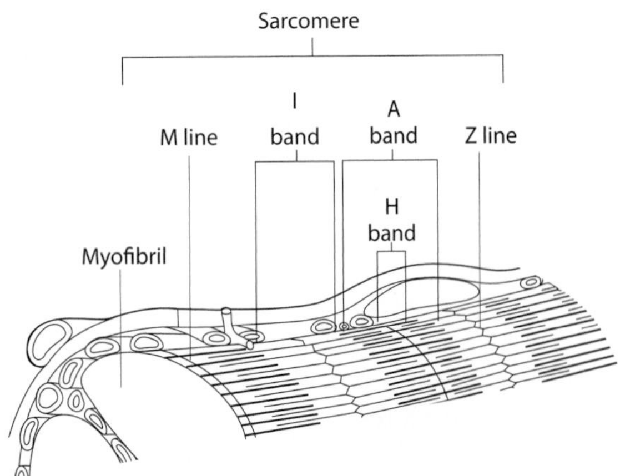

Reproduced, with permission, from USMLERx.com.

(A) Lengthening of A band; no change in H band; shortening of I band
(B) No change in A band; lengthening of H band; lengthening of I band
(C) No change in A band; shortening of H band; shortening of I band
(D) Shortening of A band; no change in H band; shortening of I band
(E) Shortening of A band; shortening of H band; no change in I band

37. A 38-year-old man comes to the clinic with a swollen, sausage-like left middle finger along with diffuse joint swelling of his left hand and right foot over the past three days. The patient also has scaly plaques with well-defined borders along the skin just distal to both elbows. His uric acid level is within normal limits. Which of the following is most likely to be seen in this patient?

(A) Antigliadin antibodies
(B) Elevated erythrocyte sedimentation rate
(C) Negatively birefringent crystals in joint fluid
(D) Positive rheumatoid factor
(E) Weakly positively birefringent crystals in joint fluid

38. A 20-year-old man presents to the physician with a nontender indurated mass over his mandible. He has had this mass for four months after undergoing oral surgery and decided to come to the physician because the mass started to ooze a thick yellow exudate. Yellow granules are seen on microscopic examination of the discharge and an antibiotic is prescribed. Which of the following best describes the mechanism of action of the antibiotic most likely prescribed?

(A) Binds ergosterol, forming pores in the membrane
(B) Block bacterial cell wall synthesis by inhibiting transpeptidase crosslinking
(C) Block bacterial nucleotide synthesis
(D) Block bacterial protein synthesis
(E) Inhibits ergosterol synthesis

39. A 74-year-old man presents to his physician with a bulge in his scrotum. He is diagnosed with an inguinal hernia on his left side, and undergoes surgery two days later to repair the hernia. On postoperative day two he complains of numbness and tingling of his scrotum. Which nerve root contributes to the affected nerve?

(A) L1-L2
(B) L2-L3
(C) S1-S3
(D) S2-S4

40. The diagram shows a cross-section of normal human skin. Pemphigus vulgaris patients suffer from production of autoantibodies against which of the following labeled layers in this image?

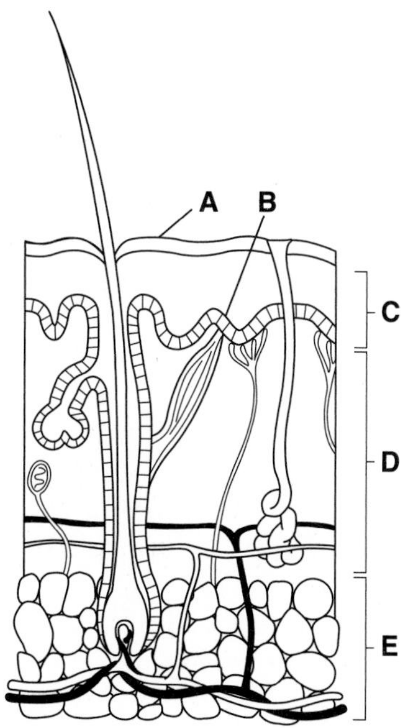

Reproduced, with permission, from USMLERx.com.

(A) A
(B) B
(C) C
(D) D
(E) E

41. A 25-year-old man develops acute onset of fever, malaise, muscle pain, hypertension, abdominal pain, bloody stool, and prerenal failure six months after recovering from an acute hepatitis B infection. Which of the following disease processes is most likely responsible for the patient's findings?

(A) Buerger disease
(B) Giant cell (temporal) arteritis
(C) Kawasaki syndrome
(D) Polyarteritis nodosa
(E) Takayasu arteritis

42. A 36-year-old woman presents to the clinic with a new complaint of fatigue of several months' duration. She also reports stiffness in both hands that is worse in the morning and decreases after soaking them in her warm morning bath each day. Physical examination reveals a low-grade fever. Subcutaneous nodules are palpated along her forearm bilaterally. What type of hypersensitivity reaction is causing this patient's arthritis?

(A) Arthus reaction
(B) Delayed cell-mediated hypersensitivity reaction
(C) Immune complex hypersensitivity reaction
(D) Type I hypersensitivity reaction
(E) Type II hypersensitivity reaction

43. A 27-year-old man comes to the physician's office with a six-month history of low back pain and stiffness that wakes him up during the night and is worst in the morning. The patient was diagnosed with bilateral sacroiliitis four months ago because of his tenderness to percussion of the sacroiliac joints and pain on springing the pelvis up. He has severe limitation of motion of his lumbar spine. Laboratory tests are most likely to be positive for which of the following?

(A) Human leukocyte antigen B27
(B) Antinuclear antibodies
(C) Anti-neutrophil cytoplasmic antibodies
(D) IgM antibodies to *B burgdorferi*
(E) Rheumatoid factor
(F) Vertebral compression fracture

44. A visibly upset 15-year-old boy is brought to the emergency department because he punched a wall and now has pain in his hand. The physician tells the patient that he has broken his hand. Which of the following is the most likely site of this patient's fracture?

(A) Distal radius
(B) Hamate
(C) Metacarpals
(D) Phalanges
(E) Scaphoid

45. A 38-year-old woman presents to the emergency department complaining of increasing muscle weakness and pain. She first noticed the muscle weakness approximately one month ago, and it has gradually worsened since then. During the same time she has had increasing difficulty swallowing her meals. Two weeks prior to this visit, she recalls swelling and a rash over her eyelids. On physical examination, deltoid and quadriceps strength are 2/5 bilaterally. Creatine kinase, lactate dehydrogenase, and aldolase levels are elevated. Which auto-antibody would diagnostic testing find to be elevated?

(A) Anti-dsDNA
(B) Anti-Jo-1
(C) Anti-IgG
(D) Anti-microsomal
(E) Anti-mitochondrial

ANSWERS

1. **The correct answer is A.** The image demonstrates osteoblastic lesions of the pelvis secondary to metastatic cancer. Prostate cancer, the most common cause of cancer in men, is notorious for producing osteoblastic lesions upon metastasis. Prostate cancer may often be detected on physical examination through the use of a digital rectal examination. Digital rectal examination can also be useful in detecting a small number of colorectal cancers, though most bony lesions of metastatic colorectal cancer are osteolytic.

   Answer B is incorrect. Palpation of the abdomen may assist in the detection of leukemia or lymphoma, as splenomegaly is a common presenting symptom. These cancers occur much less frequently than prostate cancer, and more often produce osteolytic lesions.

   Answer C is incorrect. Signs of renal cell cancer include flank pain (noted upon palpation of the costovertebral angle), the presence of a flank mass, hematuria, and/or weight loss. Renal metastases are more commonly osteolytic.

   Answer D is incorrect. Palpation of the neck may be helpful in detecting thyroid cancer. Thyroid metastases are more often lytic.

   Answer E is incorrect. A thorough skin examination would be vital in detecting a melanoma. However, melanoma is much less common than prostate cancer, and most often produces osteolytic lesions when it metastasizes to bone.

2. **The correct answer is E.** Osteosarcoma is the most common primary malignant bony tumor. These tumors are seen predominantly in males <20 years old and occur at the metaphyseal region of long bones. Plain films of the affected bone often reveal a characteristic "sunburst" pattern. Genetic mutations of the *Rb* gene are associated with both osteosarcoma and retinoblastoma, which was likely present in this patient's sister.

   Answer A is incorrect. Chondrosarcomas are malignant cartilaginous tumors that occur most commonly in men 30-60 years old, usually in the pelvis, spine, scapula, humerus, tibia, or femur.

   Answer B is incorrect. Enchondromas are benign cartilaginous tumors found in intramedullary bone, and are most often found in the distal extremities.

   Answer C is incorrect. Ewing sarcoma is the second most common primary bone cancer. Most patients present at the onset of puberty (average is between 10 and 15 years old). Ewing sarcoma most commonly occurs in the diaphyses of long bones, pelvis, scapula, and ribs.

   Answer D is incorrect. Osteochondromas are benign growths that are often first diagnosed in late adolescence or early adulthood. They are the most common benign bone tumor.

3. **The correct answer is B.** Direct inguinal hernias protrude directly through the abdominal wall in Hesselbach's triangle, which is bordered by the inguinal ligament (inferiorly), rectus abdominis muscle (medially), and inferior epigastric vessels (laterally). Direct versus indirect distinguishes where the hernia enters the inguinal canal, either through the internal ring (indirect) or straight through the abdominal wall (for *direct* hernias, think *directly* through the wall). In this case the abdominal contents pierced through the abdominal wall and through the external inguinal ring. Direct hernias often are discovered in older patients as a result of pressure and tension exerted over time that eventually leads the abdominal wall to give way. Direct hernias are less common and have less risk of strangulation than indirect hernias.

   Answer A is incorrect. Diaphragmatic hernias are serious birth defects that are lethal unless repaired soon after birth. A defective development of the diaphragm leads to herniation of abdominal contents into the thorax, displacing the lung. Even after repair of such lesions, children may have poor pulmonary function due to poor lung development in utero.

Answer C is incorrect. Femoral hernias protrude inferior to the inguinal ligament and do not go through the external inguinal ring. They protrude below and lateral to the pubic tubercle and are more common in women.

Answer D is incorrect. Hiatal hernias are hernias of the stomach protruding superiorly through the diaphragm. This is common in premature neonates and the elderly.

Answer E is incorrect. Indirect inguinal hernias occur when abdominal contents enter the internal inguinal ring through a patent processus vaginalis, exit the inguinal canal through the external ring, and usually descend into the scrotum. These hernias are the most common type found both in men and in women, but overall occur more commonly in men. They are found often in young individuals. They should be repaired when they are discovered to avoid the complications of strangulation and bowel infarction.

4. **The correct answer is A.** This patient has Guillain-Barré as a result of his gastroenteritis. The important message here is that Guillain-Barré syndrome is thought to be primarily an autoimmune disorder against peripheral nerves and the cells that myelinate them (Schwann cells). Thus, it makes sense that an excessive immune response to an infection (such as from a pathogen like *Campylobacter jejuni*) can lead to an autoimmune process. Histologically, this disease is characterized by perivenular and endoneurial infiltration with lymphocytes, macrophages, and plasma cells.

Answer B is incorrect. Guillain-Barré syndrome is a disease that primarily attacks peripheral nerves and Schwann cells. The ascending paralysis and muscle weakness that occur as a consequence are secondary to the neuropathy.

Answer C is incorrect. The mechanism suggested in this answer choice is not thought to be the primary disease process in Guillain-Barré syndrome.

Answer D is incorrect. Guillain-Barré syndrome is a disease that primarily attacks peripheral nerves and Schwann cells. The ascending paralysis and muscle weakness that occur as a consequence are secondary to the neuropathy.

Answer E is incorrect. While *Campylobacter jejuni* does produce an enterotoxin, the mechanism described in this answer choice is not the major hypothesized pathogenesis of Guillain-Barré syndrome.

5. **The correct answer is F.** Molluscum contagiosum is a member of the poxvirus family that causes a localized infection consisting of nonerythematous, pearly, dome-shaped papules on the skin of an infected individual. Children and immunosuppressed patients are often infected with this virus. The infection is usually self-limited and spontaneously resolves after a few months.

Answer A is incorrect. Adenovirus is a common cause of upper respiratory infections.

Answer B is incorrect. Hepadnavirus causes hepatitis B with jaundice being a possible dermatologic sequela.

Answer C is incorrect. The various herpes simplex viruses (HSVs) cause several different diseases resulting in rash. HSV-1 and HSV-2 cause genital herpes and cold sores. Varicella-zoster virus causes chickenpox, which can reactivate and result in shingles. The lesions are painful vesicles with an erythematous base.

Answer D is incorrect. Papillomavirus causes warts, which can be flat, raised, or resemble a cauliflower.

Answer E is incorrect. Reactivation of polyomavirus results in progressive multifocal leukoencephalopathy in immunosuppressed patients.

6. **The correct answer is C.** This patient has systemic lupus erythematosus (SLE), which is diagnosed by the presence of four of the following 11 findings designated by the American Rheumatism Association, and summarized by the mnemonic "**BRAIN SOAP, MD:**" Blood

dyscrasias (such as hemolytic anemia or thrombocytopenia), **R**enal disorder, **A**rthritis (in two or more peripheral joints), **I**mmunologic disorder (such as anti-DNA antibody and anti-Smith antibody), **N**eurologic disorder, **S**erositis (such as pleuritis or pericarditis), **O**ral ulcers, **A**ntinuclear antibody (elevated titers in the absence of drugs associated with drug-induced lupus syndrome), **P**hotosensitivity, **M**alar rash, and **D**iscoid rash. Many patients with SLE have antiphospholipid antibodies, which actually are believed to be antibodies against proteins that complex to phospholipids. Because these antibodies also bind to the cardiolipin antigen used in syphilis serology, patients with SLE may have a false-positive result for syphilis. Whereas antinuclear antibodies are sensitive for SLE, anti-Smith and anti-double-stranded DNA are the most specific. Many other autoantibodies may be present in SLE that are not necessarily sensitive or specific for the condition.

Answer A is incorrect. Anti-IgG, or rheumatoid factor, is associated with rheumatoid arthritis (RA). Although arthritis can be a symptom of SLE, a patient with RA classically will present with morning stiffness, systemic inflammatory symptoms, and symmetric swelling, particularly in the metacarpophalangeal and proximal interphalangeal joints.

Answer B is incorrect. Anti-Jo-1 antibodies are associated with inflammatory myopathies such as polymyositis and dermatomyositis. These conditions are characterized by proximal muscle weakness and, in dermatomyositis, skin involvement and increased incidence of malignancy.

Answer D is incorrect. Anticentromere antibodies are associated with **CREST** syndrome, a more limited type of scleroderma characterized by **C**alcinosis (tissue deposits of calcium), **R**aynaud phenomenon, **E**sophageal dysmotility, **S**clerodactyly (tightness and thickening of digits), and **T**elangiectasia.

Answer E is incorrect. Antimicrosomal antibodies are associated with Hashimoto thyroiditis. Clinically this would present with symptoms of hypothyroidism and a moderately enlarged, nontender thyroid.

7. **The correct answer is A.** The main adverse reactions to cyclosporine therapy are renal dysfunction, tremor, hirsutism, hypertension, and gum hyperplasia. Cyclosporine can damage renal tubules irreversibly, thus decreasing the kidney's ability to excrete potentially toxic metabolites. This patient is suffering from acute gouty arthritis secondary to impaired renal excretion of uric acid and thus increased serum levels of urate, which can precipitate as monosodium urate crystals in joints. Gout classically presents with a warm, red, painful joint. The most common joint affected in gout is the great toe. Other potential adverse effects of cyclosporine that occur secondary to renal failure include hyperkalemia, hypophosphatemia, hypomagnesemia, hypercalciuria, and metabolic acidosis. Allopurinol is used to prevent gouty arthritis by inhibiting xanthine oxidase, an enzyme involved in uric acid synthesis. The mainstay of therapy for acute gout is nonsteroidal anti-inflammatory drugs (NSAIDs) and corticosteroids.

Answer B is incorrect. Calcitonin counteracts the action of parathyroid hormone (PTH), thus reducing serum calcium level. Whereas cyclosporine is known to cause hypercalciuria, it is not associated with the formation and precipitation of calcium pyrophosphate crystals in joints and connective tissues, also known as pseudogout. The development of pseudogout is associated with joint trauma, familial chondrocalcinosis, hemochromatosis, and certain other metabolic or endocrine disorders. Thus calcitonin would not prevent acute gouty arthritis.

Answer C is incorrect. Collagenase is an enzyme involved in collagen degradation. It is key to pathogenesis of various bacteria, but it also can be induced during an immune response and lead to indirect tissue damage. Cyclosporine does not affect collagen turnover in joints. Collagenase would not counteract the effects of cyclosporine and should not lead to deposition of crystals in joint fluid.

Answer D is incorrect. Furosemide is a loop diuretic used in treatment of congestive heart failure and acute renal failure. Loop diuretics may be used to increase calcium diuresis in hypercalcemic states. However, loop diuretics are known to cause hyperuricemia, which may precipitate gout in some patients and should be avoided in this patient specifically.

Answer E is incorrect. Warfarin is an anticoagulant that inhibits vitamin K-dependent clotting factors II, VII, IX, and X. Neither elevated uric acid levels nor cyclosporine itself predisposes patients to thrombus formation; therefore antithrombotic therapy is unnecessary.

8. **The correct answer is A.** The lateral ligaments of the foot are more commonly injured than the medial ligaments, since they are weaker. The anterior talofibular ligament is the most common of the lateral ligaments to be injured. Injuries to the ligaments about the ankle usually result from inversion and internal rotation of the foot combined with ankle plantar flexion. With complete disruption of the anterior talofibular ligament, forward displacement of the talus in the ankle mortise is present. Lateral ankle sprains represent 16%-21% of all sports-related traumatic lesions. The anterior talofibular ligament is the weakest ligament and therefore the most frequently torn. There is usually a predictable pattern of injury involving the anterior talofibular ligament followed by the calcaneofibular ligament and the posterior talofibular ligament. First-degree sprain is characterized by a partial or complete tear of the anterior talofibular ligament. In second-degree sprain both the anterior talofibular and calcaneofibular ligaments are either partially or completely torn. Third-degree sprain consists of injuries to the anterior talofibular, calcaneofibular, and posterior talofibular ligaments.

Answer B is incorrect. The calcaneofibular ligament is a lateral ligament that is injured frequently, but less frequently than the anterior talofibular ligament.

Answer C is incorrect. The lateral ligaments are more commonly injured than the medial ligaments, since they are weaker. The talonavicular ligament is a medial ligament so it is much less likely to be injured.

Answer D is incorrect. The lateral ligaments are more commonly injured than the medial ligaments, since they are weaker. The tibiocalcaneal ligament is a medial ligament so it is much less likely to be injured.

Answer E is incorrect. The lateral ligaments are more commonly injured than the medial ligaments, since they are weaker. The tibiotalar ligament is a medial ligament so it is much less likely to be injured.

9. **The correct answer is C.** Osteogenesis imperfecta, or "brittle bone disease," is a group of hereditary disorders characterized by abnormal type I collagen synthesis. In this disease a number of mutations can result in either defective synthesis or secretion of type I collagen. The result is increased bone fragility, abnormal dentition, hearing loss, and a blue appearance to the sclera, as seen in this child.

Answer A is incorrect. Deletion of the dystrophin gene results in Duchenne muscular dystrophy, which causes accelerated muscle breakdown, proximal muscle weakness, and pseudohypertrophy of muscles due to fatty infiltration.

Answer B is incorrect. Marfan syndrome results from a defect in fibrillin, the major component of microfibrils found in the extracellular matrix. Although more than 100 distinct mutations in this gene can result in Marfan syndrome, these patients usually have problems with their eyes, skeleton, and cardiovascular system. These patients display bilateral lens subluxation, or dislocation, due to weakness in the suspensory ligaments. These patients also manifest distinctive skeletal abnormalities. They have a slender elongated habitus, arachnodactyly, high arched palate, and hyperextensibility of joints. Finally, as the result of a weakened extracellular matrix, these patients tend to display aortic aneurysms, dilation of the aortic ring resulting in aortic incompetence, and incompetent mitral and tricuspid valves.

Answer D is incorrect. Ehlers-Danlos syndrome is characterized by defects in collagen synthesis or structure. Accordingly, patients with this disorder have collagen that lacks tensile strength, and patients can have hyperextensible skin and hypermobile joints. Because of a defect in connective tissue, patients with this disorder are more susceptible to berry aneurysms.

Answer E is incorrect. Fractures do occur in many instances of child abuse. However, isolated long-bone fracture is considered a low-specificity fracture. Fractures more suggestive of child abuse include metaphyseal corner fractures and posterior rib fractures. In addition, this patient does not display other features such as abnormal bruising, retinal dislocations, or retinal hemorrhages that would be more consistent with this diagnosis.

Answer F is incorrect. Hemophilia A is an X-linked deficiency in factor VIII. These patients demonstrate prolonged partial thromboplastin times, easy bruising, and massive hemorrhage after trauma. Bleeding into joint spaces (hemarthroses) are the primary skeletal manifestation.

10. **The correct answer is C.** This patient has fractured his distal humerus, which is a common way to injure the ulnar nerve. Remember, the ulnar nerve courses through the medial epicondyle of the humerus just below the skin, so it is not well-protected at all. This vulnerability is famous with the so-called "funny bone" injuries. Our patient's radiograph shows a much more serious injury—a completely fractured humerus, so it should come as no surprise that muscles innervated by the ulnar nerve would have decreased function. Of the muscles listed here, only the flexor carpi ulnaris is innervated by the ulnar nerve, and on exam the patient would not be able to flex his fingers.

Answer A is incorrect. The first and second lumbrical muscles are innervated by the radial nerve, which is more classically injured by a mid-humeral frature. The third and fourth lumbricals are innervated by the ulnar nerve, though, so their function would likely be compromised for this patient.

Answer B is incorrect. The brachioradialis is innervated by the radial nerve, which is more classically damaged by a mid-humeral fracture.

Answer D is incorrect. The opponens pollicis muscle is innervated by the recurrent branch of the median nerve, so it would not be affected by an ulnar nerve injury.

Answer E is incorrect. The palmaris longus muscle is innervated by the median nerve, so it would not be affected by an ulnar nerve injury.

Answer F is incorrect. The pronator teres muscle is innervated by the median nerve, so it would not be affected by an ulnar nerve injury.

11. **The correct answer is C.** This patient is suffering from pemphigus vulgaris, an autoimmmune blistering disorder. This disease most commonly presents in the fourth to sixth decades of life. It is characterized by fragile blisters over the face, axilla, trunk, and mucosa. Large lesions can jeopardize fluid balance and temperature regulation, and can be sources of infection; thus severe cases may be life-threatening. The disease is caused by an autoimmune reaction against desmoglein 3, a component of desmosomes (also called macula adherens). Desmosomes are "spot-junctions" that attach epithelial cells to one another. Immunoglobulin is deposited in a net-like pattern surrounding keratinocytes. This condition is treated with corticosteroids and other immunosuppressive medications.

Answer A is incorrect. Gap junctions, comprised of connexons, allow for communication between adjacent cells, classically in cardiac muscle cells. These are not involved in pemphigus vulgaris.

Answer B is incorrect. Hemidesmosomes are similar to desmosomes, but are found exclusively between the basal layer of keratinocytes and the basement membrane. Autoimmune disease targeting hemidesomsomes causes bullous pemphigoid, a separate, milder disease characterized by tense bullae that do not easily rupture. Bullous pemphigoid tends to occur in the elderly, and oral involvement is less common. Direct immunofluorescence imaging in this condition demonstrates a linear pattern along the basement membrane, rather than the net-like pattern seen in the case above.

Answer D is incorrect. Zona adherens, or intermediate junctions, are found just deep to the zona occludens. These junctions are not involved in pemphigus vulgaris.

Answer E is incorrect. Zona occludens, or tight junctions, are located close to the surface of epithelial cells. They prevent diffusion between cells. These junctions are not involved in pemphigus vulgaris.

12. **The correct answer is B.** This patient has erythema nodosum, an inflammation of subcutaneous fat that is often accompanied by fever and malaise that is described clinically and pathologically in this vignette. The exact mechanism is unknown, but it often occurs together with inflammatory-bowel diseases (IBDs) such as Crohn disease or ulcerative colitis (UC); sarcoidosis; certain drugs (such as oral contraceptives and sulfonamides); certain malignant neoplasms; and certain infections (such as tuberculosis (TB), β-hemolytic streptococci, coccidioidomycosis, histoplasmosis, and leprosy).

Answer A is incorrect. Acne vulgaris is a disorder of the epidermis that has both inflammatory and noninflammatory variants. It is associated with the bacterium *Propionibacterium acnes*.

Answer C is incorrect. Eczema is an inflammatory skin disorder that is associated with contact allergies, asthma, ultraviolet light exposure, repeated physical skin rubbing, and certain drugs. It is not associated with erythema nodosum.

Answer D is incorrect. Pancreatitis, which is associated with many cases of biliary tract disease and alcoholism, is not associated with erythema nodosum.

Answer E is incorrect. Psoriasis is a nonpruritic inflammatory skin disorder associated with arthritis, enteropathy, spondylitic disease, and certain human leukocyte antigen (HLA) types, including HLA-B27, HLA-13, and HLA-17.

13. **The correct answer is D.** This image depicts a berry aneurysm. Berry aneurysms are congenital and associated with several syndromes. In this patient, the combination of a berry aneurysm, work as a contortionist (implying hyperextensible joints), and a history of easy bruising and bleeding suggests a collagen disorder, specifically Ehlers-Danlos syndrome (EDS). EDS is a group of disorders resulting from defects in collagen synthesis and processing. This patient likely had vascular EDS (type IV), which is associated with a defect in type III procollagen, a precursor of the collagen found in many tissues.

Answer A is incorrect. Marfan syndrome, caused by a mutation of the fibrillin-1 gene on chromosome 15, is associated with long, thin extremities, loose and occasionally hyperextensible joints, and aortic aneurysms. Mucocutaneous bleeding and bruising are not frequently seen with Marfan syndrome; EDS is a better answer.

Answer B is incorrect. Patients with epidermolysis bullosa have mutations in either keratin 14 or keratin 5, two of the major keratins in basal epithelial cells, resulting in skin that readily breaks and forms blisters with minor trauma. Epidermolysis bullosa is not associated with hyperextensible joints or berry aneurysms.

Answer C is incorrect. Osteogenesis imperfecta (OI), caused by mutations in the pro-α_1(I) chain or pro-α_2(I) chain in type I procollagen, is characterized by multiple spontaneous bone fractures, retarded wound healing, and characteristically blue sclerae. Although caused by defective collagen synthesis, OI is not associated with berry aneurysms.

Answer E is incorrect. A defect in type IV collagen is the underlying etiology for Alport syndrome. Alport syndrome is characterized by nephritis with hematuria, hearing loss, and eye disorders. Although it is commonly inherited in an X-linked pattern, autosomal-dominant and autosomal-recessive inheritance has been exhibited. Alport syndrome is not associated with the above pathology.

14. **The correct answer is D.** A spiral fracture is one that is caused by a twisting, rotational force to the bone. While child abuse may manifest with any kind of fracture, a spiral fracture should raise increased suspicion of intentionally inflicted injury. The mechanism of injury is usually the twisting of the bone by an angry adult.

Answer A is incorrect. A bowing fracture, also known as a bending fracture, is one in which the cortex of the diaphysis is deformed, but without injury to the periosteum. The pediatric bone structure has greater compliance and porosity than adult bone, resulting in injuries that deform or bend the bone rather than causing a line fracture. Bowing fractures are common pediatric fractures. While a bowing fracture could be caused by child abuse, it is not the most likely of the listed choices to suggest that etiology.

Answer B is incorrect. A buckle fracture, also known as a torus fracture, is caused by compression, resulting in a bulging or buckling of the periosteum, rather than a complete fracture line. Buckle fractures are one of the more common pediatric fractures and are frequently caused by accidents. While a buckle fracture could be caused by child abuse, it is not the most likely of the listed choices to suggest that etiology.

Answer C is incorrect. A greenstick fracture is an incomplete cortical fracture in which cortical disruption and periosteal tearing occurs on the convex aspect of the bone, but the concave aspect has an intact periosteum. Greenstick fractures are one of the more common pediatric fractures and are frequently caused by accidents. While a greenstick fracture could by caused by child abuse, it is not the most likely of the listed choices to suggest that etiology.

15. **The correct answer is D.** Conjunctivitis in a patient who has had both urethritis (or cervicitis) and arthritis for at least one month is suggestive of reactive arthritis. Most patients are in their 20s or 30s, and 80% are positive for HLA-B27. Reactive arthritis is thought to be caused by an autoimmune reaction to a gastrointestinal (GI) or genitourinary infection.

Answer A is incorrect. Ankylosing spondylitis is an inflammatory disease of the spine and sacroiliac joints causing stiffening of the back, and it often is accompanied by uveitis and aortic regurgitation. It is strongly associated with the HLA-B27 allele.

Answer B is incorrect. Lyme arthritis, usually caused by a bite from a tick harboring the spirochete *Borrelia burgdorferi*, presents with a local skin rash followed by arthralgias and arthritis (usually mono-articular). Its late sequelae include myocardial, pericardial, and neurologic changes.

Answer C is incorrect. Patients with psoriatic arthritis can have joint pain and conjunctivitis, but the diagnosis requires the presence of psoriasis, which is characterized by nonpruritic scaly or silvery erythematous plaques with well-defined borders.

Answer E is incorrect. SLE is diagnosed by the presence of four of the 11 symptoms summarized by the mnemonic "**BRAIN SOAP, MD**:" **B**lood dyscrasias (such as hemolytic anemia or thrombocytopenia), **R**enal disorder, **A**rthritis, **I**mmunologic disorder (such as anti-DNA antibody and anti-Smith antibody), **N**eurologic disorder, **S**erositis (such as pleuritis or pericarditis), **O**ral ulcers, **A**ntinuclear antibody (elevated titers in the absence of drugs associated with drug-induced lupus syndrome), **P**hotosensitivity, **M**alar rash, and **D**iscoid rash.

16. **The correct answer is D.** The patient has a classic case of chronic gout, with intermittent attacks eventually giving rise to disfiguring tophi. Gouty arthritis is a common manifestation of hyperuricemia, and tophi form as a result of the accumulation of monosodium urate crystals surrounded by reactive fibroblasts and chronic inflammatory cells in the joints and soft tissues. Common extra-articular sites of tophus formation include the Achilles tendon and the helix of the external ear. Aspiration of the tophus usually reveals the presence of neg-

atively birefringent needle-shaped crystals seen in the question image, which are characteristic of gout. The best therapy of chronic gouty arthritis aims to lower the levels or uric acid. Allopurinol blocks xanthine oxidase and thus reduces the generation of uric acid. Therefore it should be used in patients who overproduce uric acid and in patients at risk of tumor lysis syndrome to prevent renal toxicity during therapy for malignancies. It is the most effective urate-lowering agent. However, alcohol can interfere with the effectiveness of allopurinol. Probenecid increases excretion of uric acid by the kidneys and can therefore also be used in treatment of chronic gout.

Answer A is incorrect. Colchicine binds tubulin, thereby inhibiting microtubule polymerization, which blocks mitosis as well as neutrophil migration. Colchicine is now considered to be second-line treatment of acute gout because of its narrow therapeutic window and risk of toxicity. Colchicine causes GI upset and diarrhea in 80% of people.

Answer B is incorrect. NSAIDs block the enzymes cyclooxygenase-1 and/or -2, thereby blocking production of inflammatory mediators. NSAIDs have been used successfully in treatment of acute gout. Most NSAIDs can be used in treatment of gout but care must be taken with giving indomethacin to elderly patients (central nervous system adverse effects). An agent with a quick onset of action is desired, but aspirin should not be used because it can alter uric acid levels and potentially prolong and intensify an acute attack.

Answer C is incorrect. Corticosteroids are used to treat episodes of *acute* gout in patients who cannot use NSAIDs. Steroids have specific and nonspecific anti-inflammatory functions. Steroids inhibit release of phospholipase A2, an enzyme responsible for the formation of prostaglandins, leukotrienes, and other derivatives of the arachidonic acid pathway. Intra-articular corticosteroid injections may be particularly useful in patients with mono-articular gout flare-ups.

Answer E is incorrect. Losartan, an inhibitor of angiotensin II receptor, is used traditionally to treat hypertension and may delay progression of diabetic nephropathy. It has a moderately potent uricosuric effect and thus may be used in treatment of chronic gout, but not as first-line therapy.

17. **The correct answer is D.** The supraspinatus muscle is the most frequently injured rotator cuff muscle. Patients often report pain anteriorly and superiorly to the glenohumeral joint during abduction. The primary motion of the supraspinatus is the first 15 degrees of abduction of the arm, at which point the deltoid muscle continues the motion of abduction. Therefore, as long as a patient can assist the injured rotator cuff at the beginning of abduction, he or she will be able to continue the motion unassisted thereafter. This muscle and its tendon can be torn traumatically, but it is most often injured in a more insidious manner because of repetitive movement, as is the likely cause in this case.

    Answer A is incorrect. The deltoid muscle takes over for the supraspinatus muscle in abduction of the arm after about 15 degrees of abduction. The deltoid muscle is not injured in this case, as demonstrated by the patient's ability to initiate the lift motion by lifting the arm on the injured side with his other arm and then continue the motion unassisted.

    Answer B is incorrect. The action of the infraspinatus muscle is to laterally rotate the arm.

    Answer C is incorrect. The subscapularis is responsible for medial rotation and adduction of the arm.

    Answer E is incorrect. The teres minor muscle assists in lateral rotation and adduction of the arm.

18. **The correct answer is C.** The subscapularis muscle is one of the muscles that comprise the rotator cuff. It medially rotates and adducts the arm. It is the only rotator cuff muscle that acts to medially rotate the arm.

    Answer A is incorrect. The deltoid muscle is not a muscle that comprises the rotator cuff muscles. It is primarily involved in abduction of the arm at the shoulder.

Answer B is incorrect. The infraspinatus is an adductor of the arm and a lateral rotator of the glenohumoral joint.

Answer D is incorrect. The supraspinatus is the most often injured rotator cuff muscle. It is typically described as being the initiator of abduction for the first 15° of the arc. The deltoid muscle becomes the main propagator for abducting the arm beyond 15 degrees.

Answer E is incorrect. The teres minor is a narrow, elongated muscle of the rotator cuff that works to adduct and laterally rotate the arm.

19. **The correct answer is C.** This woman has a positive purified protein derivative test, signifying possible exposure to TB and latent disease. To decrease her risk of developing an active TB infection, a 6- to 12-month regimen of isoniazid is indicated. Isoniazid causes a decrease in the synthesis of mycolic acids that make up the unique cell envelope of mycobacterium TB. One of the possible adverse effects of isoniazid is a lupus-like syndrome. Drug-induced lupus is characterized by an abrupt onset of symptoms, which may include fever, arthritis, pleural pericarditis, and rash, along with the development of anti-nuclear antibodies. Other medications that may cause a similar lupus-like syndrome include procainamide, hydralazine, minocycline, and penicillamine.

Answer A is incorrect. Dapsone is used in the treatment of Hansen disease caused by *Mycobacterium leprae*. It disrupts the synthesis of folate in a method similar to that of sulfonamides. Other inhibitors of folate metabolism such as trimethoprim-sulfamethoxazole are used as prophylactic treatment against pneumocystis pneumonia in immunocompromised patients. Neither of these medications causes a lupus-like syndrome.

Answer B is incorrect. Rifampin is used to treat TB through suppression of RNA synthesis by inhibiting bacterial DNA-dependent RNA polymerase. It induces the cytochrome P450 enzyme system, and may cause tears and urine to turn orange in color, but it is not known to cause a lupus-like syndrome.

Answer D is incorrect. Inhibitors of peptidoglycan synthesis include penicillins, cephalosporins, monobactams, carbapenems, and vancomycin. These antibiotics are not used as prophylaxis against TB, and are not associated with a lupus-like syndrome.

Answer E is incorrect. Hydralazine causes vasodilation through increased production of cGMP and may cause a lupus-like syndrome. However, it would not be used to treat TB. Other drugs that also may cause a lupus-like syndrome are procainamide and phenytoin.

20. **The correct answer is B.** Four muscles are involved in jaw movement: the lateral pterygoid, masseter, temporalis, and medial pterygoid. The lateral pterygoid opens the jaw, and the other three close the jaw. One can remember this with the mnemonic "**M**'s **M**unch" and "**L**ateral **L**owers." All four muscles are innervated by the mandibular branch of the trigeminal nerve (V_3).

Answer A is incorrect. Cranial nerve (CN) V_2, the maxillary branch of the trigeminal nerve, relays sensory information from the middle portion of the face in the palpebral fissure to the mouth. V_3 is the only branch of CN V with a motor component.

Answer C is incorrect. CN VII innervates the muscles of facial expression. A lesion to this nerve would result in Bell palsy, which would present with ipsilateral facial droop. The patient has a symmetric smile, which suggests that his CN VII is intact.

Answer D is incorrect. CN X (vagus) innervates most muscles of the soft palate (except tensor veli palatini), pharynx (except stylopharyngeus), and larynx. Patients with a lesion to CN X would have difficulty swallowing (dysphagia). This patient has symmetric palate elevation, suggesting that his CN X is intact. Damage would lead to asymmetric palate elevation with the uvula pointing away from the lesion because the damaged side is lower.

Answer E is incorrect. CN XII (hypoglossal) innervates the hypoglossus, genioglossus, styloglossus, and all intrinsic muscles of the tongue. The only tongue muscle not innervated by CN XII is the palatoglossus, which is innervated by the vagus nerve (X). Lesions to CN XII would result in difficulty eating as well as slurred speech (dysarthria). This patient's tongue is midline, which suggests that his CN XII is intact. Damage would lead to the tongue pointing to the side of the lesion when protruded.

21. **The correct answer is A.** This patient has symptoms and signs consistent with a diagnosis of myasthenia gravis (MG). MG is an autoimmune disorder characterized by the presence of acetylcholine receptor antibodies, which cause impaired signal transmission at the neuromuscular junction. Patients typically present with characteristic ocular (ptosis, diplopia) and musculoskeletal (facial muscle weakness, proximal muscle weakness) symptoms, which are classically worsened by repetitive use of the involved muscles (which is why symptoms are worse by the end of the day). Thymomas (evidenced by the widened superior mediastinum in the image) occur in approximately 10% of patients with MG. The diagnosis of MG can be confirmed by measuring acetylcholine receptor antibodies and performing electromyography (EMG) and/or a Tensilon (edrophonium) test. Treatment generally consists of an acetylcholinesterase inhibitor such as pyridostigmine.

    Answer B is incorrect. Lymphoma can present with a mediastinal mass and constitutional symptoms, but is not routinely associated with musculoskeletal weakness. A complete blood cell count is useful in making the diagnosis in suspected cases.

    Answer C is incorrect. A parathyroid gland tumor can infrequently present with a mediastinal mass and commonly with generalized weakness secondary to high serum calcium levels. Measurements of PTH level are useful in making the diagnosis in suspected cases.

    Answer D is incorrect. Hypothyroidism can present with generalized fatigue and musculoskeletal weakness, but is not routinely associated with a mediastinal mass. Measurements of the thyroid-stimulating hormone (TSH) level are useful in making the diagnosis in suspected cases.

    Answer E is incorrect. Neuroblastoma can present with a mediastinal mass and constitutional symptoms, although it is typically a pediatric malignancy. Testing of urine catecholamine levels is useful in making the diagnosis in suspected cases.

22. **The correct answer is C.** This patient has acute osteomyelitis and a history of sickle cell disease as evidenced by her multiple hospitalizations (likely for episodes of painful crises) and medication (hydroxyurea reduces the incidence of painful crises in sickle cell disease by increasing the amount of fetal hemoglobin). Osteomyelitis is an infection of the bone tissue. It is common in young children and usually results from the hematogenous spread of organisms from another site of infection (upper respiratory infection in this case). *Salmonella* species are the most common organisms responsible for osteomyelitis in patients with sickle cell disease.

    Answer A is incorrect. *Escherichia coli* causes osteomyelitis in infants, but *Salmonella* species are the most common organisms responsible for osteomyelitis in patients with sickle cell disease.

    Answer B is incorrect. *Pseudomonas aeruginosa* typically causes infections in immunocompromised hosts and patients with cystic fibrosis.

    Answer D is incorrect. *Staphylococcus aureus* is the most common cause of osteomyelitis in the general population, but not in patients with sickle cell disease.

    Answer E is incorrect. *Streptococcus pyogenes* causes osteomyelitis in children, but *Salmonella* species are the most common organisms responsible for osteomyelitis in patients with sickle cell disease.

23. **The correct answer is C.** This child has achondroplasia, which is the most common inherited form of dwarfism. This autosomal dominant disease results in a disturbance of endochondral bone formation due to a mutation in the fibroblast growth factor receptor-3 (*FGF-3* gene). This change results in abnormal growth plates and impaired cartilage maturation.

 Answer A is incorrect. Osteopetrosis is a disease characterized by reduced osteoclast resorption. This condition usually manifests as repeated skeletal fractures early in life.

 Answer B is incorrect. Osteogenesis imperfecta involves a collagen I deficiency leading to bone fragility, among other findings. It does not explain the findings in this child.

 Answer D is incorrect. Mucopolysaccharidoses are lysosomal storage diseases caused by specific enzyme deficiencies. These can present in a variety of ways with chest wall abnormalities and malformed bones, but not as the findings seen in this child.

24. **The correct answer is B.** Osteoarthritis is a disease of wear and tear leading to destruction of articular cartilage, subchondral bone formation, osteophytes, sclerosis, and other degenerative changes. It is common and progressive, and becomes more so with age. It classically presents in weight-bearing joints as pain after use, improving with rest. It commonly affects the distal interphalangeal joints as well. Common imaging findings include narrowing of the joint space, sclerosis, and the presence of osteophytes. The image reveals Heberden's nodes, representing bony enlargement of the distal interphalangeal (DIP) joints.

 Answer A is incorrect. Gout is a painful swelling of a joint, most commonly the metatarsophalangeal joint, caused by precipitation of monosodium urate crystals. It is diagnosed by viewing the crystals in the joint's synovial fluid, which are negatively birefringent. It is not associated with osteophytes or sclerosis with narrowing.

 Answer C is incorrect. Osteomyelitis is an infection in the bone. It presents most commonly with tenderness, warmth, swelling, and more acute pain, rather than joint narrowing. The pain typically is present with and without movement.

 Answer D is incorrect. Pseudogout causes symptoms that mimic those of gout, but is caused by the precipitation of calcium pyrophosphate crystals within the joint space. These crystals are positively birefringent, which means they are blue under polarized light. This disease classically affects large joints, most commonly the knee, in men over 50 years old. It is not associated with osteophytes or sclerosis with narrowing.

 Answer E is incorrect. Rheumatoid arthritis is an autoimmune arthritis caused by inflammatory destruction of synovial joints. It is associated with pain that is worst in the morning, improving with use, and classically affects the proximal interphalangeal joints. It is not associated with osteophytes or sclerosis with narrowing.

25. **The correct answer is D.** This patient has Sjögren syndrome. The vast majority of patients with this syndrome are women between the ages of 35 and 45, and the disease is characterized by dry eyes (keratoconjunctivitis sicca), dry mouth (xerostomia), and one other connective tissue or autoimmune disease (such as rheumatoid arthritis). The eye and mouth dryness is from autoimmune destruction of the lacrimal and salivary glands.

 Answer A is incorrect. CREST syndrome is a variant of scleroderma (progressive systemic sclerosis), which is a disease characterized by extensive fibrosis throughout the body (most notably of the skin). **CREST** stands for **C**alcinosis, **R**aynaud phenomenon, **E**sophageal dysfunction, **S**clerodactyly, and **T**elangiectasia.

 Answer B is incorrect. Cystic fibrosis also causes dysfunction of the exocrine glands (such as the lacrimal and salivary glands), but it is due to a mutation in the cystic fibrosis transmembrane conductance regulator gene on chromosome 7. Individuals with cystic fibrosis also tend to have pulmonary and pancreatic dysfunction.

Answer C is incorrect. When only the first two criteria are present (dry eyes and dry mouth), the disorder is called sicca syndrome.

Answer E is incorrect. Sjögren-Larsson is an autosomal-recessive syndrome characterized by congenital ichthyosis (dry and scaly, fishlike skin) and associated with mental retardation and spastic paraplegia; it is caused by a mutation in the aldehyde dehydrogenase gene on chromosome 17p.

26. **The correct answer is B.** Anterior cruciate ligament (ACL) injuries are common injuries in sports and frequently occur without contact when people change direction on a planted foot. ACL tears are commonly associated with other injuries and occur in isolation <10% of the time. The most common association is with the lateral meniscus and medial collateral ligament (MCL), which together with the ACL are referred to as the "unhappy triad" of knee injury.

    Answer A is incorrect. The valgus force of the injury described in the question is unlikely to put tension on the lateral collateral ligament, so it is less likely to be injured.

    Answer C is incorrect. Although it is possible to injure the medial meniscus, a medial meniscus injury is less likely to be associated with a concurrent MCL and ACL injury.

    Answer D is incorrect. The patellar ligament is a thick strong ligament that is unlikely to be injured in this type of mechanism.

    Answer E is incorrect. The posterior cruciate ligament is a strong ligament, but it can be injured, especially in association with collateral ligament tears; however, it is less likely to be injured via this mechanism.

27. **The correct answer is A.** The most likely diagnosis is Ewing sarcoma. Made up of anaplastic, small blue cells, Ewing sarcoma is classified as one of the primitive neuroectodermal tumors. This patient's presentation is typical in that 80% of tumors are found in patients <20 years old. Most of these are between the ages of 10 and 15 years. Males are at slightly greater risk than females, and a great proportion of patients are white. Plain film x-ray classically reveals a lytic lesion with "onion skinning" of the periosteum. This reactive process occurs as the tumor arises out of the medullary cavity and new layers of bone are deposited around it by the periosteum (hyperlucent layers seen in the radiograph). Microscopic analysis of biopsy specimens reveals sheets of uniform, small, round cells that are slightly larger than lymphocytes. Rosette formations may be seen as cells arrange themselves around a central fibrous space. Otherwise, there is very little stromal space and no normal bony matrix material.

    Answer B is incorrect. Giant cell tumors differ in their most common presentation, peaking in incidence between the ages of 20 and 40 years, and arising from the epiphyseal end of long bones. Plain film x-ray classically shows a "soap bubble" appearance, and histology shows spindle-shaped cells with multinucleated giant cells interspersed between them.

    Answer C is incorrect. Osteochondroma, the most common benign tumor of bone, is a cartilaginous cap attached to the skeleton by a mature bony stalk. Also known as exostosis, it very rarely converts to a malignant neoplastic process.

    Answer D is incorrect. Ewing sarcoma may mimic infection with systemic findings such as fever, elevated erythrocyte sedimentation rate (ESR), anemia, and leukocytosis, as well as local inflammation of the surrounding soft tissue. However, the diagnostic work-up of this patient is not consistent with infection.

    Answer E is incorrect. Osteosarcoma is the most common primary malignant tumor of bone. Like Ewing, it peaks in occurrence between the ages of 10 and 20 years, and arises most often in the metaphyseal region of long bones. However, the key difference is in the results of the imaging and biopsy studies. Classically, osteosarcomas show Codman triangle or a sunburst pattern on plain film x-ray. Histologically, cellular patterning is highly variable, with a number of subtypes. The most characteristic feature, however, is the formation of bony matrix material by the tumor cells, which does not occur in Ewing sarcoma.

28. **The correct answer is A.** This patient has symptoms and signs consistent with vitamin D-deficient rickets, which results from the decreased or absent mineralization of osteoid (bone matrix) secondary to decreased serum calcium and/or phosphorous levels. Vitamin D normally promotes absorption of calcium and phosphorous from the GI tract. In vitamin D-deficient patients, areas of bone growth (eg, wrists, ankles, costochondral junctions) contain patches of unmineralized, soft osteoid that give rise to the classically reported signs, including widened wrists and/or ankles and enlarged costochondral junctions (rachitic rosary). In cases of severe vitamin D deficiency, laboratory studies typically demonstrate decreased serum calcium, decreased serum phosphorous, decreased serum 1,25-dihydroxycholecalciferol, increased serum alkaline phosphatase, and increased serum intact PTH levels.

    Answer B is incorrect. A decreased, not increased, serum 1,25-dihydroxycholecalciferol level is characteristic of vitamin D-deficient rickets.

    Answer C is incorrect. A decreased, not increased, serum 25-hydroxycholecalciferol level is characteristic of vitamin D-deficient rickets.

    Answer D is incorrect. A decreased, not increased, serum calcium level (due to decreased GI absorption) is characteristic of vitamin D-deficient rickets.

    Answer E is incorrect. A decreased, not increased, serum phosphorous level (due to decreased GI absorption) is characteristic of vitamin D-deficient rickets.

29. **The correct answer is C.** This woman has sustained an injury to her long thoracic nerve, which innervates the serratus anterior muscle, as a complication of her surgery. The function of the serratus anterior muscle is to anchor the scapula against the thoracic cage. When the long thoracic nerve is damaged, the scapula moves away from the thoracic cage, resulting in what is referred to as winging of the scapula. Long thoracic nerve injury is an occasional complication of mastectomy. The long thoracic nerve originates from the brachial plexus, specifically from C5, C6, and C7.

    Answer A is incorrect. C3, C4, and C5 are the origins of the phrenic nerve, which innervates the diaphragm.

    Answer B is incorrect. C5 and C6 join together to form the upper trunk, and do participate in the formation of the long thoracic nerve, but C7 is also involved.

    Answer D is incorrect. The long thoracic nerve does not originate from C7 and C8.

    Answer E is incorrect. C8 and T1 join together to form the lower trunk of the brachial plexus, while C7 is a part of the middle trunk. Neither C8 nor T1 contributes to the long thoracic nerve.

30. **The correct answer is E.** Rheumatoid factor would most likely be positive in this woman, who is suffering from RA. Eighty percent of patients with RA have positive rheumatoid factor (anti-IgG antibody). This autoimmune condition causes a marked influx of inflammatory cells into the joint synovium, as seen here, resulting in destructive change, pannus formation, and eventually joint deformity. The disease is more common in women, and classically symmetrically affects the proximal interphalangeal joints, as described here.

    Answer A is incorrect. Anti-centromere antibody is associated with the CREST variant of scleroderma (progressive systemic sclerosis). In this disease patients suffer from Calcinosis, Raynaud phenomenon, Esophageal dysmotility, Sclerodactyly, and Telangiectasia. Arthritis is not associated with this syndrome.

    Answer B is incorrect. Anti-nuclear antibody is associated with SLE, an autoimmune disease with a wide variety of symptoms including fever, rash, joint pain, and photosensitivity. The joint pain in lupus is typically transient, asymmetrical, and non-deforming.

Answer C is incorrect. *Borrelia burgdorferi* is the gram negative bacteria that causes Lyme disease. While the third stage of Lyme disease can manifest as migratory polyarthritis, this patient has no other associated signs or symptoms.

Answer D is incorrect. HLA-B27 is strongly associated with joint disease without rheumatoid factor, such as ankylosing spondylitis. This condition most commonly affects men and causes severe stiffening of the spine and sacroiliac joints, as well as uveitis. The hands are not typically involved.

31. **The correct answer is C.** Poliovirus infects the Peyer patches of the intestine and the motor neurons. It is passed by the fecal-oral route and can present as a spectrum of severity, depending on the age of the patient. Younger children and infants often have a nonclinical infection or mild fever with diarrhea. Older children who have not previously been infected can develop meningitic signs. The most severe complications are respiratory muscle failure, paraplegia, and quadriplegia.

Answer A is incorrect. The neuron loss that occurs affects the motor neurons in the anterior horns, not the posterior horns.

Answer B is incorrect. Because this is a lower motor neuron disease, reflexes are lost in the affected limbs, and the limbs atrophy.

Answer D is incorrect. The poliovirus infects the motor neurons, leaving sensation spared.

Answer E is incorrect. Poliovirus does not affect short-term memory or cortical functioning. It can affect the cranial nerves, however.

32. **The correct answer is A.** The common peroneal nerve courses around the neck of the fibula, making it vulnerable to damage by a fracture at the fibular neck. It is the most frequently lesioned nerve in the lower limb. Patients experience foot drop, which results from a loss of dorsiflexion at the ankle, and a loss of eversion. Patients will have pain and paresthesia in the lateral leg and dorsum of the foot. Patients with foot drop may also have a steppage gait, as described in the vignette. Common peroneal nerve injury can occur with fracture to the fibular neck and patients will present with an inability to dorsiflex or evert, as well as a foot drop gait.

Answer B is incorrect. The femoral nerve courses in the anterior thigh and branches into the tibial nerve and the common peroneal nerve. It is not involved in fractures to the fibular neck.

Answer C is incorrect. The L4 nerve root defines the sensory dermatome to the lateral aspect of the foot and leg. Patients also can have motor weakness in the L4 myotome. However, the combination of impaired dorsiflexion and eversion is most specific for damage to a peripheral nerve (common peroneal).

Answer D is incorrect. Obturator nerve does not travel near the fibula. It is not involved in injuries to the fibula.

Answer E is incorrect. The tibial nerve is unlikely to be injured because it is well protected in the popliteal fossa, although it can be injured by deep lacerations.

33. **The correct answer is B.** This patient has osteomyelitis, most commonly caused by *Pseudomonas aeruginosa* in intravenous drug users. The image shows a bone abscess with polymorphonuclear leukocytes and foci of degraded bone collagen. Treatment would require several weeks of antipseudomonal antibiotics such as ticarcillin or piperacillin.

Answer A is incorrect. Chronic corticosteroid use can lead to immunosuppression and osteoporosis, but does not predispose one to pseudomonal osteomyelitis..

Answer C is incorrect. Patients with miliary *Mycobacterium tuberculosis* infection are at risk for vertebral osteomyelitis, known as Pott disease. It is uncommon for tubercular osteomyelitis to affect the humerus.

Answer D is incorrect. Multiple sexual partners would put the patient at increased risk of *Neisseria gonorrhoeae* infection, which can cause osteomyelitis. More commonly, the patient would have urethritis, epidydimitis, or perhaps Fitz-Hugh-Curtis syndrome, which is the formation of postinfection adhesions on the liver capsule, leading to chronic upper right quadrant pain.

Answer E is incorrect. Patients with sickle cell anemia are at risk for osteomyelitis due to *Salmonella* or *Staphylococcus*, but not to pseudomonal osteomyelitis.

34. **The correct answer is B.** This patient suffers from lateral epicondylitis, better known as tennis elbow. This condition stems from overuse of the superficial extensor muscles of the forearm and wrist, including the extensor carpi radialis muscle. This muscle also inserts at the lateral epicondyle. The repeated forced extension and flexion of the forearm at the elbow causes an inflammation of the common extensor tendon. Patients exhibit pain over the lateral epicondyle that may radiate down the posterior aspect of the forearm. Treatment options include rehabilitation, which may include exercises, motion analysis, and straps or braces; medication; open surgery; and arthroscopic (minimally invasive) surgery.

Answer A is incorrect. The biceps muscle functions to supinate and flex the forearm.

Answer C is incorrect. The extensor carpi ulnaris muscle functions to extend and adduct the hand at the wrist but does not extend the forearm.

Answer D is incorrect. The flexor carpi ulnaris muscle functions to flex and abduct the hand at the wrist.

Answer E is incorrect. The pronator teres muscle functions to pronate and flex the forearm.

35. **The correct answer is E.** *Yersinia pestis* is the organism responsible for the plague, also known as the Black Death. The bacterium can be spread to humans by fleas from rodents, especially prairie dogs in the United States. The disease develops after two-eight days of incubation and is characterized by the presence of exquisitely tender lymph nodes called buboes. Unlike in the case of anthrax, the skin ulcers seen in *Y pestis* infection are painful. Furthermore, prolonged infection and spread of *Y pestis* can lead to disseminated intravascular coagulation.

Answer A is incorrect. *Babesia microti* is transmitted to humans through the bite of a tick. It causes a sickness similar to malaria with symptoms of fever and anemia.

Answer B is incorrect. *Bacillus anthracis* can cause cutaneous anthrax, which is characterized by a painless ulcer with a black scab.

Answer C is incorrect. *Leishmania donovani* is transmitted through the bite of a sandfly and causes visceral leishmaniasis. This disease is characterized by abdominal pain and distention, anorexia, weight loss, and fever.

Answer D is incorrect. A person infected with *Trichinella spiralis* presents with fever, periorbital and facial edema, myalgia, and eosinophilia.

36. **The correct answer is C.** A sarcomere, the basic functional unit of skeletal muscle, extends from one Z line to an adjacent Z line. Upon muscle contraction, the power stroke results from actin sliding on myosin, causing Z lines to move closer together. The absolute length of the thin (actin) and thick filaments (myosin) in a myofibril does not change during contraction, but rather the overlap of the filaments increases. Thus, the A band, which is the length of myosin, does not change upon contraction. The H band and I band are the two areas where there is no overlap of actin and myosin; both bands will then decrease when the overlap increases with contraction.

Answer A is incorrect. The A band, which is composed of myosin, does not change with contraction. H shortens and I shortens.

Answer B is incorrect. This is what will occur upon relaxation. The A band will again remain the same length, but as myosin and actin decrease their overlap, both the H and I bands will increase in length.

Answer D is incorrect. The A band, which is composed of myosin, does not change with contraction. H shortens and I shortens.

Answer E is incorrect. The A band, which is composed of myosin, does not change with contraction. H shortens and I shortens.

37. **The correct answer is B.** This patient has psoriatic arthritis, which presents with psoriasis (nonpruritic scaly or silvery erythematous plaques with well-defined borders) and joint symptoms that are of acute onset in one-third of patients. Psoriatic arthritis is an inflammatory arthritis and signs of inflammation, such as an elevated ESR, are commonly seen in patients with this condition. More than 50% of patients have an asymmetric distribution of joint swelling in the distal interphalangeal joints of the hands and feet. Some patients may develop a sausage-like finger from inflammation of the digital tendon sheaths.

Answer A is incorrect. Celiac disease is a malabsorption syndrome in which patients produce autoantibodies to gluten (gliadin). Dermatitis herpetiformis is a skin disorder commonly seen in patients with celiac disease; it causes pruritic papules and vesicles, not scaly plaques. Patients can present with arthralgias; however, the joints do not usually become swollen.

Answer C is incorrect. Gout is characterized by a raised serum uric acid level that leads to uric acid deposition in tissues, particularly the joint spaces. Urate crystal deposition in a joint can cause an inflammatory reaction, leading to joint pain and inflammation. Diagnosis of gout is generally based on clinical symptoms and the presence of urate crystals (which are negatively bifringent and needle-shaped) in the joint fluid. The presence of arthritic symptoms and the absence of elevated uric acid levels make the diagnosis of gouty arthritis unlikely.

Answer D is incorrect. Rheumatoid arthritis is another type of inflammatory arthritis; however, joint involvement is generally bilateral and symmetric. Joint involvement of the hand often leads to ulnar deviation of the wrist, as well as swan-neck and boutonniere deformities of the interphalangeal joints. Generalized swelling and a sausage-like appearance of the digits are not commonly seen. Patients with rheumatoid arthritis can also have cutaneous manifestations, the most characteristic being rheumatoid nodules that are usually located over bony prominences. About 80% of patients with rheumatoid arthritis are positive for rheumatoid factor.

Answer E is incorrect. Pseudogout is a rheumatologic disorder characterized by calcium pyrophosphate dihydrate deposition in connective tissues. The presentation of pseudogout is very similar to that of gout, except the joint fluid contains calcium pyrophosphate dihydrate crystals, which are weakly bifringent and rhomboidal in shape.

38. **The correct answer is B.** The infection caused by *Actinomyces israelii* typically presents as a chronic, slowly progressing mass that eventually evolves into a draining sinus tract. Characteristic sulfur granules are seen in the thick yellow exudate. Penicillin G is the first-line treatment.

Answer A is incorrect. This describes the mechanism for amphotericin B, which is used to treat systemic mycoses. While *Actinomyces* form long, branching filaments that resemble fungi, they are bacteria.

Answer C is incorrect. Sulfonamides act by inhibiting dihydropteroate synthetase, preventing nucleotide synthesis. They are first-line medications for *Nocardia* infection but not for *Actinomyces*.

Answer D is incorrect. Many antibiotics act by blocking protein synthesis including macrolides, aminoglycosides, and tetracyclines. However, none of these are first-line treatments for *Actinomyces* infection, which best explains this patient's presentation.

Answer E is incorrect. This describes the mechanism for azoles such as fluconazole and ketoconazole, which are used to treat fungal infections. While *Actinomyces* form long, branching filaments that resemble fungi, they are bacteria.

39. **The correct answer is A.** The genitofemoral nerve arises from the L1 and L2 nerve roots. In male subjects its genital branch travels through the superficial inguinal ring along with the spermatic cord, and supplies the cremaster and the scrotal skin. Severing the genitofemoral nerve during a hernia repair leads to numbness of the scrotum and/or inner thigh. The genitofemoral nerve and the ilioinguinal nerve have overlapping territory. Thus, severing one only leads to transient anesthesia.

    Answer B is incorrect. The lateral femoral cutaneous nerve originates from the L2-L3 roots of the lumbar plexus, passes deep to the inguinal ligament, and innervates the skin on the lateral aspect of the thigh.

    Answer C is incorrect. The posterior femoral cutaneous nerve originates from the S1-S3 roots of the sacral plexus, passes through the greater sciatic foramen, and innervates the skin overlying the buttock, the posterior aspect of the thigh, and the popliteal fossa.

    Answer D is incorrect. Nerve roots S2-S4 are associated with the pudendal nerve, which innervates the external genitals. Injury to this nerve would be associated with bowel or bladder incontinence and possible anesthesia in the perineum. This nerve is injured most commonly during childbirth or saddle injury. The pudendal nerve is not near the inguinal ligament

40. **The correct answer is C.** C is the epidermis. Pemphigus vulgaris is an autoimmune disorder in which pathogenic antibodies are directed against a cell-cell adhesion protein, desmoglein-3, which is expressed by the keratinocytes of the epidermis. The destruction of desmoglein leads to intraepidermal acantholysis with sparing of the basal layer. Physical exam typically shows flaccid epidermal bullae that easily slough off leaving large denuded areas of skin (Nikolsky sign), subject to secondary infection. Treatment is usually steroids.

    Answer A is incorrect. A is the stratum corneum, which is composed of enucleated, keratinized, flat keratinocytes. The autoantibodies that mediate pemphigus vulgaris are directed against desmoglein-3, a protein involved in cell-cell adhesion within the other layers of the epidermis, not within the stratum corneum.

    Answer B is incorrect. B is the dermoepidermal junction. The autoantibodies that mediate this disease are directed against a protein expressed in the epidermis.

    Answer D is incorrect. D is the dermis. The autoantibodies that mediate this disease are directed against a protein expressed in the epidermis.

    Answer E is incorrect. E is the hypodermis. The autoantibodies that mediate this disease are directed against a protein expressed in the epidermis.

41. **The correct answer is D.** Polyarteritis nodosa (PAN) is a vasculitis (ie, inflammation of a blood vessel) characterized by inflammation affecting small to medium-sized arteries, particularly the renal, cardiac, and GI-tract vessels (usually not the pulmonary vasculature). As many as 30% of patients have had prior hepatitis-B infections.

    Answer A is incorrect. Buerger disease, also known as thromboangiitis obliterans, is a vasculitis that mostly affects arteries and veins of the extremities. As such, patients often have intermittent claudication and Raynaud phenomenon. The majority of patients are men who are heavy smokers and show hypersensitivity to tobacco injected into the skin.

    Answer B is incorrect. Giant cell (temporal) arteritis is a type of vasculitis that affects the arteries of the head, especially, of course, the temporal arteries. The highlights of this disease can be remembered by the mnemonic, **JOE**: patients get **J**aw pain and **O**cular disturbances from ischemia to the arteries supplying them. Patients also often have markedly elevated **E**rythrocyte sedimentation rates. The disease is often associated with the presence of polymyalgia rheumatica.

    Answer C is incorrect. Kawasaki disease is a self-limited vasculitis that normally occurs in infants and children and is characterized by conjunctival and oral erythema, fever, erythema and edema of the palms and soles, generalized rash, and cervical lymph node swelling. About 20% of patients may go on to develop coronary artery inflammation and/or aneurysm.

Answer E is incorrect. Takayasu arteritis is a vasculitis characterized by fibrotic thickening of the aortic arch (it also affects the pulmonary arteries, the branches of the aortic arch, and the rest of the aorta in up to one-third of patients). Clinically, patients often have lower blood pressure and weaker pulses in the upper extremities than in the lower extremities; some patients have ocular disturbances as well.

42. **The correct answer is C.** This patient has RA, which is characterized by systemic symptoms of fever, fatigue, pleuritis, and pericarditis. Women are affected by RA more frequently than men. Patients with RA classically experience symmetric morning stiffness of joints that improves with use. Patients may also have subcutaneous rheumatoid nodules, ulnar deviation of the fingers, and joint subluxation. RA is mediated by a type III hypersensitivity reaction in which immune complexes form and activate complement. In RA, rheumatoid factor is an IgM autoantibody that is directed against the Fc region of the patient's IgG antibody, leading to immune complex formation and deposition. Rheumatoid factor antibodies are present in a number of asymptomatic patients; more recently, anti-CCP (citrulline-containing protein) antibodies have become more popular as sensitive and specific serological diagnostic indicators of RA.

Answer A is incorrect. The Arthus reaction is a local, subacute, antibody-mediated hypersensitivity reaction. Hypersensitivity pneumonitis from thermophilic actinomycetes, not RA, is explained by the Arthus reaction.

Answer B is incorrect. Delayed, cell-mediated hypersensitivity reactions are also type IV hypersensitivity reactions. In this type of reaction, sensitized T lymphocytes encounter antigen and release lymphokines, leading to macrophage activation. A positive TB skin test is an example of a type IV hypersensitivity reaction. In rheumatoid arthritis, CD4+ T lymphocytes stimulate the immune cascade, leading to cytokine production such as tumor necrosis factor-α and interleukin-1. However, the main mechanism of injury is believed to be the formation of immune complexes.

Answer D is incorrect. Type I hypersensitivity reactions are characterized by antigens that cross-link IgE antibodies present on presensitized mast cells and basophils. This cross-linking results in the release of vasoactive amines, like histamine.

Answer E is incorrect. Type II hypersensitivity reactions are mediated by antibody binding to a host antigen on a cell, leading to phagocytosis or lysis of the cell by complement. In Graves disease, an example of a type II hypersensitivity reaction, autoantibodies bind to and activate the TSH receptor on thyroid gland cells, causing increased triiodothyronine and thyroxine production and release.

43. **The correct answer is A.** This patient has ankylosing spondylitis, a chronic inflammatory disease of the spine and sacroiliac joints that often leads to the stiffening or consolidation of the bones that make up the joints. Common findings are low back pain, stiffness for over three months, pain and stiffness in the thoracic region, limited movement in the lumbar area, and limited chest expansion. Around 90% of patients are positive for human leukocyte antigen (HLA) B27, and common complications include uveitis and aortic regurgitation.

Answer B is incorrect. Antinuclear antibodies are most commonly found in systemic autoimmune diseases such as lupus, scleroderma, Sjögren syndrome, and rheumatoid arthritis.

Answer C is incorrect. Antineutrophil cytoplasmic antibodies (ANCA) are associated with the vasculitides, including Wegener granulomatosis and Churg-Strauss syndrome.

Answer D is incorrect. IgM antibodies to *B burgdorferi* are suggestive of acute Lyme disease, which is transmitted by a bite from an *Ixodes* tick. Initially patients suffer from a local skin infection (often in a bull's-eye pattern) that can be followed by arthralgias and arthritis (usually monoarticular). The late sequelae of Lyme disease include myocardial, pericardial, and neurologic changes.

Answer E is incorrect. Rheumatoid factor is positive in about 80% of patients with rheumatoid arthritis; it can also be positive in those with other rheumatic disorders such as Sjögren syndrome and lupus, as well as in healthy people. Rheumatoid arthritis is an autoimmune disorder of synovial joints and often presents with morning joint stiffness, subcutaneous joint nodules (particularly in the proximal interphalangeal joints), and symmetric joint involvement. The disease may also include systemic symptoms such as fever, pleuritis, and pericarditis.

Answer F is incorrect. Vertebral compression fractures are a complication of osteoporosis and present with acute back pain, loss of height, and kyphosis.

44. **The correct answer is C.** This patient most likely has a "boxer's fracture," which occurs when individuals strike a blow with a closed fist against a hard, unyielding object. The most commonly injured sites for experienced boxers are the first and second metacarpals, whereas for others, the neck of the fifth metacarpal is the most common site of injury. The metacarpals have a good blood supply and thus heal rapidly.

Answer A is incorrect. A complete transverse fracture of the distal radius is called Colles' fracture. This occurs most commonly in the elderly after forced dorsiflexion. It results in avulsion of the styloid process from the shaft of the radius. The radius may be shortened, and the styloid process of the ulna may project farther distally than the styloid process of the radius. The forearm and hand may exhibit a "dinner fork" deformity as a result of the posterior displacement of the distal part of the radius.

Answer B is incorrect. Fracture of the hamate is not common but can be complicated, as the ulnar nerve can often be injured. Patients with an ulnar nerve lesion at the wrist may have an ulnar claw hand, which is caused by a weakness of the medial two lumbricals that flex at the metacarpophalangeal joints and extend at the interphalangeal joints of the ring and little fingers. Patients will also experience weakness in the ability to abduct or adduct fingers or adduct the thumb at the metacarpophalangeal joints (interosseous muscles and adductor pollicis). They are unable to hold a piece of paper between the thumb and index finger or between adjacent fingers. Weakness of the interosseous muscles may also result in a slight clawing of the index and middle fingers. The muscles in the hypothenar eminence may also be affected; patients experience weakness in flexion, abduction, and opposition of the fifth finger. Altered sensation in skin of the medial aspect of the hand and medial digits may be evident. There are healing difficulties associated with this type of fracture.

Answer D is incorrect. Fracture of the phalanges is a common injury and is often due to crushing or hyperextension injuries.

Answer E is incorrect. Fracture of the scaphoid commonly occurs when individuals fall onto an outstretched hand. The scaphoid is the most commonly fractured carpal bone, and patients may exhibit pain and tenderness localized over the anatomic snuffbox.

45. **The correct answer is B.** Anti-Jo-1 antibody is a myositis-specific antibody most commonly associated with polymyositis and dermatomyositis. Polymyositis and dermatomyositis are diagnosed if five criteria are met: symmetric proximal muscle weakness; characteristic heliotrope rash; elevated serum muscle enzymes; myopathic changes on EMG; and muscle biopsy abnormalities with the absence of histopathologic signs of other myopathies. This patient presented with the heliotrope rash, a skin manifestation that is highly specific for dermatomyositis.

Answer A is incorrect. Anti-dsDNA autoantibodies are associated with SLE.

Answer C is incorrect. Anti-IgG autoantibodies are associated with rheumatoid arthritis. Anti-IgG is also known as rheumatoid factor.

Answer D is incorrect. Anti-microsomal auto-antibodies are associated with Hashimoto thyroiditis, not polymyositis or dermatomyositis.

Answer E is incorrect. Anti-mitochrondrial auto-antibodies are associated with primary biliary cirrhosis, not polymyositis or dermatomyositis.

CHAPTER 13

Neurology

QUESTIONS

1. Parents bring their 10-day-old infant to the emergency department because of poor feeding for the past two days. The infant is febrile and appears lethargic and irritable. Blood and cerebrospinal fluid (CSF) are taken for culture, and the infant is started on ampicillin and gentamicin. Laboratory culture of CSF reveals growth of gram-positive bacilli, with β-hemolysis on sheep blood agar. The microbiologist notes that the same organism may cause meningitis in an immunocompromised adult. What is the likely mode of pathogen transmission to the immunocompromised adult?

   (A) An ascending urinary tract infection
   (B) Direct inoculation into an open wound
   (C) Inhalation of aerosolized bacteria
   (D) Ingestion of unpasteurized milk

2. The diagram below depicts the arterial network of the brain. Infarction of the artery designated by arrow "A" would lead to which of the following deficits?

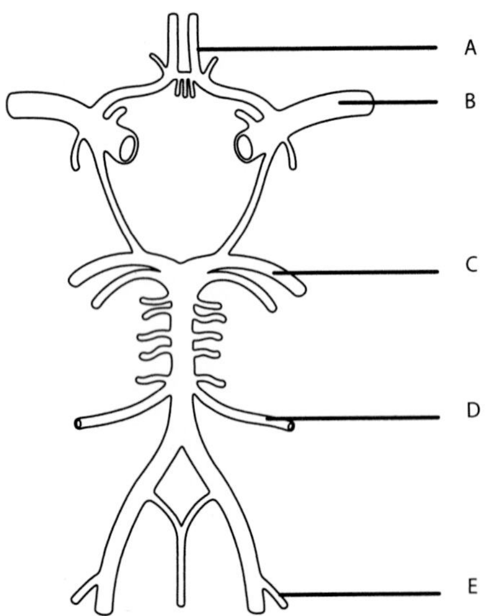

Reproduced, with permission, from USMLERx.com.

   (A) Contralateral motor deficits of the arm and hand
   (B) Contralateral motor deficits of the face
   (C) Contralateral motor deficits of the leg and foot
   (D) Ipsilateral motor deficits of the arm and hand
   (E) Ipsilateral motor deficits of the face
   (F) Ipsilateral motor deficits of the leg and foot

3. During the autopsy of a patient noted to have xanthochromia, the pathologist removes the calvarium and the attached dura. On the surface of the brain there is frank blood that cannot be removed by rubbing or scraping the surface. Which of the following most likely caused this finding?

   (A) Ruptured aneurysm
   (B) Intraparenchymal hemorrhage
   (C) Intradural hemorrhage
   (D) Tearing of bridging veins
   (E) Temporoparietal bone fracture

4. A 34-year-old man comes to the physician because of the gradual onset of involuntary limb and facial movements, mood swings, and trouble with his memory. He says that his father displayed similar symptoms when he was in his 40s. Which of the following changes would most likely be seen in this patient?

   (A) Accumulation of neuritic plaques
   (B) Copper accumulation in the basal ganglia
   (C) Gliosis of the caudate nucleus
   (D) Loss of pigmentation in substantia nigra
   (E) Scattered plaques of demyelination

5. Examination of a newborn shows a number of serious nervous system abnormalities. A diagnosis of meningohydroencephalocele is made. Which of the following descriptions is most consistent with this diagnosis?

   (A) Protrusion of the meninges, the brain, and a portion of the ventricle through a defect in the skull
   (B) Protrusion of the meninges and brain through a defect in the skull
   (C) Protrusion of the meninges and spinal cord through a vertebral defect, forming a sac

(D) Protrusion of the meninges through a defect in the skull
(E) Protrusion of the meninges through a vertebral defect, forming a sac

6. A 40-year-old man was admitted to the neurology service for evaluation of persistent numbness over his left jaw and lower face. MRI reveals a mass that is compressing a cranial nerve as the nerve exits the skull. The cranial nerve involved in this case exits the skull through which of the following foramina?

(A) Foramen ovale
(B) Foramen rotundum
(C) Foramen spinosum
(D) Jugular foramen
(E) Superior orbital fissure

7. A 47-year-old man presents with dysarthria and progressive muscle weakness of the bilateral upper and lower extremities in the absence of any history of neurologic disease or recent illness, weight loss, or trauma. Physical examination is notable for muscle atrophy and weakness in all extremities. Deep tendon reflexes are absent in the upper extremities but are 3+ in the lower extremities; some fasciculations are present. Babinski's sign is up-going bilaterally, and cranial nerves are intact. Laboratory and imaging studies are all within normal limits. Which of the following would be expected on microscopic examination of the central nervous system?

(A) Demyelination of axons in the dorsal columns and spinocerebellar tracts in the spinal cord
(B) Demyelination of axons in the posterior limb of the internal capsule in the cerebrum
(C) Neuronal loss in the region of the anterior horn cells and corticospinal tracts in the spinal cord
(D) Neuronal loss in the region of the anterior horn cells and posterior columns in the spinal cord
(E) Neuronal loss only in the region of the anterior horn cells in the spinal cord

8. A researcher studying the function of the hypothalamus ablates the supraoptic hypophyseal tract in laboratory rats. Which of the following processes will be impaired in these animals?

(A) Concentration of urine
(B) Milk synthesis
(C) Ovulation
(D) Salt retention
(E) Spermatogenesis

9. A 71-year-old woman is diagnosed with non-Hodgkin lymphoma. Soon after starting her first cycle of chemotherapy, she reports severe nausea and vomiting. Prochlorperazine is prescribed to control this adverse effect. Upon which of the following labeled areas of the brain does prochlorperazine act?

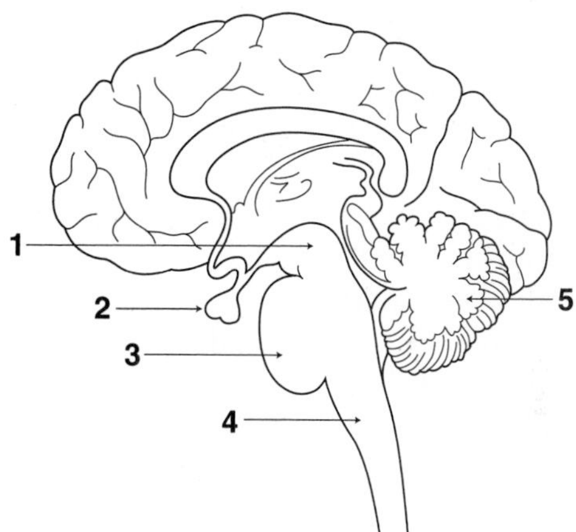

Reproduced, with permission, from USMLERx.com.

(A) 1
(B) 2
(C) 3
(D) 4
(E) 5

HIGH-YIELD SYSTEMS

Neurology

10. A patient has a sudden, almost-total occlusion of his right internal carotid artery. Brain tissue in which cerebral artery territory is likely to be affected most by the resultant ischemia?

    (A) The territory supplied by the anterior cerebral artery
    (B) The territory supplied by the middle cerebral artery
    (C) The territory supplied by the posterior cerebral artery
    (D) The watershed territory between the middle cerebral artery and the posterior cerebral artery
    (E) The watershed territory between the anterior cerebral artery and the middle cerebral artery

11. A 63-year-old homeless woman is brought to the emergency department (ED) by the police because she is disoriented and confused. On questioning the patient frequently forgets what she has been asked. She provides seemingly plausible details of the events prior to her coming to the hospital, but her accounts are entirely inconsistent with the police report. On physical examination she is emaciated and has nystagmus and an unsteady gait. ED records indicate that she has presented multiple times in the past for alcohol withdrawal and alcohol-related injuries. The lesion accounting for the patient's signs and symptoms is located in which part of the brain?

    (A) Amygdala
    (B) Basal ganglia
    (C) Broca area
    (D) Mamillary bodies
    (E) Wernicke area

12. An 89-year-old woman is brought to the clinic after suffering from a number of recent minor falls and episodes of confusion. MRI of the brain reveals a mass localized to a convexity of the left hemisphere. The patient declines treatment and dies a few months later. An autopsy slide obtained from the patient's brain lesion is shown in the image. From which type of cell does the tumor seen here typically arise?

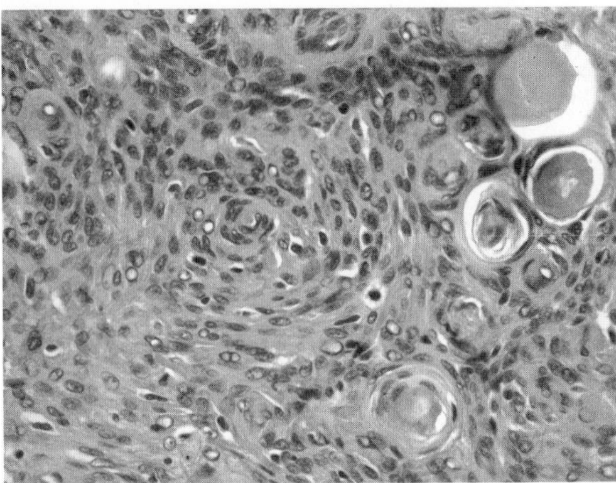

Reproduced, with permission, from USMLERx.com.

    (A) Arachnoid cells
    (B) Astrocytes
    (C) Melanocytes
    (D) Neurons
    (E) Oligodendrocytes

13. A 24-year-old woman with no significant medical history complains of double vision that began two weeks ago. Additionally, she has felt weakened after using the sauna at her local gym over the last few months. Her double vision is present only when she attempts to look to the side. On neurologic examination, when the patient attempts to look to the left, her right eye does not adduct past the midline, and her left eye exhibits beating horizontal movements. On looking to the other direction, the left eye exhibits the same signs while the right eye "beats." Her physician suspects a particular condition, and decides to send the patient for a MRI of the brain. Where is the lesion responsible for this patient's symptoms most likely located?

    (A) Arcuate fasciculus
    (B) Bilateral lesion of nuclei of Edinger-Westphal
    (C) Left medial lemniscus
    (D) Medial longitudinal fasciculus
    (E) Right medial lemniscus

14. A 55-year-old woman has received treatment for years to manage a chronic, progressive disease. Since her mid-40s the patient has had difficulty initiating movements. She has a shuffling gait, an expressionless face, and tremor in her hands and fingers at rest. Over the years she has tried many medications but with little relief of her symptoms, and instead has experienced severe adverse effects. She is referred for possible ablation surgery. The neurosurgeon explains the different pathways involved in initiation and inhibition of movement, the foundation of her disease. The neurosurgeon explains that by nullifying or accentuating some of the pathways, some of her symptoms may be alleviated. The introduction of an ablative lesion into which structure labeled in the image would be expected to improve this patient's bradykinesia?

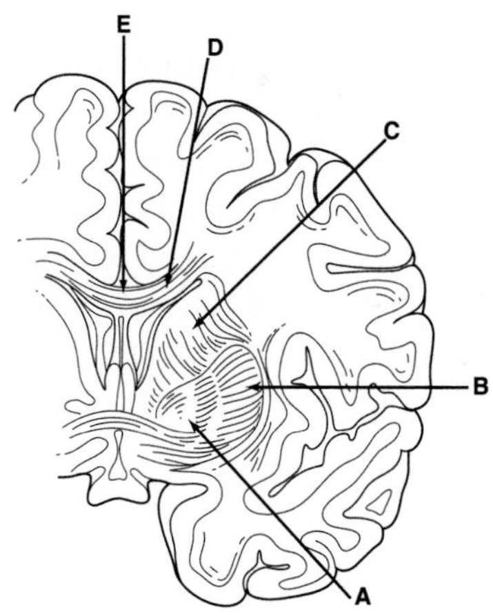

Reproduced, with permission, from USMLERx.com.

(A) A
(B) B
(C) C
(D) D
(E) E

15. A 33-year-old woman presents to the emergency department complaining of pain behind her right ear since that morning. Neurological examination is notable for paralysis of the right side of her face, decreased taste sensation on the right side of her tongue, and increased sensitivity to loud sounds in her right ear. The rest of her neurological examination is normal. The physician suspects a short course of steroids will improve her facial weakness over the next few weeks. In addition to the symptoms described above, this patient may also develop:

(A) Decreased sensation over her left upper cheek
(B) Decreased sensation over her right upper cheek
(C) Deviation of the uvula and soft palate to the left when the patient is asked to say "Ahh"
(D) Deviation of the uvula and soft palate to the right when the patient is asked to say "Ahh"
(E) Dryness in her left eye
(F) Dryness in her right eye

16. Both neostigmine and physostigmine act as acetylcholinesterase inhibitors. Although they share many of the same effects, only physostigmine is used to treat anticholinergic toxicity, whereas neostigmine is preferentially used to treat myasthenia gravis. What is the justification for using physostigmine over neostigmine as an antidote for anticholinergic toxicity?

(A) Physostigmine does not enter the central nervous system, whereas neostigmine does cross the blood-brain barrier
(B) Physostigmine enters the central nervous system, whereas neostigmine does not cross the blood-brain barrier
(C) Physostigmine has a greater effect on skeletal muscle, whereas neostigmine has a greater effect on the bladder
(D) Physostigmine has a greater effect on the bladder, whereas neostigmine has a greater effect on skeletal muscle
(E) Physostigmine irreversibly binds acetylcholinesterase, whereas neostigmine acts as a reversible inhibitor
(F) Physostigmine reversibly binds acetylcholinesterase, whereas neostigmine acts as an irreversible inhibitor

17. The high-power micrograph shown in the image demonstrates a key histologic finding obtained from the brain of a 75-year-old man at autopsy. In the years leading up to his death, the patient had exhibited the gradual onset of motor symptoms including bradykinesia, resting tremor, shuffling gait, and stooped posture. His medical history was otherwise unremarkable. Which of the following best describes the pathology underlying this patient's disease process?

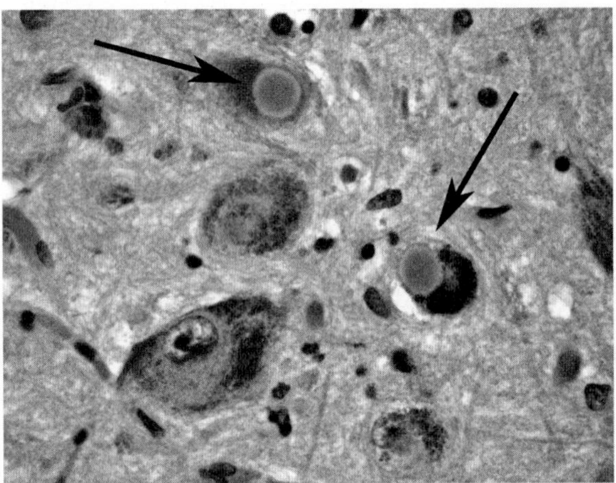

Reproduced, with permission, from USMLERx.com.

(A) Cortical atrophy associated with β-amyloid plaques, neurofibrillary tangles, and decreased cholinergic activity
(B) Defective copper transport leading to the accumulation of copper in tissues
(C) Loss of γ-aminobutyric acidergic neurons causing atrophy of the caudate nucleus
(D) Loss of pigmented dopaminergic neurons in the substantia nigra
(E) Malignant tumor cells derived from the neural crest leading to metastatic disease of the brain

18. A 67-year-old woman presents to the physician with right-sided Horner syndrome and face pain, a hoarse voice, dysarthria, diplopia, numbness, and ataxia with contralateral impairment of pain and temperature sensation in her arm and leg. No other motor or hearing deficits are evident. Which parts of the central nervous system are involved in this patient?

(A) Caudal lateral pontine tegmentum, including spinal tegmental tract of cranial nerve V, and the inferior surface of the cerebellum
(B) Cochlea and vestibular apparatus
(C) Dorsolateral quadrant of the medulla and the inferior surface of the cerebellum
(D) Internal capsule, caudate nucleus, putamen, and globus pallidus
(E) Lateral geniculate body, globus pallidus, and posterior limb of the internal capsule

19. A 26-year-old man presents with four days of progressive, bilateral, lower extremity weakness and dysesthesia. The patient denies any history of trauma, but states that he stayed home from work last week because of a fever accompanied by diarrhea. Neurologic examination demonstrates the absence of reflexes in the lower extremities with no cranial nerve deficits. What is the best therapy for this patient's condition?

(A) Plasmapheresis and immunoglobulin
(B) Glucocorticoids
(C) Acetaminophen
(D) Radiation therapy
(E) Rest and elevation of the lower extremities

20. A 70-year-old woman presents to her physician with a history of memory loss and occasionally becoming lost and disoriented in her own home. Brain biopsy of another patient suffering from the same disease process is shown in the image. What is the most appropriate therapy?

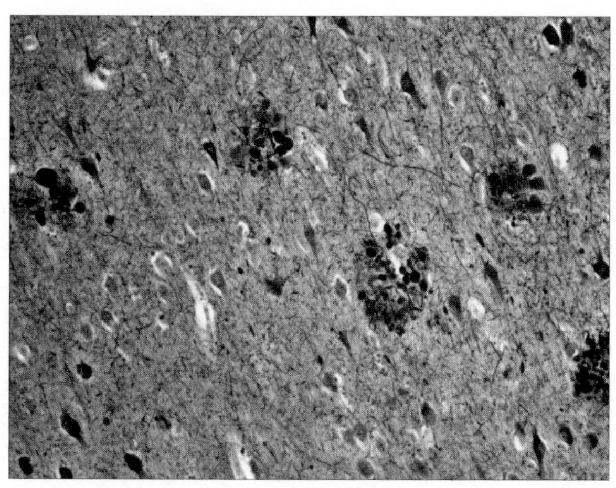

Reproduced, with permission, from USMLERx.com.

(A) Bromocriptine
(B) Diazepam
(C) Donepezil
(D) Levodopa/carbidopa
(E) Selegiline

21. A 27-year-old man presents to his primary care physician for a pre-employment physical examination. The patient states that he has been healthy and has no complaints except that he has been drinking a lot of water for what feels like an unquenchable thirst for the past couple of weeks. He reports that he has also been urinating excessively and is unable to sleep through the night due to his thirst and frequent urination. Urine analysis is significant only for a specific gravity of 1.002. Serum analysis is significant for an osmolality of 320 mOsm/L and a serum glucose level of 120 mg/dL. The patient is admitted to the hospital, where subcutaneous vasopressin is administered. Subsequent urine analysis revealed a specific gravity of 1.009, and serum analysis reveals an osmolality of 300 mOsm/L and a serum glucose level of 124 mg/dL. The patient is most likely to benefit from treatment with which of the following?

(A) Desmopressin
(B) Fluid restriction
(C) Hydrochlorothiazide
(D) Insulin
(E) Metformin

22. A 43-year-old man who is HIV positive presents to emergency department complaining of vision problems for the past two days. He has not been seeing a physician regularly, and his CD4 cell count is 24/mm³. Neurologic examination reveals problems with speech, memory, and coordination. He is admitted to the hospital but his symptoms rapidly worsen, and three weeks after admission the patient dies. What is the most likely cause of death in this patient?

(A) *Cryptococcus neoformans*
(B) Herpes simplex virus
(C) JC virus
(D) *Pneumocystis jiroveci*
(E) *Toxoplasma gondii*

23. A 71-year-old man is brought in to a dementia clinic for a neurologic evaluation. His wife reports his memory has been deteriorating for the past several years, but that she is particularly concerned about his behavioral changes. The man has become impulsive and aggressive, occasionally striking out when family members try to prevent him from doing something unsafe. Physical examination reveals obvious cognitive deficits, and the patient is uncooperative. In addition, he displays a habit of putting everything he holds into his mouth. There is no evidence of gait or movement abnormalities. Two years later, the man dies of pneumonia and an autopsy is performed. There is a complete absence of senile plaques and neurofibrillary tangles; however, there are spherical, silver-staining protein tangles and occasional ballooned neurons. Which of the following diseases is most likely?

(A) Creutzfeldt-Jakob disease
(B) Dementia with Lewy bodies
(C) Normal-pressure hydrocephalus
(D) Pick disease
(E) Wilson disease

24. A 7-year-old boy is brought to the emergency department after falling off his grandparents' deck; an x-ray film shows that he has a mid-shaft fracture of the humerus. Which of the following defects is most likely to occur with this type of fracture?

(A) A protruding scapula
(B) Inability to fully abduct the arm
(C) Inability to hold a piece of paper between fingers
(D) Pain over the palmar aspects of the first three and a half digits
(E) Weakness in wrist extension

25. A 27-year-old man is thrown from a motorcycle into a tree. He is taken to the emergency department, where he is alert and awake but in severe pain. On physical examination, he has very limited abduction of his left shoulder and flexion of his left elbow. On observation, the left shoulder is externally rotated. His forearm is pronated, and his elbow is extended. Which of the following muscles is most likely paralyzed in this patient?

(A) Flexor carpi ulnaris
(B) Flexor digitorum superficialis
(C) Latissimus dorsi
(D) Teres minor
(E) Trapezius

26. A 32-year-old man comes to the physician because of headaches that occur at night and without warning. They begin in his left eye and then generalize to the left side of his face. Alcohol can precipitate the attacks, which last for less than one hour. The patient rates the pain as a 10/10, and multiple over-the-counter analgesics have resulted in minimal benefit. He is given a prescription for sumatriptan to treat his symptoms and is prescribed verapamil for prophylaxis. Which of the following is the most likely diagnosis?

(A) Cluster headache
(B) Medication-overuse headache
(C) Migraine headache
(D) Temporomandibular joint dysfunction syndrome
(E) Tension headache

27. A 42-year-old man is brought to the emergency department by police after they found him walking unsteadily in the middle of a busy street harassing other pedestrians. On presentation the patient appears minimally responsive and his temperature is 36.8°C (98.2°F), respiratory rate is 8/min, heart rate is 54/min, and blood pressure is 101/54 mm Hg. The patient is unresponsive to glucose and naloxone administration. Laboratory tests show:

Na^+: 137 mEq/L
Cl^-: 100 mEq/L
Glucose: 69 mg/dL
WBC count: 8000/mm^3
Hemoglobin: 14.6 g/dL
Vitamin B_1: 59 pg/dL (normal: 140-820 pg/mL)

Which of the following findings is most likely to be present upon physical examination?

(A) Fruity odor to breath
(B) Miosis
(C) Nystagmus
(D) Pill-rolling tremor
(E) Shaking chills

28. A 40-year-old woman with Crohn disease presents with a tingling sensation in her fingers and toes and a recent history of fatigue. A complete history reveals that three years ago she underwent resection of her terminal ileum, but since then, she has been feeling well and eating a normal diet. Physical examination demonstrates weakness in all four extremities, hyperreflexia, and a positive Romberg sign. CBC count reveals a hematocrit of 22% and a hemoglobin level of 6 g/dL. Which of the following sets of laboratory results is most likely to be seen in this patient?

Choice	Mean corpuscular volume (fL)	Folate level	Hypersegmented PMNs on blood smear?
A	<100	normal	no
B	100	normal	no
C	>100	low	yes
D	>100	normal	no
E	>100	normal	yes

Reproduced, with permission, from USMLERx.com.

(A) A
(B) B
(C) C
(D) D
(E) E

29. A 15-year-old girl is brought to the emergency department by her mother after experiencing a first-time seizure. The thin-appearing girl has a heart rate of 55/min, signs suggestive of dehydration, and fine, velvety hair covering her arms and legs. The physician calculates her body mass index to be 16.4 kg/m². When the patient's mother leaves the room for a moment, the patient admits to the physician that she has been feeling depressed recently and that for the past week she has been self-medicating with normal daily doses of one of her friend's antidepressant medications. What antidepressant is the patient most likely taking?

(A) Amitriptyline
(B) Bupropion
(C) Fluoxetine
(D) Mirtazapine
(E) Selegiline

30. A 26-year-old woman is brought to the hospital by ambulance after an automobile accident. She sustained no injuries in the collision but is adamant that she did not see the car that hit her from the side as it approached. On neurologic examination she has bilateral visual field defects affecting nearly half of her lateral vision. On further questioning about recent changes in her health, she notes that she has not menstruated in 10 months. From which embryologic layer does this woman's neoplasm most likely originate?

(A) Endoderm
(B) Mesoderm
(C) Neural crest
(D) Neuroectoderm
(E) Surface ectoderm

ANSWERS

1. **The correct answer is D.** The organism described *Listeria monocytogenes*, causes meningitis and sepsis in neonates and the immunocompromised. Other bacteria causing neonatal meningitis include *Escherichia coli* and Group B streptococci (GBS). GBS are the most common cause of neonatal meningitis. Ingestion of poorly pasteurized milk, soft cheeses, coleslaw, and ready-to-eat turkey and pork products are implicated in the pathogenesis of listeriosis in the immunocompromised population and pregnant women.

   Answer A is incorrect. While *Escherichia coli*, a common gram-negative bacterial cause of neonatal meningitis, can produce urinary tract infections in both well and immunocompromised adults, the organism described in the clinical case is the gram-positive bacilli *Listeria monocytogenes*.

   Answer B is incorrect. Direct inoculation is a common route of transmission of infection, including gas gangrene produced by *Clostridium perfringens*, as well as tetanus caused by *Clostridium tetani*. In contrast, listeriosis in the immunocompromised is most often from ingestion of poorly pasteurized milk, soft cheeses, coleslaw, and ready-to-eat turkey and pork products.

   Answer C is incorrect. *Listeria monocytogenes*, a gram-positive, β-hemolytic, catalase-positive bacillus, causes meningitis and sepsis in neonates as well as the immunocompromised. While neonatal listeriosis may be contracted by passage through the birth canal, inhalation of infected amniotic fluid, or nosocomial infection, listeriosis in the immunocompromised is most often from ingestion of poorly pasteurized milk, soft cheeses, coleslaw, and ready-to-eat turkey.

2. **The correct answer is C.** The specimen in the photo is the circle of Willis. The artery designated by the arrow "A" is the anterior cerebral artery, which supplies the medial surface of the brain, the area responsible for the contralateral leg and foot areas of the motor and sensory cortices. Thus, a lesion in the artery would lead to deficits in contralateral motor function of the leg and foot.

   Answer A is incorrect. The artery in question does not supply the arm and hand; the middle cerebral artery does.

   Answer B is incorrect. The artery in question does not supply the face; the middle cerebral artery does.

   Answer D is incorrect. The artery in question does not supply the arm and hand; the middle cerebral artery does so in a contralateral fashion.

   Answer E is incorrect. The artery in question does not supply the face; the middle cerebral artery does so in a contralateral fashion.

   Answer F is incorrect. The artery in question supplies the medial side of the brain responsible for contralateral motor function, not ipsilateral leg and foot motor functions.

3. **The correct answer is A.** The layers of the head from superficial to deep are skin, periosteum, bone, dura mater, arachnoid, pia, and brain parenchyma. The meningeal layers consist of the dura, arachnoid, and pia. The subarachnoid space, which contains cerebrospinal fluid (CSF), is between the arachnoid and pia as the name suggests. Subarachnoid hemorrhages are usually caused by rupture of congenital berry aneurysms, and less commonly from arteriovenous malformations. Berry aneurysm rupture releases blood into the subarachnoid space and covers the surface of the brain with blood. However, the blood cannot be scraped off since it is trapped under the arachnoid mater. CSF obtained in subarachnoid hemorrhages via spinal taps will appear yellow (this indicates the presence of bilirubin in the CSF, a sign of hemorrhage and blood cell breakdown) because the subarachnoid space is continuous with the spinal space. This finding is called xanthochromia. Patients with sub-

arachnoid hemorrhages will often present with the "worst headache ever" and nuchal rigidity.

Answer B is incorrect. An intraparenchymal hemorrhage such as those caused by chronic hypertension would not appear as blood on the surface of the brain. It would likely be deeper in the brain, commonly affecting the basal ganglia and thalamus. An intraparenchymal hemorrhage appears more like a bruise of the brain tissue and less like a frank pool of blood, as described in the vignette.

Answer C is incorrect. The dura mater is a thick, fibrous structure of dense connective tissue without space for a significant amount of blood to pool. Blood collects either above or below the dura but not within it.

Answer D is incorrect. A subdural hemorrhage is defined as a hemorrhage under the dura mater that is caused by damage to bridging veins. There is a potential space between the dura mater and the arachnoid mater. When the calvarium (and its adherent dura) is removed, this space is exposed, and any blood there should be readily scraped off. Blood that cannot be scraped off must be under the arachnoid, which is under the dura. Subdural hemorrhages are commonly caused by blunt trauma, especially in the elderly, alcoholics, and children, who have atrophied or underdeveloped brains that causes extra strain on the bridging veins.

Answer E is incorrect. An epidural hemorrhage is caused by temporoparietal bone fractures that damage the middle meningeal artery. If the bony calvarium and the dura are removed, an epidural (above the dura) hemorrhage would be removed, and one would not see blood on the surface of the brain. The blood in an epidural hemorrhage is between the dura and the cranium.

4. **The correct answer is C.** Huntington disease is characterized by chorea, dystonia, altered behavior, and dementia. It is an autosomal dominant disease caused by CAG triplet repeats on chromosome 4p. It is the classic example of genetic anticipation, in disease severity increases and age of onset becomes earlier with each generation. The caudate and putamen are mainly affected, altering the indirect pathway of the basal ganglia, which results in loss of motor inhibition. Gliosis refers to the proliferation of astrocytes in areas of central nervous system (CNS) damage. On imaging the lateral ventricles may appear dilated because of the caudate atrophy. Reserpine has been shown to minimize the motor abnormalities observed in Huntington disease.

Answer A is incorrect. Alzheimer disease is the most common cause of dementia in the elderly. It is marked by progressive memory loss and cognitive impairment. Pathophysiologically, this disease is associated with deposition of neuritic plaques (abnormally cleaved amyloid protein) and neurofibrillary tangles (phosphorylated tau protein) in the cerebral cortex. Donepezil/vitamin E therapy has been shown to slow down but not prevent the progression of the disease.

Answer B is incorrect. Wilson disease, an autosomal recessive disease, is caused by failure of copper to enter circulation bound to ceruloplasmin due to a problem with excretion of copper from the liver. This disorder results in copper accumulation in the liver, corneas, and basal ganglia. Symptoms include asterixis, parkinsonian symptoms, cirrhosis, and Kayser-Fleischer rings (corneal deposits of copper). Penicillamine, a chelating agent, has been used for treatment with some success. Although Wilson disease can cause chorea and dementia, it is less likely in this scenario as it is inherited in an autosomal recessive fashion and other expected manifestations are not present.

Answer D is incorrect. Parkinson disease results from loss of dopaminergic neurons and therefore loss of pigmentation in the substantia nigra. These changes alter the direct pathway of the basal ganglia, resulting in loss of excitation. Patients with Parkinson disease present with difficulty initiating movement, cogwheel rigidity, shuffling gait, and pill-rolling tremor, not chorea. A levodopa/carbidopa combination is used for treatment.

Answer E is incorrect. Multiple sclerosis (MS) is characterized by scattered plaques of demyelination that can occur anywhere in the CNS. Periventricular areas and the optic nerve are commonly affected because of their high degrees of myelination. Oligodendrocytes, which are responsible for CNS myelination, are the specific targets of this autoimmune disease. The classic patient with MS is a white woman who presents in her 20s or 30s. Patients typically present with recurring multifocal lesions that are separated in time (intervening periods of recovery) and space and diagnosed by MRI. Common complications include optic neuritis, internuclear ophthalmoplegia (difficulty with horizontal eye movements), sensory and motor changes, and Lhermitte sign (an "electric shock" felt down the spine with neck flexion). Treatments are aimed at immunosuppression.

5. **The correct answer is A.** The diagnosis of meningohydroencephalocele is extremely rare and involves protrusion of the meninges, the brain, and a portion of the ventricle through a defect in the skull. The prognosis is extremely poor.

   Answer B is incorrect. Protrusion of the meninges and brain through a defect in the skull is consistent with a diagnosis of meningoencephalocele, which also carries a grave prognosis. Seventy-five percent of these infants die or are severely mentally retarded.

   Answer C is incorrect. Protrusion of the meninges and spinal cord through a vertebral defect to form a sac is consistent with a diagnosis of spina bifida with meningomyelocele.

   Answer D is incorrect. Protrusion of the meninges through a defect in the skull is consistent with a diagnosis of meningocele.

   Answer E is incorrect. Protrusion of the meninges through a vertebral defect to form a sac is consistent with a diagnosis of spina bifida with meningocele. In this condition, the spinal cord remains in its normal position.

6. **The correct answer is A.** The foramina of the trigeminal nerve divisions can be remembered with the mnemonic **S**tanding **R**oom **O**nly (**SRO**) for the **S**uperior orbital fissure, foramen **R**otundum, and foramen **O**vale, which transmit cranial nerves (CNs) V_1, V_2, and V_3, respectively. This patient has a schwannoma of the mandibular division of the trigeminal nerve (CN V_3) as the nerve exits the skull through the foramen ovale. Compression of CN V_3 causes numbness over the ipsilateral jaw and lower face.

   Answer B is incorrect. The maxillary division of the trigeminal nerve (CN V_2) exits the skull through the foramen rotundum, and compression would cause decreased sensation over the cheek and middle face.

   Answer C is incorrect. The meningeal (recurrent) branch of the mandibular nerve (CN V_3) exits the skull through the foramen spinosum, along with the middle meningeal artery. This nerve innervates the dura mater and is responsible for pain sensation.

   Answer D is incorrect. The jugular foramen transmits the glossopharyngeal (CN IX), vagus (CN X), and spinal accessory (CN XI) nerves. The glossopharyngeal nerve is responsible for motor innervation of the stylopharyngeus muscle, parasympathetic innervation of the parotid gland, and sensory innervation of the pharynx, middle ear, and posterior third of the tongue. It also innervates the chemoreceptors and baroreceptors of the carotid body. The vagus nerve is responsible for motor innervation of the pharyngeal and laryngeal muscles, parasympathetic innervation to visceral organs, and sensory innervation to the pharynx and meninges. It also innervates the chemoreceptors and baroreceptors of the aortic arch. The spinal accessory nerve innervates the sternomastoid and upper part of the trapezius muscles.

   Answer E is incorrect. CN III (oculomotor), CN IV (trochlear), CN V_1 (ophthalmic), and CN VI (abducens) exit the skull through the superior orbital fissure, together with the superior ophthalmic vein. Lesions of these nerves would lead to ipsilateral extraocular muscle paralysis (CNs III, IV, and VI) and numbness of the ipsilateral forehead and upper face (CN V_1).

7. **The correct answer is C.** This patient presents with signs and symptoms consistent with amyotrophic lateral sclerosis (ALS), which affects both anterior horn cells in the spinal cord and upper motor neurons in the spinal cord. ALS results in a combination of upper and lower motor neuron signs, although the deficits may be asymmetric. More males are affected than females, and the incidence rises after age 40. Riluzole (Rilutek) is the only FDA-approved treatment for the disorder, and it prolongs life by only three-six months; it is thought to function by reducing the presynaptic release of glutamate.

   Answer A is incorrect. Demyelination of axons in the dorsal columns and spinocerebellar tracts occurs in subacute combined degeneration of the spinal cord, which is also known as vitamin B_{12} neuropathy. It is associated with pernicious anemia and results in loss of vibration and position sense (dorsal columns) and arm/leg ataxia (spinocerebellar tracts).

   Answer B is incorrect. Demyelination of axons in the posterior limb of the internal capsule would cause contralateral spastic paralysis secondary to disruption of the descending fibers of the corticospinal tract, resulting in upper motor neuron signs.

   Answer D is incorrect. Neuronal loss in the region of the anterior horn cells and posterior columns in the spinal cord occurs in Charcot-Marie-Tooth disease, also known as peroneal muscular atrophy. It results in loss of conscious proprioception (posterior columns) and lower motor neuron signs (anterior horn motor neurons).

   Answer E is incorrect. Neuronal loss in the region of the anterior horn cells in the spinal cord occurs in poliomyelitis, an acute inflammatory viral infection that affects the lower motor neurons and results in a flaccid paralysis (pure lower motor neuron disease).

8. **The correct answer is A.** ADH (vasopressin) and oxytocin are synthesized by the neurons of the supraoptic and paraventricular nuclei in the hypothalamus, respectively. These hormones are transported to the *posterior* pituitary gland via the supraoptic hypophyseal tract, where they are stored and eventually released into the capillaries draining into the hypophyseal vein. ADH mediates water absorption at the renal collecting ducts via V2 receptors, allowing translocation of aquaporins, thus concentrating the urine. Oxytocin facilitates milk secretion but not synthesis, and also stimulates uterine contractions during parturition. Think "pituitary" when you see "hypophysis/hypophyseal." Also remember that the important connection between the hypothalamus and the *anterior* pituitary is the hypothalamic-hypophyseal portal system. Unlike the neuronal connection of the supraoptic hypophyseal tract, the hypothalamic-hypophyseal portal system is a capillary system that transports hormones synthesized in the hypothalamus that act on the anterior pituitary. Secretion of ADH in response to reduced plasma volume is activated by pressure receptors in the veins, atria, and carotids. Secretion of ADH in response to increases in plasma osmotic pressure is mediated by osmoreceptors in the hypothalamus.

   Answer B is incorrect. Milk synthesis is mediated by prolactin, which is secreted by the anterior pituitary gland and hence would be unaffected by ablation of the transport tract from the hypothalamus to the posterior pituitary gland. Although oxytocin does not have a role in milk synthesis, it allows milk letdown in lactating women.

   Answer C is incorrect. Ovulation is stimulated by the surge of luteinizing hormone (LH) just prior to the midpoint of the menstrual cycle. LH is secreted by the anterior pituitary gland and hence would be unaffected by ablation of the transport tract from the hypothalamus to the posterior pituitary gland.

   Answer D is incorrect. Salt retention is a primary action of aldosterone, acting at the renal distal tubules to increase sodium and chloride reabsorption as well as increase potassium and hydrogen secretion. Aldosterone is produced from cholesterol in a multistep pathway in response to ACTH stimulation. ACTH is secreted by the anterior pituitary gland and hence would be unaffected by ablation of the transport tract from the hypothalamus to the posterior pituitary gland.

Answer E is incorrect. Spermatogenesis is stimulated by follicle-stimulating hormone, which is secreted by the anterior pituitary gland and hence would be unaffected by ablation of the transport tract from the hypothalamus to the posterior pituitary gland.

9. **The correct answer is D.** The area postrema of the medulla contains the chemoreceptor trigger zone (CTZ), which controls vomiting. The CTZ is located on the floor of the fourth ventricle and communicates with the vomiting center. It is important to note that the CTZ is located outside of the blood-brain barrier, which is critical to its role in detecting toxic substances in the circulation. Prochlorperazine is a typical anti-psychotic agent that is more often used for its anti-emetic properties. It functions as a dopamine blocker at the CTZ.

   Answer A is incorrect. The midbrain helps regulate motor control, control of eye movements, and acoustic relay. It contains several essential nuclei of auditory and visual systems.

   Answer B is incorrect. The pituitary plays many roles in autonomic and endocrine control. A helpful mnemonic is "**TAN HATS**": **T**hirst, **A**denohypophysis control via releasing factors (gonadotropin hormone-releasing hormone, thyroid hormone-releasing hormone), **N**eurohypophysis and median eminence, **H**unger, **A**utonomic regulation, **T**emperature regulation, and **S**exual urges.

   Answer C is incorrect. The pons plays a role in many vital functions such as respiratory and urinary bladder control. It also contains the reticular activating system, which is responsible for regulating sleep-wake cycles and level of arousal, as well as contributing vestibular control of eye movements. It also conveys motor information from the cerebral hemispheres to the cerebellum.

   Answer E is incorrect. The cerebellum regulates movement and posture by providing constant feedback in order to allow for correction during voluntary movement. It also aids in motor learning.

10. **The correct answer is E.** The right internal carotid artery supplies blood to both the right anterior cerebral artery and the middle cerebral artery. Decreased blood supply to both the anterior and middle cerebral arteries would most severely damage the tissue that lies between the distributions of the two arteries. This area is known as the watershed zone, the zone supplied by the most distal sections of two different arteries.

    Answer A is incorrect. During occlusion of the internal carotid artery, blood supply would decrease to tissue supplied by the anterior cerebral artery. However, tissue in the watershed zone would be more susceptible to infarction and ischemia because this area is downstream of the tissue that is purely in the anterior cerebral artery distribution.

    Answer B is incorrect. During occlusion of the internal carotid artery, blood supply would decrease to tissue supplied by the middle cerebral artery. However, tissue in the watershed zone would be more susceptible to infarction and ischemia because this area is downstream of the tissue that is purely in the middle cerebral artery distribution.

    Answer C is incorrect. The internal carotid artery does not supply the posterior cerebral artery; therefore, tissue in the distribution of the posterior cerebral artery would not be infarcted.

    Answer D is incorrect. The internal carotid artery supplies the middle cerebral artery, but does not supply the posterior cerebral artery. Therefore during occlusion of the internal carotid artery, the watershed zone between the middle and posterior cerebral arteries would still be supplied by the posterior cerebral artery.

11. **The correct answer is D.** The patient presents with signs of Wernicke-Korsakoff syndrome, which is caused by thiamine (vitamin B_1) deficiency. Malnourished chronic alcohol abusers are thus particularly prone to this disease.

Thiamine pyrophosphate serves as a cofactor for several enzymes that are needed in key glucose metabolic pathways. Wernicke encephalopathy presents first, and may progress to Korsakoff psychosis if left untreated. The classic triad of Wernicke encephalopathy is confusion, ataxia, and ophthalmoplegia (weakness of eye muscles that may result in diplopia and/or nystagmus). Whereas Wernicke encephalopathy may be reversible if treated early, Korsakoff psychosis is an irreversible condition characterized by anterograde amnesia, confabulation, and personality changes. Anterograde amnesia is the inability to create new memory, and confabulation is the act of filling in gaps in one's memory with fabrications that are believed to be true. The lesion in Wernicke-Korsakoff syndrome is located in the mamillary bodies.

Answer A is incorrect. Bilateral lesions of the amygdala causes Klüver-Bucy syndrome, which is characterized by hyperorality, hypersexuality, and disinhibition. Hyperorality means placing inappropriate objects into one's mouth.

Answer B is incorrect. Lesions in the basal ganglia are associated with movement disorders such as Parkinson disease.

Answer C is incorrect. Broca area is located in the inferior frontal gyrus. Patients with lesions here have motor/nonfluent/expressive aphasia, meaning that although they can understand what others are saying, they have difficulty producing coherent speech.

Answer E is incorrect. Wernicke area is located in the superior temporal gyrus. Patients with lesions here have sensory/fluent/receptive aphasia, meaning that they can speak fluently but cannot understand what others or they themselves are saying.

12. **The correct answer is A.** The autopsy slide demonstrates psammoma bodies, which are lamellated mineral deposits formed via calcification of whorled clusters of cells found inside the tumor. Psammoma bodies are associated with several neoplasms: meningioma, papillary adenocarcinoma of the thyroid, ovarian serous papillary cystadenocarcinoma, and mesothelioma (mnemonic: **PSaMMoma** (**P**apillary [thyroid], **S**erous [ovary], **M**eningioma, **M**esothelioma). Given the CNS tumor and absence of any clues to suggest metastatic disease, meningioma is the most likely culprit. Meningiomas are the second most common type of primary brain tumor; they frequently occur in the convexities of cerebral hemispheres and in the parasagittal regions. Meningiomas arise from arachnoid cells external to the brain. Know what psammoma bodies look like and with which tumors they are associated.

    Answer B is incorrect. Astrocytes give rise to a variety of tumors, most notably gliomas. None of the astrocyte-derived tumor types contain dystrophic calcifications such as psammoma bodies.

    Answer C is incorrect. Melanocytes give rise to melanomas, which do not present with psammoma bodies.

    Answer D is incorrect. Neurons give rise to neuromas, which do not undergo calcification to form psammoma bodies.

    Answer E is incorrect. Oligodendrocytes give rise to oligodendrogliomas, which tend to occur in the cerebral hemispheres in middle-aged people, and the histology shows large, round nuclei with a clear halo of cytoplasm ("fried egg") cells. Oligodendrogliomas do not contain psammoma bodies.

13. **The correct answer is D.** This patient presents with internuclear ophthalmoplegia (INO). In young patients, bilateral INO is highly indicative of the development of MS. On gaze to the left, the primary movement is started in the left CN VI nucleus, and cannot be transmitted to the right CN III nucleus via the right medical longitudinal fasciculus (MLF) because of demyelination secondary to the underlying disease process. As a consequence, the right eye cannot adduct. The reverse is true for gaze directed to the right. However, convergence is usually intact as this maneuver does not utilize the MLF pathway.

Answer A is incorrect. The arcuate fasciculus is the tract of neurons connecting Broca area and Wernicke area in the left cerebral hemisphere. Lesions of the arcuate fasciculus most often manifest as impaired repetition. While MS can theoretically affect any white-matter tract in the brain, this patient does not present with any language deficits, thus her current lesion is not located here.

Answer B is incorrect. The Edinger-Westphal nucleus supplies preganglionic parasympathetic fibers to the eye that run on the outside of CN III. Its main function is to regulate pupillary constriction and lens accommodation. Despite its close association with the oculomotor nerve, it does not itself participate in movement of the globe.

Answer C is incorrect. The medial lemniscus is the tract in the brain stem that carries sensory information on light touch, proprioception, and vibration in the extremities from the nucleus gracilis and cuneatus to the thalamus. Although it could be affected by MS, it is not involved in the coordination of extraocular movements and thus cannot be responsible for this patient's symptoms.

Answer E is incorrect. The medial lemniscus is the tract in the brain stem that carries sensory information on light touch, proprioception, and vibration in the extremities from the nucleus gracilis and cuneatus to the thalamus. Although it could be affected by MS, it is not involved in the coordination of extraocular movements, and thus cannot be responsible for this patient's symptoms.

14. **The correct answer is A.** The patient in this question suffers from refractory Parkinson disease (PD). In this disease the internal segment of the globus pallidus produces excessive inhibition of the ventral lateral nucleus of the thalamus, making it difficult for patients to initiate movements (bradykinesia). Normally, dopaminergic neurons from the substantia nigra induce striatal neurons to inhibit the globus pallidus, thereby lifting the inhibition of the thalamus. Because of decreased dopaminergic signaling from the substantia nigra in PD, this pathway is ineffective. Ablating part of the internal segment of the globus pallidus (pallidotomy) would reduce its tonic inhibition of the thalamus and improve the patient's parkinsonian symptoms. Note that first-line treatment for PD is pharmacologic, most classically with levodopa, which is converted into dopamine in the brain.

    Answer B is incorrect. The putamen is one of the components of the striatum. It contains neurons with dopamine receptors that are responsive to projections from dopaminergic neurons of the substantia nigra. Some of the striatal neurons provide inhibitory input to the internal segment of the globus pallidus, which is necessary for the initiation of movement. Ablating the putamen may therefore make the patient's bradykinesia worse.

    Answer C is incorrect. The internal capsule is a white-matter tract that transmits the axons of upper motor neurons to the brainstem and spinal cord. Ablating the internal capsule would cause devastating hemiplegia with upper motor neuron symptoms (eg, spasticity, hyperreflexia).

    Answer D is incorrect. The caudate nucleus is one of the components of the striatum. It contains neurons with dopamine receptors that are responsive to projections from dopaminergic neurons of the substantia nigra. Some of the striatal neurons provide inhibitory input to the internal segment of the globus pallidus, which is necessary for the initiation of movement. Ablating the caudate nucleus might therefore make the patient's bradykinesia even worse.

    Answer E is incorrect. The corpus callosum is a white-matter tract that transmits axons from one side of the cerebral cortex to the other, allowing the two halves of the brain to communicate. Ablating the corpus callosum could cause perceptual abnormalities but would not improve the patient's parkinsonian symptoms.

15. **The correct answer is F.** This patient's history and physical exam findings are consistent with Bell palsy, an acute peripheral facial nerve palsy of unknown etiology. The symptoms seen in this patient can be understood if one

remembers the different nerve fibers carried by the facial nerve (cranial nerve VII): Afferent taste fibers from the anterior two-thirds of the ipsilateral tongue (decreased taste sensation), general touch and pain sensory fibers from a small area around the ipsilateral ear (retroauricular pain), and motor fibers to the muscles of facial expression (ipsilateral facial paralysis) and stapedius muscle (increased sensitivity to noise in the ipsilateral ear due to weakness of the stapedius muscle, which normally prevents excessive movement of the stapes). This patient may also experience dryness in her ipsilateral (right) eye and mouth because the facial nerve carries parasympathetic fibers to the ipsilateral lacrimal gland and submandibular/sublingual glands, which provides lubrication to the eye and mouth, respectively. In addition, weakness of the facial muscles prevents complete eye closure, exacerbating the eye dryness. Patients with facial nerve paralysis should be given lubricating eye drops and instructed to tape their eye closed at night. While facial nerve paralysis can be caused by head trauma, AIDS, Lyme disease, sarcoidosis, or brain stem lesions, in most cases no cause is discovered and the diagnosis of Bell palsy is made.

Answer A is incorrect. Decreased sensation of the left upper cheek could be caused by lesion of the left maxillary division of the trigeminal nerve (cranial nerve V_2); however, this patient shows signs of facial nerve palsy but no signs of trigeminal nerve involvement.

Answer B is incorrect. Decreased sensation on the right upper cheek could be caused by lesion of the right maxillary division of the trigeminal nerve (cranial nerve V_2); however, this patient shows signs of facial nerve palsy but no signs of trigeminal nerve involvement.

Answer C is incorrect. Lesion of the right vagus nerve would lead to deviation of the uvula and soft palate to the left; however, all signs and symptoms in this case suggest damage to the facial nerve (CN VII) and not the vagus nerve (CN X).

Answer D is incorrect. Unilateral lesions of the vagus nerve or nucleus ambiguous prevent elevation of the uvula on that side and thus cause the uvula and soft palate to deviate away from the side with the lesion due to unopposed action from the normal side. A lesion of the left vagus nerve would cause the uvula and soft palate to deviate to the right; however, the patient in this case has symptoms indicating palsy of the facial nerve (cranial nerve VII), not the vagus nerve (cranial nerve X).

Answer E is incorrect. The facial nerve (cranial nerve VII) carries sensory and motor fibers that innervate the ipsilateral face; thus a lower motor nerve palsy of the facial nerve would cause dryness of the ipsilateral (right), not contralateral (left), eye.

16. **The correct answer is B.** Physostigmine and neostigmine, both of which are amines, are reversible anticholinesterases. Both compounds act as substrates for acetylcholinesterase, thereby preventing the esterase from breaking down acetylcholine in the neuromuscular junction or synapse. Physostigmine has better CNS penetration, whereas neostigmine has better peripheral action (especially on skeletal muscle). Neostigmine does not cross the blood-brain barrier. Thus physostigmine is used as an antidote for anticholinergic toxicity because of its ability to cross the blood-brain barrier and treat central anticholinergic toxicity (delirium, agitation) as well as peripheral anticholinergic toxicity.

Answer A is incorrect. Neostigmine does not cross into the CNS, whereas physostigmine does.

Answer C is incorrect. Neostigmine has a greater effect on skeletal muscle than does physostigmine. Neither compound has much effect on the bladder.

Answer D is incorrect. Neostigmine does have a greater effect on skeletal muscle than does physostigmine. Neither compound has much effect on the bladder.

Answer E is incorrect. Both physostigmine and neostigmine are reversible anticholinesterases. Isoflurophate and other organophosphates irreversibly bind acetylcholinesterases, permanently preventing the breakdown of acetylcholine until the protein can be replaced with a new one.

Answer F is incorrect. Both physostigmine and neostigmine are reversible anticholinesterases. Isoflurophate and other organophosphates irreversibly bind acetylcholinesterases, permanently preventing the breakdown of acetylcholine until the protein can be replaced with a new one.

17. **The correct answer is D.** This specimen is taken from the patient's substantia nigra and demonstrates a typical melanin-containing neuron with pink-staining inclusions known as Lewy bodies. Lewy bodies are aggregations of the protein α-synuclein that are seen primarily in two neurologic diseases: Parkinson disease and Lewy body dementia. This patient's symptoms are characteristic of Parkinson disease, and this answer choice describes the process underlying this disease. Other common symptoms of Parkinson disease are cogwheel rigidity, postural instability, micrographia, and masked facies.

Answer A is incorrect. The pathology described in this answer choice is characteristic of Alzheimer disease, the most common cause of dementia in the elderly. This answer choice can be definitively ruled out, because Alzheimer disease is not associated with Lewy bodies.

Answer B is incorrect. The pathology described in this answer choice is consistent with Wilson disease, an autosomal recessive defect in copper transport that leads to the accumulation of copper in tissues. Wilson disease can be associated with parkinsonian symptoms, as well as chorea, psychiatric symptoms, liver disease, and the characteristic Kayser-Fleischer ring. Although some aspects of this answer choice are possible, this patient's symptoms are most consistent with Parkinson disease. Furthermore, Wilson disease is not associated with Lewy bodies.

Answer C is incorrect. This answer choice describes the pathologic process associated with Huntington disease, an autosomal dominant disease caused by a trinucleotide repeat on chromosome 4. Huntington disease is commonly associated with chorea, athetosis, and changes in personality. This disease generally presents in the third to fifth decades and is not associated with Lewy bodies.

Answer E is incorrect. This answer choice is likely referring to metastatic melanoma of the brain. This choice may be appealing because of the pigmentation of the histology shown in the image. Ultimately, though, Lewy bodies are seen only in Parkinson disease and Lewy body dementia.

18. **The correct answer is C.** The stroke syndrome described is the lateral medullary syndrome, also known as the posterior inferior cerebellar artery (PICA) syndrome or Wallenberg syndrome. This syndrome results in numbness of the ipsilateral face and contralateral limbs, diplopia, dysarthria, and an ipsilateral Horner syndrome. It classically results from disruption of the PICA, which supplies blood to the dorsolateral quadrant of the medulla, including the nucleus ambiguus and the inferior surface of the cerebellum. The infarcted dorsolateral quadrant of the medulla contains the tract of cranial nerve V (face pain), vestibular nuclei (dysequilibrium), nucleus ambiguus (palate problems and hoarse voice), the spinothalamic tract (contralateral pain and temperature loss), and descending sympathetic fibers (Horner syndrome). Limb weakness and reflex changes are not found because corticospinal fibers are in the ventral medulla at this location.

Answer A is incorrect. This vascular territory is supplied by the anterior inferior cerebellar artery. Disruption in blood flow typically causes ipsilateral deafness from involvement of the labyrinthine artery, ipsilateral facial weakness, and ataxia. It is the second most common brainstem stroke syndrome.

Answer B is incorrect. The cochlea and vestibular apparatus are perfused via the labyrinthine artery, and an isolated disruption of this end artery would result in isolated dysfunction of these two structures.

Answer D is incorrect. The internal capsule, caudate nucleus, putamen, and globus pallidus are perfused by the penetrating branches of the middle cerebral artery known as the lateral striate arteries. They are commonly involved with lacunar strokes.

Answer E is incorrect. The lateral geniculate body, globus pallidus, and posterior limb of the internal capsule are supplied by the anterior choroidal artery. Syndromes affecting this artery represent less than 1% of anterior circulation strokes and typically occur in the setting of symptomatic internal carotid artery occlusion.

19. **The correct answer is A.** Guillain-Barré syndrome is an acute, autoimmune, demyelinating polyradiculoneuropathy affecting the peripheral nervous system, usually triggered by an acute infectious process (most notably infection with *Campylobacter jejuni*). It is frequently severe and usually manifests as an ascending paralysis noted by weakness in the legs that spreads to the upper limbs and the face, along with complete loss of deep tendon reflexes. With prompt treatment by plasmapheresis followed by immunoglobulins and supportive care, most will regain full functional capacity. However, death may occur if there is paralysis of the musculature used for respiration.

Answer B is incorrect. Glucocorticoids would be indicated in the setting of acute injury to the CNS (eg, cauda equina syndrome, metastatic bone disease, or spinal cord injury). Steroid therapy reduces edema secondary to inflammation.

Answer C is incorrect. Acetaminophen is a non-narcotic analgesic and anti-pyretic. Given the pathophysiologic basis of Guillain-Barré syndrome, plasmapheresis and intravenous immune globulin are the best therapy.

Answer D is incorrect. Radiation therapy is a treatment used for CNS tumors or metastatic brain cancer. Radiation is not useful in patients with Guillain-Barré syndrome.

Answer E is incorrect. Rest and lower extremity elevation is indicated in the setting of mild trauma to the lower extremity (eg, sprain or strain).

20. **The correct answer is C.** This patient has symptoms of dementia, and the brain biopsy shows neurofibrillary tangles and senile plaques, which are characteristic of Alzheimer disease. People suffering from Alzheimer disease often have >90% loss of acetylcholine in their brains. Initial treatment of this disease is acetylcholinesterase inhibitors, which increase the amount of acetylcholine in the presynaptic space. Donepezil is an acetylcholinesterase inhibitor that is often used for this purpose.

Answer A is incorrect. Bromocriptine is a dopamine receptor agonist used to treat Parkinson disease.

Answer B is incorrect. Diazepam is a benzodiazepine. It increases the frequency of GABA channel opening and is used to treat anxiety, status epilepticus, and alcohol withdrawal.

Answer D is incorrect. Levodopa/carbidopa is a combination that increases levels of dopamine in the brain. It is used to treat Parkinson disease.

Answer E is incorrect. Selegiline is an inhibitor of monoamine oxidase type B, which increases dopamine availability and is used to treat Parkinson disease.

21. **The correct answer is A.** The patient has central diabetes insipidus (DI), a disorder in which the kidneys fail to concentrate urine due to a lack of ADH secretion by the posterior pituitary. Causes of central DI include head injuries, hypothalamic or pituitary tumors, and idiopathic causes. Without ADH, the principal cells of the distal tubule and collecting ducts remain impermeable to water. Nephrogenic DI is a related condition in which ADH is secreted by the posterior pituitary, but the principal cells of the kidneys do not respond to ADH because of defective ADH receptors. Causes include lithium toxicity and hypercalcemia. Both conditions are characterized by low urine specific gravity and high serum osmolality. The two are differentiated by a test dose of

vasopressin, which corrects serum and urine osmolalities in central DI, but not in nephrogenic DI. Desmopressin is an ADH analog that is taken nasally to treat central DI.

Answer B is incorrect. Fluid restriction is not indicated for, and is actually detrimental to, this patient because his renal system is unable to reabsorb water. In some clinical settings the fluid deprivation test may be used as part of the work-up for DI. In central DI, testing reveals low ADG levels and highly concentrated serum, yet lack of concentrated urine.

Answer C is incorrect. Although it seems counterintuitive, hydrochlorothiazide is a diuretic used to treat nephrogenic DI. Its exact mechanism of action is unclear. Desmopressin would have no effect on nephrogenic DI, because exogenous ADH is futile if its receptors are defective.

Answer D is incorrect. Insulin is used to treat type 1 diabetes mellitus (DM) and the later stages of type 2 DM. It has no indication in the treatment of DI. Although DM is part of the differential diagnosis of this patient, normal glucose levels and the positive vasopressin challenge point toward DI.

Answer E is incorrect. Metformin is an oral hypoglycemic agent used to treat type 2 DM by decreasing hepatic gluconeogenesis and increasing peripheral utilization of glucose.

22. **The correct answer is C.** This patient is presenting with progressive multifocal leukoencephalopathy (PML), which is caused by the JC virus in patients with AIDS. PML is a reactivation of a dormant virus to which the patient has previously been exposed. Initial findings include neurological deficits of speech, memory, and coordination. Vision problems are also common. The disease causes a very rapid decline in neurological function resulting in coma and death. The three-week course for this patient is not uncommon. The disease causes multiple areas of demyelination throughout the white matter of the CNS. There is no specific treatment for PML, but some patients have shown some clinical improvement with the initiation of highly active antiretroviral therapy.

    Answer A is incorrect. *Cryptococcus neoformans* is a common cause of meningitis is patients with HIV/AIDS. The classic meningitis triad of fever, headache, and nuchal rigidity are usually present. Abnormalities on CSF examination would also be present.

    Answer B is incorrect. Herpes simplex virus can cause temporal lobe encephalitis in patients with HIV/AIDS. It is also seen in the general population but at a lower frequency. Rapid onset of fever and focal neurological deficits are the most common presenting features. Deficits often stem from damage to the temporal lobe and can include memory problems, personality changes, and potentially seizures.

    Answer D is incorrect. *Pneumocystis jiroveci* (formerly *carinii*) is a common cause of pneumonia in patients with HIV whose CD4+ cell counts are <200/mm^3. On x-ray of the chest, the classic picture is one of "ground glass," although other radiological features are also common.

    Answer E is incorrect. Toxoplasmosis is the most common cause of encephalitis in patients with HIV/AIDS and is seen mostly in patients with a CD4+ cell count <100/mm^3. The most common manifestation of toxoplasmosis is seizures and headache, although other focal neurological deficits may be seen. The classic radiological picture is one or more ring-enhancing lesions with surrounding edema.

23. **The correct answer is D.** Although cognitive decline is common to all forms of dementia, the patient's increased impulsivity and hyperoral habits are suggestive of a frontotemporal dementia, such as Pick disease. This diagnosis is confirmed by the observation of intracytoplasmic, silver-staining Pick bodies on autopsy and occasional balloon neurons. The loss of neurons in the frontal lobe causes extreme changes in personality and a decline in executive functioning. Movement disorders are less prominent compared to the other dementia diagnoses listed here.

Answer A is incorrect. Creutzfeldt-Jakob disease is characterized by spongiform changes throughout the cerebral cortex. It is a rapidly progressive neurodegenerative disease characterized by severe dementia, myoclonus, and ataxia. Death generally occurs within 6-12 months of the onset of symptoms. This disease is believed to be caused by infectious prions derived from aberrant proteins.

Answer B is incorrect. In dementia with Lewy bodies, the patient's cognitive decline is frequently combined with extrapyramidal symptoms reminiscent of Parkinson disease, and visual hallucinations. As in Pick disease, intracytoplasmic inclusions (Lewy bodies) can be observed histologically. Dementia with Lewy bodies can also present with a fluctuating course, hallucinations, and prominent frontal signs. This patient's lack of parkinsonian movement abnormalities makes this diagnosis unlikely.

Answer C is incorrect. Normal-pressure hydrocephalus is characterized by the triad of urinary incontinence, progressive dementia, and ataxic gait (the "3 Ws:" Wet, Wacky, and Wobbly). In this disorder, head imaging reveals enlarged ventricles, but lumbar puncture does not reveal markedly elevated intracranial pressure. Unlike most forms of dementia, it is responsive to treatment, such as the placement of a shunt to remove excess CSF. Since this patient has no ataxia or incontinence, this diagnosis is very unlikely.

Answer E is incorrect. Wilson disease is an autosomal recessive disorder of copper metabolism that can cause dementia and psychotic symptoms as a result of accumulation of copper in different parts of the body. Because the putamen is particularly affected by the toxic accumulation of copper, extrapyramidal symptoms are common. The finding would be an accumulation of copper in the putamen; however, it would be unlikely for this disease to present so late in life. The gene for Wilson disease is located on chromosome 13, and this disease typically presents in childhood. There is a decrease in ceruloplasmin on laboratory testing, and Kayser-Fleischer rings are present in the iris of the eye.

24. **The correct answer is E.** A midshaft fracture of the humerus can cause injury to the structures found in the radial groove, which are the radial nerve and the deep brachial artery. The radial nerve is known as the great extensor nerve. Radial nerve injury results in "wrist drop," an inability to extend the wrist and metacarpophalangeal joints of all digits.

Answer A is incorrect. The long thoracic nerve innervates the serratus anterior muscle, and can be damaged in breast surgery through injury to the axilla or lateral wall of the thorax. The result is a "winged scapula," or protrusion of the scapula from the back when the person pushes forward against resistance.

Answer B is incorrect. The axillary nerve is damaged by injury to the surgical neck of the humerus or by anterior dislocation of the shoulder. It innervates the deltoid muscles, of which the middle fibers along with the supraspinatus are responsible for arm abduction.

Answer C is incorrect. The ulnar nerve can be damaged by injury to the medial epicondyle of the humerus. Motor deficits include weakness in abduction and adduction of fingers, adduction of the thumb, and extension of fingers (resulting in "claw hand").

Answer D is incorrect. The median nerve is damaged by injury to the distal end of the humerus in the supracondylar area. Median nerve injury results in the inability to flex fingers and abduct and oppose the thumb, as well as pain or paresthesia over the palmar side of the thumb, index, middle finger, and half of the ring finger. Atrophy of the thenar muscles may also occur. Similar changes are seen with carpal tunnel syndrome, in which the median nerve is compressed between the flexor tendons and the flexor retinaculum.

25. **The correct answer is D.** This patient most likely has an Erb palsy, which is characterized by the "waiter's tip" position of the affected upper extremity. It is due to downward compression of the shoulder and damage to the C5

and C6 nerve roots of the brachial plexus. Of the choices, the teres minor is innervated by the axillary nerve (C5, C6) and therefore likely to be paralyzed in this patient.

Answer A is incorrect. The flexor carpi ulnaris is innervated by the ulnar nerve (C7, C8) and is not affected in an Erb palsy.

Answer B is incorrect. The flexor digitorum superficialis is innervated by the median nerve (C7, C8, T1) and is not affected in an Erb palsy.

Answer C is incorrect. The latissimus dorsi is innervated by the thoracodorsal nerve (C6, C7, C8) and is not affected in an Erb palsy.

Answer E is incorrect. The trapezius is innervated by the spinal accessory nerve (cranial nerve XI) and is not affected in an Erb palsy.

26. **The correct answer is A.** This patient is suffering from cluster headaches, which are repetitive headaches that occur for weeks to months at a time, with intervening periods of remission. Men are affected more than women, with a peak incidence in persons 25-50 years old. Attacks begin without any prodromal symptoms (such as the vision changes characteristic of migraines), typically around the eye or temple, and are excruciating. They are always unilateral and may last for minutes to hours, with a mean duration of 45 minutes. In contrast to patients with migraines, who prefer remaining in a dark, quiet room, cluster headache patients typically prefer to stay active. Treatment can be difficult because of the short duration of symptoms, but effective options include oxygen, intranasal lidocaine, and triptans. Prophylaxis may consist of treatment with prednisone, verapamil, or methysergide for one-two months.

Answer B is incorrect. Medication-overuse headaches are secondary to excessive use of analgesics and may occur in patients who have tension, migraine, or cluster headaches. The diagnosis should be considered in patients who have frequent or daily headaches despite the use of medications. Although this patient is taking over-the-counter medications, the periodicity of the headaches precludes the regular administration of analgesics, which would be necessary for the consideration of this diagnosis.

Answer C is incorrect. Migraine headaches are typically preceded by prodromal symptoms and can also be bilateral in nature. Typically, the headaches increase in severity and can last from 10-12 hours. They may be associated with nausea and vomiting. Frequently such patients have a family history of migraine. Effective treatment involves use of triptans as an abortive agent and β-blockers for prophylaxis.

Answer D is incorrect. A headache induced by temporomandibular joint dysfunction syndrome frequently presents with unilateral ear or auricular pain radiating to the jaw. The pain is deep and continuous, is most severe in the morning, and can be associated with jaw dysfunction. Treatment is aimed at the underlying joint malfunction.

Answer E is incorrect. Tension headaches are the most common headache syndrome but typically present with pain that is bifrontal, "squeezing," and constant. They may be accompanied by nausea, but not usually by either vomiting or photophobia, and are not preceded by prodromal symptoms. Acetaminophen and nonsteroidal anti-inflammatory drugs are typically effective for relief.

27. **The correct answer is C.** The vitamin B_1 (otherwise known as thiamine) deficiency in this patient, accompanied by his gait ataxia is highly suggestive of Wernicke encephalopathy, a serious disorder. The classic triad of Wernicke encompasses encephalopathy, ataxic gait, and some variant of oculomotor dysfunction, most notably nystagmus. However, all three features of the triad are recognized in only about one-third of cases. It is important to consider Wernicke encephalopathy in the setting of alcohol abuse or malnutrition and acute confusion, decreased level of consciousness, ataxia, ophthalmoplegia, memory disturbance, hypothermia with hypotension, or delirium tremens.

Answer A is incorrect. A fruity odor to the breath is indicative of diabetic ketoacidosis (DKA), a pathophysiologic state of inadequate insulin levels resulting in high blood sugar levels and accumulation of organic acids and ketones in the blood. It is also common in DKA to have severe dehydration and significant laboratory abnormalities, including hyperglycemia, hypernatremia, and anion gap metabolic acidosis. None of these laboratory abnormalities is evident in this patient.

Answer B is incorrect. The presence of miosis (constricted pupils), which is indicative of increased parasympathetic tone, may suggest opioid intoxication. This patient presents with bradycardia and decreased respiratory rate, two other signs suggestive of opioid use. However, the patient was not responsive to naloxone administration. In patients with heroin (or other opioid) intoxication, naloxone (an opioid-receptor antagonist) rapidly reverses the effects of opioid intoxication.

Answer D is incorrect. Pill-rolling tremor is suggestive of Parkinson disease, a disorder of the basal ganglia caused by degeneration of dopaminergic neurons in the substantia nigra. These patients are usually >60 years old and present with a shuffling gait, masked facies, resting pill-rolling tremor, and bradykinesia. This patient is rather young to have Parkinson disease and does not demonstrate the classic syndrome associated with this disease.

Answer E is incorrect. Shaking chills is indicative of bacteremia and sepsis. Although this patient is hypotensive, a normal temperature and WBC count do not indicate any evidence of infection.

28. **The correct answer is E.** This patient presents with subacute combined degeneration, a neurologic condition associated with vitamin B_{12} deficiency that leads to abnormal myelin. Vitamin B_{12} deficiency causes macrocytic, megaloblastic anemia (mean corpuscular volume >100 fL) with hypersegmented neutrophils on blood smear. This patient likely has an isolated vitamin B_{12} deficiency secondary to surgical resection of the terminal ileum. When vitamin B_{12} is ingested, it combines with intrinsic factor secreted by the parietal cells in the stomach. This complex is then absorbed in the terminal ileum. It is likely that she avoided this deficiency for some time due to the large pool of vitamin B_{12} stored in the liver. Folate deficiency also presents with a macrocytic, megaloblastic anemia with hypersegmented neutrophils. However, it is not associated with neurologic problems. In this patient, folate levels would be expected to be normal, inasmuch as loss of the terminal ileum does not affect the intestinal absorption of folate, and this patient has been eating a normal diet, which should provide adequate folate levels.

Answer A is incorrect. These laboratory values are consistent with a microcytic anemia (ie, iron deficiency, thalassemia, or lead poisoning). Microcytic anemias are not associated with subacute combined degeneration. They can present with fatigue and pallor, and are most often due to some form of blood loss.

Answer B is incorrect. These laboratory values could be from a healthy patient or from someone with a normocytic anemia such as anemia of chronic disease, autoimmune hemolytic anemia, or anemia following an acute hemorrhage.

Answer C is incorrect. These laboratory values are consistent with folate deficiency. Folate deficiency is not associated with the neurologic symptoms observed in this patient, and this patient appears to be receiving adequate amounts of folate in her diet. Folate deficiency is most often seen with chronic alcohol use and malnutrition.

Answer D is incorrect. These laboratory values are consistent with a macrocytic, nonmegaloblastic anemia, which can result secondarily to liver disease, hypothyroidism, or drugs that impair DNA synthesis. Macrocytic, nonmegaloblastic anemias are not associated with subacute combined degeneration.

29. **The correct answer is B.** This patient has physical signs consistent with anorexia nervosa, most notably a low body mass index, bradycardia, evidence of hypotension, lanugo, and con-

comitant depression. Anorexia nervosa is a serious condition that requires intensive mental health care, as well as close medical monitoring of weight, electrolyte levels, and hydration status. The mainstay of therapy is a combination of cognitive behavioral therapy and selective serotonin reuptake inhibitors (SSRIs). Use of the antidepressant bupropion is contraindicated in patients with anorexia nervosa because it increases the risk of seizure in this population.

Answer A is incorrect. Amitriptyline is a tricyclic antidepressant (TCA). TCAs, although effective, are not first-line therapy in the management of anorexia nervosa, given the potential for cardiac adverse effects in anorexic patients already suffering from bradycardia and electrolyte abnormalities. TCAs are not known to increase the risk of seizure in anorexic patients.

Answer C is incorrect. Fluoxetine is an SSRI most commonly used as an antidepressant. It has also been used to treat anorexia nervosa, although with questionable efficacy. SSRIs are not known to increase the risk of seizure in anorexic patients.

Answer D is incorrect. Mirtazapine in an atypical antidepressant that induces weight gain, which may be beneficial in patients with weight control issues, although this has not yet been studied rigorously. Mirtazapine is not known to increase the risk of seizure in anorexic patients.

Answer E is incorrect. Selegiline is a monoamine oxidase (MAO) inhibitor most commonly used as an antidepressant; it is not typically used to manage anorexia nervosa. MAO inhibitors are not known to increase the risk of seizure in anorexic patients.

30. **The correct answer is E.** This patient shows the classic signs of a functional anterior pituitary adenoma, namely bitemporal hemianopsia and amenorrhea due to prolactin hypersecretion. These tumors are typically benign and slow-growing. The anterior pituitary develops from Rathke pouch, which is composed of surface ectoderm that abuts the sella turcica.

Answer A is incorrect. The gut tube epithelium and its derivatives originate from endoderm.

Answer B is incorrect. Most of the body's connective tissues are derived from mesoderm.

Answer C is incorrect. The parafollicular cells of the thyroid are derived from the neural crest.

Answer D is incorrect. The posterior pituitary is derived from neuroectoderm.

CHAPTER 14

Psychiatry

QUESTIONS

1. A 27-year-old man with a history of panic disorder and generalized anxiety disorder is brought to the emergency department after being found unconscious in his room by his parents. He is lethargic and can barely be aroused. He nods "yes" when asked if he has had any alcohol and "yes" when asked if he has taken any pills. His parents are sure the only pills in the house are those prescribed by his psychiatrist. His vital signs are normal, and his pupils are dilated to 2 mm and normally reactive. His blood alcohol level is 100 mg/dL. Results of the urine toxicology screen are pending. All of a sudden, his breathing slows and his oxygen saturation drops significantly. What should the physician give to treat this patient's condition?

   (A) Benztropine
   (B) Flucytosine
   (C) Flumazenil
   (D) Naloxone
   (E) Naltrexone

2. A 22-year-old man presents to his family physician with complaints of insomnia. He was recently honorably discharged from the army after finishing an 18-month tour of duty in Iraq. He states that the insomnia began about seven months ago after a fierce night-time battle. He reports having nightmares and flashbacks of the battle and is easily startled by loud noises. Which of the following pharmacologic agents, along with psychotherapy, would be most appropriate to treat this patient's condition?

   (A) Buspirone
   (B) Carbamazepine
   (C) Fluoxetine
   (D) Propranolol
   (E) Trazodone

3. A 42-year-old man presents to the local crisis center requesting alcohol detoxification. He has a 20-year history of heavy drinking, with the longest period of abstinence being four months. His last drink was two nights ago, and he now complains of discomfort and anxiety. Physical examination reveals coarse tremors, facial flushing, palmar erythema, and spider angiomas. His blood pressure is 145/95 mm Hg, his pulse is 115/min, and his temperature is 38.3°C (100.9°F). Thiamine is administered. Which of the following drugs is indicated for the treatment of this patient's condition?

   (A) Chlordiazepoxide
   (B) Disulfiram
   (C) Haloperidol
   (D) Methadone
   (E) Naltrexone

4. A 24-year-old woman is brought to the emergency department by ambulance after she is found collapsed and unresponsive on the street. It is not known how long she was lying on the street. Physical examination reveals constricted pupils and a heart rate of 55. Administration of which of the following drugs would be most appropriate?

   (A) Chlordiazepoxide
   (B) Flumazenil
   (C) Fomepizole
   (D) N-acetylcysteine
   (E) Naloxone
   (F) Naltrexone
   (G) Phenobarbital

5. After several failed trials of various antipsychotic drugs, a 46-year-old woman is switched to a new medication for her schizophrenia. However, a few weeks later, she develops pneumonia. A complete blood count is ordered and reveals a significantly reduced number of neutrophils, basophils, and eosinophils. Which of the following agents is the most likely cause of this clinical picture?

   (A) Chlorpromazine
   (B) Clozapine
   (C) Haloperidol
   (D) Risperidone
   (E) Thioridazine

6. A 60-year-old African-American man has been reclusive, rarely leaving his home for the past 40 years. His family describes him as an emotionally cold person with few friends. Growing up, he preferred solitary activities like reading to engaging in activities with others. Members of his church have delivered groceries to his front door once a week for the past 20 years, but he never opens the door to greet them. Which of the following is the most likely diagnosis?

(A) Avoidant personality disorder
(B) Paranoid personality disorder
(C) Schizoid personality disorder
(D) Schizophrenia
(E) Schizophreniform disorder
(F) Schizotypal personality disorder

7. A 27-year-old man is brought to the emergency department by ambulance. Paramedics report that he was found sitting on the sidewalk speaking as though engaged in a heated argument, but nobody else was around. They say that the patient appeared to be in distress and that he was quite disheveled. The man is evaluated by a psychiatrist, admitted to the hospital, and started on a medication to treat his symptoms. Two days later a medical student notices that the patient has painful spasms in his neck muscles. Which of the following is the most appropriate treatment for this man's condition?

(A) Benztropine
(B) Dantrolene
(C) Diazepam
(D) Fluphenazine
(E) Prochlorperazine

8. A 19-year-old man is brought to the emergency department by his friends after suffering a seizure. He is sweating, paranoid, tachycardic, and his pupils are dilated. His friends say that he has a history of using illicit drugs. What is the mechanism of action of the drug that is causing the patient's symptoms?

(A) Blocks NMDA receptors
(B) Increases GABA activity by increasing the duration of chloride channel opening
(C) Prevents reuptake of norepinephrine, dopamine, and serotonin by presynaptic pumps
(D) Prevents the fusion of the presynaptic vesicle with the presynaptic surface membrane
(E) Prevents the uptake of acetylcholine at cholinergic synapses

9. A 45-year-old man who has received long-term treatment for schizophrenia recently has been displaying involuntary facial movements that include lateral deviations of the jaw and "fly catching" motions of the tongue. Which of the following agents is the most likely cause of his involuntary movements?

(A) Clozapine
(B) Fluphenazine
(C) Lithium
(D) Selegiline
(E) Ziprasidone

10. A 28-year-old man who has been experiencing delusions, hallucinations, and thought disorders for the past six months now begins to display flattening affect, lack of motivation, and social withdrawal. Which of the following agents would address his newest symptoms?

(A) Olanzapine
(B) Haloperidol
(C) Lithium
(D) Fluphenazine
(E) Phenelzine

11. A 35-year-old man with depression has been treated with medication for the past seven years. Recently he began seeing a new psychiatrist who suggested changing this medication to a newer class of antidepressants that has proven effective for many of her patients. Two weeks later he presents to the emergency department because of flushing, diarrhea, sweating, and muscle rigidity. During the physical examination, he admits that he was a bit suspicious of the new medication he was given to treat his depression since he was told he no longer needed to avoid certain foods. He decided to use both medicines just to "make sure" the new one was working. Which of the following medications did the new doctor most likely prescribe for this patient?

    (A) Lithium
    (B) Nortriptyline
    (C) Phenelzine
    (D) Sertraline
    (E) Trazodone

12. A 20-year-old man is seen by a physician for the third time in three months. At the first visit he was brought to the emergency department by his mother after swallowing toilet bowl cleaner. He told the doctor that he took the cleaning product to "cleanse his body from the aliens" that had "forced their entry" and "possessed" him. Today the patient appears unclean and disheveled, and his mother reports that he has become progressively withdrawn and expressionless. Four months ago the patient witnessed the gruesome death of his father in a drive-by shooting incident. Prior to this incident, he had a normal and healthy life. Which of the following is the most likely diagnosis?

    (A) Factitious disorder
    (B) Schizophreniform disorder
    (C) Schizophrenia
    (D) Schizoaffective disorder
    (E) Shared delusional disorder

13. A 43-year-old woman comes to the clinic with complaints of pruritus and burning of both forearms that initially looked like sunburn. On physical examination the affected skin appears thickened and hyperpigmented. A similar lesion is seen on the neck. The patient states that she has recently began to have diarrhea, and at times during the interview she forgets what she was saying. For the past six months she has been following a new low-calorie fad diet. A defect in the absorption of which amino acid would cause similar symptoms?

    (A) Arginine
    (B) Histidine
    (C) Phenylalanine
    (D) Tryptophan
    (E) Tyrosine

14. A 28-year-old woman presents to her primary care provider complaining of difficulty sleeping. Although she reports trouble falling asleep despite waking up "before the sun" every morning, her major complaint is awakening from sleep multiple times each night. She also complains of decreased energy and motivation to complete tasks at work. Polysomnography reveals >25% of total sleep time is spent in REM sleep and <25% of total sleep time is spent in stages 3 and 4 sleep. Which of the following is the most appropriate treatment?

    (A) Avoidance of caffeine
    (B) Continuous positive airway pressure
    (C) Fluoxetine
    (D) Methylphenidate
    (E) No intervention is necessary; these are normal polysomnographic findings in a young adult

15. A 23-year-old man is brought to the emergency department because his friends heard him say that he was talking to president Kennedy about a secret spy mission in the Soviet Union. He appears quite anxious, agitated, and restless. Physical examination reveals dilated pupils. His pulse is 80/min and his blood pressure is 120/80 mm Hg. What is the most likely cause of his symptoms?

    (A) Alcohol
    (B) Cocaine
    (C) Lysergic acid diethylamide
    (D) Marijuana
    (E) Phencyclidine

16. The parents of an 8-year-old boy bring him to see a psychiatrist because they are frustrated with his behavior. In the last two years he has become increasingly restless and moody, interrupts other children in the classroom, and often runs into the street without looking out for cars first. The psychiatrist prescribes a medication that works through which of the following mechanisms?

(A) Increases release of norepinephrine
(B) Inhibits acetylcholine activity
(C) Inhibits reuptake of serotonin
(D) Stimulates dopamine receptors
(E) Stimulates serotonin receptors

17. A 15-year-old girl is brought to the emergency department by her mother after experiencing a first-time seizure. The thin-appearing girl has a heart rate of 55/min, signs suggestive of dehydration, and fine, velvety hair covering her arms and legs. The physician calculates her body mass index to be 16.4 kg/m². When the patient's mother leaves the room for a moment, the patient admits to the physician that she has been feeling depressed recently and that for the past week she has been self-medicating with normal daily doses of one of her friend's antidepressant medications. What antidepressant is the patient most likely taking?

(A) Amitriptyline
(B) Bupropion
(C) Fluoxetine
(D) Mirtazapine
(E) Selegiline

18. The image depicts a biochemical pathway occurring in the nervous system. An "X" marks the effect of a certain class of medications on this pathway. For which condition is this class of medications an effective first-line treatment?

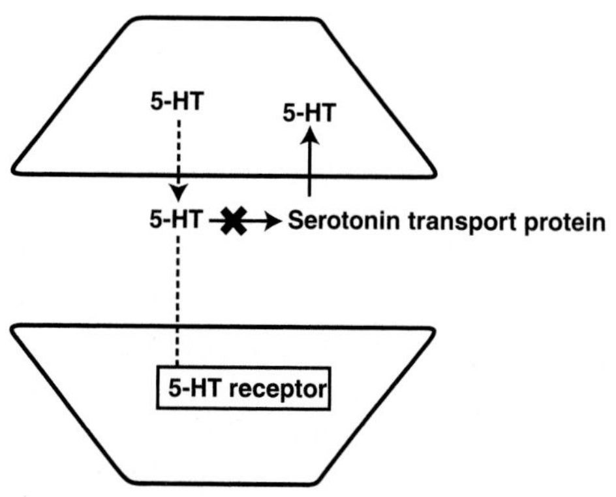

Reproduced, with permission, from USMLERx.com.

(A) Bipolar disorder
(B) Delerium tremens
(C) Dissociative identity disorder
(D) Obsessive-compulsive disorder
(E) Schizophrenia

19. An 18-year-old woman complains of weakness, fatigue, decreased appetite, and insomnia over the past month. She is no longer interested in her favorite activities, and has been unable to concentrate in school. She also reports feeling guilty about not hanging out with her friends even though they ask her out almost every weekend. As part of her treatment plan, her physician prescribes a medication. On a follow-up visit, she reports that her mood has improved, but she now feels that her face flushes more frequently and she is more sensitive to the hot weather outside. She is also worried that at times she feels like her heart is racing. On further questioning, she admits to some constipation. Which of the following drugs was most likely prescribed for this patient?

(A) Amitriptyline
(B) Clonazepam
(C) Lithium
(D) Sertraline
(E) Venlafaxine

20. A 20-year-old woman is brought to the emergency department by her roommate because she was "walking funny," had difficulty breathing, and slurred her speech. She was recently diagnosed and given medication for panic disorder. Her blood pressure is 110/75 mm Hg, pulse is 58/min, and respiratory rate is 8/min. She is afebrile. Her mucous membranes are moist and pupil size is normal. Serum laboratory studies are negative for evidence of ethanol, organophosphate, or opioid ingestion. The agent that would be used to reverse the effects of the patient's anxiety medication works by which of the following mechanisms?

(A) Activating an enzyme responsible for the termination of a drug's inactivation
(B) Amplifying the effect of an endogenous neurotransmitter by inhibiting its breakdown
(C) Displacement of the drug from its binding site
(D) Inhibiting the formation of a toxic metabolite
(E) Inhibiting the storage of a neurotransmitter

ANSWERS

1. **The correct answer is C.** This patient is exhibiting symptoms of central nervous system (CNS) depression that cannot be explained by his blood alcohol level alone (this level of CNS depression would typically be seen in a nonchronic drinker at blood alcohol levels of 250-300 mg/dL). It is reasonable, based on his psychiatric diagnoses, to think he may have ingested a benzodiazepine along with the alcohol, resulting in a synergistic effect. To reverse the effect of the benzodiazepine, the drug of choice is flumazenil, a competitive GABA antagonist.

   Answer A is incorrect. Benztropine is a centrally acting anticholinergic agent that acts as an acetylcholine receptor antagonist. It is used to treat parkinsonism as well as extrapyramidal and dystonic reactions. It is not used to treat benzodiazepine overdose.

   Answer B is incorrect. Flucytosine is a potent antifungal.

   Answer D is incorrect. Naloxone is used to reverse opioid overdose.

   Answer E is incorrect. Naltrexone, an opioid receptor antagonist, is used to treat opiate addiction.

2. **The correct answer is C.** This patient meets the criteria for diagnosis of posttraumatic stress disorder (PTSD). He has experienced an event that involved actual death of or threatened death to self or others; the traumatic event is persistently re-experienced through nightmares and flashbacks; he suffers from insomnia; and he has an exaggerated startle response. Other symptoms of PTSD include difficulty concentrating, hypervigilance, and dissociative symptoms. In PTSD, symptoms are present for longer than one month, whereas in acute stress disorder, symptoms last between two days and one month. Selective serotonin reuptake inhibitors such as fluoxetine are first-line medications for the treatment of PTSD. Side effects include nausea, headache, anxiety, agitation, insomnia, and sexual dysfunction.

   Answer A is incorrect. Buspirone is a partial agonist at the 5-HT_{1S} receptor that is commonly used as an alternative to benzodiazepines in the treatment of generalized anxiety disorder. Although its onset of action is slower than that of benzodiazepines, it does not potentiate the CNS depression of alcohol, and has little potential for abuse and addiction.

   Answer B is incorrect. Carbamazepine is an anticonvulsant medication that also can be used as a mood stabilizer in bipolar mood disorder.

   Answer D is incorrect. Propranolol is a nonspecific β-blocker. It is useful in the treatment of panic disorder and simple phobia.

   Answer E is incorrect. Trazodone is a heterocyclic antidepressant with sedative qualities that is used in the treatment of depression complicated by insomnia. It works by inhibiting serotonin reuptake, but also acts as a partial serotonin agonist. Male patients should be warned of its potential to cause priapism.

3. **The correct answer is A.** This patient is showing signs of alcohol withdrawal, manifested by tachycardia, fever, nausea, vomiting, tremors, and hypertension, and is at risk for delirium tremens. Delirium tremens is an extreme and life-threatening form of withdrawal characterized by perceptual disturbances and confusion. Intravenous benzodiazepines, such as chlordiazepoxide, are indicated in the treatment of both mild withdrawal and delirium tremens. Used early, they can prevent progression to withdrawal-induced seizures, psychosis, and coma. Chlordiazepoxide is a long-acting benzodiazepine that works via stimulation of GABA receptors. Other drugs in the same class include lorazepam, oxazepam, and diazepam, each of which could be used in this scenario.

   Answer B is incorrect. Disulfiram inhibits acetaldehyde dehydrogenase, which causes accumulation of acetaldehyde with ingestion of alcohol. This buildup of alcohol byproducts leads to extremely unpleasant adverse effects, including flushing, headache, diaphoresis, nausea, and vomiting. This drug is given to alcoholics to help them maintain sobriety.

Answer C is incorrect. Haloperidol is a typical antipsychotic. It can be used in patients withdrawing from alcohol who suffer psychotic symptoms such as hallucinations.

Answer D is incorrect. Methadone is a potent, long-acting opioid agonist used in the treatment of opioid addiction. This patient is an alcoholic and does not require a methadone taper.

Answer E is incorrect. Naltrexone is an opioid antagonist used to help maintain opioid sobriety. It also is used to help prevent alcohol relapses in alcohol dependence. This patient, however, requires acute care, not maintenance treatment.

4. **The correct answer is E.** This patient has signs indicating opioid overdose: she is comatose with miosis and bradycardia. Naloxone, an opioid antagonist given intravenously, should quickly reverse the effects of the overdose.

Answer A is incorrect. Chlordiazepoxide is a long-acting benzodiazepine used in the management of alcohol withdrawal. Though patients with alcohol intoxication can become unresponsive, alcohol tends to cause pupillary dilation, not constriction as seen with this patient. Additionally, there is no mention of the smell of alcohol on the patient's breath or clothing, which can be a clue to alcohol intoxication in an unresponsive patient.

Answer B is incorrect. Flumazenil is an antagonist at benzodiazepine receptors and is used to reverse benzodiazepine intoxication. Though benzodiazepines can cause pupillary changes, respiratory depression along with hypotension are more likely to be noted in a patient with overdose.

Answer C is incorrect. Fomepizole is an inhibitor of alcohol dehydrogenase, and is used to prevent the conversion of ethylene glycol and methanol to the toxic substances oxalic acid and formic acid, respectively. Thus it is mainly used as an antidote for methanol or ethylene glycol poisoning. There is no evidence that this patient ingested methanol or ethylene glycol.

Answer D is incorrect. N-acetylcysteine is used in cases of acetaminophen poisoning. It also has an indication for relieving mucus thickening in cystic fibrosis patients.

Answer F is incorrect. Naltrexone, like naloxone, is an opioid receptor antagonist; however, it is not indicated for reversal of acute opioid overdose. Naltrexone is more commonly used to treat alcohol and opioid dependence.

Answer G is incorrect. Phenobarbital is a long-acting barbiturate useful in patients with seizure disorders.

5. **The correct answer is B.** Clozapine is an atypical antipsychotic used to treat schizophrenia that is refractory to traditional therapy. It is considered atypical because it blocks serotonin receptors, in addition to the dopamine blockade common to all typical antipsychotics. This dual action may be useful in the treatment of the positive and negative symptoms of schizophrenia. Perhaps the most dangerous adverse effect of clozapine is bone marrow suppression, specifically agranulocytosis. This necessitates frequent monitoring of the WBC count for all patients who are started on this drug. A sudden increase in infections or bouts of illness in a patient on clozapine should raise concern about the development of agranulocytosis. If laboratory tests indicate this is the case, the drug must be discontinued immediately and the patient should be monitored carefully.

Answer A is incorrect. Chlorpromazine, a traditional antipsychotic, has a adverse-effect profile similar to that of haloperidol. Agranulocytosis can occur with its use, but occurs much more commonly as an adverse effect of clozapine.

Answer C is incorrect. Haloperidol is a traditional antipsychotic that acts by blocking dopamine receptors and is not associated with agranulocytosis. It is best known for causing extrapyramidal adverse effects.

Answer D is incorrect. Risperidone, another atypical antipsychotic agent, has a mechanism of action similar to that of clozapine. It does not, however, produce the adverse effect of agranulocytosis. Significant adverse effects of risperidone include QT-interval prolongation and metabolic aberrations.

Answer E is incorrect. Thioridazine is a traditional antipsychotic that has an adverse-effect profile similar to that of haloperidol and chlorpromazine. Although agranulocytosis is possible, it is much less frequent than with clozapine.

6. **The correct answer is C.** This man has schizoid personality disorder, marked by a lifelong pattern of social withdrawal. Patients with this disorder experience discomfort with human interaction, so they avoid close relationships, and engage in solitary activities. These patients often are viewed as eccentric, isolated, lonely, and emotionally cold. Unlike those with other cluster A personality disorders, which are schizotypal and paranoid, those with schizoid personality disorder are not more likely to have relatives with schizophrenia. Men are twice as likely as women to be affected.

   Answer A is incorrect. Avoidant patients are like schizoid patients in their pervasive pattern of social inhibition. However, they do desire companionship; an intense fear of rejection leads to avoiding any situation where there is a perceived risk of rejection. Think avoidant personality disorder in patients inhibited by feelings of inadequacy and social ineptness to the extent they will participate socially only when they are certain to be liked.

   Answer B is incorrect. Patients with paranoid personality disorder tend to be more socially engaged than those with schizoid personality disorder, even though they have a lifelong history of suspiciousness and mistrust of other people. Examples include recurrent suspicion of a sexual partner's fidelity or blaming others for their problems.

   Answer D is incorrect. Patients with schizophrenia exhibit a formal thought disorder with hallucinations, or delusional thinking. In contrast, patients with schizoid personality disorder have intact reality testing.

   Answer E is incorrect. Schizophreniform disorder is identical to schizophrenia except that symptoms last for at least one month but less than six months. Patients with schizophreniform disorder have a better prognosis than do most patients with schizophrenia, and may return to their baseline mental functioning.

   Answer F is incorrect. Schizotypal and schizoid personality disorder are rather similar, but the former is distinguished in that these patients tend to be more similar to schizophrenics. Patients with schizotypal disorder are strikingly odd, with peculiar notions, ideas of reference, illusions, magical thinking, and derealization.

7. **The correct answer is A.** The patient has classic signs of schizophrenia and was likely given haloperidol, a typical antipsychotic agent that acts by blocking dopamine receptors. Haloperidol has a high affinity for the D_2-dopaminergic receptor. The patient is experiencing an acute dystonic reaction soon after receiving the medication. The painful muscle spasm of the neck is known as torticollis. This acute extrapyramidal adverse effect is the result of unopposed cholinergic activity in the CNS following blockade of dopaminergic transmission. The treatment for this adverse effect is initiation of an anticholinergic agent such as benztropine.

   Answer B is incorrect. Dantrolene is effective in the treatment of neuroleptic malignant syndrome. Dantrolene acts by preventing the release of calcium from the endoplasmic reticulum.

   Answer C is incorrect. Diazepam can be used as an hypnotic, a sedative, an anticonvulsant, and a muscle relaxant. As a muscle relaxant, diazepam is used to treat chorea, an involuntary abnormal movement disorder or dyskinesia that is a hallmark of Huntington disease.

   Answer D is incorrect. Fluphenazine, like haloperidol, can induce potent D_2-dopaminergic receptor blockade. It is a high-potency typical antipsychotic that is sometimes used as an alternative to haloperidol for patients suffering from schizophrenia or bipolar disorder. Administration of fluphenazine will likely exacerbate this patient's symptoms rather than alleviate them.

Answer E is incorrect. Prochlorperazine is a typical antipsychotic agent with potent antidopaminergic effects. It can also be used to treat nausea because of its weak anticholinergic and antihistaminic effects. In this case it would be of no benefit for the patient, and could make his symptoms worse.

8. **The correct answer is C.** The patient's symptoms are caused by cocaine. Cocaine prevents the reuptake of norepinephrine, dopamine, and serotonin by presynaptic transporter pumps in the central and peripheral nervous systems.

Answer A is incorrect. Phencyclidine causes aggressive and impulsive behavior, nystagmus, and tachycardia. It acts as an NMDA receptor antagonist.

Answer B is incorrect. Barbiturates cause respiratory depression and act by increasing GABA activity by increasing the duration of chloride channel opening.

Answer D is incorrect. Bretylium and guanethidine prevent the fusion of presynaptic vesicles with the presynaptic membrane, resulting in an inhibition of the release of norepinephrine into the synapse.

Answer E is incorrect. Cocaine works on noradrenergic neurons; it does not work on cholinergic neurons.

9. **The correct answer is B.** This patient is displaying signs of tardive dyskinesia, a complication of long-term antipsychotic use thought to be the result of increased dopamine receptor synthesis in response to long-term receptor blockade by antipsychotics. Abnormal movements such as tongue-thrusting and jaw deviations, as seen in this patient, are the result of relative dopamine excess affecting motor pathways. This complication is encountered more commonly with use of older, typical antipsychotic medications such as fluphenazine and haloperidol.

Answer A is incorrect. Clozapine, an atypical antipsychotic that modulates both serotoninergic and dopaminergic neurons in the CNS, has a relatively low risk of inducing tardive dyskinesia. The most concerning adverse effect of clozapine is agranulocytosis, which can be fatal if left untreated.

Answer C is incorrect. Lithium is a mood stabilizer that is used primarily to treat episodes of mania in patients with bipolar disorder. Adverse effects of lithium include nephrogenic diabetes insipidus, nausea, anorexia, and mild diarrhea.

Answer D is incorrect. Selegiline is a monoamine oxidase B inhibitor that is used to treat Parkinson disease by decreasing the breakdown of dopamine. It has no role in the treatment of schizophrenia. Selegiline has the opposite effect of antipsychotics; it blocks the effects of dopamine. Adverse effects of selegiline include gastrointestinal (GI) upset, nausea, heartburn, and dry mouth.

Answer E is incorrect. Ziprasidone, like clozapine, is an atypical antipsychotic and has a lower incidence of tardive dyskinesia when compared to typical antipsychotics. More often than other atypical antipsychotics, it has been associated with QT prolongation and the risk of malignant ventricular arrhythmias.

10. **The correct answer is A.** Olanzapine is an atypical antipsychotic that blocks both serotonin and dopamine receptors. Drugs in this class are noted for their ability to treat both positive symptoms of schizophrenia (ie, hallucinations and delusions) and negative symptoms (ie, blunted affect and social withdrawal). With the onset of negative symptoms, addition of an atypical antipsychotic such as olanzapine, can effectively treat both positive and negative symptoms of this disorder.

Answer B is incorrect. Haloperidol, another typical agent, would be less effective at mitigating the patient's negative symptoms compared to olanzapine.

Answer C is incorrect. Lithium is a mood stabilizer that is used to treat the acute manic phases of bipolar disorder. It is not used in the treatment of schizophrenia and thus would have no effect on this patient's negative symptoms.

Answer D is incorrect. Fluphenazine is a typical antipsychotic that blocks only dopamine receptors. Agents in this class are more effective at mitigating positive symptoms of schizophrenia, but are less effective at relieving the negative symptoms such as flattened affect and catatonia.

Answer E is incorrect. Phenelzine, a monoamine oxidase (MAO) inhibitor, is used to treat depression in patients who are unresponsive to tricyclic antidepressants or who experience concomitant anxiety. Such agents are not used to treat schizophrenia.

11. **The correct answer is D.** This patient has likely been taking a MAO inhibitor for the past seven years since he was told he had to avoid certain foods. Sertraline is a selective serotonin reuptake inhibitor (SSRI) that can lead to serotonin syndrome when taken in conjunction with MAO inhibitors. Serotonin syndrome is the result of excess serotonin in the nervous system and is characterized by mental status changes, autonomic changes (eg, fever, diaphoresis, tachycardia), and neuromuscular changes (eg, tremor or rigidity). The treatment of serotonin syndrome consists of prompt discontinuation of the implicated agent(s) and supportive care including intravenous fluids, benzodiazepines for control of delirium, cooling measure for hyperthermia, and neuromuscular blockers such as dantrolene for hyperthermia, muscle rigidity, and the prevention of rhabdomyolysis.

Answer A is incorrect. Lithium is typically used to treat bipolar disorder. Its use has been associated with tremor, hypothyroidism, and nephrogenic diabetes insipidus. While lithium is considered an effective adjunctive therapy for depression in combination with a second antidepressant, lithium prescribed as monotherapy for depression is not recommended.

Answer B is incorrect. Nortriptyline is a tricyclic antidepressant associated with the "3 Cs:" Convulsions, Coma, and Cardiotoxicity (conduction defects and arrhythmias). Tricyclic antidepressants primarily have anticholinergic adverse effects as well, including dry mouth, mydriasis, constipation, and urinary retention.

Answer C is incorrect. Phenelzine is an MAO inhibitor. There is no evidence that two MAO inhibitors lead to serotonin syndrome when taken together. Adverse effects of phenelzine include postural hypotension, headache, dry mouth, sexual dysfunction, weight gain, and sleep disturbances.

Answer E is incorrect. Trazodone is a heterocyclic associated with sedation, nausea, priapism, and postural hypotension.

12. **The correct answer is B.** Over the course of two visits, the patient has exhibited psychotic and residual symptoms characteristic of schizophrenia and related disorders. A diagnosis of schizophrenia, however, requires active phase ("positive") symptoms, and may include "negative" ones as well, over a period of >6 months. In this case, the patient's symptoms have lasted <4 months, and were potentially incited by a traumatic event and its repercussions. If the symptoms had lasted <1 month, a diagnosis of brief psychotic disorder would be accurate; in such a diagnosis, most patients make a full recovery. In this patient, symptoms with a duration of >1 month but <6 months yield a diagnosis of schizophreniform disorder. Negative symptoms, as seen here, worsen the prognosis of a patient with schizophreniform disorder.

Answer A is incorrect. There is no evidence that either the patient or his mother is actively seeking the attention of medical personnel, or that the symptoms experienced were falsified for secondary gain of tangible items such as food, shelter, or money, as would be the case in malingering.

Answer C is incorrect. Explicit in the diagnosis of schizophrenia is the presence of "positive" and (but not always) "negative" symptoms of >6 months' duration. Many patients with a prior diagnosis of schizophreniform disorder eventually receive a diagnosis of schizophrenia.

Answer D is incorrect. The diagnosis of a schizoaffective disorder requires the symptoms of schizophrenia (often both "positive" and "negative" symptoms) as well as those of a mood disorder (ie, depression, mania). These patients typically have less cognitive impairment than those with strict psychotic disorders.

Answer E is incorrect. Delusions are fixed, false beliefs or ideas by a patient that are not shared by other individuals. Delusional disorder refers to a pathologic state whereby construct(s) of delusions impair one's social and/or cognitive functioning. Shared delusions are those transmitted from one person to another in a parent-to-child or spouse-to-spouse relationship. There is no evidence presented that the patient's mother shares the false beliefs of her son.

13. **The correct answer is D.** The patient has pellagra due to niacin (vitamin B_3) deficiency. Niacin is found in unrefined and enriched grains, cereal, milk, and lean meats. Niacin is required for adequate cellular function and metabolism as an essential component of nicotinamide adenine dinucleotide and nicotinamide adenine dinucleotide phosphate. Because cellular functions in multiple organs and tissues are impacted by niacin deficiency, there is a systemic clinical expression of pellagra involving the skin, GI tract, and CNS. The symptoms of pellagra progress through the 3 D's: **D**ermatitis, **D**iarrhea, and **D**ementia. If untreated, it can result in the fourth **D**: **D**eath. Pellagra is Italian for thickened skin, and it is usually seen in sun-exposed areas of the body. Since niacin is derived from tryptophan, a decrease in tryptophan absorption or an increase in tryptophan metabolism can produce similar symptoms.

Answer A is incorrect. Arginine is a precursor of creatine, urea, and nitric oxide.

Answer B is incorrect. Histidine is a precursor of histamine.

Answer C is incorrect. Phenylalanine is a precursor of tyrosine, dopamine, norepinephrine, and epinephrine.

Answer E is incorrect. Tyrosine is a precursor of dopamine, norepinephrine, and epinephrine.

14. **The correct answer is C.** Depression is often associated with disrupted sleep. Specifically, sleep studies performed in patients with depression reveal increased time spent in REM sleep, decreased REM latency, and decreased delta waves, which are characteristic of stages 3 and 4 sleep. Patients with depression often experience decreased daytime energy and motivation to complete tasks; these are commonly misdiagnosed as side effects of poor sleep rather than warning signs of depression. Fluoxetine, an SSRI, is an appropriate first-line agent for patients with depression. This provider should also consider referral to a psychiatrist for management of this patient's depression.

Answer A is incorrect. Avoidance of caffeine is particularly helpful in patients with insomnia, defined as difficulty falling asleep or staying asleep three times per week for at least one month. Although avoidance of caffeine may help this patient with her sleep disturbances, her specific sleep patterns indicate concern for depression. Thus, further evaluation and treatment with an SSRI should be considered.

Answer B is incorrect. Continuous positive airway pressure would be helpful in a patient suffering from sleep apnea, which occurs when a patient briefly stops breathing during the night and awakens from sleep. Patients with severe sleep apnea might awaken hundreds of times per night. This patient's polysomnographic tracing is not consistent with sleep apnea.

Answer D is incorrect. Methylphenidate is used to treat narcolepsy, or sudden sleep attacks during the day despite normal nighttime sleep.

Answer E is incorrect. Normal sleep patterns in young adults include 25% of total sleep time spent in REM sleep and 25% of total sleep time is spent in delta wave (stages 3 and 4) sleep.

15. **The correct answer is C.** This patient is experiencing hallucinations, delusions, and dilated pupils, but very few observable behavioral changes. These are symptoms consistent with lysergic acid diethylamide (LSD) abuse. LSD is a hallucinogenic drug that can cause marked anxiety, depression, nausea, weakness, and paresthesias.

    Answer A is incorrect. Alcohol abuse is characterized by a general disinhibition, slurred speech, and ataxia. It does not usually cause patients to hallucinate or become delusional. Benzodiazepines can be used to prevent delirium tremens and other signs of alcohol withdrawal.

    Answer B is incorrect. Cocaine can cause many of the symptoms this patient is experiencing. However, patients with recent cocaine use are usually hypertensive and tachycardic because of its stimulant effects.

    Answer D is incorrect. Marijuana can cause many of the symptoms this patient is experiencing. However, patients with recent marijuana use usually have an increase in appetite and dry mouth as well.

    Answer E is incorrect. Phencyclidine is a hallucinogenic drug that is often associated with belligerence and acting out impulsively.

16. **The correct answer is A.** The boy exhibits the characteristic emotional lability and impulsivity seen in patients with attention deficit/hyperactivity disorder (ADHD). Methylphenidate is a first-line treatment for ADHD. It works similarly to amphetamines by increasing the presynaptic release of norepinephrine.

    Answer B is incorrect. Antimuscarinic drugs like benztropine can be used in conjunction with typical antipsychotics in the treatment of schizophrenia to alleviate extrapyramidal symptoms.

    Answer C is incorrect. Selective serotonin reuptake inhibitors can be used to treat depression, anxiety, and obsessive-compulsive disorder.

    Answer D is incorrect. Drugs that stimulate dopamine receptors are used in the treatment of Parkinson disease.

    Answer E is incorrect. Buspirone is a serotonin receptor agonist that is used in the treatment of anxiety.

17. **The correct answer is B.** This patient has physical signs consistent with anorexia nervosa, most notably a low body mass index, bradycardia, evidence of hypotension, fine body hair (called lanugo), and concomitant depression. Anorexia nervosa is a serious condition that requires intensive mental health care, as well as close medical monitoring of weight, electrolyte levels, and hydration status. The mainstay of therapy is a combination of cognitive behavioral therapy and SSRIs. Use of the antidepressant bupropion is contraindicated in patients with anorexia nervosa because it increases the risk of seizure in this population.

    Answer A is incorrect. Amitriptyline is a tricyclic antidepressant (TCA). TCAs, although effective, are not first-line therapy in the management of anorexia nervosa, given the potential for cardiac adverse effects in anorexic patients already suffering from bradycardia and electrolyte abnormalities. TCAs are not known to increase the risk of seizure in anorexic patients.

    Answer C is incorrect. Fluoxetine is an SSRI most commonly used as an antidepressant. It has also been used to treat anorexia nervosa, although with questionable efficacy. SSRIs are not known to increase the risk of seizure in anorexic patients.

    Answer D is incorrect. Mirtazapine in an atypical antidepressant that induces weight gain, which may be beneficial in patients with weight control issues, although this has not yet been studied rigorously. Mirtazapine is not known to increase the risk of seizure in anorexic patients.

    Answer E is incorrect. Selegiline is a MAO inhibitor most commonly used as an antidepressant; it is not typically used to manage anorexia nervosa. MAO inhibitors are not known to increase the risk of seizure in anorexic patients.

18. **The correct answer is D.** SSRIs block the reuptake of serotonin (5-hydroxytryptamine [5-HT]) by the serotonin transport protein (STP) in presynaptic neurons; the result is an effective increase in serotonin within the synaptic space. SSRIs act at the "X" in the image by inhibiting the binding of 5-HT to STP. SSRIs have demonstrated efficacy for numerous medical and psychiatric conditions, most notably depression, anxiety, obsessive-compulsive disorder, and eating disorders.

    Answer A is incorrect. SSRIs are not first-line treatment for bipolar disorder; a mood stabilizing agent (eg, lithium or valproic acid) would be the treatment of choice.

    Answer B is incorrect. SSRIs are not first-line treatment for delirium tremens; a long-acting benzodiazepine (eg, chlordiazepoxide) would be the treatment of choice.

    Answer C is incorrect. SSRIs are not first-line treatment for multiple personality disorder; an antipsychotic (eg, haloperidol or risperidone) would be the treatment of choice.

    Answer E is incorrect. SSRIs are not first-line treatment for schizophrenia; an antipsychotic (eg, haloperidol or risperidone) would be the treatment of choice.

19. **The correct answer is A.** This patient is being treated for depression. Amitriptyline, a tricyclic anti-depressant, is as effective as the selective serotonin reuptake inhibitors, but often is not prescribed as a first-line agent because of its many adverse effects. These include sedation, α-blocking effects, and, most commonly, anticholinergic effects such as dry mouth, blurry vision, tachycardia, urinary retention, constipation, confusion, and dry, hot skin. These adverse effects can be remembered with the following: red as a beet (flushing), dry as a bone (anhidrosis), hot as a hare (overheating secondary to anhidrosis), blind as a bat (blurry vision), mad as a hatter (hallucinations or delirium), and full as a flask (urinary retention). Of note, MAO inhibitors, another class of antidepressants, do not have anticholinergic properties, but can cause adverse effects similar to those of anticholinergic medications, including dry mouth and urinary retention. MAO inhibitors often are associated with tyramine crises on the USMLE exam, especially when the patient described has consumed tannin-rich foods, such as red wines and aged cheeses.

    Answer B is incorrect. Clonazepam is a benzodiazepine sometimes prescribed as an anxiolytic at the initiation of anti-depressant therapy. The most commonly reported adverse effects are those associated with CNS depression, such as sedation or respiratory depression at higher doses. Dependence and rebound anxiety can result from benzodiazepine abuse.

    Answer C is incorrect. Lithium is a mood stabilizer used to treat bipolar affective disorder. It indirectly inhibits the reuptake of serotonin and norepinephrine by inhibiting the phosphatidylinositol second messenger system. Adverse effects include CNS depression, dizziness, nephrogenic diabetes insipidus, acne, edema, and hypothyroidism, as well as many others.

    Answer D is incorrect. Sertraline and other SSRIs are associated with adverse effects related to CNS stimulation such as headache, anxiety, tremor, insomnia, anorexia, nausea, and vomiting. Weight gain and sexual dysfunction are also frequently reported with SSRI use.

    Answer E is incorrect. Venlafaxine is a serotonin/norepinephrine reuptake inhibitor. It has adverse effects similar to those of selective serotonin reuptake inhibitors, plus additional adverse effects due to the norepinephrine, such as dizziness and diaphoresis. Venlafaxine is also known to cause hypertension.

20. **The correct answer is C.** This patient has evidence of benzodiazepine intoxication. This is the most likely scenario given her recent diagnosis and treatment for panic disorder, in addition to the exclusion of other causes with similar presentations. Benzodiazepines are relatively safe in overdose; however, shorter-

acting benzodiazepines such as temazepam, triazolam, and alprazolam pose a greater risk for morbidity and mortality. Competitive antagonists work by displacing a drug from its binding site. Flumazenil is a competitive antagonist that can be used in the case of benzodiazepine overdose, and naloxone is a competitive antagonist that is used to reverse symptoms of opiate overdose. When using flumazenil, be aware that rapid reversal of benzodiazepine overdose may lead to rebound seizure activity. In clinical practice flumazenil is rarely used except in children.

Answer A is incorrect. Pralidoxime, a cholinesterase regenerator, is indicated in cases of organophosphate poisoning. Organophosphates such as parathion and malathion are indirect-acting cholinomimetics that inhibit acetylcholinesterase by forming a very stable bond with it. This results in general cholinergic CNS stimulation (incontinence, bronchoconstriction, miosis, and bradycardia). Pralidoxime has a greater affinity for binding to organophosphates than acetylcholinesterase. As such, it is thought of as an organophosphate "chemical antagonist."

Answer B is incorrect. Physostigmine is an indirect-acting cholinomimetic that inhibits the action of acetylcholinesterase, thereby amplifying the effect of endogenous acetylcholine. It is indicated in cases of anticholinergic (but not tricyclic) poisoning, which would present with the classic picture described by the mnemonic "red as a beet, blind as a bat, mad as a hatter, dry as a bone, and hot as a hare." One would expect fever, flushing, delirium, dry mucous membranes, and miosis on physical exam.

Answer D is incorrect. Ethanol is indicated in cases of toxic alcohol ingestion (eg, methanol or ethylene glycol). Toxic metabolites are formed when alcohol dehydrogenase metabolizes methanol or ethylene glycol. Ethanol works by inhibiting the formation of these harmful substances by competing for binding sites on alcohol dehydrogenase.

Answer E is incorrect. Reserpine inhibits the storage of norepinephrine in adrenergic nerve terminals, thereby depleting the neuron of its stores. It has been classified as a postganglionic sympathetic nerve terminal blocker, and is rarely used as an antihypertensive medication.

CHAPTER 15

Renal

QUESTIONS

1. A patient presents with the chief complaint of an unrelenting headache of several months' duration. Her vital signs are significant for a blood pressure of 200/100 mm Hg. Abdominal ultrasound confirms the cause of her hypertension. Decreased perfusion of which of the following structures results in the renin release that is responsible for this patient's condition?

   (A) Adrenal medulla
   (B) Afferent arteriole
   (C) Distal convoluted tubule
   (D) Loop of Henle
   (E) Zona glomerulosa

2. The following graph was obtained by collecting and assaying urine from a healthy volunteer given varying amounts of glucose by intravenous infusion. Which statement concerning the graph is most accurate?

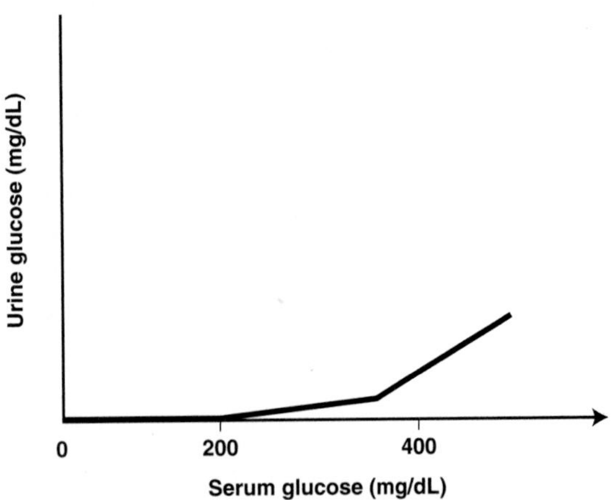

Reproduced, with permission, from USMLERx.com.

   (A) Glomerular filtration of glucose is saturated at 375 mg/dL
   (B) Proximal convoluted tubule glucose reabsorption is saturated at 375 mg/dL
   (C) Proximal convoluted tubule glucose secretion begins at 200 mg/dL
   (D) Proximal convoluted tubule glucose secretion begins at 375 mg/dL
   (E) Urine glucose begins to be detectable at 375 mg/dL

3. A 17-year-old boy with insulin-dependent diabetes is brought to the emergency department unconscious with a fruity odor on his breath. Upon his admission, insulin is administered and serum potassium levels are monitored closely. Potassium balance is essential for the normal function of excitable tissues such as muscles and nerves. Which of the following clinical situations could also put a patient at risk for hypokalemia?

   (A) High-K^+ diet
   (B) Hypoaldosteronism
   (C) Metabolic acidosis
   (D) Overuse of amiloride
   (E) Overuse of hydrochlorothiazide

4. A 66-year-old woman with acute renal insufficiency and unremarkable medical history undergoes a renal biopsy that reveals glomerular capillary subendothelial deposits. Which of the following symptoms often occurs in patients with this disease?

   (A) Achalasia
   (B) Aortic aneurysm
   (C) Esophageal reflux
   (D) Malar rash
   (E) Morbilliform rash

5. Nonsteroidal anti-inflammatory drugs (NSAIDs) are associated with the development of acute renal failure in patients living in states of effective volume depletion, such as heart failure, cirrhosis, and true volume depletion. What is the mechanism by which NSAIDs are believed to mediate this harmful effect on the kidney?

   (A) Increased prostaglandin synthesis constricts preglomerular vessels
   (B) Inhibition of prostaglandin synthesis decreases glomerular capillary permeability

(C) Inhibition of prostaglandin synthesis decreases preglomerular resistance
(D) Inhibition of prostaglandin synthesis increases preglomerular resistance
(E) The drug has direct toxic effects on the renal tubules

6. Immune complex-mediated glomerular disease can be classified according to the site of complex formation. The site also partly dictates whether the disease would give rise to either a nephritic or a nephrotic clinical presentation. Where does the immune complex deposition form in membranoproliferative glomerulonephritis?

   (A) Between the glomerular basement membrane and visceral epithelium
   (B) Between the glomerular basement membrane and the podocytes
   (C) Between the glomerular basement membrane and the visceral epithelial cells
   (D) Between the endothelium and the mesangium
   (E) Between the visceral epithelial cells and the parietal epithelium

7. A 58-year-old man with nephrotic syndrome is brought by ambulance to the emergency department with altered mental status. His wife reports that this morning he had difficulty moving the right side of his body, and that she couldn't arouse him from an afternoon nap. On physical examination the patient is obtunded and has absent right-sided movement. His International Normalized Ratio (INR) is = 0.5. CT angiogram of the brain is shown in the image. What is the most likely etiology of this patient's symptoms?

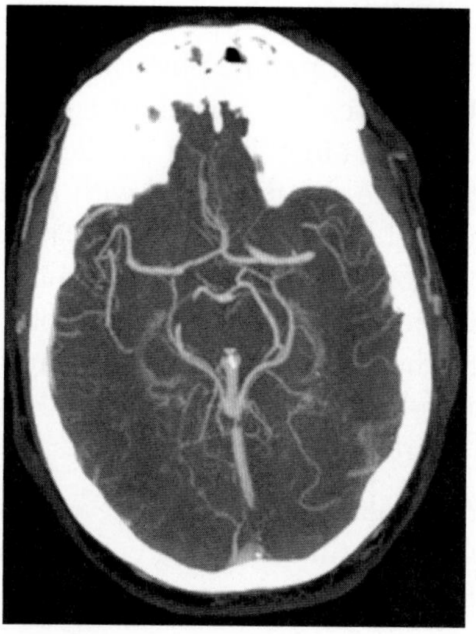

Courtesy of Dr. Per-Lennart Westesson, University of Rochester Medical Center.

   (A) Decreased antithrombin III levels
   (B) Decreased factor II levels
   (C) Decreased fibrinogen levels
   (D) Increased protein C levels
   (E) Increased protein S levels

8. A 28-year-old woman with a history of asthma presents to the emergency department with a temperature of 38.2°C (100.8°F) and complains of shaking chills and pain on her right side, which she locates by pointing to the area above her right iliac crest. She notes that she has never had this occur before. During the examination, there is tenderness to percussion at the junction of the lower ribs and the thoracic vertebrae. Urinalysis reveals WBC casts. What is the organism most likely causing her condition?

   (A) *Escherichia coli*
   (B) *Klebsiella pneumoniae*
   (C) *Proteus mirabilis*
   (D) *Staphylococcus saprophyticus*
   (E) *Ureaplasma urealyticum*

9. A 64-year-old man presents to his primary care physician for a routine physical. He is in good health, smokes half a pack of cigarettes daily, and has no other known medical problems. However, he was diagnosed with hypertension in the past. The physician notes a blood pressure of 160/100 mm Hg and 1+ pitting edema to his knees. The physician also notes bilateral bruits when auscultating the abdomen. Which of the following is contraindicated in this patient's care?

   (A) Angioplasty
   (B) Angiotensin-converting enzyme inhibitor
   (C) Diuretics
   (D) Smoking cessation
   (E) Surgical management

10. A 2-month-old boy is brought to the physician after his parents palpated an abdominal mass while bathing him. They deny any fevers, chills, decreased urine output, or hematuria. On physical examination a large mass is palpated in the midline. Abdominal ultrasound shows pelvic kidneys fused at their lower poles. Which structure prevents this abnormal kidney from occupying its appropriate position?

    (A) Aorta
    (B) Celiac trunk
    (C) Inferior mesenteric artery
    (D) Inferior vena cava
    (E) Superior mesenteric artery

11. A 23-year-old man is beginning chemotherapy for leukemia when he develops severe intermittent left flank pain that soon migrates to the pelvis. Three days later, the patient's creatinine level rises and he is diagnosed with acute renal failure. His fractional excretion of sodium (FENa) is >4% with a urine osmolality of <350 mOsm/kg. Blood and urine cultures are negative for bacteria and eosinophilia. An abdominal radiograph fails to locate any pathology. Which of the following is the most likely location of the lesion causing this patient's renal failure?

    (A) Glomeruli
    (B) Interstitium of the kidney
    (C) Kidney tubules
    (D) Spleen
    (E) Urethra

12. A 68-year-old woman with a history of diabetes and hypertension, who is recovering from a total hip replacement, is given ketorolac, a nonsteroidal anti-inflammatory drug, for the management of pain. Twenty-four hours later, her urine production decreases, and her serum blood urea nitrogen and creatinine levels rise to 44 mg/dL and 3.1 mg/dL, respectively. What is the effect of this medication on glomerular filtration rate, renal plasma flow, and filtration fraction?

    (A) Decreased renal plasma flow, decreased glomerular filtration rate, no change in filtration fraction
    (B) Decreased renal plasma flow, increased glomerular filtration rate, increased filtration fraction
    (C) Increased renal plasma flow, decreased glomerular filtration rate, increased filtration fraction
    (D) No change in renal plasma flow, decreased glomerular filtration rate, decreased filtration fraction
    (E) No change in renal plasma flow, increased glomerular filtration rate, increased filtration fraction

13. A 56-year-old man with a 60 pack-year smoking history and normal fluid intake presents to his physician with two months of fatigue and weakness accompanied by cough and mild dyspnea. The patient's vital signs are normal, but a lower left lobe mass is noted on X-ray of the chest. Biopsy leads to the diagnosis of small cell carcinoma. Results of laboratory tests are shown below.

    Plasma sodium: 125 mEq/L
    Plasma potassium: 3.9 mEq/L
    Plasma carbon dioxide: 24 mEq/L
    Plasma osmolality: 253 mOsm/L
    Urine sodium: 48 mEq/L
    Urine osmolality: 280 mOsm/L

The hormone most likely responsible for this patient's abnormal laboratory values has which of the following direct effects?

(A) Activation of G-protein coupled receptors in the adrenal cortex elevates cAMP levels and leads to increased production and secretion of corticosteroids
(B) Activation of G-protein coupled receptors in the hypothalamus results in elevated cAMP levels and inhibition of hypothalamic-induced thirst mechanism
(C) Activation of V2 receptors leads to an increase in total peripheral resistance; activation of V1 receptors results in the concentration of urine
(D) Activation of V2 receptors results in the insertion of aquaporins into the collecting duct; activation of V1 receptors leads to a decrease in total peripheral resistance
(E) Activation of V2 receptors results in the insertion of aquaporins into the renal collecting duct; activation of V1 receptors leads to an increase in total peripheral resistance
(F) Cleavage of angiotensinogen to angiotensin I leads to an increase in both aldosterone levels and total peripheral resistance

14. A hospitalized patient is given methicillin for a suspected staphylococcal infection around a central line insertion site. Approximately one week after beginning treatment, the patient develops signs of acute renal failure, including an increased serum creatinine level. A urine sample shows microscopic hematuria and WBCs, but no bacteria. Methicillin is withdrawn and the patient's renal symptoms soon improve. Administration of which of the following drugs would most likely also cause this condition?

(A) Cyclophosphamide
(B) Diphenhydramine
(C) Hydrochlorothiazide
(D) Isoniazid
(E) Lithium

15. A 50-year-old man with a history of large-bowel obstruction is diagnosed with colon cancer and undergoes resection of his colon. At check-up, he feels well except that over the past three weeks he has had significant swelling in his legs. Physical examination reveals 2+ pitting edema and a blood pressure of 155/94 mm Hg. Urinalysis shows 4+ protein with no RBCs or casts. Which of the following would most likely be present on a kidney biopsy from this patient?

(A) A spike-and-dome pattern of deposition on electron microscopy
(B) A tram-track pattern on light microscopy
(C) Lumpy subepithelial deposits on electron microscopy
(D) Nonlinear mesangial staining with IgA immunofluorescence
(E) "Splintering" of the lamina densa

16. A 5-year-old girl is brought to the pediatrician because of generalized edema. Laboratory testing reveals proteinuria of 5 gm/day, and podocyte foot process effacement is seen on electron microscopy of a kidney biopsy. Disruption of which of the following components of the filtration barrier is contributing to this patient's proteinuria?

(A) Brush border
(B) Endothelial cell
(C) Heparan sulfate
(D) Integrin
(E) Type IV collagen

17. A 67-year-old woman with osteoporosis is given a diuretic to treat her hypertension. This particular diuretic has the adverse effect of limiting calcium excretion by the kidney. Referring to the image, where along the nephron does this drug act?

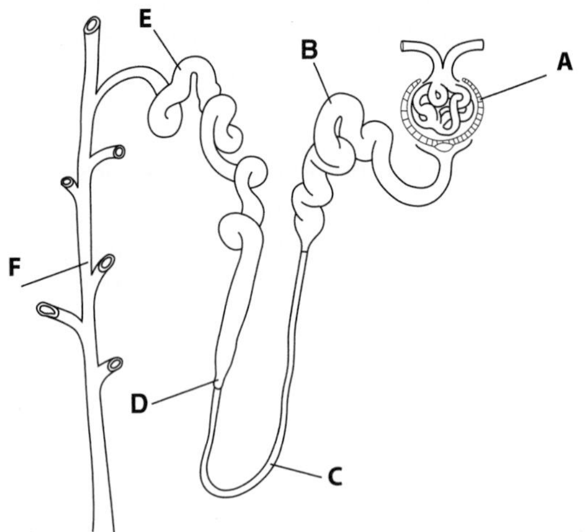

Reproduced, with permission, from USMLERx.com.

(A) A
(B) B
(C) C
(D) D
(E) E
(F) F

18. A 22-year-old college student is brought to the emergency department after he began complaining of ants crawling over his body and his friends noted increasing agitation and threatening gestures. On physical examination he is febrile, restless, and tachycardic, and his pupils are markedly dilated. His friends report he has been studying "at all hours" for his upcoming final examinations. Appropriate treatment includes which of the following?

(A) Acidifying urine to increase renal clearance
(B) Alkalinizing urine to increase renal clearance
(C) Treating with flumazenil
(D) Treating with naloxone
(E) Treating with water to dilute drug effects

19. A 28-year-old woman who received no prenatal care gives birth at 37 weeks' gestation. The fetus is stillborn and has a number of anomalies including a flattened face, large and low-set ears, and clubbed feet. What other condition would result in an amount of amniotic fluid similar to that found in this situation?

(A) Anencephaly
(B) Chronic uteroplacental insufficiency
(C) Duodenal atresia
(D) Maternal diabetes
(E) Trisomy 18

20. A 6-month-old girl is brought to the emergency department by her mother after ingesting a bottle of unmarked pills from the family medicine cabinet. On examination the child appears agitated and tachypneic. Urgent blood chemistry measurements are taken and reveal the following:

Na^+: 143 mEq/L
K^+: 4.0 mEq/L
Cl^-: 104 mEq/L
HCO_3^-: 19 mEq/L
pH: 7.28

Which of the following medications did this patient most likely ingest?

(A) Aldosterone antagonist
(B) Antacid
(C) Iron supplement
(D) Loop diuretic
(E) Opiate analgesic

21. A 16-year-old boy comes to the physician because of a one year history of intermittent, painless hematuria without dysuria or increased frequency of micturition. He notes that the hematuria becomes more prominent when he is also suffering from a respiratory infection. Which of the following is most likely to be found if the boy is diagnosed with IgA nephropathy (Berger disease)?

(A) Increased antistreptolysin O titer
(B) Lumpy-bumpy electron-dense deposits
(C) Mesangial deposits
(D) Proteinuria exceeding 3.5 gm/24 h
(E) Subepithelial deposits

22. A 34-year-old woman comes to the hospital to deliver a full-term infant. Labor is complicated by an amniotic fluid embolism, and subsequent blood tests show the presence of fibrin split products. The next day the patient abruptly develops anuria, gross hematuria, and flank pain accompanied by rapidly increasing blood urea nitrogen and creatinine levels and a new cardiac friction rub. The patient's ultrasound demonstrates hypodensities within the renal cortex. Which of the following is the most appropriate treatment?

(A) Aggressive fluid support
(B) Biopsy to evaluate for malignancy
(C) Broad-spectrum antibiotics
(D) Dialysis
(E) No treatment is necessary at this time

23. A 40-year-old man presents with hematuria and sharp, sudden, sporadic pain in his lower back. His blood pressure is normal, and his physical examination is significant for flank pain that comes in waves. A plain film of the abdomen and pelvis shows focal, marked densities bilaterally in the mid-abdomen. A follow-up noncontrast CT scan demonstrates several large stones in the ureters, bilaterally. Which of the following is the most likely cause of this man's symptoms?

(A) A full rectum, and bilateral calcified common iliac arteries
(B) A large stool passing through the small bowel
(C) Hyperparathyroidism
(D) Hyperuricemia
(E) Staphylococcal infection of the bladder

24. A man is chopping wood outside when he accidentally chops into his arm, causing it to bleed profusely. A friend drives him to the hospital, 30 minutes away. Although pressure is applied to the wound, there is continued blood loss. Upon arrival to the emergency department, he appears lethargic and pale. Which of the following set of vital signs would most likely be seen in this patient as he is being transported to the hospital?

Choice	Heart rate	Total peripheral resistance	Renin	Vasopressin
A	↓	↑	↑	↑
B	↑	↓	↑	↑
C	↑	↑	↓	↑
D	↑	↑	↑	↓
E	↑	↑	↑	↑

Reproduced, with permission, from USMLERx.com.

(A) A
(B) B
(C) C
(D) D
(E) E

25. A 72-year-old retired man recently diagnosed with heart disease arrives at the emergency department complaining of sudden-onset abdominal pain, diarrhea, and vomiting, with mild pain and swelling throughout his face, lips, and mouth. The patient denies any pruritus. On questioning he says his primary care physician recently put him on a regimen of drugs to control his high blood pressure and cholesterol. He also mentions that he sometimes gets a rash after taking antibiotics and usually gets "hives" every spring. The physician suspects that these symptoms are related to one of the patient's medications. The accumulation of what substance is most likely causing the patient's symptoms?

(A) Bradykinin
(B) Histamine
(C) Prostacyclin
(D) Prostaglandin E_2
(E) Serotonin

26. A 56-year-old woman who has been taking cefoxitin for treatment of *Klebsiella* pneumonia is found to still have *Klebsiella* organisms in her blood one week after beginning treatment. Another drug is added to the patient's regimen. Two days later, the following laboratory values are obtained:

    Na^+: 141 mEq/L
    K^+: 4.3 mEq/L
    Cl^-: 102 mEq/L
    HCO_3^-: 24 mEq/L
    Blood urea nitrogen: 65 mg/dL
    Creatinine: 4.4 mEq/L

    Which of the following medications was most likely added to this patient's regimen?

    (A) Azithromycin
    (B) Aztreonam
    (C) Clindamycin
    (D) Piperacillin
    (E) Tobramycin

27. A 2-year-old boy is brought to the emergency department (ED) with complaints of fever, chills, and flank pain. His immunizations are up to date and his mother states that this is the second time he has been to the ED because of these symptoms. His temperature is 39.1°C (102.2°F) and physical examination is unremarkable except for costovertebral angle tenderness on the right. A complete blood cell count shows leukocytosis, and urinalysis demonstrates the presence of WBCs and RBCs in the urine. What is the most likely mechanism of this patient's recurrent complaints?

    (A) Immunoglobulin deficiency
    (B) Nephroblastoma
    (C) Poststreptococcal glomerulonephritis
    (D) Vesicoureteral reflux

28. A patient suffering from an upper respiratory infection presents to his physician with complaints of body aches, urinary frequency, and "strange-colored urine." His previous medical history is significant only for recently beginning treatment with a statin drug for high cholesterol. His serum creatinine level is 2.0 mg/dL. A histologic section of the patient's kidney is shown in the image. Which of the following is the most likely diagnosis?

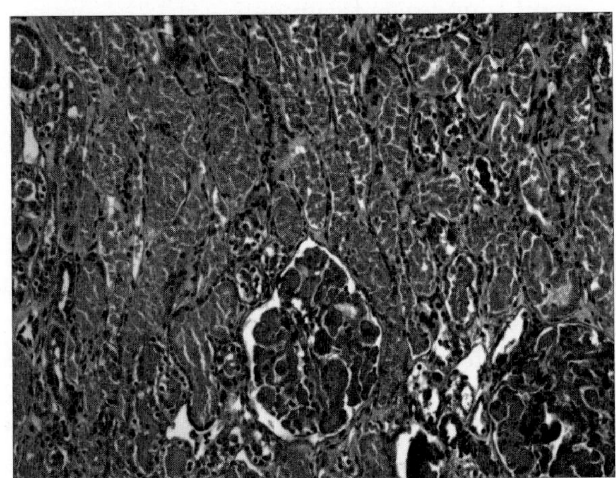

Reproduced, with permission, from USMLERx.com.

    (A) Acute tubular necrosis
    (B) Amyloidosis
    (C) Analgesic nephropathy
    (D) Focal segmental glomerulosclerosis
    (E) Pyelonephritis

29. A 40-year-old woman presents to the emergency department after five days of profuse vomiting. She has a history of rheumatoid arthritis, which is treated with celecoxib. She complains of joint pain at present. Which of the reasons below describes why celecoxib would be contraindicated in this patient at presentation?

(A) Because of its effects on platelet function
(B) Because of its effects on the arterioles of the kidney
(C) Because of its effects on the gastrointestinal mucosa
(D) Because of its effects on the macula densa
(E) Because of its effects on the production of inflammatory cytokines

30. A 57-year-old man with a 15-year history of type 2 diabetes mellitus and hypertension who is on insulin therapy presents with complaints of fatigue and swollen feet. Physical examination reveals 3+ pitting edema bilaterally in his feet as well as loss of pain and temperature sensation in all of his toes. Vital signs are within normal limits except for a blood pressure of 150/95 mm Hg. Blood tests show an LDL level of 154 mg/dL, blood glucose level of 213 mg/dL, and a hemoglobin A_{1c} level of 9.2%. A basic metabolic panel shows a blood urea nitrogen level of 67 mg/dL and creatinine level of 2.6 mg/dL. Urinalysis shows 4+ protein with no casts. Which of the following antihypertensive medications may have helped prevent this patient's current condition?

(A) A selective β-blocker
(B) An antagonist of cardiac and vascular calcium channels
(C) An inhibitor of a thick ascending limb transport protein
(D) An inhibitor of the sodium-chloride symporter in the distal convoluted tubule
(E) Angiotensin receptor blocker

31. A 27-year-old HIV-positive man presents to the emergency department with swollen legs. He states that his urine has been very foamy. Urinalysis shows massive proteinuria. Treatment with corticosteroids is initiated but is not successful. Immunofluorescence shows deposition of IgM in the affected segments. Which of the following is most likely to be seen on biopsy?

(A) Extensive glomerular crescent formation
(B) IgA deposition in the glomerular mesangium
(C) Immune complex deposition in subepithelial space
(D) Large focal hyaline deposits
(E) No deposits on immunofluorescence, some retraction of epithelial foot processes on electron microscopy

32. A large body of epidemiologic research has shown that a diet high in sodium can contribute to hypertension, resulting in left ventricular hypertrophy. The Intersalt Epidemiology Study relates increased sodium intake to higher blood pressures across diverse populations. Also, rigorous prospective clinical trials demonstrate that lowering sodium intake can lower arterial pressure in normotensive and hypertensive individuals. Which of the following is a mechanism of how the kidney responds to high sodium intake?

(A) Increase in atrial natriuretic peptide and dilation of glomerular afferent arterioles
(B) Increased release of renin due to chemoreceptor recognition of increased plasma osmolarity
(C) Increased secretion of potassium into the urine
(D) Mechanoreceptor detection of constriction of glomerular afferent arterioles
(E) Mechanoreceptor detection of dilation of glomerular afferent arterioles

33. A 72-year-old man presents to his physician complaining of pain in his lower abdomen, increased difficulty urinating, and decreased urine output for the past couple days. The physician notes an enlarged prostate on digital rectal examination. Serum creatinine level is 2.5 mg/dL. Renal ultrasound is performed, and the image shows what is visualized bilaterally. Which of the following would most likely be expected on urinalysis?

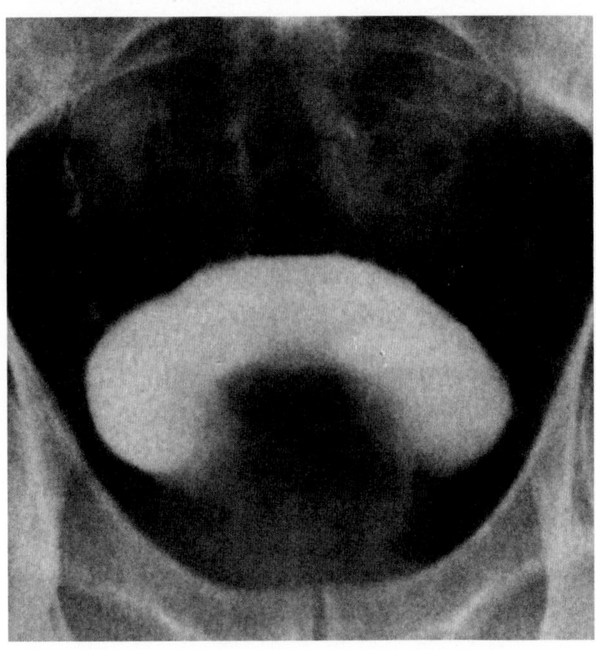

Reproduced, with permission, from Tanagho EA, McAninch JW. *Smith's General Urology*, 17th ed. New York: McGraw-Hill, 2008: Figure 6-12A.

(A) Blood urea nitrogen:creatinine ratio <15
(B) Epithelial casts
(C) Fractional excretion of sodium <1%
(D) Urine Na^+ <10 mmol/L
(E) Urine osmolality <350 mmol/kg

34. Nephrotic syndrome is characterized by severe proteinuria, a decreased serum albumin level, and edema. This results from damage to the glomerular capillary wall. In particular, the glomerular basement membrane is essential for maintaining serum oncotic pressure. In non-pathologic states, which of the following properties of the glomerular basement membrane prevent albumin from being freely filtered into the urine?

(A) A combination of small pore size and negatively charged pore-forming molecules prevents albumin filtration
(B) A combination of small pore size and positively charged pore-forming molecules prevents albumin filtration
(C) Albumin is freely filtered across the basement membrane but is readily reabsorbed along the nephron
(D) The positive charge of proteoglycans in the basement membrane repels albumin
(E) The small size of the glomerular basement membrane pores excludes albumin molecules

35. A 54-year-old homeless woman is found unconscious under a bridge. On admission to the emergency department, her laboratory tests show:

Sodium: 137 mEq/L
Potassium: 3.3 mEq/L
Chloride: 112 mEq/L
Bicarbonate: 15 mEq/L
Arterial blood gas on room air: pH 7.28
Partial pressure of carbon dioxide: 28 mm Hg
Partial pressure of oxygen: 90 mm Hg

Which of the following most likely caused her acidosis?

(A) An aspirin overdose
(B) Diabetic ketoacidosis
(C) Severe diarrhea
(D) Severe underperfusion of her peripheral muscles
(E) Uremia

36. A patient with hepatocellular carcinoma develops severe ascites such that 3-5 L of fluid must be drained from her peritoneal cavity every three days. This procedure may have detrimental effects on kidney function that necessitates monitoring of glomerular filtration rate. Laboratory values are as follows:

Creatinine clearance: 120 mL/min
Glomerular capillary hydrostatic pressure: 40 mm Hg

Plasma inulin: 1.5 mg/mL
Urinary inulin: 50 mg/mL

Which of the following is her urine flow rate?

(A) 1.6 mL/min
(B) 3.6 mL/min
(C) 4.5 mL/min
(D) 36 mL/h
(E) 450 mL/day

37. Mountain climbers sometimes take acetazolamide to help the body rapidly acclimatize to higher altitudes. Which of the following is the mechanism by which acetazolamide does this?

(A) It causes a mixed metabolic acidosis and respiratory alkalosis
(B) It causes metabolic acidosis
(C) It causes metabolic alkalosis
(D) It causes respiratory acidosis
(E) It causes respiratory alkalosis

38. A longtime patient returns to visit her rheumatologist with complaints of headaches and blood in her urine. Her blood pressure is 152/88 mm Hg. Further testing reveals protein in the urine as well as RBC casts. The rheumatologist orders a renal biopsy, which is shown in the image. The pathology seen in the image is most likely caused by which of the following processes?

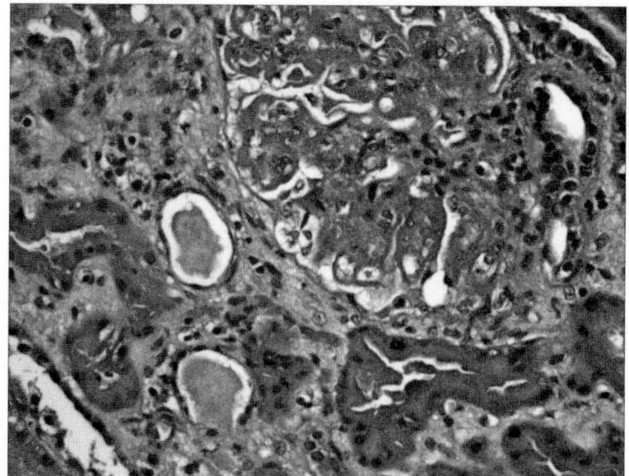

Reproduced, with permission, from USMLERx.com.

(A) Alport syndrome
(B) Membranous glomerulonephritis
(C) Minimal change disease
(D) Poststreptococcal glomerulonephritis
(E) Systemic lupus erythematosus nephritis

39. A 36-year-old man presents for his annual flu shot. He has been treated for hypertension with an angiotensin-converting enzyme inhibitor since age 30 years. He denies smoking and alcohol use. Family history is notable for his father requiring dialysis at age 50. An older brother recently underwent unilateral nephrectomy to decompress intra-abdominal organs. On examination, the patient appears barrel-chested and has a sitting blood pressure of 135/90 mm Hg. His likely genetic renal pathology is associated with an increased incidence of which of the following?

(A) Cerebral aneurysm
(B) Horseshoe kidney
(C) Macular cherry-red spots
(D) Potter syndrome
(E) Pott disease

40. A 48-year-old man is hospitalized after a motor vehicle accident. He is hypotensive and is given several units of packed RBCs by transfusion. He is kept in the intensive care unit for monitoring. On the patient's second day in the hospital, his blood urea nitrogen (BUN) and creatinine levels begin to rise and he develops pitting edema to his knees. His BUN:creatinine ratio is 12:1. A subsequent urinalysis shows numerous muddy brown epithelial and granular casts. Which of the following is another common cause of this man's condition?

(A) Ascending urinary tract infection
(B) Crush injury
(C) Diabetes mellitus
(D) Nonsteroidal anti-inflammatory drug toxicity
(E) Septic shock

41. Nephrolithiases, or kidney stones, can obstruct the flow of urine and cause pain. Stones are more likely to cause an obstruction at a junction or location where the tract is constricted. Which of the following describes a location where stones are most likely to cause an obstruction?

(A) In the bladder
(B) In the penile urethra
(C) In the prostatic urethra
(D) In the renal calyx
(E) In the ureter over the iliac vessels

42. A 53-year-old woman is undergoing renal function testing to evaluate proteinuria detected by her primary care physician at a routine visit. The patient's glomerular filtration rate (GFR) is initially estimated at 100 mL/min by inulin clearance. Subsequently, as part of a research study, the patient's GFR is determined using a novel marker (compound X) and is found to be 125 mL/min. Which mechanism most likely explains the difference noted between these two GFR estimates?

(A) Compound X is not freely filtered at the glomerulus
(B) Compound X is reabsorbed in the descending limb of the loop of Henle
(C) Compound X is reabsorbed in the proximal convoluted tubule
(D) Compound X is secreted in the proximal convoluted tubule
(E) Inulin is reabsorbed in the proximal convoluted tubule

43. The kidneys of a 65-year-old patient with long-standing diabetes mellitus are examined at autopsy and one kidney is shown in the image. In the later stage of his disease, this patient frequently required a Foley catheter to adequately drain his bladder. What condition most likely caused the anomalous appearance of his kidneys?

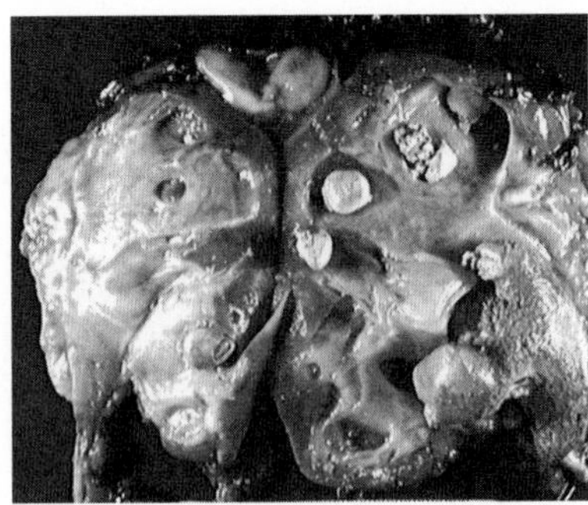

Reproduced, with permission, from USMLERx.com.

(A) Acute pyelonephritis
(B) Chronic reflux-associated pyelonephritis
(C) Drug-induced interstitial nephritis
(D) Hypertension
(E) Minimal change disease

44. A 52-year-old postmenopausal woman sees her physician because she is worried about osteoporosis. Her physician decides that he should investigate her calcium reabsorption in the thick ascending limb of Henle. Which of the following interventions would most effectively increase her calcium reabsorption in the thick ascending limb of the loop of Henle?

(A) Administration of exogenous parathyroid hormone
(B) Discontinuation of her loop diuretic
(C) Discontinuation of her thiazide diuretic
(D) Increasing serum calcium by administration of a vitamin supplement
(E) Maintenance of negative charge in the lumen

45. A 67-year-old man with a history of mild hypertension has a severe heart attack while walking to his car. When he arrives at the emergency department he is pale, cold, and diaphoretic. On physical examination he is tachycardic and hypotensive, and his ECG shows ST-segment elevations. He is treated with morphine, oxygen, and aspirin and is sent to the cardiac catheterization laboratory. The next

day he has low urine output, his blood urea nitrogen level is 35 mg/dL, his creatinine level is 1.3 mg/dL, and his blood pressure is 85/55 mm Hg. Urinalysis reveals few hyaline casts. Which of the following is the most likely cause of his low urine input?

(A) A blockage of the ureters or urethra
(B) Acute tubular necrosis
(C) Interstitial nephritis
(D) Low urine output is normal in times of stress
(E) Poor perfusion of the kidneys

46. A 13-year-old boy is brought to the emergency department with periorbital edema, hypertension, and tea-colored urine. His parents say that he had a sore throat about three weeks ago. Urinalysis shows RBCs with casts. A positive antistreptolysin O titer and decreased levels of complement are also noted. What findings would be expected in this patient's glomeruli?

(A) Granular subendothelial deposits
(B) Linear subendothelial pattern
(C) Mesangial deposits
(D) Subepithelial humps

47. A 55-year-old man admitted to the hospital because of complications of alcoholic cirrhosis and concurrent hepatitis C infection progressively develops an increase in serum blood urea nitrogen and creatinine levels, followed closely with urine output of <300 mL/day. Urinalysis reveals a sodium concentration of 5 mEq/L and the presence of benign urinary sediment. No proteinuria or hematuria is present. Imaging of this patient's kidneys is likely to reveal which of the following?

(A) Enlarged cystic kidneys
(B) Enlarged kidneys with severe hydronephrosis
(C) Horseshoe kidneys
(D) Normal kidneys with "flea-bitten" infarcted appearance
(E) Normal size and shape

48. A 22-year-old man with no significant past medical history presents to the emergency department with hemoptysis. He has never had an episode like this before. He does recall having a cold approximately three weeks earlier and has been experiencing increased fatigue and breathlessness since then, but he denies any current symptoms of rhinorrhea, sore throat, nausea, vomiting, or diarrhea. X-ray of the chest shows diffuse opacities in both lower lung fields, and urinalysis reveals RBCs in the urine. Which of the following is the most likely diagnosis?

(A) Acute poststreptococcal glomerulonephritis
(B) Alport syndrome
(C) Berger disease
(D) Goodpasture syndrome
(E) Minimal change disease

49. A 63-year-old man is seen by his doctor after measuring his blood pressure at home and finding it to be 168/100 mm Hg. The patient is concerned because he has had high blood pressure for the past 12 months that has not improved with dietary changes, exercise, or medication. A physical examination is unremarkable except for a thrill heard when auscultating the abdomen just to the left of the midline. What is the most likely cause of the patient's hypertension?

(A) Decreased levels of ADH
(B) Decreased levels of angiotensin II
(C) Elevated levels of aldosterone
(D) Excessive production of cortisol
(E) Increased levels of angiotensin-converting enzyme

50. A newborn with hypercalciuria and hypokalemic alkalosis is diagnosed with neonatal Bartter's syndrome, a rare inherited dysfunction of the thick ascending limb of the nephron. Which diuretic may mimic these symptoms by blocking a cotransporter found in this part of the nephron?

(A) Acetazolamide
(B) Furosemide
(C) Hydrochlorothiazide
(D) Mannitol
(E) Triamterene

ANSWERS

1. **The correct answer is B.** The juxtaglomerular (JG) cells in the afferent arteriole and the macula densa in the distal convoluted tubule together make up the JG apparatus, which is responsible for controlling renal blood flow via renin release. This patient's condition is confirmed by abdominal ultrasound, suggesting that renal artery stenosis is the cause of hypertension. In renal artery stenosis, the blood flow to the kidney is impeded. This low pressure is detected by JG cells in the afferent arteriole, which then secrete renin to raise blood pressure and renal perfusion through the renin-angiotensin-aldosterone axis.

   Answer A is incorrect. The adrenal medulla is responsible for the release of catecholamines and is composed of chromaffin cells. Whereas catecholamines can increase blood pressure, decreased perfusion to the adrenal medulla would result in a **decrease** in catecholamine production. This would result in a lower blood pressure. Recall that the two catecholamines of interest are epinephrine and norepinephrine, of which epinephrine is the principal hormone produced in the adrenal medulla. Lastly, it should be noted that a pheochromocytoma is a tumor of the adrenal medulla and would result in paroxysms of hypertension. However, this patient complains of an "unrelenting" headache, which is not associated with a pheochromocytoma.

   Answer C is incorrect. The distal convoluted tubule contains the macula densa cells that sense low sodium flow inside the nephron, another sign that the kidney is not well perfused. The macula densa cells are in intimate contact with the JG cells, and although the macula densa cells help in sensing low perfusion, it is the JG cells that both sense perfusion and secrete renin. Furthermore, it is the afferent arterioles that most directly sense a decrease in perfusion, as these structures receive blood directly from the renal artery.

   Answer D is incorrect. The loop of Henle is primarily responsible for concentrating urine, not for sensing perfusion or secreting renin. Recall that the descending loop of Henle is permeable to water, while the ascending loop is not.

   Answer E is incorrect. The zona glomerulosa is the outermost layer of the adrenal cortex and is responsible for the production of aldosterone. Decreased perfusion of the zona glomerulosa would result in atrophy and decreased production of aldosterone, which would lead to a decrease in blood pressure. Recall that aldosterone is responsible for sodium retention in the collecting duct.

2. **The correct answer is B.** Glucose is freely filtered at the glomerulus and, in healthy individuals, is completely reabsorbed in the proximal convoluted tubule (PCT). However, as the filtered load of glucose increases, the reabsorption ability of the nephron is eventually saturated, and glucose begins to be excreted in the urine. Due to significant variability in nephron physiology, certain nephrons are saturated at lower filtered loads than others. Thus, between 200 and 375 mg/dL glucose begins to appear in the urine, but not all nephrons are saturated. Above 375 mg/dL, all nephrons' transport maxima are reached, and any additional glucose is excreted in the urine.

   Answer A is incorrect. Glomerular filtration is never saturated because it does not depend on carrier-mediated transport. Furthermore, even if glucose were being incompletely filtered, this would tend to decrease (not increase) urine glucose levels.

   Answer C is incorrect. To whatever extent possible, the kidney attempts to fully reabsorb glucose in the proximal tubule. Thus, it is never secreted in the PCT.

   Answer D is incorrect. To whatever extent possible, the kidney attempts to fully reabsorb glucose in the proximal tubule. Thus, it is never secreted in the PCT.

Answer E is incorrect. The graph shows that the urine glucose level begins to rise at a serum glucose level of 200 mg/dL and is therefore detectable well before 375 mg/dL.

3. **The correct answer is E.** Thiazide diuretics inhibit Na^+-Cl^- reabsorption in the early distal tubule. Increased distal Na^+ delivery to the principal cells of the late distal tubule causes an increase in Na^+ reabsorption paired with an increase in K^+ secretion to maintain electroneutrality. Prolonged thiazide diuresis can cause hypokalemia.

   Answer A is incorrect. A high-K^+ diet will cause increased K^+ secretion as the filtered load of K^+ is increased.

   Answer B is incorrect. Aldosterone leads to increased synthesis of luminal Na^+ channels and basolateral Na^+/K^+-ATPase in the principal cells of the collecting duct. Decreased Na^+/K^+-ATPase activity results in increased intracellular K^+ levels.

   Answer C is incorrect. In metabolic acidosis, excess protons enter the principal cells of the late distal tubule and collecting duct. Proton entry forces the exit of K^+ ions to maintain electroneutrality. With decreased intracellular K^+ concentration, the driving force for K^+ secretion is lost and hyperkalemia results.

   Answer D is incorrect. Amiloride falls into the class of potassium-sparing diuretics. It acts on the Na^+ channels of the collecting duct to prevent Na^+ reabsorption and consequently, K^+ secrection. The potassium-sparing diuretics are used often in combination with a thiazide or a loop diuretic to prevent the excessive K^+ loss that can occur with these other agents.

4. **The correct answer is D.** Subendothelial deposits in the glomerular capillaries are indicative of lupus nephritis, a complication of systemic lupus erythematosus (SLE) that largely dictates the patient's prognosis. SLE classically presents with a malar "butterfly" rash on exposure to sunlight. Various manifestations of SLE can affect different aspects of the body, such as the cardiovascular (pericarditis), respiratory (pleural effusion), musculoskeletal (arthralgias), and hematologic (anemia, various cytopenias) systems. Treatment generally consists of immunosuppressive drugs such as prednisone.

   Answer A is incorrect. Achalasia is not particularly associated with lupus. It can be associated with Chagas disease, as a result of infection with *Trypanosoma cruzi*.

   Answer B is incorrect. Aortic aneurysms are not particularly associated with lupus. They can be associated with Marfan syndrome.

   Answer C is incorrect. Esophageal reflux is not particularly associated with lupus.

   Answer E is incorrect. Morbilliform rashes are more commonly associated with viral infections.

5. **The correct answer is D.** Nonsteroidal anti-inflammatory drugs (NSAIDs) are cyclooxygenase inhibitors. Because cyclooxygenase catalyzes the initial step in the metabolism of arachidonic acid, NSAIDs inhibit prostaglandin and thromboxane production. In healthy people, prostaglandins (which are vasodilators) are secreted at a low basal rate and have little effect on renal perfusion. In patients with states of effective volume depletion such as heart failure and cirrhosis, there is increased secretion of the vasoconstrictors angiotensin II and norepinephrine. In these cases, there is increased secretion of prostaglandins (mostly prostacyclin and prostaglandin E_2) to maintain renal blood flow by counteracting the vasoconstrictive effects of these hormones at preglomerular vessels (eg, the afferent arteriole). When prostaglandin synthesis is inhibited by NSAIDs in these patients, preglomerular resistance increases and renal blood flow (and thus glomerular filtration rate) is reduced. This ischemia can lead to acute renal failure.

   Answer A is incorrect. NSAIDs act to inhibit, not increase, prostaglandin synthesis.

   Answer B is incorrect. Prostaglandins act as vasodilators and do not have an effect on glomerular capillary permeability.

Answer C is incorrect. Inhibiting the vasodilatory effects of prostaglandins acts to increase preglomerular resistance, causing renal ischemia.

Answer E is incorrect. Although NSAIDs can also induce acute renal failure by causing an acute interstitial nephritis or minimal change disease, they have not been associated with direct toxic effects on the tubules or acute tubular necrosis.

6. **The correct answer is D.** Membranoproliferative glomerulonephritis (MPGN) can present as a nephrotic syndrome (more common) or as an acute nephritic syndrome. In MPGN, deposits are found in the subendothelial and mesangial space. The afferent and efferent vessels are lined by fenestrated endothelium, which is then partially lined by basement membrane. Beyond the basement membrane lie the visceral epithelial cells and podocytes. The glomerular basement membrane does not completely surround the capillary, especially the endothelium adjoining the mesangial area. As such, circulating immune complexes can deposit in the mesangium and subendothelial space without having to cross the negatively charged glomerular basement membrane.

   Answer A is incorrect. Immune complex deposits do not form in the subepithelial space between the basement membrane and the visceral epithelium.

   Answer B is incorrect. This describes the subepithelial space. Examples include membranous nephropathy.

   Answer C is incorrect. This describes the subepithelial space. The foot processes of podocytes and the visceral epithelial cells together entangle the side of the glomerular basement membrane opposite from the endothelium.

   Answer E is incorrect. This describes Bowman space and is the site of filtration. This space is contiguous to the collecting duct.

7. **The correct answer is A.** This patient is suffering from a massive left middle cerebral artery stroke that occurred secondary to a hypercoagulable state. Patients with nephrotic syndrome are at increased risk for thromboembolic events due to renal losses of antithrombin III, protein C, and protein S, all of which normally function as anticoagulants. Patients with nephrotic syndrome also commonly have other factors contributing to a hypercoagulable state, including hemoconcentration, increased fibrinogen, and thrombocytosis. Mental status or neurologic changes in patients with nephrotic syndrome should be taken very seriously. An INR of <1 indicates that a patient is prone to clot formation, whereas an INR >1 indicates that a patient is at increased risk of hemorrhage.

   Answer B is incorrect. Patients with decreased factor II levels have an increased risk of hemorrhagic events; nephrotic syndrome is not associated with decreased factor II levels.

   Answer C is incorrect. Patients with nephrotic syndrome have increased fibrinogen levels, which predispose them to thromboembolic events.

   Answer D is incorrect. Patients with nephrotic syndrome have decreased protein C levels, which predispose them to thromboembolic events.

   Answer E is incorrect. Patients with nephrotic syndrome have decreased protein S levels, which predispose them to thromboembolic events.

8. **The correct answer is A.** Pyelonephritis is an infection of the kidneys caused by an ascending infection from the lower urinary tract, most often caused by *E coli* from the periurethral/perianal area. The classic symptoms are fever, chills, flank pain, and costovertebral angle tenderness, all of which are demonstrated by this patient. Casts indicate that the origin of the WBCs is the kidney, which confirms the clinical suspicion of pyelonephritis. *E coli* is the major cause of pyelonephritis in uncomplicated cases, accounting for 82% of cases in women and 73% of cases in men.

   Answer B is incorrect. *K pneumoniae* accounts for approximately 3% of cases in women and 6% of cases in men. It more commonly causes community-acquired pneumonia or secondary infections in patients with chronic obstructive pulmonary disease (COPD). However, it can cause emphysematous urinary tract infections, especially in diabetics.

Answer C is incorrect. *P mirabilis* is an uncommon cause of pyelonephritis. It is a gram-negative bacterium that can be diagnosed because of its swarming motility and positive urease activity. It is a more common cause of infected nephrolithiasis.

Answer D is incorrect. *S saprophyticus* is a causative agent of pyelonephritis in approximately 3% of cases. More commonly, it causes localized cystitis. Studies have found this pathogen in 5%-20% of cases of cystitis. Localized cystitis usually is not accompanied by systemic symptoms such as fever. However, cystitis may be present in conjunction with the pyelonephritis, as it is an ascending infection. Symptoms of cystitis include urinary frequency and dysuria. Casts would not be seen if the infection were localized to the urinary bladder.

Answer E is incorrect. *U urealyticum* can cause recurrent episodes of pyelonephritis, but is uncommon in uncomplicated episodes such as in this patient.

9. **The correct answer is B.** This patient is most likely suffering from bilateral renal artery stenosis, indicated on physical exam by renal bruits. Stenosis of the renal arteries leads to a decrease in perfusion of the kidney. The result is a drop in intraglomerular pressure and glomerular filtration rate (GFR). The underperfused kidneys respond by upregulating the renin-angiotensin-aldosterone system. Angiotensin-converting enzyme (ACE) inhibitors prevent the vasoconstrictive effect of angiotensin II on the efferent arterioles. Dilation of the efferent arterioles eliminates the body's attempt to increase effective GFR. ACE inhibitors therefore should be avoided in patients with renal stenosis.

   Answer A is incorrect. Angioplasty is a minimally invasive procedure that involves placing intravascular stents in the renal artery, thereby restoring blood flow to the kidney. This form of therapy is the primary treatment for renal stenosis in symptomatic patients. Patency rates after angioplasty are strongly dependent on the size of the vessel treated and the quality of inflow and outflow through the vessel.

   Answer C is incorrect. In patients with hypertension caused by bilateral renal artery stenosis, both kidneys will be underperfused, so both will retain sodium and water by activating the renin-angiotensin/aldosterone system. Diuretics can counteract this effect and control blood pressure; therefore they are appropriate in this clinical scenario.

   Answer D is incorrect. Smoking is a risk factor for development of atherosclerotic plaques that may occlude vessels such as the renal arteries. Quitting may lower the rate of atherosclerotic build-up. This recommendation is appropriate for this patient.

   Answer E is incorrect. Surgery is another therapeutic option for renal stenosis. It is indicated particularly when angioplasty cannot be performed, as in completely occluded renal vessels.

10. **The correct answer is C.** The existence of a single kidney that has not migrated from the pelvis suggests a horseshoe kidney. A horseshoe kidney forms when the inferior poles of two kidneys fuse during development. As the kidneys rise from the pelvis, they encounter the inferior mesenteric artery and cannot rise to the normal level in the abdomen. These patients are typically asymptomatic if they have no other abnormalities, but they do have increased risks of obstruction, infection, and stones.

    Answer A is incorrect. The aorta would not obstruct the path of a rising horseshoe kidney during development.

    Answer B is incorrect. The celiac trunk leaves the aorta at a level above the location of normally developed kidneys, and thus cannot be responsible for the low location of a horseshoe kidney.

Answer D is incorrect. The inferior vena cava would not obstruct the path of a rising horseshoe kidney during development.

Answer E is incorrect. The superior mesenteric artery leaves the aorta at the level where normally developing kidneys are located, and thus it cannot be responsible for the low level of a horseshoe kidney.

11. **The correct answer is E.** The history of being started on chemotherapy for leukemia is strongly suggestive of tumor lysis syndrome. Tumor lysis syndrome occurs when leukemic cells die and release potassium, phosphate, and uric acid. Uric acid stones are radiolucent, so they may not appear on x-ray films. It is likely that this patient's presentation has been caused by a kidney stone that has passed into the left ureter and now into the urethra, causing postrenal failure. The FENa >4% tells you that the obstruction is starting to damage the nephrons as they are not conserving sodium.

Answer A is incorrect. Kidney failure as a result of glomerular dysfunction presents with a prerenal azotemia. There is an effective decrease in glomerular filtration rate, and sodium and water are retained by the kidney. The fractional excretion of sodium in prerenal failure is normally less than 1% with an osmolality that is >350 mOsm/kg.

Answer B is incorrect. Acute interstitial disease of the kidney is commonly caused by an allergic reaction to medicine (eg, penicillin, NSAIDs) or infection. In an acute setting, it presents with an intrinsic renal picture as is seen in this patient. In the setting of an infection, urine cultures are usually positive; in the setting of an allergic reaction, eosinophilia is common.

Answer C is incorrect. Kidney failure as a result of tubular dysfunction presents with an intrinsic renal picture. This is most commonly due to acute tubular necrosis or ischemia/toxins. Patchy necrosis leads to debris obstructing the tubules and fluid backflow, leading to a drop in glomerular filtration rate. The fractional excretion of sodium in intrinsic renal failure is normally >2% with an osmolality that is <350 mOsm/kg (similar to postrenal). However, the presentation of severe intermittent pelvic pain in the context of leukemia therapy is more likely to be caused by a kidney stone.

Answer D is incorrect. The spleen can be involved in leukemia, but the presence of acute renal failure in this case makes a urethral obstruction more likely.

12. **The correct answer is A.** Renal prostaglandin synthesis produces a vasodilatory effect on the afferent arterioles, whereas angiotensin II vasoconstricts primarily efferent arterioles. NSAIDs, such as ketorolac, inhibit renal prostaglandin synthesis. This results in a reduced ability to dilate the afferent arterioles. The patient may have underlying renal disease as a result of her hypertension and diabetes. Without adequate afferent arteriolar vasodilation, the GFR and renal plasma flow (RPF) are reduced, leading to acute renal failure. The blood urea nitrogen (BUN):creatinine (Cr) ratio in the question stem is consistent with an intrinsic cause of renal failure. There is no change in the filtration fraction because both RPF and GFR decrease proportionately.

Answer B is incorrect. Constriction of the efferent arteriole would serve to decrease RPF and increase GFR. NSAIDs cause constriction of the afferent arteriole, not the efferent arteriole. Both filtration fraction and GFR are increased and RPF is decreased.

Answer C is incorrect. Increased RPF, decreased GFR, and increased filtration fraction (FF) comprise an invalid combination, because FF = GFR/RPF. Therefore, if GFR decreases and RPF increases, FF also should decrease.

Answer D is incorrect. No change in RPF, decrease in GFR, and decrease in FF occur with increased plasma protein concentration or with constriction of the ureter, such as with either acquired or congenital urethral strictures or with prostate hypertrophy, a common condition in men over 60 years.

Answer E is incorrect. No change in RPF, increased GFR, and increased filtration fraction occur with decreased plasma protein concentration.

13. **The correct answer is E.** In healthy people, osmoreceptors in the wall of the third ventricle sense increased body fluid osmolarity and trigger the release of ADH from the posterior pituitary. ADH exerts its main effects on the V2 receptors located in the principal cells of the late distal tubule and collecting duct, where a G_s protein-coupled mechanism directs the insertion of aquaporin water channels into the luminal wall. These channels are permeable only to water and result in a reabsorption of water, concentration of urine, and dilution of body fluids. Activation of the V1 receptor found in the vascular smooth muscles results in activation of G_q protein second-messenger cascade and contraction of vascular smooth muscle, leading to an increase in total peripheral resistance. In patients with the syndrome of inappropriate ADH secretion (SIADH), which can be caused by central nervous system (CNS) disturbances (eg, stroke, hemorrhage, infection), small cell lung carcinoma, intracranial neoplasms, and occasionally by pancreatic tumors, the unregulated release of ADH leads to the persistent excretion of concentrated urine high in sodium. This causes hyponatremia and decreased serum osmolality without potassium or acid-base disturbances.

Answer A is incorrect. ACTH is secreted by the anterior pituitary in response to the presence of corticotropin releasing hormone produced in the hypothalamus. It can also be secreted by pituitary tumors or small cell lung carcinomas, but would present with Cushing syndrome (hypertension, weight gain, buffalo hump, truncal obesity, striae, hyperglycemia, and osteoporosis) rather than hyponatremia.

Answer B is incorrect. Neuronal signals from the osmoreceptors of the third ventricle stimulate the production of ADH as well as stimulate the sensation of thirst.

Answer C is incorrect. V2 receptors are coupled to the insertion of aquaporins; V1 receptors are coupled to the contraction of vascular smooth muscle.

Answer D is incorrect. Activation of V1 receptors leads to an increase in total peripheral resistance.

Answer F is incorrect. Renin is secreted by smooth muscle cells in the afferent arteriole and acts to cleave angiotensinogen to angiotensin I. This activates the renin-angiotensin-aldosterone axis, leading to increased salt and water retention. A patient with persistent activation of this axis would present primarily with hypertension and edema with relatively low urine sodium levels.

14. **The correct answer is C.** This patient has drug-induced acute tubulointerstitial nephritis, which manifests histologically as edema and inflammation of the renal tubules and interstitium with sparing of the glomeruli. Tubulointerstitial nephritis can be caused by infections and autoimmune phenomena, but is associated most commonly with drug toxicity. The typical picture is that of acute renal failure after drug administration. Patients classically present with the triad of low-grade fever, rash, and arthralgias, although some studies indicate <10% of patients report all three symptoms. Other symptoms include those associated with acute renal failure, such as oliguria, malaise, anorexia, and vomiting. Common findings on urinalysis are sterile pyuria, microscopic hematuria, and eosinophiluria. Drugs that have been associated with tubulointerstitial nephritis include sulfonamides (including thiazide diuretics and most loop diuretics), methicillin, ciprofloxacin, cephalosporins, allopurinol, proton pump inhibitors, rifampin, cimetidine, and nonsteroidal anti-inflammatory agents. Withdrawal of the causative agent is often the best treatment, but it may take months for a patient to fully recover renal function. Hydrochlorothiazide is a thiazide diuretic and a first-line antihypertensive drug that is especially useful in the elderly and African-American populations. Adverse effects of hydrochlorothiazide include electrolyte disturbances such as hypokalemia and hypercalcemia.

Answer A is incorrect. Cyclophosphamide is an alkylating agent that cross-links DNA and prevents DNA synthesis and cell division. It is used as an anti-neoplastic agent or as an immunosuppressant in transplant recipients and patients with autoimmune disease. Common adverse effects include alopecia, myelosuppression, nausea and vomiting, and hemorrhagic cystitis. Cyclophosphamide also can cause renal tubular necrosis, but it is not associated with tubulointerstitial nephritis.

Answer B is incorrect. Diphenhydramine is a first-generation H_1-antagonist used to treat allergic reactions, motion sickness, and dystonic reactions. It may cause sedation, anticholinergic effects, and anti-α-adrenergic effects. It is not associated with acute tubulointerstitial nephritis.

Answer D is incorrect. Isoniazid decreases the synthesis of mycolic acids and is used to treat tuberculosis (TB). It is associated with neurotoxicity, hepatotoxicity, a lupus-like syndrome, and hemolysis in patients with glucose-6-phosphate dehydrogenase deficiency. Isoniazid is not associated with acute tubulointerstitial nephritis.

Answer E is incorrect. Lithium is a mood stabilizer used to treat bipolar affective disorder. It indirectly inhibits the reuptake of serotonin and norepinephrine by inhibiting the phosphatidylinositol second messenger system. Adverse effects include CNS depression, dizziness, nephrogenic diabetes insipidus, acne, edema, and hyperthyroidism, as well as many others. Lithium has been associated with chronic tubulointerstitial nephritis, which presents after years of chronic lithium therapy. Proteinuria, hypertension, and anemia may be seen in these patients, along with other signs of chronic lithium poisoning such as thyroid abnormalities or ECG changes.

15. **The correct answer is A.** This vignette describes a nephrotic syndrome. Spike-and-dome deposits are found only in membranous glomerulonephritis. Membranous glomerulonephritis is an immune complex-mediated disease. Immunofluorescence shows a granular pattern of IgG and complement along the basement membrane. Membranous glomerulonephritis is the most common cause of adult-onset nephrotic syndrome. Patients with this disease normally present with a nephrotic picture of generalized edema due to massive loss of albumin and other proteins.

Answer B is incorrect. This is a finding of membranoproliferative glomerulonephritis, an uncommon autoimmune renal disorder that normally affects young individuals (8-30 years of age). The diagnosis is based on a histologic presentation that includes mesangial proliferation and a tram-track appearance on light microscopy. As this patient is 50 years old, this diagnosis is less likely.

Answer C is incorrect. This is a description of the findings in acute poststreptococcal glomerulonephritis, an autoimmune disease most frequently seen in children. It normally presents a few weeks after a streptococcal infection (throat or skin) with peripheral and periorbital edema, dark, tea-colored urine, and proteinuria. These symptoms are caused by circulating anti-streptococcal antibody-antigen complexes that deposit in the glomerular basement membrane, leading to complement activation and glomerular damage. As the patient has been otherwise healthy and is 50 years old, this diagnosis is unlikely.

Answer D is incorrect. This is the main finding in IgA nephropathy (Berger disease). This disease presents within several days of an infection (as opposed to poststreptococcal glomerulonephritis, which presents weeks after infection) with a nephritic picture due to IgA deposition in the mesangium. It is the most common global nephropathy, but it is a mild disease with minimal clinical significance. As this patient has not had a recent infection, this diagnosis is unlikely.

Answer E is incorrect. This is a finding of Alport syndrome, a heterogeneous (although most commonly X-linked) genetic disorder with either absent or mutated collagen IV, which leads to a nephritic renal disease and to sensorineural hearing loss and ocular disorders. This patient has no other complaints, and the edema is a fairly recent finding, making this diagnosis less likely.

16. **The correct answer is C.** The glomerular filtration barrier is composed of endothelial cells, glomerular basement membrane, and epithelial podocytes. It is responsible for the filtration of plasma according to size, shape, and net charge. The distances between the podocyte foot processes (filtration slits), the pores of the glomerular basement membrane, and the fenestrations between the endothelial cells limit the size and shape of the filtrate. The negatively charged heparan sulfate coating the filtration barrier prevents negatively charged molecules, such as albumin, from being filtered into the urine. This patient has minimal change disease manifested by nephrotic syndrome, in which the negatively charged heparan sulfate is lost, thereby allowing plasma protein to be lost in the urine.

    Answer A is incorrect. A brush border is characteristic of the proximal tubules and refers to the thickened appearance of the apical surface of these tubules due to the presence of microvilli covered by a dense glycocalyx. It is not part of the glomerulus and is not affected in minimal change disease.

    Answer B is incorrect. The endothelial cell, as previously mentioned, makes up part of the glomerular filtration barrier. However, it is intact in minimal change disease.

    Answer D is incorrect. Integrins are transmembrane proteins that serve as cell adhesion molecules, allowing cells to adhere to the underlying extracellular matrix. In leukocyte adhesion deficiency type 1, a deficiency in β-2 integrin results in an inability on the part of leukocytes to adhere to the endothelium for transmigration into the tissue, resulting in recurrent infections. Integrins are not involved in the glomerular filtration barrier and play no role in the etiology of minimal change disease.

    Answer E is incorrect. Type IV collagen is the collagen component of the basement membrane and is not compromised in nephrotic syndrome. When mutated, however, it gives rise to a form of basement membranopathy known as Alport syndrome. This syndrome is characterized by lens displacement, cataracts, and nerve deafness and is associated with hematuria.

17. **The correct answer is E.** The only diuretics that specifically limit calcium loss are the thiazides. They act in the early distal tubule, which is marked as region E in the image.

    Answer A is incorrect. There are no diuretics that act at the glomerulus.

    Answer B is incorrect. Carbonic anhydrase inhibitors, which act in the proximal convoluted tubule, do not affect calcium excretion.

    Answer C is incorrect. Osmotic diuretics act in the loop of Henle (as well as the proximal convoluted tubule and collecting duct), but they do not affect ion channels.

    Answer D is incorrect. Loop diuretics, which encourage calcium excretion, act in the thick ascending limb.

    Answer F is incorrect. Potassium-sparing diuretics and ADH antagonists such as lithium and demeclocycline act along the collecting tubule, although neither class affects calcium excretion.

18. **The correct answer is A.** This patient is suffering an acute overdose of amphetamine. He should be treated with ammonium chloride to acidify his urine and increase renal clearance of the weak base. This phenomenon, called ion trapping, occurs because increasing the ratio of ionized to non-ionized drug species in the renal tubule allows more of the drug to be retained in the urine and excreted. Weak bases in acidic environments have high ratios of ionized species, which are water-soluble and do not cross membranes. When urine is acidified, the levels of ionized amphetamine are high, and therefore more of the drug is trapped in the renal tubule.

    Answer B is incorrect. Alkalinization with bicarbonate is used to increase renal clearance of weak acids such as phenobarbital, methotrexate, tricyclic antidepressants, and aspirin.

Answer C is incorrect. Flumazenil is a treatment for acute benzodiazepine overdose.

Answer D is incorrect. Naloxone is a treatment for opioid overdose.

Answer E is incorrect. Treatment with water would have no effect on this patient's acute intoxication.

19. **The correct answer is B.** The neonate described above is suffering from Potter syndrome, a constellation of abnormalities including flattened facies, large and low-set ears, and limb deformities. The hallmark of this syndrome, however, is that these fetuses have bilateral renal agenesis, which is incompatible with life. As a result of bilateral renal agenesis, the fetus cannot urinate. This results in oligohydramnios. Another very common cause of oligohydramnios is chronic uteroplacental insufficiency (UPI). In cases of UPI, oligohydramnios occurs, because the fetus does not receive the proper nutrients or blood volume to maintain an adequate glomerular filtration rate. As a result, the fetus does not make urine and oligohydramnios develops.

    Answer A is incorrect. Anencephaly is a common neural tube defect. It is defined as partial or complete absence of the fetal brain or cranial vault. This condition is lethal, and most fetuses are stillborn. It can be diagnosed using ultrasound to identify the neural tube defect. Polyhydramnios also is commonly found in anencephaly, because the fetus is unable to swallow amniotic fluid.

    Answer C is incorrect. Duodenal atresia would lead to polyhydramnios. Polyhydramnios refers to excessive amounts of amniotic fluid. Conditions that cause polyhydramnios include fetal malformations that impair swallowing such as esophageal atresia and anencephaly. Polyhydramnios can be diagnosed with ultrasound imaging, but determining the etiology may require additional clinical work-up. This condition is not associated with bilateral renal agenesis, which would prevent the fetus from urinating and result in oligohydramnios.

    Answer D is incorrect. Maternal diabetes has been associated with polyhydramnios. The pathophysiology behind this phenomenon is that increased serum glucose in the mother is transmitted to the fetus. Just as in any other diabetic patient, increased blood glucose acts as an osmotic diuretic, causing an increased production of urine. Any cause of increased urination in the fetus will lead to polyhydramnios.

    Answer E is incorrect. Trisomy 18, or Edwards syndrome, also can present with facial deformities such as low-set ears and limb deformities such as clenched hands. It is, however, not associated with a flattened facies. Instead, the pathognomonic features of this syndrome are micrognathia and a prominent occiput, along with the aforementioned anomalies in the ears and limbs. Edwards syndrome is the most common trisomy resulting in live birth after Down syndrome, and has not been associated with oligohydramnios in utero.

20. **The correct answer is C.** This patient is suffering from a severe metabolic acidosis, as indicated by low serum pH, a low plasma bicarbonate level, and compensatory hyperventilation manifested as tachypnea. Next, note that the anion gap is elevated at 20 mmol/L (normal: 3-11 mmol/L). Of the choices, only iron toxicity (the **I** in the mnemonic **MUDPILES**) is associated with elevated anion gap metabolic acidosis.

    Answer A is incorrect. Aldosterone normally functions to increase sodium reabsorption, potassium excretion, and proton excretion in the distal nephron. Thus, aldosterone antagonists cause diminished proton excretion and metabolic acidosis. However, unlike this case, the acidosis would be expected to occur in the setting of a normal anion gap.

    Answer B is incorrect. Most simple antacids are alkaline and operate by neutralizing the low pH of the stomach. Thus, overdose would be expected to cause a metabolic alkalosis, not an acidosis.

    Answer D is incorrect. Loop diuretic toxicity is associated with metabolic alkalosis, not acidosis.

Answer E is incorrect. Ingestion of opiates results in reduced respiratory drive and subsequent hypoventilation. In this situation, a respiratory acidosis would have been expected, and tachypnea would not be observed.

21. **The correct answer is C.** IgA nephropathy (Berger disease) occurs within several days of an infection, as opposed to poststreptococcal glomerulonephritis, which presents weeks afterward. Classically, patients present with a nephritic picture due to IgA deposition in the mesangium. Berger disease is the most common global nephropathy and is generally a mild disease. IgA nephropathy usually presents in children with recurrent hematuria that is of minimal clinical significance. Nonlinear mesangial deposits of IgA are evident on immunofluorescence. Treatment is with ACE inhibitors and corticosteroids. Patients with IgA nephropathy have a risk of disease recurrence.

Answer A is incorrect. Increased antistreptolysin O (ASO) titers are associated with acute poststreptococcal glomerulonephritis rather than IgA nephropathy. The classic findings include RBCs and casts in the urine (causing the tea-colored appearance), elevated ASO titers, decreased complement levels, and "lumpy-bumpy" electron-dense deposits in the glomerulus.

Answer B is incorrect. Acute poststreptococcal glomerulonephritis is an autoimmune disease most frequently seen in children. It normally presents a few weeks after a streptococcal infection with a nephritic picture of peripheral and periorbital edema, dark urine, and proteinuria. These symptoms are caused by circulating antistreptococcal antibody-antigen complexes that deposit in the glomerular basement membrane, leading to complement activation and glomerular damage. The classic findings are RBCs and casts in the urine (which cause the characteristic tea-colored urine), a positive ASO titer, decreased levels of complement, and "lumpy-bumpy" electron-dense deposits in the subepithelium of the glomerulus. Recovery is spontaneous and treatment is supportive.

Answer D is incorrect. IgA nephropathy usually presents with a nephritic picture, which does not involve the massive proteinuria that is seen in nephrotic syndromes.

Answer E is incorrect. IgA deposition in Berger disease is primarily in the mesangium and not the subepithelium.

22. **The correct answer is D.** This patient has diffuse cortical necrosis: generalized infarctions of the cortices of both kidneys, which is a common complication of disseminated intravascular coagulation (DIC). DIC commonly occurs after a complication of pregnancy such as amniotic fluid embolus and placental abruption, and affected patients develop the abrupt onset of the triad of anuria, gross hematuria, and flank pain. The diagnosis can usually be established by ultrasonography, which will demonstrate hypodense areas in the renal cortex. Although many patients can be sustained on dialysis, only 20%-40% have partial recovery of kidney function. Indications for acute dialysis in DIC include (1) **A**cidosis refractory to bicarbonate, (2) severe **E**lectrolyte abnormalities refractory to medical intervention (especially high potassium levels), (3) **I**ntoxication with some drugs, (4) volume **O**verload refractory to diuretics, and (5) **U**remic symptoms (eg, cardiac friction rub and altered mental status), making up the mnemonic **AEIOU**. The fact that this patient has a new-onset pericardial friction rub indicates uremia and makes dialysis imperative.

Answer A is incorrect. Aggressive fluid support is not beneficial for kidney recovery after the development of diffuse cortical necrosis. The kidney has been severely damaged by the microthrombi of DIC. Aggressive fluid resuscitation is contraindicated due to (1) the lack of hypotension, and (2) the renal failure. Fluids will only cause volume overload if they cannot be excreted.

Answer B is incorrect. While renal malignancy can cause hematuria, it is less likely to cause renal failure. In this case a biopsy to look for renal malignancy is not necessary because the cause of the patient's symptoms is already known. The first treatment should be dialysis to counteract renal failure and allow any remaining renal tissue to recover.

Answer C is incorrect. Broad-spectrum antibiotics are indicated in cases of shock due to sepsis. This patient has DIC caused by an amniotic embolus, and since there is no infection, antibiotics will not be beneficial. Additionally, as the patient is experiencing renal failure, any antibiotic that is renally metabolized should be renally dosed to account for the patient's creatinine clearance rate.

Answer E is incorrect. This patient is in severe acute renal failure. Failure to treat will result in death.

23. **The correct answer is C.** Calcium stones are the most common cause of kidney stones (80%-85%). Therefore, states that lead to increased calcium (such as hyperparathyroidism, or other destructive bone diseases) can lead to their formation. The stones are made of calcium oxalate or calcium phosphate, and are radiopaque; thus large, numerous stones would likely be seen on a plain film as well as noncontrast CT. Other risk factors are increased vitamin D and milk-alkali syndrome. Remember, parathyroid hormone (PTH) brings calcium from bones into the bloodstream. Calcitonin "tones down" the bloodstream ("channels") of calcium and puts it on bone.

Answer A is incorrect. Calcified arteries are unlikely to be mistaken for ureters, and a full rectum would not cause peristaltic pain.

Answer B is incorrect. A large stool is unlikely to cause flank pain, and pain would not come in the waves of pain this patient is experiencing.

Answer D is incorrect. Normally hyperuricemia leads to kidney stones that are radiolucent and therefore not seen on X-ray. They would, however, be seen on noncontrast CT. These stones are often seen in the setting of diseases with increased cell proliferation and turnover, such as leukemia and myeloproliferative disorders. Remember that uric acid is a metabolite of nucleic acid turnover, which is heightened in the setting of cell destruction.

Answer E is incorrect. Urinary tract infection with urease-positive microorganisms such as *Staphylococcus saprophyticus* can form large struvite calculi that are radiopaque, but would not backflow into the ureters.

24. **The correct answer is E.** The man is going into hypovolemic shock due to hemorrhage. The body's normal response to hypovolemia in the short term results from a decreased blood volume that is sensed by baroreceptors, which leads to an increased sympathetic output. The response is an increased heart rate and vasoconstriction to increase cardiac output so that the body can continue to perfuse vital organs. The kidney senses decreased volume and increases renin production, which will lead to increased angiotensin II and aldosterone levels. In addition, the body will increase levels of vasopressin, or ADH, which will conserve sodium and water by facilitating water reabsorption in the distal collecting duct.

Answer A is incorrect. The heart rate will be increased in hypovolemic shock, not decreased.

Answer B is incorrect. The peripheral resistance will be increased in response to hypovolemia in order to increase effective cardiac output to the vital organs.

Answer C is incorrect. In a normal patient, renin is secreted in response to low blood pressure, so it should increase not decrease.

Answer D is incorrect. Vasopressin levels will not be decreased in hypovolemic shock.

25. **The correct answer is A.** The patient's symptoms are of angioedema, a well-known adverse effect of ACE inhibitors. These drugs are generally prescribed to patients with hypertension. Angioedema is caused by the secondary activity of ACE on the degradation of kinins, including, most commonly, bradykinin. The blockage of ACE, and the commensurate accumulation of high levels of bradykinin, account for increased vessel permeability and

subsequent edema in the face, lips, mouth, and subglottic tissues, typically without pruritus. Intestinal edema accounts for the patient's gastrointestinal symptoms of diarrhea, vomiting, and abdominal pain. Older patients with a prior history of drug-induced hypersensitivity and environmental allergies are particularly susceptible to ACE inhibitor-induced angioedema.

Answer B is incorrect. Histamine is a biogenic amine that has a variety of functions, including inflammation, smooth muscle and vascular dilatation, and neurotransmission. Histamine released by mast cells is primarily responsible for the hypersensitivity reaction, although in this case histamine levels are not affected by the use of ACE inhibitors.

Answer C is incorrect. Prostacyclin (or prostaglandin I_2) is an arachidonic acid derivative, produced by the vascular endothelial cells from PGH_2. Its major function is to prevent platelet aggregation during coagulation. Prostacyclin is also a potent vasodilator, although its metabolism is not affected by ACE, and thus prostacyclin levels are not affected by the use of ACE inhibitors.

Answer D is incorrect. Prostaglandin E_2 (PGE_2) is an arachidonic acid derivative that controls smooth muscle contraction, dilatation, and constriction of blood vessels, as well as the modulation of inflammation. It is also implicated in the induction of fever. However, PGE_2 has no relationship to ACE inhibitors and the kinin-related effects of ACE.

Answer E is incorrect. Serotonin is primarily a neurotransmitter produced by the CNS and certain peripheral neurons (enteric neurons). It is not involved in vascular dilatation and inflammation, and has no relationship to ACE inhibitors.

26. **The correct answer is E.** Tobramycin is an aminoglycoside, and like other drugs in this family (eg, gentamicin, streptomycin) it can cause nephrotoxicity. This is the result of acute tubular necrosis, and leads to a reduction in the glomerular filtration rate and a rise in the serum creatinine level, as seen in this patient. When aminoglycosides are combined with cephalosporins such as cefoxitin, the nephrotoxic effects are greatly increased. Renal failure is usually reversible when the drugs are discontinued.

Answer A is incorrect. Azithromycin is a macrolide that is not an appropriate treatment for *Klebsiella pneumoniae* infection. It is used mostly against infection by gram-positive organisms. Although it can be associated with allergic hepatitis and thrombophlebitis, it does not cause nephrotoxicity.

Answer B is incorrect. Aztreonam shows strong activity against gram-negative organisms, and it is highly resistant to β-lactamase degradation. It is not associated with nephrotoxicity.

Answer C is incorrect. Clindamycin use is typically limited to anaerobic abscesses. It is known to cause pseudomembranous colitis in up to 20% of patients, but it does not cause nephrotoxicity.

Answer D is incorrect. Piperacillin, although effective against *Klebsiella*, is associated with hypersensitivity reactions in about 10% of patients. It is not associated with nephrotoxicity.

27. **The correct answer is D.** This patient presents with pyelonephritis, which is characterized by costovertebral angle tenderness, fever, and chills. Symptoms of lower urinary tract infection (UTI) may also be present, such as dysuria, increased frequency of urination, and urgency. The onset of symptoms of pyelonephritis often occurs approximately one week after the onset of a lower UTI. In children, recurrent UTIs suggest an anatomic abnormality and warrant further investigation. Lower UTIs may ascend to the kidneys through incompetent ureterovesical sphincters, leading to pyelonephritis, dilatation of the ureters, and renal pelves, potentially causing renal scarring. Thus urologic repair is often recommended to prevent renal damage in children with vesicoureteral reflux.

Answer A is incorrect. Immunoglobulin deficiency, such as Bruton X-linked agammaglobulinemia, is associated with recurrent bacterial infections that in this age group typically affect the lungs, ears, skin, and sinuses.

Answer B is incorrect. Nephroblastoma, or Wilms tumor, is the most common solid renal tumor in children and usually presents with a palpable abdominal mass. Vesicoureteral reflux is more prevalent than nephroblastoma.

Answer C is incorrect. Poststreptococcal glomerulonephritis typically presents one-two weeks after an infection with Group A β-hemolytic streptococci. The vignette does not provide any evidence of a recent streptococcal infection.

28. **The correct answer is A.** This patient is suffering from acute tubular necrosis (ATN) as a result of rhabdomyolysis brought on by statin use. Myoglobin released by the muscles is toxic to the kidney tubule cells, especially those of the proximal tubule. In this image, all of the tubules are necrotic with sloughed pink epithelial cells and debris and loss of nuclear detail. It is commonly associated with oliguria, but ATN actually presents with increased urine output in 50% of patients. Rhabdomyolysis is an adverse effect of statins that is more likely with higher doses of statins. In addition, statins are metabolized by cytochrome P450 enzymes. If some of this patient's cold medications inhibited the P450 enzymes, then the risk of rhabdomyolysis would be increased through increasing statin levels above normal.

Answer B is incorrect. Amyloidosis has a number of causes, but is characterized histologically by deposits of cotton candy-like material in the blood vessel walls and the glomeruli.

Answer C is incorrect. Analgesic nephropathy is a type of tubulointerstitial nephritis that is associated with the long-term use of NSAIDs. The histologic appearance shows interstitial fibrosis and inflammation. Although this patient has been taking over-the-counter cold remedies (which often contain NSAIDs), it usually takes many years of high-level exposure to develop this condition.

Answer D is incorrect. Focal segmental glomerulosclerosis is associated with a number of conditions, and it is often presents with nephrotic syndrome. It is recognized histologically by the sclerosis of parts of a minority of the glomeruli.

Answer E is incorrect. Pyelonephritis is usually caused by an ascending infection. It is characterized by tubular necrosis, as seen here, but it is seen on a background of inflammation, with numerous neutrophils present in the tubule lumen.

29. **The correct answer is B.** When the amount of fluids in the body contracts, the body attempts to compensate by releasing angiotensin II, a potent vasoconstrictor. In order to protect the kidney from losing its perfusion due to this vasoconstriction, the kidney simultaneously releases prostaglandins at both the afferent and efferent arterioles, where they act as vasodilators. By inhibiting cyclooxygenase (COX)-1 and/or COX-2 enzymes, the pathway that produces the prostaglandins that keep the kidneys perfused becomes blocked, leading to decreased blood flow to the kidneys and resulting in a prerenal cause of renal failure. Celecoxib is a selective COX-2 inhibitor that affects the arterioles of the kidney and can cause renal failure in dehydrated patients.

Answer A is incorrect. Inhibition of the COX-2 enzyme will lead to a decrease in the production of prostacyclin, causing a possible increase in platelet aggregation as they continue to produce thromboxane, which is produced mainly by the COX-1 pathway. However, this effect is not the reason why COX-2 inhibitors are contraindicated in the context of volume contraction.

Answer C is incorrect. Celecoxib is a selective COX-2 inhibitor that is effective because it spares the gastric mucosa the damaging effects of COX-1 inhibition.

Answer D is incorrect. The macula densa is a specialized portion of the thick ascending limb adjacent to the hilus of the glomerulus. The cells of the macula densa sense changes in sodium and chloride concentrations as well as a drop in blood pressure, and they secrete renin in response. This patient's vomiting will activate the renin-angiotensin pathway due to fluid and electrolyte loss, but the celecoxib will have little impact on the macula densa itself.

Answer E is incorrect. Inhibition of the COX-2 enzyme will lead to a decrease in the production of prostaglandins, thromboxane, and prostacyclins, which affect platelet function and small vessel diameter. This effect is not contraindicated in the context of volume contraction.

30. **The correct answer is E.** This patient has nephropathy, as evidenced by the lower-extremity swelling (as a result of hypoalbuminemia), hyperlipidemia, and proteinuria. In this case the most likely explanation is diabetic nephropathy. This is caused by constant vasoconstriction of the efferent arteriole of the nephron by angiotensin II. Initially this serves to preserve glomerular filtration rate and kidney function in the face of hypertension, but over time, hyperfiltration injury to the glomerulus, in addition to hyperglycemic injury (this patient clearly has suboptimal glucose control) to the glomerulus by non-enzymatic glycosylation, led to the development of nephritic disease. One of the main therapies aimed at prevention of diabetic nephropathy is the use of an ACE inhibitor or angiotensin receptor blocker such as losartan to prevent hyperfiltration injury to nephrons and to treat hypertension.

    Answer A is incorrect. Metoprolol is a specific β_1-receptor blocking agent used to treat hypertension and congestive heart failure (CHF). Blockade of β_1-receptors leads to the inhibition of sympathetic stimulation of heart rate, then to a slower heart rate and decreased cardiac muscle contractility. It does not have any renal protective effects.

    Answer B is incorrect. Amlodipine is a calcium channel blocker that is used often as first-line antihypertensive therapy. Inhibition of calcium channels leads to decreased ability of vascular smooth muscle to contract, leading to less vasoconstriction and lower blood pressure. However, it does not offer renal protective effects in diabetic patients.

    Answer C is incorrect. Furosemide is a loop diuretic that acts by inhibiting sodium reabsorption in the loop of Henle. It is used in the treatment of volume overload in patients with CHF as well as in drug-resistant hypertension. It does not offer diabetics any renal protective effects.

    Answer D is incorrect. Hydrochlorothiazide is a thiazide diuretic that works by inhibiting sodium reabsorption in the distal convoluted tubule. It is used often as first-line treatment of hypertension. However, it offers no renal protective effects in diabetic patients or others.

31. **The correct answer is D.** Focal hyaline deposits are characteristic of focal segmental glomerulosclerosis (FSGS). FSGS presents as nephrotic syndrome (massive proteinuria, hypoalbuminemia, generalized edema, hyperlipidemia, and lipiduria) and often occurs in patients with HIV infection.

    Answer A is incorrect. Rapidly progressive glomerulonephritis is characterized by the presence of crescents in most glomeruli. The description of this patient indicates that many glomeruli are spared, making this syndrome unlikely.

    Answer B is incorrect. IgA nephropathy (Berger disease) is characterized by the presence of prominent IgA, not IgM, deposits in the mesangial region of the glomerulus. As it causes the nephritic syndrome, mild proteinuria usually is present, and hematuria usually is found.

    Answer C is incorrect. Although membranous glomerulonephritis is the most common cause of nephrotic syndrome, it is characterized by diffuse thickening of capillary walls and deposits of IgG in the glomerular basement membrane. Thus it is an unlikely the cause of this patient's symptoms.

    Answer E is incorrect. Minimal change disease is the most common cause of the nephrotic syndrome in children. It usually responds well to corticosteroids, however, and appears normal on light microscopy. Retraction of foot processes is consistently seen on electron microscopy.

32. **The correct answer is E.** Increased sodium intake leads to volume expansion and increased stretch in mechanoreceptors located in the afferent arteriole. The mechanoreceptor response to increased plasma volume is decreased renin secretion, which causes vasodilation of glomerular afferent arterioles. This increases the GFR while also decreasing sodium reabsorption in the proximal tubule.

    Answer A is incorrect. Atrial natriuretic peptide is secreted by the atria in response to increased extracellular fluid volume and causes dilation of the glomerular afferent arterioles. However, this is a physiologic response by cells in the atria of the heart to high sodium intake and volume expansion, not a response intrinsic to the kidney.

    Answer B is incorrect. Increased delivery of sodium and water to the macula densa would lead to a decrease in renin release from the juxtaglomerular apparatus, as renin would otherwise lead to aldosterone release and further sodium retention.

    Answer C is incorrect. Increased plasma sodium and water leads to increased sodium chloride delivery to the macula densa, leading to the suppression (not the increase) of renin release by the juxtaglomerular apparatus. Decreased renin levels lead to decreased aldosterone, which would result in increased potassium reuptake, not potassium wasting.

    Answer D is incorrect. This is the opposite response to the correct answer. High sodium intake leads to volume expansion, dilation of afferent arterioles, and increased stretch in baroreceptors, which leads to decreased renin release. Constriction of the afferent arteriole would cause a decrease in the GFR.

33. **The correct answer is E.** This clinical presentation is classic for benign prostatic hyperplasia obstructing the urethra and causing bilateral hydronephrosis (seen on ultrasound as dilation of the collecting ducts), thereby leading to renal failure. Renal failure can be divided into prerenal (due to lack of perfusion of the kidney), intrinsic renal (due to acute tubular necrosis from ischemia or toxins), and postrenal (due to obstruction of outflow). Each type of renal failure has distinct characteristics, allowing differentiation by urinalysis. In postrenal failure, the kidneys are unable to effectively concentrate the urine, so the urine osmolality would be <350 mmol/kg.

    Answer A is incorrect. A BUN:Cr ratio <15 is seen with intrinsic renal failure because renal damage causes decreased BUN reabsorption. In postrenal failure, reduced flow causes increased BUN reabsorption without increased Cr reabsorption, therefore the BUN:Cr ratio is >15.

    Answer B is incorrect. Epithelial casts are seen in acute tubular necrosis, a cause of intrinsic renal failure.

    Answer C is incorrect. The fractional excretion of sodium (FeNa) is a measure of the amount of sodium in the urine compared to the amount of sodium in the plasma, and can be calculated by [(UNa × PCr) / (PNa × UCr)] × 100. A FeNa <1% would be expected in prerenal failure, where the kidney is working to reabsorb as much sodium as possible to increase plasma volume and thereby improve perfusion. In postrenal failure, the kidney is unable to effectively reabsorb sodium, and therefore the FeNa would commonly be >4%.

    Answer D is incorrect. A urine sodium level of <10 mmol/L would be expected in prerenal failure, where the kidney is working to reabsorb as much sodium as possible to increase plasma volume and thereby improve perfusion. In postrenal failure, the kidney is unable to effectively reabsorb sodium, and therefore the urine sodium level would commonly be >40 mmol/L.

34. **The correct answer is A.** The glomerular basement membrane is composed of endothelial fenestrae with filtration slits lined with anionic glycoproteins on the lamina rara interna and externa. The small diameter of the filtration slits partially blocks albumin filtration physically, but the anionic charge of the barrier pro-

vides the largest obstacle to filtration by electrostatically repelling the negatively charged albumin molecules.

Answer B is incorrect. This choice is incorrect because the filtration slits are lined with negatively charged anionic glycoproteins and are not positively charged. Positive charges would attract albumin and conglomerate, thereby impeding further filtration.

Answer C is incorrect. Albumin is neither freely filtered by the glomerulus nor reabsorbed along the nephron.

Answer D is incorrect. Basement membrane proteoglycans are negatively charged, as is albumin.

Answer E is incorrect. The size selectivity of the endothelial filtration slits provides an obstacle to albumin filtration, but size selectivity alone does not account for the complete absence of albumin filtration in non-pathologic states.

35. **The correct answer is C.** To understand this metabolic abnormality, first look at the pH and then the bicarbonate (HCO_3^-) and partial pressure of carbon dioxide (PCO_2). Her pH is 7.28, which indicates a form of acidosis. Metabolic acidosis is the presence of low pH with low plasma HCO_3^-, in this case 15 mEq/L (normal = 22-26 mEq/L); she is suffering from metabolic acidosis. Her lungs are blowing off more carbon dioxide in order to raise the pH. The causes of metabolic acidosis are events that either increase acid levels (eg, diabetic ketoacidosis, uremia, hypovolemic shock) or decrease the amount of base present (eg, diarrhea, kidney failure). Metabolic acidosis can be subdivided further into non-anion gap and anion gap metabolic acidosis. A normal anion gap is 8-12. This patient's anion gap is 10, so there is no anion gap acidosis. If the primary cause of acidosis is a loss of HCO_3^-, there will be an increase in chloride and the anion gap will be normal, as is the case with severe diarrhea. Of the answers listed, only diarrhea can cause a non-anion gap acidosis.

Answer A is incorrect. Salicylate overdose causes an anion gap acidosis (ingested salicylic acid is the unmeasured anion).

Answer B is incorrect. Diabetic ketoacidosis (DKA) causes a severe anion gap acidosis (the unmeasured anions in this case are ketoacids). A helpful way to remember the causes of anion gap acidosis is the mnemonic **MUDPILES**: **M**ethanol, **U**remia, **D**iabetic ketoacidosis, **P**araldehyde or **P**henformin, **I**ron tablets or **I**soniazid, **L**actic acidosis, **E**thylene glycol, and **S**alicylates. In this case the patient has no anion gap so DKA would not be correct.

Answer D is incorrect. Underperfusion causes anion gap acidosis (the anion in this case is lactic acid). This patient has a non-anion gap acidosis.

Answer E is incorrect. Uremia indicates renal failure. The inability of the kidney to excrete organic acids leads to an anion gap acidosis. Renal failure also causes hyperkalemia, because the kidney is unable to excrete potassium.

36. **The correct answer is B.** Inulin is freely filtered across the glomerular capillary wall and is neither reabsorbed nor secreted. It is therefore used to calculate the GFR, otherwise known as clearance of inulin. Creatinine clearance can also be used as a physiologic approximation of GFR. GFR is calculated as: urinary concentration of inulin × urinary flow rate/plasma concentration of inulin. Using this equation, urine flow rate = GFR × plasma concentration of inulin/urinary inulin concentration = 120 mL/min × 1.5 mg/mL / 50 mg/mL = 3.6 mL/min. Glomerular capillary hydrostatic pressure, listed in the table of laboratory values, is a distracter that is not used in the equation.

Answer A is incorrect. This answer underestimates the patient's urine flow rate, which is 3.6 mL/min.

Answer C is incorrect. This answer overestimates the patient's urine flow rate, which is 3.6 mL/min.

Answer D is incorrect. This answer translates into a value of 0.6 mL/min, which underestimates the patient's urine flow rate, which is 3.6 mL/min.

Answer E is incorrect. This answer translates into a value of 0.3 mL/min, which underestimates the patient's urine flow rate, which is 3.6 mL/min.

37. **The correct answer is B.** Acetazolamide can be taken prophylactically or to alleviate symptoms of acute mountain sickness. It acts by inhibiting carbonic anhydrase, which is important for bicarbonate reabsorption in the proximal tubule of the kidney. This leads to alkalinization of the urine and a metabolic acidosis. The drop in the plasma pH results in an increased breathing drive and higher oxygen levels in the body, helping to reverse the effects of hypoxemia. Acetazolamide should be avoided in patients with an allergy to sulfa drugs.

Answer A is incorrect. Acetazolamide does not cause a mixed metabolic acidosis and respiratory alkalosis. This combination can be seen with aspirin toxicity, but respiratory alkalosis is not an effect of acetazolamide.

Answer C is incorrect. Acetazolamide does not cause metabolic alkalosis. Loop diuretics and thiazides both cause metabolic alkalosis. Furosemide is the opposite of acetazolamide in that it lowers urine pH and raises blood pH.

Answer D is incorrect. Acetazolamide does not cause respiratory acidosis. Respiratory acidosis results from impaired respiration and can be seen with COPD, sedatives/opiates, pneumothorax, acute respiratory distress syndrome, etc.

Answer E is incorrect. Respiratory alkalosis results from respiratory carbon dioxide output in excess of normal for the metabolic production of carbon dioxide by tissue. This can be seen with hyperventilation in a patient with anxiety or pain, salicylate toxicity, or CNS lesions, among other factors.

38. **The correct answer is E.** This patient has nephritis due to SLE. Up to 60% of adults with SLE eventually develop nephritis. Circulating immune complexes in the serum deposit in the glomerulus and activate complement, leading to leukocyte infiltration and membrane damage. Signs and symptoms can include proteinuria, hematuria, hypertension, and RBC casts in the urine sediment. Biopsy will show a characteristic "wire-loop" appearance along the glomerular membrane.

Answer A is incorrect. Alport syndrome is an inherited connective tissue disorder that is diagnosed by the findings of hematuria, sensorineural deafness, and anterior bulging of the ocular lenses. Biopsy and visualization with electron microscopy would show a thickened basement membrane, with a split and distorted lamina densa.

Answer B is incorrect. Membranous glomerulonephritis is a nephrotic syndrome that presents with heavy proteinuria, but not typically obvious hematuria. Other symptoms include edema, hyperlipidemia, and hypertension. On biopsy light microscopy shows a uniform thickening of the basement membrane and electron microscopy shows subepithelial deposits.

Answer C is incorrect. Minimal change disease is a nephropathy that occurs most often in the pediatric population, but it can also present in adults. The clinical presentation includes proteinuria, marked edema (especially periorbitally), hyperlipidemia, and hypoalbuminemia. Urinary sediment is usually acellular. On biopsy light microscopy reveals no obvious abnormality, but electron microscopy shows effacement of the foot processes along the epithelium.

Answer D is incorrect. Poststreptococcal glomerulonephritis is typically seen a few weeks after a streptococcal infection causing pharyngitis or impetigo, and would present with similar symptoms of hematuria, RBC casts, hypertension, and headaches. However, histologic section of a renal biopsy would show hypercellularity of mesangial cells as well as subepithelial deposits of immunoglobulins and complement, giving a "humpy" appearance, rather than the wire-loop appearance seen in this patient's biopsy specimen.

39. **The correct answer is A.** Autosomal dominant polycystic kidney disease (ADPKD) is associated with berry aneurysms in the circle of Willis and with cyst formation not only in the kidneys but in the liver, pancreas, and spleen. Hypertension is a common early finding, with an average age at onset of 30 years. Later in the course, kidneys can reach sizes triple their normal volumes, often resulting in disabling symptoms due to pressure on intra-abdominal organs. ADPKD does not present at a young age. Autosomal recessive polycystic kidney (ARPKD) disease is diagnosed most often in pediatric patients; it is associated less often with cyst formation in multiple visceral organs and with the formation of berry aneurysms.

    Answer B is incorrect. Horseshoe kidney is associated with many renal diseases, but it does not involve the extra-renal findings described in the question.

    Answer C is incorrect. Children with inborn errors of metabolism can present with ophthalmologic findings such as cherry-red spots in the macula. An example is Niemann-Pick disease, a lysosomal storage disease in which a sphingomyelinase deficiency results in accumulation of sphingomyelin. The disease is characterized by varying degrees of splenomegaly and neurologic deficits.

    Answer D is incorrect. Potter syndrome is a condition involving renal agenesis, and it is not associated with any cystic changes.

    Answer E is incorrect. Pott disease is a TB infection of the vertebrae.

40. **The correct answer is B.** This man's urinalysis indicates he is suffering from acute tubular necrosis secondary to ischemia of the epithelial cells of the renal tubules. Granular casts on urinalysis are pathognomonic for acute tubular necrosis. Due to their high metabolic rate, these particular renal cells are particularly sensitive to a drop in blood pressure such as that experienced in hemorrhagic shock. Another common cause of acute tubular necrosis is a crush injury, in which the patient undergoes rhabdomyolysis, or muscle death. When the muscle breaks down, myoglobin is released into the bloodstream. Myoglobin is nephrotoxic and causes acute tubular necrosis. Toxins such as chemotherapeutic agents and aminoglycoside antibiotics also may cause this condition.

    Answer A is incorrect. An ascending urinary tract infection, most commonly with a gram-negative rod such as *Escherichia coli*, causes pyelonephritis. Pyelonephritis generally affects the renal cortex, with relative sparing of the vessels and glomeruli. Patients present with fever, costovertebral angle tenderness, nausea, and vomiting. On urinalysis, these patients often present with WBC casts, which differ from the muddy brown epithelial casts seen in acute tubular necrosis.

    Answer C is incorrect. When causing kidney injury, diabetes generally manifests as renal papillary necrosis. This disease manifests as gross hematuria and proteinuria caused by sloughing of the renal papillae. Diabetes is not associated with muddy brown casts on urinalysis. The hallmark of diabetic nephropathy is the presence of acellular, eosinophilic deposits, known as Kimmelstiel-Wilson nodules, on renal biopsy.

    Answer D is incorrect. NSAID toxicity leads to acute interstitial nephritis, not acute tubular necrosis. This syndrome is associated with pyuria (typically eosinophils) and azotemia occurring one-two weeks after administration of the medication. It is also associated with fever, rash, hematuria, and costovertebral angle tenderness. It is not typically associated with granular casts on urinalysis.

    Answer E is incorrect. Septic shock results in diffuse cortical necrosis of the kidneys, possibly as a result of a combination of vasospasm and DIC caused by the release of the bacterial endotoxin into the bloodstream. Patients with this syndrome generally present with abrupt onset of oliguria or anuria accompanied by hematuria, flank pain, and hypotension. Diffuse cortical necrosis of the kidneys is generally a much more severe disease than acute tubular necrosis, and can be diagnosed by ultrasonography or CT scanning, which reveals hypoechoic or hypodense areas in the renal cortex. Renal cortical necrosis has also been associated with obstetric catastrophe, such as placental abruption.

41. **The correct answer is E.** Renal stones typically obstruct constricted areas of the urinary tract.

Answer A is incorrect. Stones may develop in the bladder, but these do not typically cause obstruction.

Answer B is incorrect. While passing stones through the penile urethra can be painful, it does not typically cause an obstruction.

Answer C is incorrect. The prostatic urethra is not a typical location for renal stones to obstruct flow.

Answer D is incorrect. While staghorn calculi may develop in the renal pelvis or calyces, they do not typically produce obstructive symptoms until they have grown to a considerable size.

42. **The correct answer is D.** Inulin clearance is an accurate estimate of GFR because it is freely filtered and neither reabsorbed nor secreted in the nephron. Because it overestimates true GFR, compound X must therefore undergo net secretion in the nephron. That is, more compound X is excreted in the urine than is filtered at the glomerulus. Indeed, it is precisely this mechanism that is responsible for the characteristic overestimation of GFR by measuring creatinine clearance.

Answer A is incorrect. If compound X were not freely filtered at the glomerulus, its clearance would underestimate GFR.

Answer B is incorrect. The descending limb of the loop of Henle is poorly permeable to solute and instead allows passive efflux of water from the filtrate. Furthermore, compound X cannot undergo net reabsorption in the nephron.

Answer C is incorrect. The proximal convoluted tubule is responsible for most ultrafiltrate reabsorption. However, if compound X underwent net reabsorption, its clearance would underestimate, not overestimate, the inulin-calculated GFR.

Answer E is incorrect. Inulin is freely filtered and neither reabsorbed nor secreted in the nephron. It is these characteristics that allow its use as an accurate measure of GFR.

43. **The correct answer is B.** Long-time diabetes in this patient most likely caused a neurogenic bladder. Overfilling of the bladder could have caused vesicoureteral reflux to the kidneys. Renal damage results when a bacterial urinary tract infection is superimposed on the reflux. Chronic pyelonephritis results in a kidney that grossly shows blunting and thickened dilation of the calyces and uneven scarring. The condition may happen unilaterally if due to some congenital anatomic abnormality. In the image above, there is a staghorn calculus filling calyces of kidney with chronic pyelonephritis; the cortex and medulla is atrophic and the calyces are dilated. Staghorn calculi (struvite stones) can be seen in association with chronic infection and are classically associated with urease producing organisms such as *proteus* species. The classic diagnostic clue for a struvite stone is alkaline urine.

Answer A is incorrect. While diabetic patients are susceptible to acute pyelonephritis from increased instrumentation and neurogenic bladder, the kidney shown in the image is not characteristic of acute pyelonephritis. In the acute condition, the kidney surface is frequently studded with microabscesses, indicating a recent infection.

Answer C is incorrect. There is nothing in this patient's history to indicate acute tubulointerstitial nephritis. Acute tubulointerstitial nephritis is often caused by hypersensitivity to a drug (eg, methicillin, rifampin, thiazide diuretics, and NSAIDs). It is characterized by fever, rash, eosinophilia, and renal anomalies (hematuria, increased serum creatinine, and oliguria).

Answer D is incorrect. While hypertension may be a sign of the chronic renal failure being caused by chronic pyelonephritis, hypertension alone would not cause the pathology shown in the image.

Answer E is incorrect. Minimal change disease is a glomerular disease most frequently seen in pediatric patients. It is a cause of the nephrotic syndrome in a healthy patient. Most patients respond to steroid therapy although a small fraction are at risk for chronic renal failure years later.

44. **The correct answer is B.** Calcium is reabsorbed in three areas along the nephron: the proximal tubule, the thick ascending limb of the loop of Henle, and the distal tubule. In the proximal tubule, calcium reabsorption is coupled to sodium reabsorption. In the distal tubule, calcium reabsorption is controlled by PTH. In the thick ascending limb, however, calcium reabsorption is dependent on the function of the Na^+-K^+-$2Cl^-$ co-transporter. Calcium reabsorption occurs paracellularly, driven by the electrochemical gradient created by this transporter. The cell's ATPase surface creates an electro-negative environment inside the cell by transferring three cations out (Na^+) for every two cations in (K^+). Because loop diuretics (such as furosemide) inhibit this transporter, discontinuation of the patient's loop diuretic would increase functionality of this channel and thus increase calcium resorption in this segment.

Answer A is incorrect. PTH controls calcium reabsorption in the distal tubule.

Answer C is incorrect. Thiazide diuretics inhibit the sodium chloride symporter in the distal convoluted tubules.

Answer D is incorrect. Calcium delivery plays a role in driving calcium reabsorption, but the transluminal gradient established by the sodium-potassium-chloride co-transporter is more important. Moreover, calcium's effect would not be specific for the ascending limb of the loop of Henle.

Answer E is incorrect. The triple transporter maintains a lumen positive charge; positive ions are reabsorbed to maintain electroneutrality.

45. **The correct answer is E.** This patient has experienced cardiogenic shock, as evidenced by his hypotension (systolic blood pressure <90 mm Hg) after a myocardial infarction. This has led to decreased renal perfusion, which has, in turn, led to prerenal failure. Prerenal failure is defined by a BUN:Cr ratio of >20:1. When the glomerular filtration rate drops, there is an increase in sodium and water reabsorption in the proximal tubule. This leads to an increase in tubular urea concentration, which favors increased reabsorption of urea. This will raise the BUN (remember, this is urea in the blood) and, therefore, the BUN:Cr ratio will rise.

Answer A is incorrect. Blockage of the ureters is a postrenal cause of renal failure. It would present with pain on urination and is unlikely in the setting of cardiogenic shock.

Answer B is incorrect. This patient's BUN:Cr ratio of >20:1 indicates that this is a prerenal process, not an intrarenal one. An acute tubular necrosis would present with renal failure in the setting of a BUN:Cr ratio of 10-15:1 with muddy brown granular and epithelial cell casts, as well as free renal tubular epithelial cells in the urine.

Answer C is incorrect. Although interstitial nephritis can occur from the use of NSAIDs, it usually occurs only after sustained chronic use. Signs and symptoms include rash, fever, eosinophilia, eosinophiluria, and elevated IgE levels.

Answer D is incorrect. Urine output is controlled mainly by two factors: the hydration state of the body and the level of kidney function. Therefore, low urine output is seen only in the setting of dehydration or kidney dysfunction. Stress by itself will not cause low urine output unless it is coupled with dehydration or an acute renal disease process.

46. **The correct answer is D.** Acute poststreptococcal glomerulonephritis is an autoimmune disease most frequently seen in children. Under light microscopy, the glomeruli appear enlarged and hypercellular, with neutrophils and subepithelial immune complex depositions described as "lumpy-bumpy." Under electron

microscopy, the large irregular deposits are observed in the subepithelium of the glomerulus. This condition normally presents a few weeks after a streptococcal infection with peripheral and periorbital edema, dark urine, and proteinuria. These symptoms are caused by circulating antistreptococcal antibody-antigen complexes that deposit in the glomerular basement membrane, leading to complement activation and glomerular damage. The classic findings are RBCs and casts in the urine (which cause the characteristic tea-colored urine), a positive ASO titer, and decreased levels of complement.

Answer A is incorrect. Granular subendothelial deposits are usually seen in SLE.

Answer B is incorrect. Linear subendothelial patterns are seen in vasculitides such as Goodpasture syndrome.

Answer C is incorrect. Mesangial deposits are usually seen in IgA nephropathy.

47. **The correct answer is E.** The patient described in this vignette has hepatorenal syndrome, which is a progressive functional renal failure caused by a reduction in the glomerular filtration rate due to declining hepatic function. It is characterized by splanchnic vasodilation and concomitant vasoconstriction in the renal vascular beds due to the production of mediators and to the activation of the renin-angiotensin system. The combination of these two factors causes a prerenal type azotemia that develops, most commonly, without severe oliguria. One of the features of hepatorenal syndrome is that kidney anatomy is completely unaffected, and thus visualization of the kidneys by most modalities would reveal normal size and shape.

Answer A is incorrect. Enlarged cystic kidneys can be a feature of polycystic kidney disease, but usually do not present with prerenal azotemia.

Answer B is incorrect. Enlarged kidneys with hydronephrosis can be caused by obstruction from stones in the renal calyx or ureters. However, the other clinical findings in this patient implicate a hepatorenal (prerenal) cause of renal failure.

Answer C is incorrect. Horseshoe kidney is a pediatric abnormality that is generally asymptomatic if not associated with other abnormalities. Horseshoe kidneys are caused by the embryonic blastemas (embryonic kidneys) partially fusing at their inferior poles and becoming trapped against the inferior mesenteric artery during their migration. In children it is sometimes associated with Wilms tumor.

Answer D is incorrect. A flea-bitten appearance in kidneys is usually seen in patients with malignant hypertension.

48. **The correct answer is D.** Goodpasture syndrome is a rare autoimmune disorder in which antibodies directed against glomerular basement membrane (GBM) antigen cause a rapidly progressive glomerulonephritis. The antibodies can also deposit in the alveolar basement membranes, resulting in hemoptysis. It is most often seen in young men. This condition can be diagnosed by the detection of the anti-GBM antibodies in the blood, in combination with a kidney biopsy that demonstrates a linear staining pattern on immunofluorescence. Because this condition may rapidly lead to a compromised airway or declining kidney function, immediate airway protection, plasmapheresis (to remove the autoantibodies from circulation), and treatment with corticosteroids and cyclophosphamide is indicated.

Answer A is incorrect. Poststreptococcal glomerulonephritis typically affects 2-14 year olds who have recently suffered from either impetigo or pharyngitis caused by particular M types of streptococci (nephritogenic strains). Poststreptococcal glomerulonephritis is an immune-mediated disease that develops two-six weeks after skin infection and one-three weeks after streptococcal pharyngitis. The classic presentation is an acute nephritic picture with hematuria, pyuria, RBC casts, edema, hypertension, and oliguric renal failure. This patient's age and gender in combination with his symptoms of lung hemorrhage and hematuria make Goodpasture syndrome the most likely diagnosis.

Answer B is incorrect. Alport disease is an inherited disorder caused by a mutation in collagen type IV, which is an important structural component in the basement membranes of the eyes, ears, and kidneys. Patients with this syndrome usually present in childhood with a combination of ocular defects, deafness, and hematuria. Given this patient's age and clinical presentation, Goodpasture syndrome is a more likely diagnosis than Alport syndrome.

Answer C is incorrect. Berger disease, otherwise known as IgA nephropathy, is the most common cause of glomerulonephritis worldwide. It is caused by the deposition of IgA antibodies in the mesangium of the kidney and is often triggered by a recent upper respiratory infection. Classically patients with Berger disease present with new onset frank hematuria, usually within days of an upper respiratory tract infection. Although the hematuria may persist for several days, renal function usually remains normal, and the long-term prognosis is relatively favorable. Given the patient's lung involvement, Goodpasture syndrome is a more likely diagnosis than Berger disease.

Answer E is incorrect. In the pediatric population, nephrotic syndrome (characterized by proteinuria, hypoalbuminemia, hyperlipidemia, and edema) is most commonly caused by minimal change disease (MCD). MCD is definitively diagnosed on renal biopsy, which reveals effacement of the foot process supporting the epithelial podocytes with weakening of slit-pore membranes on electron microscopy, but normal findings on light and immunofluorescent microscopy. The pathophysiology of this lesion is uncertain, although most agree there is a circulating cytokine that alters capillary charge and podocyte integrity. Treatment with steroids is indicated based on clinical suspicion of MCD; renal biopsy is not necessary before treatment is initiated. Given this patient's age and clinical presentation, Goodpasture syndrome is a more likely diagnosis than MCD.

49. **The correct answer is C.** The patient most likely has hypertension as a result of the unilateral stenosis of a renal artery. Renal artery stenosis is usually caused by atherosclerosis or fibromuscular dysplasia, and the affected kidney usually becomes atrophic. The decreased perfusion of the kidney causes juxtaglomerular cells to release renin, which cleaves angiotensinogen into angiotensin I. ACE in alveolar capillaries converts angiotensin I to angiotensin II, which stimulates the secretion of aldosterone and which is itself a vasoconstrictor. Increased levels of aldosterone lead to sodium and water retention. All of these things combined lead to hypertension.

Answer A is incorrect. Renal artery stenosis would lead to an increased level of angiotensin II, which in turn would cause increased release of ADH from the posterior pituitary.

Answer B is incorrect. Renal artery stenosis would lead to increased levels of angiotensin II.

Answer D is incorrect. Cushing syndrome, which can be of pituitary or adrenal origin, is marked by the excessive production of cortisol, which can cause hypertension. The thrill heard in the patient, however, is indicative of renal artery stenosis.

Answer E is incorrect. Renal artery stenosis would not have an effect on the levels of ACE in the lungs; however, more angiotensin I would be available and therefore there would also be an increase in angiotensin II.

50. **The correct answer is B.** The only diuretics acting along the thick ascending limb of the nephron are loop agents (eg, furosemide, torsemide, ethacrynic acid). These drugs work by inhibiting the sodium-potassium-chloride cotransporter. It is worth noting that ethacrynic acid is unique because it is not a sulfonamide and therefore can be used in individuals with an allergy to sulfa drugs.

Answer A is incorrect. Acetazolamide, which acts in the proximal convoluted tubule, blocks resorption of sodium bicarbonate.

Answer C is incorrect. Hydrochlorothiazide inhibits sodium chloride resorption in the early distal tubule.

Answer D is incorrect. Osmotic agents act in three places along the nephron: the proximal convoluted tubule, the thin descending limb, and the collecting tubule. They do not, however, act on any of the ion pumps.

Answer E is incorrect. Triamterene, a potassium-sparing diuretic, blocks sodium channels in the cortical collecting tubule.

CHAPTER 16

Reproductive

QUESTIONS

1. A 53-year-old woman calls her primary care physician because she wants to begin hormone replacement therapy (HRT). She has read that estrogen replacement therapy is supposed to ease the transition to a postmenopausal state, and that HRT can be cardioprotective, decrease cancer risk, and promote healthy bones. Which of the following is an indication for this woman to start HRT?

    (A) To decrease risk of breast cancer
    (B) To decrease risk of deep venous thrombosis and stroke
    (C) To decrease risk of myocardial infarction
    (D) To decrease risk of osteoporosis
    (E) To treat vasomotor symptoms

2. A 42-year-old woman presents to her gynecologist for a check-up. She states that this is her first gynecologic appointment in five years. As such, her physician conducts a full history and physical examination. Her medical history is significant for hyperlipidemia treated with simvastatin, and her only surgery was an appendectomy at age 21. Her family history is significant for an aunt who had breast cancer diagnosed at age 36, and a cousin with breast cancer diagnosed at age 29. On social history, she reports being happily married, never having had any children, drinking one-two glasses of wine every evening, and smoking about five cigarettes a week. She reports occasional irregular periods, and has never had a mammogram. On physical examination, the physician palpates a discrete, 1.5-x-2-cm mass in the upper outer quadrant of the left breast. There are no palpable lymph nodes in the left axilla. The patient is concerned, and asks about the chances the mass could represent breast cancer. Which of the following features of this patient's history most increases her risk of breast cancer?

    (A) One-two glasses of wine per week
    (B) Age of 42 years
    (C) Family history of breast cancer
    (D) Never having had a mammogram
    (E) Occasional irregular periods

3. A 29-year-old woman presents to the gynecologist complaining of a "fishy"-smelling vaginal odor noticeable during intercourse. Pelvic examination reveals a homogenous gray-white discharge, and a saline wet mount of vaginal epithelial cells is obtained (see image). What is the morphology of the organism that is causing this patient's symptoms?

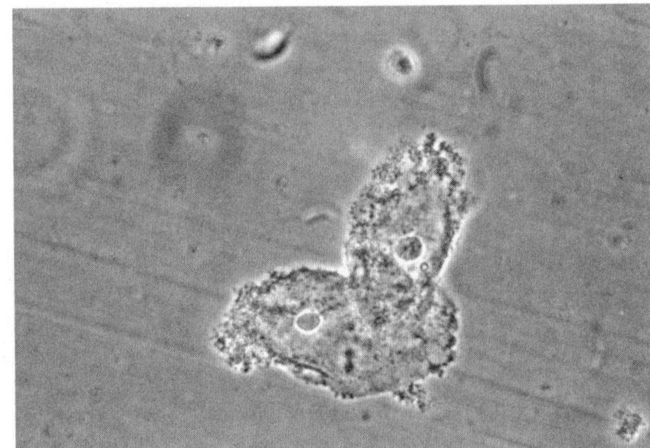

Courtesy of Dr. M. Rein, Centers for Disease Control and Prevention.

    (A) Budding yeast and/or hyphae
    (B) Gram-negative diplococci
    (C) Gram-positive rod
    (D) Obligate intracellular parasite
    (E) Pleomorphic, gram-variable rod

4. A 24-year-old woman presents with severe right lower quadrant pain. She has a history of multiple sexual partners but has been married and faithful to her husband for the last three years. A urine β-human chorionic gonadotro-

pin test is positive, but no gestational sac is visualized on transvaginal ultrasound imaging of the uterus. During the examination, her pain increases and she is becoming tachycardic. Which of the following best characterizes the organism most likely predisposed this woman to her current clinical picture?

(A) It is a gram-negative bacillus
(B) It is a gram-variable bacillus
(C) It is a spirochete
(D) It is a teardrop-shaped trophozoite
(E) It is an obligate intracellular organism

5. A 29-year-old woman in her third trimester of pregnancy is brought by her husband to the emergency department with contractions. The husband informs the nurse that "her physician said something about being at risk for seizures." Her blood pressure is 195/123 mm Hg and she is afebrile. Laboratory tests show a platelet count of 5000/mm^3, a lactate dehydrogenase level of 699 U/L, aspartate aminotransferase of 89 U/L, and alanine aminotransferase of 90 U/L. Urinalysis reveals proteinuria. The patient is given a medication and taken to the labor and delivery room. Which of the following is associated with the drug this patient most likely received?

(A) Alteration of sleep cycles
(B) Decreased tendon reflexes
(C) Epidermal erythema and sloughing
(D) Extensor plantar reflex
(E) Tetany of facial nerve when tapped

6. A 29-year-old African-American woman with menometrorrhagia undergoes ultrasound of the pelvis, which reveals uterine masses. Biopsy shows a whorled pattern of smooth muscle. A gross specimen from a patient with similar pathology is shown below. These masses are most commonly associated with which of the following conditions?

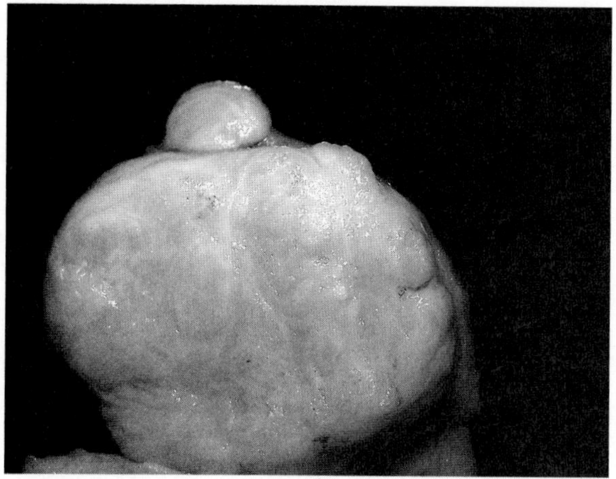

Reproduced, with permission, from USMLERx.com.

(A) Enlargement during pregnancy
(B) Formation of chocolate cysts
(C) Malignant transformation
(D) Pelvic inflammatory disease
(E) Postmenopausal metastasis

7. An endocrine research laboratory is investigating the regulation of the hypothalamic-pituitary axis through pharmacologic means in the brains of chimpanzees. They find that administering extremely high doses of chlorpromazine causes parkinsonism, amenorrhea, lack of positive reward trainability, and decreased cognitive ability test scores in female chimpanzees. These findings allow them to identify specific neural tracts in the brain that are interrupted by chlorpromazine. Interruption of what neural tract is responsible for the amenorrhea observed in the studied chimpanzees?

(A) Mesocortical tract
(B) Mesolimbic tract
(C) Nigrostriatal tract
(D) Tuberoinfundibular tract

8. A 24-year-old man presents for his annual physical and is noted to have a nontender right testicular nodule. After an initial ultrasound, he is sent for CT imaging of his abdomen and pelvis, which shows enlarged para-aortic lymph nodes that are greater on the right side. What testicular pathology does this patient most likely have?

   (A) Epididymitis
   (B) Leydig cell tumor
   (C) Seminoma
   (D) Testicular torsion

9. An 8-year-old boy presents to the clinic with a complaint of a runny nose and difficulty breathing. His mother says the boy has had recurrent respiratory infections, often with a productive cough. The child's symptoms are tolerable in the morning, but seem to become progressively worse as the day continues. Chest auscultation reveals crackles and wheezing, but the physician is unable to auscultate a normal S_1 and S_2 heart sound. Radiographic examination reveals pulmonary hyperinflation, bronchiectasis, and a complete left/right reversal of his circulatory system. What other complication(s) is this patient likely to have?

   (A) Flushing and diarrhea
   (B) Infertility
   (C) Panacinar emphysema
   (D) Pulsus paradoxus
   (E) Simple partial seizures

10. A young couple is trying to conceive their first child. The woman speaks to her mother, who tells her that she should take her temperature to determine when she ovulates. The action of which of the following hormones is responsible for this change in body temperature?

   (A) Estrogen
   (B) Human chorionic gonadotropin
   (C) Luteinizing hormone
   (D) Progesterone
   (E) Prolactin

11. A 57-year-old woman is scheduled for elective hysterectomy. Severing which of the following structures during surgery would most severely disrupt blood flow to the ipsilateral ovary?

   (A) Cardinal ligament
   (B) Fallopian tube
   (C) Round ligament
   (D) Suspensory ligament
   (E) Ureter

12. A 68-year-old retired furniture mover comes to the doctor for the first time in years because of constant backaches that radiate down his legs. He also reports fatigue, a 9.1-kg (20-lb) weight loss over the past few months, and trouble urinating, including decreased force of stream, hesitancy, and intermittency. He smokes two packs of cigarettes per day and drinks at least three beers per day, and has done so for the past 15 years. Laboratory tests show:

   Hemoglobin: 10.1 g/dL
   Hematocrit: 28%
   WBC count: 8500/mm^3
   Platelet count: 240,000/mm^3
   Na^+: 135 mEq/L
   K^+: 4.2 mEq/L
   HCO_3^-: 24 mEq/L
   Cl^-: 101 mEq/L
   Blood urea nitrogen: 18 mg/dL
   Creatinine: 1.3 mg/dL

   A radionucleotide bone scan was also performed; results are shown in the image. What is the most important risk factor for this patient's most likely current condition?

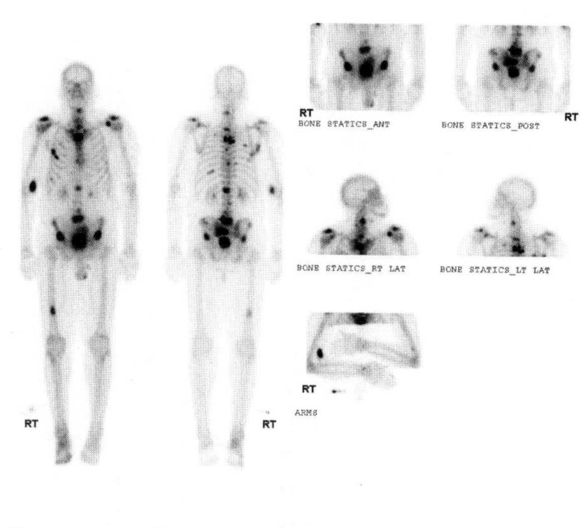

Reproduced, with permission, from USMLERx.com.

(A) Advanced age
(B) Alcohol use
(C) History of physical labor
(D) Lack of regular primary care
(E) Smoking history

13. An asymptomatic 30-year-old woman presents to her physician's office for a routine health maintenance examination. Papanicolaou smear indicates high-grade dysplasia. What is the mechanism by which the responsible agent causes disease?

(A) Arrest of blood vessel growth
(B) Continuation of cell cycle after DNA damage
(C) Inhibition of DNA replication
(D) Inhibition of mitogenic signal transduction
(E) Inhibition of RNA-dependent DNA polymerization

14. Following a normal pregnancy and labor, a baby is born to a young couple. The baby cries immediately and has Apgar scores of 9 at both one and five minutes. While examining the baby, the pediatrician present at delivery notes that the baby has ambiguous genitalia and labial fusion. The baby is also hypotensive and hypovolemic. Genotyping reveals a karyotype of 46,XX. Which of the following is the most likely cause of the patient's physical findings and symptoms?

(A) 11β-Hydroxylase deficiency
(B) 17α-Hydroxylase deficiency
(C) 21α-Hydroxylase deficiency
(D) 5α-Reductase deficiency
(E) Mutation in the androgen receptor gene

15. A 50-year-old postmenopausal G5P5 woman sees her gynecologist for a yearly well-woman check-up. Her body mass index is 34 kg/m². Results of a bimanual examination and a breast examination are normal. The patient mentions that her grandmother died of endometrial cancer, and claims that she will stop drinking and smoking if it will save her from the agony her grandmother experienced. The physician reviews the patient's medical history with her and discusses her risk factors for endometrial cancer. Which of the following interventions would have best decreased the risk for developing endometrial cancer in this patient?

(A) Avoidance of alcohol and cigarette use
(B) Delaying sexual activity
(C) Diet and exercise
(D) Nulliparity
(E) Use of a combined progesterone-estrogen birth control product

16. A 64-year-old man visits his physician for an annual examination. He complains of a recent 9.1-kg (20-lb) unintentional weight loss and pain in his back and pelvis. Otherwise, he has no complaints. His examination is notable for point tenderness along his spine and pelvis. He also had firm prostate nodules palpated on digital rectal examination. Which of the following laboratory values would be expected in this patient?

Choice	Prostate specific antigen	Calcium	Alkaline phosphatase
A	↓	↓	↓
B	↓	↓	↑
C	↑	↓	↓
D	↑	↓	↑
E	↑	↑	↓

Reproduced, with permission, from USMLERx.com.

(A) A
(B) B
(C) C
(D) D
(E) E

17. A 63-year-old man with a history of a myocardial infarction, chronic stable angina, hypertension, and diabetes presents to his physician with a complaint of erectile dysfunction. He asks about the use of a medication he saw on a TV commercial. He is currently taking metoprolol, nitroglycerin, lisinopril, and metformin. His physician informs him that it is unsafe for him to take medication for erectile dysfunction. What is the mechanism of the medication that is contraindicated in this situation?

(A) Blocks sodium channel
(B) Decreases the level of cGMP
(C) Decreases the level of nitric oxide
(D) Increases the level of cGMP
(E) Increases the level of nitric oxide

18. A patient presents two weeks after giving birth to her first child. For the past two weeks she admits to feeling "hopeless" and "helpless." She has not slept well and attributes this to frequent nighttime awakenings because she worries about the baby. She feels like she "can't handle a child right now." She sometimes feels angry at the baby and finds herself bursting into tears "for no apparent reason." She used to enjoy reading, even up to the baby's birth, but finds no joy in this presently. She assures the physician that she is taking good care of the baby, but has recently asked her mother to come stay with her for assistance. A review of her medical record reveals that she had an uncomplicated spontaneous vaginal delivery of a healthy baby boy weighing 7 lb 7 oz (3.37 kg) at 39 3/7 weeks' gestation. There was moderate loss of blood during the delivery. Her hemoglobin level following the delivery was 12.0 g/dL. What is the most likely diagnosis?

(A) Iron deficiency anemia
(B) Postpartum blues
(C) Postpartum major depression
(D) Postpartum psychosis
(E) Sheehan syndrome

19. A 28-year-old woman presents to her physician with concerns that she is unable to produce breast milk, despite having given birth approximately one month ago. On further questioning she indicates she has been exceptionally thirsty lately, and describes feelings of fatigue and cold intolerance. Physical examination reveals no abnormalities except a scarcity of axillary hair. Laboratory tests reveal a serum sodium level of 150 mEq/L and urinalysis reveals a urine osmolality of 220 mOsmol/kg. Which of the following most likely increased the patient's risk of developing this condition?

(A) Abnormalities of the placenta
(B) Alcohol intake during pregnancy
(C) Endometriosis
(D) Gestational diabetes
(E) Incorrect use of tampons
(F) Multiple sexual partners
(G) Pelvic inflammatory disease

20. A 46,XY infant is born with a nonsense mutation in the *SRY* gene. The product of the *SRY* gene is most directly responsible for which of the following normal processes in the sexual development of male fetuses?

(A) Development of internal male genitalia from the mesonephric duct
(B) Development of testes from indifferent gonads
(C) Development of the genital tubercle into the glans penis
(D) Development of the urogenital sinus into the prostate gland
(E) Involution of paramesonephric ducts

21. A woman in labor continues to be dilated 2 cm after two hours in labor. She is given a synthetic version of a hormone to help dilate her cervix. Where is the endogenous version of this hormone stored within the body?

(A) Adrenal cortex
(B) Anterior pituitary gland
(C) Hypothalamus
(D) Mammary glands
(E) Posterior pituitary gland

22. A biotechnology firm is developing a new small protein drug designed to prevent the spread of a sexually transmitted infection. Scientists want to block the infectious step of the bacteria's reproductive cycle. A Giemsa-stained smear of a patient's urethral discharge shows cytoplasmic inclusions similar to those shown in the image. During which stage of this pathogen's life cycle is it most infectious?

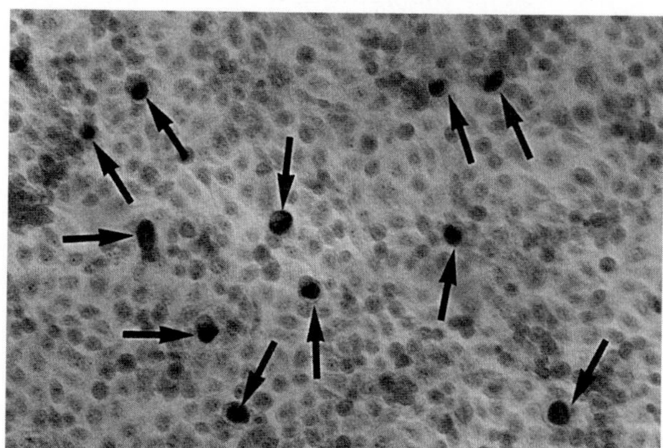

Courtesy of Dr. E. Arum and Dr. N. Jacobs, Centers for Disease Control and Prevention.

(A) Cytoplasmic inclusion body
(B) Extracellular elementary body
(C) Intracellular elementary body
(D) Multiplication of reticulate bodies
(E) Reticulate body

23. A 30-year-old woman finds a lump in her right breast during a monthly self-examination. Diagnostic mammography reveals a 2-cm mass with uneven borders and spiculated calcifications; this finding is suspicious for malignancy. A biopsy is performed. The report identifies ductal carcinoma in situ, and a lumpectomy is performed. The pathology report further states that the malignant tissue is positive for human epidermal growth factor 2/*neu* receptor, but negative for estrogen and progesterone receptors. Which of the following therapies is specifically targeted to treat this patient's breast cancer?

(A) Bevacizumab
(B) Cyclophosphamide
(C) Doxorubicin
(D) Tamoxifen
(E) Trastuzumab

24. A 19-year-old mother of two rushes to her obstetrician's office at 35 weeks' gestation because of cramping abdominal pain and mild vaginal bleeding. Both cramps and bleeding started about two hours ago. Pain is constant, with intermittent episodes of severe cramping. Bleeding has been sufficient to soak through four to five pads within the past few hours. She denies a history of trauma or leakage of clear fluid. She does admit to using cocaine three times within the past month, most recently last night. She is afebrile, blood pressure is 155/95 mm Hg, and heart rate is 100/min. Bi-manual examination reveals tenderness over the fundus and a nondilated cervix. Ultrasound reveals a normally implanted placenta with no visible abnormalities. Fetal heart rate is in the 170-180/min range. Which of the following is the most likely diagnosis?

(A) Abruptio placentae
(B) Concealed abruption
(C) Labor
(D) Placenta accreta
(E) Placenta previa

25. A 14-year-old boy is brought to the clinic by his parents who are concerned because he has not yet begun puberty. Laboratory results indicate hypogonadism secondary to failure of the hypothalamic-pituitary-gonadal axis. Which of the following are possible adverse effects of the treatment for this patient's condition?

(A) Anemia
(B) Decreased serum LDL cholesterol levels
(C) Increased spermatogenesis
(D) Leukocytosis
(E) Premature closing of the epiphyseal plates

26. A 33-year-old G1P0 woman with no previous prenatal care visits a gynecologist for a prenatal triple screen. The triple screen reveals an α-fetoprotein level 0.5 times the mean, a β-human chorionic gonadotropin level twice the mean, and an estriol level 0.75 times the mean. From which birth defect will the baby most likely suffer?

(A) Aortic coarctation
(B) Endocardial cushion defect
(C) High-pitched, cat-like cry
(D) Prominent occiput
(E) Tuft of hair at the small of the back

27. Vasectomies can be done in an outpatient setting through a small incision in the scrotum. A vasectomy involves bilateral excision of a segment of the ductus deferens between the exit from the epididymis and the entrance to the pelvis. After the ductus deferens is cut, spermatozoa can no longer travel into the urethra and the sperm degenerate in the epididymis and ductus deferens. When excising the ductus deferens segments, the surgeon takes care not to injure which anatomic structure that crosses directly posterior to the ductus as it courses from scrotum to urethra?

(A) Efferent ductules
(B) Spermatic cord
(C) Sympathetic nerve fibers
(D) Testicular artery
(E) Ureter

28. A 70-year-old woman presents to her primary care physician for a check-up after undergoing repair of a broken hip due to a minor fall. Which of the following is the most likely hormonal profile of this woman?

Choice	Estrogen	Luteinizing hormone	Follicle-stimulating hormone	Gonadotropin-releasing hormone
A	↓	↓	↓	↑
B	↓	↓	↓	↓
C	↓	↑	↑	↑
D	↑	↑	↑	↑
E	↑	↑	↑	↓

Reproduced, with permission, from USMLERx.com.

(A) A
(B) B
(C) C
(D) D
(E) E

29. A 23-year-old athletically built woman comes to the physician complaining of multiple red, ring-like lesions on her body. A careful history and physical reveals the woman has tinea corporis acquired while working on poorly cleaned yoga mats at a local gym. The physician prescribes a medicine to clear her erythematous lesions. After 15 days of treatment the lesions she returns to the office. While the lesions are clearing, she has noticed that patches of her skin have become darker than normal. Which of the following drugs did this patient most likely receive?

(A) Amphotericin B
(B) Fluconazole
(C) Flucytosine
(D) Itraconazole
(E) Ketoconazole

30. A 26-year-old man presents to the urologist because he and his wife have failed to conceive for 14 months. His total and free testosterone levels are normal, and initial semen analysis shows significantly decreased volume and no

detectable sperm. Testicular fine-needle biopsy demonstrates normal sperm motility and normal sperm morphology. His medical history is significant for hypercholesterolemia and a surgical bilateral inguinal hernia repair at 8 years of age. He also admits to smoking marijuana four-five times/week during college, and to drinking three-four alcoholic beverages/day until recently. Which of the following aspects of his work-up is the most likely cause of the patient's infertility?

(A) Four year history of heavy marijuana use
(B) Decreased semen volume
(C) History of drinking three-four alcoholic beverages/day
(D) Hypercholesterolemia
(E) Surgical inguinal hernia repair

31. After 11 days in the intensive care unit following an automobile accident, an 18-year-old woman develops increased urinary urgency, burning during urination, and lower abdominal pain. When her urine is cultured, a red pigment is observed in the Petri dish. What is the most likely organism causing these symptoms?

(A) *Escherichia coli*
(B) *Klebsiella pneumoniae*
(C) *Proteus mirabilis*
(D) *Serratia marcescens*
(E) *Staphylococcus saprophyticus*

32. A 25-year-old woman comes to her physician complaining of pain with intercourse and dysmenorrhea that worsens one-two days before her period starts. Ultrasonography reveals unilateral adnexal masses, and laparoscopy shows reddish-brown cysts on the ovaries. This patient is at increased risk for developing which of the following conditions?

(A) Carcinoma
(B) Infertility
(C) Intracranial hemorrhage
(D) Masculinization
(E) Obesity

33. Pathologic examination of bilateral ovarian masses reveals round, mucin-secreting cells as seen in the image. Which of the following is most likely to be seen on physical examination in this case?

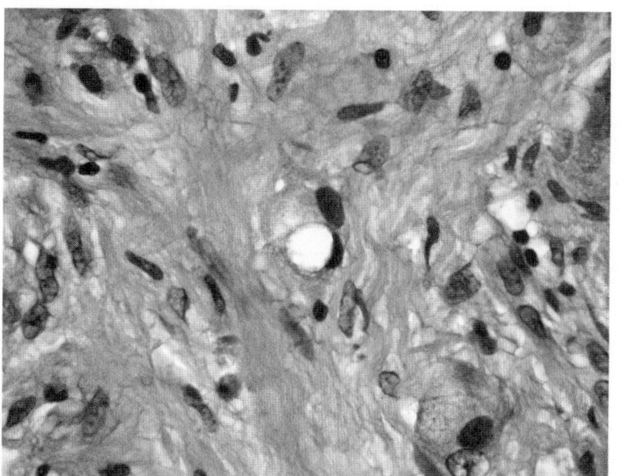

Reproduced, with permission, from USMLERx.com.

(A) Galactorrhea
(B) Hematochezia
(C) Palpable gallbladder
(D) Pearly papules on the face
(E) Supraclavicular lymphadenopathy

34. A previously healthy 25-year-old man comes to the physician because of a tingling sensation on his penis for the past day. Physical examination reveals a slightly raised, erythematous area on the head of the penis. He has not been sexually active for over a year. When his lesion is scraped with a microscope slide and Giemsa dye applied, multinucleated giant cells can be seen. Which of the following mechanisms is involved in the pathogenesis of the infective agent?

(A) Direct invasion into the bloodstream
(B) Exotoxin production
(C) Invasion of CD4+ cells
(D) Migration to the peripheral nervous system by anterograde axonal transport
(E) Migration to the peripheral nervous system by retrograde axonal transport

35. A 15-year-old who has been healthy and meeting normal developmental milestones presents with a painless, homogenous testicular mass. Following removal, the family is informed that the mass is a common germ cell tumor that is highly sensitive to radiotherapy. They are told their son has a good prognosis. Which of the following pathologies was most likely seen?

(A) A glandular/papillary morphologic pattern
(B) Cowdry type A nuclear inclusions
(C) Large cells in lobules, with watery cytoplasm
(D) Reinke crystals
(E) Structures resembling primitive glomeruli

36. A 32-year-old woman presents to her gynecologist with oligomenorrhea. On examination she is found to have enlarged, nontender ovaries bilaterally. The patient's body mass index is 31 kg/m². What other symptom or finding is this patient likely to have?

(A) Decreased estrogen levels
(B) Epicanthal folds
(C) Hirsutism
(D) Increased bleeding time
(E) Numerous spontaneous abortions

37. A 35-year-old man comes to the physician complaining of painful genital vesicles. On further questioning, he admits to unprotected sex with multiple partners. To confirm the diagnosis, the physician performs a specific test. Results are shown in the image. Which of the following is the pathognomonic finding on this patient's test?

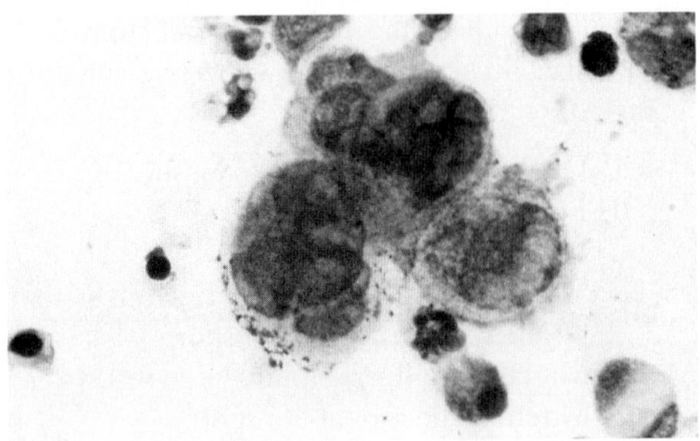

Courtesy of Dr. Joe Miller, Centers for Disease Control and Prevention.

(A) Auer rods
(B) Call-Exner bodies
(C) Lewy bodies
(D) Mallory bodies
(E) Multinucleated giant cell

38. A 32-year-old pregnant woman presents to the emergency department with vaginal bleeding. She reports that her last menstrual period was 24 weeks ago. She denies any pain or recent trauma. Transabdominal ultrasound confirms the presence of a gestational sac and an intrauterine fetal heartbeat. Which of the following in this patient's past medical or surgical history would have increased her risk for this complication?

(A) History of endometriosis
(B) History of pelvic inflammatory disease
(C) Prior cesarean section delivery
(D) Prior ectopic pregnancy
(E) Use of assisted reproductive technologies

39. A woman who has had four previous spontaneous, first-trimester pregnancy losses is found to have a uterus with the structure illustrated in the image. What is the cause of this variation?

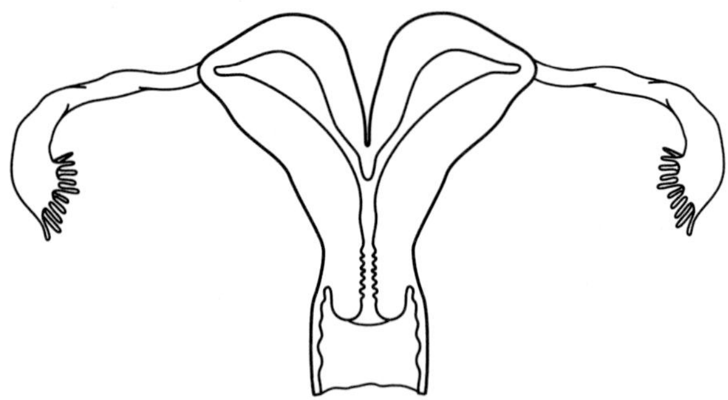

Reproduced, with permission, from USMLERx.com.

(A) Complete failure of fusion of the paramesonephric (müllerian) ducts
(B) Failure of resorption of the midline uterine septum
(C) Maternal diethylstilbestrol exposure
(D) Partial failure of fusion of the paramesonephric (müllerian) ducts

40. A 1-year-old infant is noted by his parents to have a gradually enlarging scrotal mass. There is no history of trauma. On physical examination no scrotal skin lesions are noted, and the mass is not painful on palpation. However, the scrotum is enlarged, boggy, and soft bilaterally. Results of a transillumination test are positive. Where is the site of fluid accumulation in this patient?

(A) Body of the testis
(B) Epididymis
(C) Inguinal lymphatics
(D) Pampiniform plexus
(E) Tunica vaginalis

41. A 24-year-old bartender returning from Mexico presents to the clinic because of a painful penile lesion that appeared about one week after having unprotected sex with a new female partner. On examination the ulcer is 1.5 cm in diameter with an erythematous base and clearly demarcated borders. The base of the ulcer is covered with a yellow purulent exudate and bleeds when scraped. Gram stain of the exudates shows gram-negative rods in chains in a school-of-fish appearance. Otherwise, examination is notable only for tender inguinal lymphadenopathy. Which of the following is the most appropriate treatment at this time?

(A) A 10-day course of oral acyclovir
(B) Highly active retroviral therapy until the lesion resolves
(C) Nystatin powder to the lesion daily for at least one week
(D) One high dose of intramuscular penicillin G
(E) One high dose of oral azithromycin

42. A 32-year-old woman with a history of hypertension and cocaine abuse presents at 32 weeks' gestation because of vaginal bleeding and painful abdominal cramps. She denies trauma. Her blood pressure is 105/60 mm Hg, blood oxygen saturation is 97% on room air, and her heart rate is 110 bpm. Urinalysis shows no protein, leukocytes, or bacteria, with few RBCs. Pelvic examination reveals dark-red blood in the vaginal vault and a hypertonic uterus. Fetal heart tones indicate fetal distress. Which of the following is the most appropriate course of action?

(A) Administer magnesium
(B) Await spontaneous vaginal delivery
(C) Do an abdominal FAST (focused assessment with sonography in trauma) to assess for free blood in the peritoneum
(D) Perform cesarean section
(E) Perform urgent CT of the chest to assess for amniotic fluid embolism

43. A normal woman is on day 19 of her menstrual cycle, as measured from the first day of her most recent period. Which of the following accurately describes the changes in progesterone and estrogen levels occurring at this time, as well as the feedback of these two hormones on luteinizing hormone (LH) and follicle-stimulating hormone (FSH) release at this stage of the menstrual cycle?

Choice	Progesterone	Estrogen	Feedback on LH and FSH
A	↓	↓	negative
B	no change	↑	negative
C	no change	↑	positive
D	↑	↓	negative
E	↑	↑	negative

(A) A
(B) B
(C) C
(D) D
(E) E

44. A 65-year-old man visits his physician because of increasingly difficult urination. He has trouble initiating a stream and experiences postvoid dribbling. He wakes from sleep three times per night to urinate. His baseline creatinine level was 1.0 mg/dL, and it is now 1.5 mg/dL. Which treatment is most feasible to immediately improve this patient's creatinine level?

    (A) Administration of fluid boluses
    (B) Dialysis
    (C) Placement of a Foley catheter
    (D) Prostatectomy

45. A 15 year-old girl presents to the clinic because of primary amenorrhea and recent masculinization of her genitalia. Her mother reports that the patient was born phenotypically female with clitoromegaly. On initial laboratory testing as an infant, the patient had a testosterone level of 482 ng/dL (normal: 437-707 ng/dL), an estrogen level of 12 pg/mL (normal: 10-60 pg/mL) and a luteinizing hormone level of 8 U/L (normal: 7-24 U/L). On physical examination at this visit, testes are found to be present. Which of the following disorders does this patient most likely have?

    (A) 5α-reductase deficiency
    (B) Complete androgen insensitivity
    (C) Double Y syndrome
    (D) Female pseudohermaphroditism
    (E) True hermaphroditism

46. A 35-year-old woman presents to her physician with complaints of monthly, recurring bilateral breast pain in the upper outer quadrants that radiates to the arms and shoulders, as well as discrete lumps in the upper outer quadrants of her breasts. She reports that her symptoms are most prominent prior to each menstrual cycle. The patient adds that she has one daughter and chose to bottle-feed. A mammogram is performed and shows clusters of calcifications in both breasts. She underwent core needle biopsy and the pathology demonstrated nonproliferative lesions. Which of the following is true regarding the patient's diagnosis?

    (A) This condition has no malignant potential
    (B) This condition is associated with a family history of *BRCA1*
    (C) This condition is associated with purulent nipple discharge
    (D) This condition is most common in women under 25 years old
    (E) This patient likely had breast trauma

47. A 24-year-old woman with a history of diabetes presents to her gynecologist, because she and her husband have been trying to conceive for more than a year without success. Laboratory samples were drawn and her ovarian ultrasound image is shown. Which of the following laboratory results is expected?

    (A) Decreased estrogen
    (B) Decreased testosterone
    (C) Excess follicle-stimulating hormone
    (D) Excess luteinizing hormone
    (E) Excess progesterone

48. A 23-year-old woman presents to the emergency department because of vaginal bleeding. She says that she is in her ninth week of pregnancy according to her last menstrual period. Laboratory studies show a β-human chorionic gonadotropin level of 103,000 mIU/L. The sample shown in the image is retrieved from the patient's uterus. There are no recognizable fetal parts. Which of the following describes the most likely genotype and parental source of DNA in this mass?

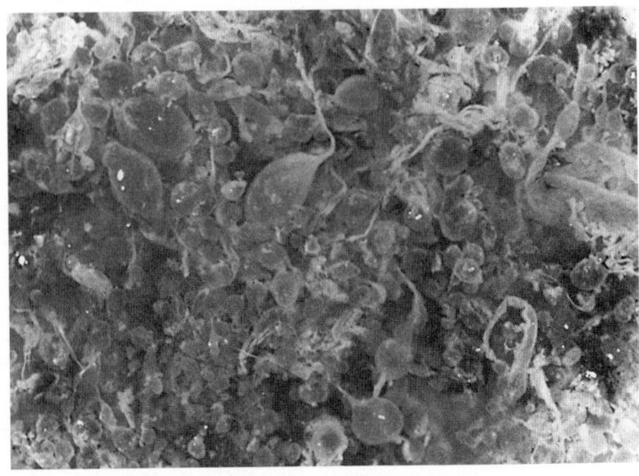

Courtesy of Armed Forces Institute of Pathology.

(A) 46,XX; maternal
(B) 46,XX; paternal
(C) 46,XX; maternal and paternal
(D) 69,XXX; maternal and paternal
(E) 69,XXY; maternal and paternal

49. After fertilization of the ovum, implantation occurs in the endometrium. At this time the developing placenta begins to produce a hormone necessary for embryonic viability. Which of the following best describes this hormone's action?

(A) Increases the production of milk by the mammary glands
(B) Increases the threshold for uterine contraction
(C) Initiates parturition at the end of pregnancy
(D) Stimulates the corpus luteum to produce estriol and progesterone
(E) Stimulates the placenta to produce estriol and progesterone

50. A 38-year-old oncology patient comes to the physician complaining of vaginal burning and itching. On physical examination a whitish, curd-like vaginal discharge and inflammation of the walls of the vagina and vulva are observed. Which of the following is another manifestation of infection with this organism?

(A) Chronic lung disease resembling tuberculosis
(B) Esophagitis
(C) Lesions in lung cavities
(D) Meningoencephalitis
(E) Migrating synovitis

ANSWERS

1. **The correct answer is E.** Menopause occurs when a woman has no menstrual cycles for one year. The two-eight years leading up to this time are called peri-menopause. During this time, hormones fluctuate tremendously, eventually leading to a decrease in estrogen, an increase in follicle-stimulating hormone (FSH), an increase in luteinizing hormone (LH), and an increase in gonadotropin-releasing hormone (GnRH). Associated symptoms include **H**ot flashes, **A**trophy of the **V**agina, **O**steoporosis, and **C**oronary artery disease (remember, menopause causes **HAVOC**). All of these hormone fluctuations can result in vasomotor symptoms, which are more commonly known as "hot flashes." Combinations of estrogen and progestin are used as HRT to decrease hot flashes, vaginal dryness, and mood swings in postmenopausal women. Unfortunately, HRT has recently been associated with an increased risk of breast cancer, stroke, myocardial infarction (MI) in the first year after starting therapy, and deep venous thrombosis that leads to pulmonary embolism.

   Answer A is incorrect. The risk of breast cancer is increased by 26% in women receiving HRT. Breast cancer has been shown to be an estrogen-dependent disease. Women who have never been exposed to estrogen, through a lack of ovarian function and absence of hormone treatment, do not develop breast cancer.

   Answer B is incorrect. The risk of deep venous thrombosis and pulmonary embolism is doubled in women receiving HRT. It was initially thought that estrogen's beneficial effects on the patient's lipid profile would decrease thromboembolic risk, but it appears that the paradoxical thrombotic risks outweigh the benefits to the lipid profile. Increased cardiovascular risk is due to hepatic estrogen receptor agonist activity upregulating protein synthesis, including clotting factors. The risk of stroke is increased by 41% in women receiving HRT. As such, HRT is not indicated to clinically reduce risk of stroke.

   Answer C is incorrect. The risk of MI is increased by 29% in women receiving HRT. It was initially thought that estrogens would have a beneficial effect on the patient's lipid profile, and thus decrease the risk of MI, but it seems that the thrombotic risks outweigh the beneficial lipid profile effects. Cardiovascular risk is due to the fact that hepatic estrogen receptor agonist activity upregulates protein synthesis, including clotting factors. As such, HRT is not indicated as a clinically cardioprotective treatment.

   Answer D is incorrect. Although HRT does have a beneficial effect in warding off bone demineralization, this is not currently an indication by itself for HRT in a postmenopausal woman.

2. **The correct answer is C.** You do not need to memorize all the risk factors for breast cancer to answer this question. One thing that should immediately jump out in this patient's history is her strong family history of breast cancer at a young age (<40 years). This should raise red flags in your mind for a genetic predisposition to breast cancer, such as the *BRCA1* or *BRCA2* gene.

   Answer A is incorrect. While consumption of alcohol does increase one's risk for breast cancer, this is not a significant amount, and is not more important than this patient's family history of breast cancer.

   Answer B is incorrect. While breast cancer increases in incidence with age, this does not raise this patient's risk more than her family history.

   Answer D is incorrect. Having never had a mammogram does increase the chance this patient has an undetected cancer; however, her significant family history is a bigger risk factor.

   Answer E is incorrect. Occasional irregular periods may mean this patient has begun menopause; however, it does not significantly increase her risk for breast cancer, and certainly is not more important than her family history.

3. **The correct answer is E.** The term pleomorphic, gram-variable rod is used to describe *Gardnerella vaginalis*, which causes vaginosis that is characterized by a gray-white vaginal discharge with a fishy odor. Clue cells on saline wet mount are diagnostic and appear as vaginal epithelial cells covered with bacteria. Inflammatory cells often are present as well.

   Answer A is incorrect. Budding yeast and/or hyphae are used to describe *Candida albicans*, a fungus that causes "yeast infection," a vulvovaginitis that presents with vulvar pruritus, dysuria, and a thick, adherent "cottage cheese-like" discharge. The organism is visualized on wet mount after addition of potassium hydroxide.

   Answer B is incorrect. The term gram-negative diplococci is used to describe *Neisseria gonorrhoeae*, which can cause urethritis, cervicitis, and pelvic inflammatory disease. Presenting symptoms often include pain and mucopurulent vaginal discharge. These organisms often are found within surrounding neutrophils.

   Answer C is incorrect. The term gram-positive rod is used to describe *Lactobacillus*, which comprises part of the normal vaginal flora in adults.

   Answer D is incorrect. The term obligate intracellular parasite is used to describe *Chlamydia trachomatis*, which can cause urethritis, cervicitis, and pelvic inflammatory disease. Presenting symptoms often include pelvic pain with mucopurulent vaginal discharge, and inclusion bodies within epithelial cells can be seen on Giemsa stain or fluorescent antibody smear.

4. **The correct answer is E.** The woman is presenting with classic signs of ectopic pregnancy. Once the β-human chorionic gonadotropin (β-hCG) is above 1500, and intrauterine pregnancy should be visible on transvaginal ultrasound imaging. If it is not, ectopic pregnancy must be suspected. If embedded in the fallopian tube, the growing fetus will eventually rupture the organ, leading to life-threatening intra-abdominal bleeding or it will die and spontaneously abort. One risk factor for the development of ectopic pregnancy is previous pelvic inflammatory disease (PID) due to its associated damage to fallopian tubes. Scarring of the lining of the tubes renders them unable to propel the fertilized ovum toward the uterus. Organisms associated with PID are *Chlamydia trachomatis*, an obligate intracellular bacterium, and *Neisseria gonorrhoeae*, a gram-negative diplococcus.

   Answer A is incorrect. *Escherichia coli*, a gram-negative bacillus, is a common cause of urinary tract infections in women, but is not associated with PID or ectopic pregnancy.

   Answer B is incorrect. *Gardnerella vaginalis*, a bacillus that has variable Gram staining, is a cause of bacterial vaginosis, which is not associated with an increased risk of PID or ectopic pregnancy.

   Answer C is incorrect. *Treponema pallidum*, a spirochete, causes the sexually transmitted disease syphilis, which is not associated with PID or ectopic pregnancy.

   Answer D is incorrect. *Trichomonas vaginalis* is a teardrop-shaped trophozoite that is spread through sexual contact. In females, it colonizes the vagina and produces a greenish, watery, and foul-smelling vaginal discharge and pruritus.

5. **The correct answer is B.** This patient has preeclampsia, which is characterized by hypertension and proteinuria. If seizures are present, the diagnosis of eclampsia is made. Preeclampsia generally occurs during the second or third trimester, and common symptoms include headache, blurred vision, abdominal pain, edema of face and extremities, altered mentation, and hyperreflexia. Thrombocytopenia and hyperuricemia may also occur. It is associated with **HELLP** (**H**emolysis, **E**levated **L**iver function tests, **L**ow **P**latelets) syndrome, which is associated with higher morbidity and mortality for both mother and fetus. The primary treatment for preeclampsia is delivery of the

fetus. Patients may be managed expectantly with bed rest and frequent monitoring of blood pressures if remote from term and no evidence of severe disease. Intravenous (IV) magnesium is administered to prevent eclamptic seizures. Alternative medications include diazepam and phenytoin, but these are second-line agents. Administration of magnesium may cause depressed tendon reflexes. If toxic levels are reached, then respiratory paralysis or cardiac arrest can occur.

Answer A is incorrect. Alteration of sleep cycles is seen in some patients taking phenobarbital. Another potential yet significant adverse effect of this medication is dependence. Neither has been demonstrated in patients given magnesium sulfate.

Answer C is incorrect. The development of erythematous papules and plaques, progressing to epidermal necrosis and sloughing, is called Stevens-Johnson syndrome (SJS). It can occur following exposure to a number of medications, including the anticonvulsants carbamazepine, phenytoin, and lamotrigine. It is generally preceded by malaise and fever, and symptoms begin after two weeks. However, magnesium sulfate is administered for seizure prophylaxis in preeclampsia, and no association has been found between magnesium sulfate and SJS.

Answer D is incorrect. An extensor plantar reflex, also known as Babinski's sign, can occur from a number of conditions, including hypomagnesemia. On the contrary, this patient would have hypermagnesemia from administration of magnesium sulfate, resulting in decreased tendon reflexes.

Answer E is incorrect. In patients with hypocalcemia, tapping the facial nerve at the angle of the jaw results in ipsilateral contraction of the facial muscles. This is known as Chvostek sign. A patient with preeclampsia, however, would be treated with magnesium. Clinical modulation of calcium levels is not indicated.

6. **The correct answer is A.** Leiomyomas, or fibroids, are common smooth muscle tumors that are most often seen in African-American women and present with multiple masses. These tumors are benign and can be associated with dysmenorrhea (menstrual pain), menorrhagia/menometrorrhagia (heavy prolonged bleeding), infertility, and abnormal pelvic exams including palpable masses extending from the uterus. Because they are estrogen sensitive, they tend to increase in size during menses or pregnancy and decrease in size after menopause. Treatment of fibroids is solely dependent on the severity of symptoms and the desire of the woman to preserve or not preserve fertility. Myomectomy can be performed in a woman wishing to preserve fertility, whereas hysterectomy is used in women with severe symptoms not wishing to preserve fertility. Medical therapy can be tried with monotherapy or combinations of GnRH analogs (leuprolide), combined oral contraceptives, progestins, and/or GnRH antagonists (centrorelix).

Answer B is incorrect. Chocolate cysts and "powder burns" are most often associated with endometriosis (nonneoplastic ectopic endometrial tissue outside the uterus). Endometriosis is often associated with severe menstrual-related pain and infertility, but this patient's masses are confined to the uterus, and the biopsy shows smooth muscle proliferation rather than the glandular and stromal proliferation at ectopic sites that would be expected with endometriosis.

Answer C is incorrect. Leiomyomas are benign tumors that are very rarely associated with malignant transformation. Malignant leiomyosarcomas most typically arise de novo with areas of necrosis and hemorrhage, not from leiomyomas.

Answer D is incorrect. Leiomyomas are not the cause of PID, but rather occur independently of the development of PID. PID is the end result of a polymicrobial infection of the genital tract, most commonly caused by untreated *Neisseria gonorrhoeae* and *Chlamydia trachomatis*. PID commonly presents with odiferous vaginal discharge, pain with sexual intercourse, urinary symptoms, and dysmenorrhea as well as a history of multiple unprotected sexual encounters. However, PID can also be asymptomatic. Treatment of PID is aimed at treating the most likely microbial pathogen(s). PID does not cause proliferation of the smooth muscle cells leading to benign tumors.

Answer E is incorrect. Leiomyomas, or fibroids, are estrogen-sensitive benign tumors and thus frequently regress in size after menopause. Also, they are not malignant nor do they metastasize. A metastatic mass in a postmenopausal woman should warrant further evaluation of a neoplastic process, and should lessen the suspicion of uterine fibroids.

7. **The correct answer is D.** Chlorpromazine is a typical antipsychotic agent that works as a D_2-receptor antagonist in all of the four major dopamine tracts listed as choices. In the normal hypothalamic-adrenal axis, all hormones are regulated by increasing or decreasing releasing hormones except prolactin. Prolactin secretion is regulated by a negative feedback system that is controlled by the dopaminergic neurons. An inverse relationship is seen, where an increase in dopamine causes a decrease in prolactin secretion and vice versa. Knowing that the typical antipsychotics act as D_2-receptor antagonists in the tuberoinfundibular tract causes hyperprolactinemia is the first step to answering this question. Combining this with the fact that hyperprolactinemia causes abnormal menstruation and/or amenorrhea leads us to choose the tuberoinfundibular tract as the interrupted tract leading to prolactin disinhibition by D_2-receptor antagonism.

Answer A is incorrect. The mesocortical tract is thought to be related to cognition, and D_2-receptor antagonism by typical antipsychotics in this tract are thought to produce and/or exacerbate the negative symptoms of schizophrenia such as decreased cognition, avolition, and alogia. This explains why atypical antipsychotics are preferred as they more effectively target dopamine receptors in this tract, resulting in fewer of the negative symptoms commonly seen in schizophrenia.

Answer B is incorrect. D_2-receptor antagonism by chlorpromazine in the mesolimbic tract causes a decrease in positive reward trainability and a decrease in the positive symptoms of schizophrenia such as hallucinations, delusions, and frank psychosis. Both typical and atypical antipsychotics act as D_2-receptor antagonists in this tract to curb the positive symptoms of schizophrenia.

Answer C is incorrect. The nigrostriatal tract is a part of the basal ganglia that is involved in the production of movement. D_2-receptor antagonism in this area by typical antipsychotics produces Parkinson-like movements and tardive dyskinesia. The atypical antipsychotics tend to have less D_2-receptor blockade in this tract and thus cause less movement-related adverse effects compared to the typical antipsychotics. Interestingly, atypical antipsychotics work more effectively antagonizing 5-HT receptors than D_2-receptors in this tract.

8. **The correct answer is C.** Testicular cancer is most often diagnosed in men who are between 15 and 35 years old, and seminomas are the most common type, accounting for approximately 40% of testicular cancers. The lymphatic spread of testicular cancers is often seen in the paraaortic chain of lymph nodes.

Answer A is incorrect. Epididymitis is an inflammation of the epididymis, which is posterior to the testis. This condition would be painful, and it is unlikely to have grossly evident lymphadenopathy in the para-aortic chain.

Answer B is incorrect. A Leydig cell tumor is a form of testicular cancer, but it is much less common than the seminoma.

Answer D is incorrect. Testicular torsion is a urologic emergency, and it would present with acute, high-intensity pain as a result of ischemia.

9. **The correct answer is B.** Kartagener syndrome is an inherited disease that results in immotile cilia caused by a dynein arm defect. The clinical symptoms that result from this defect include bronchiectasis, recurrent sinusitis, and male and female infertility. Situs inversus occurs in approximately 50% of those with the

syndrome and usually has no serious adverse health consequences.

Answer A is incorrect. Flushing and diarrhea are symptoms of a carcinoid tumor. Additional symptoms include wheezing and salivation. The peak incidence is between ages 50 and 70 years.

Answer C is incorrect. Panacinar emphysema is a symptom of α_1-antitrypsin deficiency. α_1-Antitrypsin deficiency may also present with liver disease due to accumulation of variant α_1-antitrypsin molecules within the hepatocytes.

Answer D is incorrect. Pulsus paradoxus is an exaggerated fall in systemic blood pressure during inspiration as felt in a peripheral pulse. This condition may be caused by asthma and, in this case, is not the most likely answer.

Answer E is incorrect. Simple partial seizures in children can be caused by genetic, infectious, traumatic, congenital or metabolic causes. They are not associated with Kartagener syndrome.

10. **The correct answer is D.** Progesterone is produced by the corpus luteum shortly after ovulation. One of its locations of action is the hypothalamic thermoregulatory center, leading to a slightly elevated basal body temperature (up to 1°F). Therefore it is possible to assess when ovulation has occurred by checking one's basal body temperature on a daily basis.

    Answer A is incorrect. Estrogen does have some effect at the hypothalamic thermoregulatory center during menopause, contributing to "hot flashes," but it does not affect body temperature during the normal menstrual cycle.

    Answer B is incorrect. Human chorionic gonadotropin has no effect on body temperature following ovulation. It is present during pregnancy and is the hormone detected during a pregnancy test.

    Answer C is incorrect. LH surge causes ovulation to occur but has no physiologic effects on body temperature.

    Answer E is incorrect. Prolactin has no effect on body temperature following ovulation. It is responsible for the production of breast milk, and high levels of prolactin cause anovulation.

11. **The correct answer is D.** The suspensory ligaments (also known as the infundibulopelvic ligaments) contain the ovarian arteries and veins, which are responsible for the direct blood supply to the ovaries. The ovaries also receive collateral flow from the uterine arteries that travel in the cardinal (transverse cervical) ligament at the base of the broad ligament.

    Answer A is incorrect. The cardinal (transverse cervical) ligament carries descending branches of the uterine artery. Although the uterine arteries provide collateral blood flow to the ovaries, severing the cardinal ligament should not significantly decrease blood flow to the ovary if the ovarian arteries remain intact.

    Answer B is incorrect. The fallopian tubes carry the ova from the ovary to the uterus during ovulation. Severing this structure would disrupt normal fertilization but would not significantly affect blood flow to the ovary.

    Answer C is incorrect. The round ligament runs inferior to the ovary before attaching to the uterus. It contains no important structures and is not a source of blood for the ovary.

    Answer E is incorrect. The ureters run directly inferior to the uterine arteries before feeding into the bladder. Remember: "Water under the bridge." Severing this structure would not affect ovarian blood flow.

12. **The correct answer is A.** Advancing age is the most important risk factor for prostate carcinoma. It is the most common cancer in adult males and the second most common cause of death due to cancer in adult males. This condition is more common in African-American men and is usually asymptomatic until advanced. Advancing age, family history, race, and smoking are all risk factors. The screening test for prostate cancer is prostate-specific antigen level (PSA) and subsequent biopsy. Prostate cancer can invade locally or spread via the lymphatics or bloodstream to bone, lung, and liver. The bone scan in this patient shows diffuse bony metastases.

Answer B is incorrect. There is no evidence that links prostate cancer and alcohol use.

Answer C is incorrect. This patient has a history of physical labor and may have sought medical care for back pain earlier in life. Given his current symptoms of weight loss, fatigue, and trouble urinating, he most likely has prostate cancer that has metastasized to bone, not simply a back problem.

Answer D is incorrect. Lack of primary care can be a risk factor for prostate cancer, but in this patient it is not the most important risk factor.

Answer E is incorrect. Smoking is a risk factor for prostate carcinoma, but it is not the most important risk factor.

13. **The correct answer is B.** The causative agent of cervical dysplasia and cancer is the human papillomavirus. Its critical *E6* and *E7* gene products downregulate p53 and pRb, respectively, allowing the cell to cycle out of control despite any damage to cellular DNA.

Answer A is incorrect. Blood vessel growth is an important component of many, if not all, tumors. However, the arrest of blood vessel growth is not known to be inhibited directly by human papillomavirus.

Answer C is incorrect. DNA replication (as by DNA polymerase) is not inhibited by human papillomavirus. Rather, the downstream effect of its oncogenes is an upregulation of DNA replication.

Answer D is incorrect. Mitogenic signal transduction is commonly increased by oncogenes, such as *myc*, *src*, or *bcr-abl*. Inhibition of these proteins would not cause tumorigenesis.

Answer E is incorrect. RNA-dependent DNA polymerization is an essential component of telomerase, which has been implicated in the limitless replicative potential of tumor cells. Telomerase elongates the DNA caps at the end of each chromosome, preventing the gradual erosion of genetic material that ultimately forces the cell to cease dividing. Inhibiting this process would stop the cancer cells' uncontrolled divisions and is an area of emerging cancer therapy research.

14. **The correct answer is C.** This female baby has masculinization of her external genitalia due to congenital adrenal hyperplasia (CAH). CAH is caused by deficiencies in enzymes required for adrenocortical steroid synthesis, such as 21-hydroxylase and 11β-hydroxylase. 21-Hydroxylase deficiency results in an inability to synthesize aldosterone or cortisol, resulting in shuttling of the intermediates to generate androgens, leading to an elevation of androgen levels and masculinization. Additionally, the lack of aldosterone leads to salt wasting, which can present with hypovolemia and hypotension. Blood tests will reveal hyperkalemia. Treatment includes IV saline and steroid hormone replacement.

Answer A is incorrect. 11β-Hydroxylase deficiency is a cause of CAH, but it does not result in hypotension or hypovolemia. Instead, it can result in hypertension because the deficient enzyme allows an accumulation of an aldosterone precursor (11-deoxycorticosterone) that acts as a mineralocorticoid to cause salt retention and hypervolemia. This precursor is not able to be formed with 21-hydroxylase deficiency. 11β-Hydroxylase deficiency typically presents with masculinization (due to shuttling of the intermediates to generate androgens) and hypertension.

Answer B is incorrect. 17α-Hydroxylase deficiency results in a phenotypically female newborn who will not undergo sexual maturation later in life. This enzyme has a role in the conversion of progesterone and progenolone to precursors that will go on to form cortisol, testosterone, and estrogen. The intermediates that build up will produce an excessive amount of aldosterone, resulting in hypertension and hypokalemia. This deficiency, and the resulting lack of testosterone and estrogen, result in a phenotypically female 46,XY baby with no internal reproductive organs, or a phenotypically female 46,XX baby who will not undergo normal pubertal development.

Answer D is incorrect. 5α-Reductase deficiency occurs in 46,XY newborns that have phenotypically female external genitalia (although clitoromegaly may be present) and male internal reproductive organs. Normally, 5α-reductase converts testosterone to dihydrotestosterone (DHT). DHT is essential in the development of the male external genitalia, and a lack of DHT results in feminization of the penis and scrotum with normal internal male reproductive organs. At puberty these patients may suddenly experience virilization of the external organs due to the increase in testosterone.

Answer E is incorrect. Complete androgen insensitivity is a result of a mutation in the androgen receptor gene. These 46,XY patients develop testes, which are usually undescended or found in the labia majora, and female external genitalia and vagina with no internal reproductive organs. They typically present as normal-appearing girls, with normal breast development and body habitus, who consult their physician when they do not begin menstruation. These patients typically have decreased or absent axillary and pubic hair and are taller than average.

15. **The correct answer is C.** Obesity (especially when 22.7 kg [50 lb] or more overweight) increases risk for the development of endometrial cancer five to ten-fold. The increased risk in obese patients is from increased aromatization in peripheral tissues, resulting in higher levels of circulating estrogen. Endometrial tissue is estrogen sensitive, and higher levels of circulating estrogen lead to increased glandular proliferation and increased risk for dysplastic transformation. Because weight is one of the modifiable risk factors for endometrial cancer, lowering the body mass index in patients at risk for developing endometrial cancer is a good method of primary prevention.

Answer A is incorrect. Alcoholism has little relation to endometrial cancer, but is strongly associated with chronic pancreatitis, pancreatic adenocarcinoma, and cirrhosis of the liver. Smoking is also a risk factor for these conditions, but tobacco use is actually protective against endometrial cancer to a certain extent.

Answer B is incorrect. Early sexual activity has little relation to endometrial cancer but is a major risk factor for cervical cancer. Other risk factors for cervical cancer include multiple sex partners, human papillomavirus infection, coinfection with other sexually transmitted diseases, smoking, and low socioeconomic status.

Answer D is incorrect. Nulliparity (not multiparity) is a risk factor for endometrial cancer. Multiparity protects against endometrial cancer, because it gives the endometrium a "resting period" in which it is not actively proliferating through the menstrual cycle. By the same logic, menopause occurring at or after 53 years of age would put the patient at increased risk because of an increased amount of endometrial active proliferation.

Answer E is incorrect. Although progesterone has a protective effect, estrogen-progesterone synthetic birth control products have not shown any benefit in reducing the incidence of endometrial cancer.

16. **The correct answer is D.** The firm prostate nodules and weight loss suggest prostate cancer. The prostate-specific antigen level is typically elevated in prostate cancer. Calcium levels should be low because calcium is being used to build new bone in the areas of metastases. The alkaline phosphatase level should be increased because this is a marker of bone formation.

Answer A is incorrect. Prostate-specific antigen should be elevated in prostate cancer, and the alkaline phosphatase level should be high.

Answer B is incorrect. Prostate-specific antigen should be elevated in prostate cancer.

Answer C is incorrect. In prostate cancer, because bone is being made, the alkaline phosphatase level should increase.

Answer E is incorrect. The calcium level should be low in prostate cancer because it is being used to make new bone. The alkaline phosphatase level should be elevated as a marker of bone formation.

17. **The correct answer is D.** Combining an erectile dysfunction medication such as sildenafil with a nitrate can lead to severe hypotension. Formation and maintenance of an erection requires both nitric oxide (NO) and cGMP. These mediate increased arterial blood flow and pressure in the corpora cavernosa and corpus spongiosum such that the penile venous outflow becomes obstructed. NO acts as a local neurotransmitter that relaxes trabeculae within the corpora cavernosa and allows maximal engorgement. It also activates guanylyl cyclase to promote the formation of cGMP, which is necessary for vasodilation. Sildenafil and other emergency department medications belong to a class called phosphodiesterase-5 (PDE-5) inhibitors. PDE-5 metabolizes cGMP and prevents NO-induced vasodilation. Sildenafil and other PDE-5 inhibitors prevent this metabolism, thereby increasing the level of cGMP and permitting the maintenance of an erection. Nitrates that are used intermittently for angina are contraindicated within 24 hours of the ingestion of sildenafil because the two drugs act by a similar mechanism. Nitrates are metabolized to NO and nitrosothiols, which activate guanylyl cyclase to produce cGMP and cause vasodilation. When combined, severe hypotension can ensue because blood pressure may drop by as much as 50/25 mm Hg.

Answer A is incorrect. Sildenafil is a drug that inhibits PDE-5, thus causing increased levels of cGMP; this drug has no action on sodium channels.

Answer B is incorrect. PDE-5 metabolizes cGMP and prevents NO-induced vasodilation. Sildenafil and other PDE-5 inhibitors prevent this metabolism, thereby increasing (not decreasing) the level of cGMP.

Answer C is incorrect. Sildenafil and other PDE-5 inhibitors do not directly affect the level of NO; rather, they enhance the effect of NO by increasing levels of cGMP.

Answer E is incorrect. PDE-5 inhibitors such as sildenafil prevent the degradation of cGMP, thus enhancing the effect of NO. However, NO levels are not increased by sildenafil.

18. **The correct answer is C.** Postpartum major depression (PMD) occurs in 10% of women after the birth of a child, and begins anywhere from 24 hours to several months after delivery. Symptoms of postpartum depression (PPD) are identical to the *Diagnostic and Statistical Manual of Mental Disorders*, Fourth Edition, Text Revision (DSM-IV-TR) symptoms for major depression, which can be recalled using the mnemonic **SIGECAPS**: **S**leep disturbances, loss of **I**nterest, **G**uilt, loss of **E**nergy, difficulty with **C**oncentration, loss of **A**ppetite, **P**sychomotor agitation or retardation, and **S**uicidal ideation. PMD can be difficult to diagnose because many symptoms can be confused with normal sequelae of labor and delivery.

Answer A is incorrect. Hemorrhage may cause iron deficiency anemia, which may present with a picture similar to that of major depression. Psychiatric diseases normally require that medical conditions with overlapping symptomatology have been excluded before the diagnosis is made. The patient's prominent psychiatric symptoms and normal hemoglobin rule out iron deficiency anemia as a cause of her illness.

Answer B is incorrect. Twenty-five to 85% of women experience minor mood fluctuations after delivery. These "postpartum blues" tend to peak around day five postpartum and resolve by day 10. Persistence of symptoms beyond postpartum day 10 warrants further investigation. Postpartum blues is a risk factor for the development of PMD.

Answer D is incorrect. Less than 0.5% of child-bearing women experience postpartum psychosis, usually within one month of delivery. It is characterized by a manic-like episode of agitation, expansive or irritable mood, no sleep for several nights, and avoidance of the infant. Delusions and hallucinations are present and often involve the baby (eg, command hallucinations to harm the infant).

Answer E is incorrect. The most common presentation of postpartum hypopituitarism (Sheehan syndrome) is failure to lactate, and it is caused by severe puerperal hemorrhage. Eventually the patient experiences the symptoms of hypothyroidism (fatigue, constipation, and non-resumption of menses), and hypoadrenalism (hyponatremia and hyperkalemia due to decreased aldosterone, and loss of pubic and axillary hair because androgens in women are produced in the adrenal cortex).

19. **The correct answer is A.** This patient is presenting with Sheehan syndrome or postpartum pituitary necrosis, caused by hemorrhage during delivery. Risk factors include pregnancy with multiples (twins or triplets) and abnormalities of the placenta. Peripartum hemorrhage predisposes the already enlarged pituitary to ischemia, leading to necrosis of parts of the anterior and/or posterior pituitary. The most common clinical feature of Sheehan syndrome is an inability to lactate, caused by damage to the anterior pituitary and decreased prolactin production. Other symptoms include those associated with hypothyroidism (as seen by the patient's cold intolerance), along with central diabetes insipidus (DI) caused by decreased production of ADH. DI presents with polyuria and dilute urine in the presence of elevated serum sodium levels. Decreased FSH and LH levels often lead to amenorrhea and scant pubic and axillary hair growth. Treatment involves lifelong hormone replacement therapy of all deficient hormones, along with estrogen and progesterone supplementation.

Answer B is incorrect. Alcohol intake during pregnancy is not associated with any of the symptoms seen in this patient. Instead, it is associated with growth and developmental defects in the offspring, such as microcephaly, facial dysmorphism, and malformations of the brain, cardiovascular system, and genitourinary system. Fetal alcohol syndrome is the leading cause of mental retardation and is easily preventable by maternal abstinence from alcohol during pregnancy.

Answer C is incorrect. Endometriosis is a common condition characterized by growth of ectopic endometrial tissue outside the uterus. It generally presents in women 20-40 years old, but its pathogenesis is poorly understood. Although its clinical presentation varies, endometriosis can present with pelvic pain associated with the menstrual cycle, dysmenorrhea, and dyspareunia, or it can be asymptomatic. Endometriosis is a risk factor for ectopic pregnancy and infertility, and many women who have endometriosis first present with problems getting pregnant. It is not associated with Sheehan syndrome.

Answer D is incorrect. Gestational diabetes is a form of diabetes that is present during pregnancy and is often transient, although overt nongestational diabetes may later develop. Gestational diabetes is associated with increased fetal birth weight, increased fetal mortality, and increased incidence of neonatal respiratory distress syndrome. In addition, increased fetal insulin levels created in response to maternal glucose levels can cause a hypoglycemic crisis after birth, when the maternal supply of glucose is no longer present. Gestational diabetes is not a known risk factor for Sheehan syndrome and would not cause this patient to present with the symptoms seen.

Answer E is incorrect. Incorrect use of tampons is associated with toxic shock syndrome (TSS), originally associated with the use of highly absorbent tampons left in the vagina for long periods of time. TSS is caused by an exotoxin produced by *Staphylococcus aureus*, which grows on the tampon. This toxin is a superantigen that allows nonspecific binding of MHC class II with T-lymphocyte receptors, resulting in polyclonal T-lymphocyte activation and systemic symptoms. TSS generally presents acutely with fever, hypotension, and desquamation of the palms and soles, nausea, vomiting, and diarrhea.

Answer F is incorrect. Having multiple sexual partners is associated with an increased risk of various sexually transmitted diseases (STDs), including HIV and human papillomavirus, the virus associated with cervical cancer. STDs present with various symptoms depending on the underlying infectious agent, but none would cause the symptoms seen in this patient.

Answer G is incorrect. PID is most commonly caused by infection with *Chlamydia trachomatis* or *Neisseria gonorrhea*, the latter presenting more acutely. Symptoms include fever, cervical motion tenderness, lower abdominal pain, and painful intercourse, although PID is often asymptomatic. Treatment of the underlying cause is important because PID is a risk factor for ectopic pregnancy and infertility. It is not associated with Sheehan syndrome.

20. **The correct answer is B.** The *SRY* (sex-determining region on Y) gene on the Y chromosome encodes a transcription factor called testis-determining factor. This transcription factor binds DNA, inducing a pattern of gene expression that ultimately results in development of the testes from indifferent gonads. The testes secrete both testosterone and müllerian-inhibiting factor, triggering a sequence of changes that give rise to a male phenotype. Without a functional *SRY* gene (as one might see in the setting of a nonsense mutation), this process is derailed, and the fetus will progress along the default pathway of sexual development (that of a female). The mesonephric (Wolffian) ducts will regress spontaneously, and the paramesonephric ducts will develop as they normally do in females. Such individuals will be born with a female phenotype, and they may not have any symptoms until puberty, at which point they often present with primary amenorrhea. These women may have other abnormalities including underdevelopment of both breasts and the internal female reproductive organs. Mutations in the *SRY* gene lead to XY females with gonadal dysgenesis, also known as Swyer syndrome.

Answer A is incorrect. The mesonephric (Wolffian) duct develops into the internal male genitalia that connect the testes to the prostate. Exposure to testosterone, produced by Leydig cells, during embryogenesis is critical to proper development.

Answer C is incorrect. Development of external male genitalia is controlled most directly by DHT. Insufficient levels of DHT results in male pseudohermaphroditism, where the individual has internal male genitalia but are female externally. One cause is a deficiency in 5α-reductase, the enzyme responsible for producing DHT from testosterone. Other causes leading to a male pseudohermaphrodite include partial androgen insensitivity and defects in testosterone production.

Answer D is incorrect. Development of the urogenital sinus into the prostate gland is controlled most directly by DHT. In the presence of estrogen and absence of DHT, the urogenital sinus develops into the urethral and paraurethral glands (Skene glands) instead.

Answer E is incorrect. The involution of paramesonephric (müllerian) ducts is controlled by the presence of müllerian-inhibiting factor, produced by Sertoli cells. In the female they develop to form the fallopian tubes, the uterus, and the upper portion of the vagina.

21. **The correct answer is E.** Oxytocin is a polypeptide hormone that is responsible for the dilation of the cervix and contraction of the uterus during labor, as well as the let down of milk during breastfeeding. When labor is arrested, a synthetic analog may be applied topically onto the cervix to facilitate dilation. Endogenously, oxytocin is produced in the cell bodies of hypothalamic neurons in the paraventricular nucleus. After synthesis, it is stored in terminal swellings of these neurons in the posterior pituitary, known as herring bodies.

Answer A is incorrect. The adrenal cortex mediates the production and release of hormones related to the stress response as well as sexual development. It is divided into three layers: (from superficial to deep) zona glomerulosa, which produces mineralocorticoids such as aldosterone; zona fasciculata, which produces glucocorticoids such as cortisol; and zona reticularis, which produces androgens. The adrenal cortex is not responsible for the storage of oxytocin.

Answer B is incorrect. Whereas secretion of hormones from the posterior pituitary is controlled by neurons in the hypothalamus, the anterior pituitary is a glandular secretory organ that receives releasing/inhibiting factors via a capillary plexus that connects it with the hypothalamus. Hormones released by the anterior pituitary include ACTH, thyroid-stimulating hormone, FSH, LH, growth hormone, and prolactin.

Answer C is incorrect. Oxytocin is produced, not stored, in the cell bodies in the paraventricular nucleus of the hypothalamus.

Answer D is incorrect. Oxytocin acts at receptors in the mammary glands to induce milk let down in breastfeeding mothers. Stimulation of the nipple will trigger the release of oxytocin from the posterior pituitary. Oxytocin is not stored in the mammary glands themselves.

22. **The correct answer is B.** *Chlamydia trachomatis* infection causes urethritis, cervicitis, and PID in women, as well as conjunctivitis and Reiter syndrome, although it is frequently asymptomatic. Cytoplasmic inclusions can be seen on Giemsa- or fluorescent antibody-stained urethral or cervical smear, but diagnosis can also be made from a urine sample using nucleic acid amplification techniques. Treatment of *Chlamydia* infection requires a course of either doxycycline or erythromycin. The extracellular elementary body is the infectious form of *Chlamydia* as it can attach to host cells and enter them.

Answer A is incorrect. The cytoplasmic inclusions are collections of elementary bodies in the host cell before their release. Because they are intracellular, they are not infectious.

Answer C is incorrect. The intracellular elementary body does not have access to host cells, and therefore is not infectious.

Answer D is incorrect. The multiplication of reticulate bodies is an important step in the reproduction of *Chlamydia*. Because this process is intracellular, however, it is not an infectious step in the life cycle of this bacterium.

Answer E is incorrect. The reticulate body is solely intracellular. This is the stage in which the bacteria replicate within the cell.

23. **The correct answer is E.** Trastuzumab is a monoclonal antibody against human epidermal growth factor receptor 2 (HER2) that can kill breast cancer cells over-expressing HER2. This patient's breast cancer is positive for HER2/neu receptor, thus she is likely to have a positive response to the chemotherapeutic agent trastuzumab.

Answer A is incorrect. Bevacizumab, like all drugs ending in "mab," is a monoclonal antibody. This drug binds to vascular endothelial growth factor, a cytokine frequently produced by cancer cells to promote angiogenesis. It was approved by the Food and Drug Administration in 2004 to treat metastatic colon cancer and non-small cell lung cancer. It also has been used off-label by ophthalmologists to slow the progression of macular degeneration and diabetic retinopathy, diseases that occur through abnormal proliferation of blood vessels in the eye. It is not indicated for the treatment of breast cancer.

Answer B is incorrect. Cyclophosphamide is an alkylating agent that cross-links DNA, leading to apoptosis. Cyclophosphamide is commonly used to treat non-Hodgkin lymphoma and breast/ovarian cancer, but is not specifically targeted to a HER2/neu receptor-positive tumor.

Answer C is incorrect. Doxorubicin is an antitumor antibiotic commonly used to treat breast cancer. It acts by intercalation into DNA, inhibiting topoisomerase II and resulting in DNA damage and cell death. Doxorubicin is associated with congestive heart failure. Doxorubicin might be helpful for this patient, but is not specifically targeted to an HER2/neu receptor-positive tumor.

Answer D is incorrect. Tamoxifen as a chemotherapeutic agent is useful only in estrogen receptor-positive breast cancer. It is a selective estrogen receptor modulator with estrogen receptor antagonist effects whose mechanism of action relies on binding, and thereby blocking, estrogen receptors to impede the production of estrogen-responsive genes. Tamoxifen is not useful in a breast cancer that is negative for estrogen receptor.

24. **The correct answer is A.** Abruptio placentae typically presents as bleeding along with uterine contractions and pain due to premature separation of the placenta from the uterus, despite its implantation in a normal location. It is caused most often by a rupture of defective maternal vessels in the decidua basalis. This patient is at high risk for abruptio placentae because of her known hypertension and cocaine use. Other risk factors include short umbilical cord, trauma, prior abruption, cigarette smoking, uterine fibroids, advanced age, sudden uterine decompression, preterm premature rupture of the membranes, and a bleeding diathesis. Whereas ultrasound can reveal abruptio placentae, it is not very sensitive and will be positive in only 25% of cases of abruption confirmed at delivery.

    Answer B is incorrect. Concealed abruption refers to abruptio placentae that occurs near the center of the placenta. By definition, there is no external bleeding because the blood forms a hematoma that is hidden behind the placenta. Thus this case cannot represent a concealed abruption.

    Answer C is incorrect. Labor is defined as regular uterine contractions that result in cervical change. This patient does not describe contractions at regular intervals, but rather a constant pain with intermittent cramping. In addition, her cervix remains closed, so she has not started labor.

    Answer D is incorrect. Placenta accreta refers to the abnormally strong adherence of the placenta to the uterine wall. This happens because the placental villi attach directly to the myometrium as a result of a defect in the decidua basalis layer. Placenta accreta manifests as incomplete separation of the placenta after delivery and can result in severe postpartum hemorrhage. Risk factors include placenta previa, prior cesarean delivery, and prior intrauterine manipulation or surgery. The most common setting for accreta involves a placenta previa after a prior cesarean delivery.

    Answer E is incorrect. Placenta previa occurs when the placenta overlies the internal cervical os. The distinction between placenta previa and abruptio placentae is classically made based on the presence (abruptio placentae) or absence (placenta previa) of pain.

25. **The correct answer is E.** Androgenic steroids are used to treat hypogonadism either due to failure of the hypothalamic-pituitary-gonadal axis (secondary hypogonadism) or due to Leydig cell dysfunction (primary hypogonadism). Patients should be warned that androgens cause premature closing of the epiphyseal plates by promoting calcium deposition in the bones.

    Answer A is incorrect. Androgenic steroids can cause polycythemia rather than anemia. This adverse affect is another risk factor for premature coronary artery disease and thrombosis.

    Answer B is incorrect. Some androgenic steroids increase, rather than decrease, LDL cholesterol levels. The lipid profile disturbance increases the possibility of atherosclerotic change and raises the risk of early coronary artery disease.

    Answer C is incorrect. Excess androgens can cause decreased spermatogenesis by downregulating GnRH. Decreased GnRH causes decreased release of LH and FSH, which are necessary for spermatogenesis.

    Answer D is incorrect. A serious adverse reaction to some androgens is not leukocytosis, but rather leukopenia because of decreased marrow production or decreased WBC survival.

26. **The correct answer is B.** A decreased α-fetoprotein (AFP) level indicates that this fetus may develop Down syndrome due to trisomy of chromosome 21. (Remember the phrase: "AFP goes down in Down syndrome.") Individuals with Down syndrome have excessive skin at the nape of the neck, upslanting palpebral fissures, and epicanthic folds, among other characteristic features. In addition, it is associ-

ated with multiple congenital anomalies including ventricular septal defects (VSDs), endocardial cushion defects, and omphalocele. Cardiac disease is an important cause of death in these patients.

Answer A is incorrect. Coarctation of the aorta is a characteristic defect in Turner syndrome, caused by a 45,XO genotype. Additional defects include ovarian dysgenesis and horseshoe kidney. Turner syndrome is diagnosed on karyotyping, rather than by the triple screen.

Answer C is incorrect. Deletion of 5p causes cri-du-chat syndrome. These patients demonstrate hypotonia, downslanting of the lateral portion of the palpebral fissures, and microcephaly.

Answer D is incorrect. A prominent occiput is a sign of Edwards syndrome, due to trisomy 18. This syndrome can affect nearly any organ system, with hypertonia, micrognathia, and VSDs being common signs. More than 90% of these children do not survive past 12 months, and those who do are severely mentally retarded.

Answer E is incorrect. This choice describes spina bifida occulta, a specific type of neural tube defect. Neural tube defects are characterized by an increased AFP level in the triple screen and are dramatically reduced in frequency by maternal intake of folate during pregnancy.

27. **The correct answer is E.** The ureters are muscular ducts with narrow lumina that carry urine from the kidneys to the urinary bladder. These retroperitoneal structures cross the external iliac artery just beyond the bifurcation of the common iliac artery and pass under the ductus deferens and testicular vessels ("water under the bridge").

Answer A is incorrect. Efferent ductules transport sperm from the rete testis to the epididymis, where they are stored. The tail of the epididymis is continuous with the ductus deferens, the next sperm destination during ejaculation. The efferent ductules are located inferior, not posterior, to the ductus.

Answer B is incorrect. The spermatic cord contains the ductus deferens, testicular artery, pampiniform plexus, and lymphatic vessels. It does not cross posterior to ductus deferens.

Answer C is incorrect. Sympathetic nerve fibers are constituents of the spermatic cord that run with the testicular arteries. They run parallel to the ductus deferens but do not cross posteriorly.

Answer D is incorrect. The testicular artery arises from the aorta and supplies the testis and epididymis. It runs parallel to, but does not cross, the ductus deferens to enter the spermatic cord. The testicular artery crosses the ureter.

28. **The correct answer is C.** This patient most likely suffers from osteoporosis, or weakened bones, as a complication of menopause. Estrogen regulates bone resorption, maintaining proper bone mass in women. At menopause, estrogen production ceases due to a decreased number of ovarian follicles. The reduction in estrogen results in increased bone resorption. Along with low estrogen levels, postmenopausal women have high levels of LH, FSH, and GnRH due to the lack of negative feedback of estrogen on the anterior pituitary gland and hypothalamus.

Answer A is incorrect. While estrogen levels are indeed low in postmenopausal women, levels of LH and FSH are high due to the lack of negative feedback on the anterior pituitary. This profile suggests that the problem is in the anterior pituitary, which is receiving GnRH stimulation but is unable to produce enough LH and FSH to stimulate the ovaries. Menopause, however, is a primary dysfunction of estrogen production in the ovaries, with a normally functioning anterior pituitary gland.

Answer B is incorrect. While estrogen levels are indeed low in postmenopausal women, LH, FSH, and GnRH levels are high due to the lack of negative feedback on the anterior pituitary and hypothalamus. This profile suggests a problem in the hypothalamus, resulting in low GnRH, which leads to suboptimal stimulation of the anterior pituitary causing low FSH and LH. The low FSH and LH levels cause decreased stimulation of the ovaries, resulting in low estrogen levels. Menopause, however, is a primary dysfunction of estrogen production in the ovaries, with a normally functioning anterior pituitary gland.

Answer D is incorrect. Menopause is a primary dysfunction of estrogen production in the ovaries. Thus estrogen levels are low in postmenopausal women.

Answer E is incorrect. Menopause is a primary dysfunction of estrogen production in the ovaries. Thus estrogen levels are low in postmenopausal women.

29. **The correct answer is E.** Ketoconazole is an antifungal drug used to treat tinea corporis that acts by blocking the formation of fungal membrane sterols. It also has an endocrine effect because it blocks the enzyme desmolase/CYP-450scc, which is necessary for adrenal production of testosterone and cortisol from cholesterol. Free cortisol is responsible for feedback inhibition of the *POMC* gene, which codes for synthesis of ACTH, lipotropin, melanocyte-stimulating hormone, and some endogenous endorphins. Without desmolase activity to create cortisol, this feedback inhibition is removed and thus the *POMC* gene products are freely transcribed. Excessive melanocyte-stimulating hormone can cause increased integumentary pigmentation such as in patients with Addison disease. Other endocrine effects include decreased libido, impotence, and gynecomastia in men.

Answer A is incorrect. Amphotericin B is an antifungal drug used to treat systemic mycoses. It acts by disrupting fungal wall synthesis by binding to ergosterol (a component of the cell wall). Adverse effects include fever and chills, decreased creatinine clearance, hypotension, and anemia.

Answer B is incorrect. Fluconazole is an antifungal drug with the same mechanism of action as ketoconazole, but without the endocrine side effects. It has good penetration into the cerebrospinal fluid and is used to treat *Cryptococcus neoformans*. Adverse effects include nausea and vomiting.

Answer C is incorrect. Flucytosine is an antifungal drug used solely in combination with amphotericin B to treat systemic *Cryptococcus neoformans* and systemic *Candida*. Adverse effects include pancytopenia, elevated liver enzyme levels, nausea, and vomiting.

Answer D is incorrect. Itraconazole is an antifungal that lacks the endocrine effects of ketoconazole. It is used to treat blastomycosis and AIDS-associated histoplasmosis. Adverse effects include nausea and vomiting, as well as rash in immunocompromised patients.

30. **The correct answer is E.** The history of inguinal hernia repair strongly suggests an obstructive abnormality of the vas deferens, leading to disordered sperm transport. The vas deferens can be ligated accidentally during hernia repair, or scar tissue can make passage of the sperm through the vas deferens impossible. In the case of vas deferens obstruction, the semen volume will be low with decreased or absent sperm. In these cases testicular biopsy can confirm normal sperm production, and sperm can be collected for intracytoplasmic sperm injection with in vitro fertilization.

Answer A is incorrect. Like excessive alcohol intake, heavy marijuana smoking has been associated with decreased sperm production in men. In this particular case, however, sperm production appears to be normal. Sperm transport abnormalities appear to be causing this man's infertility.

Answer B is incorrect. Although vas deferens obstruction usually causes semen volumes to decrease, it is not the decreased semen volume itself that has produced this patient's primary infertility but the obstructive azoospermia caused by his prior inguinal hernia repair.

Answer C is incorrect. Alcoholic beverage ingestion that exceeds two drinks/day has been associated with decreased sperm production in men. In this particular case, however, sperm production appears to be normal. It is the impairment in sperm transport that appears to be causing this man's infertility.

Answer D is incorrect. Hypercholesterolemia never has been shown to be associated with dysfunctional sperm transportation.

31. **The correct answer is D.** *Serratia* is a common cause of nosocomial urinary tract infections, along with *E coli*, *Proteus*, *Klebsiella* and *Pseudomonas*. Some strains produce a red pigment. Nosocomial infections generally are more resistant than community acquired infections. *Serratia* is a gram-negative, facultatively anaerobic bacillus.

    Answer A is incorrect. *Escherichia coli* is the number-one cause of urinary tract infections in ambulatory patients, accounting for about 80% of patients without catheters, urologic abnormalities, or calculi. *E coli* is not associated with red pigmentation.

    Answer B is incorrect. *Klebsiella* species are common etiologic agents of urinary tract infection that predispose to stone formation through the production of extracellular slime and polysaccharide, and are frequently found in patients with calculi. Urease-positive bacteria such as *Klebsiella* and *Proteus* species can form ammonium magnesium phosphate (struvite) stones that can be a nidus for future recurrent infections. *Klebsiella* is not associated with red pigmentation.

    Answer C is incorrect. *Proteus mirabilis* predisposes to stone formation because of its urease production, and is found more frequently in patients with calculi. *Proteus* is a gram-negative, facultatively anaerobic, urease-positive bacillus. *Proteus* is not associated with red pigmentation.

    Answer E is incorrect. *Staphylococcus saprophyticus* is the second most common cause of urinary tract infection in young ambulatory women (10-15%). *S saprophyticus* is coagulase negative and resistance to novobiocin.

32. **The correct answer is B.** A blood-filled cyst (a so-called chocolate cyst) is characteristic of endometriosis, a condition that results in non-neoplastic endometrial glands/stroma being abnormally located outside the endometrial cavity. The ovary and the pelvic peritoneum are the most common sites. The cysts are formed during cyclic bleeding from the tissue, mimicking menstruation. Severe menstrual-related pain (dysmenorrhea), pain during sexual intercourse (dyspareunia), and infertility are possible complications of endometriosis.

    Answer A is incorrect. Common cancers in the reproductive tract include endometrial carcinoma, which can arise from endometrial hyperplasia caused by excess estrogen stimulation, and cervical carcinoma, associated with human papillomavirus infection. Endometriosis does not progress to cancer.

    Answer C is incorrect. Autosomal dominant (adult) polycystic kidney disease (ADPKD) is characterized by bilaterally enlarged kidneys with multiple cysts. Cysts can also involve the liver, pancreas, heart, and brain. This disease manifests as renal abnormalities that progresses to end stage renal disease. In patients with ADPKD there is usually a family history, bilateral involvement, and constant pain that does not wax and wane in conjunction with menstrual cycles. Another manifestation of ADPKD is the emergence of intracranial berry aneurysms that can rupture and produce intracranial hemorrhage. Endometriosis is not associated with ADPKD.

    Answer D is incorrect. Polycystic ovarian syndrome (PCOS or Stein-Leventhal syndrome) has many causes. The main characteristics of PCOS are irregular or anovulation and hyperandrogenism. Features seen in PCOS include ovarian cysts, amenorrhea, infertility, obesity, and hirsutism caused by excess LH and androgens. In some women this is associated with insulin resistance and hyperinsulinemia, which increases androgen production in the ovarian theca cells and, secondarily, LH production. The insulin resistance also leads to hyperglycemia and suppresses hepatic steroid hormone binding globulin (SHBG) synthesis. The decrease in SHBG along with the increase in androgen production leads to a vicious cycle of amenorrhea and infertility. Endometriosis is not associated with masculinization and PCOS.

Answer E is incorrect. Endometriosis is not associated with obesity.

33. **The correct answer is E.** Krukenberg tumors are stomach cancer metastases to the ovaries that are described as mucin-secreting "signet-ring" cells. Stomach cancer is often adenocarcinoma that can spread aggressively to lymph nodes and the liver. A classic sign of metastatic stomach cancer is involvement of the left supraclavicular lymph node, called Virchow node. Involvement is on the left side because the thoracic duct drains all structures on the left in the thoracic cavity and all structures below the diaphragm on both sides.

Answer A is incorrect. Galactorrhea is leakage from the breasts that is not associated with normal lactation but is associated with elevated prolactin levels secondary to prolactinomas in the anterior pituitary. Prolactin stimulates breast development and milk production while also inhibiting ovulation and spermatogenesis by inhibiting the release of GnRH and subsequently suppressing LH and FSH. Galactorrhea is not associated with stomach or ovarian cancers. Prolactinomas rarely metastasize.

Answer B is incorrect. Hematochezia is bright red, bloody stool and is often an early sign of colorectal carcinoma. Risk factors for colorectal carcinoma include villous adenomas, inflammatory bowel disease, low-fiber diet, familial adenomatous polyposis, hereditary nonpolyposis colorectal cancer, and a positive family history. Hematochezia is not associated with stomach or ovarian cancers. Colorectal carcinomas usually metastasize to the liver.

Answer C is incorrect. A palpable gallbladder (Courvoisier sign) is associated with pancreatic duct obstruction secondary to pancreatic adenocarcinoma. Other signs and symptoms of pancreatic cancer include abdominal pain radiating to the subscapular area, weight loss, anorexia, and migratory thrombophlebitis (Trousseau syndrome). A palpable gallbladder is not associated with stomach or ovarian cancers.

Answer D is incorrect. Basal cell carcinoma (BCC) often presents as "pearly papules" on sun-exposed areas, such as the face and arms. Papules are not associated with stomach or ovarian cancers. BCC is locally invasive but almost never metastasizes.

34. **The correct answer is E.** The history is suspicious for the prodrome of an HSV outbreak. The pathology procedure in the vignette describes a Tzanck stain, which was positive for multinucleated giant cells, suggesting an active HSV infection. Herpes simplex virus (HSV) is an enveloped virus with a double-stranded linear DNA genome. After the primary outbreak, HSV travels in a retrograde fashion along the axon via microtubular-dependent transport to the neuronal cell body and remains latent in dorsal root ganglia. Over time, the virus can be reactivated, causing recurrent outbreaks that are usually less severe in symptoms, duration, and viral shedding than the primary infection.

Answer A is incorrect. HSV can disseminate and cause systemic illness; however, it is very unlikely in immunocompetent individuals.

Answer B is incorrect. HSV does not produce an exotoxin. Exotoxins are important in the pathogenesis of some bacteria, such as *Campylobacter jejuni*, some *Staphylococcus* infections, and some group A streptococcal infections.

Answer C is incorrect. HSV does not infect CD4+ cells. This is characteristic of HIV, which can initially present with an acute illness with symptoms that resemble infectious mononucleosis. This is usually followed by complete resolution of symptoms followed by an asymptomatic carrier state, which can last many years before infection with AIDS-defining pathogens occurs.

Answer D is incorrect. After the primary outbreak of genital herpes, HSV travels via retrograde, not anterograde, transport along neuronal axons to the cell bodies of the peripheral nerves, where it remains latent until reactivation.

35. **The correct answer is C.** This boy likely has a seminoma. Seminomas are the most common testicular neoplasm in young men (ages 15-35), and they present without pain as in this case. Histologically, seminomas are characterized by large cells in lobules, a watery cytoplasm, and a "fried egg" appearance.

Answer A is incorrect. This describes an embryonal carcinoma. These lesions are typically painful.

Answer B is incorrect. Cowdry type A nuclear inclusions are associated with cytomegalovirus infection rather than a testicular neoplasm.

Answer D is incorrect. Reinke crystals are commonly seen with Leydig cell tumors. These lesions usually produce androgens, resulting in gynecomastia in men or precocious puberty in boys. Additionally, they are a nongerm cell tumor.

Answer E is incorrect. Yolk sac tumors have structures resembling primitive glomeruli. They are called Schiller-Duval bodies.

36. **The correct answer is C.** This patient has polycystic ovarian syndrome. It consists of a constellation of findings, including enlarged polycystic ovaries, anovulation, oligomenorrhea or amenorrhea, obesity, and hirsutism.

Answer A is incorrect. Patients with polycystic ovarian syndrome are anovulatory, so they have elevated estrogen and testosterone levels.

Answer B is incorrect. Epicanthal folds are associated with several congenital genetic abnormalities, including Down syndrome, but they are not associated with polycystic ovarian syndrome.

Answer D is incorrect. Polycystic ovarian syndrome is not associated with increased bleeding time.

Answer E is incorrect. Ovulatory dysfunction in patients with polycystic ovarian syndrome typically results in infertility and the need to induce ovulation with agents such as clomiphene in order to conceive.

37. **The correct answer is E.** A Tzanck test is a smear of an opened skin lesion to detect multinucleated giant cells and assay for the HSV. The Tzanck test can detect HSV-1 and -2 and the varicella-zoster virus. Epidermal cells in the vesicles sometimes develop eosinophilic intranuclear viral inclusions, or several cells may fuse to produce giant cells (multinucleate polykaryons), changes that are demonstrated by the diagnostic Tzanck test based on microscopic evaluation of the vesicle fluid. The vesicles usually clear within three-four weeks, but the virus travels along the regional nerves and becomes dormant in the local ganglia.

Answer A is incorrect. Auer rods are rod-shaped bodies in myeloid cells. They are found in acute myelogenous leukemia (AML). They represent abnormal azurophilic granules and are particularly numerous in AML associated with the t(15;17) translocation.

Answer B is incorrect. Call-Exner bodies are spaces between granulosa cells in ovarian follicles and in granulosa cell tumors.

Answer C is incorrect. Lewy bodies are abnormal aggregates of protein that develop inside nerve cells. On microscopy of affected brain tissue, these spherical masses displace other cell components. The main disease associated with the presence of Lewy bodies is Parkinson disease. Lewy bodies also are present in patients with dementia

Answer D is incorrect. Mallory bodies are eosinophilic intracytoplasmic inclusions found in hepatic cells and seen in a variety of diseases, including alcoholic liver disease.

38. **The correct answer is C.** This patient has placenta previa, or the attachment of the placenta to the lower uterine segment, often occluding the internal cervical os. Placenta previa typically presents with painless vaginal bleeding after 20 weeks' gestation. Risk factors include history of a prior cesarean section delivery, increased number of prior pregnancies, and history of prior curettage (scraping of the uterine lining to remove fetal and placental tissue) for spontaneous or elective abortion.

Answer A is incorrect. A history of endometriosis may lead to increased risk of infertility and epithelial ovarian cancer, but it does not increase a patient's risk for placenta previa.

Answer B is incorrect. History of pelvic inflammatory disease leads to increased risk of ectopic pregnancy, but does not increase a patient's risk for placenta previa.

Answer D is incorrect. History of a prior ectopic pregnancy leads to increased risk of future ectopic pregnancies, but does not increase a patient's risk for placenta previa.

Answer E is incorrect. Use of assisted reproductive technologies leads to increased risk for multiple gestations, but does not increase a patient's risk for placenta previa.

39. **The correct answer is D.** Although genetically different from the moment of conception, male and female differentiation does not begin until around the eighth week of development, when the gonads secrete hormones that influence the development of either the paramesonephric ducts in the female or the mesonephric ducts in the male. In the absence of the testis-determining factor located on the Y chromosome, the mesonephric ducts begin to degenerate and form a matrix for the developing paramesonephric ducts. The paramesonephric ducts fuse at their inferior margin, forming the single lumen of the uterovaginal canal. Failure of complete fusion of these ducts can result in a bicornuate uterus, as shown in the image. This anatomic variation is associated with recurrent pregnancy loss.

Answer A is incorrect. Complete failure of fusion of the paramesonephric (müllerian) ducts leads to uterus didelphys, in which there are two separate uterine cavities that each have a cervix and vagina.

Answer B is incorrect. Failure of resorption of the midline uterine septum results in a septate or arcuate uterus.

Answer C is incorrect. Diethylstilbestrol (DES) is a synthetic nonsteroidal estrogenic compound given to women in the mid-1900s for a variety of indications, including the prevention of spontaneous abortions in pregnant women. However, it was later found to be a teratogen, as it causes a variety of structural changes of the cervix of female fetuses in utero and predisposes them to adenocarcinoma of the vagina as young women. Bicornuate uterus is not associated with DES exposure.

40. **The correct answer is E.** A positive transillumination test suggests that this child has a cystic mass, and a testicular hydrocele is one of the most common causes of painless scrotal enlargement in newborns. It is composed of a collection of serous fluid between the parietal and visceral layers of the tunica vaginalis. Most cases are idiopathic.

Answer A is incorrect. Fluid here would suggest orchitis, which is testicular inflammation typically caused by viral (especially mumps and rubella) or bacterial infection. Pain, tenderness, and erythema of the overlying skin would typically be seen.

Answer B is incorrect. Fluid here would suggest epididymitis, which is inflammation of the epididymis. Typical causes of this infection are *Chlamydia*, *Neisseria gonorrhoeae*, and *Escherichia coli*. Pain is usually present, along with urinary frequency, dysuria, and urethral discharge.

Answer C is incorrect. This is typically seen in elephantiasis as a complication of a parasitic filarial infection, which blocks lymphatic drainage and can cause severe swelling.

Answer D is incorrect. This is the location of a varicocele, which is a collection of dilated and tortuous veins in the pampiniform plexus surrounding the spermatic cord in the scrotum. It typically has a "bag of worms" texture on physical examination.

41. **The correct answer is E.** This patient has chancroid, a painful genital ulcer caused by *Haemophilus ducreyi*. Chancroid is relatively uncommon in the United States, but is more common in sub-Saharan Africa and Latin America. Chancroid presents with a painful exudative ulcer with lymphadenitis, and

the most appropriate treatment for this gram-negative organism is single-dose azithromycin.

Answer A is incorrect. A 10-day course of oral acyclovir would be appropriate treatment for genital herpes viral infection. Herpes lesions are also painful, but are commonly multiple, and microscopic examination (Tzanck test) shows multinucleated giant cells with viral inclusion bodies.

Answer B is incorrect. Highly active antiretroviral therapy (HAART) is appropriate treatment for HIV infection in the absence of fulminant concomitant opportunistic infections. Although chancroid and HIV are often found in the same patients, chancroid also frequently occurs in immunocompetent hosts. This particular patient shows no evidence of immunodeficiency, and HAART will not be effective for his penile lesion. However, he is clearly at high risk for HIV infection, and his HIV status should be further discussed.

Answer C is incorrect. Nystatin powder is effective treatment for candidal intertrigo in moist areas such as inguinal folds. Although this patient has inguinal lymphadenopathy, he has no reported skin changes in this area consistent with candidal intertrigo.

Answer D is incorrect. Intramuscular penicillin G is appropriate treatment for syphilis. However, genital ulcers in syphilis are typically painless, and Gram stain is unrevealing.

42. **The correct answer is D.** In a patient with antepartum hemorrhage (hemorrhage after 20 weeks' gestation), the two diagnoses that must be considered first are placental abruption (the cause in 30% of cases of antepartum hemorrhage) and placenta previa (the cause in 20% of cases). Abruptio placentae is premature separation of the placenta, most commonly during the third trimester after week 30 of gestation. It results in painful vaginal bleeding, uterine contractions, and possible fetal death secondary to uteroplacental insufficiency. Risk factors for placental abruption include hypertension, cocaine use, pelvic trauma, uteroplacental insufficiency, submucosal fibroids, cigarette smoking, and preterm premature rupture of membranes. Complications include premature delivery, hyrdrops fetalis, uterine tetany, and hypvolemic shock. In contrast to placenta previa, placental abruption is a clinical diagnosis, because ultrasound is not sensitive for abruption inasmuch as the clot has the same texture as the placenta and is easily missed. In any case, this patient is hemodynamically unstable and there is fetal distress, so an emergency cesarean section is indicated regardless of the underlying diagnosis.

Answer A is incorrect. Pre-eclampsia usually presents during the third trimester of pregnancy with hypertension, proteinuria, and edema. It can also be associated with **HELLP** syndrome (**H**emolysis, **E**levated **L**iver enzyme levels, and **L**ow **P**latelet count). Treatment would be administration of magnesium and delivery of the baby. This patient does not meet all the criteria for pre-eclampsia. A few RBCs in the urine would be normal in a patient with vaginal bleeding.

Answer B is incorrect. Spontaneous delivery is preferable to cesarean section, as it has fewer sequelae for future pregnancies. However, in a setting where the life of both the mother and fetus are threatened, cesarean section's benefits outweigh its risks and should be undertaken immediately.

Answer C is incorrect. FAST assesses for free fluid in the pericardium and abdominal cavity. It is a tool used to look for internal bleeding as may be the case in a ruptured ectopic pregnancy. However, ectopic pregnancies usually become symptomatic within the first few weeks of pregnancy and are hence unlikely in this patient. FAST will most likely produce negative results in this patient, as the bleeding is intrauterine, not extrauterine.

Answer E is incorrect. Amniotic fluid embolism is also referred to as anaphylactoid syndrome of pregnancy and is characterized by hypoxia, respiratory distress, cardiogenic shock, and disseminated intravascular coagulation. It occurs with tearing of maternal vessels and can result in maternal respiratory distress. Unless the clinician is quickly observant, it is usually diagnosed on autopsy. Amniotic fluid embolisms are very rare and occur in about 4/100,000 deliveries. Treatment is usually supportive, and includes emergent cesarean section to reduce maternal oxygen demand and prevent more amniotic fluid from entering maternal circulation

43. **The correct answer is E.** This woman is in the secretory (also called luteal) phase of her menstrual cycle, which occurs after ovulation (approximately day 14 of a typical menstrual cycle) through the end of the cycle. Progesterone increases after ovulation (as it is produced by the corpus luteum) and usually peaks around day 21-22. Progesterone is responsible for the increased glandular production of glycogen and the differentiation and maintenance of the endometrium. The estrogen level is high just prior to ovulation (it induces the LH peak), but falls dramatically around the time of ovulation (when the follicle becomes the corpus luteum). After ovulation the estrogen levels begin to rise again, returning to a relative peak during the luteal phase (around day 21). The high levels of estrogen and progesterone act in negative feedback during the luteal phase, inhibiting the release of FSH and LH. Thus during the secretory phase, progesterone and estrogen levels are high and FSH and LH levels are low due to negative feedback.

    Answer A is incorrect. This combination of hormone changes is seen during the end of the menstrual cycle, when the corpus luteum degenerates. Decreasing progesterone levels initiate the menstrual phase in the endometrium, while low levels of estrogen disinhibit FSH release (ie, a negative feedback mechanism), which is required for the recruitment of follicles to begin a new cycle.

    Answer B is incorrect. This combination is characteristic of the follicular phase of the menstrual cycle, during which estrogen increases slowly due to the maturation of the follicle(s) under the influence of FSH. Estrogen inhibits further FSH release, ultimately allowing a single follicle to develop fully. During this time, progesterone levels are low and stable due to the lack of a corpus luteum, which is responsible for secretion of the hormone later in the cycle.

    Answer C is incorrect. This combination predominates in the days prior to ovulation. During this time, the now mature and sizable ovarian follicle secretes a burst of estrogen that stimulates LH (and FSH) release from the anterior pituitary; thus the feedback mechanism of estrogen on the anterior pituitary is positive, a reversal of the negative feedback relationship that occurred during the earlier parts of the follicular phase. Progesterone levels remain low and stable, due to the lack of a corpus luteum, which is responsible for the secretion of the hormone later in the cycle.

    Answer D is incorrect. This combination of hormone changes is seen immediately following ovulation, when estrogen levels are decreasing (prior to increasing again during the luteal phase) and progesterone levels are increasing (since the hormone is secreted by the newly formed corpus luteum). FSH and LH levels are decreasing at this time due to the negative feedback exerted by estrogen and progesterone on their release.

44. **The correct answer is C.** This patient has symptoms consistent with benign prostatic hyperplasia (BPH), including difficulty initiating a stream, post-void dribbling, and frequent nighttime urination. In this case, the large prostate encasing the prostatic urethra caused urinary obstruction, leading to a decline in renal function reflected by an increase in creatinine level. On ultrasound one may be able to see dilation of the urinary collection system. A well-placed Foley catheter definitively relieves the obstruction.

    Answer A is incorrect. Giving fluids would improve renal function if the patient were hypovolemic. The patient's symptoms point to an obstructive reason for his rise in creatinine level rather than to a prerenal cause.

    Answer B is incorrect. Dialysis would be appropriate if the patient were in renal failure. However, his creatinine level is not severely elevated, and he is still making urine. Placing a Foley catheter directly addresses the cause of the patient's declining renal function.

Answer D is incorrect. While BPH represents an overgrowth of cells, it is distinctly not a malignant process. Therefore removal of the prostate is not indicated, as it might be for some cases of prostate cancer.

45. **The correct answer is A.** 5α-reductase converts testosterone to dihydrotestosterone. Dihydrotestosterone is required for the development of the penis and scrotum during embryogenesis. An infant with 5α-reductase deficiency is phenotypically female, with normal levels of testosterone, estrogen, and LH. However, the infant will have bilateral testes and a normal male internal urogenital tract. The dramatic increase in testosterone levels during puberty causes the external genitalia to be masculinized. Because the patient is genotypically male with male internal genital organs, the phenotypically female patient will fail to menstruate and may present to the physician complaining of primary amenorrhea.

    Answer B is incorrect. Complete androgen insensitivity, or testicular feminization syndrome, is caused by a defect in the gene that encodes the androgen receptor. These XY individuals are phenotypically female, but have bilateral testes that are undescended or located in the labia majora. Levels of testosterone, estrogen, and LH are high.

    Answer C is incorrect. Males with the genotype XYY are phenotypically normal males.

    Answer D is incorrect. Female pseudohermaphroditism occurs when ovaries are present and the external genitalia are virilized or ambiguous. This condition is usually due to exposure to androgens early in gestation.

    Answer E is incorrect. True hermaphroditism occurs only when both ovarian and testicular tissues are present in the same patient; this is rare in humans.

46. **The correct answer is A.** This patient's condition is consistent with fibrocystic changes of the breast. Fibrocystic changes have no malignant potential and are the most common breast mass in women from 25 years old to menopause.

    Answer B is incorrect. Fibrocystic changes are not associated with any familial breast cancer genes like *BRCA1* and *BRCA2*.

    Answer C is incorrect. Purulent nipple discharge is associated with breast-feeding and lactation, and it is often due to *Staphylococcus aureus*. Since this woman is not lactating or breast-feeding, her diagnosis cannot be acute mastitis.

    Answer D is incorrect. This patient has fibrocystic change, which is the most common breast mass in women <50 years old. Fibroadenoma usually presents with a small, mobile, rubbery mass with sharp edges, which can change size with a woman's menstrual cycle.

    Answer E is incorrect. Breast trauma can lead to traumatic fat necrosis, which can produce a painful indurated mass with possible skin retraction, simulating cancer. Given this patient has no history of breast trauma and this condition only occurs sporadically, it is most likely not traumatic fat necrosis.

47. **The correct answer is D.** This patient has PCOS, which is characterized by excessive androgen production (hirsutism and severe acne in this patient), menstrual irregularities, polycystic ovaries, and obesity. The exact pathogenesis of the disease is often debated, but excess LH is thought to play a role by stimulating ovarian theca cells to increase androgen production and secretion. These excess androgens can be converted into testosterone by most peripheral tissues, leading to hirsutism, acne, or male pattern alopecia. Also, consistently high levels of LH can lead to anovulation due to down-regulation of the LH receptors at the ovaries. On ultrasound imaging, the common appearance is that of multiple ovarian "cysts"; these are actually immature follicles with arrested development due to ovarian dysfunction. They usually are located along the periphery, appearing as a "string of pearls" on imaging

Answer A is incorrect. The majority of patients with PCOS have elevated or normal estrone and estradiol levels.

Answer B is incorrect. Serum androgen levels, including testosterone, androstenedione, and dehydroepiandrosterone sulfate, are increased in the majority of patients with PCOS.

Answer C is incorrect. FSH levels may be normal or low in PCOS, contributing to the elevated LH:FSH ratio seen in many patients.

Answer E is incorrect. Elevated LH levels and frequent anovulation leads to decreased ovarian progesterone secretion. Patients with PCOS at an increased risk for endometrial hyperplasia and carcinoma due to the unopposed estrogen stimulation of the endometrium.

48. **The correct answer is B.** A hydatidiform mole is a noninvasive tumor caused by aberrant fertilization, leading to cystic swelling of chorionic villi and proliferation of the trophoblast. It results in a mass that can look like a "cluster of grapes," as seen in the image. Hydatidiform moles can be complete or partial. The genotype of a complete mole is usually 46,XX, completely consisting of paternal DNA. It results when two sperm fertilize an empty egg. There is no associated fetus despite the elevated levels of β-hCG.

    Answer A is incorrect. Maternally derived 46,XX would not cause a hydatidiform mole. Moles are derived from "empty" ova that are then fertilized by sperm.

    Answer C is incorrect. 46,XX describes the genotype of a normal fetus, receiving one set of chromosomes from each parent.

    Answer D is incorrect. Paternally derived 69,XXX describes another possible DNA make-up of a partial mole. A partial mole contains more than two sets of chromosomes that usually consist of two paternal and one maternal set of chromosomes, resulting in triploidy or tetraploidy. Partial moles may present with a similar grapelike mass but are also associated with fetal parts.

    Answer E is incorrect. Maternally and paternally derived 69,XXY describes one possible DNA make-up of a partial mole. A partial mole contains more than two sets of chromosomes that usually consist of both paternal and maternal sets, resulting in triploidy or tetraploidy. Partial moles may present with a similar grapelike mass and are associated with fetal parts.

49. **The correct answer is D.** β-hCG is produced by the placenta immediately after implantation in the endometrium of the uterus. β-hCG acts on the corpus luteum to rescue it from regression. It stimulates the corpus luteum to produce estriol and progesterone to maintain the pregnancy until the placenta takes over this role in the second and third trimesters. β-hCG levels peak at week nine of gestation and then begin to decline until reaching a steady state around week 25.

    Answer A is incorrect. Prolactin, not β-hCG, is responsible for stimulating production of milk by the mammary glands.

    Answer B is incorrect. Progesterone, not β-hCG, raises the threshold for uterine contraction. This helps prevent spontaneous abortion of the fetus.

    Answer C is incorrect. β-hCG does not initiate parturition at the end of pregnancy. The actual initiating event is unknown.

    Answer E is incorrect. Estrogen and progesterone are produced by the corpus luteum in the first trimester and by the placenta in the second and third trimesters. The developing placenta starts producing β-hCG after implantation, which stimulates the corpus luteum to produce estrogen and progesterone until the placenta takes over.

50. **The correct answer is B.** This patient has symptoms of *Candida albicans* vulvovaginitis. Infection with this organism also can cause thrush, usually in immunocompromised patients. Candidal esophagitis is common in patients with HIV infection. *C albicans* also can cause disseminated disease of any organ.

Answer A is incorrect. Chronic lung disease resembling tuberculosis (TB) is suggestive of infection with *Histoplasma* organisms, among others. Histoplasmosis typically does not present symptomatically, although some patients experience a flu-like illness with fever, cough, headaches, and myalgias. In addition to causing lung disease resembling TB, histoplasmosis can disseminate, affecting the liver, spleen, adrenal glands, mucosal surfaces, and meninges. Histoplasmosis occurs most commonly in the Mississippi and Ohio River valleys.

Answer C is incorrect. Lesions in lung cavities ("fungus balls") are typical of *Aspergillus fumigatus* infection. In the lungs A *fumigatus* also can cause a patchy pneumonia or pulmonary nodules. A *fumigatus* is a non-dimorphic mold with septate hyphae that branch at a V-shaped 45-degree angle.

Answer D is incorrect. In immunocompromised hosts, several fungi cause meningoencephalitis, most notably *Cryptococcus neoformans*. *Cryptococcus* is a non-dimorphic, heavily encapsulated yeast found in soil and pigeon droppings. In an immunocompetent host, infection often is asymptomatic.

Answer E is incorrect. Migrating synovitis is a feature of disseminated gonococcal infection with *Neisseria gonorrhoeae*. N *gonorrhoeae* is a gram-negative diplococcus that causes urethritis in both sexes and pelvic inflammatory disease in women. It is treated with ceftriaxone.

CHAPTER 17

Respiratory

QUESTIONS

1. A 25-year-old woman with a history of asthma is brought to the emergency department by emergency medical services (EMS) after ingesting a full bottle of theophylline in a suicide attempt. At presentation, she is having a tonic-clonic seizure. Her blood pressure is 80/40 mmHg, respiratory rate is 30 breaths/minute, and her heart rate is 160/minute. The EMS personnel report that she has been seizing for at least 15 minutes. What is the mechanism of action of the most appropriate drug to counteract her intoxication?

   (A) Decreasing intracellular cAMP
   (B) Increasing intracellular cAMP through β_2-adrenergic receptors
   (C) Increasing intracellular cAMP through nonselective adrenergic receptors
   (D) Inhibiting the Na^+-K^+-$2Cl^-$ co-transporter
   (E) Inhibiting the Na^+-K^+-ATPase pump

2. A 28-year-old smoker presents to the emergency department because of sudden onset of chest pain and dyspnea while at rest. His heart rate is 115/min, respiratory rate is 24/min, and blood pressure is 140/80 mm Hg in both arms. Lung examination shows decreased breath sounds and decreased fremitus on the right with hyperresonance to percussion. Which of the following would most likely be seen on this patient's x-ray of the chest?

   (A) A widened mediastinum
   (B) Barrel chest and flattened diaphragm
   (C) Consolidation in the right lower lobe
   (D) Contralateral deviation of the trachea
   (E) Tracheal deviation to the ipsilateral side; elevated diaphragm on the right side

3. A 35-year-old HIV-positive woman with a CD4+ count of 175/βL (normal = 500-1500/βL) presents to the clinic with a two-week history of fever, nonproductive cough, and progressive dyspnea. She has a history of sulfa allergy. Physical examination reveals diffuse crackles and rhonchi. X-ray of the chest shows diffuse, bilateral interstitial infiltrates. Laboratory studies are remarkable only for an elevated lactate dehydrogenase level. Which of the following is the best choice for prophylaxis against this infection in a patient with a sulfa allergy?

   (A) Aerosolized pentamidine
   (B) Ciprofloxacin
   (C) Fluconazole
   (D) Terbinafine
   (E) Trimethoprim-sulfamethoxazole

4. A previously healthy 41-year-old man misses several days of work as a result of a viral illness with symptoms including fever, headache, and fatigue. He also experiences a nonproductive cough and a sore throat. By the third day, his symptoms begin to subside and he is able to return to work. The next week, however, he experiences a rapid relapse. His cough returns, but now it is a productive cough with mucopurulent sputum. He also begins to experience pleuritic chest pain. On visiting a physician, x-ray of the chest is ordered and is shown in the image. Which of the following describes the structure of the viral genome that most likely caused his initial illness?

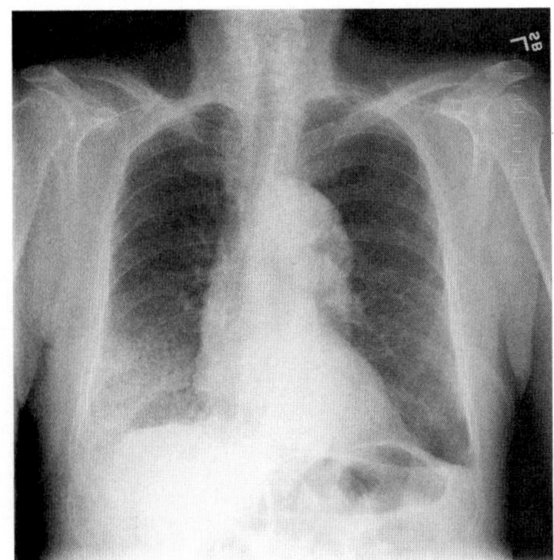

Reproduced, with permission, from Fauci AS, et al, eds. *Harrison's Principles of Internal Medicine*, 17th edition. New York: McGraw-Hill, 2008; Figure 128-1.

(A) Enveloped, double-stranded DNA
(B) Enveloped, nonsegmented, single-stranded RNA
(C) Enveloped, segmented, single-stranded RNA
(D) Non-enveloped, nonsegmented, double-stranded RNA
(E) Non-enveloped, nonsegmented, single-stranded RNA

5. A newborn baby is cyanotic and is having great difficulty breathing. The baby is tachypneic and does not improve with time. At autopsy a few days later, the lungs are wet and heavy with areas of atelectasis alternating with occasional dilated alveoli or alveolar ducts. Intra-alveolar hyaline membranes consisting of fibrin and cellular debris are also present. A patent ductus arteriosus and intraventricular brain hemorrhage are also seen at autopsy. Which of the following is the likely etiology of the baby's condition?

(A) Deficiency of hepatic glucuronyl transferase
(B) Dipalmitoyl phosphatidylcholine deficiency
(C) Full-term uncomplicated pregnancy
(D) Lecithin:sphingomyelin ratio in amniotic fluid >1.5
(E) Maternal steroid abuse prior to delivery

6. A 25-year-old medical student presents to the clinic with a nonproductive cough, low-grade fever, and malaise of three weeks' duration. A few friends in his study group have been feeling the same way. Sputum cultures are negative. The patient denies exposure to farm animals, travel, or HIV. The physician treats for an atypical pneumonia. Which of the following methods could help identify the organism responsible for this most likely causative pathogen?

(A) Acid-fast stain
(B) Cold agglutinin testing
(C) Gram stain
(D) India ink stain
(E) Serum polymerase chain reaction

7. A 2-year-old boy presents to the emergency department because of sore throat, fever, hoarseness, and stridor. The physician suspects a diagnosis of croup, but wishes to exclude epiglottitis. Compared with croup, which of the following is characteristic of epiglottitis?

(A) Epiglottitis is associated with inflammation of the larynx and subglottic trachea
(B) Epiglottitis is associated with rhinorrhea and conjunctivitis
(C) Epiglottitis often leads to respiratory distress
(D) Symptom onset is gradual in epiglottitis
(E) The barking cough of epiglottitis becomes inspiratory stridor
(F) Throat swab in epiglottitis would reveal parainfluenza virus

8. A 25-year-old man presents with new-onset hemoptysis for the past 12 hours. The patient, who recently immigrated to the United States from Vietnam, has had fever and night sweats on a daily basis for the past four years. He has no other complaints and no past medical history. The patient is diagnosed with active tuberculosis and sent home on an antimycobacterial regimen. One month later, the patient returns with new complaints of joint pain, photosensitivity, and a facial rash. Liver function tests are found to be elevated. Which of the following is the mechanism of action of the drug with the adverse effects described above?

(A) Disrupts the cell membrane's osmotic properties
(B) Inhibits arabinosyl transferases
(C) Inhibits DNA-dependent RNA polymerase encoded by the *rpo* gene
(D) Inhibits folic acid synthesis
(E) Inhibits synthesis of mycolic acids

9. A 26-year-old man presents to the emergency department with respiratory difficulty. Starting at age of 15, he began to have periodic shortness of breath. Serial pulmonary function tests revealed gradually increasing total capacity and residual volume. His renal function laboratory results were normal, but his aspartate aminotransferase and alanine aminotransferase levels were significantly elevated. He began requiring home oxygen earlier this year, but his condition continued to worsen. He died during this admission, and an autopsy was conducted. Examination of his lungs showed the pathology seen in the image. This patient's illness was most likely caused by which of the following?

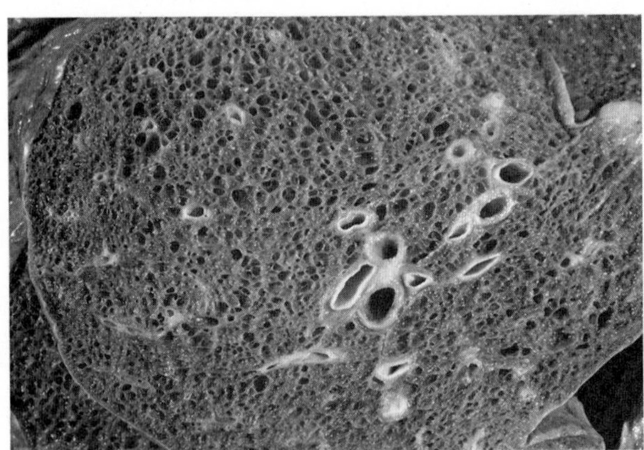

Reproduced, with permission, from USMLERx.com.

(A) Decreased levels of α_1-antitrypsin
(B) Decreased levels of elastase
(C) Increased levels of anti-neutrophil cytoplasmic autoantibodies
(D) Increased levels of copper
(E) Increased levels of iron

10. A 3-year-old boy is brought to the hospital with acute shortness of breath. He was playing with marbles in the playground when his mother noticed him cough and become acutely short of breath. Her attempt to dislodge the object on site was unsuccessful, and he was brought to the hospital. Prior to this incident he was healthy. His vaccinations are up-to-date, and he takes no medications. On chest x-ray, which portion of the lung is most likely to appear abnormal?

(A) Left lower lobe
(B) Left upper lobe
(C) Lingula
(D) Right lower lobe
(E) Right upper lobe

11. A 57-year-old man presents to his primary care physician for a routine wellness check. He denies any complaints. Social history is significant for a 50-pack-year smoking history. On physical examination, his vital signs are within normal limits except for his blood pressure, which is 170/95 mm Hg. On his previous visit, his blood pressure was 155/90 mm Hg. Which of the following antihypertensive agents is relatively contraindicated in this patient?

(A) Acebutolol
(B) Atenolol
(C) Esmolol
(D) Metoprolol
(E) Nadolol

12. A physiologist divides the lung into three zones, with the apex being zone 1, the middle region being zone 2, and the base being zone 3. In an experiment the physiologist applies a small amount of positive pressure ventilation while studying blood flow in different lung zones. Which of the following will be noted in this experiment assuming the subject is standing?

(A) Blood flow in zone 3 will be driven by the difference between alveolar and venous pressures
(B) Blood flow will be reduced in zone 1
(C) Blood flow will increase in zone 2
(D) Regional differences between blood flow will not be as great as differences in ventilation
(E) Whether supine or standing, blood flow will remain uneven throughout the lung zones

13. A 60-year-old white man comes to his physician because of a productive cough of a few months' duration. The patient reports having three of these episodes over the past two years, with each episode lasting approximately four months. Histological examination of the lung reveals hypertrophy of mucus-secreting glands in the bronchioles, with a Reid index >50%. What other changes are likely to be noted on biopsy?

    (A) Alveolar fluid and hyaline membranes
    (B) An infiltration of eosinophils and CD4+ and TH2 lymphocytes
    (C) An infiltration of monocytes and CD8+ lymphocytes
    (D) Necrotizing vasculitis and granulomatous eosinophilic tissue infiltration
    (E) Noncaseating granulomas

14. A 65-year-old man with an 80-pack-year history of smoking presents to his physician because of a cough and increasing dyspnea over the past six weeks. X-ray of the chest shows a 2-cm mass in the left lower lobe of the lung, which is biopsied, revealing squamous cell carcinoma. A sample of non-neoplastic tissue from the lung biopsy is shown in the image. Which of the following types of epithelium not normally present in the lung lines the bronchus shown in this image?

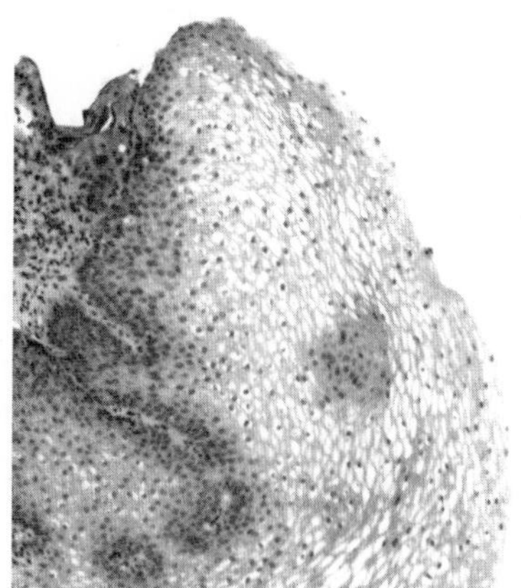

Courtesy of Wikipedia.

    (A) Pseudostratified columnar
    (B) Simple squamous
    (C) Stratified columnar
    (D) Stratified squamous
    (E) Transitional

15. The oxygen-hemoglobin dissociation curve represents the percent saturation of hemoglobin with oxygen as a function of the partial pressure of oxygen in the blood. This curve is sigmoidal in shape due to the change in affinity of heme groups for additional oxygen molecules. Which of the following in an adult would cause a shift in the curve so that it resembles that of a neonate?

    (A) Increased 2,3-diphosphoglycerate
    (B) Increased partial pressure of carbon dioxide in the blood
    (C) Increased pH
    (D) Increased temperature
    (E) Intense exercise

16. A 50-year-old woman complains of dark-colored urine and says she has not been feeling well for the past two-three weeks; she has generalized malaise and a nagging cough that occasionally is productive of blood-tinged sputum. However, she noticed changes in her urine for the first time today. Physical examination reveals an ill-appearing middle-aged woman with a blood pressure of 180/110 mm Hg. Diminished air entry in the lungs bilaterally, and an ulcerated lesion of the mucosa of the right naris, are noted. There is no history of asthma or allergies. Urinalysis is grossly positive for blood, and serum chemistry panel reveals a creatinine level of 1.7 mg/dL. What additional finding would confirm the most likely diagnosis?

    (A) Eosinophilia on WBC differential
    (B) IgA deposition in glomerular mesangium
    (C) Linear IgG deposition in the kidney
    (D) Positive for cytoplasmic anti-neutrophilic cytoplasmic antibodies
    (E) Positive for hepatitis B

17. A 35-year-old African-American woman presents to the clinic complaining of fatigue, dry cough, and dyspnea. X-ray of the chest is shown in the image. Lung parenchymal biopsy reveals a noncaseating granuloma. Which of the following cutaneous manifestations is associated with this condition?

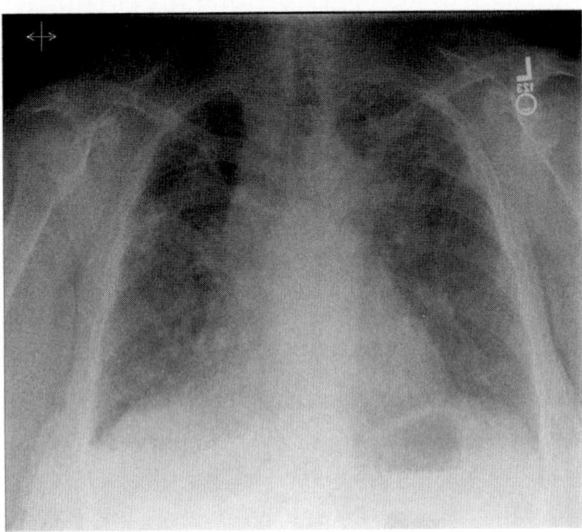

Reproduced, with permission, from USMLERx.com.

(A) Erythema infectiosum
(B) Erythema migrans
(C) Erythema multiforme
(D) Erythema nodosum
(E) Erythema toxicum

18. An 18-year-old man comes to the physician complaining of a runny nose, sneezing, and difficulty breathing for the past two days. He says that when he goes outside or is away from his house, his symptoms improve. On physical examination his turbinates are boggy and violaceous. This type of reaction is most similar to which of the following?

(A) Anaphylaxis
(B) Contact dermatitis
(C) Goodpasture syndrome
(D) Graft-versus-host disease
(E) Post-streptococcal glomerulonephritis

19. A patient undergoing lung transplantation because of pulmonary fibrosis had his pressure-volume curves monitored throughout the operation. The following events took place in the operating room: (1) his right lung was resected, (2) the new right lung was transplanted, and (3) positive end-expiratory pressure (PEEP) was added to prevent pulmonary edema. Which pressure-volume loop most likely represents the patient's pulmonary function when the patient was being ventilated on one lung prior to the new lung being transplanted?

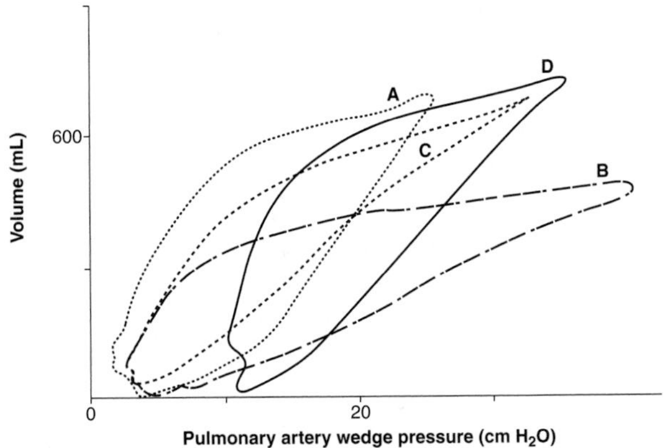

Reproduced, with permission, from USMLERx.com.

(A) Loop A
(B) Loop B
(C) Loop C
(D) Loop D

20. A 5-year-old girl visiting from Mexico is brought to the emergency department by her aunt because of a sore throat and general malaise for the past three days. Physical examination reveals temperature of 38°C (100.4°F) and a grayish-white membrane on the pharynx that bleeds on attempted dislodgement. Which of the following is the most appropriate culture media for diagnosing this patient's infection?

(A) Bordet-Gengou agar
(B) Chocolate agar with factors V and X
(C) Sabouraud agar
(D) Tellurite agar
(E) Thayer-Martin agar

21. A 57-year-old man presents to the emergency department (ED) with fever, night sweats, and a productive cough with occasional hemoptysis. He is started empirically on several medications for his underlying disease. At follow-up several months later, he reports difficulty reading the paper in the morning and has been found to wear unusual color combinations at work. Which of the following is the most likely cause of this patient's new symptoms?

(A) Ethambutol toxicity
(B) Isoniazid toxicity
(C) Pyrazinamide toxicity
(D) Rifampin toxicity
(E) Tuberculous eye infection

22. A 36-year-old woman with a history of leukemia receives a bone marrow transplant. Two and a half weeks later, she experiences fever, cough, and dyspnea. Bronchoalveolar lavage reveals large cells with prominent intranuclear inclusions, as shown in the image. What is the most likely cause of this patient's infection?

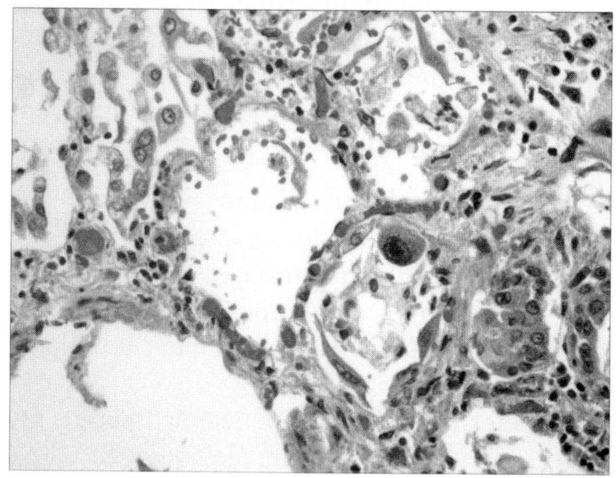

Reproduced, with permission, from USMLERx.com.

(A) *Candida albicans*
(B) Cytomegalovirus
(C) *Mycobacterium tuberculosis*
(D) *Pneumocystis jiroveci*
(E) *Toxoplasma gondii*

23. A pregnant woman who suffers from hypertension and thrombocytopenia and has elevated liver function tests suddenly has a seizure. Suspecting eclampsia, the obstetrics team performs an emergency cesarean section. The neonate is delivered at 30 weeks and is found to have bradycardia. The child also appears to have labored breathing. He is rushed to the neonatal intensive care unit, where he is intubated and treated with steroids. Which of the following is a characteristic of the alveoli of this neonate's lungs?

(A) An increased pressure is needed to collapse the lungs
(B) Increased surface tension
(C) The lungs have increased compliance
(D) The lungs lack a substance produced mainly by type I pneumocytes
(E) The lungs produce a substance with a lecithin:sphingomyelin ratio >1.5

24. A 12-year-old boy is found unconscious in his bedroom by his parents and is taken to the emergency department. On arrival the patient's skin is pale and lacks turgor, and there is a sweet scent on his breath. His parents report constant urination and weight loss in the two weeks prior to presentation. Laboratory tests show a glucose level of 610 mg/dL, sodium of 130 mEq/L, bicarbonate of 9 mEq/L, and chloride of 95 mEq/L. Which of the following would most likely be associated with this patient's condition at presentation?

(A) Calcium oxalate crystals in the urine
(B) Decreased anion gap
(C) Decreased blood partial pressure of carbon dioxide
(D) Elevated blood partial pressure of carbon dioxide
(E) Hypokalemia

25. A medical student is asked to perform a cardiovascular examination on a patient. After 10 minutes of auscultation with no success, the medical student gives up and asks his resident for help. The resident puts up the patient's anteroposterior chest radiograph (see image) and begins to explain the molecular etiology of this patient's condition. What is one respiratory complication that this patient is at increased risk of developing as a result of his condition?

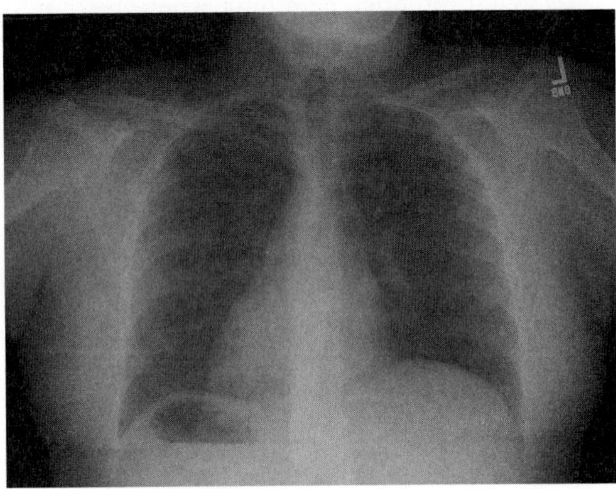

Reproduced, with permission, from Knoop KJ, et al. *The Atlas of Emergency Medicine*, 3rd ed. New York: McGraw-Hill, 2010; Fig. 7.31.

(A) Acute respiratory distress syndrome
(B) Bronchiectasis
(C) Carcinoma of the lung
(D) Exercise-induced asthma
(E) Idiopathic pulmonary fibrosis

26. A 46-year-old woman presents to the emergency department because of a one-week history of worsening nausea and lethargy. While she is waiting to see the doctor she experiences a seizure. Her past medical history is significant for tuberculosis. Laboratory values show:

Serum Na^+: 109 mEq/L
Serum osmolality: 255 mOsm/kg
Urine osmolality: 850 mOsm/kg
Hematocrit: 27%

Which of the following drugs is also known to cause the underlying disorder with which this patient presents?

(A) Cyclophosphamide
(B) Demeclocycline
(C) Hydrochlorothiazide
(D) Indomethacin
(E) Lithium

27. A 17-year-old girl involved in a car accident presents to the emergency department with penetrating chest trauma to her left side. She is having difficulty breathing and has an oxygen saturation of 86%. After x-ray of the chest is performed, a chest tube is placed, and her oxygen saturation improves. Which of the following is responsible for her difficulty breathing upon presentation?

(A) Her intrapleural pressure is equal to atmosphere pressure during inspiration
(B) Her intrapleural pressure is less than atmospheric pressure during inspiration
(C) Pain from the trauma has made it difficult to breathe
(D) Pressure within the pericardial space is increased relative to the pleural space
(E) The elastic force of the chest wall is pulling it inward

28. A 74-year-old retired shipyard laborer with a 45-pack-year smoking history and previous work in sandblasting and fiberglass operations presents with increasing shortness of breath and peripheral edema. On physical examination he is a thin, cyanotic man in moderate pulmonary distress. His chest shows an increased anteroposterior diameter, and the breath sounds are faint with a prolonged expiration. The liver edge is 3 cm below the right costal margin. There is no digital clubbing, but marked peripheral edema is present. Arterial blood gas analysis reveals a partial oxygen pressure of 43 mm Hg, a partial carbon dioxide pressure of 22 mm Hg, and a pH of 7.51. Which set of laboratory parameters is most likely to be found?

Choice	FEV_1	FVC	FEV_1:FVC	Total lung capacity
A	↓	↓	↓	↓
B	↓	↓	↓	↑
C	↓	↓	normal	↓
D	↓	normal	normal	↓
E	↓	↑	↑	↑

Reproduced, with permission, from USMLERx.com.

(A) A
(B) B
(C) C
(D) D
(E) E

29. A 74-year-old patient presents with increased shortness of breath. A sputum sample reveals golden-brown beaded fibers, which result from iron- and protein-coated fibers. On CT scan, dense fibrocalcific plaques of the parietal pleura are seen. A particular pneumoconiosis is suspected. Which of the following is the likely etiology of the patient's condition?

(A) Autoimmune attack of lung parenchyma
(B) Idiopathic (unknown) etiology
(C) Living in a polluted city for years
(D) Long-term complication of steroid abuse
(E) Reactivation of a contained primary disease
(F) Working in a coal mine for 40 years
(G) Working in a shipyard for 40 years

30. A 158.8-kg (350-lb) man with a body mass index of 40 kg/m² comes to the physician complaining of frequent fatigue, shortness of breath, general sleepiness, and an inability to concentrate. Physical examination shows an extremely obese, tired-looking man with hypertension and an elongated uvula. Which of the following metabolic findings is most likely?

(A) Decreased serum glucose
(B) Increased HDL cholesterol
(C) Increased renal H^+ reabsorption
(D) Increased renal HCO_3- reabsorption
(E) Increased renal HCO_3- secretion

31. A 68-year-old man who smokes and is alcoholic abruptly develops high fever, shakes, a severe headache, and abdominal and muscle pain. He initially has a dry, insignificant cough, but over the next few days he develops marked shortness of breath requiring assisted ventilation. X-ray of the chest demonstrates homogenous radiographic shadowing involving both the lungs extensively. Culture of bronchoalveolar lavage fluid on buffered charcoal yeast extract demonstrates a coccobacillary pathogen. What is the most likely causative organism?

(A) *Legionella pneumophila*
(B) *Listeria monocytogenes*
(C) *Spirillum minus*
(D) *Staphylococcus aureus*
(E) *Streptococcus pneumoniae*

32. A 62-year-old woman underwent bilateral knee replacement and was discharged without complications on postoperative day two. Nine days after surgery she develops severe respiratory distress and dies suddenly in the emergency department. Postmortem examination of her pulmonary artery reveals the pathology seen in the image. What medical condition could predispose to a similar pathology as observed in this patient?

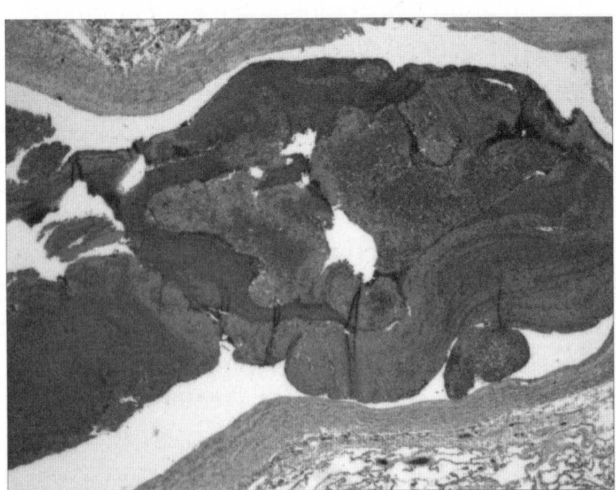

Reproduced, with permission, from USMLERx.com.

(A) Aspiration
(B) Factor V deficiency
(C) Factor VIII deficiency
(D) Protein C deficiency
(E) Thrombocytopenia

33. A 55-year-old man with a 30-pack-year smoking history presents to his physician because of a 3-month history of productive cough. He is diagnosed with chronic obstructive pulmonary disease after x-ray of the chest demonstrates hyperinflated lungs and a flattened diaphragm. The physician prescribes inhaled steroids, a β_2-agonist, and ipratropium bromide. Ipratropium bromide will produce bronchodilation through which of the following mechanisms?

(A) Blockade of acetylcholine at muscarinic receptors
(B) Inhibition of phosphodiesterase resulting in increased cAMP levels
(C) Inhibition of the degranulation of mast cells
(D) Inhibition of the synthesis of cytokines
(E) Stimulation of adenylyl cyclase resulting in increased cAMP levels

34. In an attempt to better understand the pathophysiology of obesity hypoventilation syndrome, a medical student is reviewing the ways in which the body exerts control of respiration. Which of the following is true with regard to regulation of respiration?

(A) Breathing is centrally regulated via the hypothalamus and amygdala
(B) Central chemoreceptors affect breathing by directly detecting blood levels of hydrogen ions
(C) Peripheral chemoreceptors stimulate breathing when the partial pressure of oxygen dips below 60 mm Hg
(D) Stretch, irritant, and J receptors all function outside the lung to regulate breathing
(E) The aortic and carotid bodies are considered central chemoreceptors

35. A 56-year-old man presents with fatigue, fever, weight loss, and hemoptysis of five weeks' duration. Radiography and CT of the chest reveal a centrally located mass. Results of a lung biopsy are shown in the image. Laboratory tests show:

Sodium: 130 mEq/L
Potassium: 3.9 mEq/L
Chloride: 101 mEq/L
Bicarbonate: 24 mEq/L
Calcium: 9.8 mg/dL
WBC count: 11,600/mm^3
Hemoglobin: 12 g/dL
Hematocrit: 38.1%
Platelet count: 420,000/mm^3
Blood urea nitrogen: 8 mg/dL
Creatinine: 0.8 mg/dL
Glucose: 108 mg/dL

What is the reasoning behind the best management for this patient?

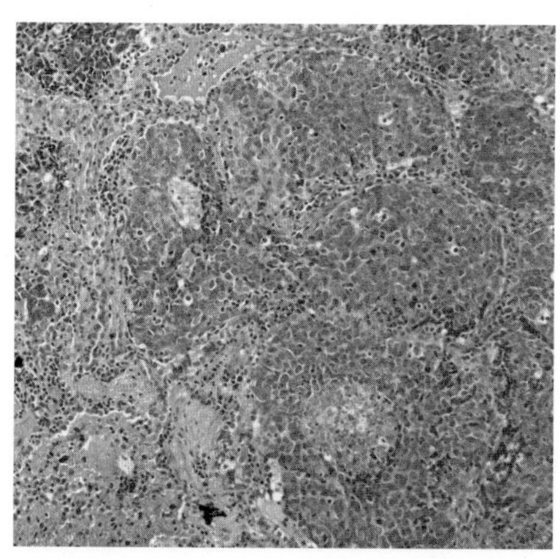

Reproduced, with permission, from USMLERx.com.

(A) Surgery carries a risk of provoking paraneoplastic syndromes on removal of the mass
(B) Surgery has not been shown to improve survival
(C) Surgery is palliative but not curative
(D) Surgery often is curative in every lung cancer without identifiable metastases
(E) This lesion is likely to regress in seven years

36. A 61-year-old man is frustrated because he is no longer able to walk up a flight of stairs without stopping to catch his breath. He has also been plagued by a dry cough for the past six months. He has not visited his primary care physician because he is not a smoker and does not believe that he could have a serious pulmonary condition. He ignores his symptoms for another eight months, during which time they continue to worsen. He finally visits his physician at the urging of his wife. While shaking hands, his physician notices that the patient has clubbing of the fingers. A clinical work-up and medical history fail to find a cause for this restrictive lung disease. What is the definitive therapy for this patient's most likely condition?

(A) Albuterol
(B) Azathioprine
(C) Cyclosporine
(D) Lung transplantation
(E) Steroids

37. Public health investigators are looking into a series of illnesses that have occurred in a small community. Many patients presented with acute-onset hyperpyrexia and a particularly severe pneumonia. Gram staining of their sputum cultures reveals neutrophils and very few organisms. Which of the following organisms is most likely to have caused this outbreak?

(A) *Bordetella pertussis*
(B) *Haemophilus influenzae* type B
(C) *Legionella pneumophila*
(D) *Mycobacterium tuberculosis*
(E) *Streptococcus pneumoniae*

38. A 26-year-old recent immigrant from Mexico presents to the emergency department with a three-week history of fevers accompanied by night sweats and chills, weight loss of 2.3 kg (5 lb), and cough that is often productive of blood-tinged sputum. Bronchoalveolar lavage is performed and an acid-fast stain of the sample reveals the organism shown in the image. Which of the following should be included in this patient's therapy to prevent a common toxicity of treatment?

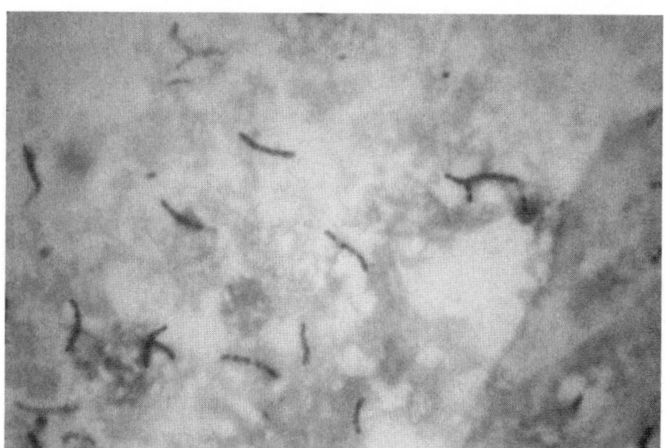

Courtesy of Dr. George P. Kubica, Centers for Disease Control and Prevention.

(A) Cobalamin
(B) Pyridoxine
(C) Vitamin B_1
(D) Vitamin C
(E) Vitamin E

39. A mother brings her 10-year-old son with fever, cough, and difficulty breathing to the emergency department. Approximately two days ago she noted the development of a rash on his face that spread downward over his body. Physical examination reveals a toxic-appearing child with a temperature of 40°C (104°F), rapid pulse, and rapid respiratory rate. The physician notes the appearance of a reddish-brown blotchy rash throughout the child's body. In his mouth he has small red spots with blue-white centers. Chest examination reveals clear breath sounds with poor inspiratory effort. CT of the chest shows diffuse interstitial involvement. Which of the following would the physician most likely see in this child's sputum?

(A) Acid-fast bacilli
(B) Cells with nuclei surrounded by halo and clear cytoplasm
(C) Cowdry-type inclusions in cells
(D) Gram-negative coccobacilli and polymorphonuclear leukocytes
(E) Gram-positive diplococci and polymorphonuclear leukocytes
(F) Multinucleated giant cells

40. A premature child is born in respiratory distress and is emergently intubated. Synthetic pulmonary surfactant is administered with no improvement in pulmonary function. After conducting a detailed physical examination, the pediatrician believes that this child's condition is related to a failure of the embryonic pleuroperitoneal folds to form and close. What physical examination finding would support the most likely diagnosis in this child?

(A) Bowel sounds in the left lower lung zone
(B) Continuous cardiac murmur
(C) Marked splenomegaly
(D) Midline deviation of the trachea

41. Which of the following letter choices represents the residual volume?

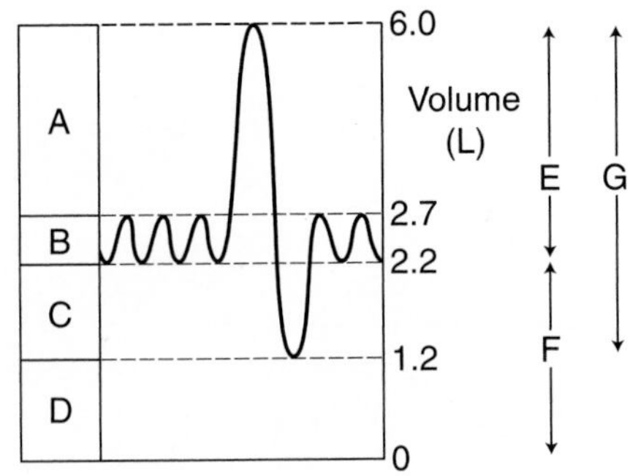

Reproduced, with permission, from USMLERx.com.

(A) A
(B) B
(C) C
(D) D
(E) E
(F) F
(G) G

42. A 63-year-old smoker visits his primary care physician because of recent weight gain and worsening coughs. On physical examination the physician notes that the patient's extremities are thinner than before, while his waist is increased in girth. The patient also has a pad of adipose tissue at the base of his neck and purple striae on his abdomen. The physician decides to run some blood tests and obtain an x-ray of the chest, which shows a central lesion. Which of the following is the most likely diagnosis?

(A) Adenocarcinoma
(B) Bronchial carcinoid
(C) Metastatic disease affecting the lung
(D) Small cell carcinoma
(E) Squamous cell carcinoma embolism

43. A 37-year-old man is brought to the emergency department after being stabbed superior to his right nipple with a knife. His blood pressure is 100/60 mm Hg, heart rate is 126/min, respiratory rate is 26/min, and oxygen saturation is 90% on 100% oxygen facemask. The wound

is bubbling, and the skin immediately around the wound is moving in and out with respirations. Which of the following will most likely be found on the right side during x-ray of this patient's chest?

(A) Hemothorax
(B) Ninth rib fracture
(C) Pleural effusion
(D) Pneumothorax
(E) Upper lobe consolidation

44. A 54-year-old woman complains about a persistent cough she has had for the past three months. The cough has been bothering her a lot and making her anxious. She thinks the anxiety is why she has lost some weight recently. She also blames the anxiety whenever she wakes up in the middle of the night and finds herself drenched in sweat. Further history reveals she has rheumatoid arthritis (RA), but her joint pains and swellings are well controlled by medications her rheumatologist has prescribed her. Following a physical examination, the physician orders an x-ray of the chest (see image). Based on the results, the physician immediately prescribes an antibiotic regimen and asks her to discontinue one of the drugs used to treat her RA. Which of the following drugs increased her risk of developing the disease shown on the radiograph?

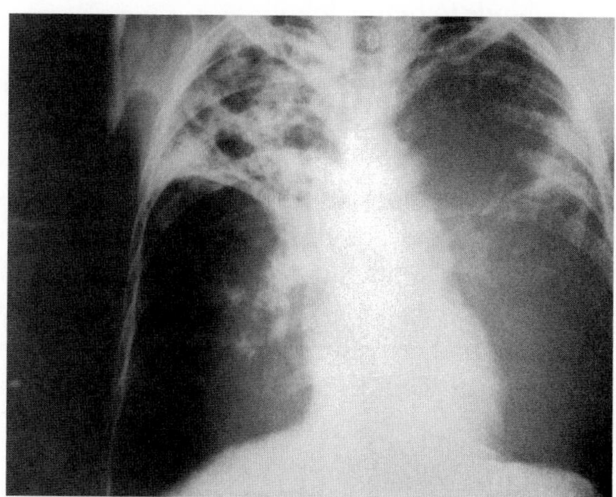

Courtesy of the Centers for Disease Control and Prevention.

(A) Etanercept
(B) Methotrexate
(C) Nonsteroidal anti-inflamatory drugs
(D) Risedronate
(E) Sulfasalazine

45. A 56-year-old man presents to the emergency department because of cough, dyspnea, and hemoptysis. X-ray of the chest shows dilation of his airways, which is confirmed by bronchoscopy. Which of the following conditions is most likely responsible for the dilation of this patient's airways?

(A) Adult respiratory distress syndrome
(B) Asthma
(C) Atelectasis
(D) Bronchiectasis
(E) Churg-Strauss syndrome

46. A 15-year-old boy with a history of severe asthma presents to the emergency department in obvious respiratory distress. After multiple nebulizer treatments and doses of intravenous corticosteroids, he develops nausea, vomiting, and weakness. Studies reveal a potassium level of 2.6 mEq/L and U waves on ECG. Which of the following medications most likely would have elicited these symptoms?

(A) Albuterol
(B) Cromolyn
(C) Ipratropium
(D) Theophylline
(E) Zileuton

47. A 32-year-old African-American woman presents to her physician complaining of a cough for the past two months and increased shortness of breath over the past year. After completing a full physical examination, her physician orders an x-ray of the chest, which shows enlarged hilar nodes bilaterally as well as lung nodules. Results of a lung biopsy are shown in the image. Which of the following treatments would be most appropriate for this patient?

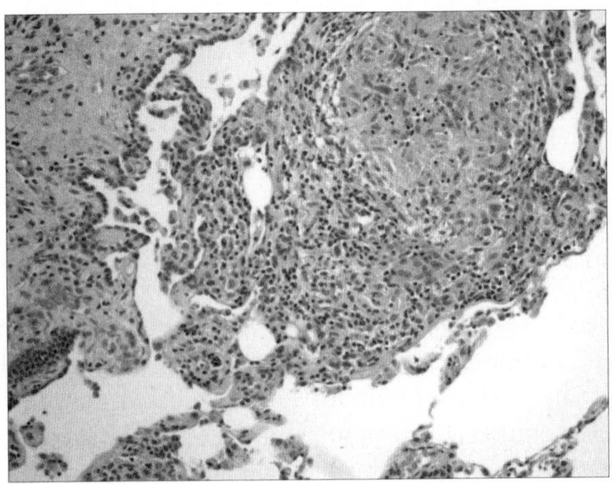

Reproduced, with permission, from USMLERx.com.

(A) Cisplatin
(B) Cyclophosphamide
(C) Dexamethasone
(D) Hydroxychloroquine
(E) Rifampin

48. A 32-year-old man returns from an in-depth tour of a sheep and goat farm. Five days later he develops fever, malaise, a dry cough, and pressure in his chest. These symptoms resolve after a few days. He then develops high fever, severe shortness of breath, chest pain, cyanosis, and diaphoresis and is rushed to the emergency department, where work-up reveals hemorrhagic mediastinitis, bloody pleural effusions, and mediastinal widening on x-ray of the chest. Within a few hours the patient develops septic shock and dies. Which of the following characterizes the most likely causative organism?

(A) Gram-negative pleomorphic aerobic coccobacilli
(B) Gram-positive rods in chains with a protein capsule
(C) Gram-negative pleomorphic coccobacilli requiring cysteine for growth
(D) Gram-positive weakly acid-fast rods forming long branching filaments
(E) Poorly stained gram-negative rods that stain best on silver stain and require iron and cysteine.

49. A 64-year-old man with sepsis has an increased peripheral metabolic rate and hypercapnia. With regard to carbon dioxide transport in this patient, which of the following physiologic processes is taking place?

(A) Bicarbonate travels in the RBCs until it reaches the lung, where it gets exhaled as carbon dioxide
(B) Carbaminohemoglobin (carbon dioxide bound to hemoglobin) becomes the primary transport carrier of the additional carbon dioxide
(C) More chloride enters the RBCs peripherally to compensate for increased carbonic anhydrase activity
(D) The acidic environment of the lungs shifts the hemoglobin-oxygen curve to the right and causes the release of carbon dioxide from hemoglobin
(E) The additional dissolved carbon dioxide becomes converted to bicarbonate, which binds to hemoglobin

50. A 65-year-old man with a 110-pack-year history of smoking presents to his primary care physician because of shortness of breath, dyspnea on exertion, and cough for three months' duration. X-ray of the chest reveals flattened diaphragms bilaterally. The doctor orders pulmonary function tests to evaluate the patient. Which of the following pulmonary function test results would most likely be found in this patient?

(A) Decreased FEV_1:FVC
(B) Decreased functional residual capacity
(C) Decreased total lung capacity
(D) Increased FEV_1
(E) Increased FEV_1:FVC

ANSWERS

1. **The correct answer is A.** The drug theophylline is a phosphodiesterase inhibitor that leads to the decreased hydrolysis of cAMP to adenosine monophosphate. An overdose of theophylline will therefore result in an elevated intracellular level of cAMP. β-blockers such as metoprolol may therefore be given to reduce cAMP levels through inactivation of adenylate cyclase. A cardioselective β-blocker must be used in cases of asthma to avoid inducing bronchial hyperreactivity.

   Answer B is incorrect. β-agonists such as albuterol would potentiate the effects of theophylline by activating adenylate cyclase and increasing the conversion of ATP to cAMP.

   Answer C is incorrect. Epinephrine would potentiate the effects of theophylline by activating adenylate cyclase and increasing cAMP formation.

   Answer D is incorrect. Furosemide is a diuretic unrelated to theophylline overdose. It works by inhibiting the Na^+-K^+-$2Cl^-$ cotransport system of the thick ascending loop of Henle.

   Answer E is incorrect. Digoxin inhibits the Na^+-K^+-ATPase pump. It is used to increase myocardial contractility in patients with congestive heart failure. It is unrelated to theophylline overdose.

2. **The correct answer is E.** This patient is most likely suffering from a spontaneous pneumothorax. Caused by the rupture of a small apical bleb on the surface of the lung, spontaneous pneumothoraces typically present in tall young men. The patient usually has sudden pain and dyspnea. Examination will show decreased breath sounds and hyperresonance on the affected side. X-ray of the chest shows overexpansion of the rib cage and an elevated hemidiaphragm on the affected side. This paradoxical abdominal motion occurs because of the negative intrathoracic pressure that causes the fatigued diaphragm to be pulled into the thorax on the right side. Spontaneous pneumothorax is treated by inserting a chest tube to remove the air from the pleural space.

   Answer A is incorrect. Aortic dissection, not a pneumothorax, would show up on x-ray of the chest as a widened mediastinum. Aortic dissection can occur in trauma, or a dissecting aortic aneurysm can occur in connective tissue diseases such as Marfan disease. The physical findings are not consistent with aortic dissection: first, the chest would not be hyperresonant to percussion and second, the blood pressure would not be equal in both arms.

   Answer B is incorrect. Barrel chests and flattened diaphragms are seen in patients with obstructive lung diseases such as chronic emphysema. Although emphysema is caused by smoking, this patient does not have a long enough smoking history. It is possible that this man could have emphysema due to an α_1-antitrypsin deficiency, but in that case it would not present this acutely.

   Answer C is incorrect. Consolidation of the right lower lobe on x-ray of the chest usually means pneumonia. The patient would present with fever, productive cough, and a high WBC count. Physical exam would show decreased resonance on the affected side and increased fremitus.

   Answer D is incorrect. In tension pneumothorax, a flap-like pleural tear allows air to enter into the pleural cavity, but prevents its exit. It can be caused by penetrating trauma to the chest resulting in increased pleural cavity pressure. Clinical findings include sudden onset of severe dyspnea, tympanitic percussion, and absent breath sounds. There is tracheal deviation and mediastinal structure deviation to the contralateral side. If tension pneumothorax occurs on the left side, there would be compression of venous return to the heart. Treatment of tension pneumothorax is emergent needle decompression into the pleural cavity to relieve the pressure.

3. **The correct answer is A.** This vignette suggests a patient with *Pneumocystis jiroveci* pneumonia based on the HIV status, physical examination and x-ray findings, and the elevated lactate dehydrogenase level. Prophylactic therapy for *P jiroveci* pneumonia is indicated for an HIV-positive patient with a CD4+ T-lymphocyte count <200/μL. The standard prophylactic therapy for *P jiroveci* pneumonia is trimethoprim-sulfamethoxazole (TMP-SMX). This combination, however, is contraindicated for patients with a sulfa allergy, because sulfamethoxazole is a sulfa drug. In these cases, the best alternative treatment is aerosolized pentamidine

   Answer B is incorrect. Ciprofloxacin is a fluoroquinolone agent used to treat urinary tract or gastrointestinal (GI) infections caused by gram-negative organisms. Adverse effects include GI upset and tendinitis.

   Answer C is incorrect. Fluconazole is an antifungal agent used to treat systemic infections. It is also indicated for treatment of hypercortisolism found in ACTH-secreting tumors and polycystic ovarian syndrome. It inhibits hormone synthesis.

   Answer D is incorrect. Terbinafine is an antifungal agent that blocks ergosterol synthesis by inhibiting squalene epoxidase. It is used to treat dermatophytoses.

   Answer E is incorrect. TMP-SMX is the initial choice for prophylactic treatment of *P jiroveci* pneumonia unless patients are unable to tolerate its harsh adverse effects, or if they have a sulfa allergy. The most common adverse effects are fever, rash, and bone marrow suppression.

4. **The correct answer is C.** From the history, it appears that this man initially experienced nonspecific viral symptoms, but there is not enough information to determine which virus he has. What is clear, however, is that his initial symptoms are distinct from what he experiences on relapse. The radiograph shows that he has lobar pneumonia (lower right lobe), which can be caused by any number of bacterial species. The question that must be asked, therefore, is, "Which viral illness predisposes to subsequent bacterial pneumonia in an otherwise healthy individual?" The classic answer is influenza. The influenza virus is an enveloped, single-stranded RNA virus with a segmented genome that permits reassortment of the genes encoding the hemagglutinin and neuraminidase proteins, resulting in the phenomenon of antigenic shift. Complications of influenza include both viral pneumonia (due to a spreading of the illness into the lower respiratory tract) and bacterial pneumonia. The latter is thought to be due largely to the fact that influenza damages the epithelium of the upper respiratory tract, compromising its ability to keep the lower respiratory tract sterile. *Streptococcus pneumoniae*, *Staphylococcus aureus*, and *Haemophilus influenzae* are the organisms most commonly seen in bacterial pneumonia secondary to influenza. This chest x-ray shows a consolidation in the right lower lobe along with a para-pneumonic effusion, highly suspicious for bacterial pneumonia.

   Answer A is incorrect. The patient's initial symptoms might be seen in a person with acute infectious mononucleosis, consistent with an infection with Epstein-Barr virus, which is an enveloped, double-stranded DNA virus. However, the symptoms of mononucleosis typically last longer than three days, and bacterial pneumonia is not a common complication.

   Answer B is incorrect. The patient's initial symptoms are consistent with an upper respiratory infection, which could be caused by coronavirus, which is an enveloped, non-segmented, single-stranded RNA virus. Infection with a coronavirus would not be expected to lead to bacterial pneumonia in a healthy individual.

   Answer D is incorrect. Non-enveloped, non-segmented, double-stranded RNA viruses include reovirus and rotavirus, neither of which is a cause of respiratory illness in adults.

   Answer E is incorrect. Another cause of upper respiratory infections in adults is rhinoviruses, which are non-enveloped, non-segmented, single-stranded RNA viruses. Rhinovirus infections are typically mild and uncomplicated in healthy individuals, and a secondary bacterial pneumonia would be atypical.

5. **The correct answer is B.** Dipalmitoyl phosphatidylcholine is a primary component of surfactant, which is deficient in neonatal respiratory distress syndrome (NRDS). Chronic hypoxemia to the fetus can result in congenital abnormalities such as a patent ductus arteriosus and intraventricular brain hemorrhage.

   Answer A is incorrect. Deficiency of hepatic glucuronyl transferase occurs in all newborns, because the enzyme is not found at adult levels in neonates. This leads to physiologic jaundice, which has nothing to do with NRDS, but could lead to kernicterus.

   Answer C is incorrect. Predisposing factors for NRDS include prematurity, maternal diabetes mellitus (DM), and birth by cesarean section.

   Answer D is incorrect. In NRDS, the lecithin:sphingomyelin ratio in the amniotic fluid is usually <1.5.

   Answer E is incorrect. Steroids are given to mothers who will deliver prematurely to try to prevent NRDS. Intratracheal administration of artificial surfactant to the newborn can also be performed.

6. **The correct answer is B.** In patients who present with insidious onset of dry cough, low-grade fever, headache, myalgias, nausea, or emesis, an atypical pneumonia should be considered. Atypical pneumonias are mostly caused by *Mycoplasma* or viruses. *Mycoplasma* cannot be cultured and is detected by the cold agglutinin test, which measures the agglutination of immunoglobulins when they are cooled. X-ray of the chest is often more impressive than physical examination findings, and is characterized by a patchy interstitial pattern. Treatment consists of antibiotic therapy with a macrolide, usually azithromycin, for five days.

   Answer A is incorrect. The acid-fast stain is used to diagnose mycobacterial illness, specifically *Mycobacterium tuberculosis*.

   Answer C is incorrect. Gram stains are used to visualize gram-positive or gram-negative bacteria. *Mycoplasma pneumoniae* is not visible on Gram stain.

   Answer D is incorrect. India ink stain can be used to visualize mucoid encapsulated yeasts such as *Cryptococcus*. This diagnostic tool is not useful in identifying *Mycoplasma* species or viruses.

   Answer E is incorrect. Serum polymerase chain reaction (PCR) can be used to diagnose viral illnesses such as HIV. PCR testing of the throat and sputum can be used to detect *Mycoplasma*, but this is not commonly performed. Cold agglutinin testing is preferred over PCR for the detection of *Mycoplasma*.

7. **The correct answer is C.** Epiglottitis is a medical emergency, and 90% of patients require surgery to reestablish an airway. At presentation patients with epiglottitis can have little or no respiratory compromise, but this can progress to life-threatening respiratory distress within a matter of hours.

   Answer A is incorrect. Epiglottitis on x-ray film of the neck reveals a "thumbs up" sign (ie, "thumbprint" on radiograph), which correlates with an inflamed epiglottis. Inflammation of the larynx and sublgottic trachea is not associated with epiglottitis.

   Answer B is incorrect. Patients with epiglottitis do not have the symptoms or physical findings of conjunctivitis or rhinorrhea. These findings are more typical of croup. Epiglottitis has additional symptoms of drooling and labored breathing.

   Answer D is incorrect. In general, the onset of symptoms is abrupt with epiglottitis and gradual with croup.

   Answer E is incorrect. A typical barking cough is seen with croup, which may eventually lead to inspiratory stridor. Epiglottitis typically presents with stridor and hoarseness.

   Answer F is incorrect. Most of the time, a throat swab in epiglottitis will reveal *Haemophilus* *influenzae*, not parainfluenza. Parainfluenza is more often seen in croup.

8. **The correct answer is E.** Of the antimycobacterial drugs, only isoniazid (INH) produces the lupus-like syndrome described above. INH decreases synthesis of mycolic acids. Furthermore, hepatotoxicity is common to many antituberculosis drugs (rifampin, pyrazinamide, and INH).

   Answer A is incorrect. Disruption of the cell membrane's osmotic properties describes the mechanism of action of polymyxins. Polymyxins are not part of the treatment for TB.

   Answer B is incorrect. Ethambutol, not isoniazid, inhibits the arabinosyl transferase-mediated synthesis of arabinogalactin for mycobacterial cell walls. The side effects of ethambutol include dose-dependent visual disturbances, decreased visual acuity, red-green color blindness, optic neuritis, and retinal damage.

   Answer C is incorrect. The mechanism of action here is that of rifampin, another antimycobacterial drug.

   Answer D is incorrect. Inhibition of folic acid synthesis is the mechanism of action of dapsone.

9. **The correct answer is A.** The image shows a gross fixed lung with focal intrapulmonary hemorrhage as a result of pulmonary emphysema. The combination of early-onset emphysema and hepatic cirrhosis suggests homozygous α_1-antitrypsin (AAT) deficiency, an uncommon autosomal-recessive disorder. AAT is normally secreted by the liver and acts to neutralize elastase activity in the lung. In patients with AAT deficiency, increased elastase activity leads to a loss of elastic fibers and increased lung compliance, resulting in panacinar emphysema. Furthermore, the accumulation of dysfunctional AAT in hepatocytes results in liver damage and cirrhosis.

   Answer B is incorrect. It is the increased levels of elastase activity resulting from AAT deficiency that causes the disease.

   Answer C is incorrect. Increased levels of antineutrophil cytoplasmic autoantibodies are associated with certain small-vessel vasculitic syndromes, including Wegener granulomatosis. Wegener granulomatosis is characterized by granulomatous inflammation of various organs resulting in acute renal failure, pulmonary disease, and other manifestations. Wegener granulomatosis is not associated with hepatic disease.

   Answer D is incorrect. Excess copper is a sign of Wilson disease, an autosomal-recessive defect that impairs the transport of copper from the liver into bile for excretion. The subsequent accumulation of copper in the liver causes cirrhosis and leakage of copper into the blood, where it damages other organs resulting in neurologic, hematologic, and renal disease. Wilson disease is also characterized by decreased serum ceruloplasmin due to a defect in the incorporation of copper into ceruloplasmin. Wilson disease is not associated with lung pathology.

   Answer E is incorrect. Excess iron is a sign of hereditary hemochromatosis, an autosomal-recessive disorder characterized by excessive dietary iron absorption due to the impaired regulation of iron stores (*HFE* gene mutation). While iron overload can cause cirrhosis in addition to DM and cardiomyopathy, it is not associated with lung disease. Diagnostically, hemochromatosis is associated with increased levels of transferrin saturation and serum ferritin.

10. **The correct answer is D.** The right main bronchus is more vertical and wider than the left, and aspirated particles are more likely to lodge at the junction of the right inferior and right middle bronchi. Because of this, aspiration pneumonia contracted when an individual is in an upright position is most common in the right lower and middle lobes. On x-ray, the right lower lobe may appear collapsed as a result of foreign object aspiration.

    Answer A is incorrect. The left main bronchus is narrower and less vertical than the right main bronchus. The right main bronchus is more vertical and wider than the left, and aspirated particles are more likely to lodge at the junction of the right inferior and right middle bronchi.

Answer B is incorrect. The left main bronchus is narrower and less vertical than the right main bronchus. The right main bronchus is more vertical and wider than the left, and aspirated particles are more likely to lodge at the junction of the right inferior and right middle bronchi.

Answer C is incorrect. The lingula is in the left lung, and the left main bronchus is narrower and less vertical than the right main bronchus. The right main bronchus is more vertical and wider than the left, and aspirated particles are more likely to lodge at the junction of the right inferior and right middle bronchi.

Answer E is incorrect. When a person is supine, aspiration pneumonia may affect the upper lobes and posterior segments of the lungs, since they become the gravity-dependent regions when a person lies flat.

11. **The correct answer is E.** Nonselective β-blockers are contraindicated in patients with lung disease because they can cause bronchoconstriction by blocking β_2-receptors responsible for relaxation of bronchial smooth muscle. Nadolol is a nonselective β-blocker and should not be used in a patient with lung disease. Other nonselective β-blockers include propranolol, timolol, and pindolol. Acebutolol, atenolol, esmolol, metoprolol, and betaxolol are cardioselective β_1-blockers that should be favored in patients with lung/airway disease. Although the stem does not specifically state that this patient has lung disease, smoking causes airway hyperreactivity and bronchoconstriction. Adding a nonselective β-blocker could exaggerate these adverse effects of smoking.

    Answer A is incorrect. Acebutolol is cardioselective and can be used in patients with asthma or other obstructive lung diseases.

    Answer B is incorrect. Atenolol is cardioselective and can be used in patients with asthma or other obstructive lung diseases.

    Answer C is incorrect. Esmolol is cardioselective and can be used in patients with asthma or other obstructive lung diseases. However, it has a very short half-life (about nine minutes), and would not be used for long-term outpatient management.

    Answer D is incorrect. Metoprolol is cardioselective and can be used in patients with asthma or other obstructive lung diseases

12. **The correct answer is B.** In zone 1, alveolar pressure is greater than arterial pressure. There is risk of blood flow obstruction in zone 1 where ventilation/perfusion (V/Q) is high (wasted ventilation). In positive pressure ventilation alveolar pressure increases, which also increases V/Q and compresses the capillaries, limiting blood flow.

    Answer A is incorrect. Normally in zone 3, arterial pressure is greatest and alveolar pressure is weakest. Thus the alveolar pressure is too weak to impact blood flow, and the difference between arterial and venous pressure determines blood flow. This will still be the case with a small amount of positive pressure ventilation.

    Answer C is incorrect. Normally in zone 2, arterial pressure is greater than alveolar pressure, which is greater than venous pressure.

    Answer D is incorrect. Regional differences between blood flow are greater than differences in ventilation, due to the effects of gravity. Positive pressure ventilation will not change this.

    Answer E is incorrect. Blood flow changes depending on whether a person is lying down or standing up. When supine, blood flow is distributed evenly throughout the lung because the effects of gravity are not present.

13. **The correct answer is C.** A diagnosis of chronic bronchitis can be made based on the patient's symptoms and biopsy results. Along with the hypertrophy of mucus-secreting

glands and goblet cells, one typically sees an inflammatory infiltrate with a lymphocytic predominance, squamous cell metaplasia, and fibrosis.

Answer A is incorrect. Alveolar fluid and hyaline membranes are characteristic of adult respiratory distress syndrome.

Answer B is incorrect. Although these cells can be found in chronic bronchitis, they are much more typical of asthma.

Answer D is incorrect. Necrotizing vasculitis and granulomatous eosinophilic tissue infiltration is characteristic of Churg-Strauss syndrome.

Answer E is incorrect. Noncaseating granulomas are typical of pulmonary sarcoid, not chronic bronchitis.

14. **The correct answer is D.** In smokers, pseudostratified ciliated columnar epithelium lining the bronchi can undergo metaplasia and transform into stratified squamous epithelium. Stratified epithelium is defined as epithelial membrane composed of more than one cell layer. Stratified squamous epithelium is classified by the flattened shape of the cells in the surface layer. Examples of tissues with stratified squamous epithelium include the skin, mouth, anus, vagina, and esophagus. While it is wrongly believed that stratified epithelium is the result of the need for additional protection from the noxious smoke, the metaplasia actually results from genetic mutation related to the developing cancer.

    Answer A is incorrect. Pseudostratified columnar epithelium is the normal respiratory epithelium on the right that is undergoing metaplasia. This type of epithelium only appears stratified; however, all cells are in contact with basal lamina and only some cells reach the surface of epithelium.

    Answer B is incorrect. Simple squamous epithelium lines alveoli, the loops of Henle, and blood vessels. Simple epithelium indicates that the epithelial membrane is composed of a single layer of cells, which helps when diffusion is important. Under the microscope, simple squamous epithelium is characterized by a single sheet of flattened cells lying on a basal lamina. It does not play a role in this case.

    Answer C is incorrect. Stratified columnar epithelium is found in only a few places in the body, namely, the conjunctivae of the eye and regions of the male urethra. It is composed of a low polyhedral to cuboidal deeper layer in contact with the basal lamina along with a superficial layer of columnar cells.

    Answer E is incorrect. The bladder is lined by transitional epithelium, not the lung. Transitional epithelium is characterized by several layers of cuboidal cells, with the surface layer being large and dome-shaped.

15. **The correct answer is C.** Neonates have high concentrations of fetal hemoglobin in their blood. Fetal hemoglobin has a higher affinity for oxygen than adult hemoglobin (to allow fetuses to extract oxygen from mother's blood), therefore fetal oxygen-hemoglobin dissociation curves are left-shifted. Other physiologic conditions that cause left shifts (higher hemoglobin affinity for oxygen) in the curve include increased pH (or reduced hydrogen ion concentration), decreased temperature, decreased 2,3-diphosphoglycerate (2,3-DPG) levels, and decreased arterial carbon dioxide pressure. Conversely, during exercise, temperature, 2,3-DPG levels, and partial pressure of carbon dioxide increase as a result of increased metabolism in the skeletal muscle. These would decrease hemoglobin affinity for oxygen, facilitating unloading of oxygen to the tissue of highest metabolic activity, and hence there would be a right shift of the oxygen-hemoglobin dissociation curve.

    Answer A is incorrect. An increase in 2,3-DPG binds to deoxygenated hemoglobin in RBCs, allosterically upregulating the ability of RBCs to release oxygen. Because it reduces RBC affinity for oxygen, increased 2,3-DPG right-shifts the oxygen-hemoglobin dissociation curve.

    Answer B is incorrect. An increase in the partial pressure of carbon dioxide in the blood right-shift the curve, allowing increased delivery of oxygen to tissues because of decreased affinity for oxygen by RBCs.

Answer D is incorrect. Increased temperature is an indicator of metabolic activity (and therefore increased oxygen demand). At high temperatures, the curve shifts to the right, indicating a decreased affinity for oxygen by RBCs.

Answer E is incorrect. The acidosis that results from the production of lactate during intense exercise causes a shift in the curve to the right, reducing the affinity of RBCs for oxygen, thereby allowing them to deliver more oxygen to tissues.

16. **The correct answer is D.** This patient's constellation of symptoms is most consistent with Wegener granulomatosis, with the triad of focal necrotizing vasculitis, necrotizing granulomas of the upper and/or lower airways, and necrotizing glomerulonephritis. Most patients have positive titers for anti-neutrophil cytoplasmic antibodies with a cytosolic staining pattern (c-ANCA). The disease is caused by systemic granulomatous inflammation, particularly of small- and medium-sized arteries such as those supplying the kidneys and lungs. If not treated with immunomodulating drugs, focal glomerulonephritis can progress to a crescentic form, with ensuing renal failure.

Answer A is incorrect. Eosinophilia is associated with Churg-Strauss syndrome, also known as allergic granulomatous angiitis. Patients often have asthma and/or allergies. Involvement can include the lungs, heart, skin, kidneys, and nerves. The lack of a history of asthma or allergies argues against Churg-Strauss syndrome.

Answer B is incorrect. IgA nephropathy (such as Berger disease), characterized by deposition of IgA in glomerular mesangium, is a highly variable entity, ranging from asymptomatic hematuria to rapidly progressive glomerulonephritis. IgA nephropathy is limited to the kidneys.

Answer C is incorrect. Goodpasture syndrome is associated with anti-basement membrane IgG antibodies that recognize an epitope on collagen IV. It is a type II hypersensitivity immune response. Like Wegener granulomatosis, Goodpasture syndrome is associated with hemorrhagic pneumonitis and glomerulonephritis. However, neither lesions of the nares and sinuses, nor positive c-ANCA titers, are characteristic of this disease. Moreover, Goodpasture syndrome more commonly affects young adults.

Answer E is incorrect. Polyarteritis nodosa is an immune complex inflammation occurring in medium-sized vessels. It is associated with hepatitis B virus in 30% of patients, is associated with lesions of various ages, and can occur in almost any organ. However, it rarely involves the lung. Patients typically have fever, weight loss, malaise, abdominal pain, melena, and hypertension, as well as cutaneous eruptions, neurologic dysfunction, and hematuria.

17. **The correct answer is D.** The patient has signs and symptoms of sarcoidosis, with classic race, pathology (noncaseating granuloma), and x-ray of the chest revealing prominent bilateral hilar lymphadenopathy, which is present in >90% of patients with sarcoidosis. Erythema nodosum, an inflammatory panniculitis, is the most common cutaneous manifestation of sarcoidosis, and frequently presents as bilateral tender red bumps on the shins. Additional features of sarcoidosis include hypercalcemia due to increased activation of vitamin D by activated macrophages.

Answer A is incorrect. Erythema infectiosum, or fifth disease, is a common childhood viral infection caused by erythrovirus or parvovirus B19. It is often associated with bright red cheeks in the early stages. It is not seen in sarcoidosis.

Answer B is incorrect. Erythema migrans is a characteristic rash that is often seen in patients with early-stage Lyme disease. It often presents as a "bull's-eye" lesion. It is not seen in sarcoidosis.

Answer C is incorrect. Erythema multiforme is a skin condition caused by inflammation of the microvasculature and mucous membranes. It is most often precipitated by herpes simplex virus infection, mycoplasma infection, or adverse drug reactions. It is not seen in sarcoidosis.

Answer E is incorrect. Erythema toxicum is a harmless rash that appears in approximately half of all newborns. It is not seen in sarcoidosis.

18. **The correct answer is A.** This patient's symptoms are characteristic of allergic rhinitis, likely due to an indoor allergen. This response is an example of a type I hypersensitivity reaction in which an allergen cross-links antigen-specific IgE on the surface of mast cells and basophils. Anaphylaxis occurs via the same mechanism. Subsequently, the mast cells and basophils release vasoactive amines such as histamine. Because antibodies are preformed in this type of hypersensitivity, the reaction develops quite rapidly.

Answer B is incorrect. Contact dermatitis is an example of type IV hypersensitivity or delayed-type hypersensitivity. In this reaction, sensitized T lymphocytes release lymphokines in response to antigen. The clinical response occurs several days after antigen exposure. Other type IV reactions include Guillain-Barré syndrome, graft-versus-host disease, and a positive purified protein derivative (PPD), or tuberculin, skin test.

Answer C is incorrect. Goodpasture syndrome is an example of a type II hypersensitivity reaction in which antibodies bind directly to antigen, leading to complement-mediated cell lysis. Other type II reactions include hemolytic anemia, idiopathic thrombocytopenia purpura, and bullous pemphigoid.

Answer D is incorrect. Graft-versus-host disease is an example of type IV hypersensitivity or delayed-type hypersensitivity. In this reaction, sensitized T lymphocytes release lymphokines in response to antigen. The clinical response occurs several days after antigen exposure. Other type IV reactions include Guillain-Barré syndrome, contact dermatitis, and a positive PPD, or tuberculin, skin test.

Answer E is incorrect. Poststreptococcal glomerulonephritis is an example of a type III hypersensitivity reaction in which antigen-antibody complexes activate complement. The complex then causes the release of lysosomal enzymes from neutrophils. Other type III reactions include serum sickness, the Arthus-type reaction, and systemic lupus erythematosus (SLE).

19. **The correct answer is B.** Loop B is notable for the decreased volume and increased pressure of respiration compared to loops A, C, and D. This loop was recorded while the patient was breathing with only one lung. The decreased volume compared to the other loops should make you think of a lung that had a large decrease in area available for oxygen exchange. The lower baseline pressures compared to loop D show that PEEP was not being used when this tracing was made.

Answer A is incorrect. Loop A shows the patient's pulmonary function after the completed transplant. There is improved volume and compliance (change in volume/change in pressure) of the pulmonary system over the baseline loop C.

Answer C is incorrect. Loop C is the patient's baseline prior to transplant. The total lung volume and pressures would be expected to be higher in a patient after total lung resection. These diseased lungs have a poorer compliance than the transplanted lungs and baseline pressures show that PEEP was not being used when these tracings were made.

Answer D is incorrect. Loop D reflects the patient's condition after transplant and maintenance on PEEP, as can be seen by the right shift of the curve on expiration (at low lung volumes) compared to the other three curves. The application of PEEP increases the volume of the alveoli and helps open collapsed alveoli, increasing the portion of ventilated lung and improving the V/Q ratio.

20. **The correct answer is D.** This patient likely has diphtheria, an infection caused by the gram-positive rod *Corynebacterium diphtheriae*. Diphtheria classically presents with a grayish-white pseudomembrane on the phar-

ynx or tonsils; this pseudomembrane should not be disrupted in order to avoid increased absorption of the lethal exotoxin. Fever is usually mild or absent. It is seen very rarely in vaccinated populations but is endemic to certain parts of the world. Culture of *C diphtheriae* requires tellurite agar (Loeffler medium) to prevent growth of normal upper respiratory tract flora. Colonies will become gray to black within 24 hours.

Answer A is incorrect. Bordet-Gengou agar is used to culture *Bordetella pertussis*. Pertussis presents with paroxysmal coughing spells and whooping sounds on inspiration.

Answer B is incorrect. Chocolate agar is used to grow *Haemophilus influenzae*. Encapsulated strains of *H influenzae* cause invasive diseases such as septicemia, meningitis, cellulitis, septic arthritis, epiglottitis, and pneumonia. Nonencapsulated strains are likely to cause otitis media, conjunctivitis, bronchitis, and sinusitis.

Answer C is incorrect. Sabouraud agar is used to grow fungi.

Answer E is incorrect. Thayer-Martin agar is a chocolate agar plate, which has VCN antibiotics (vancomycin, colistin, and nystatin) that suppress the growth of endogenous flora while supporting *Neisseria gonorrhoeae* growth. This patient does not have symptoms of gonorrhea.

21. **The correct answer is A.** Ethambutol is active against *Mycobacterium tuberculosis*, and it is among the first-line agents used to treat tuberculosis (TB) infection (others are isoniazid, rifampin, and pyrazinamide). Ethambutol's mechanism of action appears to be the inhibition of polymerization of cell-wall precursors. Although the drug generally is well tolerated, its most common adverse effects involve ocular toxicity such as loss of visual acuity and red-green color blindness, which usually appears several months after the initiation of treatment. Ethambutol usually is used in an anti-TB regimen with rifampin for patients who either cannot tolerate isoniazid or are infected with isoniazid-resistant *M tuberculosis*. For children, most literature supports a regimen of six months with isoniazid and rifampin, with additional coverage of pyrazinamide during the first two months.

 Answer B is incorrect. Although rifampin is considered the best antituberculous agent, isoniazid is used for prophylaxis in asymptomatic patients with a positive PPD test. A six-month course of isoniazid prevents activation of latent TB in 90% of patients for at least 20 years. Isoniazid blocks mycolic acid cell-wall synthesis and is bactericidal for rapidly multiplying organisms. Major adverse effects include hepatotoxicity and peripheral neuropathy, but many other adverse effects occur, such as lupus-like syndrome and optic atrophy.

 Answer C is incorrect. Like isoniazid, the spectrum of action of pyrazinamide is limited to *Mycobacterium tuberculosis*. The site of activity for pyrazinamide is thought to be a fatty acid synthase gene. The major adverse effect of pyrazinamide therapy is hepatotoxicity, but it is rare at recommended dosages. Another major adverse effect is hyperuricemia and subsequent gout.

 Answer D is incorrect. Rifampin is the most potent antituberculous agent available. Rifampin blocks DNA-dependent RNA polymerase, preventing RNA synthesis. Although it is a better agent than isoniazid for preventing active TB infection, it has a significant risk of liver toxicity that outweighs its benefits as a preventive medicine.

 Answer E is incorrect. *Mycobacterium tuberculosis* can have extrapulmonary manifestations, but the eye is not commonly involved. Miliary TB infection can affect the eye and cause chorioretinitis, uveitis, and conjunctivitis, but these manifestations are rare. Color blindness would not be associated with such an infection.

22. **The correct answer is B.** Cytomegalovirus (CMV) infection is a common complication in immunocompromised patients following bone-marrow transplantation. Histopathology shows large cells with intranuclear inclusions (so-called "owl's eyes") typical of CMV infection.

Answer A is incorrect. Histopathology would show budding cells with pseudohyphae.

Answer C is incorrect. Histopathology would show a granulomatous reaction, with the possible presence of giant cells.

Answer D is incorrect. Histopathology would show acellular, foamy material.

Answer E is incorrect. Histopathology would show cysts with bradyzoites.

23. **The correct answer is B.** This child is suffering from NRDS, which is the result of underproduction of surfactant by the immature neonatal lungs. Surfactant is produced most abundantly after week 35 of gestation. This substance, produced by type II pneumocytes, contains mainly phospholipids and apoproteins. It coats alveoli and small airways and serves to reduce surface tension over the air-water interface.

    Answer A is incorrect. According to LaPlace's law, increasing the surface tension increases the pressure required to keep the alveoli open. This results in less pressure required to collapse the alveoli.

    Answer C is incorrect. Surfactant decreases surface tension, which increases compliance. This is because, per LaPlace's law, decreasing the surface tension increases the collapsing pressure, and compliance is inversely related to the collapsing pressure. Thus, in a child lacking surfactant, the compliance of the alveoli will be decreased.

    Answer D is incorrect. This child's lungs are lacking surfactant. Surfactant is produced mainly by type II pneumocytes.

    Answer E is incorrect. In NRDS, the lungs are immature and thus do not produce mature surfactant. A hallmark of surfactant production is a lecithin:sphingomyelin ratio >1.5. Because this child has immature lungs and is not producing surfactant, this ratio is likely to be <1.5.

24. **The correct answer is C.** This patient most likely has type 1 DM and a resulting ketoacidosis. He has a metabolic acidosis with a large anion gap (>10 mEq) as calculated by the following formula: Anion gap = Na^+ - [HCO_3^- + Cl^-]. This leads to respiratory compensation by deep respiration (Kussmaul's respiration), resulting in a decrease in blood partial pressure of carbon dioxide. The large anion gap is due to the overproduction of ketones in the absence of insulin production.

    Answer A is incorrect. Calcium oxalate crystals may be seen in ethylene glycol poisoning, which can be another cause of metabolic acidosis with an increased anion gap.

    Answer B is incorrect. This case of metabolic acidosis involves an increased anion gap. Normal-gap acidosis is caused by renal loss of bicarbonate due to tubular dysfunction (caused by drug toxicity, SLE) or GI loss of bicarbonate through vomiting or diarrhea.

    Answer D is incorrect. In metabolic acidosis, respiratory compensation occurs and reduces blood partial pressure of carbon dioxide through deep respiration. Elevated blood partial pressure of carbon dioxide is seen in patients with metabolic alkalosis with respiratory compensation or respiratory acidosis.

    Answer E is incorrect. Hyperkalemia, not hypokalemia, is associated with diabetic ketoacidosis.

25. **The correct answer is B.** The reason the overwhelmed medical student could not hear any heart sounds on the left is because this patient has complete situs inversus. As can be seen from the anteroposterior chest radiograph, the cardiac outline is on the right, as is the gastric bubble. This condition is usually not harmful if the reversal of viscera is complete, but is quite debilitating if the reversal is limited to the heart. Often, situs inversus is associated with Kartagener syndrome, a condition caused by an autosomal recessive defect in the molecular motor protein dynein. This genetic defect results in immotile cilia, impairing a number of important processes. The important findings are: male infertility due to immotile sperm, female infertility due to immotile cilia in the Fallopian tube, recurrent sinusitis due to a failure in bacteria and particle clearance, and

bronchiectasis due to a nonfunctional mucociliary elevator.

Answer A is incorrect. Kartagener syndrome is not associated with acute respiratory distress syndrome.

Answer C is incorrect. Kartagener syndrome is not associated with an increased incidence of lung cancer.

Answer D is incorrect. Kartagener syndrome is not associated with exercise-induced asthma.

Answer E is incorrect. Kartagener syndrome is not associated with idiopathic pulmonary fibrosis.

26. **The correct answer is A.** The patient is suffering from the syndrome of inappropriate ADH secretion (SIADH), a condition in which excessive ADH is secreted independently of serum osmolality; this can be seen in a variety of pulmonary diseases (including TB) as well as central nervous system (CNS) disorders that enhance ADH release (eg, stroke, hemorrhage, infection, and trauma) and certain carcinomas (most commonly small cell lung carcinoma). SIADH can also be an adverse effect of some drugs, notably high-dose intravenous cyclophosphamide. Other drugs shown to cause SIADH include carbamazepine, vincristine, vinblastine, cisplatin, amitriptyline, amiodarone, and monoamine oxidase inhibitors. Excessive ADH secretion can lead to nausea, lethargy, seizures, and even coma. The patient's laboratory values are typical of someone with SIADH, showing hyponatremia, serum hypo-osmolality, urine hyperosmolarity, and decreased hematocrit secondary to dilution.

Answer B is incorrect. Like lithium, demeclocycline has been associated with nephrogenic diabetes insipidus (DI). Demeclocycline is not known to cause SIADH, the underlying disorder that accounts for this patient's presentation. In fact, demeclocycline is sometimes used to treat SIADH.

Answer C is incorrect. Hydrochlorothiazide (HCTZ) is a diuretic that may sometimes result in hyponatremia. However, this patient is presenting with SIADH, and HCTZ is not a known cause of SIADH. HCTZ would be unlikely to account for the degree of hyponatremia (as well as the other laboratory abnormalities) seen in this patient. Like indomethacin, HCTZ can be used to treat nephrogenic DI.

Answer D is incorrect. Indomethacin has not been associated with SIADH. It is, however, sometimes used to treat nephrogenic DI. Patients with nephrogenic DI typically present with serum hyperosmolality, hypernatremia, and urine hypoosmolality.

Answer E is incorrect. Lithium toxicity has been shown to cause nephrogenic DI rather than SIADH. In nephrogenic DI the kidneys are unable to absorb water appropriately in response to ADH. Patients present with production of large quantities of dilute urine, serum hyperosmolality, and hypernatremia. They report both polydipsia and polyuria. Medical treatment of nephrogenic DI may consist of hydrochlorothiazide or indomethacin.

27. **The correct answer is A.** The patient's penetrating chest wound opened her intrapleural space to the atmosphere. Therefore, as she attempts to inhale, her thoracic cavity expands but air enters through the wound, equalizing the pressure; this prevents the normal expansion of the lungs. If air is not able to escape through the wound duration exhalation, this is called a tension pneumothorax, in which the quantity of free air in the thoracic cavity increases after each breath.

Answer B is incorrect. Intrapleural pressure should be less than atmospheric pressure during inspiration, allowing air entry. The problem with this patient is that air is entering through a penetrating wound, rather than only into the lungs.

Answer C is incorrect. Pain with inspiration is a frequent complication of traumatic injury. While it may decrease the tidal volume, it would also increase breathing frequency, resulting in an oxygen saturation closer to normal. Additionally, this would not be corrected by chest tube placement.

Answer D is incorrect. Increased pressure in the pericardial space may result in a condition called cardiac tamponade, during which the heart cannot properly dilate. This may occur when blood or other fluid enters the pericardial space. This can result in decreased blood pressure, increased jugular venous distention, and distant heart sounds (called Beck's triad). None of these clinical signs was noted in this patient; furthermore, a chest tube would not relieve the symptoms in cardiac tamponade.

Answer E is incorrect. The elastic properties of the chest wall would tend to spring out, but the negative intrapleural pressure normally created during inspiration opposes this tendency. After the penetrating injury equalized the pressure of the intrapleural space and the atmosphere, the chest wall will spring out, not pull inward.

28. **The correct answer is B.** Increased anteroposterior diameter and prolonged expiration suggests the patient is suffering from chronic obstructive pulmonary disease (COPD). Reduction of FEV_1, forced vital capacity (FVC), and the FEV_1:FVC ratio are the hallmark of airway obstruction. Total lung capacity (TLC) is increased due to lung hyperinflation, secondary to expiratory flow limitation.

Answer A is incorrect. These changes are not consistent with either an obstructive or restrictive pattern. TLC will be increased in COPD.

Answer C is incorrect. In restrictive lung conditions, there is a decrease in the lung's ability to expand. The FVC is decreased more than the decrease in FEV_1; therefore, the FEV_1:FVC ratio is normal or high. TLC is decreased because there is a loss of lung tissue elasticity.

Answer D is incorrect. These changes are not consistent with either an obstructive or restrictive pattern.

Answer E is incorrect. These changes are not consistent with either an obstructive or restrictive pattern.

29. **The correct answer is G.** Working in a shipyard is associated with asbestos exposure. Chronic inhalation of asbestos fibers can result in asbestosis, which is marked histologically by ferruginous bodies that stain positively with Prussian blue. Asbestosis, unlike most other pneumoconioses, results in marked predisposition to bronchogenic carcinoma and to malignant mesothelioma. Smoking and asbestos exposure together greatly increase one's risk of developing bronchogenic carcinoma.

Answer A is incorrect. Asbestosis is not related to an autoimmune phenomenon.

Answer B is incorrect. The cause of asbestosis is the inhalation of asbestos fibers into the lungs. Idiopathic restrictive lung diseases include sarcoidosis and idiopathic pulmonary fibrosis.

Answer C is incorrect. Living in an urban area for years can cause anthracosis, which is a result of inhalation of carbon dust. It is characterized histologically by carbon-carrying macrophages and results in irregular black patches visible on gross inspection. Anthracosis is harmless.

Answer D is incorrect. Ferruginous bodies and ivory-white pleural plaques are not long-term sequelae of steroid abuse.

Answer E is incorrect. TB has Ghon complexes in primary infection. Cavitary lesions are present in secondary reactivation.

Answer F is incorrect. Working in a coal mine can cause "coal workers' pneumoconiosis" or silicosis. It involves inhalation of coal dust, which contains both carbon and silica. It is marked histologically by macrophages containing coal dust particles located around the bronchioles.

30. **The correct answer is D.** This man is likely suffering from obstructive sleep apnea (OSA) secondary to extreme obesity (Pickwickian syndrome). During the night he has intermittent cessation of airflow at the nose and mouth. During this progressive asphyxia, he has a brief arousal, restores airway patency, and returns to sleep. This patient's obesity and elongated

uvula are very good indicators of OSA, as are his daytime sleepiness, inability to concentrate, and hypertension. Periodic, recurrent asphyxia has the effect of causing a respiratory acidosis that, when present chronically, is compensated for by renal retention of HCO_3^-.

Answer A is incorrect. If anything, this patient's glucose is likely elevated.

Answer B is incorrect. This patient likely has a decreased HDL level.

Answer C is incorrect. Increased reabsorption of H^+ would worsen acidosis.

Answer E is incorrect. Renal secretion of HCO_3^- would worsen acidosis.

31. **The correct answer is A.** The patient has a severe, potentially fatal, pneumonia with prominent systemic symptoms. Culture on buffered charcoal yeast extract is the specific clue that the organism is *Legionella pneumophila*. The disease is respiratory legionellosis, also known as legionnaire's disease, so named because the disease was first described when it occurred in epidemic form after an American Legion convention at a Philadelphia hotel. Patients tend to be older and may have risk factors, including cigarette use, alcoholism, diabetes, chronic illness, or immunosuppressive therapy.

Answer B is incorrect. *Listeria monocytogenes* causes listeriosis and is not a notable cause of pneumonia.

Answer C is incorrect. *Spirillum minus* is a cause of rat-bite fever and is not a notable cause of pneumonia.

Answer D is incorrect. *Staphylococcus aureus* can cause pneumonia but is easily cultured on routine media.

Answer E is incorrect. *Streptococcus pneumoniae* can cause pneumonia but is easily cultured on routine media.

32. **The correct answer is D.** This patient most likely died from a massive pulmonary embolism; the image shows an embolus in a pulmonary artery. Immobilization postoperatively increases a patient's risk of deep vein thrombosis (DVT) due to venous stasis. Virchow's triad describes the three biggest risk factors for thromboembolism: (1) stasis, (2) hypercoagulability, and (3) endothelial damage. To prevent DVTs in postoperative, bed-bound patients, heparin is often started in the hospital and transitioned to warfarin on an outpatient basis. Once in the lungs, DVTs can cause chest pain, shortness of breath, pulmonary hypertension, right heart strain/failure, or death. Her physical exam findings are consistent with right heart strain and are related to the obstruction of the pulmonary artery, effectively forcing the right side of heart to work against increased resistance (leading to delayed, pronounced pulmonic valve closure and a split S_2). Protein C deficiency can cause a hereditary prothrombotic disorder because protein C is normally responsible for inactivating factors Va and VIIIa in the coagulation cascade.

Answer A is incorrect. The pathology shown indicates a vascular problem. It does not show signs of aspiration. Aspiration pneumonia is certainly a concern in elderly patients postoperatively. Furthermore, aspiration pneumonia would likely lead to hospitalization first, rather than sudden death caused by a pulmonary embolus.

Answer B is incorrect. Factor V deficiency does not increase the risk of coagulopathy. However, factor V Leiden, a mutation in factor V that confers resistance to activated protein C, does result in a hypercoagulable state. Essentially this mutation results in excessive factor V activity. Do not confuse factor V Leiden with factor V deficiency.

Answer C is incorrect. Factor VIII deficiency is a bleeding disorder. Congenital factor VIII deficiency occurs in hemophilia A and is X-linked recessive. Acquired factor VIII deficiency may occur in autoimmune conditions (inhibitors to clotting factors) or in liver disease (defective production of factors). Factor VIII deficiency is not associated with an increased risk of deep venous thrombosis or pulmonary embolism.

Answer E is incorrect. Thrombocytopenia, characterized by a decreased platelet count and increased bleeding time, would unlikely be the cause of a hypercoaguable state leading to a pulmonary embolus.

33. **The correct answer is A.** Ipratropium bromide is a muscarinic antagonist used to treat COPD and asthma. It competitively blocks muscarinic receptors, preventing acetylcholine-mediated bronchoconstriction. It is administered directly to the airway and is minimally absorbed, leading to few adverse events. At high doses, however, atropine-like toxicity may occur.

    Answer B is incorrect. Methylxanthines such as theophylline act by inhibiting phosphodiesterase, resulting in increased cAMP levels.

    Answer C is incorrect. Cromolyn acts by inhibiting the degranulation of mast cells.

    Answer D is incorrect. Corticosteroids such as beclomethasone and prednisone act by inhibiting the synthesis of cytokines.

    Answer E is incorrect. β-Agonists such as albuterol and salmeterol act by stimulating adenyl cyclase, resulting in increased cAMP levels.

34. **The correct answer is C.** Peripheral, not central chemoreceptors stimulate breathing in response to oxygen levels <60 mm Hg.

    Answer A is incorrect. Central control is located in the brain stem and cerebral cortex. The most important structures include the medullary respiratory center located in the reticular formation, the apneustic center in the lower pons, the pneumotaxic center in the upper pons, and the cerebral cortex.

    Answer B is incorrect. Central chemoreceptors do affect breathing with varying levels of hydrogen in the blood, but they do not directly detect levels of hydrogen in the blood. The hydrogen in blood cannot cross the blood-brain barrier. Thus, carbon dioxide in the blood crosses the cerebrospinal fluid and combines with water to form hydrogen and bicarbonate. The resulting hydrogen acts directly on the receptors.

    Answer D is incorrect. Stretch, irritant, and J receptors function within the lung to regulate breathing. Stretch receptors are located in the smooth muscle; irritant receptors are located in the airway epithelial cells; and the J (juxtacapillary) receptors are located in the alveolar walls close to the capillaries.

    Answer E is incorrect. The aortic and carotid bodies are not central chemoreceptors. They are the peripheral chemoreceptors that are able to respond to decreased partial pressure of oxygen in arterial blood.

35. **The correct answer is B.** The patient has hyponatremia, which can be attributed to the SIADH secretion from a presenting paraneoplastic phenomenon (which is more common in small-cell than non-small-cell lung cancers). Lung cancer management initially involves distinguishing small-cell from non-small-cell carcinomas. Early small-cell carcinoma management entails chemotherapy; early non-small-cell carcinomas can be treated via surgical resection. Survival time for those with untreated small-cell carcinoma is 6-17 weeks. With chemotherapy, median survival increases to 18 months.

    Answer A is incorrect. Surgery does not carry a risk of provoking para-neoplastic syndromes in small-cell carcinoma of the lung. In pheochromocytoma, however, manipulation of the tumor during surgical resection is known to stimulate catecholamine release.

    Answer C is incorrect. Surgical resection has not been shown to improve morbidity or mortality for small-cell lung cancer, and is thus contra-indicated because of increased and unnecessary morbidity. Resection may be more effective for non-small-cell lung carcinoma. Some patients with very advanced GI tumors benefit from surgical resection to relieve obstructive symptoms.

    Answer D is incorrect. Surgical resection is more effective for non-small-lung carcinoma. It leads to increased morbidity and no improvement in survival in patients with small-cell carcinoma.

    Answer E is incorrect. This explanation would suggest that *no therapy* is the best course of action, which is false. There are few masses for which nothing is done; an example is the cutaneous hemangioma seen in pediatric patients.

36. **The correct answer is D.** Interstitial (or idiopathic) pulmonary fibrosis (IPF) is a chronic, progressive fibrotic disorder of the lower respiratory tract that affects older adults. It is characterized by the abnormal proliferation of mesenchymal cells, disruption of collagen structures, and impaired gas exchange. The exact pathogenesis of IPF is still unknown. If not treated, IPF often results in death within five years. Lung transplantation is currently the only "cure" for this disease. On x-ray of the chest, IPF usually is seen best in the lower parts of both lungs as white lines in a netlike pattern.

    Answer A is incorrect. Albuterol is a β_2-adrenergic agonist used in treating patients with asthma. It is not a definitive therapy for IPF.

    Answer B is incorrect. Azathioprine may be useful in the treatment of IPF, but a patient's pulmonary status will still deteriorate despite its use.

    Answer C is incorrect. Cyclosporine is an immunosuppressive drug most commonly used after transplantation. By inhibiting T-lymphocytes from producing interleukin-2 and other lymphokines, cyclosporine is able to reduce inflammation. Although it can be useful in the treatment of IPF, a patient's pulmonary status often continues to deteriorate.

    Answer E is incorrect. Steroids may be useful in the treatment of idiopathic pulmonary fibrosis, but the patient's pulmonary status generally continues to deteriorate despite their use. The only cure for the disease is lung transplantation.

37. **The correct answer is C.** *Legionella pneumophila* is an aerobic, gram-negative rod that causes Legionnaire's disease, a condition in which patients develop acute, severe pneumonia and a high fever. Other signs and symptoms include hyponatremia (which is unique to this pneumonia) and CNS changes. Legionnaire's disease is one of the most common causes of community-acquired pneumonia but is identified as the cause in only 3% of cases. The organism is present only in water sources (eg, air conditioning systems, whirlpools, mist sprayers) and causes infection when aerosolized water droplets are inhaled. Transmission is not by person-to-person contact. Typically, more severe illness is seen in patients who are >50 years of age, those who smoke, and those whose Gram stain shows neutrophils and very few organisms, as in this case. Treatment is with erythromycin, because *L pneumophila* produces a β lactamase that renders it resistant to penicillin derivatives.

    Answer A is incorrect. *Bordetella pertussis* is a gram-negative rod that causes whooping cough, characterized by paroxysms of coughing followed by a loud inspiration, or "whoop." *B pertussis* infection does not typically cause pneumonia.

    Answer B is incorrect. *Haemophilus influenzae* type B is a gram-negative rod commonly associated with acute epiglottitis or meningitis. It is an exclusively human pathogen that is transmitted by aerosolized droplets or direct contact with secretions. The *H influenzae* type B vaccine has rendered these infections far less common, making it an unlikely agent in this scenario.

    Answer D is incorrect. *Mycobacterium tuberculosis* is an acid-fast mycobacterium that causes TB. The first exposure to *M tuberculosis*, or primary TB, is usually asymptomatic. Secondary, or reactivation, TB occurs after the bacteria have been dormant for some time and re-emerge as a result of temporary weakening of the immune system. This phase of disease is typically a chronic process characterized by low-grade fever, night sweats, weight loss, and a productive cough. This chronic picture differentiates TB from the acute picture of Legionnaires disease.

    Answer E is incorrect. *Streptococcus pneumoniae* presents acutely and is a significant cause of bacterial pneumonia in adults. Unlike *L pneumophila*, however, sputum culture in *S pneumoniae* infection would reveal significant growth of gram-positive diplococci.

S pneumoniae is transmitted by person-to-person contact.

38. **The correct answer is B.** The patient is suffering from TB, with the causative organism (*Mycobacterium tuberculosis*) seen as red on acid-fast stain. Symptoms include fever, night sweats, chills, cough, and weight loss. His treatment regimen will include isoniazid and other antimycobacterial agents. Isoniazid inhibits mycolic acid synthesis in the mycobacterial cell wall. Because of rapid development of resistance, isoniazid should never be used alone to treat active TB. Isoniazid depletes pyridoxine (vitamin B_6), which is required for the production of dopamine, epinephrine, norepinephrine, and monoamine neurotransmitters. Hence, one of the adverse effects of isoniazid therapy is peripheral neuropathy, which can be prevented by co-administration of vitamin B_6.

    Answer A is incorrect. There is no role for the administration of cobalamin (vitamin B_{12}) in the treatment of TB. Vitamin B_{12} is used to treat patients with deficiency who are showing neurologic symptoms and macrocytic anemia. Vitamin B_{12} is a coenzyme that facilitates arrangement of a hydrogen atom between two adjacent atoms and methyl group transfer between two molecules. Deficiency is seen in chronic alcoholics, pure vegans, and those with pernicious anemia.

    Answer C is incorrect. There is no role for the administration of vitamin B_1 (thiamine) in the treatment of TB. Thiamine combines with ATP to form thiamine pyrophosphate, a cofactor for oxidative decarboxylation of α-ketoacids and branched-chain amino acid dehydrogenase; it is also a cofactor for transketolase in the hexose monophosphate shunt. Thiamine deficiency leads to beriberi, Wernicke-Korsakoff syndrome, and lactic acidosis. Vitamin B_1 is used to treat alcoholics to prevent Wernicke-Korsakoff syndrome.

    Answer D is incorrect. There is no role for the administration of vitamin C in the treatment of TB. Vitamin C is used to treat scurvy.

    Answer E is incorrect. There is no role for the administration of vitamin E in the treatment of TB. Vitamin E is a potent lipid-soluble antioxidant that protects the cell membranes from lipid peroxide.

39. **The correct answer is F.** This child has measles complicated by pneumonia. Pneumonia complicates approximately 4% of measles cases in the United States and as many as 50% of cases abroad. Clinically, this child has a high fever, Koplik's spots, maculopapular rash, and CT of the chest showing diffuse interstitial involvement. Measles-infected respiratory cells will fuse and form multinucleated giant cells, which can be detected in sputum samples. Measles is a member of the Paramyxoviridae family, a group of negative-sense, single-stranded RNA viruses. In immunocompromised hosts, measles pneumonia may evolve to giant cell pneumonia, which is often fatal.

    Answer A is incorrect. Acid-fast bacilli would be expected in the sputum of a child infected with mycobacteria such as *Mycobacterium tuberculosis*.

    Answer B is incorrect. Cells with nuclei surrounded by a halo and clear cytoplasm are koilocytes and would be found in cells infected with human papillomavirus. This child has measles, which will form multinucleated giant cells.

    Answer C is incorrect. Cowdry-type inclusions in cells are suggestive of infection with CMV. Although CMV can cause pneumonia, it does so more commonly in immunocompromised hosts.

    Answer D is incorrect. Gram-negative coccobacilli and polymorphonuclear leukocytes are commonly associated with *Haemophilus influenzae*, which is a common cause of pneumonia in children. However, this child is likely infected with measles.

    Answer E is incorrect. Gram-positive diplococci and polymorphonuclear leukocytes are often seen in pneumococcal pneumonia, which would more likely present with a dense lobar pneumonia. This child has other signs and symptoms characteristic of measles.

40. **The correct answer is A.** This child suffers from a congenital diaphragmatic hernia caused by the failure of the diaphragm to properly form and close. The presence of bowel sounds in a lung zone indicates that abdominal contents have herniated past the boundary of the diaphragm into the thorax. The developing diaphragm is derived from the **S**eptum transversum, **P**leuroperitoneal folds, **B**ody wall, and **D**orsal mesentery of the esophagus. These four components can be remembered by the mnemonic "**S**everal **P**arts **B**uild the **D**iaphragm."

    Answer B is incorrect. A continuous cardiac murmur (ie, present during both systole and diastole) could be the consequence of a patent ductus arteriosus, but is not related to the pleuroperitoneal folds and is unlikely to cause the presentation in this patient.

    Answer C is incorrect. Marked splenomegaly in children has many etiologies, but is unlikely to be consistent with the features of this vignette. Causes of splenomegaly include congenital infections and metabolic genetic disorders. Congenital infections include the **ToRCHeS** infections, which include **To**xoplasmosis, **R**ubella, **C**ytomegalovirus, **He**rpesvirus/HIV, and **S**yphilis. These infections often cause hepatosplenomegaly, jaundice, mental retardation, and intrauterine growth retardation. Lysosomal storage diseases such as Gaucher disease, Niemann-Pick disease, Hunter syndrome, and Hurler syndrome also have symptoms of hepatosplenomegaly.

    Answer D is incorrect. Midline deviation of the trachea is commonly associated with pneumothorax or space-occupying lesions of the cervical region.

41. **The correct answer is D.** Choice D represents the residual volume, which is the volume that remains in the lungs after a maximal expiration. The residual volume increases dramatically in emphysema.

    Answer A is incorrect. Choice A represents the inspiratory reserve volume, which is the volume that can be inspired after inspiration of the tidal volume.

    Answer B is incorrect. Choice B represents the tidal volume, which is the volume inspired or expired with each normal breath.

    Answer C is incorrect. Choice C represents the expiratory reserve volume, which is the volume that can be expired after the expiration of the tidal volume.

    Answer E is incorrect. Choice E represents the inspiratory capacity, which is the sum of tidal volume and inspiratory reserve volume.

    Answer F is incorrect. Choice F represents the functional reserve capacity. It is the sum of the expiratory reserve volume and the residual volume, and it is the volume that remains in the lungs after a tidal volume is expired.

    Answer G is incorrect. Choice G represents vital capacity, which is the sum of tidal volume, inspiratory reserve volume, and expiratory reserve volume. Vital capacity (also called FVC) is the volume of air that can be forcibly expired after a maximal inspiration.

42. **The correct answer is D.** This patient is showing signs of Cushing syndrome with a buffalo hump and purple striae. Cushing syndrome is caused by an excess of cortisol either because of a pituitary adenoma producing excess ACTH, an adrenal adenoma producing excess cortisol, or ectopic ACTH production by a neoplasm. This man's smoking history and lung nodule shown on chest radiography point to lung cancer. Taken together with ectopic production of ACTH, this patient has paraneoplastic syndrome, with ectopic production of ACTH by the malignant lung mass. Of the different histological classifications of lung cancer listed above, small cell carcinoma is the most likely in the case for several reasons: Squamous cell and small cell carcinomas are most closely linked to smoking history (>98% are associated with smoking) and both present as central lesions such as that shown on the x-ray film. Additionally, tumors producing

ACTH or ADH are usually small cell carcinomas.

Answer A is incorrect. Adenocarcinoma is the most common lung cancer found in women and nonsmokers (although 75% are found in smokers). Adenocarcinomas are usually peripherally located, and are less likely to cause para-neoplastic conditions such as Cushing syndrome.

Answer B is incorrect. Bronchial carcinoid is a rare neuroendocrine lung tumor that is not linked to smoking. These tumors cause cough, hemoptysis, and an increase the number of respiratory infections. Some of them are capable of producing serotonin and causes the classic "carcinoid syndrome" characterized by episodic attacks of diarrhea, flushing, and cyanosis.

Answer C is incorrect. Many cancers cause metastases to the lung. These typically present as multiple discrete nodules found in all lobes. The picture shown here is that of a single solitary lesion, which is more likely to be a primary lung cancer.

Answer E is incorrect. Squamous cell carcinoma accounts for 25%-40% of lung cancers and is closely linked to smoking. Like small cell carcinoma, squamous cell carcinoma also arises centrally and is associated with paraneoplastic syndromes. However, while small cell carcinomas are responsible for Cushing syndrome and the SIADH secretion, squamous cell carcinomas usually cause hypercalcemia by producing parathyroid hormone-related peptide.

43. **The correct answer is D.** This question requires knowledge of both the anatomy and the physiology of the sucking chest wound, as described in this patient. A penetrating wound to the chest can puncture the pleura, making an opening for air to be sucked into the pleural space. With inspiration, the diaphragm descends, lowering the intrapleural pressure. If there is a communication directly between the pleural space and the outside world, air is sucked into this negative-pressure space and collapses the lung. Pneumothorax is seen on x-ray of the chest as a collapsed lung with a mediastinum shifted away from the collapsed lung. With pneumothorax, the patient should be assessed for signs and symptoms of hemodynamic compromise. This patient, for example, is hypotensive, tachycardic, and tachypnic, and therefore requires urgent management.

Answer A is incorrect. It is possible that this patient has a hemothorax, but this vignette describes a pneumothorax injury. A hemothorax is characterized by blood in the thoracic cavity.

Answer B is incorrect. The stab wound is above the nipple, which is about the level of the fourth and fifth ribs, superior to the ninth and tenth ribs. It is possible that the man has also sustained injury to his lower ribs, but this would not be related to the knife injury and is not described in this vignette. Of note is the risk that a fractured lower rib (11th or 12th) may puncture the kidney, leading to retroperitoneal bleeding.

Answer C is incorrect. A pleural effusion is seen on radiographs as a fluid collection in the dependent portions of the thorax. Pleural effusions can occur in heart failure, pneumonia, or iatrogenic fluid overload (eg, improper fluid management of a hospitalized patient).

Answer E is incorrect. Right upper lobe consolidation would be consistent with right upper lobe pneumonia, which is not described in this vignette. One would expect to see a history of fever and other signs of infection, which is not the case here. Also, radiographs would show an uninterrupted opacity.

44. **The correct answer is A.** This patient is likely suffering from a TB infection that was reactivated by her use of etanercept. The x-ray of the chest shows a dense cavitary apical lung lesion that is highly indicative of a reactivated TB infection. Etanercept is a fusion protein that contains two identical tumor necrosis factor (TNF)-receptor monomers fused to a human IgG Fc domain. Therefore, it acts as a TNF antagonist. In TB infections, TNF (secreted by activated macrophages) recruits monocytes to form the epithelioid granulomas required to contain the mycobacteria. When TNF is ef-

fectively removed from the infection site (by drugs or other forms of immunosuppression), patients face an increased risk of reactivation with caseation and cavitary lesions.

Answer B is incorrect. Methotrexate is an anti-inflamatory agent used in the treatment of RA. It inhibits dihydrofolate reductase and blocks thymine synthesis. It is not an inhibitor of tumor necrosis factor. The dosage of methotrexate used in the treatment of RA does not induce myelosuppression, although higher doses can produce this complication.

Answer C is incorrect. Nonsteroidal anti-inflammatory drugs (NSAIDs) do not impair immunity, although they do impair platelet function. These drugs can help decrease inflammation, but do not slow the progression of RA. It is quite unlikely that a patient with RA who complains of well-controlled joint pain would be relying on NSAIDs alone.

Answer D is incorrect. Risedronate is a bisphosphonate used in the prevention and treatment of osteoporosis. Bisphosphonates are not used in the treatment of RA, and do not have immunosuppressive effects.

Answer E is incorrect. Although the exact mechanism of action of sulfasalazine is not known, it is believed to suppress the activity of natural killer cells and impair lymphocyte transformation, which would not directly allow mycobacteria to overcome immune surveillance and reactivate.

45. **The correct answer is D.** Bronchiectasis can be caused by a chronic necrotizing infection of the bronchi leading to dilated airways. In addition to bronchopulmonary infections, bronchiectasis can be caused by bronchial obstructions or congenital abnormalities (bronchial cysts, tracheobronchial fistulas). Bronchiectasis is a common cause of hemoptysis and also frequently presents with cough and dyspnea.

Answer A is incorrect. Adult respiratory distress syndrome causes diffuse alveolar damage that leads to increased alveolar capillary permeability. It does not cause airway dilation.

Answer B is incorrect. Asthma is a condition associated with airway constriction, marked by wheezing. It does not present with hemoptysis or airway dilation

Answer C is incorrect. Atelectasis is alveolar collapse and is not associated with airway dilation.

Answer E is incorrect. Churg-Strauss syndrome is a multisystem disease that commonly affects the lung. It is characterized by eosinophilia and vasculitis, not airway dilation.

46. **The correct answer is A.** β-agonists such as albuterol may cause potassium to shift into cells, resulting in hypokalemia. This may lead to ECG abnormalities due to destabilization of cardiac cell membranes, the classic examples of which are U waves. Short-acting β-agonists such as albuterol are used in the treatment of acute asthma exacerbations because of their relaxing effects on bronchial smooth muscle. Long-acting β-agonists such as salmeterol are used for prophylaxis of bronchospasm.

Answer B is incorrect. Cromolyn inhibits antigen-induced bronchospasm by inhibiting mediator release from bronchial mast cells, and suppressing chemotaxis of neutrophils, eosinophils, and monocytes. It is used as a prophylactic agent in mild to moderate asthma. Cromolyn is generally well tolerated, and adverse effects are generally minor, including bronchospasm, cough, wheezing, angioedema, headache, and nausea.

Answer C is incorrect. Ipratropium is an antimuscarinic agent that is used for both asthma and COPD. Common adverse effects include cough, nausea, and dizziness. It is not known to cause hypokalemia.

Answer D is incorrect. Theophylline most likely causes bronchodilation by increasing levels of cAMP. It does this by inhibiting phosphodiesterase, an enzyme that hydrolyses cAMP to AMP. Theophylline has a narrow therapeutic window and may cause cardiotoxicity (and neurotoxicity) but does not result in hypokalemia.

Answer E is incorrect. Zileuton is an asthma medication that blocks the production of leukotrienes. Serious adverse reactions include hepatotoxicity and neutropenia. It is not known to cause hypokalemia.

47. **The correct answer is C.** This image shows noncaseating granulomas involving lung septae. Noncaseating granulomas are characteristic of sarcoidosis. Sarcoidosis is a multiorgan inflammatory disorder of unknown etiology. It is thought to be immune mediated. The lung is the most frequently involved organ, but other commonly affected organs are lymph nodes, skin, eyes, kidneys, the heart, and the CNS. Findings that might be expected in a patient with sarcoidosis include **γ** **G**lobulinemia, **R**heumatoid arthritis, elevated **A**ngiotensin-converting enzyme levels, **I**nterstitial fibrosis, and **N**oncaseating granulomas (remember the mnemonic **GRAIN**). Initial treatment of sarcoidosis includes a short course of glucocorticoids such as dexamethasone if the patient is symptomatic. For chronic disease, glucocorticoids may be continued or alternative agents such as methotrexate may be used.

Answer A is incorrect. Small cell lung cancer is recognized by numerous small blue neoplastic cells on histologic exam. The primary treatment of small cell lung cancer is operative, but in patients with stages IB and II disease, adjuvant therapy with cisplatin has shown a trend toward improved survival. The image shows noncaseating granulomas, which are characteristic of sarcoidosis and would not be treated with chemotherapy.

Answer B is incorrect. Goodpasture syndrome is caused by anti-basement membrane antibodies, which can be demonstrated on immunofluorescence. It is not associated with noncaseating granulomas. Initial treatment of Goodpasture syndrome is a five-day course of methylprednisolone followed by a long taper and maintenance. However, if the disease is particularly severe, immunosuppressive agents such as cyclophosphamide or azathioprine may be started.

Answer D is incorrect. SLE can be associated with pleuritis, but it is not associated with noncaseating granulomas. Initial treatment of non-life-threatening SLE includes analgesics and antimalarials such as hydroxychloroquine. As this patient has sarcoidosis, not lupus, hydroxychloroquine would not be an appropriate treatment for her.

Answer E is incorrect. TB is characterized by caseating granulomas, which can be recognized by the necrotic, cheese-like center in the granuloma. Bacteria within the granuloma may not be destroyed, but may rather be dormant only to be later reactivated. This is more likely if the patient is immunosuppressed at any time. TB is treated with a multidrug regimen consisting of isoniazid, rifampin, pyrazinamide, and ethambutol for two months followed by a four-month course of isoniazid and rifampin.

48. **The correct answer is B.** This describes *Bacillus anthracis*, which can cause cutaneous anthrax, inhalation anthrax, and GI anthrax. This patient had inhalation anthrax (also known as "wool-sorter's disease"), which usually has two phases: the initial phase characterized by malaise, dry cough, and chest pressure that resolve in a few days; and the second phase in which patients suddenly develop acute respiratory distress and hypoxemia followed by hemorrhagic mediastinitis and bloody pleural effusions. A classic radiologic finding is mediastinal widening. If a patient is not rapidly treated with penicillin, doxycycline, ciprofloxacin, or levofloxacin, systemic infection can cause septic shock (due to exotoxins produced by the bacteria) and death within 24 hours. Spores from sheep or goat skin are the primary mode of transmission in this kind of anthrax. Interestingly, *B anthracis* is the only medically relevant bacteria with a protein capsule.

Answer A is incorrect. This describes *Brucella*. *Brucella* is transmitted from cattle to humans who have contact with infected animal meat, milk products, or aborted animal placentas. The pathogen penetrates multiple organs, including the lungs, skin, conjunctiva, and GI tract. Patients with brucellosis have systemic symptoms such as fever (undulant fever that is worse in the evening), chills, loss of appetite, and lymphadenopathy. Brucellosis is rarely fatal, and its symptoms can last from months to years.

Answer C is incorrect. This describes *Francisella tularensis*, which causes tularemia, characterized by abrupt onset of fever, chills, malaise, and fatigue. Six clinical forms of tularemia exist: ulceroglandular, glandular, oculoglandular, oropharyngeal, pneumonic, and typhoidal (septicemic). Pulmonic tularemia is very similar to inhalational anthrax; however, hemorrhagic mediastinitis is not seen in tularemia, and death does not occur within 24 hours. Tularemia is also associated with rabbit, tick, or deerfly contact.

Answer D is incorrect. This describes *Nocardia asteroides*, which causes pulmonary infections primarily in immunocompromised individuals.

Answer E is incorrect. This describes *Legionella pneumophila*. *Legionella* is a cause of severe pneumonia, particularly in cigarette smokers and immunocompromised individuals. It is associated with environmental water sources. It does not cause mediastinitis or hemorrhagic pleural effusions.

49. **The correct answer is C.** In the tissues, more carbon dioxide is being produced because of the increased metabolic rate. The additional carbon dioxide enters the RBC and is combined with water by carbonic anhydrase to form H_2CO_3, which then dissociates into hydrogen and bicarbonate. The hydrogen ions are buffered by deoxyhemoglobin, while the bicarbonate diffuses out of the RBCs in exchange for chloride ions. This is called the chloride shift.

Answer A is incorrect. Bicarbonate travels in the plasma, not the RBCs. When it gets to the lung, it enters the RBCs, transforms back to water and carbon dioxide, and the latter is exhaled.

Answer B is incorrect. The primary transport of carbon dioxide in the blood (90%) is via bicarbonate. Carbaminohemoglobin accounts for only about 5%.

Answer D is incorrect. The lungs do not have an acidic environment; the peripheral tissues have an acidic environment. The oxygenation of hemoglobin in the lungs promotes the dissociation of hydrogen ions from deoxyhemoglobin and the equilibrium is shifted toward the production of carbon dioxide from carbonic acid.

Answer E is incorrect. While most of the carbon dioxide is converted to bicarbonate, bicarbonate does not bind to hemoglobin; hydrogen ions bind hemoglobin. Dissolved carbon dioxide that remains in the plasma accounts for about 5% of transport.

50. **The correct answer is A.** The long smoking history and presence of flattened diaphragms on radiographs are suggestive of COPD. The hallmark of obstructive lung disease is a decreased FEV_1:FVC ratio (to <80%). FEV_1 is reduced in patients with COPD because of obstruction. In restrictive lung diseases, FEV_1:FVC is normal or increased.

Answer B is incorrect. Functional residual capacity (FRC) is increased in COPD because the patient is unable to expire air fully, resulting in air trapping in the lungs. In restrictive lung disease, FRC is decreased because the lung has restricted expansion so all lung volumes are decreased.

Answer C is incorrect. The total lung capacity in patients with COPD increases. It decreases in patients with restrictive lung disease.

Answer D is incorrect. COPD has a characteristically decreased FEV_1.

Answer E is incorrect. Emphysema is an obstructive lung disease, which has a characteristically decreased FEV_1:FVC ratio. Restrictive lung diseases can have increased FEV_1:FVC ratios because FVC is reduced along with total lung volume.

SECTION III

Full-Length Examinations

Test Block 1

QUESTIONS

1. An investigator is attempting to create new treatments for patients in shock. Her premise is that increasing oxygen delivery and availability in tissue should reduce some of the tissue damage seen in most forms of shock. From a basic physiologic standpoint, which of the following steps would increase peripheral oxygen availability?

   (A) Administering high doses of norepinephrine
   (B) Administering hydroxyurea
   (C) Inhibiting synthesis of 2,3-bisphosphoglycerate receptors
   (D) Lowering the patient's core body temperature
   (E) Raising levels of partial pressure of arterial carbon dioxide

2. A 32-year-old woman with pheochromocytoma is being treated with phenoxybenzamine. After surgical excision of the tumor, the patient has an episode of hypotension requiring 30 seconds of cardiopulmonary resuscitation and subsequent treatment in the intensive care unit. The attending physician asks his intern what physiologic responses he would expect to see if the patient had been given epinephrine during resuscitation. What would have been observed following administration of epinephrine?

   (A) Decrease in blood pressure
   (B) Decrease in heart rate
   (C) Increase in blood pressure
   (D) Increase in respiratory rate
   (E) No changes in vital signs

3. On physical examination, a 5-year-old girl has hypertension in the upper extremities. She also has weak pedal and popliteal pulses. Her pediatrician is concerned and orders an echocardiogram that confirms the diagnosis. Based on this diagnosis and on the patient's characteristic physical features, the physician performs a karyotype analysis that reveals a genetic abnormality in the patient. The parents are told that the abnormalities observed in the karyotype analysis can explain the abnormal physical examination findings. What is the most likely genetic makeup of this child?

   (A) Trisomy 18
   (B) Trisomy 21
   (C) XO
   (D) XXY
   (E) XYY

4. A 66-year-old man is seen in the emergency department after an acute episode of severe hip pain that caused him to fall while walking at home. X-ray shows the presence of a pathological fracture of the pelvis. On questioning, the man reports that in recent months he has felt very fatigued and has been bothered by constant dull pain in his hips, back, and head. A radiograph of his skull is shown in the image. Laboratory studies show a serum calcium of 13.5 mg/dL and alkaline phosphatase of 60 U/L. Which of the following is an additional finding that would be likely in this patient?

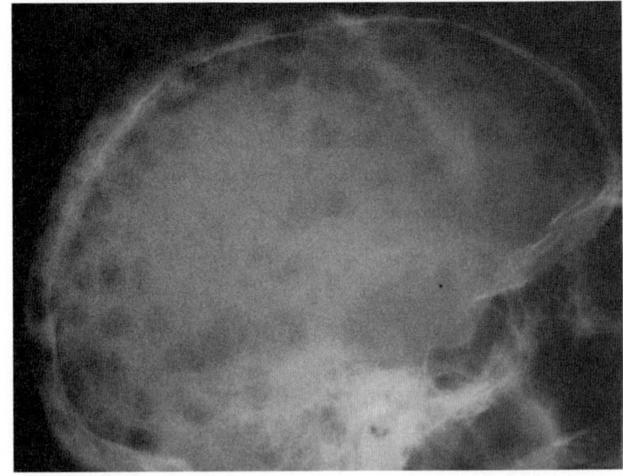

Reproduced, with permission, from USMLERx.com.

   (A) Blue sclerae
   (B) Facial muscle contraction on tapping the facial nerve
   (C) Hard prostatic nodule on digital rectal examination
   (D) Palpable parathyroid nodule
   (E) Proteinuria

5. A 33-year-old man presents to his physician because of recurrent headaches. Although his symptoms are consistent with tension headaches and are alleviated by ibuprofen, he has been conducting research on the Internet and is concerned that his headaches may be caused by a subarachnoid hemorrhage. He insists on undergoing CT of the head. Which of the following is the most appropriate next step?

(A) Address the patient's concerns about a subarachnoid hemorrhage
(B) Compromise with the patient and send him for a less costly x-ray of the head
(C) Obtain a CT scan to alleviate the patient's fears
(D) Send the patient for a neurology consult
(E) Tell him he does not have a subarachnoid hemorrhage
(F) Tell the patient ibuprofen will cure a subarachnoid hemorrhage

6. A 21-year-old woman with no family or personal history of breast cancer presents to the clinic with a small, firm mass in the lower inner quadrant of her right breast. Palpation of the mass reveals the mass is firm, nontender, and mobile, with no overlying skin changes and no nipple discharge. There is no associated palpable axillary or supraclavicular lymphadenopathy. A urine pregnancy test is negative. Which of the following would most likely be found on histological examination of this mass?

(A) Branching fibrovascular core extending from a dilated duct
(B) Fibrosing stroma around normal glandular tissue
(C) Large cells with clear "halos"
(D) Parallel arrays of small, monomorphic cells with scant cytoplasm
(E) Sheets of pleomorphic cells infiltrating adjacent stroma

7. A 16-year-old boy comes to the physician because of recurrent sinusitis that progressed to a pulmonary infection with left-sided chest pain and fever. One year ago he had an episode of *Staphylococcus aureus* pneumonia, and he had repeated oral *Candida* infections until a few years ago. The physician suspects that he has an immunodeficiency that results from abnormal NADPH oxidase activity. Which of the following would confirm the most likely diagnosis?

(A) Large lysosome vesicles in neutrophils on light microscopy
(B) Low levels of IgM but elevated levels of IgE and IgA
(C) Low levels of IgM, IgE, and IgA
(D) Negative nitroblue tetrazolium dye reduction test
(E) Positive nitroblue tetrazolium dye reduction test

8. A 79-year-old man presents to his family physician for an annual physical examination. He denies chest pain, dyspnea, fevers, or chills. He suffered a myocardial infarction five years ago. He is taking aspirin, lisinopril, and metoprolol. His ECG is shown in the image. He is admitted to the hospital for therapy consisting of rate control and anticoagulation. After successful in-patient treatment, he is discharged with new medicines. Which of the following is the mechanism of the anticoagulant used in the long-term therapy of this patient's condition?

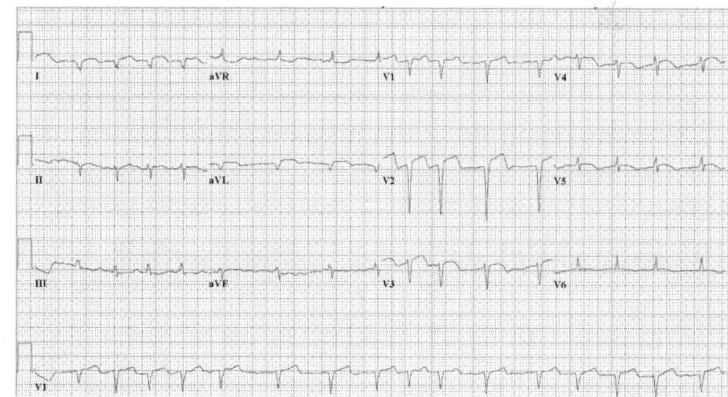

Reproduced, with permission, from USMLERx.com.

(A) Activation of antithrombin III
(B) Antibody to tumor necrosis factor-α
(C) Inhibition of γ-carboxylation of vitamin K-dependent clotting factors
(D) Inhibition of cyclooxygenase
(E) Inhibition of the ADP pathway of thrombus formation

9. A 22-year-old woman presents to her family physician because of increasing fatigue and because she looks "pale" despite spending many hours outside on her sailboat. She also states that her urine looks "cola-colored" when she first goes to the bathroom in the morning. The patient feels well otherwise. Blood analysis shows a low platelet count, a low RBC count, and a low WBC count. The patient's RBCs are mixed with acidified normal serum and compared to normal RBCs at room temperature and at 37°C (98.6°F); both temperatures cause the patient's, but not the normal, RBCs to lyse. Which of the following best describes the pathophysiology behind this patient's disorder?

   (A) Decreased respiratory rate while sleeping → respiratory acidosis → complement-mediated lysis of RBCs
   (B) Decreased respiratory rate while sleeping → respiratory acidosis → osmotic lysis of RBCs
   (C) Decreased respiratory rate while sleeping → respiratory alkalosis → complement-mediated lysis of RBCs
   (D) Decreased respiratory rate while sleeping → respiratory alkalosis → osmotic lysis of RBCs
   (E) Increased respiratory rate while sleeping → respiratory acidosis → complement-mediated lysis of RBCs
   (F) Increased respiratory rate while sleeping → respiratory alkalosis → osmotic lysis of RBCs

10. An acid-fact stain of a sputum sample taken from a 49-year-old woman who recently immigrated to the United States from Mexico is shown in the image. Which of the following should be administered to people who have come in contact with this patient and who have a positive tuberculin test but negative findings on x-ray of the chest?

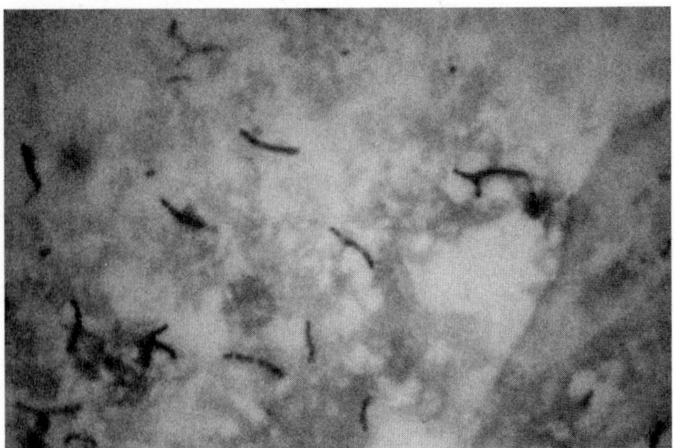

Courtesy of Dr. George P. Kubica, Centers for Disease Control and Prevention.

   (A) Cycloserine
   (B) Isoniazid and rifampin
   (C) Isoniazid and vitamin B_6
   (D) Rifampin
   (E) Rifampin and vitamin B_6

11. A 4-year-old boy has a sublingual mass. ^{99m}Tc pertechnetate scanning shows significant uptake in this region. Which of the following is the embryologic explanation for this mass?

   (A) The thymus has developed ectopically
   (B) The thymus has hypertrophied
   (C) The thyroid has failed to migrate caudally
   (D) The thyroid has migrated too far rostrally
   (E) The third and fourth branchial (pharyngeal) arches have hypertrophied

12. A 27-year-old healthy man presents because he and his wife have been repeatedly unsuccessful in conceiving a child. His wife has been tested and determined to be fertile. Upon questioning, the patient denies coronary or lipid abnormalities but admits to having multiple sinus infections and a chronic productive cough. Further analysis of his semen shows a normal number of sperm. Which of the following is the most likely etiology for the patient's infertility?

(A) Age-related increase in estradiol with possible prostate dihydrotestosterone sensitization
(B) Autosomal recessive dysfunction of a chloride ion channel
(C) Failure of testicles to descend into the scrotum
(D) Familial disease causing early atherosclerosis leading to erectile dysfunction
(E) Lack of dynein ATPase arms in microtubules of cilia

13. An anxious young woman presents to the emergency department because of acute-onset severe abdominal pain. She consumed eight or nine alcoholic drinks earlier in the evening. She also admits to using diuretics to "lose water weight." Physical examination reveals periumbilical tenderness to palpation. Her stool is guaiac negative. Arterial blood gas analysis reveals a pH of 7.55, a bicarbonate level of 21 mEq/L, and a partial pressure of carbon dioxide of 25 mm Hg. Her sodium level is within normal limits. Which of the following is the most likely cause of her acid-base disturbance?

(A) An accumulation of unmeasured anions as a result of hepatic metabolism of alcohol
(B) Electrolyte imbalance due to diuretic use
(C) Hyperventilation secondary to pain and anxiety
(D) Hypoventilation due to the respiratory depression caused by alcohol ingestion
(E) Vomiting due to alcohol toxicity

14. Below is an artist's rendition of the anatomy of the base of the brain. What is a major function of the cranial nerve indicated by the arrow?

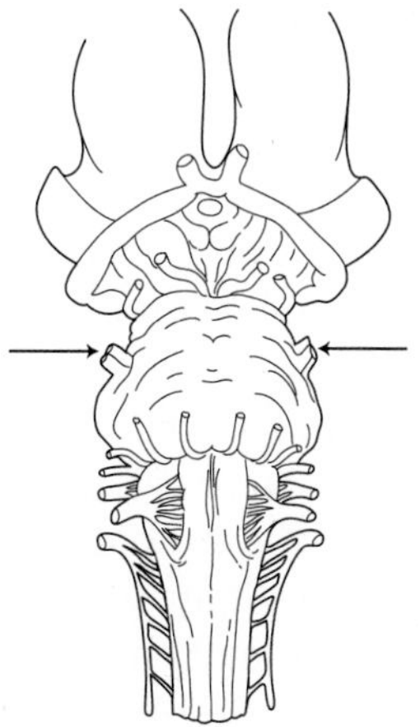

Reproduced, with permission, from USMLERx.com.

(A) Eye movement
(B) Facial movement
(C) Hearing
(D) Mastication
(E) Tongue movements

15. A 65-year-old woman with a history of anxiety presents to her doctor with renewed anxiety. She had been prescribed barbiturates in the past, but has heard that benzodiazepines are now more commonly prescribed. She wants to know how the medications are different. Which of the following statements accurately contrasts the features of benzodiazepines with barbiturates?

(A) Benzodiazepines are less safe for the treatment of anxiety
(B) Benzodiazepines have a higher incidence of respiratory depression
(C) Benzodiazepines have a shorter half-life
(D) Benzodiazepines increase the duration of the chloride channel opening
(E) Benzodiazepines increase the frequency of the chloride channel opening

16. A 3-week-old girl is brought to the emergency department by her mother, who says her daughter has suddenly developed a large, tense bulge on the top of her head and a fever. The mother also notes that the patient has become more irritable and has not been feeding well. Although her mother received limited prenatal care, the child was born at 38 weeks' gestation via spontaneous vaginal delivery without complications. The patient undergoes lumbar puncture, and a Gram stain of cerebrospinal fluid is shown in the image. Which of the following best characterizes the disease-causing agent in this patient?

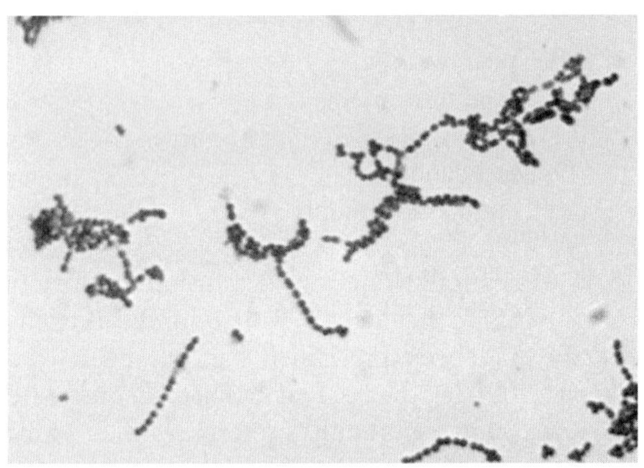

Courtesy of the Centers for Disease Control and Prevention.

(A) Gram-negative bacilli, lactose fermenter
(B) Gram-negative coccobacilli, grows on chocolate agar with factors V and X
(C) Gram-positive bacilli, facultative intracellular
(D) Gram-positive cocci, α-hemolytic, optochin-sensitive, bile-soluble
(E) Gram-positive cocci, β-hemolytic, bacitracin-resistant

17. A 34-year-old woman at 26 weeks' gestation presents with severe abdominal pain, jaundice, ascites, and mental status changes. She has a history of multiple spontaneous abortions. Ultrasonography reveals a blockage in the hepatic venous connection to the inferior vena cava and absence of any waveform in the hepatic veins. She has a positive serum antiphospholipid antibody titer. Which of the following would, if present, predispose a patient to the condition causing symptoms in this woman?

(A) Cholecystitis
(B) Chronic obstructive pulmonary disease
(C) Polycythemia vera
(D) Primary biliary cirrhosis
(E) Renal failure

18. A 42-year-old man with no medical history visits a doctor after he develops sudden, unilateral left-arm weakness after an argument with his wife. He states that he packed up a few of his things and walked out, but when he got to the garage, he could not open the car door. Physical examination findings are normal except for 0/5 strength in his left arm and 2+ deep-tendon reflexes. Sensation is intact. CT scan of the head is negative for acute bleeding. What is the most likely cause of his sudden arm weakness?

(A) Conversion disorder
(B) Factitious disorder
(C) Hypochondriasis
(D) Malingering
(E) Stroke

19. A 4-year-old boy with a history of mental retardation and seizures is brought to the physician with a three-month history of worsening shortness of breath. During physical examination, the physician notices numerous acne-like papules on the patient's face. Echocardiography shows significant left ventricular outflow obstruction. Which of the following is the most likely diagnosis for this patient's heart condition?

(A) Dilated cardiomyopathy
(B) Lipoma
(C) Myxoma
(D) Rhabdomyoma
(E) Transposition of the great vessels

20. A 26-year-old man presents with left eye pain and intermittent double vision. When at rest, his left eye is deviated downwards and laterally, as pictured in the image. Upward gaze and adduction are limited in the affected eye; how-

ever, abduction appears intact. Also, the left lid droops, and the left pupil is dilated and unresponsive to light. Which of the following cranial nerves is most likely to have been injured?

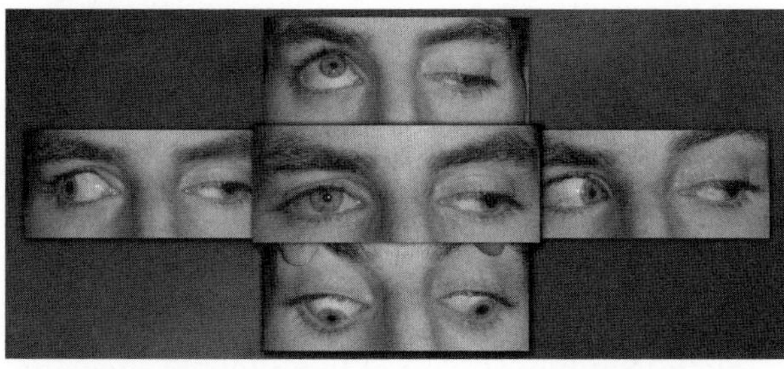

Reproduced, with permission, from USMLERx.com.

(A) Abducens nerve
(B) Oculomotor nerve
(C) Optic nerve
(D) Trigeminal nerve
(E) Trochlear nerve

21. A 61-year-old man with a medical history of cancer presents with a two-week history of constant and severe headaches that are most severe when he wakes up in the morning. He also notes changes in vision associated with the headaches. Physical examination shows a healing ecchymotic lesion on the right forearm, papilledema in the left eye, a right-sided pronator drift, and weakness of the right arm. The diagnosis of an intracranial hemorrhage is confirmed with CT of the head. Which of the following cancers is most likely to have resulted in this patient's presentation?

(A) Angiosarcoma
(B) Basal cell carcinoma
(C) Colorectal carcinoma
(D) Melanoma
(E) Prostate cancer

22. A 24-year-old man is brought to the emergency department by his mother because of a change in mental status. Physical examination reveals a febrile, dysarthric patient with retinal hemorrhages and numerous crusted puncture marks on his left forearm. Auscultation at the apex reveals a new murmur. Blood cultures reveal a gram-positive, catalase-negative organism. Which of the following culture conditions would aid in identifying the most likely single causative organism?

(A) Absence of colonies in the presence of penicillin
(B) Growth in 6.5% sodium chloride
(C) Growth of colonies in the presence of optochin
(D) Growth on chocolate agar
(E) Soluble in bile

23. A researcher is designing an in vitro experimental system to study the kinetics of GLUT 4-mediated glucose transport into mammalian cells of insulin-dependent organs. The system will measure radiolabeled glucose levels in cell culture media both before and at intervals after the addition of insulin. Which of the following cell types is the best choice for use in this experimental system?

(A) Adipocytes
(B) Cortical neurons
(C) Erythrocytes
(D) Hepatocytes
(E) Pancreatic β cells

24. Myasthenia gravis is an autoimmune disorder that affects approximately 3 in 100,000 people. Individuals with mysasthenia gravis classically present with complaints of muscle weakness and fatigue secondary to the formation of autoantibodies directed against the acetylcholine receptors at neuromuscular junctions. The most accurate method of diagnosis involves the detection of these autoantibodies. On average, this test is approximately 80% sensitive and 90% specific. If an individual has a positive test for autoantibodies against the acetylcholine receptor, what is the approximate posttest probability of having this disease, assuming a pretest probability of 50%?

(A) 80%
(B) 85%
(C) 89%
(D) 95%
(E) 99%

25. A 55-year-old alcoholic woman presents to the emergency department because of bloody emesis. She woke up that morning coughing and retching, and later vomited; she had a few more episodes of emesis throughout the day, with the most recent episode containing blood-tinged vomitus. The patient denies any history of bloody emesis, gastroesophageal reflux, or ascites. She denies trouble swallowing or recent weight loss. She does complain of some epigastric pain with inspiration. Physical examination is largely benign except for some tenderness in the epigastric area. She continues to periodically vomit bright-red content; she undergoes an endoscopic evaluation. Which of the following is a finding consistent with this patient's clinical presentation?

(A) Esophageal mass
(B) Esophageal stricture
(C) Gallbladder inflammation and pericholecystic fluid accumulation
(D) Partial-thickness tears near gastroesophageal junction
(E) Transmural esophageal tear

26. A 30-year-old man is involved in a motorcycle accident and is pronounced dead on arrival at the emergency department. A cross-section of his coronary arteries at autopsy is shown in the image. Under normal circumstances, which substance is produced in the innermost cells of the layer (ie, the layer closest to the blood) where these plaques develop?

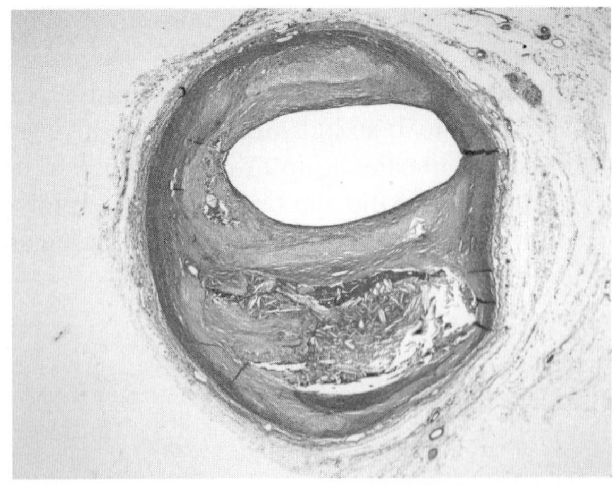

Reproduced, with permission, from USMLERx.com.

(A) Collagen
(B) Fibrillin
(C) Hemoglobin
(D) Macrophage colony-stimulating factor
(E) Nitric oxide

27. An 82-year-old woman with chronic obstructive pulmonary disease is hospitalized for an acute exacerbation and is placed on ventilatory support. During the course of her hospitalization, she becomes febrile with an associated elevation in her WBC count. X-ray of the chest shows a new infiltrate in the right lower lobe. Sputum studies of the infiltrate show that it is the gram-negative bacillus *Acinetobacter baumannii*. She is treated with intravenous (IV) antibiotics. Several hours after starting IV antibiotics, the patient has a seizure that lasts 45 seconds. A subsequent lumbar puncture is negative. Which of the following antibiotics would most likely cause this effect?

(A) Gentamicin
(B) Imipenem
(C) Levofloxacin
(D) Linezolid
(E) Rifampin

28. A 23-year old woman presents to the physician with a chief complaint of an excruciating, sharp pain in her right upper quadrant and fever. Complete physical examination is performed. Pelvic exam reveals bilateral adnexal and cervical motion tenderness and purulent discharge. Other laboratory studies reveal:

WBC count: 14,200/mm^3
Amylase: 28 U/L
Aspartate aminotransferase: 19 U/L
Alanine aminotransferase: 17 U/L
Alkaline phosphatase: 23 U/L
Hepatitis A IgG antibody: positive

Which of the following is the most likely diagnosis?

(A) Acute cholecystitis
(B) Chlamydial cervicitis
(C) Fitz-Hugh-Curtis syndrome
(D) Gonococcal urethritis
(E) Hepatitis A
(F) Tubo-ovarian abscess

29. A 60-year-old woman with a 25-year history of type 2 diabetes mellitus presents with pruritus, diffuse bone pain, and proximal muscle weakness. Laboratory studies show a serum calcium level of 6.5 mg/dL, serum phosphate of 6.0 mg/dL, serum creatinine of 2.7 mg/dL, and intact parathyroid hormone of 300 pg/mL (normal: 10-65 pg/mL). The laboratory findings in this patient are most likely due to which of the following conditions?

(A) Parathyroid adenoma
(B) Parathyroid insufficiency
(C) Renal failure
(D) Underlying malignancy
(E) Vitamin D intoxication

30. A 73-year-old man diagnosed with atrial fibrillation has been treated pharmacologically for the past 10 years. He presents to his primary care physician complaining of shortness of breath and gasping. Pulmonary function tests show that the forced expiratory volume in 1 second (FEV_1) and the forced vital capacity (FVC) are each <70% of predicted values, with an FEV_1:FVC ratio of 81%. The flow-volume curve is shown in the image. Which of the following is the most likely cause of this patient's clinical findings?

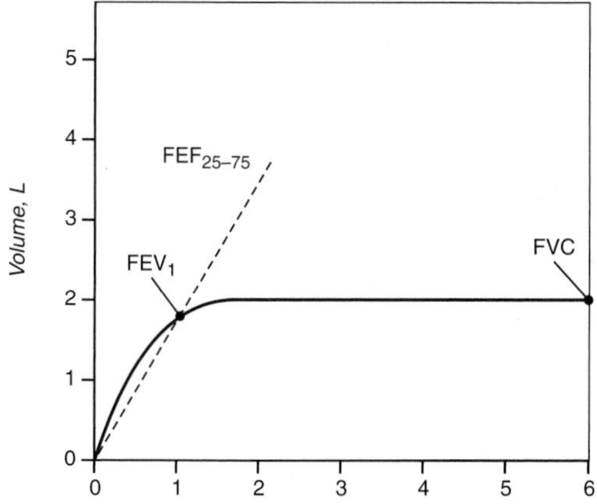

Reproduced, with permission, from USMLERx.com.

(A) Adult-onset asthma
(B) Amiodarone
(C) Diltiazem
(D) Sotalol
(E) Tobacco

31. While working in a rural village in central Mexico, a volunteer physician encounters a 7-year-old girl who presents with a 1-week history of jaundice. The patient's mother reports that, for the past few weeks, the girl has not eaten well and that she has often felt nauseated and has vomited after the few meals that she has eaten. A few days ago, the girl's urine darkened and her stool became pale. On physical examination, the physician notes a fever of 38.5°C (101.3°F), hepatomegaly, jaundice, and icterus. A liver enzyme panel reveals an alanine aminotransferase level of 10,103 IU/ml and an aspartate aminotransferase level of 8030 IU/ml. The patient and her mother deny any illicit drug use or sexual contacts or abuse of the patient. The mother also reports that 1 month ago, two of the girl's playmates had similar symptoms. Which of the following pathogens shares the route of transmission as the pathogen most likely causing this girl's symptoms?

(A) Flavivirus
(B) Hepatitis B virus
(C) Poliovirus
(D) Rabies virus
(E) Varicella-zoster virus

32. A 35-year-old man is brought to the emergency department by ambulance after having a tonic-clonic seizure at work. The patient reports that he has always been healthy and has never had a seizure before. On further questioning, the patient reports that he has been having intermittent bloody stools for the past four months. CT of the head reveals an irregular 3-cm × 4-cm mass extending from the right to the left hemisphere. CT of the abdomen shows multiple polypoid masses in the sigmoid colon. Which of the following is the most likely diagnosis?

(A) Familial adenomatous polyposis
(B) Gardner syndrome
(C) Hereditary nonpolyposis colorectal carcinoma
(D) Tuberous sclerosis
(E) Turcot syndrome

33. A 24-year-old previously healthy woman in the final stages of labor suddenly becomes short of breath. She becomes hypotensive and begins to lose large volumes of blood from her vagina. Moments later, small ecchymoses appear on her legs and near her intravenous site. Which of the following is this woman's most likely coagulation profile?

Choice	Platelet count	Bleeding time	Prothrombin time	Partial thromboplastin time
A	normal	normal	normal	↑
B	normal	normal	↑	normal
C	normal	↑	normal	normal
D	normal	↑	normal	↑
E	↓	↑	normal	normal
F	↓	↑	↑	↑

Reproduced, with permission, from USMLERx.com.

(A) A
(B) B
(C) C
(D) D
(E) E
(F) F

34. A 3-year-old boy comes to the physician because of fever and erythema in his conjunctivae, oral mucosa, palms, and soles for the past week. Physical examination is significant for fever, enlarged cervical lymph nodes, and edema of the hands and feet. Although the precise cause of the patient's disease is unknown, it is speculated that autoantibodies may play a role. Based on the known structure that is primarily affected in the patient's disease, what autoantibodies are suspected to be associated with this condition?

(A) Anti-endothelial cell antibodies
(B) Anti-IgG antibodies
(C) Anticentromere antibodies
(D) Antihistone antibodies
(E) Antinuclear antibodies

35. A 6-year-old boy arrives at the emergency department breathing rapidly and complaining of tinnitus and nausea. His parents reported he had swallowed half a bottle of aspirin accidentally. The emergency department physician decides to administer a medication that alters the pH of the boy's urine to improve excretion of the drug. How does altering the pH of the urine improve the excretion of aspirin?

(A) Acidification of urine increases the glomerular filtration of salicylate molecules
(B) Acidification of urine ionizes salicylate molecules, trapping them in the proximal tubule
(C) Acidification of urine neutralizes ionized salicylate molecules in the proximal tubule
(D) Alkalinization of urine increases the glomerular filtration of salicylate molecules
(E) Alkalinization of urine ionizes salicylate molecules, trapping them in the proximal tubule
(F) Alkalinization of urine neutralizes ionized salicylate molecules in the proximal tubule

36. A 45-year-old man visited his primary care physician one month ago because of chest pain that he had experienced four times in the past four months. The onset of the pain is sudden and radiates to his left jaw. He has experienced this pain while watching television but has never felt it during exercise. During last month's visit, the physician prescribed sublingual nitroglycerin, and the patient reports that this has shortened the duration of his episodes. Last month's ECG is shown in the image. Which of the following is the most likely cause of this patient's chest pain?

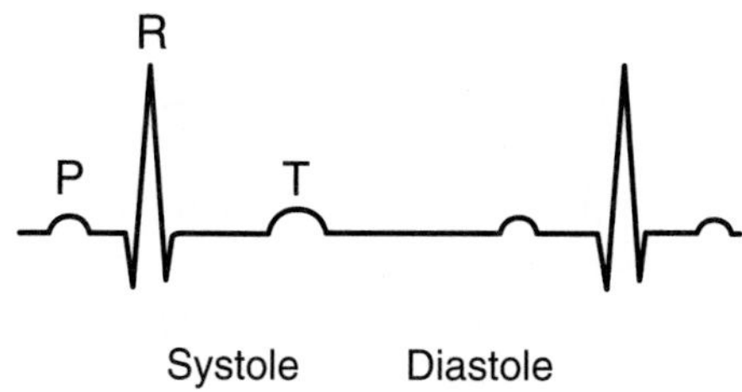

Reproduced, with permission, from USMLERx.com.

(A) Myocardial infarction
(B) Pericarditis
(C) Prinzmetal's angina
(D) Stable angina
(E) Unstable angina

37. A 7-year-old boy presents to the physician with acute-onset edema and facial swelling. Dipstick urinalysis reveals 4+ proteinuria. Renal biopsy shows no appreciable changes under light and fluorescence microscopy, but electron microscopy demonstrates glomerular epithelial cell foot process effacement. A diagnosis of minimal change disease is made. How does this disease affect the pressures governing the flow of fluid across the glomeruli?

(A) Bowman space hydrostatic pressure will be decreased
(B) Bowman space hydrostatic pressure will be increased
(C) Bowman space oncotic pressure will be decreased
(D) Glomerular capillary hydrostatic pressure will be increased
(E) Glomerular capillary oncotic pressure will be decreased

38. A 62-year-old woman who has been on dialysis for end-stage renal failure for six months comes to the physician's office. She is accompanied by her 45-year-old daughter, who is present because of their close relationship. During the visit, her daughter hears about the need for transplantation for the first time, and is visibly surprised, but declares that they will do "anything it takes." After the physician and the women discuss the possible options, the patient turns to her daughter and asks her to be the donor. For which of the following reasons should consent be obtained from the daughter at a different time?

(A) More of the family should be involved in the discussion
(B) The daughter cannot have a full understanding of the procedure
(C) The daughter is not free from coercion
(D) The emergent nature of the patient's clinical symptoms requires immediate action
(E) The patient is not competent to make health decisions due to her condition

39. A 67-year-old obese man complains of swelling in his hands, feet, and face. Physical examination is significant for 3+ edema in his lower extremities and 1+ edema in his hands and around his eyes. Urine dipstick reveals 3+ protein and no blood. Renal biopsy is shown in the image. In addition to the underlying cause of his renal disease, which of the following comorbidities is most likely present in this patient?

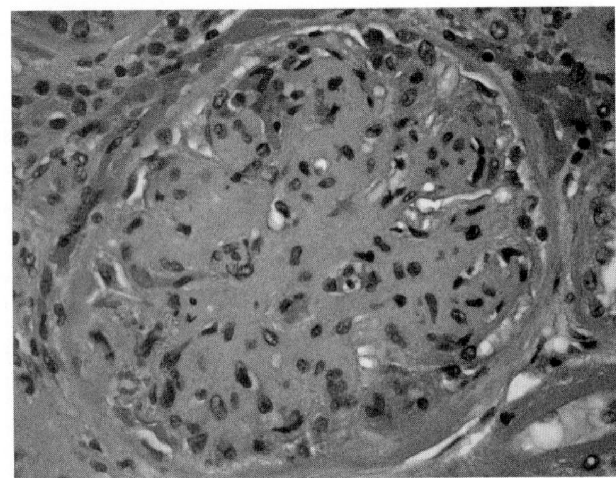

Reproduced, with permission, from USMLERx.com

(A) Arthritis
(B) Bone pain
(C) Coronary artery disease
(D) Hearing loss
(E) Hemoptysis
(F) Pharyngitis

40. A town with 1000 citizens has a 10% prevalence of disease X. A screening test for disease X just came out, with a sensitivity of 80% and a specificity of 70%. How many people with disease X will be missed by this screening test?

(A) 20
(B) 80
(C) 100
(D) 270
(E) 630

41. A 35-year-old man presents to the physician with a two-month history of non-bloody, non-mucoid, non-oily watery diarrhea. He has a diastolic murmur that gets louder with inspiration and is best heard over the left lower sternal border. His face is warm and appears to be engorged with blood for several minutes during the examination. His laboratory studies show the following:

Vanillylmandelic acid: 5 mg/day (normal 0-7 mg/day)
Metanephrine, urine: 250 μg/g of creatinine (normal 0-300 μg/g)
Homovanillic acid, urine: 14 mg/day (normal 0-15 mg/day)
5-HIAA: 28 mg/day (normal 0-9 mg/day)

Gastrointestinal endoscopy is most likely to show a lesion located near which of the following?

(A) Gastroesophageal junction
(B) Ligament of Treitz
(C) Pancreaticoduodenal junction
(D) Rectosigmoid junction
(E) Splenic flexure

42. A 46-year-old man comes to his physician after visiting his optometrist. While being fitted for new glasses, the patient was found to have persistent constriction of his right pupil. After a thorough history and physical examination, x-ray of the chest was ordered, and results are shown in the image. In which ganglion is there evidence of decreased sympathetic synapse activity?

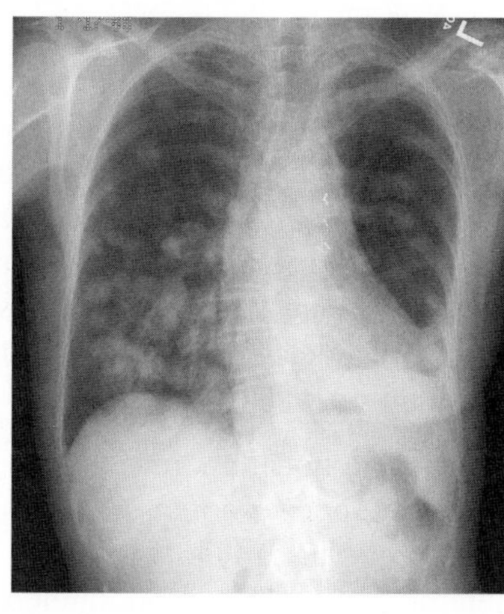

Reproduced, with permission, from Hanley ME and Welsh CH. *Current Diagnosis & Treatment in Pulmonary Medicine*, New York: McGraw-Hill, 2003; Fig. 3-8.

(A) Inferior cervical ganglion
(B) Sphenopalatine ganglion
(C) Superior cervical ganglion
(D) Superior mesenteric ganglion
(E) T4 dorsal root ganglion

43. A 38-year-old white woman presents to the physician with a two-week history of aching pain in her left calf that is made worse by dorsiflexion of her foot. On physical examination, her left calf is found to be erythematous, warm, and swollen. Which of the following measures should she take to decrease similar problems in the future?

(A) Begin taking a bile acid resin
(B) Begin taking a statin
(C) Begin taking low-dose oral contraceptives
(D) Exercise 30 minutes three times per week
(E) Quit smoking
(F) Reduce alcohol consumption to one or two glasses of red wine per week

44. A 10-year-old boy is brought to the emergency department after his parents noted that he was acting confused and lethargic following several bouts of nausea and vomiting. Upon arrival the patient is tachycardic and is breathing deeply and slowly. Laboratory studies are remarkable for a serum pH of 7.21, a serum glucose level of 700 mg/dL, a serum bicarbonate level of 16 mEq/L, and a serum anion gap of 22 (normal: 7-16). Intravenous fluids and insulin are administered. Measurement and management of which of the following electrolytes are most critical in this patient?

(A) Bicarbonate
(B) Calcium
(C) Chloride
(D) Potassium
(E) Sodium

45. A 51-year-old man presents to the emergency department (ED) 30 minutes after experiencing difficulty speaking and moving the left side of his body. The patient is alert and oriented to person and place. His wife states that he has a history of benign prostatic hypertrophy and high blood pressure. According to the wife, the patient has never experienced symptoms like this before and has never had surgery of any type. The ED physicians determine that the patient is hemodynamically stable and an initial CT scan is normal. Which of the following is the best next step in management?

(A) Echocardiogram
(B) Hemicraniectomy
(C) Heparin
(D) Insulin
(E) Tissue plasminogen activator

46. A 3-year-old girl presents to the pediatrician for her annual well child visit. She is developing well and her mother has no concerns at this time. Her temperature is 38°C (100.4°F). Physical examination reveals an enlarged, tender, erythematous left axillary lymph node. Close inspection of the skin reveals a series of small linear scratches on the left forearm, with a nearby erythematous papule. Which of the following organisms is the most likely cause of these findings?

(A) *Bartonella henselae*
(B) *Borrelia burgdorferi*
(C) *Eikenella corrodens*
(D) *Francisella tularensis*
(E) *Pasteurella multocida*

47. A 35-year-old man presents to his primary care physician with a chief complaint of palpitations and occasional chest pain. Further questioning reveals a recent history of weight loss, diarrhea, and heat intolerance. Laboratory evaluation shows anti-thyroid-stimulating hormone (TSH) receptor antibodies in the patient's serum. Which of the following best describes this patient's TSH and thyroid hormone levels relative to normal baseline values?

Choice	Thyroid-stimulating hormone	Total thyroxine	Free thyroxine
A	↑	↑	↑
B	↑	↓	↑
C	↑	↓	↓
D	↓	↑	↑
E	↓	↓	↓

Reproduced, with permission, from USMLERx.com.

(A) A
(B) B
(C) C
(D) D
(E) E

48. A 12-year-old boy who recently emigrated from Nigeria presents with a six-month history of intermittent fever, fatigue, and night sweats. He has a large mass on his right mandible. Biopsy of the mass shows an interspersed pattern of macrophages with sheets of lymphoblasts. The pathogen associated with this patient's presentation also is associated with which of the following conditions?

(A) Cervical adenocarcinoma
(B) Gastric adenocarcinoma
(C) Hepatocellular carcinoma
(D) Heterophile-negative mononucleosis
(E) Nasopharyngeal carcinoma

ANSWERS

1. **The correct answer is E.** This question is asking about the basic physiology behind the oxygen-hemoglobin dissociation curve, which shows how much oxygen is bound to hemoglobin at a given partial pressure of oxygen under normal conditions. Under abnormal conditions the curve can shift to the left, indicating increased affinity for oxygen, or shift to the right, indicating decreased affinity (lower percentage of bound oxygen at a given partial pressure of oxygen). Having a decreased affinity means that it may take higher partial pressures to bind four oxygen molecules to one molecule of hemoglobin, but in the periphery hemoglobin is quicker to release oxygen molecules. Therefore shifting the curve to the right would increase peripheral oxygen availability. pH has a direct relationship with oxygen affinity. Therefore raising partial pressure of arterial carbon dioxide, which translates into decreasing pH, in principle ought to increase peripheral oxygen availability.

   Answer A is incorrect. Norepinephrine is clinically used in shock to maintain a patient's blood pressure by inducing peripheral vasoconstriction. It maintains blood flow to the brain at the expense of the some organs and peripheral tissue. At high doses, peripheral vasoconstriction is so severe that cyanotic fingers may be seen. Therefore while norepinephrine has no direct effect on hemoglobin, it decreases peripheral oxygen availability.

   Answer B is incorrect. Hydroxyurea is an antitumor agent that is also used in sickle cell disease. It actually raises fetal hemoglobin levels. Higher fetal hemoglobin levels raise oxygen affinity which decreases peripheral availability.

   Answer C is incorrect. 2,3-Bisphosphoglycerate (BPG) has a inverse relationship with oxygen affinity. It is a by-product of glycolysis. High levels of 2,3-BPG decrease oxygen affinity. Therefore inhibiting its synthesis will increase oxygen affinity and make hemoglobin less likely to release oxygen at a given partial pressure of oxygen in the periphery.

   Answer D is incorrect. Lowering a patient's temperature shifts the oxygen-hemoglobin curve to the left reducing oxygen availability.

2. **The correct answer is A.** Phenoxybenzamine is a nonselective α-antagonist that will block both α_1- and α_2-receptors. In this patient, the administration of high-dose epinephrine (which is both an α- and a β-agonist) would result in unopposed β_1- (increased heart rate, increased contractility) and β_2- (vasodilation, bronchodilation) agonist effects because the α-effects of epinephrine are blocked by prior phenoxybenzamine administration. The net effect will be β-agonist effects, including an increase in heart rate and a decrease in blood pressure.

   Answer B is incorrect. Unopposed β-agonist effects will cause an increase in heart rate because β_1-agonists result in increased heart rate.

   Answer C is incorrect. Unopposed β-agonist effects will cause a decrease in blood pressure because β_2-agonists result in vasodilation.

   Answer D is incorrect. Unopposed β-agonist effects do not have a significant effect on respiratory rate.

   Answer E is incorrect. Unopposed β-agonist effects will cause changes in both blood pressure and heart rate.

3. **The correct answer is C.** The upper-extremity hypertension and weak pedal and popliteal pulses suggest coarctation of the aorta. Coarctation of the aorta typically is a discrete narrowing of the thoracic aorta just distal to the left subclavian artery. The major clinical finding in patients with coarctation of the aorta is a difference in systolic blood pressure between the upper and lower extremities. Coarctation of the aorta is sometimes associated with Turner syndrome. Other common features of Turner syndrome include short stature, a webbed neck, streaked ovaries, and primary amenorrhea. The genetic makeup of a person with Turner syndrome is XO.

Answer A is incorrect. Trisomy 18 is Edwards syndrome. These children have severe mental retardation, "rocker bottom" feet, and clenched hands (ie, flexion of fingers). Although patients with Edwards syndrome do have congenital heart disease, it generally is not associated with coarctation of the aorta.

Answer B is incorrect. Trisomy 21 also is known as Down syndrome. These patients have mental retardation, prominent epicanthal folds, and congenital heart disease (most often atrial septal defects). They typically do not suffer from coarctation of the aorta.

Answer D is incorrect. XXY is the karyotype in Klinefelter syndrome, which is not associated with coarctation of the aorta. Klinefelter syndrome manifests in phenotypic males as testicular atrophy, androgenous body shape, long extremities, and gynecomastia.

Answer E is incorrect. XYY is the karyotype in "double Y" males. The overwhelming majority of XYY males have normal phenotype and are unaware of their chromosomal status. Nevertheless, tall stature, acne, learning difficulties, and a tendency toward aggressive behavior are all associations drawn on the USMLE. The association between XYY and antisocial behavior is somewhat contentious if not apocryphal (prior studies suggesting a propensity toward violent criminal behavior have not been substantiated). In any case, this karyotype is not associated with coarctation of the aorta.

4. **The correct answer is E.** This patient is suffering from multiple myeloma. The x-ray shows multiple lytic "punched out" lesions in the skull, which is a classic finding for this plasma cell malignancy. Other areas of the skeleton commonly infiltrated by myeloma cells include the vertebrae, ribs, and pelvis, explaining the patient's fracture in the absence of overt trauma. The lytic bone lesions are responsible for this patient's hypercalcemia in the setting of normal alkaline phosphatase levels. Urinary protein (termed Bence-Jones proteins in this setting) is a common finding in multiple myeloma because the neoplastic plasma cells secrete an abundance of immunoglobulin proteins, with the light chains readily excreted. Excessive serum levels of immunoglobulin can lead to nephropathy or amyloidosis in these patients.

   Answer A is incorrect. Osteogenesis imperfecta results from a defect in the synthesis of collagen I and leaves patients susceptible to pathologic fractures. In addition to brittle bones, insufficient collagen I can lead to abnormal dentition, conductive hearing loss, and a bluish hue in the sclera. However, this disease does not first present in late adulthood, and would not be associated with lytic bone lesions.

   Answer B is incorrect. This is a description of Chvostek sign, which is a manifestation of neuromuscular hyperexcitability. This would be expected in a person with symptomatic hypocalcemia, not in a patient with hypercalcemia.

   Answer C is incorrect. Although adenocarcinoma of the prostate commonly metastasizes to bone, it is an unlikely cause of this patient's symptoms. Bone metastases from the prostate tend to produce dense and sclerotic osteoblastic bone lesions, rather than the lytic lesions seen on the radiograph. Moreover, one would expect an elevated alkaline phosphatase level in the setting of osteoblastic metastases.

   Answer D is incorrect. Parathyroid adenomas are a common cause of hyperparathyroidism and consequent hypercalcemia. However, alkaline phosphatase levels should be markedly elevated in hyperparathyroidism. Moreover, parathyroid neoplasms are rarely malignant, and widespread skeletal metastases would not be expected in a patient with a parathyroid adenoma.

5. **The correct answer is A.** It is appropriate to discuss the patient's concerns. Explaining the thought process behind your diagnosis and educating about the disease process may alleviate the patient's fears, and make him more comfortable with your proposed course of action. A discussion of the utility as well as the risks of CT of the head may help the patient understand your perspective.

Answer B is incorrect. This action violates the principle of non-maleficence because, although less risky than a CT scan, x-ray files are associated with a radiation dose and are unlikely to be of any benefit.

Answer C is incorrect. It is inappropriate to send this patient for CT of the head if a subarachnoid hemorrhage is not being entertained in the differential diagnosis. Unfortunately, many tests are performed upon patient request despite the associated risks, simply because it is less time consuming to order the test than to explain why it is unwarranted. Ordering CT of the head in this case would violate the principle of non-maleficence because the risks outweigh the benefits.

Answer D is incorrect. It is important to be compassionate by attempting to understand and alleviate patients' concerns rather than to pass the responsibility on to someone else.

Answer E is incorrect. Simply stating that he does not have a subarachnoid hemorrhage fails to address the patient's concerns and may ultimately lead to increased patient anxiety. It's also unlikely to change the patient's desire for a CT scan.

Answer F is incorrect. It is never appropriate to lie to a patient.

6. **The correct answer is B.** Fibroadenomas are the most common benign breast tumors and usually occur in young women 20-35 years old. They present as small, firm, mobile masses. They are not associated with malignancy progression. On histology, fibrosing interlobular stroma is seen around normal duct and gland structures. Fibroadenomas are frequently single, well-circumscribed, rubbery, and painless masses. They are hormone responsive during the menstrual cycle and often become hyalinized and can calcify, mimicking breast carcinomas on mammography. A stable fibroadenoma in a young woman is usually followed by ultrasonography; however, cytology is indicated if there is any doubt about malignancy or if mass is growing in size.

Answer A is incorrect. Intraductal papillomas are benign solitary lesions that line the lactiferous ducts. These masses present in premenopausal women with serosanguinous (serous fluid and/or blood) and unilateral nipple discharge. Usually the mass undergoes cytology to rule out invasive papillary carcinoma due to the bloody discharge associated with both. These benign masses rarely undergo malignant transformation and are treated with ice packs, the cessation of breast-feeding, and tight-fitting support bras. If the mass does not subside in a couple weeks, then excision is warranted to avoid abscess formation.

Answer C is incorrect. Paget disease of the breast is a rare manifestation of breast cancer that presents unilaterally with eczematous skin findings associated with underlying ductal carcinomas. The eczematous nipple is due to the tumor cells disrupting the tight junctions. Paget cells (cells of the underlying ductal carcinoma) are large cells with halo-like clearings.

Answer D is incorrect. Infiltrating lobular carcinomas are identified as irregular masses on palpation or serendipitously on mammography. These cells are found in clusters or in a linear formation; the histological hallmark is a pattern of monomorphic infiltrating cells usually only one cell wide. These masses are more common in postmenopausal women and present like invasive ductal carcinoma, so they must be differentiated with excisional biopsy for cytology.

Answer E is incorrect. Invasive ductal carcinoma (nonspecific type) is the most common breast mass in older women. It usually becomes clinically apparent when there are associated overlying skin changes such as pigmented dimpling (due to the carcinoma impinging on the suspensory ligaments [also referred to as peau d'orange skin]) and/or unilateral bloody nipple discharge. On palpation, they are usually firm, irregular, fixed masses; on mammography, they appear as multiple small calcifications.

7. **The correct answer is D.** This patient has chronic granulomatous disease (CGD), which

usually presents with an increased susceptibility to opportunistic bacterial and fungal infections. It results from defective neutrophil phagocytosis due to a lack of NADPH oxidase (or similar enzyme) activity. A decrease in free radical production because of this enzyme deficiency renders host neutrophils sensitive to catalase-producing organisms (notably *Staphylococcus aureus*, *Candida albicans*, *Aspergillus flavus*, *Escherichia coli*, and *Pseudomonas aeruginosa*), because catalase breaks down free radicals. To confirm the diagnosis, nitroblue tetrazolium (a yellow liquid) is added to a sample of the patient's blood. In patients with normal levels of NADPH oxidase, there is a positive result as the neutrophils reduce the nitroblue tetrazolium and a dark blue granular substance precipitates in their cytoplasm. Patients with CGD have a negative result: the cytoplasm of their neutrophils remains colorless despite the addition of nitroblue tetrazolium.

Answer A is incorrect. Large lysosome vesicles in neutrophils are characteristic of Chédiak-Higashi disease, an autosomal recessive condition that presents with recurrent streptococcal and staphylococcal infections. A defect in lysosomal emptying of phagocytic cells due to microtubular dysfunction is the underlying cause of the disease.

Answer B is incorrect. Low IgM levels with elevated IgE and IgA levels are characteristic of Wiskott-Aldrich syndrome, an X-linked disorder resulting in a cytoskeletal defect that affects immune cells and reduces the body's ability to mount an IgM response to bacteria. Recurrent pyogenic infections, eczema, and thrombocytopenia are the typical triad of symptoms. Wiskott-Aldrich syndrome does not present with any specific enzyme abnormality.

Answer C is incorrect. Low levels of IgM, IgE, and IgA are characteristic of Bruton agammaglobulinemia and of the severe combined immunodeficiency syndromes. In both instances, levels of all immunoglobulin isotypes are decreased. Bruton agammaglobulinemia is an X-linked defect in a tyrosine kinase involved in B lymphocyte development. Patients have normal T lymphocytes and a low number of B lymphocytes. Severe combined immunodeficiency is a defect in early differentiation of immune cells. Patients usually have a low number of T lymphocytes and a normal number of B lymphocytes.

Answer E is incorrect. A positive nitroblue tetrazolium dye reduction test is present in patients with normal neutrophils, which are able to reduce the nitroblue tetrazolium. This causes a dark blue precipitate in their cytoplasm.

8. **The correct answer is C.** This patient suffers from atrial fibrillation, as demonstrated by the absence of P waves on ECG, which places him at higher risks for mural thrombosis and embolic complications. Warfarin is the anticoagulant of choice. Warfarin inhibits γ-carboxylation of vitamin K-dependent clotting factors II, VII, IX, and X and proteins C and S, and is used for chronic anticoagulation. It is taken orally and has a long half-life. Measurement of the degree of anticoagulation must be followed by measurement of the International Normalized Ratio (INR).

Answer A is incorrect. Heparin works by catalyzing the activation of antithrombin III, decreasing the level of available thrombin, and inhibiting factor Xa. Heparin has a short half-life and can be monitored by using the partial thromboplastin time (PTT). Heparin is used commonly in the in-patient setting to treat thrombosis or to anticoagulate symptomatic patients before bridging them to warfarin; however, it is not used in the long-term management of atrial fibrillation.

Answer B is incorrect. Infliximab is a monoclonal antibody to tumor necrosis factor-α, thereby interfering with inflammation. It is used to treat many chronic inflammatory/rheumatologic conditions including refractory Crohn disease, rheumatoid arthritis, and ankylosing spondylitis, and to promote fistula healing.

Answer D is incorrect. Aspirin works by irreversibly inhibiting cyclooxygenase, thereby preventing the conversion of arachidonic acid to prostaglandins. The four effects of aspirin are antiplatelet, antipyretic, analgesic, and anti-inflammatory. Aspirin is a powerful antiplatelet agent; however, it is not used routinely in the management of atrial fibrillation unless the patient is low risk based on the 2006 American Heart Association guidelines.

Answer E is incorrect. Clopidogrel acts by inhibiting platelet aggregation by irreversibly inhibiting the ADP pathway involved in the binding of fibrinogen to the platelet surface. It is used in the setting of acute coronary syndrome and stenting.

9. **The correct answer is A.** This patient presents with signs and symptoms of anemia. The dark urine is due to the presence of hemoglobin, which occurs only in the setting of intravascular hemolysis. Urine color change points to paroxysmal nocturnal hemoglobinuria (PNH), a rare form of hemolytic anemia. We would expect laboratory abnormalities, including a normocytic anemia, elevated unconjugated bilirubin and LDH, and low haptoglobin. PNH classically presents as the triad of hemolytic anemia, pancytopenia, and thrombosis. In PNH, a defective protein known as glycosylphosphatidylinisotol (GPI) anchor (encoded by the *PIG-A* gene) is present on the RBC membrane. Normally, GPI attaches proteins to the surface of RBCs and prevents the attachment of complement to the membrane and subsequent lysis. Because complement preferentially attaches to the RBC membrane at acidic pH, PNH can be diagnosed by mixing the patient's RBCs and control RBCs with an acidic solution and observing for increased hemolysis of the patient's RBCs. This pH-dependent adhesion explains why RBC lysis happens selectively overnight in those with PNH: While sleeping, the decrease in respiratory rate leads to retained carbon dioxide and thus a slight acidification of the blood.

Answer B is incorrect. The mechanism of RBC damage in PNH is through the complement cascade. Other hemolytic anemias are due to osmotic lysis of RBCs, including hereditary spherocytosis.

Answer C is incorrect. Decreased respiratory rate (hypoventilation) causes excess carbon dioxide in the blood, leading to production of acid. A respiratory alkalosis would result from hyperventilation.

Answer D is incorrect. The mechanism of RBC damage in PNH is through the complement cascade. Other hemolytic anemias are due to osmotic lysis of RBCs, including hereditary spherocytosis.

Answer E is incorrect. Respiratory rate does not increase while sleeping; it decreases.

Answer F is incorrect. Respiratory rate does not increase while sleeping; it decreases.

10. **The correct answer is C.** The image reveals *Mycobacterium tuberculosis* infection. Although rifampin is considered the best anti-tuberculous agent, isoniazid is used for prophylaxis in asymptomatic patients with a positive PPD. A six-month course of isoniazid prevents active tuberculosis (TB) in 90% of patients for at least 20 years. Isoniazid blocks mycolic acid cell wall synthesis and is bactericidal for rapidly multiplying organisms. Vitamin B_6 is given with isoniazid to prevent neurotoxicity, an adverse effect of isoniazid therapy.

Answer A is incorrect. Cycloserine is a broad-spectrum antibiotic active against *Mycobacterium tuberculosis*. Adverse effects related to cycloserine include peripheral neuropathy, psychosis, and seizures. One of the reasons cycloserine is so effective is that it spreads throughout the body, including the cerebrospinal fluid.

Answer B is incorrect. Combined isoniazid and rifampin therapy is effective for treating *Mycobacterium tuberculosis*. However, the risk of liver toxicity with rifampin outweighs its benefits in patients without active infection.

Answer D is incorrect. Rifampin is the most potent antituberculous agent available. Rifampin blocks DNA-dependent RNA polymerase, preventing RNA synthesis. Although it is a better agent than isoniazid for preventing active TB infection, it has a significant risk of liver toxicity that outweighs its benefits in this population.

Answer E is incorrect. Vitamin B_6 is given with isoniazid to prevent neurotoxicity, an adverse effect of isoniazid therapy. The other major adverse effect of isoniazid is hepatotoxicity. Rifampin does not cause peripheral neuropathy, and thus coadministration of vitamin B_6 is unnecessary.

11. **The correct answer is C.** The uptake of ^{99m}Tc pertechnetate (which is captured by thyroid tissue just as iodine is) in this mass and its sublingual position strongly suggest that it is composed of ectopic thyroid tissue. Normally the thyroid diverticulum develops from the floor of the primitive pharynx and then descends into the neck. The presence of thyroid tissue attached to the tongue implies that it has failed to migrate caudally. The tongue is the most common site of ectopic thyroid tissue.

    Answer A is incorrect. The thymus is located in the anterior mediastinum, deep to the sternum. Thymic tissue would not be found in either the oropharynx or the neck. Furthermore, the uptake of ^{99m}Tc pertechnetate suggests that this mass is composed of ectopic thyroid tissue.

    Answer B is incorrect. The thymus is not normally found in the neck; it is instead located in the anterior mediastinum. Thymic hypertrophy would not explain the location of this mass. Furthermore, the uptake of ^{99m}Tc pertechnetate suggests that this mass is composed of thyroid tissue.

    Answer D is incorrect. The thyroid does not migrate rostrally during development. Instead, it develops near the tongue and migrates caudally (descends) to its normal position in the lower neck.

    Answer E is incorrect. The third and fourth branchial (pharyngeal) arches form the posterior third of the tongue. However, the ^{99m}Tc pertechnetate uptake in this mass indicates that it is composed of thyroid, and not lingual, tissue.

12. **The correct answer is E.** This patient has Kartagener syndrome, which is caused by a lack of dynein arms in microtubules in cilia, rendering them immotile. It results in infertility due to immotile sperm, as well as recurrent sinusitis due to deficient removal of bacteria and other infectious particles. It is also associated with situs inversus, in which the major organs are reversed or mirrored from their original locations.

    Answer A is incorrect. Benign prostatic hypertrophy could cause impairment of ejaculation by not allowing semen to be expelled from the body. Because the patient is without an enlarged prostate and is only 27 years old, this diagnosis is highly unlikely.

    Answer B is incorrect. Cystic fibrosis does cause infertility, but usually because of bilateral absence of the vas deferens, which would lead to lack of sperm in semen.

    Answer C is incorrect. Undescended testicles are associated with infertility and an increased risk of testicular cancer. It is usually found at a very young age and resolves by itself or is surgically corrected before serious complications occur.

    Answer D is incorrect. Familial hypercholesterolemia can cause atherosclerosis of the vessels of the male genitalia, causing erectile dysfunction. Without a history of erectile dysfunction or elevated lipid levels, this diagnosis is highly unlikely.

13. **The correct answer is C.** According to her lab data, this patient has an acute respiratory alkalosis. Respiratory alkalosis is caused by a loss of carbon dioxide, which is compensated for by increased renal excretion of bicarbonate. The key to this question is to recognize that respiratory alkalosis can be caused only by an increase in ventilation, which can be caused by low oxygen (in high altitudes) or by sympathetic stimulation such as anxiety, panic attack, or pain. This patient is described as anxious and presents with severe abdominal pain, which is most likely the result of acute alcohol-induced pancreatitis. Both the anxiety and the pain could be causing her to hyperventilate.

Answer A is incorrect. An increase in anions would be consistent with anion-gap metabolic acidosis. Metabolic acidosis is indicated by the presence of a low pH with a low plasma bicarbonate, a low carbon dioxide, and an increased anion gap. The anion gap, measured by a formula involving sodium, chloride, and bicarbonate $\{[Na^+] - ([Cl^-] + [HCO_3^-])\}$, is normally between 10 and 16 mEq/L.

Answer B is incorrect. Diuretic use can cause metabolic alkalosis by volume contraction. This causes the kidney to compensate by reabsorbing sodium and excreting hydrogen ions. A metabolic alkalosis would present with elevated pH, elevated carbon dioxide, and elevated bicarbonate.

Answer D is incorrect. Hypoventilation causes a reduction in pH due to carbon dioxide retention. The excess retained carbon dioxide leads to a respiratory acidosis. The compensatory mechanism for respiratory acidosis is an increase in bicarbonate retention by the kidneys to normalize the pH.

Answer E is incorrect. Vomiting causes a metabolic alkalosis secondary to the loss of acid and chloride from the stomach. If this were the cause, this patient's lab results would show a high pH, a high bicarbonate, and (with respiratory compensation) a high carbon dioxide. The causes of metabolic alkalosis include vomiting, diuretic therapy, and chloride restriction. The compensation for metabolic alkalosis is hypoventilation.

14. **The correct answer is D.** The arrow points to the trigeminal nerve (cranial nerve V) in the image. The major functions of the trigeminal nerve include mastication and facial sensation.

Answer A is incorrect. Eye movements are controlled by the oculomotor, trochlear, and abducens nerves (cranial nerves III, IV, and VI, respectively), rather than the trigeminal nerve.

Answer B is incorrect. Facial movement is a function of the facial nerve (cranial nerve VII) rather than the trigeminal nerve.

Answer C is incorrect. Hearing is a function of the vestibulocochlear nerve (cranial nerve VIII) rather than the trigeminal nerve.

Answer E is incorrect. Tongue movements are controlled by the hypoglossal nerve (cranial nerve XII) rather than the trigeminal nerve.

15. **The correct answer is E.** Benzodiazepines and barbiturates differ in their effect on the chloride channel adjacent to the γ-aminobutyric acid receptor. Benzodiazepines increase the frequency of the channel's opening, while barbiturates increase the duration the channel is open.

Answer A is incorrect. Benzodiazepines have largely replaced barbiturates in the treatment of anxiety because of their more favorable after-effect profile. They are less likely than barbiturates to lead to respiratory depression and central cardiac depression.

Answer B is incorrect. Barbiturates are far more likely than benzodiazepines to cause central respiratory and cardiac depression and are significantly less safe.

Answer C is incorrect. Half-life depends on the pharmacokinetics of the particular medication and not its class. Some half-lives may be longer, some shorter.

Answer D is incorrect. Barbiturates, not benzodiazepines, increase the duration of chloride channel opening.

16. **The correct answer is E.** This patient's presentation is highly suspicious for bacterial meningitis. In the neonate, clinical symptoms are nonspecific (fever, irritability, lethargy, poor feeding) when compared with those in older children or adults (nuchal rigidity). The most common cause of neonatal meningitis is group B *Streptococcus*, specifically *Streptococcus agalactiae*, a β-hemolytic, gram-positive coccus found in chains. In contrast with its group A counterparts, *S agalactiae* is bacitracin resistant. Infection with this organism occurs during vaginal delivery, as 40% of women are asymptomatic carriers of this bacterium in the gastrointestinal (GI) tract and vagina.

Escherichia coli and *Listeria monocytogenes* are the second and third most common causes of meningitis in infants <3 months old.

Answer A is incorrect. *Escherichia coli* is a gram-negative, lactose-fermenting bacillus. It is the second leading cause of neonatal meningitis.

Answer B is incorrect. *Haemophilus influenzae* type B (Hib) is a small gram-negative encapsulated coccobacillus that was once a major cause of serious bacterial infections, including meningitis, sepsis, and epiglottitis. It requires factors V and X to successfully culture on chocolate agar. However, the incidence of *H influenzae* meningitis has decreased significantly in the last 10-15 years as a result of the widespread administration of the Hib vaccine. Nevertheless, Hib still causes 5% of cases of meningitis in children ages 6 months to 6 years.

Answer C is incorrect. *Listeria monocytogenes* is the third most common cause of neonatal meningitis (2%). It is a gram-positive bacillus.

Answer D is incorrect. *Streptococcus pneumoniae* is a gram-positive coccus that is found in chains, but it is not a significant cause of meningitis in neonates. However, in children ages 6 months to 6 years, it is the leading cause of meningitis.

17. **The correct answer is C.** Budd-Chiari syndrome (BCS) is a nearly complete obstruction to blood flow by an acute clot in the hepatic veins or in the inferior vena cava. This sudden event is followed by the onset of hepatomegaly, pain, ascites, and jaundice. The patient has antiphospholipid antibody syndrome (positive antiphospholipid antibody titer, seizures, and multiple abortions), a coagulation disorder that is often associated with systemic lupus erythematosus (SLE) and is a risk factor for developing BCS. The ultrasound result further supports the diagnosis by suggesting hepatic venous occlusion. Predisposing conditions for BCS are hematologic disorders (polycythemia vera, essential thrombocytosis), thrombotic diatheses (antiphospholipid antibody syndrome, factor V Leiden), pregnancy, oral contraceptive use, and intra-abdominal neoplasms (hepatocellular carcinoma, renal cell carcinoma). Thus this patient has two conditions (pregnancy and antiphospholipid antibody syndrome) that predispose her to developing BCS.

    Answer A is incorrect. BCS leads to blockage of hepatic venous outflow, congestion, and ultimately portal hypertension. However, cholecystitis is inflammation of the gallbladder, usually due to blockage of the cystic duct by a gallstone. This condition does not predispose to BCS.

    Answer B is incorrect. Chronic obstructive pulmonary disease (COPD) does not increase the risk of developing BCS.

    Answer D is incorrect. Primary biliary cirrhosis is an intrahepatic autoimmune disease that leads to granulomatous destruction of bile ducts, ultimately causing cirrhosis due to biliary obstruction. However, BCS is a syndrome of venous, not biliary, flow obstruction. Both can lead to liver failure, but primary biliary cirrhosis would not cause the flow obstruction seen in the hepatic veins in this patient. Primary biliary cirrhosis does not increase the risk of developing BCS.

    Answer E is incorrect. Renal failure does not increase the risk of developing BCS.

18. **The correct answer is A.** A conversion disorder mimics dysfunction in the voluntary motor or sensory system. Common presentations include pseudo seizures, vocal cord dysfunction, blindness, tunnel vision, deafness, and a variety of paresthesias and paralyses. On careful clinical examination and with the aid of laboratory investigations, these symptoms lack physiologic explanation. A clinical example is the presence of normal deep-tendon reflexes and normal sensation in a person with a "paralyzed" arm. Patients with conversion disorder involuntarily have loss of function, usually in response to an unconscious conflict, and seek secondary gain in the form of assumption of the sick role.

    Answer B is incorrect. Patients with factitious disorder voluntarily have a loss of function or voluntarily do things to themselves to create illness or injury, usually in response to an unconscious conflict, and seek secondary gain in the form of assumption of the sick role.

Answer C is incorrect. Hypochondriasis is the preoccupation with fears of having a particular disease or diagnosis based on one's misinterpretation of symptoms, despite clear evidence to the contrary. It lasts >6 months.

Answer D is incorrect. Patients with malingering voluntarily have loss of function, usually consciously in response to known situations, and seek secondary gain in the form of tangible gain (monetary, housing, or avoidance of responsibilities).

Answer E is incorrect. The fact that the patient has no medical history, normal reflexes, and normal results of physical examination, other than the left-arm weakness, indicates he is unlikely to have had a stroke. The events surrounding the situation make it more likely that he has conversion disorder.

19. **The correct answer is D.** Tuberous sclerosis is a genetic condition (autosomal dominant) characterized by nodular proliferation of multinucleated atypical astrocytes. These form tubers, which are found throughout the cerebral cortex and periventricular areas. The classic triad, which is manifest in only the most severe of cases, consists of seizures, mental retardation, and facial angiofibromas (also known as adenoma sebaceum). Half of patients with tuberous sclerosis develop rhabdomyomas, primary tumors of cardiac muscle that, although benign, may compromise cardiac function, especially of the atrioventricular valves. Tuberous sclerosis is also notable for a link to angiomyolipomas of the kidney.

    Answer A is incorrect. Dilated cardiomyopathy is often idiopathic. It involves four-chamber hypertrophy and dilation, and eventually heart failure. This condition is not associated with tuberous sclerosis. Note that hypertrophic cardiomyopathy also causes ventricular outflow obstruction and is often responsible for sudden death in young athletes.

    Answer B is incorrect. Lipomas, like rhabdomyomas, are capable of obstruction. These can create ball-valve obstructions and are most often located in the left ventricle, right atrium, or atrial septum. However, in conjunction with the history suggesting tuberous sclerosis, lipoma is a less likely diagnosis.

    Answer C is incorrect. Myxomas, like rhabdomyomas, are capable of obstruction. However, these are seen in adults and are often located in the atria.

    Answer E is incorrect. Transposition of the great vessels is a situation in which the pulmonary trunk arises from the left ventricle and the aorta arises from the right ventricle. This arrangement is incompatible with life, and a compensatory anomaly such as a patent ductus arteriosus is necessary.

20. **The correct answer is B.** This patient has oculomotor palsy from disruption of cranial nerve (CN) III. This nerve innervates the medial rectus, the superior rectus, the inferior rectus, and the inferior oblique muscles of the eye. When damaged, the extraocular muscles not innervated by CN III dominate (ie, the superior oblique, which depresses and intorts the eye, and the lateral rectus, which abducts the eye). Hence the eye appears "down and out." CN III also innervates the levator palpebrae superioris, which causes ptosis. The pupil is dilated because of involvement of the parasympathetic fibers that run on the outside of the oculomotor nerve and can be compressed by structures such as tumors and aneurysms. If it is a pupil-sparing third nerve palsy, then infarction of the nerve is commonly the cause.

    Answer A is incorrect. The abducens nerve (cranial nerve VI) innervates the lateral rectus, which abducts the eye. Abduction is intact in this patients affected eye.

    Answer C is incorrect. The optic nerve does not innervate any of the extraocular muscles and therefore cannot account for the findings above.

    Answer D is incorrect. The trigeminal nerve does not innervate any of the extraocular muscles and therefore cannot account for the findings above.

Answer E is incorrect. The trochlear nerve innervates the superior oblique muscle, which depresses and intorts the eye. In trochlear nerve palsy, the affected eye is elevated and extorted, and the patient often tilts their head away from the affected eye to compensate. These abnormalities were not found here.

21. **The correct answer is D.** Intracranial metastases represent nearly half of all brain tumors, yet only 15% of tumors metastasize to the brain. Intracranial hemorrhages are a recognized but relatively uncommon complication of brain tumors and can result in intraparenchymal, subarachnoid, subdural, and epidural hematomas. Focal neurologic signs are frequently evident and are due to pressure exerted on the brain parenchyma. Because melanoma is a relatively frequent source of metastatic lesions to the brain (although less common than breast or lung carcinoma) and demonstrates a tendency to hemorrhage, melanoma is the correct answer in this case.

    Answer A is incorrect. Angiosarcomas are malignant endothelial neoplasms that resemble hemangiomas. Although these tumors may bleed, angiosarcomas rarely metastasize, and only a few case reports exist of hemorrhage of cerebral metastasis from angiosarcoma.

    Answer B is incorrect. Some cancers rarely metastasize to the brain; these include carcinomas of the oropharynx, esophagus, and prostate, as well as nonmelanoma skin cancers.

    Answer C is incorrect. Colorectal carcinoma does metastasize to the brain (though less frequently than melanoma) but does not typically result in intracranial hemorrhage. Since colorectal carcinoma is less likely than melanoma to result in brain metastases and is not as likely to hemorrhage, melanoma is a better answer.

    Answer E is incorrect. Carcinoma of the prostate almost never results in metastatic brain disease. Prostate cancer can cause malignant spinal cord compression by metastasizing to the vertebra. Thus it should be considered in an elderly man with localized back pain that is most severe in the supine position.

22. **The correct answer is B.** This patient likely has bacterial endocarditis as a result of intravenous (IV) drug use, and the dysarthria and retinal hemorrhages are suggestive of a left-sided valvular lesion showering septic emboli to the brain and retinal arteries. The blood culture points to a *Streptococcus* species; these are gram positive and catalase negative. To further characterize *Streptococcus*, evaluate the degree of hemolysis of the plate medium. α-Hemolytic streptococci demonstrate partial hemolysis, whereas β-hemolytic streptococci show complete hemolysis. γ-Hemolytic organisms show no hemolysis and include *Enterococcus* species. The only organisms of this group known to cause endocarditis are the viridans group streptococci and *Enterococcus faecalis*. Viridans streptococcus is α hemolytic, optochin resistant, and bile soluble. *E faecalis* is γ hemolytic, optochin resistant, and bile soluble, but unlike the *Streptococcus* species, it is able to grow on 6.5% sodium chloride solution. Therefore, to differentiate between the two, 6.5% sodium chloride would be the best culture condition to isolate a single organism.

    Answer A is incorrect. The absence of colonies in the presence of penicillin suggests that the organism is sensitive to penicillin. *Treponema pallidum* and any number of streptococci are sensitive to this antibiotic; therefore, this would not be best culture condition for isolating a single type of organism.

    Answer C is incorrect. Both the viridans group streptococci and *E faecalis* are optochin resistant. Therefore, use of optochin would not help you differentiate between the two strains.

    Answer D is incorrect. *Haemophilus influenzae* is cultured on chocolate agar, along with factors V (nicotinamide adenine dinucleotide) and X (hematin) for growth. However, this organism is not a common cause of bacterial endocarditis; rather, it causes epiglottitis, meningitis, otitis media, and pneumonia.

Answer E is incorrect. *Streptococcus pneumoniae* is a gram-positive bacterium that is bile soluble, but it is not a common cause of bacterial endocarditis.

23. **The correct answer is A.** Adipocytes are the cells that comprise adipose (fat) tissue. GLUT 4-mediated glucose transport occurs in only two tissue types: adipose tissue and skeletal muscle. In the fasting state, when insulin levels are low, there is decreased intake of glucose into adipose tissue and skeletal muscle, enabling glucose to be utilized by more pertinent organs. In this context, decreased glucose intake into fat and muscle cells will promote mobilization of stored precursors such as amino acids and free fatty acids. This is the only choice among those listed that could be used in the hypothetical experimental system described.

Answer B is incorrect. Cortical neurons are derived from the brain, where glucose transport occurs independent of insulin stimulation. Thus these cells could not be used in this hypothetical system. Brain and RBCs take up glucose via GLUT 1 transport.

Answer C is incorrect. RBCs take up glucose independent of insulin levels using GLUT 1 transport.

Answer D is incorrect. Insulin has no effect on glucose uptake in hepatocytes, so this cell type could not be used in this hypothetical system.

Answer E is incorrect. Pancreatic β cells express GLUT 2 transporters, which serve as glucose sensors. These cells do not express GLUT 4 transporters and would not be appropriate for use in this hypothetical system.

24. **The correct answer is C.** The positive predictive value (PPV) of the test can be calculated with the following formula, where TP is true-positive results and FP is false-positive results: TP / (TP + FP). Given the pretest probability of 50%, we need to set up a hypothetical 2 × 2 table in which the number of subjects with the disease is equal to the number not having the disease (or to be said differently, the pretest probability becomes the prevalence). If we set the number of those with the disease as 10, then TP = 8 and FP = 1, given the sensitivity of 80% and specificity of 90%. Therefore, the PPV would be calculated as 8 / (8 + 1) = 89%, or about 90%. The same answer can also be obtained by converting the pretest probability to an odds ratio (1:1) and multiplying it by the test's positive likelihood ratio (LR+), which can be calculated using the formula LR+ = sensitivity / (1 - specificity) = 0.80 / (1 - 0.90) = 8. Therefore, the posttest odds of having the disease is 8:1 or 8/9 = 89% once the figure is converted back into a probability.

Answer A is incorrect. This value is too low to be the correct answer.

Answer B is incorrect. This value is too low to be the correct answer.

Answer D is incorrect. This value is too high to be the correct answer.

Answer E is incorrect. This value is too high to be the correct answer.

25. **The correct answer is E.** This patient's clinical presentation, history of alcoholism, and hemodynamic instability suggest a rapid loss of blood related to an upper GI bleed. Boerhaave perforation is a transmural perforation that normally presents with the Mackler triad: vomiting, lower thoracic pain, and subcutaneous emphysema. Boerhaave perforation has a high mortality rate and a rate of progression much more rapid than seen in the patient in this vignette. These patients need to be treated with emergent surgical repair; the single greatest factor impacting survival is diagnosis and treatment within 24 hours.

Answer A is incorrect. A patient with an esophageal mass usually would have a more chronic evolution of symptoms that includes progressive swallowing difficulties and a history of hematemesis. The onset of this patient's symptoms is acute, without a history of dysphagia or upper GI bleeding, making esophageal mass an unlikely cause in this scenario.

Answer B is incorrect. Esophageal stricture usually does not present with hematemesis; it most often presents with complaints of solid-food dysphagia.

Answer C is incorrect. Acute cholecystitis would present typically with epigastric or right upper quadrant pain that is worse with inspiration (Murphy sign). However, patients with acute cholecystitis typically are hemodynamically stable, unlike this patient. In addition, the history of hematemesis is not consistent with acute cholecystitis, which typically presents with right upper quadrant pain, nausea, non-bloody vomiting, and fever that may be exacerbated by consumption of fatty foods.

Answer D is incorrect. This patient's history of alcohol abuse and acute onset of bright-red emesis after an episode of retching is consistent with a Mallory-Weiss tear. These nonpenetrating mucosal tears frequently are found at the gastroesophageal junction. A sudden increase in transabdominal pressure as seen in vomiting and retching is believed to be the pathophysiology. Alcoholism is a predisposing risk factor because of the violent vomiting that may follow an alcohol binge. Frequently the bleeding is self-limited; therefore the hemodynamic instability in this case most likely is due to esophageal rupture.

26. **The correct answer is E.** The plaque shown in the image is an atheroma. These lesions of extracellular lipid develop within the intima of the arterial wall. The intima lines the luminal side of the artery; it is the most "intimate" with the blood. The innermost layer of cells of the intima is therefore the endothelial cells. In a nonpathologic state, endothelial cells prevent plaque formation by releasing antithrombotic factors such as prostacyclin and nitric oxide.

Answer A is incorrect. Collagen is produced by the smooth muscle cells in the media of the arterial wall. These cells also produce elastin and proteoglycans that are the other two important components of the vascular extracellular matrix of arterial walls.

Answer B is incorrect. Fibrillin is a component of elastin, which is made by the smooth muscle cells of the media.

Answer C is incorrect. Hemoglobin is a molecule found in RBCs and is not produced by any cells in the arterial wall.

Answer D is incorrect. Macrophage colony-stimulating factor is made by macrophages, which are not part of the typical cell architecture of the arterial wall. Under pathologic conditions, macrophages invade the intima and facilitate the formation of atherosclerotic plaques.

27. **The correct answer is B.** Imipenem is a broad-spectrum, β-lactamase-resistant antibiotic of the carbapenem class. These drugs are structurally similar to β-lactam antibiotics but are β-lactamase-resistant and are administered with cilastatin to decrease renal metabolism. Imipenem can be used to treat gram-positive and gram-negative infections and it is first-line therapy in the treatment of *Acinetobacter* and *Enterobacter* species infection. Imipenem is not useful in treating methicillin-resistant *Staphylococcus aureus*, *Enterococcus faecium*, or *Staphylococcus epidermidis*. Adverse effects include GI distress, thrombophlebitis, skin rashes, and seizures.

Answer A is incorrect. Gentamicin is an aminoglycoside antibiotic used to treat gram-negative bacilli that works by inhibiting protein synthesis. Adverse effects include nephrotoxicity, ototoxicity, and neuromuscular blockade. Gentamicin is effective in treating *Acinetobacter* species infection, but it is not as efficacious as imipenem, which is the first-line choice. It is not associated with seizures.

Answer C is incorrect. Levofloxacin is a fluoroquinolone antibiotic that acts by inhibiting DNA gyrase. It is used to treat gram-negative rods and some gram-positive organisms and therefore is good for upper respiratory infections and urinary tract infections. Fluoroquinolones are generally well tolerated but are associated with anaphylaxsis, GI discomfort, headache, and phototoxicity. They are also associated with damaged cartilage in animal models, thus are contraindicated in children.

Answer D is incorrect. Linezolid is used for community acquired pneumonias and acts by binding to the bacterial 50S ribosomal RNA subunit and blocking protein synthesis. Adverse effects include GI upset, headache, and myelosuppression. It does not cause seizures.

Answer E is incorrect. Rifampin is used to treat TB and acts by inhibiting DNA-dependent RNA polymerase. Important adverse effects include a transient rise in hepatic aminotransferase levels (which usually return to normal without discontinuation of rifampin) and hepatitis, which can occur directly or due to rifampin potentiating the hepatic toxicity of other drugs. Rifampin also causes discoloration of body fluids. It does not cause seizures.

28. **The correct answer is C.** Perihepatitis, or Fitz-Hugh-Curtis syndrome, is seen in up to 25% of women with pelvic inflammatory disease (PID). PID is an ascending, polymicrobial infection of the female genital tract that can involve the endometrium, uterine tube, and/or peritoneal cavity. *Chlamydia trachomatis* and *Neisseria gonorrhoeae* cause up to half of the cases of PID. Perihepatitis is a complication that usually presents with right upper quadrant pain associated with symptoms of PID (the classic triad is fever, abdominal pain, and vaginal discharge). On laparoscopy, "violin-string" adhesions will be present in the peritoneal cavity.

Answer A is incorrect. Acute cholecystitis presents with constant, severe pain and tenderness in the right upper quadrant (RUQ) or epigastrium, nausea and vomiting, and fever and leukocytosis. The acute attack often follows a large, fatty meal. Murphy sign on physical examination will show a cessation of inspiration on simultaneous palpation of the RUQ. Liver function tests will be elevated.

Answer B is incorrect. *Chlamydia trachomatis* infection is often asymptomatic in women. The clinical silence may eventually lead to PID via ascending infection. However, symptomatic chlamydial cervicitis presents with a mucopurulent cervical discharge that may or may not have an associated vaginal discharge. Patients may complain of postcoital bleeding. The cervix will be erythematous on examination.

Answer D is incorrect. Gonococcal infection is often asymptomatic in women. A patient with urethritis will present with a mucopurulent urethral discharge, urinary frequency, dysuria, and urgency. The clinical picture may be identical to cystitis.

Answer E is incorrect. Hepatitis A (HAV) causes an acute viral hepatitis after a four-week incubation period. The disease is self-limited and presents with symptoms such as jaundice and right upper quadrant pain, along with highly elevated transaminases. The IgM antibody is useful to diagnose the disease during its presentation. However, the IgG antibody is elevated indefinitely after infection and indicates only previous exposure.

Answer F is incorrect. A tubo-ovarian abscess is a complication of PID. It is often polymicrobial, with a predominance of anaerobes. The clinical presentation will involve abdominal pain and bilateral or unilateral adnexal masses.

29. **The correct answer is C.** This patient has secondary hyperparathyroidism due to chronic renal insufficiency, or renal osteodystrophy. Chronic renal failure is the most common cause of secondary hyperparathyroidism. There are numerous etiologies of chronic renal failure; nephropathy secondary to diabetes mellitus (DM) is the most common in the United States. In renal osteodystrophy, nephron damage leads to impaired calcium reabsorption, impaired phosphate excretion, and impaired activation of vitamin D in the kidney (vitamin D normally increases the absorption of calcium in the intestines). This results in decreased serum calcium and increased serum phosphate levels. The resulting hypocalcemia stimulates secretion of parathyroid hormone (PTH; secondary hyperparathyroidism), causing increased bone turnover, which further contributes to the hyperphosphatemia and leads to an increased serum alkaline phosphatase level. The elevated creatinine level in this patient is a clue that her kidney function is abnormal. Diffuse bone pain and proximal

muscle weakness are typical symptoms of secondary hyperparathyroidism caused by the hypocalcemia and increased bone resorption. Pruritus is occasionally seen in renal insufficiency due to deposition of excess calcium.

Answer A is incorrect. Parathyroid adenoma would cause primary hyperparathyroidism with increased secretion of PTH, resulting in hypercalcemia and hypophosphatemia rather than hypocalcemia and hyperphosphatemia.

Answer B is incorrect. Parathyroid insufficiency would result in hypocalcemia, with typical symptoms of tetany and increased neuromuscular excitability and decreased serum intact PTH levels. Additionally, it cannot account for the hyperphosphatemia presented in this case.

Answer D is incorrect. Malignancy usually results in hypercalcemia due either to lytic metastases to bone (with increased serum alkaline phosphatase activity and hyperphosphatemia) or to production of PTH-related peptide (with hypophosphatemia).

Answer E is incorrect. Vitamin D intoxication results in hypercalcemia and hyperphosphatemia with decreased serum intact PTH levels, and thus would be inconsistent with the lab values presented in the vignette. However, vitamin D intoxication may indeed present with clinical findings similar to those stated above, including pruritus, weakness, and renal dysfunction.

30. **The correct answer is B.** This clinical picture is highly suggestive of restrictive lung disease; although the FEV_1:FVC ratio is near normal levels, both the FEV_1 and FVC are markedly reduced. Amiodarone is an antiarrhythmic agent that is known to cause pulmonary fibrosis, a restrictive lung disease. Additional adverse effects include interstitial pneumonitis, photosensitivity, thyroid disorders, and GI disturbances.

Answer A is incorrect. Asthma is a cause of COPD. Asthma-induced abnormalities on pulmonary function testing would not fit a restrictive pathology profile.

Answer C is incorrect. Diltiazem is an antiarrhythmic that is sometimes used in IV form to treat atrial fibrillation. It infrequently causes hypotension or bradyarrhythmias, but is not known to cause pulmonary fibrosis.

Answer D is incorrect. Sotalol works by both nonselectively antagonizing β-receptors and by prolonging action potentials. It is used to treat ventricular and supraventricular arrhythmias in children and life-threatening ventricular arrhythmias in adults. Sotalol can sometimes cause torsades des pointes when taken at higher doses. However, it does not cause pulmonary fibrosis.

Answer E is incorrect. Tobacco is a known risk factor for COPD. COPD presents with a reduced FEV_1:FVC ratio, typically <80%. There is also a convex inward sloping of the flow-volume curve on pulmonary function testing.

31. **The correct answer is C.** The patient is presenting with the classic signs and symptoms of HAV. Hepatitis often presents with a prodrome of flulike symptoms that is followed by a possible icteric phase during which patients present with jaundice, icterus, hepatomegaly, pruritus, arthralgias, and rashes. Aspartate aminotransferase (AST) and alanine aminotransferase (ALT) levels can exceed 10,000 IU/ml, with ALT > AST levels (as opposed to alcoholic hepatitis, in which AST levels > ALT levels). The next thing to do is to determine which hepatitis virus this is. The patient's demographics and contact history as well as the lack of any sexual or illicit drug abuse suggest the diagnosis of HAV. Of the viral hepatitides, the hepatitis A and E viruses are transmitted via the fecal-oral route. HAV is not common in the United States, but it is very common in Africa, Asia, and South America. Acquisition in childhood is the norm, and most adults in those areas show seropositivity for HAV. Factors that predispose this population to infection include overcrowding, poor sanitation, and lack of a clean water source. Of the answer options, the only virus that also has a fecal-oral route of transmission is poliovirus, an RNA enterovirus that causes acute flaccid paralysis in <1% of cases.

Answer A is incorrect. Flavivirus, which is the causative agent of yellow fever, is one of the arboviruses, and it is transmitted by the *Aedes* mosquito.

Answer B is incorrect. Hepatitis B virus (HBV) is transmitted sexually and parenterally; this includes both maternal-fetal and blood-borne routes.

Answer D is incorrect. Rabies virus is transmitted via the bite of an infected animal, which in the United States would most likely be a skunk or a bat.

Answer E is incorrect. Varicella-zoster virus, which causes chickenpox and shingles, is transmitted by respiratory secretions.

32. **The correct answer is E.** This patient has Turcot syndrome, an autosomal dominant disease. All familial polyposis syndromes, with the exception of Peutz-Jeghers syndrome, predispose to colorectal cancer. Turcot syndrome is associated with two separate dominant mutations. The first is a mutation of the *APC* gene leading to polyposis and medulloblastoma, and the second is associated with the *hMLH1* DNA mismatch repair gene leading to polyposis and glioblastoma multiforme.

    Answer A is incorrect. Familial adenomatous polyposis is associated with hundreds of colorectal polyps, and nearly all affected patients will develop colorectal cancer.

    Answer B is incorrect. Gardner syndrome is characterized by colorectal polyposis and osteomas or other bone and soft tissue tumors.

    Answer C is incorrect. Hereditary nonpolyposis colorectal carcinoma is associated with dozens of colorectal polyps, and a majority of affected patients will develop colorectal cancer.

    Answer D is incorrect. Tuberous sclerosis is an autosomal dominant condition characterized by mental retardation, seizures, tuberous central nervous system tumors, angiomyolipomas of the kidneys, leptomeningeal tumors, and skin lesions such as ash-leaf spots and shagreen patches.

33. **The correct answer is F.** This woman is suffering from disseminated intravascular coagulation (DIC), most likely secondary to an amniotic fluid embolism that traveled to her pulmonary circulation. Common causes of DIC are gram-negative sepsis, malignancy, pancreatitis, trauma, transfusion reactions, and obstetric complications. During DIC, there is a massive activation of the coagulation cascade that results in thrombus formation throughout the microvasculature. This results in rapid consumption of both platelets and coagulation factors. Concurrent with this consumptive coagulopathy is activation of the fibrinolytic system. Ultimately, complications in DIC result from thrombosis and bleeding and may include massive blood loss and organ failure. Laboratory findings include a decreased platelet count, elevated bleeding time, elevated prothrombin time (PT), and elevated PTT.

    Answer A is incorrect. An isolated increase in PTT indicates a problem with the intrinsic coagulation cascade. This can be caused by hemophilia A or B, both of which are X-linked disorders that result in deficiencies in factor VIII and IX, respectively.

    Answer B is incorrect. An isolated increase in PT indicates a problem with the extrinsic coagulation cascade. This can be caused by treatment with warfarin.

    Answer C is incorrect. An isolated increase in bleeding time indicates a functional defect in platelets. This can be caused by vascular bleeding and platelet defects found in diseases such as Glanzmann thrombasthenia.

    Answer D is incorrect. An increase in both bleeding time and PTTs indicates both platelet dysfunction and a problem with the intrinsic coagulation cascade. This can be caused by von Willebrand disease, an inherited bleeding disorder that affects both platelet function and factor VIII availability.

    Answer E is incorrect. Decreased platelet count and elevated bleeding time indicates thrombocytopenia. This can be caused by aplastic anemia, leukemia, immune thrombocytopenic purpura, thrombotic thrombocytopenic purpura/hemolytic-uremic syndrome, and splenic sequestration.

34. **The correct answer is A.** To answer this question, one must know that Kawasaki syndrome (also referred to as mucocutaneous lymph node syndrome) is an arteritis that primarily affects medium- and small-sized arteries. Hence, it makes sense that there is evidence suggesting the formation of anti-endothelial cell (and anti-smooth muscle cell) autoantibodies in patients with this disease. The clinical manifestations of this disease include fever for more than five days, cervical lymphadenopathy, a skin rash (which often has desquamation, or shedding of the skin), and erythema of the conjunctivae, oral mucosa, palms, and soles. Eighty percent of patients are under the age of four years. Twenty percent of patients develop cardiovascular disease, including coronary artery vasculitis and coronary artery aneurysm.

    Answer B is incorrect. Anti-IgG (rheumatoid factor) is not particularly associated with Kawasaki syndrome. Elevated levels of serum rheumatoid factor are present in 80% of patients with rheumatoid arthritis.

    Answer C is incorrect. Anticentromere antibodies, which are found in 90% of patients with the CREST variant of scleroderma, are not particularly associated with Kawasaki syndrome.

    Answer D is incorrect. Antihistone antibodies, which are found in over 95% of patients with drug-induced lupus erythematosus, are not particularly associated with Kawasaki syndrome.

    Answer E is incorrect. Antinuclear antibodies, which are present in over 95% of patients with SLE, are not particularly associated with Kawasaki syndrome.

35. **The correct answer is E.** Because aspirin is a weak acid with an acid dissociation constant (pK_a) near 3.5, it can interconvert between neutral and negatively charged forms depending on the pH. Increasing the pH of tubular fluid shifts the equilibrium toward the non-protonated charged state of the molecule. Thus neutral molecules diffusing into the tubule will become ionized. Once in the charged state, molecules cannot diffuse back across tubular epithelial membranes to the bloodstream. Thus the clearance of aspirin is increased greatly when urine pH is alkalinized.

    Answer A is incorrect. Acidification of urine has no effect on the glomerular filtration rate (GFR). GFR is affected by the difference in pressures across the glomerulus and glomerular permeability.

    Answer B is incorrect. Acidification of the urine would lower the pH and shift the equilibrium toward the protonated neutral form of aspirin. These non-ionized molecules could then move back into the bloodstream, and clearance of aspirin would be decreased.

    Answer C is incorrect. Acidification of the urine would lower the pH and shift the equilibrium toward the protonated neutral form of aspirin, but these molecules can diffuse across cell membranes back into the bloodstream and would not be excreted.

    Answer D is incorrect. Alkalinization of urine has no effect on the GFR. GFR is affected by the difference in pressures across the glomerulus and glomerular permeability.

    Answer F is incorrect. Alkalinization of urine promotes ionization of aspirin in the urine; the concentration of non-ionized molecules of aspirin in the tubule would decrease as the urine is alkalinized.

36. **The correct answer is C.** This patient has classic symptoms of cardiac ischemia: chest pain with sudden onset that radiates to his left shoulder or jaw and is relieved by sublingual nitroglycerin. However, the patient is young, and the pain is not prompted by activity but occurs at rest. Additionally, his ECG is normal, showing no evidence of infarct or ischemia. As a result, he probably suffers from coronary vasospasm, also known as Prinzmetal's (variant) angina.

    Answer A is incorrect. The absence of evidence for an infarct on ECG makes myocardial infarctions an unlikely etiology of his chest pain.

Answer B is incorrect. Pericarditis can cause sudden onset of chest pain without exertion, but the pain would be not relieved with nitroglycerin. Typically, an ECG would also show diffuse ST-segment elevations.

Answer D is incorrect. Although the patient's clinical symptoms are of cardiac ischemia, they are not induced by a specific amount of exercise, which is the classic definition of stable angina.

Answer E is incorrect. Because the patient's symptoms have not increased in frequency, changed in intensity, and are not prompted by a light amount of exercise or strain, it is unlikely that they are due to unstable angina.

37. **The correct answer is E.** Minimal change disease results in nephrotic syndrome, which is manifested primarily in the loss of significant protein in the urine. As a result of this protein loss the plasma protein concentration will decrease, thus decreasing the oncotic pressure in the glomerular capillary. According to the Starling equation (glomerular filtration rate $= K_f [(P_{GC} - P_{BS}) - (p_{GC} - p_{BS})]$), this change will lead to a higher glomerular filtration rate by decreasing the oncotic forces that normally oppose ultrafiltration.

Answer A is incorrect. Tubular hydrostatic pressures are not affected by nephrotic syndrome. The Bowman space hydrostatic pressure generally does not decrease.

Answer B is incorrect. Tubular hydrostatic pressures are not affected by nephrotic syndrome. The Bowman space hydrostatic pressure could be increased in a patient with an obstruction to urine flow.

Answer C is incorrect. Bowman space oncotic pressure will increase, not decrease, as protein is filtered into Bowman space and thus increases the protein concentration there.

Answer D is incorrect. Hydrostatic pressures are not affected in minimal change disease. The glomerular capillary hydrostatic pressure could be increased with constriction of the efferent arteriole, for example.

38. **The correct answer is C.** Informed consent requires that the patient understand the risks, benefits, and alternatives to treatment. Additionally, following discussion of pertinent information, the patient must agree to care in a setting free from coercion. In this setting, the patient of concern is the daughter. It is not clear that this setting is free from coercion. Before allowing the daughter to consent, she should be addressed alone.

Answer A is incorrect. While it is ideal to involve as much of the family as possible, the most important people involved (the patient and her potential donor) are present. Involving the rest of the family ensures a good support network should the transplant proceed.

Answer B is incorrect. There is not enough information in the question to determine whether the patient has sufficient understanding. Although this is required for informed consent, there is a better answer.

Answer D is incorrect. Transplantation is rarely an emergent procedure. Ample time should be given to both the donor and the recipient to prepare for the operation.

Answer E is incorrect. There is no information indicating that this patient is not competent to make decisions. Simply being ill does not suggest that she is incompetent.

39. **The correct answer is C.** This patient most likely has diabetic nephropathy caused by long-standing and often poorly managed DM. The patient's presentation is typical for nephrotic syndrome, with massive proteinuria and peripheral and periorbital edema. Blood tests would likely have shown hypoalbuminemia and hyperlipidemia, which are also associated with nephrotic syndrome. The image shows changes typically associated with diabetic nephropathy, including basement membrane thickening and presence of hyaline deposits in the periphery of the glomerulus (known as Kimmelstiel-Wilson nodular lesions). The increased glucose levels in diabe-

tes can lead to vascular damage, and diabetes is strongly associated with coronary artery disease. In addition to management of lipids and blood glucose, angiotensin-converting enzyme inhibitors and/or angiotensin II receptor blockers are beneficial in the treatment of diabetic nephropathy.

Answer A is incorrect. Although renal disease associated with SLE may have similar presenting symptoms (proteinuria, peripheral and periorbital edema, and hypoalbuminemia), the image shows Kimmelstiel-Wilson nodular lesions, which are characteristic of diabetic nephropathy. With SLE, there are five different patterns of renal involvement. In the membranous glomerulonephritis pattern, biopsy reveals wire-loop lesions with subepithelial deposits. In addition to arthritis, symptoms of SLE include fatigue, malar rash, photosensitivity, pleuritis, pericarditis, and many more.

Answer B is incorrect. Although renal disease associated with amyloidosis has similar presenting symptoms (proteinuria, peripheral and periorbital edema, and hypoalbuminemia), the image shows Kimmelstiel-Wilson nodular lesions, which are characteristic of diabetic nephropathy. Renal biopsy viewed under immunofluorescence with Congo red stain reveals apple-green birefringence in patients with amyloidosis. One excellent example of amyloidosis is amyloid from immunoglobulin light chains, which is produced by cancerous plasma cells in multiple myeloma. In addition to bone pain, signs and symptoms of multiple myeloma include renal failure, elevated calcium, anemia, and increased vulnerability to infection.

Answer D is incorrect. Alport syndrome is an inherited glomerular disease caused by a mutation in type IV collagen. It can be inherited in an X-linked or an autosomal recessive manner. It typically presents with recurrent episodes of gross hematuria during childhood. It is associated with sensorineural hearing loss and ocular disorders. Renal biopsy would show a split basement membrane, not the Kimmelstiel-Wilson nodular lesions shown in the image.

Answer E is incorrect. Goodpasture disease results in a rapidly progressive glomerulonephritis, with proteinuria and hematuria, and alveolar hemorrhage causing shortness of breath and hemoptysis. It is caused by antibodies directed against the glomerular basement membrane. Renal biopsy with immunofluorescence would show linear deposition of IgG along the glomerular membrane. Kimmelstiel-Wilson nodular lesions, as seen in the image, would not be observed.

Answer F is incorrect. Acute poststreptococcal glomerulonephritis is associated with recent streptococcal infection, which would present with a history of pharyngitis, low-grade fever, swollen lymph nodes, and tonsillar exudates. It is seen most often in children, and although it shares with diabetic nephropathy the presenting symptoms of peripheral and periorbital edema and proteinuria, it usually also presents with either gross or microscopic hematuria, which is not found in this patient. Additionally, renal biopsy of a patient with acute poststreptococcal glomerulonephritis would typically show a "lumpy bumpy" appearance on light microscopy, with neutrophilic infiltrate and subepithelial deposits.

40. **The correct answer is A.** Sensitivity = true-positives / (true-positives + false-negatives). False-negatives signify the people with disease X who will be missed by the screening test. In this case, 100 people have the disease, and 80% will be diagnosed correctly (80 people are the true-positive fraction). Rearranging the equation yields: false-negatives = (true-positives / sensitivity) – true-positives or (80 / .8) – 80 = 20. Thus 20 people with disease X will not be diagnosed with this screening test (ie, they will be false-negatives).

Answer B is incorrect. The figure 80 is the number of people who will have a correct positive screening test result (ie, true-positives). If 100 people have the disease (10% prevalence) and the test is 80% sensitive, then 80 people will be correctly diagnosed (true-positives).

Answer C is incorrect. The figure 100 is the number of people in the town with disease X (ie, the prevalence of disease X). This is calculated: $1000 \times 0.10 = 100$.

Answer D is incorrect. The figure 270 is the number of people who will have an incorrect positive screening test result (ie, false-positives). One way of calculating this is that there are 900 people without the disease (with a 10% incidence in 1000 people 100 will have the disease and 900 will not). If the specificity is 70% (the percentage of true-negative test results in people without the disease) then there will be 630 people who are correctly negative (true-negatives). This means that there are $900 - 630 = 270$ people without the disease that will test positive (false-positives).

Answer E is incorrect. The figure 630 is the number of people who will have a correct negative screening test result (ie, true-negatives). If 100 people have the disease (10% prevalence) then there are 900 left that don't have the disease: $1000 - 100 = 900$. Of these 900 people the test is 70% specific (meaning it's the percentage of true-negatives detected by the test in a population without the disease): $900 \times 0.70 = 630$.

41. **The correct answer is B.** This patient presents with chronic diarrhea, intermittent facial flushing, and a murmur consistent with tricuspid stenosis, a triad of findings classic for carcinoid syndrome. One-third of carcinoid tumors of the GI tract occur in the midgut-derived small bowel, which begins at the ligament of Treitz and ends at the mid-transverse colon. While adenocarcinoma is the most common type of small bowel tumor, carcinoid tumors are most likely to occur in the small bowel. Carcinoid tumors of the small intestine secrete serotonin, which is usually metabolized by the liver and doesn't cause the symptoms of the carcinoid syndrome. However, when metastases to the liver are present, the bioactive amines can no longer be metabolized and enter the systemic circulation causing diarrhea, abdominal cramps, GI bleeding, malabsorption, flushing, bronchospasm, and right heart valvular disease from serotonin-mediated fibroelastosis. Electron microscopy reveals "salt and pepper" granulation of cells, consistent with their neuroendocrine origin. An elevated urinary 5-HIAA level is diagnostic of carcinoid syndrome.

Answer A is incorrect. The gastroesophageal junction is affected by gastroesophageal reflux disease, not carcinoid tumors.

Answer C is incorrect. The pancreaticoduodenal junction is the site where pancreatic endocrine and exocrine secretions empty into the small bowel to aid in digestion. It is part of the foregut-derived intestine, and it is a rare site for carcinoid tumors.

Answer D is incorrect. The rectosigmoid junction is not a common location for carcinoid tumors.

Answer E is incorrect. The splenic flexure is a watershed area that is susceptible to ischemic damage if cardiac output becomes low. It is not, however, a common site for carcinoid tumors.

42. **The correct answer is C.** The plain film reveals a lung tumor located in the superior sulcus and lung apex. Cancers in this location, which are also termed Pancoast tumors, frequently strangulate and/or damage the sympathetic fibers that ascend to synapse in the superior sympathetic ganglion. This results in Horner syndrome: unilateral ptosis, miosis, and anhidrosis.

Answer A is incorrect. The sympathetic fibers that are damaged in Horner syndrome and cause the symptoms this man is experiencing synapse in the superior cervical ganglion and not the inferior cervical ganglion.

Answer B is incorrect. The sympathetic fibers that are damaged in Horner syndrome and cause the symptoms this man is experiencing synapse in the superior cervical ganglion and not the sphenopalatine ganglion.

Answer D is incorrect. The sympathetic fibers that are damaged in Horner syndrome and cause the symptoms this man is experiencing synapse in the superior cervical ganglion and not the superior mesenteric ganglion.

Answer E is incorrect. The sympathetic fibers that are damaged in Horner syndrome and cause the symptoms this man is experiencing synapse in the superior cervical ganglion and not the T4 dorsal root ganglion. Furthermore, the sympathetic impulses that are blocked arise from C8-T2, levels rostral to T4.

43. **The correct answer is E.** This patient presents with deep venous thrombosis (DVT). Erythematous, warm, and tender unilateral calf swelling is classic for DVT. Risk factors for DVT and subsequent pulmonary thromboembolism include Virchow's triad, which consists of stasis (eg, immobility, obesity, congestive heart failure), endothelial injury (eg, trauma, surgery, previous DVT), and hypercoagulable state (eg, pregnancy, oral contraceptive use, coagulation disorders, malignancies, smoking). This patient also has a positive Homans sign (calf pain on forced dorsiflexion), which further supports the diagnosis. Not only should this patient be anticoagulated with heparin or warfarin upon presentation, but she should quit smoking to decrease her clotting tendencies.

   Answer A is incorrect. Bile acid resins such as cholestyramine and colestipol decrease serum triglycerides and cholesterol, which may indirectly, although not directly, improve vascular health.

   Answer B is incorrect. Statins decrease LDL cholesterol but do not affect the rate of deep venous thrombosis formation.

   Answer C is incorrect. Oral contraceptives are associated with hypercoagulable state, so they would make deep venous thrombosis more likely.

   Answer D is incorrect. Moderate exercise has been linked to improved cardiovascular health and a decreased incidence of acute coronary syndromes, although it is not specifically linked to deep venous thrombosis. Stasis, however, can make deep venous thrombosis more likely.

   Answer F is incorrect. Modest alcohol consumption has been associated with improved cardiovascular health, although no specific link to deep venous thrombosis has been proven.

44. **The correct answer is D.** The pH and electrolyte profiles for this patient describe an elevated anion gap metabolic acidosis (low pH, low bicarbonate, high anion gap). Given the signs and symptoms described, the most likely cause of acidosis in this patient is diabetic ketoacidosis (DKA), which is often the presenting syndrome in type 1 DM. Typical signs and symptoms of DKA include polyuria, polydipsia, fatigue, vomiting, abdominal pain, abnormal breathing (tachypnea early in the course, Kussmaul breathing with slow, deep breaths later), drowsiness, lethargy, and coma. The initial management of DKA requires aggressive fluid resuscitation and correction of hyperglycemia with insulin. Insulin stimulates the shift of potassium from the extracellular compartment to the intracellular compartment, causing a decrease in serum potassium levels. In addition, the rise in serum pH (as a result of correcting the ketoacidosis with insulin) will cause hydrogen ions to come out of the cells, which occurs in exchange for positively charged potassium ions that move intracellularly, leading to further hypokalemia. Thus patients with an apparent low or normal serum potassium level before administering insulin are at risk of having a potentially life-threateningly low total body potassium level, which can cause cardiac conduction abnormalities and death. Hence, after the administration of insulin, judicious monitoring and administration of potassium is the most important next step in the treatment of DKA.

   Answer A is incorrect. Bicarbonate does not undergo insulin-mediated transcellular shifts as does potassium. Bicarbonate levels often normalize with the correction of hyperglycemia and fluid administration, which promotes the diuresis of serum ketoacids. Bicarbonate should be administered only in severe cases of acidosis, such as a pH <6.9.

   Answer B is incorrect. Calcium does not undergo insulin-mediated transcellular shifts as does potassium; hence, serum levels of calcium do not fluctuate to the same extent with DKA and insulin administration. Serum calcium levels are usually not a major concern in patients with DKA.

Answer C is incorrect. Chloride does not undergo insulin-mediated transcellular shifts as does potassium; hence, serum levels of chloride do not fluctuate to the same extent with DKA and insulin administration. Appropriate fluid resuscitation is generally sufficient to manage serum chloride levels in patients who may be dehydrated.

Answer E is incorrect. Sodium does not undergo insulin-mediated transcellular shifts as does potassium. However, correction of the hyperglycemia will lead to a decrease in plasma osmolality, which will cause water to move into the cells. This movement of water will lead to an increase in serum sodium concentration. However, unlike with potassium, this change in serum sodium level is usually not potentially life-threatening. Fluid resuscitation is generally sufficient to manage serum sodium levels.

45. **The correct answer is E.** The history and physical examination suggest a possible cerebrovascular accident. Before any therapeutic intervention is done, an emergent CT scan must be performed to rule out hemorrhage. In this case, we are told that the CT was normal, meaning that no hemorrhage was seen. Given the high clinical suspicion for stroke, your attention should focus on the likely possibility of an ischemic etiology. It is important to remember, however, that an ischemic infarct will often not be visible on the initial scan, especially if the scan is done within a few hours of symptom onset. Tissue plasminogen activator (tPA), a thrombolytic agent, is the best next step in management given that the patient does not have any obvious contraindications to thrombolytic therapy. Treatment with tPA has been shown to be very effective in the management of acute ischemic stroke, especially if administered within three hours of symptom onset. This form of treatment does, however, carry a risk of hemorrhage.

    Answer A is incorrect. Once a hemorrhagic stroke has been ruled out by CT scan, the possibility of a cardioembolic source should be investigated with an echocardiogram. Patients with a history of atrial fibrillation are at significantly increased risk of thromboembolism. Thrombolysis/anticoagulation, however, helps restore perfusion to the brain and therefore should be done first.

    Answer B is incorrect. Some strokes, particularly those involving the middle cerebral artery, are associated with significant parenchymal edema and subsequent mass effect, with possible sequelae including herniation and death. Hemicraniectomy is a rather novel therapeutic intervention that involves temporarily removing half of the skull over the edematous area with the goal of relieving pressure and reducing the chance of herniation. This intervention is not widely used and is not considered the standard of care in the management of acute stroke.

    Answer C is incorrect. Heparin therapy is the next step in management for patients who have contraindications to thrombolytic therapy. Such contraindications include past history of hemorrhagic stroke, active internal bleed, history of surgery within the past three weeks, and any form of coagulopathy. As with tissue plasminogen activator, it is imperative to rule out the presence of intracranial hemorrhage with a CT scan before initiating therapy.

    Answer D is incorrect. Hyperglycemia worsens functional outcomes in cases of ischemic stroke. It has been hypothesized that hyperglycemia may increase local tissue acidosis and blood-brain barrier permeability. While glucose control with insulin would help minimize the harmful effects of hyperglycemia, it is not the next step in management.

46. **The correct answer is A.** This patient presents with a primary inoculation lesion, regional lymphadenopathy, and low-grade fever characteristic of cat scratch disease, which is caused by *Bartonella henselae*. Typically (in 60% of cases) infection occurs when a child is scratched or bitten by a bacteremic young cat.

    Answer B is incorrect. The spirochete *Borrelia burgdorferi* is the cause of Lyme disease. The spirochete is carried by the *Ixodes* tick, which is most common in the northeastern United States. It initially presents with an expanding ring-shaped lesion at the site of the tick bite known as erythema migrans.

Answer C is incorrect. *Eikenella corrodens* is a gram-negative organism that is part of the normal flora of the mouth and nasopharynx. It is associated with infections resulting from human bites.

Answer D is incorrect. *Francisella tularensis* is the cause of tularemia. This disease is carried by wild rabbits and ticks in the southeastern United States. It often presents with lymphadenopathy and an ulcer at the site of entry as well as with fever.

Answer E is incorrect. *Pasteurella multocida* is caused by cat bites and dog bites. This infection causes a rapid inflammation (often within hours) and is accompanied by purulent drainage.

47. **The correct answer is D.** The vignette describes a classic history of an autoimmune hyperthyroidism, Graves disease. In this disorder, thyroid follicular cells are stimulated to synthesize and secrete thyroid hormone by anti-TSH receptor antibodies, leading to increased levels of thyroxine (T_4) and triiodothyronine (T_3) in the blood, which results in negative feedback on the anterior pituitary and suppression of TSH secretion. Thus, both free T_4 and total T_4, which includes free T_4 and T_4 bound to proteins in the blood (eg, albumin and thyroxine-binding globulin) will be increased, while blood TSH levels will be low relative to the normal baseline.

    Answer A is incorrect. An elevated TSH level is not characteristic of Graves disease, and elevated T_4 levels should result in a lower TSH level due to negative feedback on the anterior pituitary.

    Answer B is incorrect. An elevated TSH level is not characteristic of Graves disease, and an elevated free T_4 level should result in a lower TSH level due to negative feedback on the anterior pituitary. Furthermore, thyroid hormone binding to proteins in the blood should not be decreased but instead should be increased in the setting of increased free T_4. Therefore, the total T_4 level should be elevated rather than low.

    Answer C is incorrect. Graves disease is characterized by a low TSH level due to the circulating thyroid-stimulating immunoglobulins, which elevate T_3 and T_4 levels and, via negative feedback, downregulate the level of TSH. In this answer choice, the level of TSH is elevated, which would lead to elevated, not diminished, levels of T_3 and T_4.

    Answer E is incorrect. Total and free T_4 levels are expected to be low in the setting of low TSH levels. However, in Graves disease, stimulation of TSH receptors on the thyroid follicular cells by anti-TSH receptor antibodies stimulates the secretion of thyroid hormones and results in increased total and free T_4 levels in the setting of normal or even low TSH levels. The resulting negative feedback loop to the anterior pituitary leads to reduced TSH levels.

48. **The correct answer is E.** Endemic African Burkitt lymphoma frequently manifests as masses involving the mandible (and less often the kidneys, ovaries, and adrenals). Affected lymph nodes show a classic "starry-sky" pattern of neoplastic lymphoblasts and non-neoplastic "tingible body" macrophages. The neoplastic cells typically show a translocation of the *c-myc* gene on chromosome 8 onto the immunoglobulin heavy-chain gene on chromosome 14. It is more common in African children and is associated with the Epstein-Barr virus (EBV). EBV also is associated with heterophile-positive mononucleosis, oral hairy leukoplakia in patients infected with HIV, lymphoproliferative disorders in immunocompromised hosts (including Hodgkin and non-Hodgkin lymphomas), and nasopharyngeal carcinoma. Interestingly, nonendemic Burkitt lymphoma presents as an abdominal mass and is associated with HIV, not EBV.

    Answer A is incorrect. Cervical adenocarcinoma is associated with human papillomavirus.

    Answer B is incorrect. Gastric adenocarcinoma may be associated with *Helicobacter py-*

lori, but not EBV. Gastric carcinomas, 90% of which are adenocarcinomas, are more common in developing countries than in industrialized countries; they rarely occur before age 40 years; and incidence peaks in the seventh decade with a male:female ratio of 2:1. Gastric carcinoma also is associated with atrophic gastritis, post-gastrectomy states, achlorhydria, pernicious anemia, Ménétrier's disease, and adenomatous polyps.

Answer C is incorrect. Hepatocellular carcinoma is associated with chronic HBV and HCV infections. Other noninfectious associations with hepatocellular carcinoma include cirrhosis (secondary to alcohol, or cryptogenic), hemochromatosis, aflatoxin ingestion, and α_1-antitrypsin deficiency.

Answer D is incorrect. Heterophile-negative mononucleosis is associated with cytomegalovirus, acute HIV, toxoplasmosis, and human herpesvirus types 6 and 7. Although heterophile-negative mononucleosis may present with similar symptoms of fever and lymphadenopathy without pharyngitis (as in this case), these infectious agents typically would not result in the large mass on the right mandible. Heterophile-positive mononucleosis is associated with EBV.

Test Block 2

QUESTIONS

1. An oncologist recently discovered that certain cancerous cells secrete a protein named ca-1panc. Using this protein, he developed a serum test to detect this type of cancer. He performed the blood test on 1000 patients. One hundred of these patients had the cancer, and the test came back positive for 60 of them, while for the remaining 40 patients the test was negative. Nine hundred of the patients did not have the cancer; however, the test was positive for 100 of them. In the remaining 800, the test came back negative. Which of the following numbers represents how well the test identified those who had the cancer?

   (A) 10.0%
   (B) 37.5%
   (C) 60.0%
   (D) 88.8%
   (E) 90.0%
   (F) 95.2%

2. A 33-year-old pregnant woman presents to her physician with tendonitis of the left shoulder. The patient has taken nonsteroidal anti-inflammatory drugs (NSAIDs) in the past, but developed gastric ulcers associated with long-term NSAID use. A medication is available that will reduce the incidence of NSAID-associated gastric ulcers, but it is contraindicated in pregnancy. Which of the following is an adverse event associated with this medication that makes it absolutely contraindicated during pregnancy?

   (A) Induction of labor
   (B) Intrauterine growth retardation
   (C) Neural tube defects
   (D) Placenta previa
   (E) Premature fetal closure of ductus arteriosus

3. A 9-year-old girl is brought to the emergency department with an arrhythmia that started while she was sitting in class. Since birth she has had a disorder that predisposes her to arrhythmias, but because her parents were not present, the hospital staff was unable to determine her medical history. The staff attempts to treat the patient with an atrioventricular nodal block antiarrhythmic, which does not cure the problem and instead makes it worse. What congenital pathophysiology could this girl have had?

   (A) Atrioventricular accessory tract
   (B) Atrioventricular nodal re-entry
   (C) Tetralogy of Fallot
   (D) Ventricular hypertrophy
   (E) Ventricular tachycardia

4. A 57-year-old African-American man complains of lethargy, weakness, and confusion. His wife says that he also has been complaining of increasing pain in his bones, particularly in his hips, lower back, and legs. Levels of protein and calcium are elevated. Results of digital rectal examination and prostate-specific antigen testing are normal. X-ray of his skull is shown in the image. Which of the following laboratory test results are diagnostic?

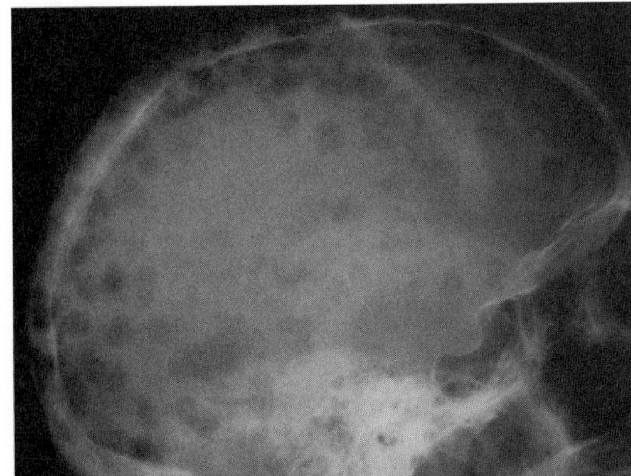

Reproduced, with permission, from USMLERx.com.

(A) Bone mineral density T score >2.5
(B) Elevated serum parathyroid hormone
(C) Fasting glucose >126 mg/dL
(D) Monoclonal M spike on protein electrophoresis
(E) Positive HLA-B27 haplotype
(F) Prostate specific antigen of 4 ng/mL

5. A 14-year-old high school freshman presents to her family doctor for a sports physical. She has not played organized sports in the past but is in good physical shape. She mentions that she experienced severe leg cramps after trying out for the soccer team last week. The night after the tryouts, she noticed that her urine had a reddish tinge. She has no other medical complaints. Her physician orders an ischemic forearm exercise test, which reveals no increase in venous lactate. Which of the following enzymes is most likely deficient in this patient?

(A) α-1,6-Glucosidase
(B) Cystathionine synthase
(C) Glucose-6-phosphatase
(D) Glycogen phosphorylase
(E) Lysosomal α-1,4-glucosidase

6. A 62-year-old woman visits her family doctor with complaints of chronic lower back pain. She has also suffered from severe rheumatoid arthritis of the knees for the past 10 years, which has significantly limited her physical activity despite appropriate medical treatment. Her mother died at age 58 years from a massive pulmonary embolus following hip replacement surgery after falling. Which of the following sets of serum laboratory findings best describes her condition?

Choice	Calcium	Phosphorus	Alkaline phosphatase
A	↓	↑	↓
B	normal	normal	normal
C	normal	normal	↑
D	↑	↓	↑

Reproduced, with permission, from USMLERx.com.

(A) A
(B) B
(C) C
(D) D

7. A 45-year-old man comes to the physician with a three-day history of a temperature of 39°C (102.2°F). He also complains of headache, neck stiffness, and a maculopapular rash on his trunk. A diagnosis of meningitis is made, and a smear and culture of his cerebrospinal fluid reveal a gram-negative diplococcus as the causative agent. Which of the following symptoms can develop as a severe complication of this infection?

(A) Acute renal failure and thrombocytopenia with hemolytic anemia
(B) Fever, migratory polyarthritis, and carditis
(C) Fever, new murmur, small erythematous lesions on the palms, and splinter hemorrhages on the nail bed
(D) Shock, widespread purpura, disseminated intravascular coagulation, and adrenal insufficiency
(E) Symmetric ascending muscle weakness beginning in the distal lower extremities

8. A 57-year-old man with a history of arthritis treated with a cyclooxygenase (COX)-2 inhibitor presents to the emergency department because of sudden shortness of breath and chest pain radiating to his jaw and left arm. Which of the following proposals best explains why the patient may have been better off using aspirin for his arthritis instead of selective COX-2 inhibitors? (PGI_2 = prostaglandin I_2, TxA_2 = thromboxane A_2)

	Choice	PGI_2	TxA_2
A	COX-2 inhibitor Aspirin	↑ ↓	-- ↓
B	COX-2 inhibitor Aspirin	-- ↓	↑ ↓
C	COX-2 inhibitor Aspirin	↓ ↓	↓ ↓
D	COX-2 inhibitor Aspirin	↓ ↑	-- ↑
E	COX-2 inhibitor Aspirin	↓ ↓	-- ↓

Reproduced, with permission, from USMLERx.com.

(A) A
(B) B
(C) C
(D) D
(E) E

9. A 30-year-old woman with systemic lupus erythematosus treated with high-dose prednisone comes to her physician complaining of easy fatigability. Blood studies reveal a hemoglobin level of 10 g/dL, a low serum iron level, elevated ferritin level, and low total iron-binding capacity. Normocytic RBCs are seen on blood smear. Which of the following is the most appropriate treatment for this patient's anemia?

(A) Erythropoietin
(B) Ferrous sulfate
(C) Folate
(D) Parenteral vitamin B_{12}
(E) Phlebotomy

10. The retinoblastoma gene on chromosome 13, which encodes the retinoblastoma tumor suppressor protein, has served as a paradigm for the study of several other tumor suppressor genes. Survivors of hereditary retinoblastoma have increased risk for the development of additional neoplasms. Which of the following is the most likely non-ocular tumor to occur in a survivor of hereditary retinoblastoma?

(A) Esophageal adenocarcinoma
(B) Femoral osteosarcoma
(C) Medullary carcinoma of the thyroid
(D) Renal cell carcinoma
(E) Serous cystadenoma of the ovary
(F) Squamous cell carcinoma of the lung
(G) Transitional cell carcinoma

11. An obese, 56-year-old African-American man with a 25-pack-year history of smoking experiences chest pain associated with myocardial infarction. The pain radiates to the man's left shoulder and down his left arm. What is the reason for referred pain to this region?

(A) Common lymphatic drainage pathways of the molecular mediators of inflammation and pain
(B) Proximity of sensory nerve fiber tracts in the anterior horn of the spinal cord
(C) Proximity of sensory nerve fiber tracts in the posterior horn of the spinal cord
(D) Shared parasympathetic pathways
(E) Shared sympathetic pathways

12. A 57-year-old man who is HIV-positive presents to his physician with headache, nausea and vomiting, and a change in mental status. No nuchal rigidity is noted. A lumbar puncture is performed and shows a high opening pressure. A preparation of his bronchoalveolar lavage fluid with India ink stain is shown in the image. Intravenous treatment is started for the acute condition. Which of the following adverse effects might occur with this patient's initial treatment?

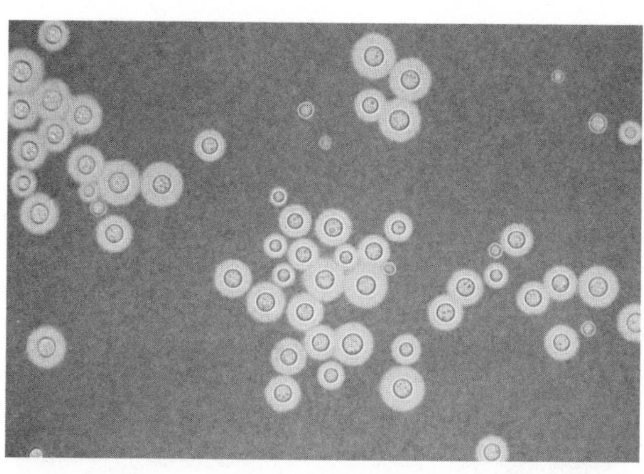

Courtesy of Dr. Leanor Haley, Centers for Disease Control and Prevention.

(A) Arrhythmia
(B) Bone marrow suppression
(C) Flushing
(D) Gynecomastia
(E) Nausea and vomiting

13. A 56-year-old obese man with unknown medical history presents to the emergency department. He was found by his wife on the floor of the bathroom, conscious but disoriented, vomiting, and clutching his abdomen. She is unsure of the name of his one oral medication, but knows he takes it regularly, twice daily. He was recently admitted to another hospital for a cholecystectomy. On examination, the patient is breathing heavily and quickly, but other vital signs are normal. Laboratory test results include:

Na^+: 142 mEq/L
K^+: 4.0 mEq/L
Cl^-: 105 mEq/L
HCO_3^-: 19 mEq/L
Blood urea nitrogen: 20 mg/dL
Creatinine: 1.6 mg/dL
Glucose: 256 mg/dL

What drug is the patient most likely taking?

(A) Glyburide
(B) Insulin
(C) Metformin
(D) Orlistat
(E) Rosiglitazone

14. A woman with a 2-year-old son comes to her physician because she has been unable to conceive a second child for more than a year. The woman is currently breastfeeding her son. Which of the following best explains the physiologic mechanism currently preventing her from getting pregnant?

(A) Prolactin inhibits secretion of estrogen from the ovaries
(B) Prolactin inhibits secretion of follicle-stimulating hormone from the anterior pituitary gland
(C) Prolactin inhibits secretion of gonadotropin-releasing hormone from the hypothalamus
(D) Prolactin inhibits secretion of luteinizing hormone from the anterior pituitary gland
(E) Prolactin inhibits secretion of progesterone from the corpus luteum

15. A neonate has apparent difficulty with feeding, including repeated episodes of choking and coughing with attempted breastfeeding and bottle-feeding. The child, when not feeding, has a normal temperature, heart rate, respiratory rate, and blood pressure. On physical examination the lungs are clear and the heart has no adventitial sounds. Facies are normal. What is the embryologic abnormality that has caused this child's feeding difficulties?

(A) Failure of the first and second branchial arches to fuse
(B) Failure of the maxillary processes to fuse
(C) Failure of the medial nasal processes to fuse
(D) Failure of the palatine processes to fuse
(E) Failure of the second and third branchial arches to fuse

16. A woman strikes her head in a car crash and is admitted to the hospital. On admission, she reports a medical history of hypertension, hypercholesterolemia, diabetes type II, fibromyalgia, and breast cancer for which she underwent a lumpectomy and chemotherapy. Her current medications include simvastatin, metformin, furosemide, hydrocodone, and tamoxifen. During the interview, she complains of severe thirst and frequent urination, and her urine bag is nearly full after only two hours. Which medication should the patient be given immediately?

(A) Demeclocycline
(B) Desmopressin
(C) Furosemide
(D) Insulin
(E) Mannitol

17. A 46-year-old man with a history of obstructive sleep apnea, hypertension, and type 2 diabetes mellitus is referred to a sleep laboratory for evaluation. On arrival he is hooked up to an electroencephalograph (EEG) and begins to fall asleep a few minutes later. During the night the patient has multiple apneic episodes preceded by very loud snoring spells. At 3 o'clock in the morning the patient has beta waves on his EEG. This patient is currently in what stage of sleep?

(A) Awake
(B) Stage 1
(C) Stage 2
(D) Stage 3
(E) Stage 4

18. A 51-year-old man visits his physician for a routine physical examination. During the examination, the physician notices cervical, axillary, inguinal, and femoral lymphadenopathy. The patient reports the size of the nodes has waxed and waned over the past several months. He never came in to get them checked because they did not cause him any pain. A lymph node biopsy is performed (see image). Which of the following oncogenes and translocations is associated with this type of lymphoma?

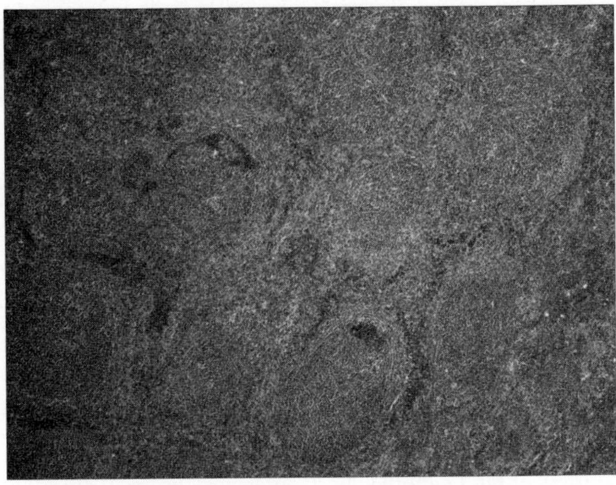

Reproduced, with permission, from USMLERx.com.

(A) *c-myc*; t(8,14)
(B) *bcl-2*; t(14;18)
(C) *erb* B2; t(11;14)
(D) *p53*; t(8:14)
(E) *ras*; t(11:14)

19. A 15-year-old girl presents to her pediatrician for her annual physical examination. She reports that she has been in good health but is somewhat concerned because, unlike all of her friends, she has not yet started to menstruate or develop breasts. On physical examination, she is 150 cm (59 in) tall and is obese with a short neck. Her genitalia and breasts are Tanner stage I. Laboratory studies show elevated serum follicle-stimulating hormone and luteinizing hormone levels and a low estradiol level. Which of the following findings is most likely to be seen in a patient with this condition?

(A) Blood pressure in upper extremity greater than that in lower extremity
(B) Carotid bruits
(C) III/IV late systolic murmur with midsystolic click
(D) Mediastinal widening on x-ray of the chest
(E) Pulsus parvus et tardus

20. A 53-year-old man with a long-standing history of allergic rhinitis and asthma presents with uveitis, mild hearing loss, numbness and tingling in his right hand, and diffuse joint pain for the past 10 days. Physical examina-

tion shows weak to absent left knee patellar reflexes (right knee reflex strong and intact). Laboratory studies show a markedly elevated eosinophil count. A diagnosis is made, and the patient is treated with cyclophosphamide. Further laboratory studies show elevated serum levels of the most common autoantibody associated with this condition. What structure is primarily targeted by the autoantibodies that are most likely elevated in this patient's serum?

(A) Acetylcholine receptors
(B) Neutrophils
(C) Oligodendrocytes
(D) RBCs
(E) Thyroid-stimulating hormone receptors

21. A 48-year-old woman is brought to the emergency department after having her first generalized seizure. When questioned, she complains of chronic early morning headaches that have increased in severity over the past six months. A neurological examination shows a slight loss of her temporal visual field on the right. Imaging studies reveal the presence of a tumor compressing the optic nerve. Biopsy results are shown in the image. Which of the following is the most likely diagnosis?

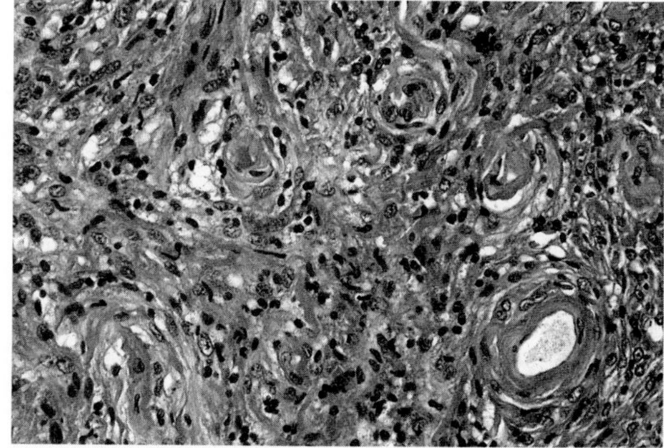

Courtesy of Wikipedia.

(A) Hemangioblastoma
(B) Meningioma
(C) Oligodendroglioma
(D) Papillary thyroid carcinoma
(E) Pituitary adenoma

22. A 32-year-old female dialysis patient visits her general internist for a health maintenance visit. She subsequently has a dual-energy x-ray absorption examination, which demonstrates significant osteoporosis. What is the most likely etiology of this patient's osteoporosis?

(A) 1,25-Dihydroxycholecalciferol excess
(B) Chronic metabolic alkalosis
(C) Hypercalcemia
(D) Hypophosphatemia
(E) Secondary hyperparathyroidism

23. A 62-year-old man arrives at his doctor's office complaining of recent onset dull pain in his left flank region. He is a retired steel plant worker with a long history of excessive smoking, hypertension, and obesity. He does not recall any history of similar illness in his family. On physical examination a firm, homogeneous, nontender movable mass is palpated deep in the left umbilical region near the lower pole of the kidney. Laboratory tests show hypercalcemia, hypophosphatemia, and moderate polycythemia. Urinalysis reveals the presence of hematuria. Which of the following is the most likely diagnosis?

(A) Adult polycystic kidney disease
(B) Angiomyolipoma
(C) Pheochromocytoma
(D) Renal cell carcinoma
(E) Wilms tumor

24. A 3-year-old boy is brought to his pediatrician's office because his parents noticed worsening protrusion of his abdomen. After thorough imaging studies and histopathologic confirmation of Wilms tumor, the physician prescribes a medication that acts by causing arrest of the cell cycle during metaphase. However, the parents are concerned about the use of that medication because of what they have read about its adverse effects. Which adverse effect are the parents most likely concerned about?

(A) Cardiotoxicity
(B) Hemorrhagic cystitis
(C) Hyperglycemia
(D) Pulmonary fibrosis
(E) Neurotoxicity

25. A 7-year-old girl has numerous vesicles on her face, particularly around her mouth after falling and scraping her face on the ground. Over a few days the vesicles turn into pustules and crust over, becoming flaky and light yellow in color. Which of the following statements about the organism most likely responsible for this girl's infection is correct?

(A) Endotoxin is present in the outer membrane of this organism
(B) Sabouraud agar is required to culture this bacterium
(C) The bacterium is β-hemolytic and resistant to bacitracin
(D) The bacterium is β-hemolytic and sensitive to bacitracin
(E) The bacterium is a facultative intracellular organism

26. An 18-year-old man presents complaining of an inability to keep his balance. A complete neurologic examination is conducted, and funduscopy reveals retinal hemangioblastomas. He reports that his mother has a history of a "brain tumor," the specifics of which he is unaware. Given the classic evolution of this patient's disease, for which of the following does this patient require close monitoring?

(A) Astrocytoma
(B) Colon cancer
(C) Depression
(D) Pheochromocytoma
(E) Renal mass

27. A 45-year-old white man presents to his doctor complaining of weakness, lethargy, and decreased libido over the past few months. He also notes that his skin seems darker than usual. The patient denies any past medical conditions and has a family history of diabetes mellitus. The patient's father died from a "long-standing liver problem." On physical examination the patient appears to have skin pigmentation, which is most evident on his face and arms. The heart and lung examination is normal. On abdominal examination, the liver edge is palpable two finger-widths below the costochondral angle. The patient is referred to a surgeon who performs a liver biopsy; findings are shown in the image. What laboratory changes can be expected with this patient's condition?

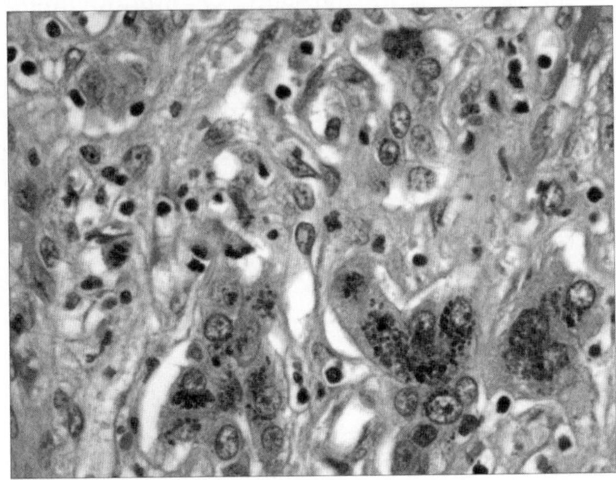

Reproduced, with permission, from USMLERx.com.

(A) Decreased serum ferritin
(B) Increased iron-binding capacity
(C) Increased transferrin saturation
(D) No change in plasma iron
(E) No change in serum ferritin

28. A 25-year-old woman presents to her family physician for a routine check-up. Physical examination reveals a mildly overweight woman, but is otherwise unremarkable. A fasting lipid panel, however, shows an LDL cholesterol level of 310 mg/dL, HDL cholesterol level of 42 mg/dL, triglyceride level of 150 mg/dL, and total cholesterol level of 382 mg/dL. Because a diagnosis of familial hypercholesterolemia is suspected, the doctor initiates treatment of her condition. Soon after starting treatment, however, she presents with myalgias. Laboratory values show elevated levels of aspartate aminotransferase, alanine aminotransferase, and creatinine kinase. Which of the following describes the mechanism of the intervention that was initiated to treat this patient's hypercholesterolemia?

(A) Inhibition of 3-hydroxy-3-methylglutaryl coenzyme A reductase enzyme
(B) Inhibition of bile-acid reuptake in the intestine

(C) Inhibition of cholesterol uptake by the intestinal brush border
(D) Reduced transfer of cholesterol from HDL to LDL and delayed HDL clearance
(E) Selective removal of LDL molecules from the blood via immunoadsorption columns

29. Informed consent is the legal demonstration of a patient's understanding of the risks, benefits, and outcomes of treatments and alternatives. As such, the patient is taking responsibility for making decisions in the medical process, but is authorizing the physician to provide the treatment. While informed consent is an important ethical principle, there are exceptions to the requirement of obtaining it. Which of the following circumstances is a valid exception to the requirement of obtaining informed consent?

(A) A competent patient's son wishes to waive his father's rights
(B) A paralyzed patient cannot speak but can nod his head for consent
(C) A patient is mentally disabled but legally competent
(D) A physician believes that informing the patient will be detrimental to the patient's health
(E) A stable patient is in the emergency department for treatment of a femur fracture

30. A 45-year-old man presents to the clinic because of severe back pain, muscle weakness, and fatigue that gradually started two months ago. Physical examination reveals slightly darkened skin and a systolic blood pressure in the 90s. Upon further questioning the patient reveals he stopped taking a medication about three months ago. Which of the following is the most likely medication?

(A) Dehydroepiandrosterone
(B) Fluconazole
(C) Hydrocortisone
(D) Metformin

31. A 78-year-old man comes to the physician for evaluation after falling five times in two months. An x-ray skeletal survey reveals no fractures, but the patient admits to worsening urinary incontinence over the previous four months. His wife states that his memory and concentration have deteriorated recently. The patient's vital signs are normal, and his physical examination is notable for a wide-based gait with short steps. A Mini-Mental State Examination results in a score of 26/30. His funduscopic examination is normal, and his neurologic examination is notable for slight bradykinesia without tremor. Laboratory tests, including serum vitamin B_{12}, folate, and thyroid-stimulating hormone, are normal. What is the most likely etiology of this patient's recent decline?

(A) Alzheimer disease
(B) Hypothyroidism
(C) Multi-infarct dementia
(D) Normal pressure hydrocephalus
(E) Parkinson disease

32. A 31-year-old woman with newly diagnosed tuberculosis is begun on a standard treatment regimen. During a follow-up appointment, it is noted as she walks into the room that her gait is markedly unsteady. Physical examination is notable for decreased sensation over the upper and lower extremities. Which of the following drugs is most likely causing this patient's symptoms?

(A) Ethambutol
(B) Isoniazid
(C) Levofloxacin
(D) Pyrazinamide
(E) Rifampin

33. A 19-year-old man who recently emigrated from Mexico comes to the emergency department because of blood in his sputum. The patient mentions he has had weight loss and night sweats. On examination, the patient has a fever and bronchial breath sounds with crepitant rales. Laboratory tests show lymphocytosis and an increased erythrocyte sedimentation rate. X-ray of the chest shows a calcified lung lesion and hilar lymphadenopathy. Of the following, which is the stain used to identify the most likely infectious organism?

(A) Congo red
(B) Giemsa
(C) India ink
(D) Periodic acid-Schiff
(E) Ziehl-Neelsen

34. A 65-year-old postmenopausal woman presents with progressive constipation and frequent, excessive urination. She reports a 40-pack-year history of smoking. On physical examination, respiratory findings prompt an x-ray film of the chest, in which a concerning circular lesion is found overlying the right hilum. Laboratory testing demonstrates a decreased phosphorus level. Which of the following is the most likely cause of this patient's symptoms?

(A) Central bronchogenic carcinoma
(B) Cervical sympathetic chain compression
(C) Chronic silica exposure
(D) Congenital chloride channel dysfunction
(E) Dynein arm defect in cilia
(F) Ectopic ADH production
(G) Solitary parathyroid adenoma

35. The image demonstrates a specialized epithelium that overlies a type of peripheral lymphoid tissue. It is thought that most disseminated *Mycobacterium avium* infections in patients with AIDS are acquired by the bacteria penetrating through this tissue-type of the immune system. What is the main class of antibodies associated with this lymphoid tissue?

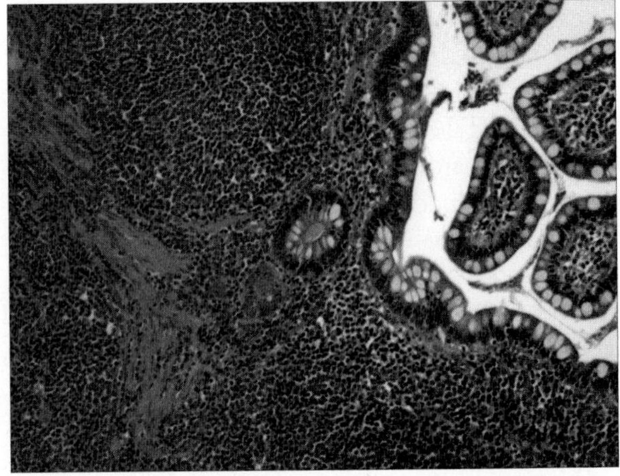

Reproduced, with permission, from USMLERx.com.

(A) IgA
(B) IgD
(C) IgE
(D) IgG
(E) IgM

36. A patient presents to the emergency department with a severe headache, palpitations, and elevated blood pressure. He is found to have elevated urinary vanillylmandelic acid levels. He is diagnosed with a pheochromocytoma with predominantly elevated norepinephrine levels. Which of the following agents will antagonize both the vascular and cardiac actions of norepinephrine?

(A) Atenolol
(B) Doxazosin
(C) Esmolol
(D) Isoproterenol
(E) Labetalol

37. A physician is caring for a hospitalized 31-year-old man with long-standing, poorly controlled type 1 diabetes mellitus. He is blind and has peripheral neuropathy with sensory loss in both feet, and his most recent hemoglobin A_{1c} level was 13.9%. He recently presented with altered mental status, polyuria, and polydip-

sia. At that time, his serum glucose level was 475 mg/dL, arterial blood pH was 6.96, and his anion gap was 27. Since then his acidosis has resolved with appropriate treatment, and fingerstick blood glucose levels have normalized. However, he has persistent nasal discharge; paranasal sinus tenderness; and new onset of periorbital edema, proptosis, facial numbness, and obtundation. Fungal stain of fluid obtained from urgent surgical sinus drainage would most likely reveal which of the following?

(A) 45-degree angle branching, septate hyphae with rare fruiting bodies
(B) 5- to 10-μm yeasts with wide capsular halo on India ink stain
(C) Broad-based budding dimorphic fungi
(D) Irregular, broad, nonseptate hyphae with 90-degree branching
(E) Pseudohyphae with budding yeasts

38. A 64-year-old woman presents to her primary care physician with fatigue, weakness, and a weight loss of 4.5 kg (10 lb) in the past four months. Also, her vision has deteriorated over that time, and she has had several severe nosebleeds. Physical examination demonstrates hepatosplenomegaly, and laboratory tests show an increased total protein level. Serum protein electrophoresis reveals a large spike in the gamma region. A skeletal survey is negative. Which of the following is the most likely diagnosis?

(A) Chronic lymphocytic leukemia
(B) Diabetes mellitus
(C) Monoclonal gammopathy of undetermined significance
(D) Multiple myeloma
(E) Waldenström macroglobulinemia

39. A pharmaceutical company has created a new drug that, when taken daily, is thought to be highly effective at preventing the onset of migraines. The company would like to market the drug and is conducting a study to look at its benefits and possible risks. In coordination with a physician at a local hospital, it enrolls 800 people for the study. The physician places 100 patients with the worst and most frequent migraines in the medication group, as he thinks that they are in most need of the drug's benefit. Which of the following best explains why the drug may not perform up to expectations?

(A) Differences in group size
(B) Late-look bias
(C) Recall bias
(D) Sampling bias
(E) Selection bias

40. A 62-year-old man with a known diagnosis of benign prostatic hyperplasia is seen at his annual physical and found to have a prostate-specific antigen level of 11.2 ng/mL, up from 6.4 ng/mL the previous year. Ultrasound-guided transrectal prostate biopsies are performed. If the biopsies are positive for prostate cancer, what zone of the prostatic tissue is most likely involved by the cancer cells?

(A) Neurovascular bundle
(B) Peripheral
(C) Periurethral
(D) Seminal vesicle
(E) Transition

41. A patient presents to the emergency department complaining of chills, cough, and malaise. His temperature is 38.6°C (101.5°F). An x-ray of his chest demonstrates consolidation of the right middle lobe. A complete blood count reveals leukocytosis with a left shift on differential. Based on the results of Gram staining and sputum culture, the patient is treated with cefazolin. Gram staining and sputum culture most likely revealed which of the following?

(A) Anaerobic, encapsulated, gram-negative rods without endotoxin
(B) Gram-positive cocci in clusters
(C) Gram-positive rods with long branching filaments
(D) Gram-positive, aerobic, spore-forming rods
(E) Oxidase-positive, non-lactose-fermenting, gram-negative rods

42. A 20-year-old woman presents to the physician because of a history of bloody diarrhea and abdominal pain. She states that she has not traveled recently or changed her eating habits. A stool culture is negative for an infectious cause of diarrhea. Flexible sigmoidoscopy shows numerous lesions in the descending colon interrupted by normal-appearing mucosa. Which of the following features would most likely be present on a tissue biopsy of the affected region?

(A) Cells with loss of mucin and hyperchromatic nuclei
(B) Crypt abscesses
(C) Hyperplastic goblet cells
(D) Noncaseating granulomas
(E) Ulcerated mucosa only

43. A 38-year-old man from rural Guatemala dies of heart failure. Notable autopsy findings include dilated large bowel. Microscopy of a blood sample taken in the emergency department before the man's death shows flagellated parasites. Which of the following parasites did this man most likely harbor?

(A) *Cryptosporidium* species
(B) *Entamoeba histolytica*
(C) *Giardia lamblia*
(D) *Toxoplasma gondii*
(E) *Trypanosoma cruzi*

44. A 27-year-old man presents to the emergency department with a cough productive of blood-tinged sputum. He also complains that in the past couple weeks he has noticed increased fatigue and some blood in his urine. A renal biopsy is performed that, upon on immunofluorescence staining, shows a linear pattern of IgG deposition along the basement membrane. Which of the following is most likely responsible for this patient's disease?

(A) Anti-type III collagen antibodies
(B) Anti-type IV collagen antibodies
(C) Antineutrophil cytoplasmic antibodies
(D) Immune complexes
(E) T lymphocytes

45. A 36-year-old man who completed a marathon six hours earlier presents to the emergency department with severe muscle pain and swelling and complaints of red urine. Laboratory tests show a creatine kinase level of 6800 U/L but no RBCs or WBCs on urinalysis. Which of the following symptoms would most likely also be present?

(A) Arrhythmia
(B) Hepatomegaly
(C) Pain in a dermatomal distribution
(D) Pain on urination
(E) Shuffling gait

46. A 43-year-old woman visits her obstetrician for her scheduled check-up at 20 weeks' gestation. Her obstetrician recommends that she have a series of screening tests. One of these tests shows an elevated serum α-fetoprotein level. Which of the following is most likely responsible for this result?

(A) Bilateral renal agenesis
(B) Failure of the ductus arteriosus to close
(C) Inadequate folic acid intake
(D) Inheritance of a recessive disorder
(E) Nondisjunction occurring during meiosis

47. The father of a 7-year-old boy is contacted by his child's schoolteacher because she is concerned about his inattentiveness during class. The teacher states that the boy appears to be daydreaming multiple times each day, during which time he blinks his eyes repeatedly. She reports that the boy's daydreaming episodes are brief and he is able to refocus shortly following the daydream. What is the most appropriate therapy for the child's underlying condition?

(A) Carbamazepine
(B) Clonazepam
(C) Ethosuximide
(D) Gabapentin
(E) Methylphenidate
(F) Tiagabine

48. A 68-year-old man with a six-month history of back pain and fatigue presents to the emergency department because of severe low back pain. MRI shows multiple lytic bone lesions scattered throughout the man's body, and laboratory results show a serum M spike and light chain proteinuria. Bone marrow biopsy demonstrates an excessive number of the cells shown in the image. Which of the following is most likely to be present in these cells?

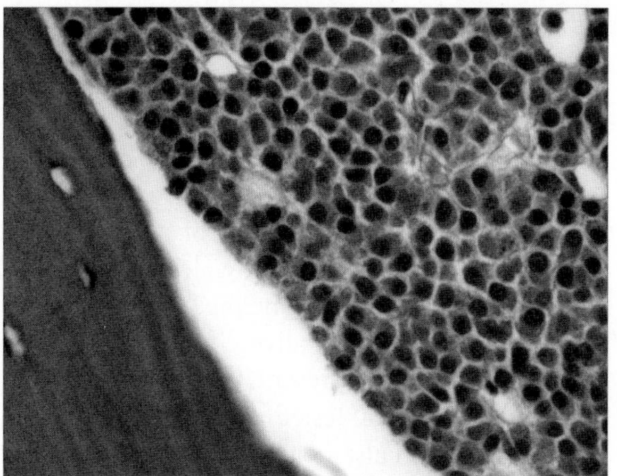

Reproduced, with permission, from USMLERx.com.

(A) Abundant mitochondria
(B) Abundant rough endoplasmic reticulum
(C) Abundant secondary lysosomes
(D) Abundant smooth endoplasmic reticulum
(E) Abundant Nissl bodies

ANSWERS

1. **The correct answer is C.** It is important to understand that the question is asking for the sensitivity, the proportion of people who have the disease and test positive out of all the people who have the disease. It is calculated by TP / (TP + FN), where TP means true-positive and FN means false-negative. The true-positives in the vignette represent those with the cancer who correctly tested positive with this new test (n = 60). False-negatives are those with the cancer who tested negative with the new test (n = 40); thus, 60 / (60 + 40) = 60%. Screening tests theoretically would aim to identify all those with the disease, and therefore high sensitivities are desired. In this case 60% represents a low number, and the ca-1panc blood test would not be a good screening test for the cancer.

   Answer A is incorrect. The 10.0% figure represents the prevalence of the disease, calculated as total cancer/total people (100/1,000).

   Answer B is incorrect. The 37.5% figure is the positive predictive value, or the probability that someone with a positive test (ca-1panc) truly does have the cancer. The predictive values vary with how prevalent a disease is in the population. It is calculated as TP / (TP + FP) (where TP means true-positive and FP means false-positive) or 60 / (60 + 100) = 37.5%.

   Answer D is incorrect. The 88.8% figure represents the specificity of the blood test, which measures the proportion of the people who don't have the disease and test negative out of all the people who don't have the disease. It is important to correctly detect those without the disease in order to prevent them from undergoing unnecessary treatment or studies that could be painful or harmful to the patient. It is calculated as TN / (TN + FP) (where TN means true-negative and FP means false-positive), or 800 / (800 + 100) = 88.8%.

   Answer E is incorrect. The 90.0% figure simply represents the percentage of people without the cancer, 900/1000.

   Answer F is incorrect. The 95.2% figure is the negative predictive value, or the probability that the person with a negative test really does not have the cancer. It is calculated as TN / (TN + FN) (where TN means true-negative and FN means false-negative), or 800 / (800 + 40) = 95.2%.

2. **The correct answer is A.** Misoprostol is a prostaglandin E_1 analog. One of its mechanisms of action consists of increased production and secretion of gastric mucous barrier. This characteristic makes the drug useful in concomitant chronic NSAID use to decrease the incidence of NSAID-induced peptic ulcers. Misoprostol, however, is contraindicated in women of childbearing potential due to its abortifacient properties. It can also be used for medical termination of pregnancy of <49 days (in conjunction with mifepristone) and off-label for ripening and labor induction. Another common adverse effect of misoprostol is diarrhea.

   Answer B is incorrect. Intrauterine growth restriction (IUGR) can result from poor maternal nutrition, hypertension, infections, congenital anomalies, and smoking. Misoprostol has not been associated with IUGR.

   Answer C is incorrect. The chance of neural tube defects is increased in women who do not take prenatal folate supplements. Misoprostol has not been associated with neural tube defects.

   Answer D is incorrect. Placenta previa results from abnormal placental implantation where placenta covers the cervical os. Placenta previa is a common cause of painless third-trimester bleeding. Some of the risk factors for this phenomenon are prior cesarean section, multiparity, advanced maternal age, multiple gestations, and prior placenta previa. Misoprostol does not appear to increase the risk of placenta previa.

   Answer E is incorrect. Misoprostol keeps the ductus arteriosus open, not closed. NSAIDs are commonly used for closure of patent ductus arteriosus.

3. **The correct answer is A.** The patient likely has an abnormal atrial re-entrant tract that bypasses the atrioventricular (AV) node and goes straight from the atrium to the ventricle. That is why the AV nodal block medication would not work and instead provided an unopposed pathway for the abnormal tract. The syndrome resulting from the presence of an accessory tract is Wolff-Parkinson-White.

   Answer B is incorrect. An abnormal tract through the AV node likely would be ablated if the patient were given an antiarrhythmic that blocked the AV node.

   Answer C is incorrect. Tetralogy of Fallot usually does not lead to arrhythmias.

   Answer D is incorrect. Hypertrophic cardiomyopathy indeed may lead to ventricular fibrillation and sudden death, but a more common presentation would be a previously healthy adolescent who suddenly collapses under extreme exertion (eg, during a sports game).

   Answer E is incorrect. Ventricular tachycardia is not a congenital heart defect. Rather, it is usually the result of other heart disorders, such as acute myocardial infarction (MI), scar from an old infarct, long-QT syndrome, or electrolyte abnormalities.

4. **The correct answer is D.** This patient's presentation is consistent with multiple myeloma. The primary pathophysiology is a neoplastic proliferation of mature plasma cells producing abnormal immunoglobulins, most commonly IgG. Characteristic features of multiple myeloma include destructive "punched-out" bone lesions (as demonstrated on the radiograph), hypercalcemia (causing the lethargy, weakness, and confusion in this case), and renal insufficiency (often causing polyuria and nocturia). Excess immunoglobulins are responsible for the increased total protein levels. Pathologic fractures also are seen commonly. Serum protein electrophoresis would demonstrate a monoclonal M spike, as opposed to a normal polyclonal distribution.

   Answer A is incorrect. The classic findings in osteoporosis are a significant loss of bone mass and vertebral fractures. Unlike multiple myeloma, osteoporosis does not produce "punched-out" lesions on radiographs. In addition, osteoporosis does not cause mental status changes, increased total protein levels, or polyuria. Diagnostic testing may include measurement of bone mineral density by dual-energy x-ray absorptiometry. In this technique the energy absorbed by dual x-ray beams is used estimate the surface area and density of mineralized tissue.

   Answer B is incorrect. Parathyroid adenoma is the most common cause of primary hyperparathyroidism, a disorder characterized by hypercalcemia, kidney stones, and bone lesions, all of which result from increased circulating parathyroid hormone (PTH) levels. However, the serum protein level typically is normal. Treatment includes surgical removal of the adenoma and biopsy of the remaining parathyroid glands to rule out parathyroid hyperplasia.

   Answer C is incorrect. Diabetes mellitus (DM) can present with several of the symptoms seen in multiple myeloma, including mental status changes, polyuria, and nocturia. However, the lytic skull lesions, hypercalcemia, and increased total protein level make multiple myeloma a far more likely diagnosis.

   Answer E is incorrect. Ankylosing spondylitis is a degenerative inflammation of the spine and sacroiliac joints, resulting in a stiff spine. Radiographs typically show forward curvature of the spine and fusion of the lumbar vertebrae, often referred to as a "bamboo spine." Though it is highly associated with HLA-B27 haploptype, this finding is not diagnostic. Patients with HLA-B27 haplotypes are more likely to have aortic regurgitation secondary to aortitis, or may develop blindness secondary to uveitis.

   Answer F is incorrect. Features of prostate cancer include a palpable mass on digital rectal examination, dysuria, nocturia, and, if metastasis has occurred, back pain due to spinal lesions. Many of these symptoms overlap with those seen in multiple myeloma; however, the increased total serum protein level and hypercalcemia seen in this patient are more typical of multiple myeloma. Screening for prostate cancer includes digital rectal examination and testing for prostate-specific antigen (PSA) yearly after age 50 years. PSA is sensitive but not specific for prostate cancer. For example, PSA between 4-10 ng/mL may be indicative of either early cancer or benign prostatic hyperplasia (BPH). In this patient, PSA was in the normal range, which means <4 ng/mL.

5. **The correct answer is D.** This patient suffers from McArdle disease, a glycogen storage disorder in which glycogen phosphorylase is deficient in muscle. The enzyme is responsible for liberating individual units of glucose-1-phosphate from branches of a glycogen molecule. Onset of the disease typically occurs in adolescence or early adulthood and is characterized by muscle cramping, rapid fatigue, and poor endurance during exertion. Severe myoglobinuria is also observed in some patients.

   Answer A is incorrect. α-1,6-Glucosidase is the enzyme responsible for the debranching of glycogen. It is implicated in Cori disease, which is a mild form of Von Gierke disease with normal blood lactate levels. It is not implicated in McArdle disease as it wouldn't cause the muscle cramping.

   Answer B is incorrect. Homocystinuria is an inborn error of metabolism caused by a defect in cystathionine synthase, the enzyme that converts homocysteine to cystathionine. In addition to Marfan-like features, these patients are at increased risk for a variety of cardiovascular derangements due to increased atherosclerosis, including premature vascular disease and early death.

   Answer C is incorrect. Glucose-6-phosphatase is the enzyme responsible for converting glucose-6-phosphate to glucose. It is a component of gluconeogenesis. A deficiency of this enzyme causes Von Gierke disease, characterized by a severe fasting hypoglycemia, increased glycogen in the liver, hepatomegaly, and increased blood lactate. These findings are inconsistent with the symptoms observed in this patient.

   Answer E is incorrect. Lysosomal α-1,4-glucosidase is the defective enzyme in Pompe disease, another glycogen storage disorder. The findings in Pompe disease typically manifest in early childhood and include respiratory difficulties (due to diaphragmatic weakness), cardiomegaly, and progressive loss of muscle tone leading to early death.

6. **The correct answer is B.** Osteoporosis is a metabolic bone disease characterized by decreased bone mass. It can be caused by impaired synthesis or increased resorption of bone matrix protein. It is clinically associated with a postmenopausal state, physical inactivity, hypercortisolism, hyperthyroidism, and calcium deficiency. This patient has several risks factors for osteoporosis: She is postmenopausal and has a family history of osteoporosis, as evidenced by her mother, who fell at age 58 and needed hip replacement surgery. The pulmonary embolism was most likely provoked by the surgery. Her history of severe rheumatoid arthritis predisposes her to hypercortisolism as a result of treatment with corticosteroids. Her lower back pain suggests the possibility of a vertebral compression fracture. Lab tests in osteoporosis reveal normal serum calcium, normal serum phosphorus, and normal or decreased alkaline phosphatase levels. Treatments for osteoporosis include weight-bearing exercise, calcium supplementation, hormone replacement therapy, and bisphosphonates.

   Answer A is incorrect. These findings describe hypoparathyroidism, which may occur congenitally (DiGeorge syndrome) or after thyroidectomy. Symptoms are related to hypocalcemia: tetany, depression, dementia, and seizures. ECG will show a prolonged QT interval, which predisposes the patient to developing torsades de pointes. This patient does not have symptoms of hypocalcemia.

   Answer C is incorrect. These lab values are seen in Paget disease, also known as osteitis deformans. This is a disease of abnormal bone architecture due to haphazard osteoblastic and osteoclastic activity. Symptoms include bony pain, increased risk for bony fractures, hearing loss, and headaches. Patients are at increased risk for osteosarcoma as well as high-output cardiac failure from multiple arteriovenous shunts. This patient does not have symptoms of Paget disease.

Answer D is incorrect. These findings describe hyperparathyroidism. PTH stimulates bone resorption, calcium reabsorption, and phosphorus excretion. Symptoms are related to hypercalcemia: osteopenia, kidney stones, polyuria, constipation, abdominal pain, depression, and psychosis. ECG will show a shortened QT interval. This patient does not have symptoms of hypercalcemia.

7. **The correct answer is D.** The causative agent in this scenario, based on the Gram stain, is *Neisseria meningitidis*. Waterhouse-Friderichsen syndrome is a possible complication of meningococcemia. In this disorder, bilateral hemorrhage into the adrenal gland causes adrenal insufficiency. This results in hypotension, tachycardia, a rapidly enlarging petechial skin lesion, disseminated intravascular coagulation, and coma.

Answer A is incorrect. Hemolytic-uremic syndrome (HUS) is characterized by acute renal failure and thrombocytopenia with hemolytic anemia. HUS can be a complication of infection caused by *E coli* O157:H7 and not *Neisseria meningitidis*.

Answer B is incorrect. Rheumatic fever is characterized by fever, migratory polyarthritis, and carditis. It may follow group A streptococcal pharyngitis.

Answer C is incorrect. Fever, a new murmur, Janeway lesions, and nail-bed hemorrhages are all signs of bacterial endocarditis. Acute endocarditis is caused by *Staphylococcus aureus* and subacute infection can be caused by *Streptococcus viridans*.

Answer E is incorrect. Guillain-Barré syndrome is characterized by rapidly progressing ascending paralysis. It is thought to follow a variety of infectious diseases, such as cytomegalovirus, Epstein-Barr virus, HIV, and gastroenteritis caused by *Campylobacter jejuni*.

8. **The correct answer is E.** PGI_2 inhibits platelet aggregation and therefore is an antithrombotic agent. On the other hand, TxA_2 increases platelet aggregation and is a prothrombotic agent. COX-2 inhibitors selectively decrease PGI_2, leaving the action of TxA_2 unopposed. This could well result in increased cerebrovascular and cardiovascular events due to the tonic, unopposed prothrombotic action of TxA_2. This patient is most likely suffering from an acute thrombus in his coronary artery causing a MI.

Answer A is incorrect. COX-2 inhibitors do not increase PGI_2. They are thought to spare the gastric mucosa because they selectively block the synthesis of other prostaglandins, not because they increase the production of PGI_2.

Answer B is incorrect. COX-2 inhibitors do not increase TxA_2. COX-2 inhibitors in general do not increase PGI_2 and TxA_2, which are downstream products.

Answer C is incorrect. COX-2 inhibitors and aspirin do not have the same actions.

Answer D is incorrect. COX-2 inhibitors do decrease PGI_2, but aspirin does not increase PGI_2 and TxA_2. Aspirin is a nonselective COX inhibitor that decreases both PGI_2 and TxA_2.

9. **The correct answer is A.** This patient's history and presentation are consistent with anemia of chronic disease (ACD) in the setting of systemic lupus erythematosus (SLE). Hepcidin, an acute-phase reactant that is elevated in SLE, impairs the transfer of iron from macrophages to erythroid precursors. Hence ACD presents with a low serum iron level, low total iron-binding capacity, an elevated ferritin level, and normochromic/normocytic RBCs. ACD resolves if the underlying condition is corrected, but in the absence of a successful primary treatment, erythropoietin can be effective in treating the anemia.

Answer B is incorrect. Iron therapy is not indicated in the treatment of ACD. In ACD the problem is iron utilization, not iron deficiency.

Answer C is incorrect. Folate supplementation is appropriate therapy in macrocytic anemia caused by folate deficiency.

Answer D is incorrect. Parenteral vitamin B_{12} is appropriate for treating pernicious anemia. In pernicious anemia, because of a lack of intrinsic factor, vitamin B_{12} is not absorbed. Macrocytic RBCs are seen on blood smear.

Answer E is incorrect. Phlebotomy is appropriate for treating significant iron overload, as seen in patients with chronic transfusion therapy and hemochromatosis.

10. **The correct answer is B.** Hereditary retinoblastoma survivors are at increased risk for soft tissue sarcomas, osteosarcomas, melanomas, and several types of brain cancer. Osteosarcoma, the most common malignant primary bone tumor, most frequently originates in the distal femur, proximal tibia, or proximal humerus. Other risk factors for osteosarcoma include Paget disease of bone, bone infarcts, and radiation. Codman triangle or sunburst pattern is seen on x-ray.

Answer A is incorrect. Esophageal adenocarcinoma is a tumor of glandular epithelium and is not associated with hereditary retinoblastoma. Risk factors for esophageal cancer include **ABCDEFG**: **A**lcohol/**A**chalasia, **B**arrett Esophagus, **C**igarettes, **D**iverticuli, **E**sophageal web (Plummer-Vinson)/ Esophagitis, and **F**amilial and **G**astroesophageal reflux disease.

Answer C is incorrect. Medullary carcinoma of the thyroid is a tumor of thyroid solid glandular epithelium and is not associated with hereditary retinoblastoma. It forms from parafollicular C cells, and produces calcitonin and sheets of cells in an amyloid stroma. It is associated with MEN 2A and 2B.

Answer D is incorrect. Renal cell carcinoma (RCC) is a tumor of renal solid glandular epithelium and is not associated with hereditary retinoblastoma. RCC manifests with hematuria, a palpable mass, and flank pain. It is associated with von Hippel-Lindau syndrome.

Answer E is incorrect. A serous cystadenoma of the ovary is a benign tumor of columnar epithelium and is not associated with hereditary retinoblastoma. It occurs in 20% of ovarian tumors and is frequently bilateral and lined with fallopian-tube-like epithelium. Risk factors include the **BRCA1** gene and hereditary nonpolyposis colorectal cancer.

Answer F is incorrect. Squamous cell carcinoma of the lung is a tumor of squamous surface epithelium and is not associated with hereditary retinoblastoma. Its characteristics include a hilar mass arising from the bronchus, cavitation, and PTH-related protein. Histologically, keratin "pearls" and intercellular bridges are seen. A major risk factor is smoking.

Answer G is incorrect. Transitional cell carcinoma is a tumor of transitional surface epithelium in the bladder and is not associated with hereditary retinoblastoma. Painless hematuria is suggestive of this diagnosis. It is associated with problems of your "**Pee SAC**": **P**henacetin, **S**moking, **A**niline dyes, and **C**yclophosphamide.

11. **The correct answer is C.** Afferent pain fibers of the heart enter the posterior horn of the spinal cord at the same level as the brachial plexus, leading to pain perceived as being located in the neck and shoulder region.

Answer A is incorrect. Lymphatic drainage does occur in the left upper quadrant, but it plays no role in the model of referred myocardial pain.

Answer B is incorrect. Sensory neurons have their origin in the dorsal root ganglion and send their axons to the posterior horn of the spinal cord instead of the anterior horn, where efferent neurons arise.

Answer D is incorrect. The heart and the neck and shoulder region do not share similar parasympathetic innervation patterns.

Answer E is incorrect. The heart and the neck and shoulder region do not share similar sympathetic innervation patterns.

12. **The correct answer is A.** Patients with AIDS are susceptible to a variety of infections that are unusual in the immunocompetent population. Among diseases that cause fever and headache in these patients are *Cryptococcus*, toxoplasmosis, and central nervous system (CDS) lymphoma. An encapsulated yeast that stains with India ink is a pathognomonic description of *Cryptococcus neoformans*, which is a yeast found in pigeon droppings. Infection occurs when patients inhale fungus particles, which can lead to pneumonia. Initial treatment of *C neoformans* is intravenous (IV) amphotericin B, followed by fluconazole once the patient's condition is stable. Amphotericin toxicity can cause fever and chills, hypotension, nephrotoxicity, and arrhythmias. The arrhythmias are due to QT prolongation, which is exacerbated by changes in potassium and magnesium levels.

    Answer B is incorrect. Bone marrow suppression is seen with a number of drugs, including flucytosine.

    Answer C is incorrect. Flushing can be caused by caspofungin, an antifungal medication used to treat aspergillosis infection. Caspofungin inhibits synthesis of the β(1,3)-D-glucan component of the fungal cell wall. Other adverse effects include gastrointestinal (GI) upset.

    Answer D is incorrect. Gynecomastia is an adverse effect of fluconazole treatment. The -azole antifungals inhibit ergosterol synthesis. They are used to treat systemic mycoses but are less effective than amphotericin B and are adjunct therapies in acute cases. In patients with AIDS, the initial amphotericin course should be followed by maintenance fluconazole therapy daily for life. Other adverse effects include liver dysfunction and fever.

    Answer E is incorrect. Nausea and vomiting (along with diarrhea and bone marrow suppression) are toxicities associated with flucytosine, which is used to treat systemic fungal infections. It is often used in conjunction with amphotericin B to treat cryptococcal meningitis, but is not first-line treatment as a single agent. Flucytosine inhibits DNA synthesis because it is converted to fluorouracil in vivo.

13. **The correct answer is C.** Given the patient's body habitus and glucose level, a diagnosis of diabetes is extremely likely. The patient is presenting after recent surgery with symptoms consistent with lactic acidosis. His low bicarbonate is concerning for an acidotic state. Calculating the anion gap ($Na - Cl - HCO_3^- =$ anion gap) gives a result of 18. The physiologic range of the anion gap in healthy adults is 8-12 mEq/L. High-anion-gap metabolic acidosis can be caused by multiple conditions and can be remembered by the mnemonic **MUDPILES**: **M**ethanol, **U**remia, **D**iabetic ketoacidosis, **P**araldehyde, **I**nfection or isoniazid, **L**actic acidosis, **E**thylene glycol, and **S**alicylates. Metformin is a biguanide that suppresses hepatic glucose production, decreases intestinal absorption of glucose, and improves insulin sensitivity. It is known to increase the risk of lactic acidosis, particularly in those with renal impairment (the patient in this case has an elevated creatinine of 1.6 mg/dL), as well as in the postoperative period if it is stopped for an extended period.

    Answer A is incorrect. Glyburide is a sulfonylurea that increases pancreatic secretion of insulin by depolarizing the β-cell membranes. Its major adverse effect is hypoglycemia, which could present as loss of consciousness, seizure, or altered mental status. However, the patient's lab values show that he is actually **hyper**glycemic, making glyburide less likely.

    Answer B is incorrect. Insulin as a pharmacologic preparation is not administered orally, but rather is subcutaneously injected. It binds the insulin receptor to increase hepatic glycogen production from glucose and promote protein synthesis in muscle. A major adverse effect of insulin treatment is hypoglycemia, weight gain, and injection-site lipodystrophy, but it is not associated with lactic acidosis.

Answer D is incorrect. Orlistat alters fat metabolism by decreasing pancreatic lipase activity. It is often used for long-term weight management, and causes GI adverse effects, such as loose and fatty stools (steatorrhea), diminished absorption of vitamins A, D, K, and E, and headache. It has not been associated with lactic acidosis.

Answer E is incorrect. Rosiglitazone is a thiazolidinedione that increases tissue sensitivity/target cell response to insulin. A major adverse effect of this medication is weight gain and edema, and it has also recently been associated with increased cardiovascular risks. However, it is not known to cause lactic acidosis.

14. **The correct answer is C.** Lactation is maintained by prolactin secretion from the anterior pituitary. Prolactin prevents ovulation by inhibiting the secretion of gonadotropin-releasing hormone (GnRH) from the hypothalamus. This decrease in GnRH leads to decreased secretion of luteinizing hormone (LH) and follicle-stimulating hormone (FSH) from the anterior pituitary gland, which prevent ovulation. This woman would likely have a better chance of becoming pregnant if she were to stop breastfeeding her son.

Answer A is incorrect. Prolactin does not directly inhibit the secretion of estrogen from the ovaries. There is a decrease in estrogen secretion due to decreased FSH levels, which is due to prolactin's direct inhibition of GnRH secretion from the hypothalamus.

Answer B is incorrect. Prolactin does not directly inhibit the secretion of FSH from the anterior pituitary gland. There is a secondary decrease in FSH secretion due to a decrease in GnRH release from the hypothalamus.

Answer D is incorrect. Prolactin does not directly inhibit the secretion of LH from the anterior pituitary gland. There is a secondary decrease in LH secretion due to a decrease in GnRH release from the hypothalamus.

Answer E is incorrect. Prolactin does not affect the secretion of progesterone from the corpus luteum. It does, however, prevent ovulation, thus preventing the formation of the corpus luteum.

15. **The correct answer is D.** This child has normal facies and is suffering from an isolated cleft palate. This orofacial defect makes it difficult to create the suction needed for proper feeding. It results in choking and coughing, as well as aspiration and poor weight gain in affected children. It is the result of the failure of the fusion of the lateral palatine processes, the medial palatine processes, and/or the nasal septum. Surgical correction is usually attempted between 9 and 12 months of age.

Answer A is incorrect. The first and second branchial arches do not fuse.

Answer B is incorrect. Failure of the maxillary processes to fuse results in cleft lip. Cleft lip and cleft palate often occur together.

Answer C is incorrect. Failure of the medial nasal processes to fuse results in cleft lip.

Answer E is incorrect. The second and third branchial arches do not fuse.

16. **The correct answer is B.** Desmopressin is 1-deamino-8-D-arginine vasopressin (dDAVP), an analog of ADH. This woman has central diabetes insipidus caused by trauma to the posterior pituitary. This inhibits secretion of ADH. Of the options given, repleting her ADH is the most appropriate.

Answer A is incorrect. Demeclocycline is used to treat the syndrome of inappropriate ADH secretion. This compound acts to inhibit ADH action and would exacerbate her condition.

Answer C is incorrect. Furosemide is a loop diuretic and is likely to exacerbate her condition.

Answer D is incorrect. Insulin is an inappropriate treatment. Central diabetes insipidus shares only the symptoms of polydipsia and polyuria with DM. The treatments and causes are completely different.

Answer E is incorrect. Mannitol is an osmotic diuretic that would exacerbate her condition.

17. **The correct answer is A.** Beta waves are seen on EEG when the patient is awake and actively concentrating. Alpha waves are seen on EEG when the patient is awake and relaxed with eyes closed.

Answer B is incorrect. Stage 1 sleep is the transition from the awake state to sleep and is characterized by theta waves in the range of 4-7 cycles per second on EEG. Stage 1 accounts for 5% of total sleep.

Answer C is incorrect. Stage 2 sleep, known as true physiologic sleep, is defined by sleep spindles and K-complexes on EEG. Stage 2 sleep accounts for 45% of total sleep.

Answer D is incorrect. Stage 3, or deep sleep, is characterized by delta waves on EEG. Delta waves are slow waves that are <3 Hz. Stage 3 accounts for 12% of total sleep.

Answer E is incorrect. Stage 4 sleep is identical to stage 3 sleep, and they are now characterized together as stage N3. Stage 4 sleep accounts for 13% of total sleep.

18. **The correct answer is B.** The image shows nodular collections of lymphoma cells in a lymph node consistent with follicular lymphoma (also known as small-cleaved-cell lymphoma). Follicular lymphoma is one of the non-Hodgkin lymphomas. This type of lymphoma is characterized by numerous irregularly sized follicles; the neoplastic cells appear similar to normal germinal center B lymphocytes. The neoplastic cells express *bcl-2*; normal cells do not. *Bcl-2*, an antiapoptotic gene, is overexpressed due to a translocation between the IgH locus on chromosome 14 and the *bcl-2* locus on chromosome 18. When you think of follicular lymphoma, you should think B lymphocytes, *bcl-2*, and t(14;18). It typically occurs in middle-aged adults, has an indolent course, and is incurable. Patients with small-cleaved-cell lymphoma often present with complaints of waxing and waning painless lymphadenopathy.

Answer A is incorrect. *c-myc* and t(8;14) are involved in Burkitt lymphoma. The t(8;14) translocation juxtaposes the *c-myc* oncogene locus and the IgH locus. On histopathology, you would expect to see a "starry sky" pattern with benign macrophages containing clear cytoplasm distributed throughout a dense field of intermediate-sized neoplastic lymphoid cells.

Answer C is incorrect. *Erb* B2 is an oncogene present in some breast cancers. The t(11;14) translocation is involved in mantle cell lymphomas. Tumor cells of mantle cell lymphoma are similar to the normal mantle zone B lymphocytes, and neoplastic cells surround germinal centers, which may be small and atrophic. *Erb* B2 is not related to the t(11;14) translocation.

Answer D is incorrect. *p53* is not an oncogene, but rather a tumor suppressor gene that is downregulated in many cancers. It is not paired with t(8:14).

Answer E is incorrect. *ras* is the oncogene implicated in many colon cancers. The t(11;14) translocation juxtaposes the cyclin D_1 and IgH loci, and is involved in mantle cell lymphoma. Tumor cells of mantle cell lymphoma are similar to the normal mantle zone B lymphocytes and neoplastic cells surround germinal centers, which may be small and atrophic. *ras* is not related to the t(11;14) translocation.

19. **The correct answer is A.** This patient has features of Turner syndrome (XO), a chromosomal disorder occurring in 1:3000 births that is associated with short stature, primary amenorrhea, and webbing of the neck. Laboratory values are consistent with the premature ovarian failure of Turner syndrome. Coarctation of the aorta is a narrowing of the aorta found in 3-10% of people with Turner syndrome. The finding of upper extremity blood pressure greater than lower extremity blood pressure would suggest that this patient has coarctation of the aorta. The narrowing of the aorta is usually distal to the three great vessels coming off the aortic arch (brachiocephalic trunk, left common carotid, and left subclavian), increasing the pressure above this narrowing and obstructing flow to the vessels distal to the narrowing. Coarctation in Turner syndrome is usually the infantile (preductal) type, with the

narrowing located between the subclavian artery and the ductus arteriosus.

Answer B is incorrect. Carotid bruits may be heard when carotid arteries are narrowed and obstructed due to atherosclerosis. This condition is not associated with Turner syndrome.

Answer C is incorrect. Aortic coarctation may produce a systolic murmur, but a late systolic murmur with a mid-systolic click is characteristic of mitral valve prolapse. This condition, while associated with other genetic disorders such as Marfan syndrome, is not associated with Turner syndrome.

Answer D is incorrect. Mediastinal widening on x-ray of the chest can be evidence of an aortic dissection, caused by a longitudinal tear within the aortic wall. This life-threatening condition is associated with genetically acquired connective tissue disorders such as Marfan syndrome, but is not associated with Turner syndrome.

Answer E is incorrect. Slowly rising and weak carotid pulses are associated with aortic stenosis. A subset of patients with Turner syndrome can have aortic valve disease, including a bicuspid valve that can calcify over time. However, in a young patient with Turner syndrome aortic coarctation is more likely.

20. **The correct answer is B.** This patient has Churg-Strauss syndrome (also known as allergic granulomatosis and angiitis), which is one of a trio of diseases (Wegener granulomatosis and microscopic polyangiitis being the others) that are commonly referred to as the ANCA (antineutrophil cytoplasmic antibody)-associated vasculitides (ie, diseases causing inflammation of blood or lymphatic vessels). Fifty to seventy percent of patients with Churg-Strauss syndrome have elevated levels of ANCA, usually the perinuclear pattern of staining type (P-ANCA). Pulmonary vasculature involvement is common and patients often have preexisting asthma and allergic rhinitis. They also present with markedly elevated eosinophil counts and mononeuritis multiplex (simultaneous deficits of two or several peripheral nerves in different areas of the body). Other symptoms include uveitis, conductive hearing loss, and muscle/joint pain. An eosinophilic gastroenteritis may precede the onset of the other symptoms.

Answer A is incorrect. Autoantibodies to acetylcholine receptors are not particularly associated with Churg-Strauss syndrome. Myasthenia gravis is characterized by an autoimmune attack on the acetylcholine receptors of the neuromuscular junction between motor neurons and skeletal muscle fibers.

Answer C is incorrect. Autoantibodies to oligodendrocytes are not particularly associated with Churg-Strauss syndrome. There is evidence suggesting that multiple sclerosis may be partially caused by autoimmune antibody attack on CNS myelin-secreting oligodendrocytes.

Answer D is incorrect. Autoantibodies to RBCs, which may be found in certain cases of immune hemolytic anemia, are not particularly associated with Churg-Strauss syndrome.

Answer E is incorrect. Autoantibodies to thyroid-stimulating hormone (TSH) receptors are not particularly associated with Churg-Strauss syndrome. Graves disease is a disorder resulting from IgG-type autoantibodies to the TSH receptor.

21. **The correct answer is B.** The whorled pattern of cell growth surrounding lamellated areas of dystrophic calcification represents psammoma bodies. This pathologic finding is most commonly seen in meningiomas, papillary thyroid tumors, and certain ovarian tumors. Given this patient's complaints of a seizure, headache, and visual-field deficit, meningioma is the most likely answer.

Answer A is incorrect. Hemangiomas are more common in children and are often located in the cerebellum. The cells tend to be "foamy," and the tumors display a high degree of vascularity. Psammoma bodies would not be expected in tumors of this type.

Answer C is incorrect. Pathology specimens of oligodendrogliomas reveal "fried egg" cells, not psammoma bodies. These fried egg cells have round nuclei amidst a halo of clear cytoplasm. Oligodendrogliomas are benign brain tumors found in the cerebral hemispheres. They tend to have areas of calcification that can be detected radiographically.

Answer D is incorrect. While psammoma bodies can be found in papillary thyroid carcinoma, this diagnosis does not fit with the patient's history and clinical presentation. Papillary thyroid carcinoma is the most common cancer of the thyroid. It is associated with psammoma bodies and "orphan Annie" nuclei. Compared to other cancers of the thyroid, this variant has the best prognosis.

Answer E is incorrect. Psammoma bodies are not associated with pituitary adenomas. Furthermore, the visual field deficit that would result from a pituitary adenoma is bilateral hemianopsia, due to pressure on the optic chiasm. This patient only had loss of her temporal visual field on the right. Additionally, some evidence of hypopituitarism or other endocrine abnormality would be likely by the time the adenoma was large enough to cause seizures.

22. **The correct answer is E.** Patients with significant renal disease are at particularly high risk for developing skeletal complications, generally known as renal osteodystrophy. Renal failure produces numerous downstream consequences that affect bone health, including increased phosphate retention (resulting in calcium phosphate deposition leading to hypocalcemia and secondary hyperparathyroidism), decreased renal conversion of 25-hydroxcholecalciferol to 1,25-dihydroxycholecalciferol (resulting in decreased intestinal calcium absorption and decreased suppression of parathyroid hormone production), and chronic metabolic acidosis (resulting in increased bone reabsorption). The resulting secondary hyperparathyroidism increases osteoclast activity and the reabsorption of bone.

    Answer A is incorrect. Patients with renal failure have decreased levels of 1,25-dihydroxycholecalciferol because of decreased renal conversion of 25-hydroxycholecalciferol to 1,25-dihydroxycholecalciferol. 1,25-Dihydroxycholecalciferol excess does not result in osteoporosis.

    Answer B is incorrect. Patients with renal failure have a chronic metabolic acidosis due to decreased renal handling of acid anions. Metabolic alkalosis does not result in osteoporosis.

    Answer C is incorrect. Patients with renal failure have hypocalcemia as a result of decreased intestinal absorption of calcium and increased calcium phosphate deposition in tissues. Hypercalcemia is not associated with renal failure and does not result in osteoporosis.

    Answer D is incorrect. Patients with renal failure have hyperphosphatemia due to decreased renal excretion of phosphorous. Hypophosphatemia does not result in osteoporosis.

23. **The correct answer is D.** This patient most likely suffers from RCC. RCC is characterized by the triad of flank pain, hematuria, and abdominal mass, although <10% of patients have all three symptoms. It occurs most commonly in men and is associated with risk factors such as obesity, hypertension, smoking, and environmental toxin exposure (this patient was a worker in a steel plant). Importantly, the major distinguishing feature of RCC is its association with paraneoplastic syndromes due to the ectopic production of hormones such as parathyroid hormone-related protein (hypercalcemia, hypophosphatemia), erythropoietin (polycythemia), and ACTH. RCC is also associated with hereditary conditions such as Von Hippel-Lindau (VHL) syndrome. In VHL-related RCC, patients usually present with bilateral tumors. RCC has a relatively poor prognosis because most tumors are asymptomatic until they have undergone metastasis.

    Answer A is incorrect. Adult polycystic kidney disease (APKD) is usually an autosomal dominant genetic disease that causes rapid cystic enlargement of the kidneys, leading to renal failure. It usually manifests with hypertension, pain, and hematuria. Patients with APKD do have occasional palpable masses, but renal masses are usually bilateral.

Answer B is incorrect. Angiomyolipomas are relatively rare, benign vascular tumors that occur in the kidney. Renal angiomyolipomas, however, have a more insidious course of progression than RCC, are more common in women, and do not cause paraneoplastic syndromes. Nevertheless, the triad of flank pain, hematuria, and palpable abdominal mass can also occur with angiomyolipomas.

Answer C is incorrect. Pheochromocytoma is a rare tumor derived of catecholamine-producing chromaffin cells of the adrenal glands. Major clinical findings usually result from the ectopic production of catecholamines, including episodic headache, palpitations, and sweating with severe hypertension. It can also be associated with café-au-lait spots and neurofibromas. These clinical features predominate in the presentation of the pheochromocytoma-affected patient, rather than the triad of flank pain, hematuria, and palpable mass and the electrolyte abnormalities seen in this patient.

Answer E is incorrect. Wilms tumor is a common pediatric malignancy and is not found in adult patients. It can be sporadic or familial. In almost all cases, Wilms tumor is caused by mutations in the *WT1* gene. In familial Wilms tumor the disease can be associated with numerous congenital abnormalities, including single, horseshoe, or ectopic kidney; hypospadias; cryptorchidism; and aniridia.

24. **The correct answer is E.** The patient has a Wilms tumor, a childhood nephroblastoma that can be treated with the MOPP regimen, which includes the plant alkaloid vincristine (Oncovin). Vincristine halts cell division by inhibiting microtubule polymerization, thus preventing formation of the mitotic spindle and causing metaphase arrest. It has the adverse effect of neurotoxicity as manifested by areflexia, peripheral neuritis, muscle weakness, and paralytic ileus. The **MOPP** regimen refers to the chemotherapeutic agents **M**echlorethamine, **O**ncovin, **P**rocarbazine, and **P**rednisone.

Answer A is incorrect. Cardiotoxicity is most often associated with the use of anthracycline antibiotics such as doxorubicin and daunorubicin. It is thought that these medications can cause toxic levels of free radicals to build up in the myocardium, leading to muscle damage, decreased left ventricular ejection fraction, and symptoms of congestive heart failure.

Answer B is incorrect. Hemorrhagic cystitis is an adverse reaction seen with the use of cyclophosphamide, an alkylating agent used to treat solid tumors and lymphoma. It is also used as an immunosuppressant to treat severe rheumatologic disorders.

Answer C is incorrect. Hyperglycemia is a common adverse effect of prednisone and other steroid drugs. Vincristine, however, does not cause hyperglycemia. Prednisone is part of the MOPP regimen. Its mechanism of action is unclear, but is thought to relate to triggering apoptosis.

Answer D is incorrect. Pulmonary fibrosis is seen with several chemotherapeutic agents including busulfan, which is used to treat chronic myelogenous leukemia, and bleomycin, which is used to treat testicular cancer and lymphoma.

25. **The correct answer is D.** This girl has impetigo, most likely caused by *Streptococcus pyogenes*, a gram-positive group A β-hemolytic organism that is bacitracin sensitive. This infection is characterized by an eruption of vesicles on the face. These vesicles later turn into pustules with a characteristic honey-colored crust. A distinctly bullous form of impetigo is caused by *Staphylococcus aureus* infection.

Answer A is incorrect. Endotoxin is a characteristic of gram-negative bacteria and *Listeria*, but not *S pyogenes*, which is the most likely causative organism in this case.

Answer B is incorrect. Sabouraud agar is required to culture fungi, not *S pyogenes*.

Answer C is incorrect. *Streptococcus agalactiae* is a group B β-hemolytic organism that is bacitracin resistant. However, it is not a common cause of impetigo.

Answer E is incorrect. *Mycobacterium, Brucella, Francisella, Listeria, Yersinia, Legionella,* and *Salmonella* are facultative intracellular organisms, but *S pyogenes* is not. None of the other bacteria are common causes of impetigo.

26. **The correct answer is E.** Patients with VHL disease, which is autosomal dominant, have hemangioblastomas, or cavernous hemangiomas of the retina, cerebellum, and medulla. The cerebellar manifestations are suggested by the difficulty keeping his balance, and the retinal hemangioblastoma. Patients with von Hippel-Lindau disease are at increased risk of developing renal cell carcinoma. Only 10% of patients develop the so-called "classic triad" of flank pain, palpable flank mass, and hematuria, but this is the classic presentation of a renal cell carcinoma that many VHL disease patients go on to develop. VHL disease is associated with the deletion of the *VHL* gene on chromosome 3.

Answer A is incorrect. Astrocytomas, CNS tumors that arise in the cranial vault, are not associated with VHL disease, but with tuberous sclerosis. The penetrance of tuberous sclerosis is incomplete, and its symptoms are variable. Among its symptoms is a retinal hamartoma. The funduscopy could be interpreted as a retinal hamartoma, but none of the other characteristics of tuberous sclerosis are present. These would include facial lesions, hypopigmented spots on the skin, and seizures.

Answer B is incorrect. The deletion of the tumor-suppressing *VHL* gene on chromosome 3p, which causes VHL disease, does not affect the appearance of colon cancer. This is more often a sequela of familial adenomatous polyposis. The deletion of the *APC* gene on chromosome 5 results in familial adenomatous polyposis, also an autosomal-dominant disease.

Answer C is incorrect. Depression is a comorbidity of many diseases, and particularly, among the autosomal-dominant disorders, of Huntington disease. But, where VHL disease is concerned, renal cell carcinoma is a better and more specific answer than depression.

Answer D is incorrect. Pheochromocytomas, "the 10% tumor," occur in the medulla of the adrenal glands, and can appear as a consequence of a mutation in the *VHL* gene, the same gene responsible for VHL disease. However, pheochromocytomas are rarer sequelae than renal carcinomas, the more specific answer to the question.

27. **The correct answer is C.** This patient has clinical findings and a biopsy consistent with hereditary hemochromatosis. The image above shows iron deposition in the liver parenchyma. Hereditary hemochromatosis is associated with a defect in a gene that encodes the protein HFE. This gene is near the MHC locus on chromosome 6. As a result of this defect, there is an increase in the efficiency of dietary iron absorption. This, coupled with the inability to excrete iron, leads to an increase in hepatic iron storage. Increased iron storage causes the liver to secrete more ferritin and serum transferrin becomes increasingly saturated with iron. Transferrin saturation is calculated as serum iron/total iron binding capacity (TIBC). TIBC is calculated as 1.4 times the serum transferrin level.

Answer A is incorrect. Serum ferritin is usually increased in hereditary hemochromatosis secondary to increasing iron loads and the inability to excrete iron.

Answer B is incorrect. The iron-binding capacity remains about the same in hereditary hemochromatosis.

Answer D is incorrect. Plasma iron levels increase in hereditary hemochromatosis.

Answer E is incorrect. Serum ferritin is usually increased in hereditary hemochromatosis secondary to increasing iron loads and the inability to excrete iron.

28. **The correct answer is A.** Dietary modification (drastically limiting saturated and trans fats and cholesterol), weight loss, and aerobic exercise are the first-line treatment options for any patient with elevated cholesterol levels, and although these lifestyle modifications should be attempted by this patient, they likely will have

only minimal effect in a patient with familial hypercholesterolemia. Statin medications are 3-hydroxy-3-methylglutaryl coenzyme A reductase inhibitors. By blocking the rate-limiting step in cholesterol synthesis, they can increase hepatic synthesis of LDL receptors, thereby lowering serum LDL levels. High-dose therapy with a statin such as atorvastatin, or combined therapy with one of the fibrate drugs, is first-line treatment for patients with familial hypercholesterolemia. The toxicity of statin medications includes myositis, which is causing this patient's symptoms, and elevated creatinine kinase levels. Rarely, patients can develop rhabdomyolysis with renal failure. Elevated liver enzyme levels also can be observed with statin treatment, although this usually is reversible.

Answer B is incorrect. Bile acid sequestrants such as cholestyramine or colesevelam inhibit reuptake of bile acids in the intestine, reducing total body LDL. Such medications can cause elevated liver enzymes, but are more commonly associated with GI bloating and diarrhea.

Answer C is incorrect. Ezetimibe inhibits cholesterol uptake by the intestinal brush border by blocking specific transporters, with no effect on the absorption of fat-soluble vitamins or minerals. Although adjunctive use with a statin does augment lipid-lowering effects, combined therapy does not reduce cardiovascular events.

Answer D is incorrect. Although niacin (vitamin B_3) can lower LDL, its primary effect is an increase in HDL levels. Niacin can be added to the regimen as a third drug (with a fibrate) or can be used in patients who are refractory to statin treatment. Its use often is limited by tolerability (it causes flushing in the majority of patients), although new formulations offer reduced adverse effects.

Answer E is incorrect. LDL apheresis is a method for selectively removing LDL molecules from the blood using immunoadsorption columns. This process takes at least three hours and is done every one-two weeks. It is very expensive and not readily available.

29. **The correct answer is D.** The therapeutic privilege is a rare case of an appropriate exception to informed consent. The principle is that informing the patient will be detrimental to his or her health. In general a physician should consult another physician not involved in the patient's care, a psychiatrist, and/or an ethics committee when invoking this principle. It does not refer to withholding information a physician believes will make a patient less likely to have a procedure performed.

    Answer A is incorrect. Only a patient can waive his or her own right to informed consent. If a patient is incapacitated such that he or she no longer retains competency, then a proxy (such as the son) may be designated, but this is not the case here.

    Answer B is incorrect. This patient has met the four basic requirements for valid informed consent: mental capacity, disclosure, understanding, and voluntariness. Consent does not have to be given verbally or in writing.

    Answer C is incorrect. Any competent adult can make informed consent.

    Answer E is incorrect. Informed consent is assumed in an emergency situation in which reasonable persons would want treatment. In this case the patient is stable and therefore capable of giving informed consent.

30. **The correct answer is C.** This patient most likely has Addison disease, which is characterized by insufficient production of adrenal hormones including cortisol, androgen, and aldosterone. Its signs and symptoms include hyperpigmentation, low blood pressure, muscle weakness, and salt cravings, among others. The condition is usually treated with oral hydrocortisone. However, sudden discontinuation of hydrocortisone can lead to severe back pain.

    Answer A is incorrect. Dehydroepiandrosterone is an androgen replacement therapy sometimes used to treat Addison disease. Discontinuation of this therapy usually would not result in the signs and symptoms found in this patient.

Answer B is incorrect. Fluconazole is an antifungal agent. Its discontinuation would not result in the signs and symptoms found in this patient.

Answer D is incorrect. Metformin sensitizes the body's response to insulin and is used to treat type 2 diabetes, not Addison disease.

31. **The correct answer is D.** This patient has a potentially reversible case of dementia: normal pressure hydrocephalus (NPH), with the classic triad of incontinence, gait difficulty, and mental decline ("wet, wobbly, and wacky"). Patients with NPH often demonstrate mild bradykinesia and their gait has been described as "magnetic" because their feet seemingly cling to the floor. The score of 26/30 on the Mini-Mental State Examination (MMSE) indicates only that some mild abnormality is present. Regardless, the patient should undergo magnetic resonance imaging to rule out a mass lesion that could cause similar symptoms. The pathophysiology of NPH is not well understood, but it is thought that neurons are stretched secondary to ventricular dilation caused by excessive cerebrospinal fluid production, decreased absorption, or both. It is imperative to identify these patients because timely intervention with a ventriculoperitoneal shunt can reverse the dementia and decline.

    Answer A is incorrect. Alzheimer disease can present with some of the symptoms in this case. However, significant physical impairment tends to occur later in the Alzheimer disease process and would thus correlate with a much lower score on the MMSE. The time course and the relatively rapid progression in symptoms are not consistent with this diagnosis.

    Answer B is incorrect. Hypothyroidism, another potential cause of reversible dementia in the elderly, should be ruled out early in the work-up. This patient's TSH level is normal, indicating euthyroidism.

    Answer C is incorrect. Multi-infarct dementia is the most common cause of cognitive decline with a stepwise drop in function in the setting of prior cerebrovascular disease and stroke. In this case, the decline has been steadily progressive in a patient with no history of vascular disease.

    Answer E is incorrect. Parkinson disease classically presents with bradykinesia, masklike facies, shuffling gait, tremor, and rigidity. This patient has mild bradykinesia and no rigidity or tremor, so this diagnosis is a less likely possibility.

32. **The correct answer is B.** This patient presents to her appointment exhibiting ataxia and paresthesias, signs of vitamin B_6 (pyridoxine) deficiency in a patient taking isoniazid. Pyridoxine is the precursor to the coenzyme pyridoxal phosphate, and isoniazid, which is used to treat tuberculosis (TB), inhibits pyridoxine. Pyridoxine plays a role in neurotransmitter production and the conversion of tryptophan to niacin (vitamin B_3). Patients taking isoniazid without supplemental vitamin B_6 can develop neuropathy as well as symptoms of depression, irritability, confusion, and convulsions. Cheilosis (cracks or sores on the lips), glossitis, and stomatitis can also be seen. Vitamin B_6 is routinely administered to TB patients taking isoniazid; deficiency rarely occurs in well-nourished adults.

    Answer A is incorrect. Ethambutol can be used in combination therapy to treat TB, but it causes optic neuropathy (change in visual acuity or red-green color blindness). Ethambutol is not recommended in children, since visual acuity and changes in color perception are difficult to assess in them.

    Answer C is incorrect. Levofloxacin, a respiratory fluoroquinolone, is used as second-line combination therapy for the treatment of TB. Potential toxicities include tendinitis or tendon rupture in adults, and cartilage damage in children.

    Answer D is incorrect. Pyrazinamide can be used in combination therapy to treat TB, and it causes hepatotoxicity.

    Answer E is incorrect. Rifampin is a first-line therapy used in the treatment of TB, but it does not cause peripheral neuropathy. Adverse effects include GI (nausea, vomiting, and diarrhea), CNS (headache and fever), dermatologic (rash, itching, and flushing), and hematologic (thrombocytopenia and acute hemolytic anemia). Patients should also be informed that rifampin causes red-orange discoloration of body fluids (eg, sweat, saliva, and tears).

33. **The correct answer is E.** This patient most likely has a *Mycobacterium tuberculosis* infection. *M tuberculosis* is an aerobic, gram-positive, acid-fast bacillus, and the Ziehl-Neelsen stain is used to reveal acid-fast bacteria. Characteristics favoring a diagnosis of TB include pulmonary symptoms, immigrant status, night sweats, weight loss, and chest x-ray findings. Primary TB is known to result in Ghon complexes, which show up as calcifications on x-ray imaging. Ghon complexes are a combination of parenchymal lesions and involved hilar and/or mediastinal lymph nodes. The lesions are calcified because of the caseating granuloma formation. Secondary TB presents with cavitary lesions and is seen more in immunocompromised patients. Other pathologies that can present with hilar/mediastinal nodes are lymphoma and sarcoidosis, making the Gram stain important in diagnosis.

    Answer A is incorrect. Congo red is used to visualize amyloid, showing apple-green birefringence in polarized light. It is used to visualize amyloidosis associated with multiple myeloma, TB, rheumatoid arthritis, and chronic conditions.

    Answer B is incorrect. Giemsa stain is used to reveal *Borrelia*, *Plasmodium*, trypanosomes, and *Chlamydia* organisms.

    Answer C is incorrect. India ink is the stain of choice for *Cryptococcus neoformans*. Mucicarmine can also be used to stain the thick polysaccharide capsule red.

    Answer D is incorrect. Periodic acid-Schiff stains glycogen and mucopolysaccharides. It is used to diagnose Whipple disease, caused by *Tropheryma whipplei*.

34. **The correct answer is A.** The patient has symptoms of hypercalcemia in combination with a history of smoking and a “coin” lesion in the lung, very suspicious of a lung tumor that produces parathyroid hormone-related peptide. Squamous cell carcinoma is a centrally located bronchogenic carcinoma.

    Answer B is incorrect. Horner syndrome is characterized by ptosis, miosis, and anhidrosis. It is a complication of lung cancer at the apex, referred to as Pancoast tumor.

    Answer C is incorrect. Chronic silica exposure is associated with increased TB susceptibility. TB usually presents with chronic cough, hemoptysis, fevers, chills, and weight loss. This patient does not demonstrate the classic signs and symptoms of silicosis.

    Answer D is incorrect. Cystic fibrosis causes respiratory, reproductive, and GI symptoms. Although not completely impossible, it would be highly unlikely for a 65-year-old patient to be afflicted with cystic fibrosis.

    Answer E is incorrect. Kartagener syndrome is associated with sinusitis, bronchiectasis, and infertility. Always think of Kartagener syndrome if situs inversus is suspected on physical exam.

    Answer F is incorrect. Ectopic ADH production, as often observed in small cell carcinoma, would cause water retention (oliguria) and fatigue.

    Answer G is incorrect. Solitary parathyroid adenoma can present with hypercalcemia and low phosphorus levels. However, the patient’s smoking history and new findings on chest imaging cannot be ignored.

35. **The correct answer is A.** The image depicts the epithelium that lies above the Peyer patches, found within the ileum. This epithelium superficial to Peyer patches has several microfold cells (known as M cells), specialized cells that function to endocytose and phagocytose particles in the lumen of the gut. Thus, they serve as immune surveillance in the intestines. In adults, B lymphocytes predominate in Peyer patches and secrete IgA, the main

antibody present within the mucosal lining of the gut. IgA is synthesized by plasma cells that reside within the lamina propria. Of note is the fact that several gut pathogens express virulence factors, known as IgA proteases, which cleave and therefore deactivate the dimeric IgA antibodies. *Mycobacterium avium* infection is common in patients with AIDS. Eighty percent to 90% acquire the infection by oral ingestion and subsequent penetration of the bacteria through Peyer patches of the ileum.

Answer B is incorrect. IgD is found only on the surface of B lymphocytes; its function is not known.

Answer C is incorrect. IgE orchestrates the type I hypersensitivity response. Cross-linking of two IgE molecules on the surface of mast cells by antigen results in mast cell degranulation and allergic reaction.

Answer D is incorrect. IgG is the main antibody produced during a secondary immune response and also the most abundant.

Answer E is incorrect. While IgM can be found within the gut lumen, IgA predominates.

36. **The correct answer is E.** Norepinephrine exerts its agonist effect at α_1, α_2, and β_1 receptors. Its vascular effects are due to its action at α (predominantly α_1) receptors, and its cardiac effects are due to its action on β receptors. Labetalol is a nonselective antagonist at α and β receptors, and therefore would prevent the action of norepinephrine at both sites.

    Answer A is incorrect. Atenolol is a β_1-selective antagonist and would only mitigate the cardiac effects of norepinephrine.

    Answer B is incorrect. Doxazosin is a selective α_1-antagonist that is used to treat hypertension and urinary retention in the setting of BPH. It would be effective at blocking norepinephrine's effect on the vasculature, but would not antagonize its action on the heart.

    Answer C is incorrect. Esmolol is a short-acting β_1-selective antagonist, and therefore would only control the cardiac effects of norepinephrine.

    Answer D is incorrect. Isoproterenol is a nonselective agonist at both β_1 and β_2 receptors. It would enhance the cardiac effects of norepinephrine via its actions on β_1 receptors, while its action on α_1 receptors (vasodilation) would antagonize the vasoconstrictive properties that norepinephrine would exert via α_1 receptors.

37. **The correct answer is D.** A feared infectious complication seen in patients with long-standing diabetic ketoacidosis is invasive rhinocerebral mucormycosis. As in this case, this infection leads to persistent sinusitis with inevitable invasion into adjacent neural structures such as the trigeminal nerve and the frontal lobe. *Rhizopus* organisms thrive in serum containing high glucose levels and low pH. Other conditions predisposing patients to this aggressive infection include iron overload/chelator treatment, AIDS, immunosuppression due to prolonged steroid use, and hematologic malignancies. Under the microscope, *Mucor* species appear as irregular, broad, nonseptate hyphae with 90-degree branching. Both *Mucor* and *Rhizopus* species can cause this condition.

    Answer A is incorrect. *Aspergillus* species appear microscopically as 45-degree angle branching, septate hyphae with rare fruiting bodies. Invasive *Aspergillus* infection occurs mainly after prolonged profound immunosuppression (as in patients with AIDS or cancer or in individuals with chronic granulomatous disease) and typically leads to bronchopulmonary aspergillosis with cavitary lesions in the lung.

    Answer B is incorrect. *Cryptococcus* species appear as 5- to 10-µm yeasts with a wide capsular halo. These infections represent an important opportunistic infection in patients with AIDS, causing cryptococcal meningitis. Cryptococcal infections are extremely rare in patients with normal CD4+ T-lymphocyte counts.

    Answer C is incorrect. *Blastomycetes* species appear as broad-based, budding, dimorphic fungi. Blastomycosis is mainly a pulmonary infection, endemic to states east of the Mississippi River and Central America. Infection of the lung leads to polygranulomatous infection with frequent hematogenous dissemination. These fungal species are cultured on Sabouraud agar.

Answer E is incorrect. Candidal species appear microscopically as pseudohyphae with budding yeasts. Candidal infections are more common in patients with poorly controlled diabetes, but they rarely cause invasive rhinocerebral infections as described in this patient. Rather, candidal infection may cause vulvovaginosis, chronic mucocutaneous infections, or disseminated candidiasis in advanced cases.

38. **The correct answer is E.** The disease that is described is Waldenström macroglobulinemia, which is characterized by weakness, weight loss, a monoclonal M spike on serum protein electrophoresis (seen as a large spike in the gamma region), and a hyperviscosity syndrome (manifesting as nosebleeds, headaches, and vision disturbances). Hyperviscosity is caused by the large amount of IgM protein in the blood that is produced by a B-cell neoplasm. These large proteins interfere with microvascular and cellular processes, causing blood vessel damage, which results in headaches due to impaired cranial blood flow and in disturbances in vision due to poor ocular blood flow. Additionally, circulating IgM proteins can bind to clotting factors and inhibit them, causing increased bleeding.

    Answer A is incorrect. Chronic lymphocytic leukemia (CLL) typically presents with lymphadenopathy, hepatosplenomegaly, a warm-antibody autoimmune hemolytic anemia, and smudge cells in the peripheral blood. The hyperviscosity syndrome is not present in CLL.

    Answer B is incorrect. Diabetes presents with nocturia, polyuria, and polydipsia. Blood tests would demonstrate increased glucose. Superficial resemblances between the hyperviscosity syndromes and diabetic retinopathy, and diabetic kidney disease with the renal insufficiency of multiple myeloma, may be misleading. However, bleeding complications due to diabetes alone would be rare.

    Answer C is incorrect. Monoclonal gammopathy of undetermined significance (MGUS) is similar to the condition described in the correct answer in that it, too, has a monoclonal spike. An important difference is that MGUS is asymptomatic as a result of a lower level of protein. Some patients may experience mild polyneuropathy, but they will not have the bone pain, renal failure, and anemia of multiple myeloma or the hyperviscosity of Waldenström macroglobulinemia. Nonetheless, MGUS may be a pre-malignant lesion that can progress to multiple myeloma.

    Answer D is incorrect. Multiple myeloma is similar to the condition described in the correct answer, but it also involves abnormal plasma cells overproducing immunoglobulin, seen as a monoclonal M spike (critical for diagnosis). Multiple myeloma typically presents with a collection of characteristic symptoms, which include lytic bone lesions causing bone pain and hypercalcemia, renal insufficiency and azotemia, increased susceptibility to infection, and anemia. Additionally, one may find Bence Jones protein (immunoglobulin light chains) in the urine and a rouleaux formation of RBCs on peripheral blood smear.

39. **The correct answer is E.** Selection bias is being displayed in this scenario. The physician is selecting his more serious cases for the treatment group (ie, those who are in most need of the benefit). The placebo group contains patients who are healthier, less symptomatic, and more likely to have a better outcome. Therefore, when it comes time for collecting data, the drug's beneficial effect compared to placebo may be blunted.

    Answer A is incorrect. Studies can still be valid if there are differences in group size. There is no evidence that there is a difference in group size in this scenario.

    Answer B is incorrect. Late-look bias occurs when information or results are gathered at an inappropriate time. Late-look bias is not displayed in this scenario.

    Answer C is incorrect. Recall bias occurs when knowledge of the presence of a disorder alters the way a subject remembers his or her history. For example, patients may over- or underestimate their consumption of a certain drug upon learning of its detrimental effect on the body. Recall bias is not displayed in this scenario.

Answer D is incorrect. Sampling bias occurs when those in the trial are not truly representative of the general population. Therefore, the results (both positive and negative) of the study cannot be truly applied to the general population. There is no evidence of sampling bias in this scenario.

40. **The correct answer is B.** Prostate cancer is present in the peripheral zone in 70% of cases. The peripheral zone has a different embryologic derivation than the transition zone, which is the most common site of BPH.

    Answer A is incorrect. The neurovascular bundle is a periprostatic structure. It may be involved in prostate cancer that spreads to adjacent structures beyond the prostate capsule.

    Answer C is incorrect. The periurethral zone is synonymous with the transition zone, which is the most common site for BPH. Periurethral involvement causes voiding problems, and this is a presenting symptom in many patients with periuretheral involvement.

    Answer D is incorrect. The seminal vesicles are organs adjacent to the prostate, but they are not made of prostatic tissue. Invasion of prostate cancer into the seminal vesicles would increase the cancer stage.

    Answer E is incorrect. The transition zone is the most common area for BPH, but not for prostate cancer.

41. **The correct answer is B.** This patient presents with a lobar pneumonia caused by *Staphylococcus aureus*. Cefazolin is a first-generation cephalosporin that has excellent coverage of gram-positive cocci. It does not cover methicillin-resistant *S aureus* or vancomycin-resistant enterococcus. It is commonly used in surgical prophylaxis and is a first-line treatment of *S aureus*. *S aureus* infection is associated with indwelling catheters, respiratory infections, and surgical wound infections as well as with endocarditis, skin infections, and toxic shock syndrome.

    Answer A is incorrect. *Bacteroides fragilis* is an anaerobic bacterium that is found in a variety of infections but is especially common in abdominal infections. It can lead to peritonitis or intraperitoneal abscesses. Treatment of anaerobic infection involves use of metronidazole or clindamycin. Abscesses may require surgical drainage. *B fragilis* is one of the few gram-negative bacteria that do not contain lipid A in its outer cell membrane; thus, it has no endotoxin.

    Answer C is incorrect. *Actinomyces* species can be identified as gram-positive rods with branching filaments. *Actinomyces* infection usually involves the cervical or facial region and is associated with abscesses, sinus tract infections, and fistulas. It is easily confused with other diseases of the head and neck, such as malignancy. Antibiotic treatment of *Actinomyces* species infections is with penicillin G or with tetracyclines in the case of penicillin allergy.

    Answer D is incorrect. *Bacillus anthracis* is a gram-positive, aerobic, spore-forming, rod-shaped bacterium. Infection can be of either the cutaneous or the inhalational form. The cutaneous form is transmitted by contact with spores and is manifested by cutaneous ulceration and eschar formation. Treatment for cutaneous infection is with penicillin, erythromycin, or ciprofloxacin. The inhalational variety, also called woolsorters' disease, presents with nonspecific symptoms of fever and malaise but progresses to respiratory failure. Treatment of the inhalational infection is with IV penicillin, although most patients will die despite treatment.

    Answer E is incorrect. *Pseudomonas aeruginosa* is an oxidase-positive, non-lactose-fermenting, gram-negative, rod-shaped bacterium that causes many different types of infection, including pneumonia, swimmer's ear, urinary tract infection, and hot-tub folliculitis. It is an aerobic gram-negative rod that produces pyocyanin, a blue-green pigment. *P aeruginosa* infection can be treated with many agents, including anti-pseudomonal penicillins, ciprofloxacin, and anti-pseudomonal cephalosporins such as fourth-generation cephalosporins like cefipime. First-generation cephalosporins (such as cefazolin) are not effective against *Pseudomonas* species.

42. **The correct answer is D.** Inflammatory bowel disease typically presents during late adolescence to early adulthood with symptoms of abdominal pain and frequent bouts of diarrhea. Types of Inflammatory bowel disease are differentiated and diagnosed on the basis of their clinical picture, their appearance on endoscopy and biopsy, and the exclusion of other intestinal infectious etiologies. In this patient, the areas of normal-appearing mucosa should immediately point to the diagnosis of Crohn disease as opposed to ulcerative colitis. Ulcerative colitis is characterized by continuous mucosal inflammation that is limited to the colon and always involves the rectum. Crypt abscesses and ulceration of the mucosa are classically seen on biopsy. Crohn disease, however, shows transmural inflammation interspersed with normal mucosa ("skip" lesions), as seen in this patient. Crohn disease can affect any part of the GI tract but usually spares the rectum. Noncaseating granulomas may be found in Crohn disease but are not found in ulcerative colitis.

    Answer A is incorrect. Cells with loss of mucin and hyperchromatic nuclei are present in colon cancer, which is more commonly associated with a long history of ulcerative colitis.

    Answer B is incorrect. Crypt abscesses are typically seen in ulcerative colitis.

    Answer C is incorrect. Hyperplasia of goblet cells is the central feature of hyperplastic polyps, the most common type of non-neoplastic polyp. Although usually asymptomatic, they may cause bleeding, abdominal pain, and, rarely, obstruction.

    Answer E is incorrect. Ulceration limited to the mucosa is a feature of ulcerative colitis. In Crohn disease the inflammation is often transmural and interspersed with areas of normal-appearing tissue, as described in this vignette. Due to the transmural quality of the inflammation, fistulas may develop more frequently in Crohn disease than in ulcerative colitis.

43. **The correct answer is E.** *Trypanosoma cruzi* infection can cause aganglionic megacolon and Chagas disease, a condition in which the heart is enlarged and flaccid. *T cruzi* is transmitted via the reduviid bug. Microscopic examination reveals flagellated trypomastigotes in the blood and non-flagellated amastigotes in cardiac muscle. *T cruzi* infection is treated with nifurtimox. The fact that this man was from Central America is a second clue to his illness; epidemiologically, *T cruzi* infections are most common among the poor in rural Central and South America.

    Answer A is incorrect. *Cryptosporidium* infection presents with severe diarrhea in HIV-positive patients and mild watery diarrhea in HIV-negative patients. *Cryptosporidium* is transmitted via cysts in water (fecal-oral transmission). Microscopically, acid-fast-staining cysts are found. Unfortunately, there is no treatment available for *Cryptosporidium* infection; however, in healthy patients, cryptosporidiosis is self-resolving.

    Answer B is incorrect. *Entamoeba histolytica* is acquired by ingestion of viable cysts from fecally contaminated water, food, or hands (fecal-oral transmission). Infection presents with bloody diarrhea, abdominal cramps with tenesmus (a feeling of incomplete defecation), and pus in the stool. It also can cause right-upper-quadrant pain and liver abscesses. On microscopy, one observes amebas with ingested RBCs. Treatment includes metronidazole and iodoquinol.

    Answer C is incorrect. *Giardia lamblia* infection presents with bloating, flatulence, foul-smelling diarrhea, and light-colored fatty stools. *G lamblia* is transmitted via cysts in water (fecal-oral transmission). On microscopy, one observes teardrop-shaped trophozoites with a ventral sucking disc or cysts. Metronidazole is used to treat *G lamblia* infection.

Answer D is incorrect. *Toxoplasma gondii* infection presents with brain abscesses in HIV-positive patients and with birth defects if infection occurs during pregnancy. Toxoplasmosis is one of the **ToRCHeS** organisms (**To**xoplasmosis, **R**ubella, **C**ytomegalovirus, **He**rpesvirus/HIV, **S**yphilis). *T gondii* is transmitted via cysts in raw meat or cat feces. The definitive stage (sexual stage) occurs in cats. The diagnosis most often is made serologically. Sulfadiazine and pyrimethamine are used to treat toxoplasmosis.

44. **The correct answer is B.** A young man presenting with hemoptysis should raise a high index of suspicion for Goodpasture syndrome. This diagnosis is supported by his fatigue and hematuria (although typically renal symptoms follow pulmonary symptoms by weeks to months). As the disease progresses, one would expect a nephritic picture with hematuria, hypertension, and oliguria. The diagnosis of Goodpasture syndrome is confirmed by the renal biopsy, which on immunofluorescence staining shows a linear pattern of IgG deposition along the basement membrane. These anti-glomerular basement membrane (GBM) antibodies are specific to the $\alpha 3$ chain of type IV collagen, and cause injury to both the glomerular and alveolar basement membranes.

Answer A is incorrect. Goodpasture syndrome is caused by anti-GBM antibodies specific to the $\alpha 3$ chain of type IV collagen. Type III collagen is found in skin, blood vessels, and other organs and is not affected by anti-GBM antibodies. The most common pathology involving type III collagen is Ehlers-Danlos syndrome, a connective tissue disorder in which patients bleed very easily and have hyperelastic skin.

Answer C is incorrect. Antineutrophil cytoplasmic antibodies (ANCA) are found in certain pauci-immune glomerulonephritides such as Wegener granulomatosis. This could account for a nephritic picture, but immunofluorescence would show an absence of any immue deposition. Furthermore, if the patient had Wegener granulomatosis, one would expect to see a specific pattern of symptoms involving the sinuses, lungs, and kidneys.

Answer D is incorrect. Immune complex deposition causes damage to the glomerulus in many diseases such as poststreptococcal glomerulonephritis and SLE. The cause can be idiopathic, due to an antigenic stimulus, or due to a systemic immune complex disorder. On immunofluorescence one would see lumpy or granular deposition of immune complexes in the glomerulus.

Answer E is incorrect. The patient's presentation is characteristic of Goodpasture syndrome, which is caused by antibodies specific to type IV collagen. Immune-related injury to the glomerulus can be separated into three categories: immune-complex glomerulonephritis, anti-GBM, and pauci-immune glomerulonephritis (no antibodies, complement, or immune deposition). It has been proposed that pauci-immune glomerulonephritis is mediated by T lymphocytes, which release cytokines and thereby recruit inflammatory cells.

45. **The correct answer is A.** The patient has experienced rhabdomyolysis secondary to extreme muscle strain. Rhabdomyolysis causes the release of muscle cell contents into the bloodstream, leading to an elevated creatine kinase level and myoglobinuria (red urine characterized by a urine dipstick test that is positive for blood but shows no RBCs on urinalysis). Release of intracellular potassium may lead to the development of significant arrhythmias and possibly death.

Answer B is incorrect. Hepatomegaly is a nonspecific sign of many medical conditions but is not a typical consequence of rhabdomyolysis.

Answer C is incorrect. Pain in a dermatomal distribution is characteristic of shingles and is unrelated to rhabdomyolysis.

Answer D is incorrect. Pain on urination would be a symptom of a urinary tract infection. Because this patient does not have WBCs in his urine, he most likely does not have a urinary tract infection.

Answer E is incorrect. A shuffling gait may be seen in Parkinson disease and is unrelated to rhabdomyolysis.

46. **The correct answer is C.** An elevated α-fetoprotein (AFP) level in amniotic fluid and maternal serum may indicate neural tube defects such as spina bifida, meningocele, and meningomyelocele. These defects are caused by the failure of the caudal portion of the neural tube to close. The AFP level is elevated because AFP is leaked into the amniotic fluid from the neural tube defect. Children with these defects suffer from a varying degree of symptoms that usually include motor and sensory defects in the lower extremities and dysfunction of bowel and bladder control. Folate deficiency during the first four weeks of pregnancy has been implicated in causing neural tube defects. Drugs that increase the risk of neural tube defect include valproate and carbamazepine.

Answer A is incorrect. Bilateral renal agenesis (Potter syndrome) is caused by disruption in the interaction between the ureteric bud and the metanephrogenic tissue. Because the fetus does not produce urine (which is a component of amniotic fluid), there is a smaller volume of amniotic fluid than normal. This is described by the term oligohydramnios. The smaller amount of protective fluid results in pulmonary hypoplasia, fetal compression with altered facies, and positioning defects of hands and feet. Bilateral renal agenesis is not compatible with life. Oligohydramnios, not increased AFP levels, would be noted in this case.

Answer B is incorrect. The ductus arteriosus is a connection between the pulmonary artery and the aorta that allows oxygenated blood from the placenta to bypass the fetal lungs and enter the systemic circulation. This pathway should be open during gestation and is not an abnormality. At birth, as the infant takes a breath, an increase in oxygen content causes a decrease in prostaglandins, resulting in closure of the connection. If the ductus arteriosus remains patent after birth, the baby can be given indomethacin to help stimulate the vessel to close.

Answer D is incorrect. It is possible that this fetus inherited a recessive disorder such as cystic fibrosis, phenylketonuria, or sickle cell anemia. However, these diseases are usually tested for in patients with a family history using DNA studies of fetal cells collected from amniotic fluid, not by measuring AFP levels.

Answer E is incorrect. Nondisjunction during meiosis is the usual cause of trisomy 21, the genetic abnormality in Down syndrome. Trisomy 21 is more common in women >35 years old, so this patient's age puts her at increased risk of having a baby with Down syndrome. However, unlike neural tube defects, Down syndrome causes a decrease in AFP levels and an increase in β-human chorionic gonadotropin levels.

47. **The correct answer is C.** The boy has a history consistent with absence seizures. On clinical examination, typical absence seizures appear as brief staring spells with no warning or postictal phase. Children are not responsive during the seizure and are amnestic of what happened during the attack. In fact, patients are generally unaware that a seizure has occurred. Classically, a regular and symmetric 3-Hz spike is found on electroencephalography. Ethosuximide is the primary treatment option in cases of absence (petit mal) seizures.

Answer A is incorrect. Carbamazepine has been associated with the exacerbation of absence seizures.

Answer B is incorrect. Clonazepam and the ketogenic or medium-chain triglyceride diet have been attempted to reduce seizure frequency. These adjunctive therapies, however, have limited efficacy.

Answer D is incorrect. Gabapentin has been associated with the exacerbation of absence seizures.

Answer E is incorrect. The teacher's concerns regarding the boy are quite common in the case of absence seizures. Often such concerns will be incorrectly attributed to inattentiveness and may even lead to a misdiagnosis of attention deficit/hyperactivity disorder (ADHD). Methylphenidate, a CNS stimulant, is the cornerstone of therapy in ADHD.

Answer F is incorrect. Tiagabine has been associated with the exacerbation of absence seizures.

48. **The correct answer is B.** This patient has multiple myeloma, a neoplastic proliferation of plasma cells in the bone marrow that often leads to lytic bone lesions and pathological fractures. The plasma cell is a differentiated B lymphocyte that can produce and secrete large amounts of antibody specific to a particular antigen. Rough endoplasmic reticulum is the site of synthesis of secretory proteins; thus antibody-secreting plasma cells are rich in RER. Normally there is a polyclonal distribution of immunoglobulins of different isotypes and antigen specificities in the serum. In multiple myeloma, however, the majority of plasma cells are producing immunoglobulin of one isotype and antigen specifically, which can be detected as an M spike by serum protein electrophoresis. The free light chains (either kappa or lambda) can often be detected in the urine; this is referred to as Bence-Jones proteinuria. Patients with multiple myeloma might also manifest anemia, increased susceptibility to infection, or clotting abnormalities secondary to the reduced production of normal blood components.

Answer A is incorrect. The primary function of mitochondria is the synthesis of ATP. They are abundant in cells that require a large amount of energy, such as myocytes.

Answer C is incorrect. Secondary lysosomes are formed when a primary lysosome, with its hydrolytic enzymes, fuses with materials for degradation. Secondary lysosomes have substrates at different stages of digestion. Cells such as macrophages, which are responsible for phagocytosis of cell debris, may contain multiple secondary lysosomes.

Answer D is incorrect. Smooth endoplasmic reticulum (SER) is the site of steroid synthesis and detoxification of drugs and poisons; thus, cells like hepatocytes and steroid-producing cells of the adrenal cortex are rich in SER.

Answer E is incorrect. Areas of rough endoplasmic reticulum in neurons are called Nissl bodies. This is the site of enzyme and peptide neurotransmitter synthesis.

Test Block 3

QUESTIONS

1. An 18-month-old child is brought to the physician by her distraught parents because of a sore throat, difficulty breathing, and a barking cough for the past day. On physical examination, the toddler is found to have some respiratory stridor and a runny nose but is not in acute distress. The rest of the examination is unremarkable. Which of the following is the most appropriate treatment for this patient?

   (A) Amantadine
   (B) Bronchoalveolar lavage
   (C) Emergency department admittance
   (D) Penicillin
   (E) Supportive therapy

2. A 32-year-old woman presents to her family doctor complaining of fatigue, myalgia, and anorexia for nearly one week. Physical examination reveals cervical lymphadenopathy and the rash seen in the image. If this illness is left untreated, which of the following symptoms or conditions is most likely to occur next?

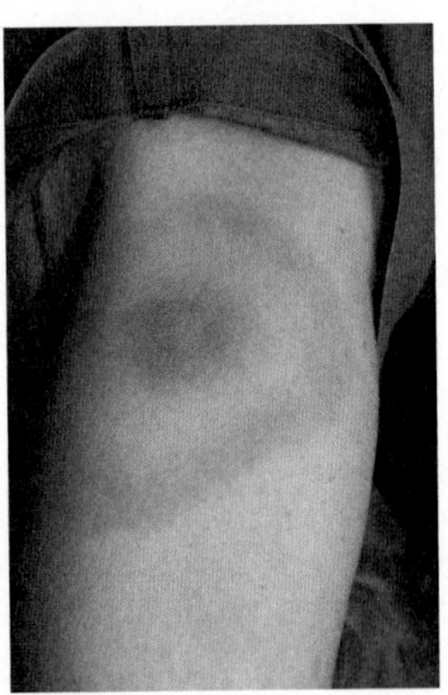

Courtesy of Dr. James Gathany.

   (A) Aortic aneurysm
   (B) Argyll Robertson pupil
   (C) Autoimmune polyarthritis
   (D) Facial nerve palsy
   (E) Opportunistic infection with *Pneumocystis jiroveci*

3. A 41-year-old man is admitted to the hospital for progressive obtundation. On admission the patient's serum sodium level is 114 mEq/L. Treatment is initiated, and seven hours later the patient's serum sodium level is 134 mEq/L. Over the next four days the patient's condition worsens with the development of dysarthria, dysphagia, and paraparesis. What pathologic process is most likely responsible for this patient's new symptoms?

   (A) Cerebral edema
   (B) Diffuse axonal injury
   (C) Intracerebral hemorrhage
   (D) Osmotic demyelination
   (E) Uncal herniation

4. A 74-year-old man with chronic renal failure has had repeated pathological fractures. Laboratory analysis reveals:

   Serum calcium: 6.3 mg/dL
   Serum phosphate: 4.7 mg/dL
   Parathyroid hormone: 750 pg/mL

   Which of the following most likely contributes to the pathogenesis of this man's bone disease?

   (A) Decreased 1,25-dihydroxycholecalciferol production
   (B) Decreased 25-hydroxyvitamin D production
   (C) Decreased calcium intake
   (D) Decreased vitamin D_2 intake
   (E) Decreased vitamin D_3 intake

5. An epidemic of a diarrhea has broken out in a city hospital. Colonoscopy of one of the affected patients reveals colonic inflammation with exudates and necrosis of the mucosal surface. Assays for toxin A and toxin B are positive. Which of the following is the microbiology laboratory likely to isolate from the affected patients?

   (A) A gram-negative facultative intracellular organism
   (B) A gram-negative lactose fermenter
   (C) A gram-negative lactose nonfermenter

(D) A gram-positive aerobe
(E) A gram-positive anaerobe

6. A 9-year-old boy is brought to the emergency department with a two-day history of abdominal pain, vomiting, and a rash. His mother reports that he had a runny nose and mild cough about a week ago. On examination there is diffuse abdominal tenderness and a rash over the arms and the legs. His complete blood cell count is within normal limits and urinalysis shows 12 RBCs/hpf, 2 WBCs/hpf, no protein, and no glucose. An image of the rash is shown in the image. What is the most likely etiology of this patient's symptoms?

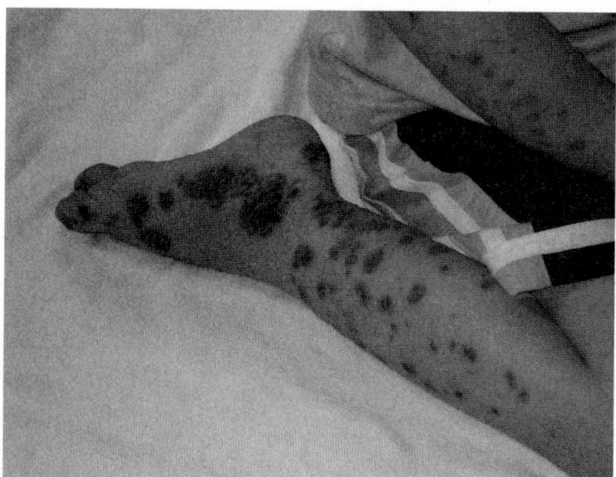

Courtesy of Wikipedia.

(A) Deficiency of von Willebrand factor-cleaving metalloproteinases
(B) IgA antibody deposition in the mesangium
(C) IgA immune complexes deposited in small vessels
(D) IgG antibodies against platelets
(E) IgG antibodies deposited in the glomerular basement membrane

7. A 68-year-old woman presents to the emergency department with altered mental status. Her temperature is 38.8°C (101.8°F), heart rate is 116/min, respiratory rate is 23/min, and blood pressure is 132/87 mm Hg. Arterial blood gas shows a pH of 7.28, partial pressure of carbon dioxide of 15 mm Hg, and a bicarbonate level of 7 mEq/L. Which of the following is the most accurate description of the patient's acid-base status?

(A) Metabolic acidosis
(B) Metabolic acidosis with respiratory alkalosis
(C) Metabolic acidosis with respiratory compensation
(D) Metabolic alkalosis with respiratory acidosis
(E) Respiratory alkalosis

8. A patient is found to have hypertension, hematuria, and oliguria. A renal biopsy specimen is obtained and reveals a focal proliferative glomerulonephritis, characterized by linear staining of the basement membrane on immunofluorescence for IgG. He is also found to have lung involvement. What pulmonary condition would present with similar respiratory function?

(A) Asthma
(B) Emphysema
(C) Kartagener syndrome
(D) Pneumothorax
(E) Sarcoidosis

9. Referring to the image, where A = afferent arteriole and B = efferent arteriole, which of the following most accurately reflects the actions of angiotensin II and prostaglandins in a dehydrated patient?

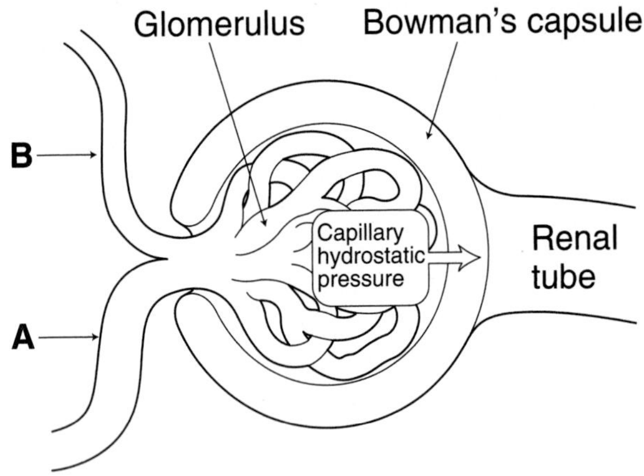

Reproduced, with permission, from USMLERx.com.

(A) Angiotensin II vasoconstricts A; prostaglandins vasodilate B; there is an overall decrease in GFR and increase in RPF
(B) Angiotensin II vasoconstricts A; prostaglandins vasodilate B; there is an overall increase in GFR and decrease in RPF
(C) Angiotensin II vasoconstricts B; prostaglandins vasodilate A; there is an overall increase in GFR and decrease in RPF
(D) Angiotensin II vasoconstricts B; prostaglandins vasodilate A; there is an overall decrease in GFR and increase in RPF
(E) Angiotensin II vasodilates B; prostaglandins vasoconstrict A; there is an overall decrease in GFR and increase in RPF

10. A 24-year-old man presents to the emergency department with hypertension, tachycardia, fever, diaphoresis, mydriasis, and severe agitation. When asked, his mother states that her son and his friends "probably used some drugs they got in the neighborhood." Which of the following agents is the most appropriate therapy for this patient?

(A) Atropine
(B) Flumazenil
(C) Fluoxetine
(D) Labetalol
(E) Naloxone
(F) Physostigmine

11. A 2-year-old child has no red reflex in the right eye. He is subsequently found to have an eye tumor that is caused by dysfunction of a specific cell-cycle regulatory gene product. What is the normal function of this gene product in a quiescent cell?

(A) Inhibits apoptosis
(B) Prevents cell-cycle progression past the G_1/S checkpoint
(C) Prevents cell-cycle progression past the G_2/M checkpoint
(D) Promotes DNA damage repair
(E) Promotes histone acetylation

12. Acute allograft rejection is mediated by cytotoxic T-lymphocytes that recognize and are activated by the major histocompatibility complex proteins expressed by the donated organ. A depleting monoclonal antibody to which of the following cell surface molecules would be most useful in reducing this immune-mediated graft rejection?

(A) CD3
(B) CD4
(C) CD14
(D) CD16
(E) CD19

13. A 67-year-old former landscaper is referred to the dermatologist for a lesion on his right forearm. The lesion is a flesh-colored pearly papule approximately 1.5 cm in diameter with a central telangiectasia. A biopsy is taken, and the results are shown in the image. Which of the following is the most likely diagnosis?

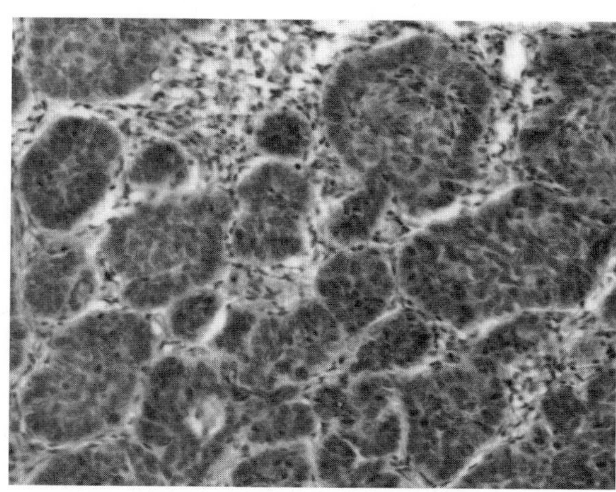

Reproduced, with permission, from USMLERx.com.

(A) Actinic keratosis
(B) Basal cell carcinoma
(C) Dermatitis herpetiformis
(D) Melanoma
(E) Seborrheic keratosis
(F) Squamous cell carcinoma

14. A 28-year-old woman with a past medical history significant for pelvic inflammatory disease presents to the emergency department with right lower quadrant abdominal pain. The pain began two hours ago, has been consistently localized to the right lower quadrant without migration, and has been associated with nausea and vomiting. Although her periods are usually regular, her last menstruation was approximately six weeks ago. On examination, she is found to be afebrile with a blood pressure of 90/60 mm Hg, a pulse of 110/min, and a respiratory rate of 26/min. Abdominal examination shows localized tenderness with guarding in the right lower quadrant. Pelvic examination is deferred due to excessive pain, but vaginal bleeding is noted. Laboratory studies show a hematocrit of 29.8% and an elevated human chorionic gonadotropin (hCG) level. Which of the following is the most likely etiology of this patient's illness?

(A) A blastocyst implanted in the ampulla
(B) A blastocyst implanted in the posterior superior uterine wall
(C) A fecalith obstructing the appendiceal lumen
(D) Ectopic endometrial tissue implanted on the ovary
(E) Two spermatozoa fertilizing a single ovum

15. A 64-year-old man with a history of hypertension, coronary artery disease, and type 2 diabetes presents to his physician because he "has trouble seeing." Visual field testing reveals a defect in the left half of the visual field for both eyes, with sparing of central acuity. Which of the following is the most likely cause of the patient's symptoms?

(A) Complete infarction of the optic chiasm
(B) Infarction of the lower division of the middle cerebral artery
(C) Left retinal artery occlusion with sparing of the vessels supplying the macula
(D) Right posterior cerebral artery infarction with sparing of Meyer's loop
(E) Right posterior cerebral artery infarction with sparing of the occipital pole

16. A 60-year-old woman is receiving chemotherapy for breast cancer. She presents to her oncologist complaining of fatigue and dyspnea on exertion. Physical examination reveals an elevated jugular venous pressure, crackles, and 4+ pitting edema bilaterally. X-ray of the chest shows an enlarged cardiac silhouette. Her oncologist believes her chemotherapeutic agent is responsible for these complaints. What is the mechanism of the chemotherapeutic agent she is most likely receiving?

(A) DNA intercalation
(B) Inhibition of dihydrofolate reductase
(C) Inhibition of microtubule formation
(D) Inhibition of purine synthesis
(E) Selective estrogen receptor modulator

17. A 22-year-old woman comes to your office complaining of vaginal itching and burning. She says she feels as if she "has the flu" and has had intermittent fevers and muscle aches over the past few days. Vaginal examination reveals the lesion seen in the image, and treatment is started. The patient subsequently develops elevated levels of blood urea nitrogen and creatinine in addition to a tremor and mental status changes. Which of the following agents did this patient most likely receive?

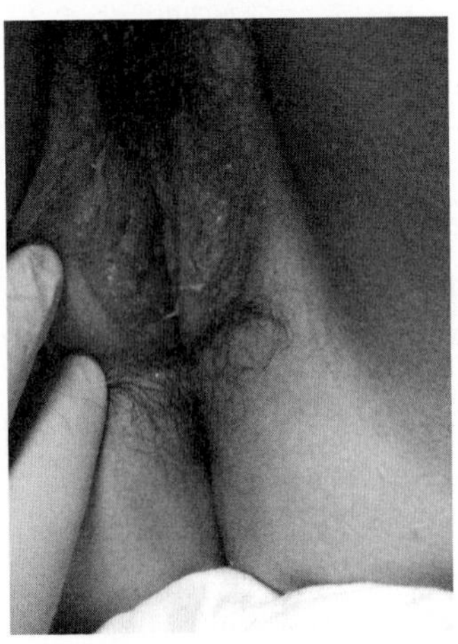

Reproduced, with permission, from USMLERx.com.

(A) Acyclovir
(B) Fluconazole
(C) Metronidazole
(D) Penicillin
(E) Ribavirin

18. A 60-year-old woman with chronic obstructive pulmonary disease (COPD) is brought into the emergency department after having a witnessed tonic-clonic seizure lasting two minutes. She is currently unresponsive. Her family states that she has been increasingly confused over the past two days or so, and has no prior history of seizures. Physical examination reveals no abnormalities, and the patient's vital signs are all within normal limits. Laboratory tests show:

Na^+: 123 mEq/L
K^+: 3.8 mEq/L
Cl^-: 100 mEq/L
HCO_3^-: 24 mEq/L
Glucose: 96 mg/dL
Serum osmolality: 250 mOsm/kg

Which of the following is the most likely cause of this patient's condition?

(A) Excessive fluid intake
(B) Glioblastoma multiforme
(C) Metastatic breast cancer
(D) Small cell lung cancer
(E) Squamous cell lung cancer

19. A 33-year-old man from upstate New York comes to his physician because of flu-like symptoms after a camping trip one week ago. He also notes a troubling rash on his leg that has moved slowly from his ankle to his midthigh over the past several days. The physician diagnoses Lyme disease and prescribes tetracycline. The patient recently lost his prescription benefits through his health insurance plan, so he uses an old bottle of tetracycline from his medicine cabinet at home. One week later the man presents to the emergency department with signs of dehydration and a creatinine level of 3.6, up from his baseline of 0.6. Which of the following renal conditions is this man most likely experiencing?

(A) Acute tubular necrosis
(B) Glomerulonephritis
(C) Kidney stones
(D) Renal papillary necrosis
(E) Renal tubular dysfunction

20. A 21-year-old woman presents to her male family practitioner complaining of sleep deprivation and severe depression. When asked about her sleeping habits in greater depth, she reports sleeping for seven-nine hours per night, but states that it is "just not right." In addition, she later claims to not have any problems with her personal life and is happy and excited about her recent promotion. Throughout the course of the visit, the patient becomes progressively more animated and begins making aggressive sexual advances toward the physician and the staff. She reports that her mood has been good, but not overly elevated, expansive, or elated. Which of the following is the most likely diagnosis?

(A) Bipolar disorder type I
(B) Histrionic personality disorder
(C) Obsessive-compulsive personality disorder
(D) Paranoid personality disorder
(E) Schizotypal personality disorder

21. A 37-year-old man complains of an unsteady gait when he walks. He has a history of drug abuse, alcohol abuse, and numerous sex partners. A myelin stain of the spinal cord is shown in the image. Which of the following organisms is responsible for this spinal cord lesion?

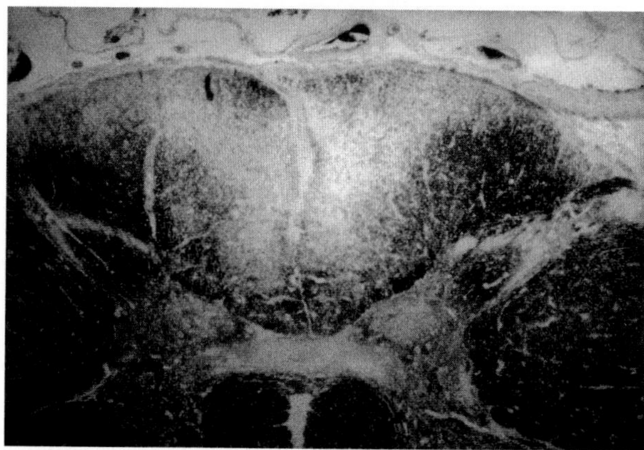

Courtesy of Dr. Susan Lindsley, Centers for Disease Control and Prevention.

(A) Herpes simplex virus
(B) HIV
(C) *Mycobacterium tuberculosis*
(D) Poliovirus
(E) *Treponema pallidum*

22. A 2-year-old boy presents to his pediatrician with hepatosplenomegaly, failure to thrive, and progressive central nervous system deterioration. Liver biopsy shows that hepatocytes and Kupffer cells have a foamy, vacuolated appearance. The pediatrician suspects that the boy will die by age three. Which of the following is the function of the metabolic enzyme deficient in this patient?

(A) Converts ceramide trihexoside to lactosyl cerebroside
(B) Converts galactocerebroside to cerebroside
(C) Converts sphingomyelin to cerebroside
(D) Converts glucocerebroside to cerebroside
(E) Converts ganglioside M_2 to ganglioside M_3

23. The following graph is a depiction of the Starling curve showing the relationship between cardiac output and ventricular end diastolic volume in a patient with congestive heart failure. If this patient is treated with a positive inotropic agent, the Starling curve would do which of the following?

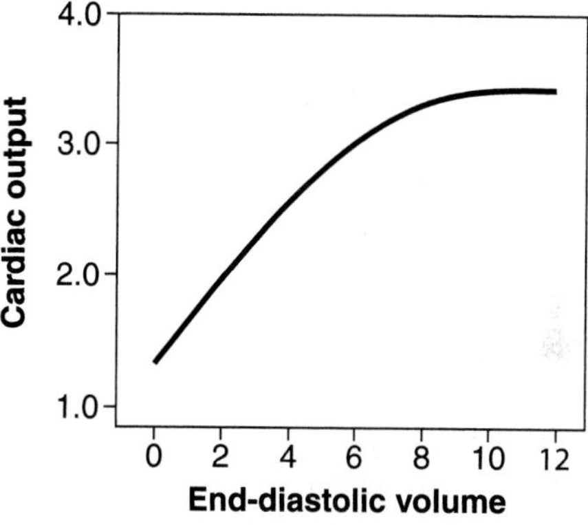

Reproduced, with permission, from USMLERx.com.

(A) Flatten out
(B) Shift down and left
(C) Shift down and right
(D) Shift right only
(E) Shift up and left
(F) Shift up and right

24. A 16-year-old girl visits her family physician with complaints of amenorrhea. Although she falls 20% below the minimum body weight expected for her height, she doesn't think she is skinny enough. After breaking up with her boyfriend a year ago, she dropped out of cheerleading and has been struggling with school, although she used to be an honors student. She admits to crying spells, feeling guilty, and thoughts of suicide. Which of the following medications is contraindicated in this patient?

(A) Bupropion
(B) Buspirone
(C) Haloperidol
(D) Phenelzine
(E) Sertraline

25. A patient with adult T-lymphocyte leukemia receives a bone marrow transplant from an unrelated donor. Despite an immunosuppressive post-transplant treatment regimen, over the course of several weeks the patient develops a severe cutaneous rash and intractable diarrhea. Blood tests were normal except for alanine aminotransferase (1032 U/L), aspartate aminotransferase (829 U/L), lactate dehydrogenase (634 U/L), and alkaline phosphatase (446 U/L). Which of the following is the most likely etiology of the patient's current symptoms?

(A) Acute graft rejection
(B) Graft-versus-host disease mediated by alloreactive donor T-lymphocytes
(C) Graft-versus-host disease mediated by alloreactive recipient T-lymphocytes
(D) Hyperacute graft rejection
(E) Recurrence of leukemia

26. An infectious disease clinician sends a serum sample to a clinical laboratory technician for HIV diagnostics. To confirm a positive enzyme-linked immunosorbent assay result, the technician performs a Western blot, assaying for the presence of antibodies to three different HIV proteins in the patient's serum. The image shows the results: tube 1 is the control for positives, tube 2 is the control for negatives, and tube 3 is the patient's sample. Which of the following is the most appropriate next step for the clinician?

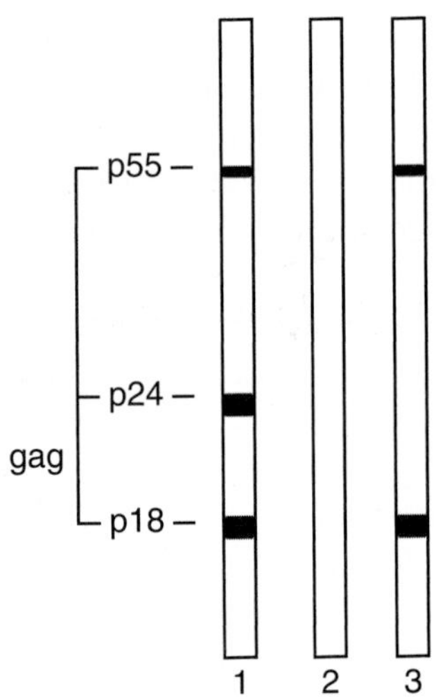

Reproduced, with permission, from USMLERx.com.

(A) Begin this patient on AZT therapy
(B) Profile this patient's T cells
(C) Repeat Western blot because of contamination
(D) Repeat Western blot because of failed positive control
(E) The patient does not have HIV

27. Vinca alkaloids such as vincristine are chemotherapeutic agents that are used for the treatment of choriocarcinoma as a part of the mechlorethamine/Oncovin/procarbazine/prednisone regimen. Vincristine's mechanism of action makes the drug specific for which phase of the cell cycle?

(A) G_0 phase
(B) G_1 phase
(C) G_2 phase
(D) M phase
(E) S phase

28. A 29-year-old reports to her obstetrician's office three months after a difficult delivery. She describes constant fatigue and recent weight loss. Her menses have not returned. She has been bottle-feeding, because breastfeeding "did not work." An endocrine abnormality is suspected. Which of the following laboratory test abnormalities would support the most likely diagnosis? (Note that normal values are as follows: total serum thyroxine, 5-12 µg/dL; serum thyroid-stimulating hormone (TSH), 0.5-5.0 µU/mL; serum ACTH, 9-52 pg/mL.)

(A) Total serum thyroxine, 0.1 µg/dL; serum TSH, 0.15 U/mL; serum ACTH, 10 pg/mL
(B) Total serum thyroxine, 0.1 µg/dL; serum TSH, 10 U/mL; serum ACTH, 25 pg/mL
(C) Total serum thyroxine, 0.1 µg/dL; serum TSH, 10 U/mL; serum prolactin, 200 ng/mL
(D) Total serum thyroxine, 1.0 µg/dL; serum TSH, 4 U/mL; serum ACTH, 250 pg/mL
(E) Total serum thyroxine, 2.5 µg/dL; serum TSH, 0.15 U/ml; serum ACTH, 25 pg/mL

29. A neonate who is born with a cleft palate and abnormal facies becomes cyanotic and hypoxic soon after birth. On physical examination, the neonatologist hears a crescendo-decrescendo murmur with a harsh systolic ejection. Further investigation shows tetralogy of Fallot. Examination of this patient's serum is likely to reveal which of the following?

(A) High IgM and normal T cell number
(B) Hypogammaglobulinemia and normal T cell number
(C) Hypogammaglobulinemia and reduced T cell number
(D) Low IgM and normal T cell number
(E) Reduced T cell number alone

30. A 3-year-old boy is brought to the pediatrician because of decreased vision and pain in his right eye. Past medical history is significant for the diagnosis of glaucoma shortly after birth that has been refractory to standard medical therapies. Focused physical examination reveals iris hamartomas. Which of the following additional signs is most likely on physical examination?

(A) Bilateral acoustic neuromas
(B) Bilateral renal cell carcinomas
(C) Cystic medial necrosis of the aorta
(D) Leptomeningeal angioma
(E) Scoliosis

31. A 10-year-old boy is brought to the emergency department after falling from his bicycle. He presents with a large, painfully swollen knee; aspiration shows gross hemarthrosis. On further questioning, the patient's parents say that he bruises easily and that he had an episode of prolonged bleeding after losing a tooth one month ago. His maternal uncle had similar bleeding difficulties. After further testing, the patient is diagnosed with an X-linked recessive disorder. Which of the following laboratory test results corresponds to the patient's disorder?

Choice	Platelet count	Bleeding time	Prothrombin time	Partial thromboplastin time
A	normal	normal	normal	↑
B	normal	↑	normal	normal
C	normal	↑	normal	↑
D	↓	↑	normal	normal
E	↓	↑	↑	↑

Reproduced, with permission, from USMLERx.com.

(A) A
(B) B
(C) C
(D) D
(E) E

32. An obese 32-year-old man presents at the clinic complaining of increasing difficulty catching his breath. He also reports that he has been wheezing and has a productive cough. He was told that his lungs are lacking a particular enzyme due to genetic mutations. Relevant social history reveals that he has been smoking cigarettes for the past 15 years. Family history is significant for a father with significant lung disease. X-ray of the chest shows basilar hyperlucency that is localized solely to the lung bases and not the apices. This patient is also at increased risk for which other condition?

(A) Cor pulmonale
(B) Liver cirrhosis
(C) Pseudomonal pneumonia
(D) Renal cysts

33. A 32-year-old woman presents to the emergency department with mental status changes, severe weakness, and multiple petechiae evolving over the past three weeks. Physical examination is also notable for pale conjunctiva. Temperature is 101.7°F (38.7°C). Laboratory studies show a severe anemia, thrombocytopenia, and leukocytosis. A peripheral blood smear is shown in the image. Which of the following chromosomal translocations is most likely involved in this disorder?

(A) t(8;14)
(B) t(9;22)
(C) t(11;22)
(D) t(11;14)
(E) t(15;17)

34. A 17-year-old girl who is six weeks pregnant presents to the emergency department because of abdominal pain and vaginal bleeding. Ultrasound imaging shows no fetal heartbeat and incomplete fetal development. The decision is made to terminate the pregnancy. On questioning, the patient reports that she has been taking high doses of her mother's ulcer medication for her own heartburn. Which of the following medications did this patient most likely take?

(A) Cimetidine
(B) Magnesium hydroxide
(C) Misoprostol
(D) Omeprazole
(E) Sucralfate

35. A 43-year-old man with a history of hypercalcemia and bitemporal hemianopsia presents to the emergency department with muscle weakness, lethargy, and watery diarrhea. He reports brief episodes of complete paralysis in his lower extremities. The pH of the patient's nasogastric suction fluid is increased. An abdominal mass is noted on CT scan. The patient's family history is positive for numerous endocrine organ abnormalities. Which of the following is the most likely cause of this patient's symptoms?

(A) Carcinoid tumor
(B) Gastrinoma
(C) Insulinoma
(D) Pheochromocytoma
(E) VIPoma

36. Patients with Paget disease of the bone usually have serum calcium levels between 8.4 and 10.5 mg/dL and phosphate levels between 2.7 and 4.0 mg/dL. During the second phase of the disease, which of the following laboratory values is most likely to be seen?

Choice	Alkaline phosphatase (U/L)	Phosphate (mg/dL)
A	20	3.7
B	50	5.2
C	100	5.4
D	400	3.5
E	1500	5.2

(A) A
(B) B
(C) C
(D) D
(E) E

37. A 40-year-old nulligravid woman visits her gynecologist because of menstrual irregularities. She also recently started producing breast milk even though she is not nursing. A pregnancy test is negative. Which of the following recent medical diagnoses is most likely related to the patient's symptoms?

(A) Menopause
(B) Parkinson disease
(C) Schizophrenia
(D) Turner syndrome
(E) Type 2 diabetes mellitus

38. A 37-year-old man with end-stage liver disease secondary to hepatitis C presents to the emergency department confused and lethargic. He has ascites, spider angiomata, and asterixis. Bowel sounds are normal. Laboratory studies show the following results:

Aspartate aminotransferase: 46 U/L
Alanine aminotransferase: 55 U/L
Alkaline phosphatase: 100 U/L
Bilirubin, total serum: 1.4 mg/dL
Prothrombin time: 38 seconds
Albumin: 2.0 g/dL (normal: 3.4-5.4 g/dL)

Which of the following is the mechanism of action of the most appropriate acute treatment of this patient's condition?

(A) Acidification of colonic contents, causing ammonium trapping
(B) Decreasing substrate for ammonia-producing reactions
(C) Eliminating colonic flora and decreasing their subsequent ammonia production
(D) Facilitating the binding of GABA to the GABA receptor
(E) Inhibiting synthesis of tumor necrosis factor-α

39. A 39-year-old man who is HIV-positive presents to the physician with fever, cough, and difficulty breathing. Physical examination shows that the patient is breathing abnormally fast, and the tips of his fingers have a slight bluish tinge. X-ray of the chest reveals diffuse interstitial pneumonia with a ground-glass appearance. Which of the following therapies should be used to treat this patient?

(A) Fluconazole or ketoconazole
(B) Itraconazole or potassium iodide
(C) Sulfadiazine and pyrimethamine
(D) Topical miconazole or selenium sulfide
(E) Trimethoprim-sulfamethoxazole

40. A 17-year-old girl with type 1 diabetes mellitus gives birth to a baby boy at 37 weeks' gestation by cesarean section. At one minute after birth, the boy is pink with blue fingers and toes. His heart rate is 80/min, and he does not respond to noxious stimuli. Muscle tone is absent, and his cry is weak. What is this child's one-minute APGAR score?

(A) 1
(B) 3
(C) 5
(D) 7
(E) 9

41. A 60-year-old Scandinavian woman presents to her doctor with a two-month history of progressive fatigue. She also reports tingling and numbness in her lower extremities and feeling "wobbly" lately. She has no significant medical history. Physical examination reveals a pulse of 101/min and decreased light touch and vibration sense on her lower extremities. Laboratory studies show a hemoglobin level of 9 g/dL and a mean corpuscular volume of 110 fL. Peripheral blood smear is shown in the image. The etiology of this patient's anemia results from which of the following?

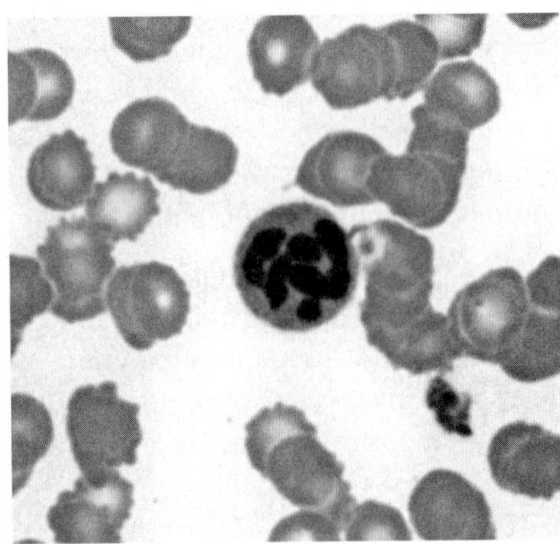

Reproduced, with permission, from USMLERx.com.

(A) Abnormal neural crest cell migration
(B) Antibodies against parietal cells
(C) Bacterial overgrowth of colon
(D) Diet deficient in leafy vegetables
(E) Embolus to the superior mesenteric artery

42. An 83-year-old retired construction worker comes to his physician because his chronic cough has gotten worse over the past year. He also notes some moderate facial swelling and bilateral arm edema. He has a 50-pack-year smoking history. X-ray of the chest shows a show large pleural-based mass in the right lower lung. A thoracoscopic-guided biopsy demonstrates malignant cells in the mesothelium. What other microscopic findings are likely to be found?

(A) Granulomas with central caseous necrosis and Langhans' giant cells
(B) Histiocytic cells with cytoplasmic inclusions resembling tennis rackets
(C) Intra-arterial thrombus with RBC extravasation
(D) Marked intra-alveolar fibrin and cellular debris
(E) Thick-walled spherules containing endospores with surrounding inflammatory cells
(F) Yellow-brown, rod-shaped bodies with clubbed ends that stain positively with Prussian blue

43. A 27-year-old man enters the emergency department in an agitated state. He complains of severe abdominal pain, but soon becomes paranoid and combative, requiring five-point restraint. His vital signs show elevated blood pressure and tachycardia. When a straight catheter is inserted, reddish urine flows into the Foley bag. The urine is negative for RBCs, and a toxicity screen result is negative. The doctor suspects a porphyria. Laboratory tests for urine porphobilinogen are positive. Which of the following enzyme deficiencies is most likely responsible for this patient's disorder?

(A) Aminolevulinate dehydratase
(B) Aminolevulinate synthase
(C) Ferrochelatase
(D) Heme oxygenase
(E) Porphobilinogen deaminase
(F) Uroporphyrinogen decarboxylase
(G) Uroporphyrinogen III cosynthase

44. A 4-year-old girl presents to her pediatrician, who obtains the peripheral blood smear shown in the image. The loss of function of what body part will cause her to become symptomatic?

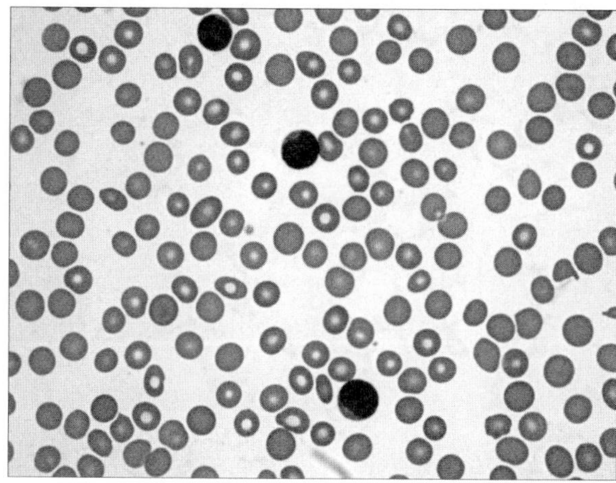

Reproduced, with permission, from USMLERx.com.

(A) Bone marrow
(B) Kidney
(C) Lining of the small intestine
(D) RBCs
(E) Spleen

45. A 59-year-old man with a history of obesity, myocardial infarction, and foot ulcers complains to his primary care physician about numbness and tingling in his lower extremities. Hemoglobin A_{1c} level is 10%. Which of the following describes the glomerular pathology most likely seen on light microscopy of this patient's kidneys?

(A) Diffuse capillary and basement membrane thickening
(B) Enlarged hypercellular glomeruli with neutrophils
(C) Nodular glomerulosclerosis with thickened basement membranes
(D) Segmental sclerosis with hyalinosis
(E) Wire-loop appearance with subendothelial basement membrane deposits

46. A 15-month-old boy sustained scald burns of his legs and feet in a bathtub. His mother, who brought him into the emergency department, says he was being lowered into the water with his knees bent when he screamed in pain, and was immediately removed from the bathtub. Physical examination reveals deep partial-thickness to full-thickness burns bilaterally on his anterior shins and ankles, the dorsa of his feet, and the plantar surfaces of the toes and distal feet. What is/are the next step(s) in the management of this child?

(A) Obtain collateral history information from other family members, neighbors, or friends
(B) Order imaging of head, chest, and extremities
(C) Provide appropriate treatment for the wounds and admit to the hospital without informing the authorities
(D) Provide appropriate treatment for the wounds and call authorities immediately
(E) Provide appropriate treatment for the wounds, complete a full physical examination, and release the patient back to guardian

47. A 45-year-old man goes to his primary care physician complaining of recent headaches. They rarely persist for more than an hour, but are sporadic and often accompanied by sudden sweating and palpitations. "Doc," he says, "it feels like my heart is racing." Acetaminophen provides minimal relief from the pain. He is afebrile and his blood pressure is 128/70 mm Hg. His physical examination is unremarkable with the exception of moist palms and pale skin. A urinalysis is notable for elevated metanephrines. This patient's most likely diagnosis is often associated with which of the following conditions?

(A) Hashimoto thyroiditis
(B) Insulinoma
(C) Parathyroid tumor
(D) Prolactinoma
(E) Zollinger-Ellison syndrome

48. A 39-year-old woman presents to her primary care physician with sporadic shooting pains across the left side of her face. She has no history of migraine headaches. On further questioning she says that three years ago she experienced several weeks of tingling in her right lower extremity, and as recently as last year, she was unable to drive her car because of bilateral arm weakness. The physician proceeds with a full neurologic work-up, including MRI of the head (see image). Given the patient's likely diagnosis, what is the best long-term therapy?

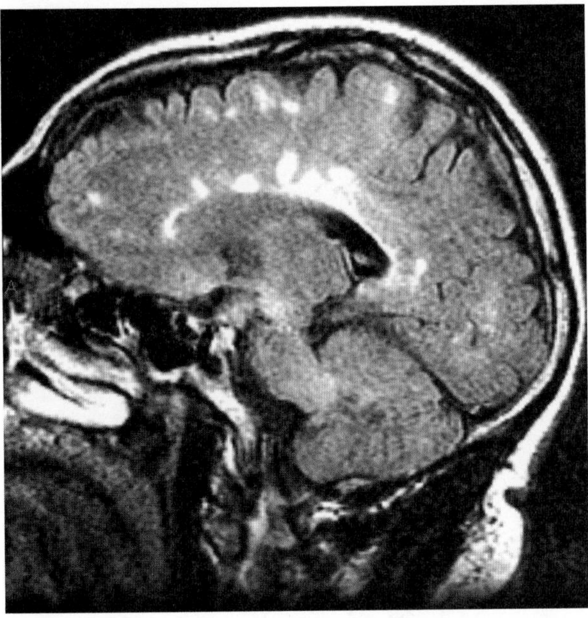

Courtesy of Dr. Per-Lennart Westesson, University of Rochester Medical Center.

(A) Acetaminophen
(B) Corticosteroids
(C) Heparin
(D) Interferon
(E) Sumatriptan

ANSWERS

1. **The correct answer is E.** The most likely diagnosis is croup, which is most commonly caused by parainfluenza virus. Croup is an infection of the upper airway causing narrowing that leads to inspiratory wheezing and a barking cough. Most cases of croup require only supportive therapy as treatment. Severe cases may require supplemental oxygen, corticosteroids, and epinephrine. While parainfluenza is the most common agent responsible for croup, it can also be caused by influenza, respiratory syncytial virus, and measles.

   Answer A is incorrect. Amantadine is an antiviral that has a narrow spectrum and is used to treat influenza type A. While influenza can cause croup, it is not the most common cause of this disease.

   Answer B is incorrect. Bronchoalveolar lavage is used to sample the lower respiratory tract in severe pneumonia, in the diagnosis of a lung tumor, and in the assessment of fibrosing alveolitis, among other indications.

   Answer C is incorrect. Admission to the emergency department may be called for if the child is in acute respiratory distress.

   Answer D is incorrect. Penicillin can be used to treat streptococcal pharyngitis, which presents with red, swollen tonsils and pharynx and a high fever.

2. **The correct answer is D.** This patient presents in the early, localized stage (stage 1) of Lyme disease, caused by infection with the spirochete *Borrelia burgdorferi*. This organism is carried by several species of the *Ixodes* tick and is common in the northeastern United States. This first stage is characterized by a flu-like illness and the erythema migrans rash, which classically spreads over time and develops a central clearing. The second stage (early disseminated disease) targets four organ systems; skin, central nervous system, heart, and joints. Bilateral cranial nerve VII palsy (Bell palsy) is a common early effect of *B burgdorferi* infection.

   Answer A is incorrect. Aortic aneurysms form in approximately 10% of patients with tertiary syphilis. The cardiac involvement typical of disseminated Lyme disease is atrioventricular nodal block, myocarditis, or left ventricular function.

   Answer B is incorrect. Argyll Robertson pupil is characteristic of tertiary syphilis. As a result of a midbrain lesion, the pupil constricts during accommodation but not in response to light.

   Answer C is incorrect. Autoimmune polyarthritis does occur in untreated Lyme disease. However, this phenomenon occurs months to years after the initial presentation of the disease (late stage).

   Answer E is incorrect. Opportunistic infection with *Pneumocystis jiroveci* is found in immunocompromised patients, such as those in the later stages of HIV infection.

3. **The correct answer is D.** Osmotic demyelination, also known as central pontine myelinolysis, can result from overaggressive treatment of hyponatremia. As hyponatremia develops, the brain prevents cerebral edema by gradually reducing its own osmolarity, thus reducing the osmotic gradient that would otherwise force water intracellularly. The brain can gradually replace these lost osmoles as the serum osmolarity is corrected, but correction of the serum sodium level at a rate faster than about 1 mEq/L/hr outpaces the brain's ability to compensate, resulting in neuronal shrinkage and death. The clinical manifestations occur several days later and include dysarthria, dysphagia, and flaccid quadriparesis that can become spastic and may progress to a "locked-in" syndrome, in which the patient retains full awareness but can move only the extraocular muscles.

   Answer A is incorrect. Cerebral edema occurs with acute hyponatremia as water flows freely across both the blood-brain barrier and cell membranes and into brain cells to compensate for the drop in serum sodium. However, cerebral edema does not typically accompany overly aggressive treatment of hyponatremia with hypertonic saline, but rather the opposite, as cell shrinkage and death occur as a result of water leaving the cells.

Answer B is incorrect. Diffuse axonal injury occurs in the setting of central nervous system trauma or angular acceleration or both and results in disruption of the axon at the nodes of Ranvier. Diffuse axonal injury does not occur with electrolyte abnormalities.

Answer C is incorrect. Intracerebral hemorrhage can occur as a result of hypertension, arteriovenous malformations, anticoagulation, thrombolysis, or amyloid angiopathy; however, it does not occur as a result of hyponatremia or the associated treatment.

Answer E is incorrect. Uncal herniation can result only from focal processes within the cranial vault, such as intracranial hemorrhage, but does not occur with diffuse processes associated with electrolyte abnormalities.

4. **The correct answer is A.** This man has renal osteodystrophy, a common complication of chronic renal insufficiency. In these patients, decreased conversion of 25-hydroxyvitamin D to the active 1,25-dihydroxycholecalciferol in kidney cells leads to decreased calcium absorption and thus a low serum calcium level. Secretion of parathyroid hormone increases to counteract the low calcium levels by increasing bone resorption. The hyperparathyroid state also decreases kidney reabsorption of phosphate. Renal osteodystrophy is treated with calcium, phosphate binders, and calcitriol (synthetic vitamin D_3) supplementation.

   Answer B is incorrect. Active vitamin D is 1,25-dihydroxycholecalciferol (1,25-OH-D) produced from two sequential hydroxylation reactions of vitamin D. The intermediate is 25-hydroxyvitamin D (25-OH-D), which is the storage form of vitamin D. The production of active 1,25-OH-D would be reduced in this patient, but production of 25-OH-D would be unaffected.

   Answer C is incorrect. Calcium intake should be increased in this patient to above-normal levels. Decreased intake, however, is not the pathogenesis of his disease.

   Answer D is incorrect. Ergocalciferol, vitamin D_2, is found in plants. Patients with renal osteodystrophy can have normal or even elevated vitamin D intake.

   Answer E is incorrect. Cholecalciferol, or vitamin D_3, is found in meats. It is also produced in humans in the dermis by ultraviolet light exposure. Patients with renal osteodystrophy can have normal or even elevated vitamin D intake.

5. **The correct answer is E.** The description of colonic inflammation with exudates and necrosis of the mucosal surface describes the pseudomembranous colitis of *Clostridium difficile*, of which there have been several outbreaks. C *difficile* is a gram-positive anaerobe spore-former that produces toxin A (which causes diarrhea) and toxin B (which is cytotoxic). Strains that produce an increased amount of these toxins have led to increased morbidity and even mortality associated with C *difficile* colitis.

   Answer A is incorrect. *Salmonella* is an example of a gram-negative facultative intracellular organism and could produce diarrhea, but only C *difficile* produces toxin A and toxin B.

   Answer B is incorrect. Gram-negative lactose fermenters that can cause diarrhea include *Escherichia coli*, but not C *difficile*.

   Answer C is incorrect. Gram-negative lactose nonfermenters that can cause diarrhea include *Shigella* and *Salmonella*, but not C *difficile*.

   Answer D is incorrect. C *difficile* is an obligate anaerobe; the other gram-positive organisms are aerobic or facultative anaerobes.

6. **The correct answer is C.** Henoch-Schönlein purpura (HSP) is a systemic vasculitis caused by the deposition of IgA immune complexes. It often follows a respiratory infection, and is characterized by the triad of purpura, abdominal pain, and glomerulonephritis. Some

children also present with arthritis in major joints. The rash of HSP is usually described as palpable purpura on the buttocks and legs. It is the most common small-vessel vasculitis in children, and rarely affects adults. The disease is self- limiting and treatment is supportive. An older adult presenting with the same symptomatology is more likely to have a vasculitis associated with antineutrophil cytoplasmic antibodies.

Answer A is incorrect. The metalloproteinase ADAMTS-13 normally cleaves von Willebrand factor (vWF) multidimers, which then enter the circulation and rest on the surface of endothelial cells. In thrombotic thrombocytopenic purpura (TTP), deficiency of ADAMTS-13 leads to large vWF multidimers in the circulation, where they bind platelets causing the formation of platelet thrombi. TTP is characterized by fever, thrombocytopenia, hemolytic anemia, and renal and neurologic impairment.

Answer B is incorrect. IgA antibody deposition in the mesangium is the characteristic pattern of nephropathy associated with Berger disease, which presents with hematuria and low-grade proteinuria during or a few days after an infection.

Answer D is incorrect. IgG antibodies against platelets is the pathophysiology of idiopathic thrombocytopenic purpura, which is characterized by thrombocytopenia leading to mucosal or skin bleeding, purpura or petechiae, and epistaxis. In children it has an acute onset after a viral infection, whereas in adults it has a gradual onset and often follows a viral infection or the administration of a new drug (eg, sulfa drugs).

Answer E is incorrect. IgG antibodies deposited in the glomerular basement membrane is the etiology of Goodpasture syndrome, which is a type II hypersensitivity reaction and presents with glomerulonephritis and pneumonitis.

7. **The correct answer is A.** The patient is experiencing a metabolic acidosis, but there is also a simultaneous respiratory alkalosis.

Answer B is incorrect. This patient is acidotic, with a pH below the normal range of 7.35-7.45. Her bicarbonate level is low, so this is a metabolic acidosis. Next we look to see if she has appropriate respiratory compensation using Winter's formula: partial pressure of carbon dioxide = 1.5 (HCO_3^-) + 8 (±2). The expected partial pressure of carbon dioxide would therefore be 16.5 mm Hg at the lowest, but the patient's level is 15 mm Hg, telling us that there is a simultaneous respiratory alkalosis. This picture of metabolic acidosis with respiratory alkalosis is seen with severe salicylate intoxication, which would explain the patient's altered mental status.

Answer C is incorrect. If the patient were experiencing metabolic acidosis with respiratory compensation, given the bicarbonate level of 7 mEq/L, we would expect to see a partial pressure of carbon dioxide of 16.5 mm Hg. However, the patient's partial pressure of carbon dioxide is 15 mm Hg, suggesting that there is a simultaneous respiratory alkalosis that is more than compensatory.

Answer D is incorrect. This patient is acidotic, and her bicarbonate level is low, so we know this is a metabolic acidosis, not a respiratory acidosis or metabolic alkalosis.

Answer E is incorrect. The patient is experiencing a respiratory alkalosis, but there is also a simultaneous metabolic acidosis.

8. **The correct answer is E.** The report of the kidney biopsy mentions a characteristic pattern of linear antibody deposition, consistent with anti-GBM disease. Anti-GBM disease, or Goodpasture syndrome, occurs when circulating auto-antibodies bind to type IV collagen in basement membranes in the lung and kidney, leading to nephritic kidney disease and a restrictive lung disease. Sarcoidosis is characterized by immune-mediated noncaseating granulomas and also produces restrictive lung pathology. Restrictive lung diseases are classified as pathologies that result in decreased lung volumes with a relative preservation of the FEV_1/FVC ratio. In contrast, obstructive lung diseases are characterized by expanded

lung volumes with a decrease in the FEV_1/FVC ratio.

Answer A is incorrect. Asthma is a characteristic obstructive respiratory disease caused by airway hyperreactivity. Goodpasture syndrome produces a restrictive lung disease.

Answer B is incorrect. Emphysema is an obstructive respiratory disease caused by alveolar destruction and airway collapse, whereas Goodpasture syndrome produces a restrictive lung disease.

Answer C is incorrect. Kartagener syndrome leads to bronchiectasis, a disease with obstructive pathology due to immotile cilia and impaired mucociliary clearance of particles from the lung. In contrast, Goodpasture syndrome produces a restrictive lung disease.

Answer D is incorrect. Pneumothorax results in a decrease of total lung capacity. It is a restrictive pattern seen because of restriction of lung expansion. However, there is not specifically destruction of lung parenchyma.

9. **The correct answer is C.** During hemorrhage, blood loss leads to an increase in the renin-angiotensin-aldosterone (RAA) system. Angiotensin II has the effect of preferentially constricting the efferent arteriole. Renal prostaglandins are produced in response to increased sympathetic activity and act to preferentially vasodilate afferent arterioles. The overall result is an increase in GFR and a decrease in RPF. It is notable that the reason angiotensin converting enzyme inhibitors are protective for the kidney is that they prevent vasoconstriction of the efferent arterioles and thereby prevent a decrease in RPF. The reason that drugs blocking the formation of prostaglandins (ie, nonsteroidal anti-inflammatory drugs) are damaging to the kidney is that they block vasodilation at the afferent arterioles and thereby cause a decrease in both GFR and RPF.

   Answer A is incorrect. Angiotensin II would cause vasoconstriction of B, while the prostaglandins would cause vasodilation of A. The overall result would be an increase in GFR and a decrease in RPF.

   Answer B is incorrect. Angiotensin II would cause vasoconstriction of B, while the prostaglandins would cause vasodilation of A. The overall result would be an increase in GFR and a decrease in RPF.

   Answer D is incorrect. Angiotensin II would cause vasoconstriction of B, while the prostaglandins would cause vasodilation of A. The overall result would be an increase in GFR and a decrease in RPF.

   Answer E is incorrect. Angiotensin II would cause vasoconstriction of B, while the prostaglandins would cause vasodilation of A. The overall result would be an increase in GFR and a decrease in RPF.

10. **The correct answer is D.** The patient described above is probably under the influence of a central nervous system (CNS) stimulant such as methamphetamine. Labetalol is a nonselective α- and β-antagonist that blocks many of the dangerous peripheral effects of CNS stimulants, such as hypertension and cardiac stimulation. Other appropriate medications that could be administered under these conditions would be neuroleptic agents (to control the agitation and psychotic symptoms) and diazepam (to control possible seizures).

    Answer A is incorrect. Atropine is a muscarinic antagonist that would be appropriate therapy for overdose of an acetylcholinesterase inhibitor. A patient presenting with acetylcholinesterase inhibitor overdose would have miotic pupils and bradycardia.

    Answer B is incorrect. Flumazenil is a benzodiazepine receptor antagonist. It is used in cases of benzodiazepine overdose. The clinical features of acute benzodiazepine intoxication include slurred speech, lack of coordination, unsteady gait, and impaired attention or memory. A severe overdose may lead to stupor or coma.

    Answer C is incorrect. Fluoxetine is a selective serotonin reuptake inhibitor. It would not be helpful in a case of CNS stimulant overdose.

Answer E is incorrect. Naloxone is an opioid-receptor antagonist that would be appropriate therapy for an opiate overdose such as with heroin or morphine. A patient who presents with opioid overdose would appear sleepy, lethargic, or comatose, depending on the degree of overdose. Pupils would be miotic, not mydriatic. Blood pressure and heart rate are typically decreased, and respiration would be depressed.

Answer F is incorrect. Physostigmine is an acetylcholinesterase inhibitor that might be used for an antimuscarinic drug overdose, such as with atropine, scopolamine, or Jimson weed. An antimuscarinic overdose can look similar to a CNS stimulant overdose, but has one important exception. The hyperthermia seen with an antimuscarinic overdose is accompanied by hot and dry skin (due to blockade of cholinergic receptors present on sweat glands); however, stimulant overdose is associated with profuse sweating. Tachycardia, hypertension, hyperthermia, and mydriasis are common to both.

11. **The correct answer is B.** This child most likely has retinoblastoma, a rapidly progressive neoplastic growth in the retina. Retinoblastoma may present in one eye, as in this patient, or bilaterally, as in approximately 30% of cases. The clinical vignette does not allude to any family history, in which case the retinoblastoma is called sporadic, in contrast with the familial form, which is associated with a family history. In either case, the disease is believed to arise from a loss-of-function mutation in the *RB1* gene. *RB1* is a tumor suppressor gene that normally binds the E2F transcription factor complex in quiescent cells, which prevents the cell from progressing through the G_1/S checkpoint. Under appropriate conditions for cell replication, E2F is released when the Rb protein becomes phosphorylated by cyclins D and E, and their associated cyclin-dependant kinases (CDK 2, 4, and 6). Loss of function of the *RB1* gene is associated with osteosarcoma and retinoblastoma. According to the two-hit hypothesis, both copies of the *RB1* gene in a single retinoblast must be mutated in order to cause cancer. In inherited cases, the first hit is carried in the germline. A second hit to any retinoblast will result in cancer, making it more likely that multiple tumors will occur. In sporadic cases, both hits have to occur in the same retinoblast. This is a rare event, therefore tumors are typically solitary and more often occur later in life.

Answer A is incorrect. p53, not Rb, plays an important regulatory role in apoptosis.

Answer C is incorrect. The G_2/M checkpoint is another important cell-cycle regulatory checkpoint. It provides another opportunity to prevent the cell from undergoing mitosis should the environment be inappropriate for cell replication or there is DNA damage. Some important regulatory proteins at the G_2/M checkpoint include the CHK1 and CHK2 kinases through interactions with G_2-specific cyclin A and CDK2.

Answer D is incorrect. The Rb protein does not promote DNA damage repair. This function is often associated with p53, which is a protein that like Rb, promotes cell-cycle arrest in the presence of DNA damage (or other factors that do not constitute a favorable environment for successful cell replication). In addition, it also initiates the apoptotic cascade in the presence of overwhelming DNA damage that cannot be repaired by the cell.

Answer E is incorrect. The Rb protein does not promote histone acetylation. In fact, the Rb-E2F complex promotes histone deacetylation on chromatin.

12. **The correct answer is A.** Anti-CD3 antibodies that bind to CD3 and trigger destruction of T-lymphocytes (via phagocytes or complement-mediated lysis) would be most useful in this scenario, as CD8+ T-lymphocytes are the main effectors mediating acute allograft rejection. Note that monoclonal antibodies may be triggering, depleting, or blocking, and therefore it is absolutely necessary to characterize which of these effector functions they elicit, as those three scenarios would have three very different therapeutic applications.

Answer B is incorrect. Cytotoxic T-lymphocytes express CD8, while helper T-lymphocytes express CD4. While targeting CD4 T-lymphocytes may be partially effective, it would be more useful to deplete all T-lymphocytes with an anti-CD3 monoclonal antibody.

Answer C is incorrect. CD14 is a common macrophage cell surface marker.

Answer D is incorrect. CD16 is a common natural killer-cell surface marker.

Answer E is incorrect. CD19 is a common B-lymphocyte surface marker.

13. **The correct answer is B.** The patient has a likely diagnosis of basal cell carcinoma. It is characterized by pink or flesh-colored pearly papules found in sun-exposed areas; the papules are locally invasive but usually nonmetastatic. Histology shows islands of tumor within mucinous dermis, as show in the image. There is a purely basaloid population with minimal stromal response. Areas of palisading nuclei, or small fusiform cells with little cytoplasm and hyperchromic dense nuclei, are characteristic of the disease.

    Answer A is incorrect. Actinic keratosis is a premalignant lesion characterized by small, rough erythematous or brownish papules. It is commonly found in sun-exposed areas and is a precursor to squamous cell carcinoma.

    Answer C is incorrect. Dermatitis herpetiformis is a dermatologic condition associated with celiac disease that is characterized by pruritic papules and vesicles.

    Answer D is incorrect. Melanoma commonly presents with a dysplastic nevus that has undergone malignant transformation. It is commonly found in sun-exposed areas. However, histology would show tumor cells with large nuclei located directly below the epidermis.

    Answer E is incorrect. Seborrheic keratosis is a benign, flat, pigmented squamous proliferation with keratin cysts.

    Answer F is incorrect. Squamous cell carcinoma commonly appears on the hands and face. It is locally invasive but nonmetastatic. Histology is characterized by keratin pearls.

14. **The correct answer is A.** This patient is presenting with a ruptured ectopic pregnancy, which occurs when a blastocyst implants in an inappropriate location, most commonly the ampulla of the uterine tube. This typically presents as described in the question stem and constitutes a medical emergency. The most common risk factors are pelvic inflammatory disease, prior appendicitis or endometriosis, and previous abdominal surgery.

    Answer B is incorrect. This describes appropriate implantation of a blastocyst in a normal pregnancy and is therefore not directly associated with pathology.

    Answer C is incorrect. This describes the likely etiology of acute appendicitis. This will present with right lower quadrant (RLQ) abdominal pain but typically begins with diffuse periumbilical pain that later migrates to the RLQ. This condition is not associated with prior PID, a missed period, or elevated hCG level, and will typically produce a fever.

    Answer D is incorrect. This describes endometriosis. Although this can be associated with irregular bleeding and abdominal/pelvic pain, it does not typically result in missed periods, shock-like signs, or elevated hCG level.

    Answer E is incorrect. When two sperm fertilize a single ovum, a partial hydatidiform mole is formed. Like a ruptured ectopic pregnancy, this will produce vaginal bleeding and an elevated hCG level but will not cause acute shock-like signs and is not associated with prior PID. It will also cause a rapid increase in uterine size.

15. **The correct answer is E.** The right posterior cerebral artery (PCA) supplies the right occipital lobe, which is responsible for perceiving the left lateral visual field in both eyes. The occipital pole is the extreme posterior end of the occipital lobe, which houses the fibers that originate from the macula. The macula is responsible for central vision. Thus PCA infarcts that spare the occipital pole cause hemianopia

(in this case, left homonymous hemianopia) with sparing of central vision.

Answer A is incorrect. A lesion in the optic chiasm would cause bitemporal hemianopia, not left homonymous hemianopia. The most common cause of optic chiasm lesions is a pituitary adenoma.

Answer B is incorrect. Infarction of the lower division of the middle cerebral artery would cause defects of the temporal lobe, including the lower optic radiations (Meyer's loop). Such lesions would cause contralateral superior quadrantanopia, or "pie in the sky" defects.

Answer C is incorrect. A left retinal artery occlusion with sparing of the vessels supplying the macula could cause a hemianopia of the left eye, with macular sparing, but "left homonymous hemianopia" means that the left visual field of *both* eyes is defective.

Answer D is incorrect. Meyer's loop refers to the inferior division of optic radiations as they pass through the temporal lobe. Meyer's loop lesions are caused by middle cerebral artery infarcts. All PCA lesions should spare Meyer's loop. This answer choice does not support the macular sparing seen in our patient, a phenomenon caused by sparing of the occipital pole.

16. **The correct answer is A.** This patient is most likely taking doxorubicin, which is associated with cardiotoxicity. Doxorubicin and daunorubicin are DNA intercalators that act by binding to DNA and disrupting nucleic acid synthesis. The risk of heart failure is related to the current dose and cumulative dose administered to the patient. Patients can present in acute heart failure, with ECG changes, arrhythmias, pericarditis, or myocardial infarction. Chronic use of these agents can lead to congestive heart failure, as seen in this patient, particularly a dilated cardiomyopathy. Other adverse effects of doxorubicin include bone marrow suppression, local skin irritation, and red urine. Other cardiotoxic chemotherapeutic agents include fluorouracil, busulfan, cisplatin, mitoxantrone, and paclitaxel.

Answer B is incorrect. Methotrexate inhibits dihydrofolate reductase in the S phase of the cell cycle, causing decreased synthesis of purines. Adverse effects include gastrointestinal (GI) irritation, mucositis, bone marrow suppression, and renal failure. Methotrexate is also used as an anti-inflammatory agent and to induce abortion. It is not associated with cardiotoxicity.

Answer C is incorrect. Vincristine and vinblastine inhibit microtubule formation and prevent assembly of the mitotic spindle. Adverse effects include neurotoxicity, fever, vomiting, and (with vinblastine) severe bone marrow supression. These agents are not associated with cardiotoxicity.

Answer D is incorrect. 6-Mercaptopurine acts as a false metabolite and blocks purine synthesis. Adverse effects include myelosuppression, GI effects, and liver toxicity. 6-Mercaptopurine is not associated with cardiotoxicity.

Answer E is incorrect. Tamoxifen is a selective estrogen receptor modulator used as an adjuvant or preventative treatment for breast cancer. It acts as a partial agonist at the estrogen receptor. Adverse effects include endometrial hyperplasia and carcinoma, increased bone density, hypercoagulability, hot flashes, night sweats, and vaginal discharge. Tamoxifen is not associated with cardiotoxicity.

17. **The correct answer is A.** The image shows a genital herpes lesion, which is caused by the herpes simplex virus (HSV). The treatment for genital herpes is acyclovir, usually given orally. Acyclovir is activated by viral thymidine kinase to form a complex that inhibits viral DNA polymerase. Intravenous (IV) acyclovir can cause phlebitis, headache, nausea, neurotoxicity, and renal toxicity. Neurotoxicity can manifest as lethargy, confusion, tremor, delirium, or seizures. Kidney injury can take the form of a crystalluria that can lead to obstructive nephropathy or interstitial nephritis. Lesions of HSV infection consist of vesicles, pustules, and ulcers on an erythematous base. Patients complain of pain, itching, dysuria, and vaginal or urethral discharge. A primary episode is usu-

ally accompanied by fever, malaise, and myalgias. Subsequent episodes resolve faster and have fewer systemic symptoms.

Answer B is incorrect. Fluconazole is an antifungal agent that inhibits fungal steroid synthesis. It is used to treat candidiasis and cryptococcal meningitis and as prophylaxis against fungal infections in immunocompromised patients. It can cause GI upset, alopecia, elevated liver enzyme levels, and occasionally neurotoxicity. Vulvovaginal candidiasis (a yeast infection) is associated with erythematous labia with shallow ulcerations, and tiny papules ("satellite lesions") beyond the main area of erythema. Patients complain of pruritus, dysuria, and dyspareunia. The discharge classically associated with vaginal candidiasis is thick and white. Simple vulvovaginal candidiasis is not accompanied by systemic symptoms such as fever and muscle aches.

Answer C is incorrect. Metronidazole is used to treat infections caused by protozoa and anaerobic bacteria, including *Trichomonas vaginalis* and bacterial vaginosis. It works by forming DNA-damaging metabolites in the bacterial cell. Adverse effects of metronidazole include a disulfiram-like reaction with alcohol ingestion, GI distress, headache, a metallic taste, and, rarely, neurotoxicity. Infection with *T vaginalis* presents with a malodorous, frothy green discharge, vaginal pruritus, and erythema. Bacterial vaginosis, which is usually due to *Gardnerella vaginalis* infection, presents with perivaginal inflammation and irritation, dysuria, dyspareunia, and a grayish discharge with a "fishy" odor. Neither illness is usually accompanied by systemic symptoms or demarcated vaginal lesions as seen in the image.

Answer D is incorrect. Penicillin is the treatment of choice for syphilis. It is a β-lactam antibiotic and inhibits bacterial cell-wall synthesis. Adverse effects include hypersensitivity reactions and hemolytic anemia. A syphilitic chancre, indicative of primary syphilis, is usually a solitary, painless, 1- to 2-cm papule with an indurated base. Primary infection is not accompanied by systemic symptoms.

Answer E is incorrect. Ribavirin is an antiviral agent used to treat chronic hepatitis C (HCV) or respiratory syncytial virus infections. The oral form is associated with hemolytic anemia and headache, and the aerosolized form is associated with bronchospasm, rash, and conjunctival irritation.

18. **The correct answer is D.** This patient is presenting with acute mental status changes and seizures secondary to severe hyponatremia. A hyponatremia of this severity in the presence of decreased serum osmolality is highly suggestive of the syndrome of inappropriate ADH secretion (SIADH). Given this patient's history of COPD, which is almost always secondary to an extensive history of smoking, and the presence of SIADH, this patient is most likely presenting with a paraneoplastic syndrome secondary to small cell lung cancer. This cancer has a high association with smoking, and is known to present in particular with SIADH. A hint for the future: a sodium ion level in the 120s is almost always suggestive of SIADH.

Answer A is incorrect. While it is certainly possible to become hyponatremic from excessive fluid intake (polydipsia), one would not expect to see a hyponatremia of this severity purely from drinking too much fluid. In addition, a patient who is purely drinking too much should have relatively appropriate compensatory mechanisms, such as the ability to suppress ADH secretion. This would lead to water loss from the kidneys to compensate, and thus serum osmolality should not decrease. This patient clearly has a pathologically low serum osmolality, essentially ruling out polydipsia as the cause of this patient's hyponatremia.

Answer B is incorrect. A new-onset seizure in an older adult always raises concern for a primary brain process, especially tumor. While primary brain tumors can certainly present with mental status changes or seizures, and can be associated with SIADH, this patient's lung pathology and probable smoking history place her at a much higher risk of lung cancer than for primary brain cancer. So while both are certainly possible, small cell lung cancer is much more likely in this patient.

Answer C is incorrect. Mental status changes and seizures always raise concern for pathology occurring in the brain, in particular space-occupying lesions such as tumors. Metastatic tumors in the brain are much more common than primary brain tumors. While this patient's age and smoking history place her at increased risk for breast cancer, the paraneoplastic syndromes associated with breast cancer do not include SIADH. This patient's hyponatremia in the setting of COPD make small cell lung cancer far more likely.

Answer E is incorrect. While squamous cell lung cancer is clearly associated with smoking, the paraneoplastic syndrome it presents with is usually the secretion of a parathyroid-like peptide, which causes signs and symptoms relating to the resultant hypercalcemia, such as fatigue, depression, muscle weakness, abdominal pain, nausea, and constipation.

19. **The correct answer is E.** Degraded tetracycline is associated with Fanconi syndrome, a disorder of proximal tubule function that results in severe loss of protein, glucose, and essential minerals (especially calcium and magnesium). Tetracycline's primary degradation product is anhydro-4-epitetracycline, which is toxic and accumulates in the proximal tubules to cause Fanconi syndrome. Patients present with symptoms of polydipsia, polyuria, and dehydration due to excess loss of water and solutes in their urine.

Answer A is incorrect. Acute tubular necrosis is typically associated with hypoperfusion and is not associated with either Fanconi syndrome or tetracycline.

Answer B is incorrect. Glomerulonephritis is most often caused by immune complex deposition and is not associated with either Fanconi syndrome or tetracycline.

Answer C is incorrect. Kidney stones, commonly caused by hypercalciuria or infection, are not associated with either Fanconi syndrome or tetracycline.

Answer D is incorrect. Renal papillary necrosis, often caused by diabetes or acute pyelonephritis, is not associated with either Fanconi syndrome or tetracycline. Renal papillary necrosis can be caused by an overdose of analgesics such as aspirin, phenacetin, and acetaminophen. Necrosis results from a combination of decreased blood flow to the kidney, consumption of antioxidants, and subsequent oxidative damage.

20. **The correct answer is B.** Histrionic personality disorder is one of the cluster B personality disorders (the "wild" group) that presents early in adulthood. It is best characterized as a pattern of excessive emotionality and attention seeking, and it is often accompanied by somatoform disorders (somatization is a process by which an individual uses his or her body or symptoms for a range of psychologic purposes and gains). An especially important characteristic to remember about histrionic personality disorder is the often overtly sexual nature of those affected. Relationships with physicians in particular are affected by the patient's attention-seeking behavior, as is evident in this case by the patient reporting both sleep deprivation and depression without objective signs of either.

Answer A is incorrect. Type 1 bipolar disorder is characterized by manic episodes (periods of elevated or irritable mood that must last at least one week) as well as depressive syndromes and mixed syndromes. Sleep of seven-nine hours per night is not usually consistent with a manic syndrome.

Answer C is incorrect. Obsessive-compulsive personality disorder is characterized by an excessive preoccupation with control, order, and perfectionism. This patient presents none of these characteristics.

Answer D is incorrect. Paranoid personality disorder is characterized by the inherent belief that the world is a dangerous and threatening place. Upon meeting these individuals they often project strength and capability, and their distrust and suspiciousness of everyone is evident. These individuals tend to believe in various conspiracy theories.

Answer E is incorrect. Schizotypal personality disorder is characterized by interpersonal awkwardness, odd beliefs or magical thinking, and an eccentric appearance.

21. **The correct answer is E.** This patient is experiencing neurosyphilis caused by *Treponema pallidum*. Doxycycline can be used in the treatment of both syphilis and *Chlamydia* infection. When the dorsal columns are progressively demyelinated and the posterior nerve roots are sclerosed, the condition is referred to as tabes (Latin for "shriveled") dorsalis. These patients have decreased reflexes, decreased pain sensation, and decreased proprioception. In this situation the patient's chief complaint was ataxia associated with walking, which is caused by his lack of proprioception. The Romberg test is useful in this situation, because it can reveal a loss of proprioception when visual input is removed. Generally, the pathophysiology of syphilis is based on obliterative endarteritis; however, the precise cause of tabes dorsalis is not fully understood. In the spinal cord the disease is limited to the dorsal columns.

    Answer A is incorrect. HSV type 1 can cause viral encephalitis. However, the swelling and inflammation occur in the brain, not the spinal cord. Infection is treated with acyclovir.

    Answer B is incorrect. HIV can cause a myelopathy (usually in untreated patients with low T-lymphocyte counts) that can manifest as a painful or painless syndrome. This disease mimics the neuropathy associated with cobalamin deficiency. Infection is treated with a cocktail of three anti-retroviral drugs.

    Answer C is incorrect. Tuberculosis (TB) can invade the spinal column and cause bone destruction, it can compress various regions of the spinal cord, or it can do both. This often is called Pott disease, and the first symptom usually is pain rather than ataxia. TB can be treated with long-term courses of the antibiotics isoniazid and rifampin.

    Answer D is incorrect. Poliovirus has a specific trophism to motor neurons, and its lesions directly target the anterior horns of the spinal cord. Infection is prevented by vaccination.

22. **The correct answer is C.** Sphingomyelinase converts sphingomyelin to cerebroside. Deficiency of sphingomyelinase in Niemann-Pick disease causes accumulation of sphingomyelin and cholesterol in parenchymal and reticuloendothelial cells.

    Answer A is incorrect. α-galactosidase A converts ceramide trihexoside to lactosyl cerebroside. This enzyme is deficient in Fabry disease.

    Answer B is incorrect. β-galactosidase converts galactocerebroside to cerebroside. This enzyme is deficient in Krabbe disease.

    Answer D is incorrect. β-glucocerebrosidase converts glucocerebroside to cerebroside. This enzyme is deficient in Gaucher disease.

    Answer E is incorrect. Hexosaminidase A converts ganglioside M_2 to ganglioside M_3. This enzyme is deficient in Tay-Sachs disease.

23. **The correct answer is E.** A positive inotropic agent would increase the contractility of the heart, causing both stroke volume and cardiac output to increase at any given end-diastolic volume. Therefore the curve would shift up and to the left.

    Answer A is incorrect. The Starling curve does not change its shape in response to inotropic agents; rather, it shifts to the left and upward.

    Answer B is incorrect. A shift down and to the left indicates a very low end-diastolic volume and cardiac output, which would occur in instances of decreased blood volume such as in severe hemorrhage.

    Answer C is incorrect. A shift of the Starling curve down and to the right would indicate an increasingly failing heart. A positive inotropic agent would affect the heart in the opposite manner and ameliorate the effects of heart failure.

    Answer D is incorrect. The Starling curve shifts left, not right, as end-diastolic volume decreases.

Answer F is incorrect. A shift up and to the right would indicate that there is an extremely high cardiac output along with a high end-diastolic volume. This would occur in the presence of an extremely high blood volume, not an increase in contractility.

24. **The correct answer is A.** Anorexia nervosa is an eating disorder characterized by excessive dieting, excessive exercising, and body image disturbances. It is most common in adolescents and young adults. Physiologic consequences of the condition include severe weight loss, amenorrhea, lanugo (downy body hair on the trunk), melanosis coli (a blackened area on the colon as a result of laxative abuse), an increased risk of osteoporosis, mild anemia, leukopenia, and electrolyte disturbances. This patient's amenorrhea and very low body weight indicate that she may be suffering from anorexia. She also has symptoms of depression: sadness, anhedonia, feelings of guilt, and suicidal ideation. Although she may benefit from therapy and an antidepressant medication, her electrolyte disturbances put her at risk for seizures, and contraindicate the use of bupropion, which is an atypical antidepressant. Bupropion functions as a norepinephrine and dopamine reuptake inhibitor, and unlike other selective serotonin reuptake inhibitors, it does not carry sexual adverse effects.

Answer B is incorrect. Buspirone is a serotonin 5-hydroxytryptamine$_{1A}$-receptor partial agonist used to treat depression and generalized anxiety disorder. This drug does not cause addiction or sedation, and does not interact with alcohol. Seizure is not a contraindication against its use.

Answer C is incorrect. Haloperidol is a high-potency, typical anti-psychotic drug. It is a dopamine receptor antagonist used for the treatment of schizophrenia. It is not indicated for the treatment of depression. It is associated with a relatively high incidence of extrapyramidal symptoms, such as dystonia and ultimately tardive dyskinesia. However, seizure is not a contraindication against its use.

Answer D is incorrect. Phenelzine is a monoamine oxidase (MAO) inhibitor. Seizure is not a contraindication to its use. Tyramine crisis, a potentially lethal condition, may occur when patients taking MAO inhibitors ingest tyramine-rich foods (eg, certain cheeses and wine). However, it is not contraindicated in patients who have seizures.

Answer E is incorrect. Sertraline is selective serotonin reuptake inhibitor. It is not contraindicated in patients with seizures. Concomitant use of a MAO inhibitor may precipitate a dangerous complication known as serotonin syndrome.

25. **The correct answer is B.** Graft-versus-host disease (GVHD) is an unwanted side effect of bone marrow transplantation whereby donor T-lymphocytes recognize the recipient as foreign and mount an immune response. The organs most often affected are the gut, skin, and liver. Human leukocyte antigen matching of the donor and recipient can help reduce the severity of GVHD, but the disease may still occur due to a minor histocompatibility mismatch.

Answer A is incorrect. Acute graft rejection is a potential side effect of solid organ transplant and is mediated by the recipient's cytotoxic T-lymphocytes. The recipient of a bone marrow transplant undergoes myeloablative therapy before transplant, and therefore it is not expected that the patient would have significant numbers of T-lymphocytes.

Answer C is incorrect. GVHD is mediated by donor T-lymphocytes; recipient T-lymphocytes are ablated before transplant.

Answer D is incorrect. Hyperacute graft rejection is a potential side effect of solid organ transplant and is mediated by preformed recipient antibodies. It occurs within minutes to hours post-transplant.

Answer E is incorrect. The clinical scenario described is more suggestive of GVHD than recurrence of leukemia.

26. **The correct answer is B.** Enzyme-linked immunosorbent assay has a high false-positive

rate, and its result must be confirmed by Western blot. The Western blot is a highly specific test with a very low false-positive rate, such that a positive reaction for two of the three commonly tested HIV antigens indicates disease. Positive and negative controls are commonly used in the same batch to ensure that the assay was successful. The most appropriate next step is to establish a risk profile for this patient by obtaining the CD4+ count.

Answer A is incorrect. Once a CD4+ count is established and viral load obtained, this patient should begin appropriate prophylactic treatment for opportunistic infections such as *Pneumocystis jiroveci* pneumonia. For anti-retroviral treatment, a combination of highly active anti-retroviral therapy (also known as HAART) is the appropriate approach, not AZT monotherapy.

Answer C is incorrect. There is no reason to believe contamination has occurred. In fact, if the positive control antibodies were mistakenly loaded in the patient's sample lane, one would expect that there would be three bands present in that lane.

Answer D is incorrect. Both the positive and negative controls worked well, as three bands are clearly present in the positive control lane, and no bands are evident in the negative control lane.

Answer E is incorrect. The Western blot is confirmatory for HIV.

27. **The correct answer is D.** Vincristine and other vinca alkaloids block the polymerization of microtubules, thereby preventing the formation of a mitotic spindle. The mitotic spindle is necessary for mitosis; thus, vincristine is specific to the M phase.

Answer A is incorrect. Vincristine prevents the formation of the mitotic spindle through the blockage of microtubule polymerization. Therefore, it is specific to the M phase.

Answer B is incorrect. Vincristine prevents the formation of the mitotic spindle through the blockage of microtubule polymerization. Therefore, it is specific to the M phase.

Answer C is incorrect. Podophyllotoxins and bleomycin are specific to the G_2 phase of the cell cycle.

Answer E is incorrect. Antimetabolites and podophyllotoxins are S-phase specific.

28. **The correct answer is A.** This patient is exhibiting classic symptoms of Sheehan syndrome, or postpartum hypopituitarism. Although Sheehan syndrome is thought to result from infarction of the pituitary gland from severe bleeding and hypotension during delivery, most patients do not experience hypotension or severe blood loss in delivery. Patients exhibit signs of global hypopituitarism and often present complaining of fatigue, anorexia, poor lactation, and loss of pubic and axillary hair. Treatment includes replacement of all deficient hormones.

Answer B is incorrect. These lab values suggest primary hypothyroidism. Patients with hypothyroidism can present with weight gain, cold intolerance, weakness, myxedema and fatigue. Primary hypothyroidism can result from iodine deficiency, surgical removal of the thyroid gland, pharmacologic thyroid ablation, or autoimmune attack, as in Hashimoto thyroiditis.

Answer C is incorrect. Primary hypothyroidism can present with these lab values. Increased thyrotropin-releasing hormone can cause elevated prolactin levels as well as elevated levels of thyroid-stimulating hormone (TSH). Patients can, therefore, present with galactorrhea in addition to normal symptoms of hypothyroidism, such as weight gain, cold intolerance, weakness, myxedema, and fatigue.

Answer D is incorrect. In this set of lab values, serum ACTH is elevated while thyroxine and TSH are normal, indicating Cushing syndrome. Cushing can be caused by a primary pituitary adenoma, an adrenal neoplasm, ectopic ACTH production, or exogenous administration of corticosteroids. Patients with Cushing syndrome present with hypertension, weight gain, moon facies, increased truncal obesity, hyperglycemia, amenorrhea, immune suppression, and skin changes, such as skin thinning and abdominal striae.

Answer E is incorrect. In this set of lab values, thyroxine is elevated, while TSH is decreased. This represents the hormone levels present in primary hyperthyroidism, such as Graves disease, which results from stimulation of the thyroid gland by autoimmune antibodies. Symptoms of hyperthyroidism include heat intolerance, hyperactivity, weight loss, heart palpitations, diarrhea, increased reflexes, and exophthalmia.

29. **The correct answer is E.** This patient has thymic aplasia (DiGeorge syndrome), in which the third and fourth pharyngeal pouches, and thus the thymus and parathyroid glands, fail to develop. This disease often presents with congenital defects such as cardiac abnormalities, cleft palate, and abnormal facies. Patients suffer frequent viral and fungal infections because of T-cell deficiency.

    Answer A is incorrect. High IgM levels and normal T cell number are suggestive of hyper-IgM syndrome, in which B cells are unable to class switch because of a defect in helper T cells. Patients have normal numbers of T cells and high IgM levels; levels of IgA, IgE, and IgG are low.

    Answer B is incorrect. Hypogammaglobulinemia with normal T cell number is characteristic of Bruton agammaglobulinemia, an X-linked defect in a tyrosine kinase that is necessary for B cell maturation. After six months of age, when the levels of maternal antibodies have declined, patients with the disease tend to present with recurrent bacterial infections.

    Answer C is incorrect. Hypogammaglobulinemia with reduced T cell numbers is suggestive of severe combined immunodeficiency (SCID). SCID presents with recurrent viral, bacterial, fungal, and protozoal infections due to a total lack of cellular immunity secondary to a stem cell deficit in the bone marrow. SCID does not present with the congenital defects described in the vignette.

    Answer D is incorrect. Low IgM levels and normal T cell numbers are typical of Wiskott-Aldrich syndrome, an X-linked defect associated with elevated IgA levels, elevated IgE levels, normal IgG levels, and low IgM levels. It involves a defect in the body's ability to mount an IgM response to bacteria. Patients have a normal number of T cells, but their T cells respond ineffectively to antigens. Recurrent pyogenic infections, eczema, and thrombocytopenia are the typical symptoms. Wiscott-Aldrich syndrome does not present with any specific enzyme abnormality.

30. **The correct answer is E.** This patient demonstrates several characteristics classic for neurofibromatosis type 1 (also known as von Recklinghausen disease). Potential findings include café au lait spots, two or more neurofibromas, optic glioma, iris hamartomas (Lisch nodules), a positive family history (autosomal dominant inheritance), and a distinctive bony lesion such as sphenoid dysplasia or scoliosis. Patients with this disease generally demonstrate 95% of the criteria by age 8 years and all of the criteria by age 20. These patients are also at increased risk for tumors. The gene is located on the long arm of chromosome 17.

    Answer A is incorrect. Bilateral acoustic neuromas are characteristic of neurofibromatosis type 2. It is much less common than type 1 and typically manifests with multiple central nervous system tumors. The *NF2* gene is located on chromosome 22.

    Answer B is incorrect. Bilateral renal cell carcinoma occurs in von Hippel-Lindau disease, an autosomal dominant disease that is characterized by hemangioblastomas of the retina, cerebellum, and medulla. About half of patients develop bilateral renal cell carcinomas. The disease is associated with the deletion of the *VHL* gene located on chromosome 3, which is a tumor suppressor gene.

    Answer C is incorrect. Cystic medial necrosis of the aorta leading to aortic insufficiency and dissecting aortic aneurysm is associated with Marfan syndrome, a connective tissue disorder caused by the autosomal dominant inheritance of a defective fibrillin gene.

Answer D is incorrect. Leptomeningeal angioma is associated with Sturge-Weber syndrome (SWS), which is a rare congenital vascular disorder of unknown etiology affecting capillary-sized blood vessels. Its characteristic features include angiomas and a facial port-wine stain. Only a small portion of patients with port-wine stains at birth have SWS.

31. **The correct answer is A.** Hemophilia (types A and B) is an X-linked recessive disorder, with affected male individuals inheriting a defective copy of the X chromosome from heterozygous (asymptomatic) mothers. It is caused by a deficiency in factor VIII (hemophilia A) or factor IX (hemophilia B) of the clotting cascade. Platelet number and bleeding time are normal because there is no deficiency of platelet function. Prothrombin time (PT) measures activity of factors VII, X, V, prothrombin, and fibrinogen, thus it is also normal in hemophilia. Partial thromboplastin time (PTT) measures activity of factors VIII, IX, XI, and XII in addition to factors X, V, prothrombin and fibrinogen. PTT is therefore elevated in the case of factor VIII or IX deficiency.

Answer B is incorrect. This profile describes qualitative platelet defects such as Bernard-Soulier disease and Glanzmann thrombasthenia. Since there is no clotting factor deficiency, PT and PPT are normal.

Answer C is incorrect. This profile describes von Willebrand disease, an autosomal dominant disease. Von Willebrand factor promotes platelet adhesion to damaged endopthelium, therefore its deficiency prolongs bleeding time. It also serves as a carrier for factor VIII, so PTT is also prolonged in this disorder.

Answer D is incorrect. This profile describes thrombocytopenia. Since there is no clotting factor deficiency, PT and PPT time are normal. Since platelets are low, bleeding time is prolonged.

Answer E is incorrect. This profile describes disseminated intravascular coagulation (DIC). In this disorder, widespread intravascular coagulation consumes platelets and clotting factors, resulting in lab findings indicative of a deficiency in all elements of the clotting machinery. In DIC one would also see an increase in fibrin split products and D-dimers.

32. **The correct answer is B.** In the lung, α_1-antitrypsin deficiency predisposes to chronic obstructive pulmonary disease, specifically panacinar emphysema. Additionally, misfolded gene products of α_1-antitrypsin can be deposited in the hepatocellular endoplasmic reticulum. Therefore, patients with α_1-antitrypsin deficiency are at increased risk for developing end-stage liver disease like cirrhosis.

Answer A is incorrect. Cor pulmonale can present with dyspnea and is the result of dysfunction of the right ventricle caused by pulmonary hypertension in diseases affecting the lung or its vasculature. Patients with α_1-antitrypsin deficiency are not known to have increased risk of cor pulmonale.

Answer C is incorrect. *Pseudomonas aeruginosa* is commonly associated with nosocomial infections through contaminated ventilators or bronchoscopes. In the community, immunocompromised patients (eg, HIV-positive and transplant patients) are most susceptible to *Pseudomonas* infection. α_1-antitrypsin deficiency is not known to increase the risk of pseudomonal pneumonia.

Answer D is incorrect. Renal cysts are associated with inheritable renal conditions such as autosomal-dominant polycystic kidney disease, tuberous sclerosis, and Von Hippel-Lindau syndrome. α_1-antitrypsin is not present in the kidney and thus is not associated with development of renal cysts.

33. **The correct answer is E.** The disease described in this patient is acute myelogenous leukemia (AML). This condition is characterized by acute onset of myelosuppression and the presence of increased myeloblasts in the peripheral smear and bone marrow. One subtype of AML is acute promyelocytic leukemia with abnormal presence of t(15;17), which en-

codes for a fusion protein of the retinoic acid receptor with the promyelocytic leukemia gene. Auer rods, as shown in the image, are often present in this condition.

Answer A is incorrect. In general, translocations involving chromosome 14 occur in B-cell lymphomas, as the locus for immunoglobulin production is on chromosome 14. Translocation t(8:14) is associated with Burkitt lymphoma and induces overproduction of the *c-myc* oncogene.

Answer B is incorrect. Translocation t(9;22), also known as the Philadelphia chromosome, which encodes the Bcr-Abl fusion protein, is found in more than 90% of cases of chronic myelogenous leukemia (CML). If this translocation is found in an acute leukemia, it is associated with a poor prognosis. The Bcr-Abl fusion protein is a constitutively active tyrosine kinase that drives the cells to express a cancerous phenotype.

Answer C is incorrect. Translocation t(11;22), found in Ewing sarcoma of bone, results in production of the EWS transcription factor, which induces the overexpression of various oncogenes such as *bcl-1*.

Answer D is incorrect. Translocation t(11;14) is associated with mantle cell lymphoma, a type of lymphoma with a very poor prognosis. The translocation produces increased activity of cyclin D1, which causes rapid progression of the cell cycle.

34. **The correct answer is C.** Misoprostol is a prostaglandin E_1 analog that can be used to prevent ulcers produced by nonsteroidal anti-inflammatory drug use. It is also used as a medical abortifacient in many countries, particularly Latin American countries, and is therefore strictly contraindicated in pregnant women. Prostaglandins E_1 (misoprostol) and E_2 have been successfully used to induce labor by activating the dissolution of collagen bundles, increasing the submucosal water content of the cervix and potentiating effects of endogenous oxytocin. As an antacid, misoprostol acts on parietal cells to inhibit acid secretion and stimulate bicarbonate and mucus production.

Answer A is incorrect. Cimetidine is an H_2-antagonist and is associated with headache, confusion, gynecomastia, thrombocytopenia, and inhibition of the cytochrome P450 system. It is not considered a teratogen and can be taken safely by pregnant women.

Answer B is incorrect. Magnesium hydroxide is an antacid that is not absorbed and does not exhibit any systemic adverse effects. It is associated with diarrhea, but it is not considered a teratogen and can thus be taken safely by pregnant women.

Answer D is incorrect. Omeprazole is an irreversible proton pump inhibitor. It is used to treat hypersecretory states, recurrent ulcers, gastroesophageal reflux disease, and stress-related gastritis. It is associated with headache and GI disturbances. It is not considered a teratogen and can be taken safely by pregnant women.

Answer E is incorrect. Sucralfate is a polysaccharide combined with aluminum hydroxide. It binds to ulcers, providing a physical protective barrier. It has been known to cause constipation and nausea, but it is not considered a teratogen and can be taken safely by pregnant women.

35. **The correct answer is E.** This patient has clinical evidence of multiple endocrine neoplasia (MEN) type I, which can cause tumors in the "3 P's": the **P**ituitary gland, the **P**arathyroid gland, and the **P**ancreas. The MEN I syndrome follows an autosomal dominant pattern of inheritance, thus this patient's family history of multiple endocrine organ abnormalities further supports this diagnosis. In this patient, parathyroid involvement is suggested by hypercalcemia; and a pituitary adenoma is most likely causing his bitemporal hemianopsia. This patient has signs and symptoms consistent with elevated levels of vasoactive intestinal peptide (VIP). VIP acts on the gut mucosa to promote Na^+ secretion, causing a secretory diarrhea. VIP also stimulates K^+ secretion in the colon, causing hypokalemia, which can lead to the muscle weakness, tetany, and even periodic paralysis seen in this patient. Finally,

VIP inhibits gastric acid secretion, leading to hypochlorhydria, which can be tested by an elevated pH on nasogastric suction fluid. The majority of VIPomas arise within the pancreas and are one type of pancreatic tumor seen in MEN I.

Answer A is incorrect. Carcinoid tumors are malignant neuroendocrine tumors that tend to arise in the GI tract. These tumors may secrete substances such as serotonin and, when they metastasize, they may cause carcinoid syndrome (symptoms include bronchoconstriction, cutaneous flushing, diarrhea, and right-sided valvular heart disease). Carcinoid tumors are not known to be associated with any of the MEN syndromes.

Answer B is incorrect. Gastrinomas are non-β islet cell tumors that commonly arise from the pancreas and secrete gastrin, leading to hypersecretion of hydrochloric acid. Although gastrinomas do cause diarrhea and are associated with MEN I, the pH of the nasogastric suction fluid would be decreased, not increased, in a patient with a gastrinoma.

Answer C is incorrect. Insulinomas are islet cell tumors that secrete insulin. These tumors are associated with Whipple triad: hypoglycemia, symptoms of hypoglycemia that include mental status changes, and relief of symptoms upon glucose administration.

Answer D is incorrect. Pheochromocytoma is a tumor arising from the chromaffin cells of the adrenal medulla. It is associated with MEN types II and III (but not MEN type I), and its symptoms include episodic palpitations, hypertension, and other adrenergic symptoms.

36. **The correct answer is D.** Paget disease of the bone is characterized by three stages: an initial osteolytic lesion involving marked bone resorption, a period of disorganized bone formation, and a final sclerotic or burned-out phase. The primary abnormality is the overproduction and overactivity of osteoclasts, which are derived from the bone marrow. Alkaline phosphatase is a marker of bone formation, whereas hydroxyproline signifies bone resorption. During the period of haphazard bone formation, bone-specific alkaline phosphatase levels are elevated. Rarely, the total alkaline phosphatase level is normal while the bone-specific alkaline phosphatase level is elevated. The level of elevation of alkaline phosphatase rarely exceeds 10 times the upper limit of normal. The serum phosphate level stays normal, while the calcium level may be normal or slightly elevated.

Answer A is incorrect. A value of 20 U/L is an abnormally low level of alkaline phosphatase. It would not be found in a patient who was forming large amounts of bone. The phosphate level is within normal limits.

Answer B is incorrect. A value of 50 U/L is within the normal range of alkaline phosphatase, and it is not likely to be found during the osteoblastic phase of the disease. The phosphate level is elevated; Paget disease is associated with a normal level of phosphate.

Answer C is incorrect. A value of 100 U/L is within the normal range of alkaline phosphatase. It is not likely to be found during the osteoblastic phase of the disease. Furthermore, the phosphate level in this choice is elevated; Paget disease is associated with a normal level of phosphate.

Answer E is incorrect. A value of 1500 U/L is >10 times the normal level of alkaline phosphatase, and it is not likely to be found, even in patients with highly active Paget disease. Highly elevated alkaline phosphatase levels are typically found in patients with involvement of the skull and at least one other site. In addition, this phosphate level is elevated, which is not typically seen in Paget disease.

37. **The correct answer is C.** The patient most likely has hyperprolactinemia. Increased secretion of prolactin explains the lactation in the absence of recent pregnancy and breastfeeding. Also, because prolactin inhibits gonadotropin-releasing hormone synthesis and release, the patient is experiencing menstrual irregularities. Hyperprolactinemia commonly is caused by tumors or anti-psychotic drugs. Anti-psychotic agents are dopamine antagonists and lead to increased secretion of prolactin (dopa-

mine inhibits prolactin release). The patient has most likely been diagnosed with a psychiatric disorder such as schizophrenia that requires dopamine suppression.

Answer A is incorrect. Premature menopause is associated with loss of ovarian function before the age of 40 years. The cause usually is idiopathic. Lab tests will reveal high levels of follicle-stimulating hormone and luteinizing hormone, with low levels of estrogen. However, with premature menopause we would not expect to see high levels of prolactin and lactation.

Answer B is incorrect. Parkinson disease is a movement disorder characterized by four cardinal signs: resting tremor, rigidity, bradykinesia, and postural instability. Because the disorder stems from a lack of dopamine (which functions in the basal ganglia to stimulate the motor cortex), one type of medication used to treat Parkinson disease is the dopamine agonist. However, dopamine downregulates prolactin. Thus, we would not expect to see effects of hyperprolactinemia if the patient were taking a medication to treat Parkinson disease.

Answer D is incorrect. Turner syndrome is a chromosomal disorder (45,XO). It frequently is diagnosed via amniocentesis during pregnancy. Typical physical features include a webbed neck, short stature, low-set ears, low hairline, and lymphedema. Females with Turner syndrome may be infertile and may have primary amenorrhea, unlike this patient, who has menstrual irregularities (secondary amenorrhea).

Answer E is incorrect. Drugs for treating type 2 diabetes include metformin, sulfonylureas, glitazones, and α-glucosidase inhibitors. None of these drugs would produce hyperprolactinemia. Notably, sulfonylureas can cause hypoglycemia. Metformin rarely causes lactic acidosis. Glitazones may cause weight gain and hepatotoxicity. α-glucosidase inhibitors may cause GI disturbances.

38. **The correct answer is A.** This patient has developed cirrhosis of the liver from chronic HCV infection. In addition to the physical exam findings suggestive of cirrhosis (jaundice, spider angiomata, ascites), the patient has decreased liver synthetic function (elevated PT, low albumin). This patient also manifests signs of hepatic encephalopathy, including asterixis (flapping tremor), confusion, and lethargy. The etiology of hepatic encephalopathy is not entirely understood, but it is thought that ammonia acts as a toxin to the central nervous system when it is not converted into urea by the cirrhotic liver. Lactulose, when digested by colonic bacteria, acidifies the colonic contents. This acidification then converts ammonia into a nonabsorbable protonated form. It also changes the bowel flora so that fewer ammonia-forming organisms are present.

Answer B is incorrect. Although a restricted protein diet should be standard in all patients with end-stage liver disease, it will not acutely decrease ammonia concentrations.

Answer C is incorrect. Although neomycin can be used as an adjunct to decrease ammonia production by gut flora, it is not first-line therapy. Neomycin works by destroying the gut flora that normally produce ammonia. Neomycin is more appropriate for prophylactic treatment of hepatic encephalopathy.

Answer D is incorrect. Lorazepam, as well as other benzodiazepines that are metabolically cleared by the liver, should not be used and can actually worsen the encephalopathy.

Answer E is incorrect. Pentoxifylline is a methylated xanthine derivative that acts as a competitive, nonselective phosphodiesterase inhibitor. Ultimately it decreased tumor necrosis factor-α and leukotriene synthesis, and thus reduces inflammation. It is useful in treating patients with advanced cirrhosis, as it can decrease complications such as hepatic encephalopathy and GI hemorrhage.

39. **The correct answer is E.** *Pneumocystis jiroveci* (formerly *carinii*), like most fungal infections, does not present with symptoms in the immunocompetent host. In children or patients afflicted with HIV, cancer, or inherited immune deficiencies, *P jiroveci* can present with pneumonia. Symptoms begin suddenly. The

patient develops a fever and begins to cough and breathe abnormally fast. Often the patient's lips, fingernails, and skin turn blue or gray because the patient has difficulty drawing in air. On chest x-ray, the diffuse interstitial pneumonia gives a ground-glass appearance. *P jiroveci* infection is treated with trimethoprim-sulfamethoxazole.

Answer A is incorrect. Fluconazole or ketoconazole is used for the treatment of local blastomycosis infections, and amphotericin B is used for the treatment of systemic infections. Blastomycosis can present with flu-like symptoms, fevers, chills, productive cough, myalgia, arthralgia, and pleuritic chest pain. Some patients will fail to recover from an acute infection and develop chronic pulmonary infection or widespread disseminated infection.

Answer B is incorrect. Itraconazole or potassium iodide is used for the treatment of *Sporothrix schenckii* infection. *S schenckii* is the cause of sporotrichosis. When *S schenckii* is introduced into the skin, usually by a thorn prick, it causes a local pustule or ulcer with nodules along draining lymphatics (ascending lymphangitis). *S schenckii* is a dimorphic fungus that has cigar-shaped budding yeast visible in pus.

Answer C is incorrect. Sulfadiazine and pyrimethamine are used to treat toxoplasmosis. *Toxoplasma gondii* infection presents with brain abscesses in HIV-positive patients and with birth defects. *T gondii* is transmitted via cysts in raw meat or cat feces. The definitive stage (sexual stage) occurs in cats. Microscopically, acid-fast staining cysts are found.

Answer D is incorrect. Topical miconazole or selenium sulfide are treatments for *Malassezia furfur*. *M furfur* is the cause of tinea versicolor. Symptoms of this infection include hypopigmented skin lesions that occur in hot and humid conditions.

40. **The correct answer is B.** The **APGAR** scoring system evaluates newborns' general health as a measure of likely survival in the immediate period surrounding birth. Five areas are evaluated on a scale of 0-2 to produce a 10-point score. Values of 7 or higher indicate survival is highly likely; values of 4 or lower indicate greater mortality risk. This child scores one point each for **A**ppearance, **P**ulse, and **R**espiration; he scores 0 points for **G**rimace (ie, no response to noxious stimuli) and **A**ctivity (absence of muscle tone). Thus, his one-minute APGAR score is 3.

Answer A is incorrect. This child has a higher APGAR score than 1.

Answer C is incorrect. This APGAR score is too high for this child.

Answer D is incorrect. This APGAR score is too high for this child.

Answer E is incorrect. This APGAR score is too high for this child.

41. **The correct answer is B.** This patient has neurologic symptoms consistent with vitamin B_{12} (cobalamin) deficiency caused by demyelination of the dorsal columns, spinocerebellar tract, and lateral corticospinal tract. Pernicious anemia is a vitamin B_{12} deficiency associated with chronic atrophic gastritis. Autoantibodies are directed against gastric parietal cells, leading to an intrinsic factor deficiency. Without intrinsic factor, vitamin B_{12} cannot be absorbed in the ileum. Patients may present with fatigue, dyspnea, and tachycardia. A peripheral blood smear will show macrocytic RBCs with hypersegmented polymorphonuclear leukocytes, consistent with megaloblastic anemia (as seen in the image). It is imperative to check folate and vitamin B_{12} levels before beginning treatment with vitamin B_{12} injections.

Answer A is incorrect. Abnormal neural crest cell migration leads to Hirschsprung disease, which is a congenital aganglionic motility disorder affecting the large bowel. Patients present with obstructive symptoms such as constipation, abdominal distention, and bilious emesis.

Answer C is incorrect. The colon is not the site of vitamin B_{12} absorption, and bacterial overgrowth there, such as with *Clostridium difficile*, will produce symptoms such as diarrhea, flatulence, and weight loss.

Answer D is incorrect. Green leafy vegetables contain folate, not vitamin B_{12}. Folate is an essential cofactor in nucleic acid synthesis, and its deficiency commonly leads to megaloblastic anemia as seen in the image. Therapy with folate should not be started until vitamin B_{12} deficiency is ruled out. However, folate deficiency does not explain the neurologic symptoms experienced by this patient

Answer E is incorrect. An embolus to the superior mesenteric artery can lead to an acute bowel infarction, a life-threatening problem. Patients typically present with abdominal pain, bloody stools, fever, and peritoneal signs. Anemia in a patient with acute blood loss is typically a normocytic anemia (normal mean corpuscular volume).

42. **The correct answer is F.** This answer choice is a description of a ferruginous body, which is consistent with asbestosis. The patient's career as a construction worker makes asbestos exposure likely. Asbestosis results in a marked predisposition to bronchogenic carcinoma, and specifically increases the risk of malignant mesothelioma of the pleura or peritoneum. Cigarette exposure, as in this patient, further increases the risk of lung cancer.

Answer A is incorrect. This answer is a characteristic description of the microscopic appearance of pulmonary TB. While the patient has a history of a progressive cough, other nonspecific symptoms of TB are not present, including symptoms of fever, hemoptysis, pleural effusions, night sweats, or generalized wasting.

Answer B is incorrect. This answer is a histologic description of intracellular Birbeck granules, a feature of eosinophilic granuloma. This interstitial lung disease is caused by a localized proliferation of histiocytic cells that are closely related to the Langerhans' cells of the skin. An eosinophilic granuloma does not share features or a common etiology with bronchogenic carcinoma.

Answer C is incorrect. This answer is a histologic description of a pulmonary embolus. While many cancers produce a hypercoagulable state, this patient has no symptoms of respiratory distress and no history of stasis, trauma, or deep venous thrombosis. In this regard, the histologic finding of a pulmonary embolus is unlikely.

Answer D is incorrect. Marked intra-alveolar fibrin and cellular debris is a histologic feature of acute respiratory distress syndrome (ARDS). There is nothing in this patient's presentation to suggest severe hypoxia or an etiology for ARDS. Causes of ARDS are varied and include shock, sepsis, trauma, uremia, and acute pancreatitis.

Answer E is incorrect. This answer is a histologic description of coccidoidomycosis. The patient has no history of an influenza-like illness, arthralgias, or erythema nodosum (red, tender nodules on extensor surfaces). The patient has no known history of exposure and no demonstrated positive skin test.

43. **The correct answer is E.** Acute intermittent porphyria (AIP) and porphyria cutanea tarda (PCT) are the two most common porphyrias seen clinically. AIP results from a defect in the enzyme porphobilinogen (PBG) deaminase, also called uroporphyrinogen (URO) I synthase. PBG deaminase is the third enzyme in the heme synthetic pathway, and its absence leads to an aberrant accumulation of aminolevulinate (ALA) and PBG. In contrast, PCT is a defect in the enzyme URO decarboxylase, the fifth step in the heme pathway, which causes an accumulation of URO but not ALA or PBG. In this case the patient presents with symptoms most consistent with AIP: neurovisceral symptoms (most commonly abdominal pain, muscle weakness, and psychiatric manifestations such as anxiety, paranoia, and depression) and high PBG levels in urine. In severe cases the PBG can cause the urine to appear the color of port wine.

Answer A is incorrect. ALA dehydratase, the enzyme responsible for condensing ALA into PBG, is absent in ALA dehydratase porphyria. Whereas this porphyria clinically resembles AIP, deficiency of ALA dehydratase is extremely rare, making AIP a more likely diagnosis in this patient.

Answer B is incorrect. ALA synthase deficiency is associated with X-linked sideroblastic anemia. ALA synthase is the first and rate-limiting step in heme synthesis.

Answer C is incorrect. Ferrochelatase incorporates iron into protoheme, the last step of heme biosynthesis. Deficiency of ferrochelatase results in erythropoietic porphyria, a disorder that usually begins with marked photosensitivity in childhood.

Answer D is incorrect. Heme oxygenase catalyzes the oxidation of heme to biliverdin.

Answer F is incorrect. PCT is seen frequently in the clinical setting. PCT results from a deficiency in URO decarboxylase. This deficiency may be inherited or acquired, the latter due to the inactivation of URO decarboxylase by iron, alcohol, estrogens, and infection with HCV or HIV. In contrast to AIP, patients with PCT present with photosensitivity, chronic, blistering lesions on sun-exposed skin, and an absence of neuropsychiatric signs.

Answer G is incorrect. URO III cosynthase deficiency can result in congenital erythropoietic porphyria, and is associated with hemolytic anemia and photosensitive cutaneous lesions.

44. **The correct answer is A.** This blood smear shows abundant lymphoblasts typical of acute lymphocytic leukemia (ALL). Lymphoblasts can be distinguished from normal mature lymphocytes by their fine, homogenous chromatin, irregular nuclear borders, and scant cytoplasm. ALL is a neoplasm that originates from a single B- or T-lymphocyte progenitor cell. Blast cells proliferate and accumulate in the marrow, crowding out other blood cell lines and resulting in suppression of hematopoiesis. Eventually, patients develop symptomatic anemia, thrombocytopenia, and neutropenia.

    Answer B is incorrect. If this child suffered from chronic kidney disease, she may become anemic due to decreased erythropoietin secretion from the kidneys. Her blood smear would not correlate with that in the image.

    Answer C is incorrect. One important function of the small intestine is to absorb nutrients. If the image showed hypochromic, microcytic RBCs without WBC abnormalities, it would be suggestive of iron-deficiency anemia. Conversely, a macrocytic anemia would suggest folate or vitamin B_{12} deficiency. These findings could be due to intestinal dysfunction.

    Answer D is incorrect. If this blood smear showed RBCs infected with parasites, we could diagnose malaria. Diagnosis is made using both thin and thick blood smears because the former reveals the species of *Plasmodium*, and the latter quantifies the percentage of RBCs that are infected (parasite density). One important function of the RBC is to carry hemoglobin-bound oxygen to tissues. The loss of functioning RBCs can lead to symptomatic anemia in patients with malaria.

    Answer E is incorrect. Loss of function of the spleen would show Howell-Jolly bodies (clusters of DNA) in RBCs on a blood smear. A functioning spleen usually removes these protein aggregates. The spleen's function is similar to that of lymph nodes, the major difference being that the spleen is the major site of immune responses to blood-borne antigens, whereas lymph nodes respond to antigens in the lymph. The spleen is also important in the defense against encapsulated organisms. An example of loss of splenic function is seen in children with sickle cell disease who are at risk for sepsis, meningitis, and pneumonia from encapsulated bacteria such as pneumococcus and *Haemophilus influenzae*.

45. **The correct answer is C.** This patient has a history consistent with uncontrolled type 2 diabetes mellitus. Long-term hyperglycemia in these patients, reflected by the increased hemoglobin A_{1c}, may result in diabetic nephropathy. The pathogenesis of diabetic nephropathy involves non-enzymatic glycosylation of the glomerular and tubule basement membranes, thereby increasing permeability to proteins; hence, microalbuminuria is an early sign of diabetic nephropathy. Nonenzymatic glycosylation is a ubiquitous process in poorly controlled diabetes, and this patient's neuropathic

lower extremity pain likely is due to nonenzymatic glycosylation of nerve fibers. Glomerular hypertrophy also occurs due to cytokine release. On light microscopy, early changes show diffuse mesangial expansion in the glomeruli, whereas more advanced diabetic nephropathy (as might be seen in this patient) demonstrates nodular glomerulosclerosis (Kimmelstiel-Wilson nodules). Nodular glomerulosclerosis is characterized by increased cellularity and mesangial matrix deposition, as well as hyaline masses and thickening of the lamina densa. Diabetic nephropathy can present with either a nephrotic or a nephritic syndrome, although nephrotic is more common.

Answer A is incorrect. Diffuse capillary and basement membrane thickening is associated with membranous glomerulonephritis.

Answer B is incorrect. Enlarged hypercellular glomeruli with neutrophils can be found in acute poststreptococcal glomerulonephritis.

Answer D is incorrect. Segmental sclerosis with hyalinosis is seen in focal segmental glomerulosclerosis.

Answer E is incorrect. Glomeruli demonstrating a wire-loop appearance with subendothelial basement membrane deposits are seen in lupus nephropathy.

46. **The correct answer is D.** The pattern and location of the child's wounds are consistent with the mother's description. However, burns of the depth described in the question stem could only be caused by a much longer duration of contact with hot water than the mother indicates. The physical findings suggest this child has been forcibly held in deeper, much hotter water, which suggests child abuse. Suspected child abuse requires further investigation by authorities once immediate attention to wounds is provided.

    Answer A is incorrect. Collateral information may be important in the investigation of the potential abuse of this child, but it should be obtained only after treating the child's wounds and contacting appropriate authorities.

    Answer B is incorrect. Imaging may be part of the work-up of a child in cases of suspected abuse, but in this situation the child's scald burns should be treated initially, prior to obtaining imaging to look for further evidence of abuse (eg, old, healed fractures). In addition, the authorities need to be contacted.

    Answer C is incorrect. This answer choice outlines appropriate, but incomplete, actions. The child needs to be treated for his wounds, and a full physical examination should be conducted to look for other signs of child abuse. In cases of suspected child abuse such as this one, the appropriate authorities must be contacted. This answer is incorrect because it does not reflect the need to contact the appropriate personnel.

    Answer E is incorrect. Given the inconsistencies between the patient's wounds and the history provided, further investigation by authorities is necessary before the child is released back to his mother.

47. **The correct answer is C.** Intermittent headaches, sweating, and palpitations in an otherwise healthy man are suggestive of a pheochromocytoma, a catecholamine-secreting tumor most commonly found in the adrenal glands. Episodes are limited in duration, but blood pressure during these events can reach dangerously high levels. High urinary catecholamines, metanephrine, and vanillylmandelic acid confirm the diagnosis. Pheochromocytomas are associated with parathyroid tumors as part of the MEN type II syndrome, which also includes medullary carcinomas of the thyroid.

    Answer A is incorrect. Hashimoto thyroiditis is an autoimmune disorder resulting in hypothyroidism. Antimicrosomal and antithyroglobulin antibodies are present and diagnostic. During the initial phase of glandular injury, a transient state of hyperthyroidism may result from cellular rupture. Hashimoto thyroiditis is not associated with pheochromocytomas.

    Answer B is incorrect. Insulinomas are associated with parathyroid and pituitary tumors as part of the MEN type I complex. Insulinomas are insulin-secreting tumors of the pancreas that produce symptoms due to hypoglycemia. They are not associated with pheochromocytomas.

Answer D is incorrect. Prolacintomas are associated with pancreatic tumors (Zollinger-Ellison syndrome, insulinomas, and VIPomas) and parathyroid tumors as part of the MEN type I syndrome. Prolactinomas cause excessive secretion of prolactin, resulting in secondary amenorrhea in women and galactorrhea. Prolactinomas are not associated with pheochromocytomas.

Answer E is incorrect. Zollinger-Ellison syndrome is associated with parathyroid and pituitary tumors as part of the MEN type I complex. Zollinger-Ellison syndrome is caused by a gastrin-secreting tumor (gastrinoma), resulting in recurrent upper GI ulcers that are resistant to medical treatment. Zollinger-Ellison syndrome is not associated with pheochromocytomas.

48. **The correct answer is D.** Multiple sclerosis (MS) is a chronic inflammatory demyelinating disease of unknown etiology. It typically has a relapsing-remitting course and is most commonly seen in female patients with peak age of onset between 20 and 40 years. MS usually presents with weakness and/or numbness in one or more extremities. Another common presentation is visual loss secondary to optic neuritis and unilateral shooting facial pain secondary to trigeminal neuralgia. MRI is the most sensitive radiographic technique for imaging MS, with sensitivity of nearly 85%. Classic findings on MRI are periventricular white matter lesions known as "Dawson's fingers," as seen in the image. These lesions appear as "finger like" projections around the ventricles and are easiest to see with a sagittal image. Commonly, foci identified on MRI imaging are clinically silent. A combination of history, physical examination, laboratory tests such as cerebrospinal fluid oligoclonal banding, and imaging findings is used to diagnose MS. Interferon beta-1a is indicated for the long-term treatment of patients with relapsing forms of the disease to slow the accumulation of physical disability and decrease the frequency of clinical exacerbations. Patients with MS in whom interferon's efficacy has been demonstrated include patients who have experienced a first clinical episode and have MRI features consistent with MS.

Answer A is incorrect. The patient presents with trigeminal neuralgia in the setting of several other past neurologic complaints. While trigeminal neuralgia is characterized by unilateral shooting facial pains, it is important to distinguish this pain from that of a headache (eg, migraine, cluster, or tension). Acetaminophen may be considered in the initial treatment of tension headache.

Answer B is incorrect. Short courses of IV corticosteroids are commonly used to treat acute MS flares associated with neurologic deficits. However, interferon or glatiramer, not corticosteroids, are appropriate for the long-term treatment of MS.

Answer C is incorrect. Heparin would be an appropriate therapeutic intervention in the case of an ischemic stroke. Given that the patient's neurologic signs and symptoms are separated both by time and space, a stroke is not likely. Moreover, the patient is quite young and an ischemic stroke in such a young patient would be exceedingly rare.

Answer E is incorrect. Unilateral facial pain is more characteristic of trigeminal neuralgia (a common feature of MS) than of migraine headache. Triptans are used as initial treatment in the case of cluster and migraine headache.

Test Block 4

QUESTIONS

1. A 6-year-old boy was brought to a pediatrician two weeks ago because his teacher noticed he had begun "blanking out" in the classroom, staring into space, failing to respond to his name, and occasionally drooling. The pediatrician prescribed a drug for these episodes one week ago. The boy's parents bring him to the emergency department because he has worsening gastrointestinal upset, pain on swallowing, and blistering around his nose and mouth. Which drug most likely caused this boy's symptoms?

   (A) Carbamazepine
   (B) Ethosuximide
   (C) Lamotrigine
   (D) Phenytoin
   (E) Valproic acid

2. A 30-year-old man presents with a seven-month history of fatigue, weight loss, depression, and abdominal pain worsened by eating. He recently experienced two episodes of kidney stones, which he has never had before, and reports decreased libido over the past couple years. He was adopted at an early age, has no children, and is unsure of his family history. What is the most likely mode of inheritance of this man's condition?

   (A) Autosomal dominant
   (B) Autosomal recessive
   (C) Mitochondrial inheritance
   (D) X-linked dominant
   (E) X-linked recessive

3. A 29-year-old woman presents to the obstetrician-gynecologist with complaints of amenorrhea for the past two months. She notes that she is sexually active with her boyfriend of six months, and they do not use any form of contraception. She is worried about pregnancy, despite several negative home pregnancy tests a few days ago. She also complains about feeling increasingly anxious, "hot all the time," and weight loss, but she attributes these symptoms to increased stress at work, where she was recently promoted to a project manager position. On physical examination, the physician finds fine hair growth on her face and extremities, with body mass index of 16.5 kg/m^2. Which of the following autoantibodies is responsible for this woman's condition?

   (A) Antimicrosomal antibodies
   (B) Thyrotropin receptor inhibitory antibodies
   (C) Thyrotropin receptor stimulatory antibodies
   (D) Thyrotropin-releasing hormone receptor inhibitory antibodies
   (E) Thyrotropin-releasing hormone receptor stimulatory antibodies

4. A 59-year-old woman was recently admitted to the hospital because of oral ulcers and diffuse, crusted, erythematous plaques on her torso and upper arms (see image). She has tested positive for anti-epithelial cell antibodies. Which of the following is the most likely diagnosis?

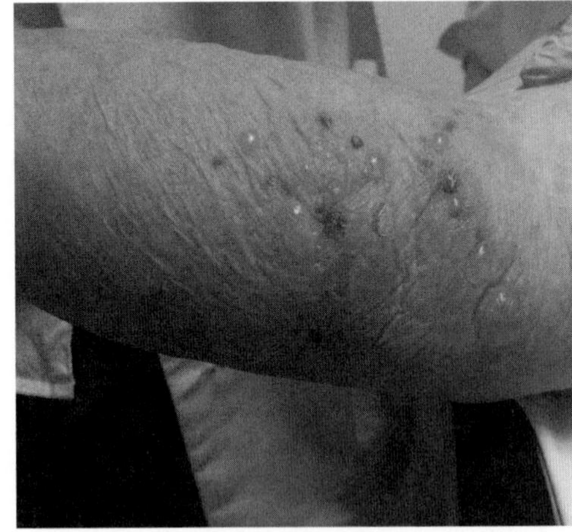

Reproduced, with permission, from USMLERx.com.

   (A) A disease associated with a type II hypersensitivity reaction to type IV collagen
   (B) A disease associated with a type IV hypersensitivity reaction to poison ivy
   (C) A disease associated with anti-scl-70 autoantibodies

FULL-LENGTH EXAMS

Test Block 4

(D) A disease associated with linear deposits of IgG in the epidermal basement membrane
(E) A disease associated with the HLA-B27 histocompatibility complex allele

5. A 40-year-old woman develops bloody mucoid diarrhea with abdominal cramping after eating fresh fruit in a small Mexican village. Four months later, she still has intermittent abdominal pain. A CT scan of the abdomen shows evidence of a necrotic liver lesion. Her laboratory studies show the following results:

Aspartate aminotransferase (AST), serum: 18 U/L
Alanine aminotransferase (ALT), serum: 20 U/L
Alkaline phosphatase: 300 U/L
Bilirubin, total serum: 1.1 mg/dL
Bilirubin, direct: 0.3 mg/dL

Which of the following is the best treatment for this patient?

(A) A course of ampicillin, gentamicin, and clindamycin
(B) A course of metronidazole
(C) Core needle biopsy of the hepatic lesion
(D) Surgical excision of the hepatic lesion
(E) Ultrasound-guided aspiration of the hepatic lesion

6. A 46-year-old man comes to the clinic with a cough that is occasionally productive of blood, diffuse muscle and joint pain in the upper extremities, and blood in his urine for the past several days. On further questioning the patient reveals that he has had chronic sinusitis for the past several years. Laboratory studies show a markedly elevated erythrocyte sedimentation rate, and staining for antibodies to cytoplasmic antigens of neutrophils is positive. Which of the following is the most likely finding on kidney biopsy?

(A) A split basement membrane
(B) Normal glomeruli with foot process effacement
(C) Segmental necrotizing glomerulonephritis
(D) Smooth linear staining on immunofluorescence
(E) Wire-loop lesion with subepithelial deposits

7. A peripheral T-helper lymphocyte engages peptide-bound class II major histocompatibility complex molecules on the surface of an antigen-presenting cell (APC). No other contact is made between cell surface molecules present on the T lymphocyte and the APC. Which of the following can be concluded about this peripheral T lymphocyte?

(A) The T lymphocyte will be activated and fully able to perform effector functions
(B) The T lymphocyte will be activated but unable to perform effector functions
(C) The T lymphocyte will cause the APC to undergo apoptosis
(D) The T lymphocyte will undergo anergy
(E) The T lymphocyte will undergo clonal expansion

8. A 27-year-old man is brought to the emergency department after he was found shuffling unsteadily around a busy intersection for several hours. The patient is unreliable in providing his medical history. His vital signs are within normal limits. On physical examination his liver edge is palpable 6 cm below the costal margin and truncal spider angiomata are noted. Ophthalmologic examination reveals dark rings around the iris. His abdomen is soft and non-tender. Which of the following is the most likely diagnosis?

(A) Drug intoxication
(B) HIV infection
(C) Parkinson disease
(D) Schizophrenia
(E) Wilson disease

9. A 22-year-old man with metastatic testicular carcinoma is undergoing treatment with high doses of cisplatin and experiences severe nausea after each treatment. What class of drug could be added to his chemotherapeutic regimen to reduce his nausea?

(A) 5-Hydroxytryptamine$_3$ antagonist
(B) Anticholinergic
(C) Benzodiazepine
(D) Glucocorticoid receptor agonist
(E) Histamine receptor antagonist

10. An elderly woman with a history of atrial fibrillation is admitted to the hospital because of congestive heart failure. Laboratory studies show:

Na^+: 140 mEq/L
K^+: 4 mEq/L
HCO_3^-: 25 mEq/L
Cl^-: 104 mEq/L
Glucose: 100 mg/dL
Blood urea nitrogen: 18 mg/dL
Creatinine: 2.1 mg/dL

A complete blood count is within normal limits. She develops the arrhythmia shown in the image. Which of the following antiarrhythmic agents is associated with the arrhythmia shown in the image?

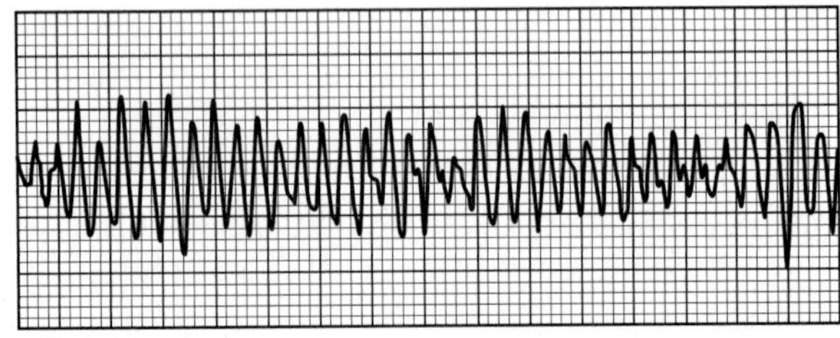

Reproduced, with permission, from USMLERx.com.

(A) Adenosine
(B) Esmolol
(C) Lidocaine
(D) Propranolol
(E) Quinidine
(F) Verapamil

11. A patient presents two weeks after a severe upper respiratory infection complaining of increasing weakness in his legs. Strength is 2/5 in his bilateral lower extremities, 4/5 in his bilateral upper extremities. Sensation in the upper and lower extremities is intact. Which of the following is a consequence of this disease process?

(A) A descending paralysis beginning in the proximal parts of the lower extremities
(B) Demyelination of the basal ganglia
(C) Demyelination of white matter tracts in the spinal cord
(D) Hyperreflexia and bilateral positive Babinski reflexes
(E) Slower conduction velocity of action potentials in nerves myelinated by Schwann cells

12. A 58-year-old East Asian man with recently diagnosed type 2 diabetes mellitus presents to the emergency department because of the acute onset of flushing, tachycardia, nausea, and hyperventilation. The drug he recently started taking to treat his diabetes works by stimulating the release of endogenous insulin. Which of the following drugs did the patient recently start taking?

(A) Acarbose
(B) Glargine
(C) Metformin
(D) Tolbutamide
(E) Troglitazone

13. A 4-year-old boy is brought to his pediatrician's office by his mother because he has been "acting out" for the past six months. The child's past medical history is unremarkable, and he has reached all of his developmental milestones on time. The pediatrician inquires about the parent's disciplinary methods. The mother says that she and her husband "reason" with the child when he misbehaves. According to Piaget's theory of cognitive development, this 4-year-old patient is able to process information in which of the following ways?

(A) He can deal with abstract ideas
(B) He can formulate and test hypotheses
(C) He has some limited logical thought processes
(D) He possesses an awareness of conservation
(E) He understands symbolic representations of the world

14. A 27-year-old woman is brought to the emergency department with an intense headache, left-sided weakness, and blurred vision that began after she was ejected from her car in a

motor vehicle accident. Paramedics report that she was ambulatory and cooperative at the scene of the crash but was unable to recall the events leading up to the accident. While in the ambulance, the patient had an episode of projectile vomiting and has displayed steadily deteriorating mental status. CT of the head shows extra-axial fluid collection on the right side and a temporal bone fracture on the same side. Injury to which of the following is the most likely cause of the patient's presentation?

(A) Inferior cerebral veins
(B) Middle meningeal artery
(C) Posterior ethmoidal artery
(D) Sigmoid sinus
(E) Superior sagittal sinus

15. An infant with severe jaundice that is not corrected by phototherapy is in danger of developing kernicterus. This can occur in infants with Crigler-Najjar syndrome, a genetic disorder in which there is a near-complete deficiency of glucuronyl transferase. Which of the following laboratory findings would be expected in blood tests in an infant with Crigler-Najjar syndrome?

(A) Decreased hematocrit
(B) Decreased indirect bilirubin
(C) Increased direct bilirubin
(D) Increased indirect bilirubin
(E) Increased reticulocyte count

16. A 3-year-old girl is brought to her pediatrician because of a progressive loss of motor function and a decline in her cognitive abilities. On physical examination, it is noted that the patient has decreased deep tendon reflexes, truncal ataxia, and a decreased attention span in comparison to the child's last visit six months ago. The physician knows that her pathology is due to an abnormal accumulation of cerebroside sulfate in her brain, peripheral nerves, kidney, and liver. A deficiency of which of the following enzymes leads to this condition?

(A) α-Galactosidase A
(B) β-Galactosidase
(C) Arylsulfatase A
(D) Hexosaminidase A
(E) Sphingomyelinase

17. A 65-year-old African-American man presents with increasing difficulty swallowing over the past three months. Upper gastrointestinal endoscopy reveals an annular mass with ulceration in the lower third of his esophageal wall, similar to the gross specimen depicted in the image. Histologic examination reveals increased mitosis, dysplasia, and nuclear atypia of glandular columnar epithelial cells. Which of the following is a risk factor for this variant of esophageal cancer, but not the other common morphologic variant of esophageal cancer commonly found in the upper to middle third of the esophagus?

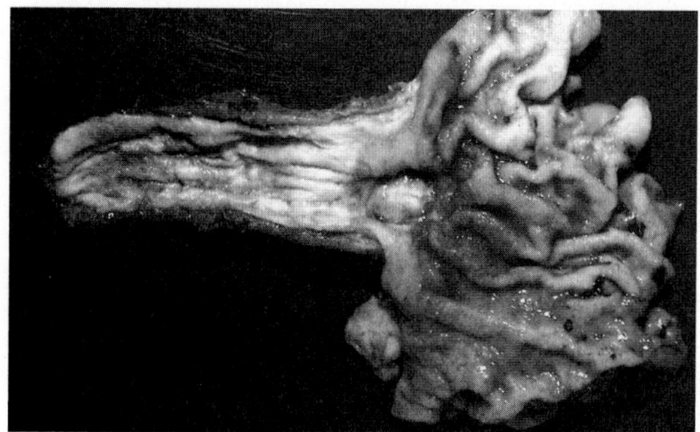

Reproduced, with permission, from USMLERx.com.

(A) Achalasia
(B) African-American decent
(C) Male gender
(D) Obesity
(E) Tobacco use

18. A 27-year-old man presents to the physician with fever, malaise, cough, and wheezing. During the physical examination, the patient intermittently coughs up brownish-colored mucus. The rest of the physical examination is unremarkable. Mucus cultures are taken and the results are pending. An x-ray shows a mass within a cavity in his left lung. If the causative agent is a fungus, which of the following will most likely be seen on microscopic observation of the mucus?

    (A) A cyst with a thick cell wall and intracystic bodies
    (B) A heavily encapsulated yeast that is not dimorphic
    (C) A mold with irregular nonseptate hyphae branching at wide angles (more than 90 degrees)
    (D) A mold with septate hyphae that branch at a V-shaped 45-degree angle
    (E) Cigar-shaped budding yeast visible in pus

19. A 65-year-old obese man with a 60-pack-year smoking history presents with partial loss of vision after suffering a stroke. Physical examination reveals a bilateral defect in the upper left visual quadrants. Where is this patient's lesion most likely located?

    (A) Dorsal optic radiation in the left parietal lobe
    (B) Dorsal optic radiation in the right parietal lobe
    (C) Left optic tract
    (D) Meyer's loop in the left temporal lobe
    (E) Meyer's loop in the right temporal lobe
    (F) Right optic tract

20. A 44-year-old woman with end-stage renal disease and on hemodialysis presents to the physician with abdominal pain. Laboratory tests are positive for hepatitis B surface antigen (HBsAg), anti-hepatitis B core antibody (HBcAb), and hepatitis B early antigen (HBeAg), but negative for anti-hepatitis B surface and anti-hepatitis B early antibodies (anti-HBsAb and anti-HBeAb, respectively). Which of the following is the appropriate treatment for this patient's disease?

    (A) Do not treat, because this patient's laboratory tests are most consistent with previous hepatitis B vaccination
    (B) Lamivudine and interferon-α
    (C) Lamivudine and interferon-β
    (D) Ribavirin and lamivudine
    (E) Ribavirin and pegylated interferon-α

21. A 40-year-old woman presents to her physician with complaints of blood in her urine and decreased urine output for the past week. She had a sore throat three weeks ago, which has since resolved. Her temperature is 37°C (98.6°F), heart rate is 70/min, and blood pressure is 147/93 mm Hg. Physical examination reveals bilateral pedal edema to the mid-calf. In addition to several serologic tests, the patient undergoes renal biopsy (see image). Which of the following is the most accurate diagnosis?

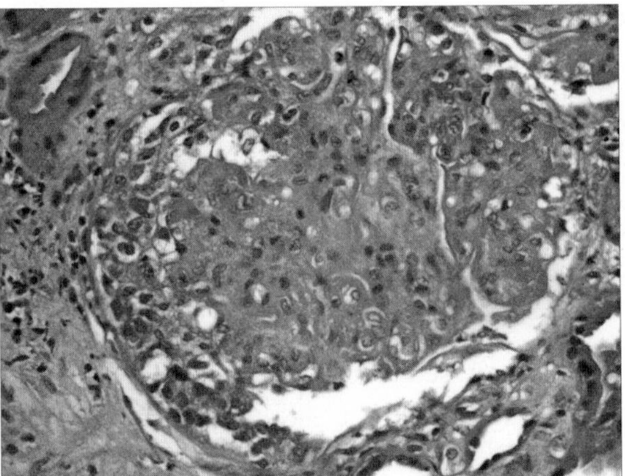

Reproduced, with permission, from USMLERx.com.

    (A) Diabetic nephropathy
    (B) Goodpasture syndrome
    (C) IgA nephropathy
    (D) Lupus nephritis
    (E) Poststreptococcal glomerulonephritis
    (F) Rapidly progressive glomerulonephritis
    (G) Renal amyloidosis

22. A 38-year-old woman at 24 weeks' gestation undergoes prenatal ultrasonography. Results show a male fetus with bilateral hydroureteronephrosis. Soon after birth, laboratory values show a moderately elevated creatinine. A voiding cystourethrogram reveals posterior urethral valves in the prostatic urethra. The etiology of posterior urethral valves remains unclear, but failure of regression of the developmental structure that comprises the prostatic urethra has been postulated. Anomalous development of what structure may give rise to posterior urethral valves?

(A) Genital tubercle
(B) Mesonephric duct
(C) Paramesonephric duct
(D) Urogenital folds
(E) Urogenital sinus

23. An 8-year-old boy is brought to his pediatrician for a school physical. His parents report that he is in good health. They are concerned, however, because occasionally they find dark brown urine in the toilet when their son forgets to flush. Urinalysis is ordered; while his urine initially appears normal, it turns dark after standing. Which of the following enzymes is defective in this child?

(A) Branched-chain α-ketoacid dehydrogenase
(B) Homogentisic acid oxidase
(C) Phenylalanine hydroxylase
(D) Phytanic acid oxidase
(E) Tyrosinase

24. A 2-year-old child has required frequent transfusions throughout his life because of anemia. A peripheral blood smear demonstrates microcytic, hypochromic red cells, with target cells and anisopoikilocytosis. After further genetic testing, the child's spleen is removed to lessen the need for transfusions. When his genetic code is sequenced, the mutation in the image is seen at the 5' end of one of his introns. This change is most likely to affect which of the following processes?

Normal	5′ TTCGUTCCGACT 3′
Mutant	5′ TTCAUTCCGACT 3′

Reproduced, with permission, from USMLERx.com.

(A) Capping
(B) Hybridization
(C) Polyadenylation
(D) Splicing
(E) Transcription

25. A 20-year-old college student presents complaining of severe fatigue and lethargy. She experienced a recent mononucleosis infection that has resolved. Physical examination shows scleral icterus, cervical lymphadenopathy, and splenomegaly. The tips of her fingers are purple. Laboratory testing shows a decreased hemoglobin level, an appropriate reticulocyte count, and a positive heterophile test. Which of the following is the most likely diagnosis?

(A) Aplastic anemia
(B) Disseminated intravascular coagulation
(C) IgG-mediated (warm) hemolytic anemia
(D) IgM-mediated (cold) hemolytic anemia
(E) Paroxysmal nocturnal hemoglobinuria

26. A new growth factor, XGEF, has been found to be upregulated in breast carcinomas. This growth factor appears to activate a seven-transmembrane-domain cell surface receptor on endothelial cells. The binding of the receptor results in the increase of calcium in the cell cytosol. By what mechanism does XGEF exert its effect on endothelial cells?

(A) Activation of G_i
(B) Activation of G_q
(C) Activation of G_s
(D) Upregulation of cGMP

27. A 71-year-old Russian man comes to the physician complaining of a four-month history of fatigue, low-grade fevers, night sweats, and cough. He became extremely worried yesterday when he noticed blood in his sputum. On physical examination, he is extremely thin, with enlarged, nontender left-sided cervical lymph nodes. His x-ray film of the chest is shown. The physician prescribes medication not only for the patient, but also for those who may have been in close contact with the patient. Which of the following is an important adverse effect of the first-line medication for the prevention of this disease?

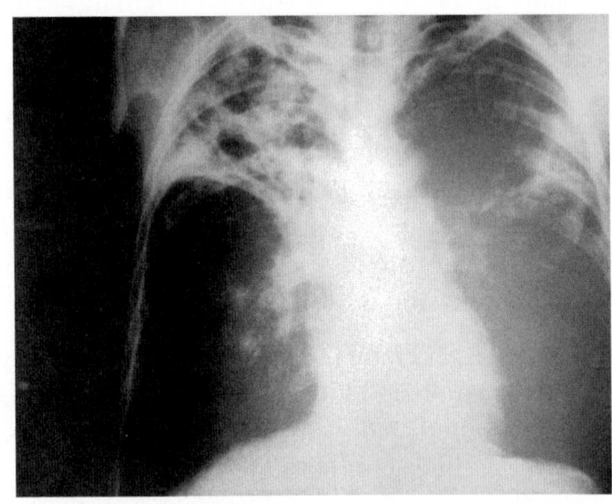

Courtesy of the Centers for Disease Control and Prevention.

(A) A disulfiram-like reaction with alcohol
(B) Aplastic anemia
(C) Hepatotoxicity
(D) Inhibition of bone growth in children
(E) Nephrotoxicity

28. A 47-year-old woman presents to her physician complaining of weight gain, fatigue, and lethargy. Her appetite has decreased recently and she has been constipated. Physical examination reveals an enlarged, symmetric, and firm thyroid. A thyroid biopsy is significant for a lymphocytic and plasma cell infiltrate with occasional germinal center formation. The follicles contain little colloid, and the follicular epithelial lining shows enlarged epithelial cells containing acidophilic cytoplasm. Which of the following antibodies is most likely to be found in this patient?

(A) Anti-smooth muscle
(B) Anti-U1 RNP
(C) Anticentromere
(D) Antimicrosomal
(E) Antimitochondrial

29. A couple brings their 3-year-old daughter to her doctor because she has not behaved normally in the past month. The physician notes that the girl is quiet and less expressive than she was at her well-child visit several months ago. She was previously able to name four colors, but she now stutters and recalls only one. Furthermore, she responds to questions with one- or two-word sentences, which is uncharacteristic of her usually articulate personality. What other symptom might be expected in this patient?

(A) Hand wringing
(B) Hearing loss
(C) Hyperactivity
(D) Psychosis
(E) Repetitive behaviors
(F) Tics

30. The peripheral blood smear shown in this image is from a patient who has taken phenytoin for five years for a seizure disorder. The patient has a well-balanced diet and is taking no other medications. Which of the following conditions most likely caused the abnormality seen in this image?

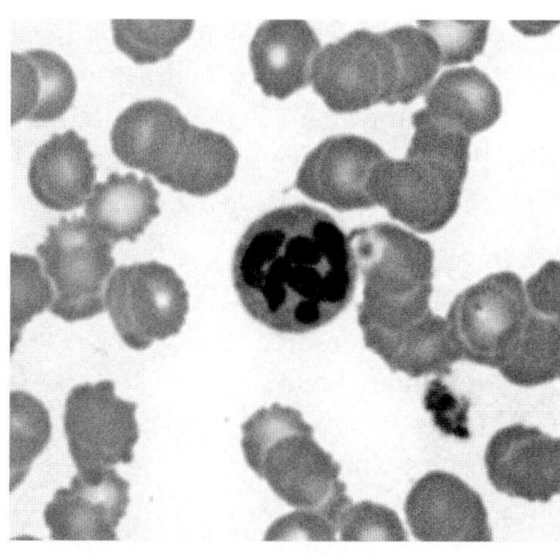

Reproduced, with permission, from USMLERx.com.

(A) Decreased β-hemoglobin synthesis
(B) Folic acid deficiency
(C) Iron deficiency
(D) Vitamin B_{12} deficiency
(E) Vitamin B_6 deficiency

31. A 28-year-old woman begins taking a drug to treat her schizophrenia. The patient misses her subsequent psychiatric appointments and is lost to follow-up. Two weeks later she is admitted to the hospital with fever, dyspnea, and a productive cough. Cultures are consistent with *Streptococcus pneumoniae*. Laboratory tests show a WBC count of 3000/mm³ and an absolute neutrophil count of 1000/mm³ (normal: <1500/mm³). The physician suspects a drug interaction when he sees that the patient is not taking other medication and is HIV negative. What is the prescribed drug's main mechanism of action?

(A) D_1- and D_2-receptor agonist
(B) D_1- and D_2-receptor antagonist
(C) GABA receptor agonist
(D) GABA receptor antagonist
(E) N-methyl-D-aspartate receptor antagonist

32. Tertiary syphilis may lead to cardiovascular complications, resulting in aortic aneurysm and death. Patients with this pathology may have a cardiac abnormality that causes a high-pitched diastolic murmur. This murmur is caused by a valvular defect similar to the type of defect found in which condition?

(A) Chronic rheumatic heart disease
(B) Congenital bicuspid aortic valve
(C) Congenital pulmonary stenosis
(D) Marfan syndrome

33. A 48-year-old woman with amenorrhea visits her doctor. Her last menstrual period was 12 months ago. Results of physical and pelvic examinations are normal. Blood test levels show:

Estrogen: 35 pg/mL (normal: 150-200 pg/mL)
Follicle-stimulating hormone: 60 IU/L (normal: <12 IU/L)
Luteinizing hormone: 40 IU/L (normal: <12 IU/L)

What is the most likely underlying physiologic mechanism explaining the hormonal changes seen in this woman?

(A) Decrease in negative feedback
(B) Decrease in positive feedback
(C) Down-regulation of nuclear receptors
(D) Increase in negative feedback
(E) Increase in positive feedback
(F) Up-regulation of nuclear receptors

34. A 3-week-old infant presents with failure to thrive, poor feeding, and lethargy. A physical examination reveals an enlarged liver and jaundice. Laboratory analysis reveals an elevated blood galactitol level and increased urinary reducing substance. Which of the following could correctly describe the levels of intermediates of galactose metabolism in this patient?

(A) Decreased galactose
(B) Decreased uridine diphosphoglucose
(C) Elevated glucose-1-phosphate
(D) Increased galactose-1-phosphate
(E) Increased glycogen

35. A 25-year-old white woman of Ashkenazi Jewish descent presents to the physician with a three-week history of lower abdominal cramps and intermittent bloody stools two times per day. She has not been febrile and reports no sick contacts, unusual food exposures, or travel history. She has an aunt with similar symptoms. Gross pathologic findings from a patient with similar symptoms are shown in the image. Her laboratory studies show the following results:

Hemoglobin: 13.0 g/dL
Hematocrit: 39%
WBC count: 6000/mm^3
Platelet count: 200,000/mm^3
Erythrocyte sedimentation rate: 35 mm/h

Which of the following is the most appropriate treatment for this patient's condition?

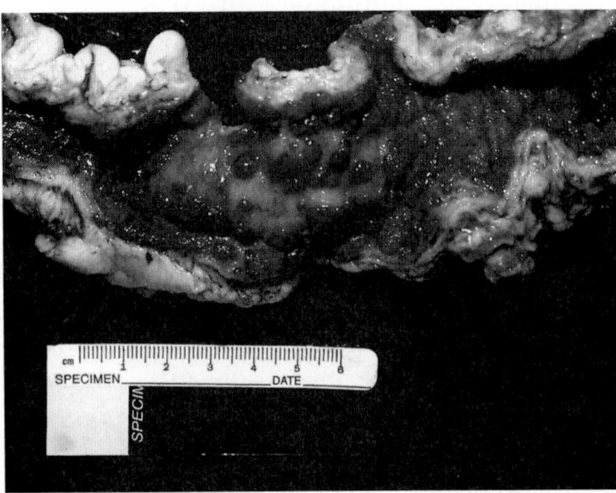

Reproduced, with permission, from USMLERx.com.

(A) Ciprofloxacin
(B) Emergent surgery
(C) Infliximab
(D) Loperamide
(E) Oral steroids
(F) Sulfasalazine

36. A 32-year-old man presents with progressive dementia and sudden, jerky, purposeless movements. On evaluation the patient is noted to be depressed. The patient states that his father, who died at age 50 years, had a similar condition as a young man. Which of the following is the most likely location of this man's brain lesion?

(A) Amygdala
(B) Caudate nucleus
(C) Lateral corticospinal tracts
(D) Mammillary bodies
(E) Nucleus basalis of Meynert
(F) Substantia nigra

37. To assess the efficacy of a new bronchodilator drug X, the peak expiratory flow rate of a population of asthmatics is measured during an asthma attack under three conditions: after no intervention, after the administration of albuterol, or after the administration of drug X. The graph shows the mean peak flow and 95% confidence intervals for each condition. Which is the best statement regarding the results of the study?

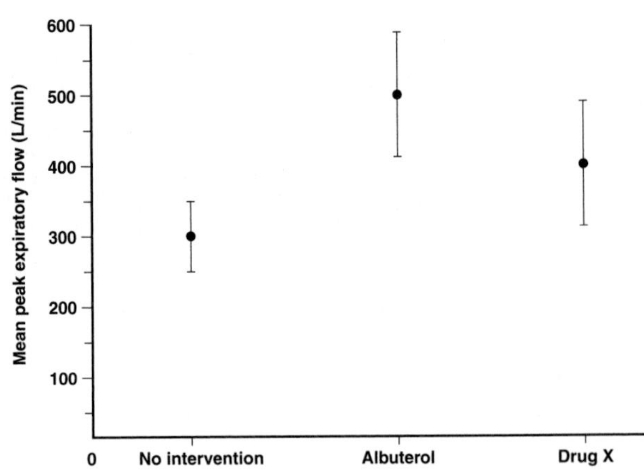

Reproduced, with permission, from USMLERx.com.

(A) There is likely a significant difference between the mean peak expiratory flow rate of albuterol versus drug X
(B) There is likely a significant difference between the mean peak expiratory flow rate of albuterol versus no intervention
(C) There is likely a significant difference between the mean peak expiratory flow rate of drug X versus no intervention

(D) There is not likely a significant difference between the mean peak expiratory flow rate of albuterol versus drug X because the ratio of these two means is close to 1
(E) There is not likely a significant difference between the means of any of the conditions because the confidence intervals are too wide

38. A 51-year-old man with HIV infection presents to the clinic with a four-month history of increasing cognitive decline characterized by increasing apathy and mental slowing. His medical history is significant for several infections with *Pneumocystis jiroveci* (formerly *carinii*) pneumonia, and a recent CD4+ cell count was 112/mm³. Physical examination is notable for impaired saccadic eye movements, diffuse hyperreflexia, frontal release signs, and dysdiadochokinesia. Lumbar puncture reveals a total protein level of 72 mg/dL and an elevated IgG level. MRI of the brain shows global cerebral atrophy with multiple ill-defined areas of signal hyperintensity on T2-weighted images. Which of the following is the most likely cause of this patient's cognitive decline?

(A) Central nervous system lymphoma
(B) Cytomegalovirus encephalitis
(C) Disseminated *Mycobacterium avium* complex infection
(D) HIV-associated dementia
(E) Toxoplasmosis

39. A 62-year-old man presents to his physician complaining of a milky discharge from his nipples. The physician determines that the patient is suffering from a prolactinoma. What is the embryologic derivative of the region of the pituitary gland responsible for prolactin secretion?

(A) Endoderm
(B) Mesoderm
(C) Neural crest cells
(D) Neuroectoderm
(E) Oral ectoderm

40. An 8-week-old boy is brought to his pediatrician because his mother notes abnormal limb movements. Although both pregnancy and birth were not complicated, and there is an unremarkable family history and healthy siblings, this child has had developmental delay since birth. On examination the child has normal vital signs, coarse facial features, diffuse joint stiffness, claw hand deformities, and kyphoscoliosis. Muscle biopsy reveals numerous intracytoplasmic inclusions in cells. What is the pathophysiology of this disease?

(A) Congenital herpes infection
(B) Congenital rubella infection
(C) Failure to cross-link collagen fibrils
(D) Improper protein trafficking
(E) Mutations in the structural protein fibrillin

41. A 35-year-old woman presents with a fever of 38°C (100.8°F), night sweats, fatigue, and a weight loss of 4.5 kg (10 lb) over the past six months. CT scan demonstrates mediastinal lymphadenopathy in multiple contiguous nodes. A photomicrograph of the biopsy specimen of the nodes is shown in the image. Which of the following is the most likely diagnosis?

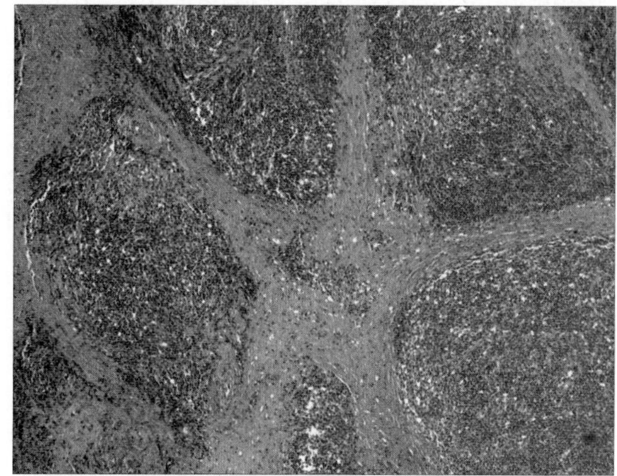

Reproduced, with permission, from USMLERx.com.

(A) Acute myelogenous leukemia
(B) Burkitt lymphoma
(C) Lymphocyte-depletion Hodgkin disease
(D) Mixed-cellularity Hodgkin disease
(E) Nodular-sclerosing Hodgkin disease

42. A 22-year-old man presents to the emergency department complaining of itching over his palms and soles and recent onset of diarrhea. The patient received an unrelated donor bone marrow transplant six weeks ago. He denies eating different foods and has no allergies. On physical examination, a maculopapular rash is present over his neck, shoulders, palms, and soles. Laboratory studies show:

WBC count: 7000/mm^3
Hemoglobin: 10.2 g/dL
Hematocrit: 32%
Platelet count: 125,000/mm^3
Aspartate aminotransferase: 432 U/L
Alanine aminotransferase: 356 U/L
Alkaline phosphatase: 400 U/L

Which of the following is the most likely diagnosis?

(A) ABO incompatibility
(B) Acute graft-versus-host disease
(C) Chronic graft-versus-host disease
(D) Graft rejection
(E) Hyperacute rejection

43. After three days of flu-like symptoms, a patient is feeling unsteady on her feet and dizzy when she attempts to stand up. During her illness she has eaten very little and has had frequent emesis. Blood tests reveal an arterial pH of 7.5 and a partial pressure of carbon dioxide of 53 mm Hg. What is the most likely etiology of this acid-base disturbance?

(A) Consumption of antacids
(B) Decreased hydrogen excretion in the distal tubule
(C) Increased bicarbonate reabsorption by the proximal tubule
(D) Production of ADH
(E) Volume depletion and increased hydrogen excretion in the distal tubule

44. A 63-year-old man with a history of malignant hypertension presents to the emergency department with severe chest pain radiating to his back. An ECG is performed immediately but does not reveal the typical patterns of a myocardial infarction. Unfortunately, the patient dies before further tests can be initiated. On autopsy, the pathologist will most likely detect abnormalities in which area?

(A) Aorta
(B) Esophagus
(C) Left coronary artery
(D) Left ventricular wall of the heart
(E) Pericardium

45. An obese 35-year-old woman presents to her physician with a six-month history of amenorrhea. She is concerned particularly because she and her husband have been trying for more than one year to conceive, with no success. Results of physical examination are normal, except the patient has noticed darkly pigmented periareolar hair since she stopped menstruating. Test results show:

Blood pressure is 128/88 mm Hg
Luteinizing hormone level: 300 mIU/mL
Follicle-stimulating hormone level: 5 mIU/mL
Thyroid-stimulating hormone level: 0.7 μU/mL

Results of a urine pregnancy test are negative. An ultrasound shows enlarged ovaries bilaterally. Which of the following additional findings is associated most commonly with her condition?

(A) Anosmia
(B) Galactorrhea
(C) Hyperglycemia
(D) Polycystic kidneys
(E) Weak pulses in the lower extremities deposits

46. A 4-year-old girl is brought to the emergency department by ambulance late at night. Her caretaker reports that the child has been unable to bear weight on her left leg and that she fell down the stairs this morning. She was brought to the emergency department two other times in the past year, each time with trauma after falling down at home. Her examination is mostly unremarkable, but there are several bruises at varying stages of healing. X-ray of the leg shows a spiral fracture of her left femur. Which of the following is the appropriate course of action?

(A) Ask about family history of brittle bones
(B) Consult ophthalmology department for urgent retinal examination
(C) Contact child protective services
(D) Request a private meeting with the family
(E) Talk to the child about being more careful at home

47. The image shows one anatomic variation that can occur from abnormal development of this paired, embryonic, mesodermally derived organ. In the presence of müllerian inhibiting factor, the embryonic organ giving rise to the structure below will develop into which of the following?

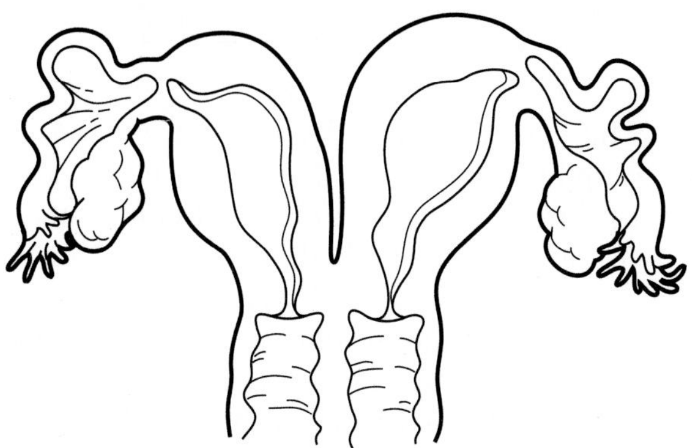

Reproduced, with permission, from USMLERx.com.

(A) Appendix epididymis
(B) Appendix testes
(C) Bulbourethral glands
(D) Paradidymis
(E) Skene glands

48. A 35-year-old woman presents to her physician at the first sign of painful genital ulcerations. She requests a treatment to shorten the course of her illness. Which of the following medications is her physician most likely to prescribe as first-line treatment?

(A) Acyclovir
(B) Didanosine
(C) Foscarnet
(D) Ganciclovir
(E) Zanamivir

ANSWERS

1. **The correct answer is B.** Based on the description of this boy's "episodes," he is suffering from absence seizures. Ethosuximide is the only drug that is both used to treat absence seizures and associated with Stevens-Johnson syndrome. Ethosuximide is an antiepileptic indicated for absence seizures that works by blocking T-type calcium channels. A rare but severe adverse effect is drug-induced Stevens-Johnson syndrome. This is characterized by extensive shedding of the epidermis, blistering of the nasal, oral, and genital mucosa as well as the conjunctivae. This results in complaints of severe pain on swallowing and dehydration. Erythema, palpable purpura, and epidermal necrolysis also may ensue. Ethosuximide also causes gastrointestinal (GI) disturbances, fatigue, dizziness, and, in rare cases, blood dyscrasias. Stevens-Johnson syndrome is treated by stopping the offending agent, managing fluid balance, preventing secondary infections of the skin and possibly administering corticosteroids, although this last measure is controversial.

   Answer A is incorrect. Carbamazepine is used to treat partial and tonic-clonic seizures, but not absence seizures. It acts by increasing sodium channel inactivation. Carbamazepine can cause diplopia, induction of the cytochrome P450 system, blood dyscrasias, liver toxicity, and Stevens-Johnson syndrome.

   Answer C is incorrect. Lamotrigine is used to treat partial and tonic-clonic seizures, but not absence seizures. It acts by blocking voltage-sensitive sodium channels. Lamotrigine can cause GI upset, dizziness, diplopia, amnesia, and Stevens-Johnson syndrome.

   Answer D is incorrect. Phenytoin is used to treat partial and tonic-clonic seizures, but not absence seizures. It acts by increasing sodium channel inactivation. Phenytoin toxicity causes nystagmus, diplopia, ataxia, gingival hyperplasia, and hirsutism. Like ethosuximide, it is associated with Stevens-Johnson syndrome.

   Answer E is incorrect. Valproic acid also is indicated for absence seizures, and adverse effects include GI distress and a rare, but fatal, hepatotoxicity. It acts by elevating concentrations of GABA in the brain. Valproic acid is not associated with Stevens-Johnson syndrome.

2. **The correct answer is A.** Multiple endocrine neoplasia type I (MEN type I) is an autosomal dominant disorder that typically involves tumors of the **P**arathyroid glands, anterior **P**ituitary, and **P**ancreatic islet cells (the three **P**s). The patient's complaints of fatigue, weight loss, depression, and kidney stones are related to hypercalcemia secondary to increased parathyroid hormone (PTH) secretion from a tumor of the parathyroid gland. MEN type I can also involve the anterior pituitary, which in this case manifests as a prolactinoma leading to decreased libido and infertility. Pancreatic neoplasias of MEN type I include insulinomas, VIPomas, and Zollinger-Ellison syndrome, as in this patient, which involves increased gastrin secretion that may manifest with multiple peptic ulcers producing abdominal pain that is worse after eating food.

   Answer B is incorrect. MEN type I is inherited in an autosomal dominant fashion, not autosomal recessive. Important diseases to know that are inherited in an autosomal recessive fashion include cystic fibrosis, phenylketonuria, thalassemias, sickle cell anemias, glycogen storage diseases, infant polycystic kidney disease, and hemochromatosis.

   Answer C is incorrect. MEN type I is inherited in an autosomal dominant fashion. Individuals inherit all of their mitochondrial DNA from their mother because unlike the sperm, the ovum is large enough to house a multitude of copies of mitochondrial DNA. Thus, mitochondrial diseases are passed only from mother to offspring.

   Answer D is incorrect. MEN type I is inherited in an autosomal dominant fashion. X-linked dominant inheritance is rare; some examples include hypophosphatemic rickets and adrenomyeloneuropathy.

Answer E is incorrect. MEN type I is inherited in an autosomal dominant fashion. X-linked recessive diseases include glucose-6-phosphate dehydrogenase deficiency, Duchenne muscular dystrophy, hemophilia A and B, Fabry disease, and Hunter syndrome.

3. **The correct answer is C.** Graves disease is caused by autoantibodies to the thyrotropin (thyroid-stimulating hormone) receptor. The autoantibodies activate the receptor, stimulating thyroid hormone synthesis and secretion and growth of the thyroid gland. Hence, Graves disease most commonly presents with the signs and symptoms of hyperthyroidism, including heat intolerance, sweating, weight loss, tremor, anxiety, weakness, and diarrhea as well as exophthalmos and pretibial myxedema.

   Answer A is incorrect. Antimicrosomal antibodies are present in >90% of patients with Hashimoto thyroiditis and in 50%-80% patients with silent thyroiditis.

   Answer B is incorrect. Thyrotropin (thyroid-stimulating hormone) receptor inhibitory autoantibodies lead to Hashimoto thyroiditis and thus signs and symptoms consistent with hypothyroidism.

   Answer D is incorrect. Graves disease does not involve thyrotropin-releasing hormone receptor inhibitory antibodies, but rather is a result of stimulatory autoantibodies to the thyrotropin (thyroid-stimulating hormone) receptor.

   Answer E is incorrect. Graves disease does not involve thyrotropin-releasing hormone receptor stimulatory antibodies, but rather is a result of stimulatory autoantibodies to the thyrotropin (thyroid-stimulating hormone) receptor.

4. **The correct answer is D.** This patient has bullous pemphigoid, a subepidermal blistering disease that is most commonly seen in the elderly. Patients with bullous pemphigoid have skin vesicles that are filled with a clear fluid and may rupture, but not as easily as the vesicles of pemphigus vulgaris; usually the skin heals without scarring. Oral mucosal lesions are found in 10%-40% of patients with bullous pemphigoid. The disease is characterized by IgG autoantibodies against the epidermal basement membrane, and deposits of antibody or complement are seen on electron microscopy.

   Answer A is incorrect. A type II hypersensitivity reaction against collagen type IV is characteristic of Goodpasture syndrome, which classically presents with hemoptysis and hematuria, not skin lesions.

   Answer B is incorrect. Contact dermatitis is a type IV hypersensitivity reaction that occurs following exposure to allergens such as poison ivy and nickel. These can form blisters in the epidermis similar to the ones seen in the photo, but tend to be localized only to the area that came into contact with the allergen. Furthermore, patients would not test positive for anti-epithelial antibodies.

   Answer C is incorrect. Systemic scleroderma is associated with anti-scl-70 autoantibodies. Patients with this disease present with thickened, indurated skin.

   Answer E is incorrect. Several autoimmune diseases are associated with the HLA-B27 allele. These include Crohn disease and the spondyloarthropathies, but not pemphigus vulgaris.

5. **The correct answer is B.** This patient has amebiasis due to infection with *Entamoeba histolytica*. She has classic features of amebiasis, including bloody mucoid diarrhea, recent travel to a developing country, and hepatic abscess. Amebic hepatic abscesses may show liver function tests consistent with an infiltrative pattern of liver injury (ie, increased alkaline phosphatase with near-normal AST, ALT, and bilirubin). The treatment of hepatic abscess due to *E histolytica* infection consists of a course of metronidazole, which usually leads to complete resolution of pathology. Metronidazole is an antibiotic used for anaerobic infections such as *Giardia*, *Entamoeba*, and *Trichomonas*. Metronidazole is well tolerated but can cause adverse effects, including abdominal

discomfort, nausea, and a disulfiram-like effect when combined with alcohol.

Answer A is incorrect. Ampicillin, gentamicin, and clindamycin are used for broad coverage of GI infections with gram-negative rods. Gram-negative rod infections typically present with GI symptoms in the absence of liver lesions.

Answer C is incorrect. Core needle biopsy is a technique that is rarely used in the workup of liver lesions.

Answer D is incorrect. Surgical excision of hepatic lesions is the standard treatment for *Echinococcus* infection causing a hydatid cyst in the liver. Hydatidosis is often caused by eating contaminated meat. It presents as a granulomatous liver lesion, not a necrotic liver lesion. Hydatidosis lesions are walled off and potentially anaphylactic if they burst; thus, careful surgical removal is first-line treatment.

Answer E is incorrect. Aspiration is the first-line technique for hepatic cysts and lesions suspicious for cancer or other unknown pathology. An infectious etiology is more likely than cancer because the patient has diarrheal symptoms, a recent history of foreign travel, and crampy abdominal pain.

6. **The correct answer is C.** This patient has Wegener granulomatosis, a disease characterized by necrotizing, granulomatous vasculitis affecting several organs, most notably the upper respiratory tract, lung, and kidney. The elevated erythrocyte sedimentation rate (ESR) also points toward a rheumatologic cause. Furthermore, elevated serum cytoplasmic antineutrophil cytoplasmic antibody (C-ANCA) is found in 90% of patients with Wegener granulomatosis and is highly specific for the disease. Blood in the urine indicates renal involvement, and Wegener granulomatosis is associated with a segmental necrotizing glomerulonephritis, sometimes with crescents, on kidney biopsy.

   Answer A is incorrect. This finding on kidney biopsy is consistent with Alport syndrome. Patients with Alport syndrome may have hematuria, but the hallmarks are ocular disorders and nerve deafness due to defective synthesis of collagen type IV. Furthermore, C-ANCA is not associated with Alport syndrome.

   Answer B is incorrect. This finding on kidney biopsy is consistent with minimal change disease, which occurs most commonly in children and is associated with edema rather than blood in the urine.

   Answer D is incorrect. This finding on kidney biopsy is consistent with Goodpasture syndrome. Goodpasture syndrome is a type II hypersensitivity reaction against collagen type IV, causing the smooth linear staining on immunofluorescence. While this disease does commonly present with concurrent hemoptysis and hematuria, Goodpasture is not associated with C-ANCA nor is it characterized by arthralgias or sinusitis.

   Answer E is incorrect. This finding on kidney biopsy is associated with systemic lupus erythematosus (SLE), specifically a membranous glomerulonephritis (Type V) pattern. While SLE can present with varied symptoms, antinuclear antibodies and anti-double-stranded DNA antibodies are usually present and not C-ANCA, as in this patient.

7. **The correct answer is D.** This is a phenomenon known as peripheral tolerance. It is an important factor because deletion of self-reactive T lymphocytes within the thymus ("central tolerance") is not completely efficient at removing all self-reactive T lymphocytes. Thus, one mechanism of peripheral tolerance is that of anergy: When a T lymphocyte receives the first signal (peptide-major histocompatibility complex) but no second signal (costimulation, such as CD28-B7 ligation), that T lymphocyte undergoes a reprogramming known as anergy, wherein it is subsequently made refractory to any future stimulation. Note that an anergic T lymphocyte cannot be activated later even if costimulation is present.

   Answer A is incorrect. For a T lymphocyte to become activated and fully able to perform its effector functions, it must receive a second or costimulatory signal. Without a costimulatory signal, the T lymphocyte cannot be activated and instead becomes anergic.

Answer B is incorrect. A T lymphocyte that becomes anergic does not undergo activation.

Answer C is incorrect. Causing cells to undergo apoptosis is a function of an activated T-cytotoxic lympocyte.

Answer E is incorrect. The T lymphocyte will not clonally expand. Clonal expansion is more typical of B lymphocytes and requires a costimulatory signal to first activate the lymphocyte.

8. **The correct answer is E.** The patient presents with several classic features of Wilson disease. Wilson disease, a genetic condition caused by an absolute decrease in the body's production of a copper-binding protein called ceruloplasmin, is characterized by basal ganglia degeneration (producing parkinsonian-like symptomatology), elevated plasma copper levels, Kaiser-Fleischer rings (corneal copper deposits), micronodular cirrhosis of the liver, and neuropsychiatric symptoms.

   Answer A is incorrect. While the strange nature in which the patient was initially found in the street and his unwillingness to provide his medical history puts drug intoxication on the differential, the presence of other signs and symptoms (eg, corneal deposits, angiomata, and hepatomegaly) supports the diagnosis of a metabolic disorder. In addition, pupillary changes (ie, dilation and constriction) and an abnormal respiratory rate would likely be present in the case of drug intoxication.

   Answer B is incorrect. The patient's age puts him in the highest risk group for HIV infection. Given the patient's lack of cooperation and the physician's lack of knowledge regarding his sexual activity, HIV should always be considered in a young patient presenting with altered mental status. However, the variety of other clinical findings supports a different diagnosis. In addition, most patients newly infected with HIV present with a mononucleosis-like syndrome characterized by low-grade fever, myalgias, generalized rash, fatigue, and lymphadenopathy. The patient does not have any of these symptoms.

   Answer C is incorrect. Parkinson disease tends to affect older adults, with a mean age of onset around 60 years. Given that Wilson disease is characterized partly by basal ganglia degeneration, both diseases may present with a rather unsteady, shuffling gait. A more convincing scenario for Parkinson disease would involve an older man with bradykinesia, masked facies, and resting tremor.

   Answer D is incorrect. Schizophrenia is the classic psychotic disorder with an onset that closely correlates with this patient's age (age of onset: males, 15-25 years; females 20-30 years). In order to fulfill the diagnosis of schizophrenia, the patient must exhibit positive (eg, hallucinations, delusions, and disorganized speech and behavior) and negative (eg, poverty of speech and avolition) symptoms. None of these symptoms is present in this patient.

9. **The correct answer is A.** The most effective class of drug for the treatment of chemotherapy-induced nausea is the serotonin 5-hydroxytryptamine$_3$ antagonist, which includes ondansetron, dolasetron, and granisetron. These drugs can cause mild fatigue, headache, constipation, urinary retention, and dizziness.

   Answer B is incorrect. The anticholinergic class of anti-emetics includes scopolamine. These drugs are used for motion sickness, not for the treatment of chemotherapy-induced nausea.

   Answer C is incorrect. Benzodiazepines include lorazepam and diazepam. They may be effective in treatment of the anticipatory nausea associated with chemotherapy, but they are not as effective as the 5-hydroxytryptamine$_3$ antagonists.

   Answer D is incorrect. Glucocorticoids (such as dexamethasone) can suppress nausea, but are not routinely used for this indication because of their myriad other effects in the body (which may or may not be desirable).

   Answer E is incorrect. Histamine receptor antagonists include diphenhydramine and promethazine. They are used for acid reflux and allergies. Promethazine also is prescribed as an anti-emetic, but usually in the postoperative setting to combat post-narcotic nausea, or for motion sickness.

10. **The correct answer is E.** The rhythm strip shows torsades de pointes, a potentially fatal rapid ventricular rhythm. The rate is variable between 250 and 350/min and is usually transient. Torsades de pointes can be caused by a low potassium level (this patient's potassium level is within normal limits), potassium channel blockers such as sotalol, congenital abnormalities such as long QT syndrome, and, in this case, quinidine. Quinidine is notable because induced torsades de pointes occurs at therapeutic or even subtherapeutic levels. In addition, quinidine induces cinchonism, a syndrome that includes headaches and tinnitus.

    Answer A is incorrect. Adenosine is not known to cause torsades de pointes. Adenosine can cause flushing, dyspnea, and chest pain, as well as sinus bradycardia and ventricular ectopy following paroxysmal supraventricular tachycardia conversion.

    Answer B is incorrect. Esmolol, a β-blocker, is not known to cause torsades de pointes. Because esmolol is extremely short acting (15-20 minutes), there are few major adverse effects if used as indicated.

    Answer C is incorrect. Lidocaine, a sodium channel blocker, is not known to cause torsades des pointes. The possible adverse effects of lidocaine are third-degree atrioventricular (AV) heart block, altered AV node conduction, and depressed sinoatrial node automaticity.

    Answer D is incorrect. Propranolol, a β-blocker, is not known to cause torsades de pointes. Propranolol can cause bradycardia and hypotension.

    Answer F is incorrect. Verapamil, a calcium channel blocker, is not known to cause torsades des pointes. Verapamil can cause transient hypotension if incorrectly administered. This can be countered by pretreatment with calcium.

11. **The correct answer is E.** Guillain-Barré syndrome (GBS), also known as acute inflammatory demyelinating polyradiculopathy (*radiculopathy* means a disease of the spinal nerve roots and spinal nerves), is characterized morphologically by segmental demyelination of areas of peripheral nerves; inflammation of the axons themselves may also occur. Because myelin (produced by Schwann cells in the peripheral nervous system) acts physiologically as a nerve insulator to increase conduction velocity, GBS causes slower conduction velocity of action potentials through peripheral nerves and spinal nerve roots. GBS is often associated with viral infection, so this patient's recent upper respiratory infection is suspicious for the syndrome. With proper respiratory support, the mortality rate has fallen from 25% in the past to 2%-5% in 2001. Most deaths are due to paralysis, autonomic instability, or cardiac arrest.

    Answer A is incorrect. The clinical hallmark of GBS is an **ascending motor paralysis**, which begins in the distal extremities and spreads proximally. The most common causes of death from this disease are respiratory paralysis, complications of tracheostomy, and autonomic instability.

    Answer B is incorrect. GBS primarily causes demyelination of peripheral nerves, not demyelination of the basal ganglia.

    Answer C is incorrect. GBS primarily causes demyelination of peripheral nerves, not demyelination of tracts in the spinal cord.

    Answer D is incorrect. Hyperreflexia and a positive Babinski reflex are hallmarks of an upper motor neuron lesion, which occurs in the central nervous system (CNS). GBS primarily affects peripheral nerves.

12. **The correct answer is D.** Tolbutamide is a first-generation sulfonylurea that acts by stimulating the closing of potassium channels expressed in the cell membrane of pancreatic acinar β cells. It causes cellular depolarization and then calcium influx, which in turn triggers insulin release. An adverse effect of the first-generation sulfonylureas is a disulfiram-like reaction, including flushing, tachycardia,

nausea, and hyperventilation. Tolbutamide is ineffective in conditions in which there is an absolute deficiency of insulin, such as type 1 diabetes.

Answer A is incorrect. Acarbose is an α-glucosidase inhibitor that acts at the intestinal brush border to decrease the absorption of starches and other polysaccharides. This agent would be effective in maintaining glycemic control in someone with type 2 diabetes.

Answer B is incorrect. Glargine is a long-acting synthetic insulin that provides a continuous baseline level of insulin in the blood. This agent would be appropriate for use in a patient with type 1 diabetes, where it can be used in combination with a short- or intermediate-acting insulin to cover the glycemic loads associated with meals and snacks. This agent would also be suitable for a patient with type 2 diabetes, where it can be used in combination with sulfonylurea.

Answer C is incorrect. Metformin is an oral hypoglycemic agent that is thought to decrease gluconeogenesis and increase glycolysis, resulting in decreased blood glucose levels. This agent would be effective in helping to maintain glycemic control in someone with type 2 diabetes.

Answer E is incorrect. Troglitazone is a thiazolidinone that acts to sensitize peripheral tissues to insulin and increase target cell response; it does not act on pancreatic acinar cells. This agent would be effective in helping to maintain glycemic control in someone with type 2 diabetes.

13. **The correct answer is E.** According to Piaget, children from the ages of two-seven years are in the preoperational stage of cognitive development. According to Piaget, preoperatory thought includes any procedure for mentally acting on objects. At this age the procedures are typically logically inadequate. The parents in this vignette have an unreasonable expectation of their 4-year-old child's abilities to reason and think logically. Children in the preoperational stage are not capable of sustained logical thought.

    Answer A is incorrect. Dealing with abstract ideas occurs in the formal operational stage around age 12 years into adulthood. Once children reach this stage, they are able to reason logically and abstractly.

    Answer B is incorrect. Formulation and testing of hypotheses is a skill achieved in the formal operational stage, around age 12 years though adulthood. Children can play with possibilities at this stage and can see the potential strengths and weaknesses of different ideas.

    Answer C is incorrect. Children in the concrete stage, around ages 7-11 years, are capable of limited logical thought processes. They can see the relationships between thoughts and ideas and can classify them in a rational manner.

    Answer D is incorrect. Awareness of conservation is a skill from the concrete stage of cognitive development that occurs during ages 7-11 years.

14. **The correct answer is B.** This patient's presentation is consistent with intracranial injury sustained from the significant force caused by the ejection from her car. The patient was able to talk with the police at the scene of the accident but was unable to recall how the accident occurred, which likely demonstrates an initial loss of consciousness followed by normal mentation and subsequent deterioration of consciousness. While different types of intracranial bleeds can occur with trauma, this "lucid interval" is classically seen with an epidural hematoma. An overlying skull fracture is also most consistent with an epidural hematoma with rupture of the middle meningeal artery. An urgent neurosurgical consult is indicated for immediate evacuation of the expanding hematoma, which can lead to herniation.

    Answer A is incorrect. Injury to the inferior cerebral veins would result in subarachnoid bleeding. Bleeding from the inferior cerebral veins does not result from a fracture of the temporal bone and is unlikely to cause the rapid deterioration evident in this case because it has a slower rate of bleeding. However, subarachnoid bleeding is frequently seen in the setting of trauma and could be an associated finding with the epidural hematoma.

Answer C is incorrect. The posterior ethmoidal artery supplies the anterior superior nose and nasal septum with blood; its tearing would not result in an epidural hematoma secondary to a temporal bone fracture.

Answer D is incorrect. Injury to the sigmoid sinus would result in a subarachnoid hemorrhage. Thus such a finding is inconsistent with an injury to the temporal bone, the lucid interval in this patient's history, and the CT findings.

Answer E is incorrect. Injury to the superior sagittal sinus would also result in a subarachnoid hemorrhage, but this is a far less likely cause of this patient's deterioration than an epidural hematoma.

15. **The correct answer is D.** In Crigler-Najjar syndrome, the absence of glucuronyl transferase results in an inability to conjugate bilirubin, leading to an unconjugated hyperbilirubinemia (high indirect bilirubin). The jaundice will become more severe as bilirubin accumulates, and at high levels will result in brain damage. Two entities have been identified: type 1 (autosomal recessive) and type 2 (autosomal dominant). A partial glucuronyl transferase deficiency is found in Gilbert syndrome.

    Answer A is incorrect. While the patient may have abnormalities in hematocrit, they would not be due to a glucuronyl transferase deficiency.

    Answer B is incorrect. If an enzyme for conjugation is lacking, unconjugated (indirect) bilirubin will increase, not decrease.

    Answer C is incorrect. Because the enzyme missing is used for conjugating bilirubin, direct bilirubin will decrease, not increase.

    Answer E is incorrect. A hemolytic anemia would cause an increased reticulocyte count and also increase bilirubin level, which would result in jaundice. While this would further complicate the infant's condition, hemolytic anemia is not the cause of Crigler-Najjar syndrome, nor is it associated with that syndrome.

16. **The correct answer is C.** Arylsulfatase A converts sulfatide to galactocerebroside. This enzyme is deficient in patients with metachromatic leukodystrophy, an autosomal recessive lysosomal storage disease in which patients cannot degrade sulfatides, leading to accumulation of cerebroside sulfate in both neuronal and non-neuronal tissues. There is abnormal myelination with widespread loss of myelination in the CNS and peripheral nerves, leading to the clinical signs. Metachromatic granules can be seen on histologic examination.

    Answer A is incorrect. α-galactosidase A converts ceramide trihexoside to lactosyl cerebroside. This enzyme is deficient in Fabry disease.

    Answer B is incorrect. β-galactosidase converts galactocerebroside to cerebroside. This enzyme is deficient in Krabbe disease.

    Answer D is incorrect. Hexosaminidase A converts ganglioside M_2 to ganglioside M_3. This enzyme is deficient in Tay-Sachs disease.

    Answer E is incorrect. Sphingomyelinase converts sphingomyelin to cerebroside. This enzyme is deficient in Niemann-Pick disease.

17. **The correct answer is D.** The specimen from this patient indicates adenocarcinoma, which typically develops in the lower third of the esophagus near the gastric cardia. Chronic gastroesophageal reflux disease leads to Barrett esophagus, metaplasia of the squamous epithelium of the distal esophagus to columnar epithelium as a result of chronic acid exposure. Obesity increases the risk of esophageal adenocarcinoma by exacerbating reflux esophagitis. Other risk factors include known Barrett esophagus, tobacco use, and prior radiation therapy.

    Answer A is incorrect. Achalasia is caused by esophageal hypomotility and defective relaxation of the lower esophageal sphincter, leading to dysphagia, chest pain, and regurgitation of food. It is associated with squamous cell carcinoma of the esophagus, most likely as a result of chronic irritation from food abnormally retained in the esophagus.

Answer B is incorrect. The other common variant of esophageal cancer is squamous cell carcinoma. It presents similarly to adenocarcinoma with dysphagia, odynophagia, and weight loss, but is differentiated on the basis of histology and location of focus in the esophagus (the upper to middle third). Whereas adenocarcinoma of the esophagus is more common in white men, squamous cell carcinoma is typically found in African-American men. The higher incidence is most likely due to poverty and increased rates of alcohol and tobacco use.

Answer C is incorrect. Both types of esophageal cancer are more common in male patients. Squamous cell carcinoma of the esophagus is four times more common, and adenocarcinoma seven times more common, in men than in women.

Answer E is incorrect. Tobacco use is associated with both morphologic variants of esophageal cancer.

18. **The correct answer is D.** This patient's history is suggestive of infection with *Aspergillus fumigatus*, a ubiquitous fungus that can cause lung cavity aspergillomas ("fungus balls"), usually in patients with preexisting cavities in their lungs. Treatment for these lesions is by surgical removal, if they are causing significant hemoptysis; otherwise itraconazole is commonly given. *A fumigatus* can also cause bronchopulmonary aspergillosis and invasive aspergillosis, the latter almost exclusively in patients who are immunocompromised. *A fumigatus* is a non-dimorphic mold with septate hyphae that branch at a V-shaped 45-degree angle.

    Answer A is incorrect. *Pneumocystis jiroveci* recently was identified as a fungus and typically infects HIV-positive patients and other immunocompromised individuals. Symptoms include fever, malaise, dyspnea, and a nonproductive cough. Microscopy shows cup-shaped cysts with intracystic bodies. However, chest films will normally show a ground-glass appearance, not cavitations.

    Answer B is incorrect. *Cryptococcus neoformans* infection often does not present with any symptoms in an immunocompetent host. However, in an immunocompromised individual, it can present with meningoencephalitis. *Cryptococcus* is a heavily encapsulated yeast that is not dimorphic. The fungus is found in soil and pigeon droppings.

    Answer C is incorrect. *Mucor* species are molds with irregular nonseptate hyphae branching at wide angles (more than 90 degrees). Symptoms of *Mucor* pulmonary infection include an allergic reaction and infarction of distal tissue due to fungal proliferation in the walls of blood vessels. The disease is typically seen in patients with diabetic ketoacidosis and other causes of diminished immune function (eg, hematologic malignancies). Surgery and high doses of amphotericin B are used to treat pulmonary mucormycosis.

    Answer E is incorrect. *Sporothrix schenckii* is the cause of sporotrichosis. When *S schenckii* is introduced into the skin, usually by a thorn prick, it causes a local pustule or ulcer with nodules along draining lymphatics (ascending lymphangitis). *S schenckii* is a dimorphic fungus that has cigar-shaped budding yeast visible in pus. Itraconazole or potassium iodide is used for the treatment of *S schenckii* infection.

19. **The correct answer is E.** Meyer's loop is located in the temporal lobe. It carries fibers from the inferior retina that are responsible for the contralateral upper quadrant of vision. The fibers first pass through the ipsilateral optic tract. Damage to Meyer's loop on the right temporal lobe would result in bilateral left upper quadrant anopsia.

    Answer A is incorrect. The dorsal optic radiation carries fibers from the superior retina that are responsible for the contralateral lower quadrant of vision. Damage to the left dorsal optic radiation causes bilateral right lower quadrant anopsia.

Answer B is incorrect. The dorsal optic radiation carries fibers from the superior retina that are responsible for the contralateral lower quadrant of vision. Damage to the right dorsal optic radiation causes bilateral left lower quadrant anopsia.

Answer C is incorrect. The optic tract carries fibers from the temporal retina of the ipsilateral eye and from the nasal retina of the contralateral eye. Damage to the left optic tract would cause right homonymous hemianopia.

Answer D is incorrect. Damage to Meyer's loop in the left temporal lobe would result in bilateral right upper quadrant anopsia.

Answer F is incorrect. The optic tract carries fibers from the temporal retina of the ipsilateral eye and from the nasal retina of the contralateral eye. Damage to the right optic tract would cause left homonymous hemianopia.

20. **The correct answer is B.** This patient recently acquired acute hepatitis B virus (HBV) infection. Abdominal pain, positive HBsAg, and presence of IgM anti-HBcAb are consistent with the diagnosis. Up to 15 weeks after exposure, patients with HBV infection are positive for HBV DNA, HBsAg, anti-HBcAb, and HBeAg, but they are negative for anti-HBeAb and anti-HBsAb. The correct combination therapy for hepatitis B is lamivudine and interferon-α. Lamivudine is a cytidine analog that inhibits reverse transcription and therefore blocks hepatitis replication. It also is used as an HIV medication. Interferon-α is thought to block viral replication and thereby inhibit hepatitis replication.

    Answer A is incorrect. The presence of HBeAg in the patient's serum indicates an active HBV infection. HBeAg levels often are used as a marker of infectivity of the patient. A patient previously vaccinated for HBV would have only anti-HBsAb and no other markers.

    Answer C is incorrect. Interferon-β is not used in the treatment of hepatitis.

    Answer D is incorrect. Ribavirin in combination with pegylated interferon-α_2 is used in the treatment of hepatitis C. Lamivudine in combination with interferon-α_2 is used in the treatment of hepatitis B.

    Answer E is incorrect. Ribavirin in combination with pegylated interferon-α is used in the treatment of hepatitis C.

21. **The correct answer is F.** The image shows a crescent of epithelial cells and fibrin as well as a hypercellular glomerulus, which together are characteristic of rapidly progressive glomerulonephritis (RPGN). Furthermore, the clinical scenario demonstrates a nephritic syndrome, with hematuria, oliguria, and hypertension, which one would expect with RPGN. In about 50% of cases, RPGN is caused by deposition of immune complexes, but it can also be caused by pauci-immune glomerulonephritis and anti-glomerular basement membrane (GBM) disease (called Goodpasture syndrome when associated with pulmonary hemorrhage).

    Answer A is incorrect. The most common cause of end-stage renal disease in the United States is diabetic nephropathy, which causes a nephrotic syndrome. A renal biopsy would show Kimmelstiel-Wilson lesions, which are nodules of mesangial matrix.

    Answer B is incorrect. Patients with Goodpasture syndrome present with pulmonary hemorrhage and glomerulonephritis. The syndrome is caused by anti-GBM antibodies. On immunofluorescence, renal biopsy would show a linear pattern tracing the basement membrane of the glomeruli. Anti-GBM antibodies are implicated in the pathogenesis of type 1 RPGN.

    Answer C is incorrect. IgA nephropathy, or Berger disease, often presents in children as hematuria following infection. Renal biopsy shows mesangial expansion due to deposition of IgA.

    Answer D is incorrect. Lupus nephritis is the most serious symptom of SLE and often determines the prognosis of the disease. Additional symptoms of SLE included malar rash, discoid rash, photosensitivity, oral ulcers, arthritis, serositis, neurologic disorders, and immunologic disorders. Lupus nephritis causes a nephrotic syndrome with proteinuria, hypoalbuminemia, edema, and hyperlipidemia; many patients also develop hypertension. Renal biopsy is important to determine treatment, and histologic findings are classified in five patterns, including mesangial and subendothelial deposits (called "wire-loop" lesions).

Answer E is incorrect. Poststreptococcal glomerulonephritis is a common cause of nephritic syndrome that occurs about 10 days after pharyngitis. On light microscopy one would see diffuse proliferative glomerulonephritis without crescents. Electron microscopy would show subepithelial humps. Most cases are subclinical, and usually patients recover on their own, but some go on to develop RPGN, like the patient in this vignette.

Answer G is incorrect. Renal amyloidosis is associated with chronic inflammatory diseases and causes nephrotic syndrome. Glomerular amyloid deposits can be seen on renal biopsy by staining with Congo red and examining the specimen under polarized light.

22. **The correct answer is E.** The urogenital sinus in the male gives rise to the bladder, prostate, prostatic and membranous parts of the urethra and bulbourethral glands.

Answer A is incorrect. The genital tubercle gives rise to the glans penis and corpus spongiosum in the male, or the glans clitoris in the female. In contrast, posterior urethral valves may be due to failure of regression of the urogenital sinus, which normally gives rise to the prostatic urethra.

Answer B is incorrect. The mesonephric (wolffian) duct develops into the seminal vesicles, epididymis, ejaculatory duct, and vas deferens. In contrast, posterior urethral valves may be due to failure of regression of the urogenital sinus, which normally gives rise to the prostatic urethra.

Answer C is incorrect. The paramesonephric (müllerian) duct develops into the fallopian tube, uterus, and superior third of the vagina in the female. In contrast, posterior urethral valves may be due to failure of regression of the urogenital sinus, which normally gives rise to the prostatic urethra.

Answer D is incorrect. The urogenital folds make up the ventral shaft of the penis and penile urethra in the male. In contrast, posterior urethral valves may be due to failure of regression of the urogenital sinus, which normally gives rise to the prostatic urethra.

23. **The correct answer is B.** This patient suffers from the autosomal recessive disorder alkaptonuria, a deficiency in homogentisic acid oxidase. This enzyme is responsible for degradation of tyrosine. As a result of the deficiency, there is an accumulation of alkapton bodies (homogentisic acid) in urine and cartilage. The lack of homogentisic oxidase blocks the metabolism of phenylalanine-tyrosine at the level of homogentisic acid. The homogentisic acid accumulates and a large amount is excreted, imparting a black color to the urine if allowed to stand and undergo oxidation. Dark spots can also be observed in the eyes of some patients. Affected patients are usually asymptomatic in childhood other than the change in urine color upon standing. In adulthood, the build-up of pigment in cartilage and its calcification can cause arthritic changes. By an unknown mechanism, the pigment causes the cartilage to lose its resiliency and become brittle and fibrillated. The arthropathy develops slowly and usually does not manifest until the patient is >30 years old. Although it is not life-threatening, it may be severely disabling.

Answer A is incorrect. A deficiency of branched-chain α-ketoacid dehydrogenase would result in maple syrup urine disease, an inability to break down branched-chain amino acids.

Answer C is incorrect. Phenylketonuria is caused by a deficiency in phenylalanine hydroxylase.

Answer D is incorrect. Refsum disease is a deficiency of phytanic acid oxidase and is characterized by an inability to break down branched-chain fatty acids.

Answer E is incorrect. Tyrosinase is the enzyme responsible for the synthesis of tyrosine. This deficiency results in albinism because patients are unable to make melanin, a derivative of tyrosine.

24. **The correct answer is D.** Introns are noncoding regions of RNA that are spliced out of mature mRNA. Almost all introns begin and end with 5'-GU——AG-3'. A mutation in one of those nucleotides affects splicing. This type of mutation is one of those found in the thalassemia picture, as described in this patient.

    Answer A is incorrect. Capping of the mRNA occurs at the 5' end as it is being transcribed. A mutation at the 5' end of an intron would not affect capping.

    Answer B is incorrect. Hybridization is a process in which single-stranded DNA base-pairs with a complementary sequence. A mutation at the 5' end of an intron would not affect hybridization

    Answer C is incorrect. A poly (A) tail is added to the 3' end of heterogeneous nuclear RNA (hnRNA, the initial RNA transcript) after transcription. Poly(A) polymerase uses ATP as a precursor for adding adenosine one molecule at a time. A mutation at the 5' end of an intron would not affect polyadenylation.

    Answer E is incorrect. Transcription of the DNA into RNA would not be affected by this mutation.

25. **The correct answer is D.** This patient's presentation suggests an IgM-mediated (cold) hemolytic anemia, an anemia often encountered after a recent Epstein-Barr virus (EBV) infection. Infectious mononucleosis (which is caused by EBV) is associated with IgM antibodies directed at the i (lower case) antigen found on RBCs. In contrast, *Mycoplasma pneumoniae* infection typically yields a hemolytic anemia in which IgM antibodies are directed at the I (upper case) antigen. Following either infection, IgM binds both complement and RBCs at lower temperatures (ie, as found in the extremities), but falls off the RBCs as the cells return to the central circulation. Agglutination of RBCs in the periphery can lead to gray/purple discoloration of the fingers, as seen in this patient.

    Answer A is incorrect. Aplastic anemia results in pancytopenia, malaise, and severe infection. This disorder is a hypoproliferative anemia in which an appropriate reticulocytosis, as seen in this patient, is absent.

    Answer B is incorrect. Acute disseminated intravascular coagulation (DIC) results in bleeding and shock. Chronic DIC results in thrombosis and clotting. DIC typically is not associated with mononucleosis, but instead with gram-negative sepsis, acute myelogenous leukemia (AML), and obstetric complications.

    Answer C is incorrect. Coombs test for IgG-mediated (warm) hemolytic anemia is positive for IgG that preferentially binds RBCs at warmer temperatures. Warm hemolytic anemia is associated with autoimmune disease, lymphoproliferative disorders, and drug abuse.

    Answer E is incorrect. Paroxysmal nocturnal hemoglobinuria is caused by a defect in the RBC's protective mechanism against complement-mediated lysis. Loss of the *PIGA* gene product, required for the surface anchoring of decay-accelerating factor, results in episodic acute intravascular hemolysis and thrombosis.

26. **The correct answer is B.** Seven-transmembrane-domain receptors on cell surfaces are G-coupled receptors. Many drugs bind to G-protein-coupled receptors. Activation of G_q leads to activation of phosphatidylcholine, which breaks down phosphatidylinositol bisphosphate into inositol 1,4,5-triphosphate (IP_3) and diacylglycerol (DAG). IP_3 activates IP_3 receptors in the endoplasmic reticulum, leading to release of calcium from intracellular stores, while DAG activates protein kinase C.

    Answer A is incorrect. Activation of G_i leads to downregulation of adenylyl cyclase and subsequent decrease in cAMP and downregulation of protein kinase A. Activation of G_i is not linked to a rise in intracellular calcium.

    Answer C is incorrect. Activation of G_s leads to upregulation of adenylyl cyclase and an increase in cAMP, which then would lead to activation of protein kinase A. Activation of G_s is not related to a rise in intracellular calcium.

Answer D is incorrect. Upregulation of cGMP does not lead to an increase in intracellular calcium.

27. **The correct answer is C.** The symptoms of fever, fatigue, night sweats, lymphadenopathy, and hemoptysis are consistent with the diagnosis of tuberculosis (TB). The causative agent of TB is *Mycobacterium tuberculosis*. Primary TB infections are only rarely symptomatic in patients with normal immune function due to rapid containment by resident alveolar macrophages and infiltrating monocytes and lymphocytes. Symptomatic primary infection is mostly seen in the elderly, children, and immunocompromised individuals. Primary TB resembles an acute bacterial pneumonia, is typically located in the lower and middle lobes, and rarely causes cavitation. Secondary TB often localizes to the apex/upper lobes of the lungs, as shown in the x-ray film. A caseating granuloma is formed in which necrotic tissue and bacteria are surrounded by macrophages and giant cells. TB is initially treated with isoniazid, rifampin, ethambutol, pyrazinamide, and streptomycin, while isoniazid can be used alone to prevent TB or to treat suspected cases of latent TB. The adverse effects of isoniazid include neurotoxicity and hepatotoxicity.

   Answer A is incorrect. This is an adverse effect of metronidazole, which is not used to treat or prevent TB.

   Answer B is incorrect. Aplastic anemia is not commonly associated with isoniazid.

   Answer D is incorrect. This effect has been associated with tetracyclines, which are not used as first-line treatment or for prevention of TB.

   Answer E is incorrect. Nephrotoxicity, ototoxicity, and teratogenic effects are associated with aminoglycosides, which are often used to treat gram-negative infections, not to prevent or treat TB.

28. **The correct answer is D.** The patient is suffering from Hashimoto thyroiditis, an autoimmune disorder that is a common cause of hypothyroidism. Other classic signs and symptoms of hypothyroidism include cold intolerance, hypoactivity, weakness, diminished reflexes, dry and cool skin, and coarse hair. Laboratory studies would reveal increased thyroid-stimulating hormone (TSH) levels (the most sensitive laboratory test for primary hypothyroidism) and decreased total triiodothyronine and thyroxine levels. In patients with Hashimoto thyroiditis, the thyroid gland is usually enlarged and firm, while histology reveals a significant lymphocyte and plasma cell infiltrate with germinal center formation, colloid-sparse follicles, and Hörthle cells (the acidophilic cells described in the vignette). Patients with Hashimoto thyroiditis frequently have a personal or family history of autoimmune disease, and there is an increased incidence of in the disease among individuals with HLA-DR5 and -B5 haplotypes. Antimicrosomal antibodies, also called antithyroid peroxidase antibodies, are associated with Hashimoto thyroiditis. Antithyroglobulin antibodies may also be seen.

   Answer A is incorrect. Anti-smooth muscle antibodies may be seen in the setting of autoimmune hepatitis.

   Answer B is incorrect. Anti-U1 RNP antibodies are associated with mixed connective tissue disease.

   Answer C is incorrect. Anticentromere antibodies are associated with CREST syndrome.

   Answer E is incorrect. Antimitochondrial antibodies are associated with primary biliary cirrhosis.

29. **The correct answer is A.** This is a typical clinical picture of Rett syndrome, a rare pervasive developmental disorder nearly always affecting girls 4 years old or younger. The hallmark features include decelerating social, cognitive, and verbal development that slowly progress to degeneration in these areas. Children become mentally retarded, expressionless, and nonverbal over the course of several years. Character-

istic hand-wringing movements begin at about the same time as the developmental decline.

Answer B is incorrect. Although language and social degeneration occurs in patients with Rett syndrome, gross hearing is unaffected.

Answer C is incorrect. Hyperactivity is not associated with Rett syndrome; in fact, children with Rett syndrome are typically withdrawn, apathetic, and solemn.

Answer D is incorrect. Psychosis is not a feature of Rett syndrome.

Answer E is incorrect. Repetitive and compulsive behaviors such as self-injury and purposeless movements characterize autism and Asperger's disorder. They are not associated with Rett syndrome.

Answer F is incorrect. Tics are characteristic of Tourette syndrome, which typically begins in childhood. Loss of social and cognitive function is not associated with this disorder.

30. **The correct answer is B.** The image shows hypersegmented neutrophils, which are commonly seen in megaloblastic anemia. Causes of megaloblastic anemia are folate and vitamin B_{12} deficiency. By an unknown mechanism, phenytoin blocks absorption of folate and increases utilization of folate by the body, leading to folic acid deficiency.

    Answer A is incorrect. β-thalassemias are hereditary disorders of hemoglobin that result in decreased β-chain synthesis. This disorder results in a microcytic anemia.

    Answer C is incorrect. Iron deficiency results in a microcytic anemia with small, hypochromic RBCs on peripheral blood smear.

    Answer D is incorrect. While vitamin B_{12} deficiency can cause a megaloblastic anemia, phenytoin is not a cause of vitamin B_{12} deficiency.

    Answer E is incorrect. Vitamin B_6 (pyridoxine) deficiency can cause dermatitis, glossitis, stomatitis, a microcytic anemia, and peripheral neuropathy in adolescents and adults. Younger children will suffer from encephalopathy and seizures.

31. **The correct answer is B.** This woman is suffering from bacterial pneumonia, but despite her infection, her WBC count and absolute neutrophil count are low. The most likely explanation for her laboratory results is agranulocytosis, an adverse effect of clozapine use. Clozapine antagonizes D_1- and D_2-receptor. Patients taking clozapine must have regular blood panel testing to monitor for abnormalities.

    Answer A is incorrect. Bromocriptine, pergolide, pramipexole, and ropinirole are dopamine receptor agonists working mainly at D_1 to D_3 receptors in the brain. They are used as adjunctive treatment to levodopa in Parkinson disease. Dopamine receptor agonists are not associated with agranulocytosis, but neurologic adverse effects include dyskinesias, hallucinations, and confusion.

    Answer C is incorrect. GABA receptor agonists, such as benzodiazepines, ethanol, or barbiturates, inhibit the CNS, causing relaxation and sedation. They are not associated with agranulocytosis or other hematologic abnormalities.

    Answer D is incorrect. The GABA receptor antagonist flumazenil is used as an antidote to benzodiazepine overdose. Flumazenil competitively binds at the site on the GABA receptor where benzodiazepines usually bind, thus reversing their sedating effects. It does not antagonize the CNS effects of other GABA agonists. Flumazenil does not have any hematologic adverse effects.

    Answer E is incorrect. N-methyl-D-aspartate (NMDA) receptors open in response to binding glutamate, allowing an influx of cations. NMDA receptors play an important role in learning and memory. NMDA receptor antagonists are most often used as anesthetics for animals and are rarely used in humans. More commonly, humans use NMDA receptor antagonists as recreational drugs because of their hallucinogenic effects; examples include ketamine and phencyclidine. NMDA receptor antagonists have a number of neurologic and psychiatric adverse effects, but they do not have hematologic adverse effects.

32. **The correct answer is D.** *Treponema pallidum*, the bacterium that causes syphilis, produces an endarteritis obliterans of the vasa vasorum, which supplies blood to the arch of the aorta. This can lead to ischemia of the tissue, weakening and dilation of the aorta, and subsequent aortic regurgitation. The murmur described is generally associated with this type of pathology. Marfan syndrome, an autosomal dominant genetic disorder resulting in defects in the fibrillin-1 protein, is also associated with aortic regurgitation, due both to instrinsic valvular degeneration and to dilation of the aortic root.

    Answer A is incorrect. Chronic rheumatic heart disease can lead to various types of valvular damage, most commonly mitral stenosis. Although it can lead to aortic valvular damage, it would almost always be accompanied by symptoms of mitral stenosis as well.

    Answer B is incorrect. Congenital bicuspid aortic valves generally lead to calcification of the valves and aortic stenosis, not aortic regurgitation. Aortic stenosis is associated with a crescendo-decrescendo systolic ejection murmur that follows an ejection click.

    Answer C is incorrect. Congenital pulmonary stenosis is not associated with aortic insufficiency. It is associated with right ventricular hypertrophy, increased jugular venous pressure, and poor oxygenation of blood.

33. **The correct answer is A.** This patient presents with amenorrhea due to menopause, defined by 12 months of amenorrhea that results from ovarian follicular depletion with consequent decrease in estrogen. Because of a lack of a maturing follicle, there is decreased estrogen secretion. Normally, estrogen feeds back to the pituitary to decrease gonadotropin-releasing hormone, follicle-stimulating hormone (FSH), and luteinizing hormone (LH). Without estrogen there is a decrease in the negative feedback. Thus FSH and LH levels increase without estrogen's suppression.

    Answer B is incorrect. Positive feedback is a rare regulatory mechanism. One example of its use is when estrogen has positive feedback on the pituitary, causing the estrogen-dependent estrogen surge right before the LH surge of ovulation. Although a decrease in estrogen may lead to less estrogen to cause this normal positive feedback mechanism, this is not the most likely explanation of menopause.

    Answer C is incorrect. There would be no down-regulation of nuclear receptors in menopause.

    Answer D is incorrect. There is a decrease, not an increase, in the negative feedback of estrogen on the pituitary that leads to increases in LH and FSH.

    Answer E is incorrect. There is no increase in positive feedback as would be seen during ovulation of a normal non-menopausal cycle.

    Answer F is incorrect. Another mechanism of increasing the sensitivity of hormonal changes is in up-regulating and down-regulating hormone receptors. Although in theory this might be expected as menopause ensues and there is less estrogen, this is not the best answer to explain the increases in FSH and LH.

34. **The correct answer is D.** Elevated galactitol levels is the cause of clinical symptoms in patients with galactosemia. Galactose is converted in two steps to glucose-1-phosphate. The first step is catalyzed by the enzyme galactokinase, which phosphorylates galactose to galactose-1-phosphate. The second step is catalyzed by galactose-1-phosphate uridyl transferase (G1PUR), which converts galactose-1-phosphate to glucose-1-phosphate. In the absence of G1PUR, upstream intermediates in galactose metabolism accumulate, including galactose-1-phosphate and galactitol. A deficiency in enzymes involved in other aspects of galactose metabolism leads to a much milder presentation (ie, only infantile cataracts). Although treatment is not available, prevention of disease progression involves excluding galactose-containing foods from the diet, including breast milk and lactose-containing formulas.

Answer A is incorrect. Galactose is upstream from G1PUR and ts levels would be elevated.

Answer B is incorrect. Classic galactosemia is caused by a deficiency of this uridyltransferase and would theoretically lead to a build up of galactose-1-phosphate, uridine diphosphoglucose, and galactose, and decreased glucose-1-phosphate.

Answer C is incorrect. Glucose-1-phosphate is a downstream product of G1PUR, and would be decreased in galactosemia.

Answer E is incorrect. Glucose-1-phosphate is an intermediate in glycogen pathways. However, galactosemia does not affect glycogen levels.

35. **The correct answer is F.** Based on the presenting symptoms of abdominal pain, bloody stools, Ashkenazi Jewish ancestry, and family history, this patient is suffering from inflammatory bowel disease (IBD), most likely ulcerative colitis. The image shows classical diffuse mucosal inflammation with pseudopolyps. Pseudopolyps are areas where mucosa has been eroded away such that only islands of intact mucosa remain; given their polypoid shape, these islands are referred to as pseudopolyps. However, they are actually the only "normal" parts of mucosa left, and the pathology is the ulcerative lesions all around these pseudopolyps. Infectious etiologies of diarrhea are less likely given the patient's absence of fever, left shift, sick contacts, and foreign travel. Increased ESR is also consistent with diagnosis of IBD. Sulfasalazine is first-line therapy for ulcerative colitis. It is metabolized to 5-aminosalicylic acid in the digestive tract and decreases inflammation locally. Adverse effects include renal insufficiency and increased risk of bleeding.

    Answer A is incorrect. Ciprofloxacin may be useful in the treatment of ulcerative colitis complicated by strictures and infections of the GI tract; however, it is not first-line treatment for inflammatory bowel disease.

    Answer B is incorrect. Surgery, specifically colectomy in the case of ulcerative colitis, should be reserved for patients who have failed medical therapy.

    Answer C is incorrect. Infliximab, a monoclonal antibody against tumor necrosis factor α, is used for the treatment of severe ulcerative colitis following failure of more conservative therapies.

    Answer D is incorrect. Loperamide, an antidiarrheal, should be used only in mild ulcerative colitis. While it may be useful for treatment of mild symptoms, it is not first-line therapy. Caution for development of fulminant colitis and/or toxic megacolon should preclude the use of antidiarrheals in patients with severe disease.

    Answer E is incorrect. Oral steroids are used for treatment of moderate-severity ulcerative colitis that is refractory to first-line therapy. This patient is suffering from mild disease and may benefit from the addition of oral steroids if sulfasalazine therapy fails.

36. **The correct answer is B.** Huntington disease is inherited in an autosomal dominant manner. It is caused by the expansion of CAG repeats on chromosome 4, which is associated with the progressive degeneration of the caudate nucleus and subsequent loss of GABAergic neurons. A primary function of the caudate is to modulate motor action plans arising from the frontal cortex. Patients typically present in the third or fourth decades of life with symptoms of chorea, depression, and dementia.

    Answer A is incorrect. Klüver-Bucy syndrome, clinically manifested by hyperorality, hypersexuality, and disinhibited behavior, is associated with bilateral obliteration of the amygdala.

    Answer C is incorrect. Amyotrophic lateral sclerosis, more commonly known as Lou Gehrig's disease, is associated with degeneration of the lateral corticospinal tracts.

    Answer D is incorrect. Wernicke encephalopathy, which is most commonly seen in malnourished alcoholics, is associated with atrophy of the mammillary bodies.

Answer E is incorrect. Alzheimer disease is marked by a decreased number of neurons in the nucleus basalis of Meynert.

Answer F is incorrect. Parkinson disease is characterized histologically by neuronal depletion and depigmentation of cells in the substantia nigra.

37. **The correct answer is B.** Confidence intervals (CIs) specify a lower and upper limit of variability around a specific probability in which data points are likely to fall. Frequently, the 95% CI is used; this means that in 95% of cases, the true value for the population will fall within the given CI. Generally, if the 95% CIs do not overlap, the means of the groups differ significantly. If the CI overlap considerably, it is less likely that there is a significant difference between the means of the two groups. However, one must be careful with this assumption because if two CI come very close but do not overlap, there may not be significant difference at the $p = 0.05$ level. Conversely, a small overlap of CI does not preclude the possibility of difference between the means, but the chance that this difference is significant at the $p = 0.05$ level is much less likely. In this case, the CI of the mean for no intervention does not overlap the CI of the mean for albuterol. Thus, there is likely a significant difference between these means.

Answer A is incorrect. Because there is overlap in the CI of the mean peak expiratory flow rate with albuterol and drug X, it is unlikely that there is a significant difference between the means of these two conditions.

Answer C is incorrect. Because there is overlap in the CIs of the mean peak expiratory flow rate with albuterol and no intervention, it is unlikely that there is a significant difference between the means of these two conditions.

Answer D is incorrect. When assessing odds ratio or relative risk, if the 95% CI includes the value 1, the null hypothesis cannot be rejected. This means that the data do not confirm a significant difference between the odds of having a disease based on the odds ratio or the risk of getting a disease based on the relative risk versus the unexposed population. However, in this case, the CI refers to means of the population, not to odds ratio or relative risk, and these values cannot be determined simply by dividing the two means. Thus, it is unlikely that there is a significant difference between the means of albuterol and drug X because the CI of the means overlap.

Answer E is incorrect. The CI of the mean for no intervention does not overlap the CI of the mean for albuterol. Thus, there is likely a significant difference between these means. Although the width of the CIs signifies increased variability within the population, this does not preclude significant differences between the means.

38. **The correct answer is D.** HIV-associated dementia (also known as AIDS dementia complex) presents with memory loss, gait disorder, and spasticity. It represents the most common direct CNS complication of HIV disease and generally occurs later in the course of illness. Early symptoms may be subtle and may include depressive symptoms and apathetic withdrawal; later symptoms include global dementia and motor deficits. As the dementia progresses, patients experience difficulty with smooth limb movement, dysdiadochokinesia (impairment in performing rapid, alternating movements), impaired saccadic eye movements, hyperreflexia, and frontal release signs. Imaging studies are imperative to rule out mass lesions; 20%-40% of patients will demonstrate non-enhancing, poorly demarcated areas of increased T2 signal intensity in the deep white matter. The symptoms must be distinguished from typical focal neurologic signs and symptoms that may be evident in patients with mass lesions. Elevated levels of protein and IgG on cerebrospinal fluid (CSF) examination are present in approximately 45% and 80% of cases, respectively.

Answer A is incorrect. CNS lymphoma typically affects patients with AIDS whose CD4+ cell counts are <50/mm^3 with one or more enhancing lesions on MRI (50% multiple; 50% single). It can present with many signs and symptoms that overlap with HIV-associated dementia, but it is less insidious and typically causes more focal signs earlier in the course of the illness. CNS lymphoma can present with a positive polymerase chain reaction for Epstein-Barr virus within the CSF.

Answer B is incorrect. Cytomegalovirus (CMV) encephalitis can mimic HIV-associated dementia, but is usually more rapidly progressive and is typically concurrent with more generalized CMV infections. MRI typically demonstrates enhancing periventricular white matter lesions in cortical and subependymal regions.

Answer C is incorrect. Disseminated *Mycobacterium avium* complex infection is a late-stage complication of AIDS and is associated with CD4+ cell counts <50/mm^3. It typically presents with constitutional signs and symptoms that include fever, night sweats, lymphadenopathy, hepatosplenomegaly, weight loss, and pancytopenia. The symptoms are more generalized and severe than those in HIV-associated dementia.

Answer E is incorrect. Space-occupying lesions secondary to toxoplasmosis infection begin to occur with CD4+ cell counts <100/mm^3 and typically appear as enhancing CNS lesions (which may be multiple) on MRI, with positive serologies. Treatment is typically with sulfadiazine and pyrimethamine, with imaging studies repeated after a few weeks. If no regression has occurred, the diagnosis should be reconsidered, and CNS lymphoma should be considered the most likely diagnosis.

39. **The correct answer is E.** The hormone prolactin is secreted by the anterior pituitary. In contrast to the posterior pituitary, which is derived from neuroectoderm and considered an extension of the brain, the anterior pituitary is derived from oral ectoderm on the roof of the mouth.

Answer A is incorrect. Neither the anterior nor the posterior pituitary is derived from endoderm. The patient's adenoma developed in the anterior pituitary, which is derived from oral ectoderm.

Answer B is incorrect. Neither the anterior nor the posterior pituitary is derived from mesoderm. The patient's adenoma developed in the anterior pituitary, which is derived from oral ectoderm.

Answer C is incorrect. Neither the anterior nor the posterior pituitary is derived from neural crest cells. The patient's adenoma developed in the anterior pituitary, which is derived from oral ectoderm.

Answer D is incorrect. Neuroectoderm gives rise to the posterior pituitary, but the patient's adenoma is a prolactin-secreting tumor that develops in the anterior pituitary. The anterior pituitary is derived from oral ectoderm.

40. **The correct answer is D.** I-cell disease is an autosomal recessive disorder that results from improper intracellular trafficking. This impaired trafficking results from the failure to add a mannose-6-phosphate residue to proteins that should be directed to lysosomes. On a cellular level, this results in the presence of numerous intracytoplasmic inclusions in cells of mesenchymal origin. These inclusions are membrane-bound vacuoles that are filled with fibrillogranular material, including a variety of lipids, mucopolysaccharides, and oligosaccharides. Clinically this deficiency results in a select group of identifying features. Be on the lookout for coarse facial features in a baby that is developmentally delayed and has restricted joint movement.

Answer A is incorrect. Congenital herpes infection is characterized by acute CNS findings; keratoconjunctivitis, vesicles on the skin, eyes, and mucous membranes.

Answer B is incorrect. Congenital rubella infection is a devastating disease. It is characterized by cataracts, glaucoma, pigmented retinopathy, cardiac malformations and deafness. None of these symptoms is evident in this child.

Answer C is incorrect. Ehlers-Danlos syndrome is not explained by this mechanism. This baby does not demonstrate any of the symptoms of this disease; furthermore, this disease is not usually diagnosed until the end of the first decade of life.

Answer E is incorrect. Fibrillin mutations account for Marfan syndrome, not a likely diagnosis in this baby.

41. **The correct answer is E.** As seen in the image the presence of many lymphocytes and few Reed-Sternberg cells with collagen bands that circumscribe the lymphoid tissue into discrete nodules is consistent with the nodular-sclerosing subtype of Hodgkin disease. This is the subtype with the best prognosis, and it also is the most common. Nodular-sclerosing Hodgkin lymphoma is more common in women. This histologic picture also resembles the lymphocyte-predominance subtype, which is much less common but has an excellent prognosis; it also is found in women.

Answer A is incorrect. AML does not affect the lymph nodes but, rather, produces abnormalities in the blood and bone marrow. This disease usually affects patients of middle age (35-50 years) and is characterized by the presence of numerous myeloid precursor cells with the presence of Auer's rods.

Answer B is incorrect. Burkitt lymphoma is a non-Hodgkin type of lymphoma that predominantly is a B-lymphocyte lymphoma. It is associated with Epstein-Barr virus infections that can lead to activating mutations of *c-myc* caused by chromosomal translocation t(8;14). Histologically Burkitt lymphoma is characterized by sheets of lymphocytes with interspersed macrophages; this is referred to commonly as a "starry sky" appearance.

Answer C is incorrect. Any type of Hodgkin disease (HD) involving many Reed-Sternberg cells and no or few lymphocytes describes the rare lymphocyte-depletion subtype. This has the worst prognosis of any type of HD and generally is present in elderly men with disseminated disease.

Answer D is incorrect. The heterogeneous mixture of many mononuclear cells, many Reed-Sternberg cells, and many lymphocytes is consistent with mixed-cellularity HD. This subtype is more common in men and more likely to be diagnosed at a later stage. The overall prognosis is good.

42. **The correct answer is B.** This patient is undergoing acute graft-versus-host disease (GVHD), which classically has a triad of dermatitis, hepatitis, and gastroenteritis. GVHD is a serious complication of allogeneic blood or marrow transplantation, and is mediated by donor lymphocytes reacting against major or minor histocompatibility antigens on recipient cells that are recognized as foreign.

Answer A is incorrect. ABO incompatibility occurs when there is transfusion of incompatible blood types. If patients are exposed to blood that is incompatible with their own blood type, they may undergo an immune-mediated hemolytic anemia that could eventually lead to jaundice. The most common example is Rh incompatibility in pregnant patients.

Answer C is incorrect. By definition, chronic graft-versus-host disease occurs >100 days after transplant and can affect any organ system.

Answer D is incorrect. Primary graft rejection occurs when neutrophil and platelet recovery does not occur in the usual time frame expected after transplantation, and is mediated by the recipient immune system against alloantigens expressed on donor stem cells. Patients in acute rejection do not present with dermatitis, hepatitis, and gastroenteritis as in graft-versus-host disease.

Answer E is incorrect. Hyperacute rejection is seen only in solid organ transplants. Hyperacute graft-versus-host disease is an entity that may occur within minutes of the time of engraftment.

43. **The correct answer is E.** This patient has a metabolic alkalosis as her pH is >7.4 and partial pressure of carbon dioxide is > 40 mm Hg. This is secondary to her dehydration (which is apparent by her symptoms of orthostatic hypotension). Her frequent emesis results in the loss of large quantities of protons from the body in the form of stomach acid. In addition, rapid loss of bicarbonate-free fluids such as

stomach contents or urine can result in a net increase in plasma bicarbonate concentration; this effect is termed "contraction alkalosis." Finally, volume depletion leads to stimulation of the renin-angiotensin-aldosterone system (RAAS), causing (1) an angiotensin-mediated increase in hydrogen secretion via the sodium-hydrogen antiporter in the proximal tubule, and (2) an aldosterone-triggered influx of sodium (and water) and an efflux of potassium and protons in the distal tubule. The loss of protons and build-up of bicarbonate in this patient causes metabolic alkalosis.

Answer A is incorrect. Consumption of antacids can contribute to metabolic alkalosis but is not the cause in this patient.

Answer B is incorrect. Dehydration causes an increase, not decrease, in hydrogen excretion in the distal tubule.

Answer C is incorrect. Total bicarbonate reabsorption in the setting of metabolic alkalosis and volume depletion is likely to be reduced. Acutely, volume depletion will result in a net decrease in the filtered load of bicarbonate, despite an increase in bicarbonate concentration. In addition, increased plasma levels of bicarbonate will impair the ability of the proximal tubule cells to secrete acid necessary for bicarbonate reabsorption. Although angiotensin II stimulation serves to partially counteract these effects, the proximal tubule is not the primary site of acid loss in this patient.

Answer D is incorrect. ADH does not have direct effects on acid-base status because the aquaporin channels it mobilizes to the cell membrane are permeable only to water.

44. **The correct answer is A.** The patient suffered a thoracic aortic dissection. Malignant hypertension predisposes to this sudden tear along the aorta. In fact, aortic dissections often present with a tearing pain along the patient's back. Because the symptoms of aortic dissection are similar to those of a myocardial infarction (MI), and because dissections are often not recognized on ECG, they are often either misdiagnosed or not recognized at all.

Answer B is incorrect. Gastrointestinal reflux disease (GERD) can often mimic the symptoms of MI and cause pathologic abnormalities in the esophagus. GERD, however, rarely results in the sudden death of a patient.

Answer C is incorrect. An occlusion of the left coronary artery is a very common cause of MI that is detectable on ECG.

Answer D is incorrect. Acute thrombosis due to coronary artery atherosclerosis results in myocyte necrosis of the ventricular wall. This would be an MI with a typical and strongly detectable pattern on ECG.

Answer E is incorrect. Changes in the pericardium may evolve over time as a result of an MI. Fibrinous pericarditis (friction rub) can occur three-five days after an MI. Dressler syndrome (an autoimmune phenomenon) may occur several weeks after an MI in a surviving patient.

45. **The correct answer is C.** The condition described is polycystic ovarian syndrome (PCOS, or Stein-Leventhal syndrome). The main characteristics of PCOS are oligoovulation or anovulation and hyperandrogenism. Features seen in PCOS include ovarian cysts, amenorrhea, infertility, obesity, and hirsutism caused by excess LH production and androgens. In some women PCOS is associated with insulin resistance and hyperinsulinemia, which increases androgen production in the ovarian theca cells and, secondarily, LH production. Insulin resistance leads to hyperglycemia and also suppresses hepatic steroid hormone-binding globulin (SHBG) synthesis. The decrease in SHBG along with the increase in androgen production leads to a vicious cycle of amenorrhea and infertility.

Answer A is incorrect. Patients with Kallmann syndrome present with hypogonadotrophic (decreased levels of gonadotropin-releasing hormone) hypogonadism (decreased LH and FSH levels) along with anosmia (lack of smell).

Answer B is incorrect. Amenorrhea and galactorrhea are signs of hyperprolactinemia.

Prolactin is controlled by dopamine secretion from the hypothalamus and inhibits gonadotropin secretion. Patients with hyperprolactinemias typically have pituitary microadenomas that secrete prolactin. They present with visual field defects, nipple discharge bilaterally, and hypogonadism. This leads to decreased levels of LH and FSH, oligomenorrhea or amenorrhea, infertility, and galactorrhea. This would not explain the high level of LH, elevated androgen levels, or enlarged ovaries seen in this patient.

Answer D is incorrect. Polycystic kidney disease (PKD) is an autosomal dominant disease. Patients generally present in their 40s-50s with abdominal discomfort, hematuria, urinary tract infections, hypertension, and renal insufficiency. On gross pathology, the kidneys are enlarged and the normal parenchyma is replaced by dozens of cysts. Although PKD is associated with berry aneurysms and cardiac anomalies, this disease is not associated with polycystic ovarian syndrome.

Answer E is incorrect. Weak pulses in the lower extremities may be a sign of coarctation of the aorta, which is associated with Turner syndrome. Turner syndrome is the most common cause of primary amenorrhea, and patients present with short stature, webbed neck, and infantile genitalia. Ovaries are replaced with fibrous streaks, and appear small and fibrotic on ultrasound, as opposed to enlarged and cystic.

46. **The correct answer is C.** The suspicion of child abuse arises when the injury and the story of the injury do not match. Spiral fractures generally do not occur with a simple fall down the stairs. Another indication of abuse is multiple bruises at varying stages of healing and this patient's history of trauma occurring in the home. Suspicion of child abuse must be reported in all 50 states.

Answer A is incorrect. Children with osteogenesis imperfecta can present with spiral fractures as a result of seemingly benign accidents. In this case, however, the history and evidence strongly support child abuse.

Answer B is incorrect. Retinal hemorrhage and detachment also are seen frequently in cases of child abuse. If there is suspicion of retinal damage, the child should then see an ophthalmologist, but an urgent retinal examination is not necessary at this time.

Answer D is incorrect. Although confronting the family and offering assistance may be well intended, it is not the appropriate course of action in this situation.

Answer E is incorrect. The possibility of child abuse should not be taken lightly. Normal or even careless play is an insufficient explanation for a serious injury such as a spiral fracture of the femur.

47. **The correct answer is B.** The paired, mesodermally derived organs that give rise to a bicornuate uterus are the müllerian tubes, otherwise known as the paramesonephric ducts. These paired structures also develop into the fallopian tubes, and the upper, proximal portion of the vagina. In the presence of müllerian inhibiting factor, which is synthesized and secreted by Sertoli's cells (ie, in XY individuals), the müllerian tubes degenerate into a vestigial remnant called the appendix testes, or hydatid of Morgagni. These vestigial structures are most often found on the upper pole of the testes adjacent to the tunica vaginalis.

Answer A is incorrect. The appendix epididymis is a small appendage on the head of the epididymis derived from the wolffian (mesonephric) duct, which is the genital duct that develops into the seminal vesicles, epididymis, ejaculatory duct, and vas deferens in the presence of androgens.

Answer C is incorrect. The bulbourethral glands (also known as Cowper glands) are small exocrine glands found on the posterior and lateral aspect of the membranous urethra at the base of the penis. They are not derived from the müllerian ducts.

Answer D is incorrect. The paradidymis is another structure derived from the wolffian duct. It is composed of tubules located above the head of the epididymis.

Answer E is incorrect. Skene glands (also known as paraurethral glands) are small glands found on the anterior wall of the vagina. They are not derived from the müllerian ducts.

48. **The correct answer is A.** Acyclovir is a guanosine analog used in the treatment of active herpesvirus infections. Acyclovir causes premature DNA chain termination and limits the length of a herpes outbreak, although it does not change the frequency with which they occur.

Answer B is incorrect. Didanosine is a nucleoside reverse transcriptase inhibitor used in HIV therapy. It is not used in treating herpes virus infection.

Answer C is incorrect. Foscarnet is a viral DNA polymerase inhibitor that binds to the pyrophosphate binding site of the enzyme. It is used to treat CMV retinitis when ganciclovir fails. It is also used to treat acyclovir-resistant herpes simplex virus infection.

Answer D is incorrect. Ganciclovir is phosphorylated by viral kinase. It preferentially inhibits CMV DNA polymerase and is used to treat CMV retinitis, especially in immunocompromised patients. It is not first-line treatment for herpes virus infection.

Answer E is incorrect. Zanamivir inhibits influenza neuraminidase, reducing the release of progeny virus. It is used in the treatment of both influenza A and B virus infections.

Test Block 5

QUESTIONS

1. A 47-year-old man with a history of hyperparathyroidism presents to his physician because of a mass in his anterior neck. Laboratory studies show an elevated serum calcitonin level. The patient reports that multiple family members have had "thyroid problems" in the past. Which of the following is the most likely histology of this patient's neck mass?

   (A) Atrophic follicles with lymphocyte infiltrate and germinal centers
   (B) Nests of hormone-secreting tumor cells in an amyloid-filled stroma
   (C) Papillary pattern with ground-glass nuclei and psammoma bodies
   (D) Sheets of undifferentiated, pleomorphic cells
   (E) Uniform follicles with sparse colloid and a large cell lining

2. A 65-year-old cancer patient gives his best friend durable power of attorney. As his condition worsens, he goes into respiratory failure and is now on a ventilator in a coma. The friend believes the patient would have wished for life support to be withdrawn. However, the patient had previously made a living will stipulating that all measures should be undertaken to maintain his life. The patient's son believes his father's living will reflects his wishes and wants extreme measures taken to maintain his life. What action should the physician take?

   (A) Advise the friend to listen to the son's wishes
   (B) Appoint the son durable power of attorney because he is next of kin
   (C) Keep the patient on life support in accordance with the living will
   (D) Poll all family members present and follow the most supported course of action
   (E) Respect the durable power of attorney and withdraw life support

3. A 50-year-old man comes to the physician because of abdominal fullness, fatigue, and weight loss but denies any fever or night sweats. Physical examination is significant for splenomegaly. Blood tests are positive for pancytopenia and on bone marrow aspiration predominant, large white cells demonstrate tartrate-resistant acid phosphatase activity. The patient's peripheral blood smear is shown in the image. Which of the following disease processes is most likely causing this patient's problems?

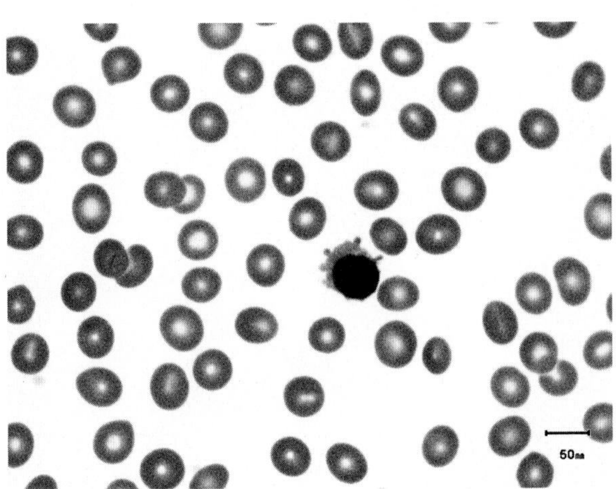

Reproduced, with permission, from USMLERx.com.

   (A) Chronic lymphocytic leukemia
   (B) Follicular lymphoma
   (C) Hairy cell leukemia
   (D) Mantle cell lymphoma
   (E) Nodular sclerosis Hodgkin lymphoma

4. A 55-year-old white woman with type 2 diabetes mellitus has the following lipid profile on routine laboratory testing:

   Total cholesterol: 280 mg/dL
   LDL cholesterol: 170 mg/dL
   HDL cholesterol: 23 mg/dL
   Triglycerides: 320 mg/dL

A treatment strategy is initiated. A few weeks later, the patient develops hip pain and weakness. Laboratory analysis reveals normal liver markers and a creatine kinase of 3000 mg/dL. Which of the following medication(s) places this patient at the greatest risk of developing these adverse effects?

(A) Ezetimibe alone
(B) Gemfibrozil alone
(C) Simvastatin and ezetimibe
(D) Simvastatin and gemfibrozil
(E) Simvastatin and niacin

5. A 42-year-old African-American woman with a history of sarcoidosis presents to a neurologist with a sudden onset of a unilateral inability to close the eye and decreased tearing. When she wrinkles her forehead or smiles, the affected side of her face remains relaxed. The muscles involved in this condition are derived from which of the following embryologic structures?

(A) First branchial (pharyngeal) arch
(B) Second branchial (pharyngeal) arch
(C) Third branchial (pharyngeal) pouch
(D) Fourth branchial (pharyngeal) pouch
(E) Thyroglossal duct

6. A 43-year-old man presents to his physician with fatigue. The patient says he is concerned about his fatigue because he has a strong family history of cancer. He thinks that if his parents did not drink, smoke, and eat such poor diets they would have lived longer lives. He says that because of all this, he never drinks alcohol or smokes tobacco. He has also followed a strict vegan diet for 10 years. He says that all of his meals are high in leafy green vegetables. Laboratory tests show a hematocrit of 35% with a normal RBC distribution width. Results of a peripheral blood smear are shown in the image. Which of the following laboratory tests will most definitively determine the likely cause of his abnormal blood smear?

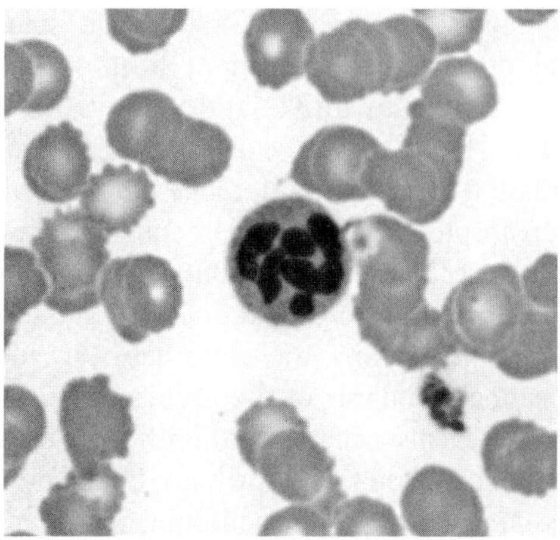

Reproduced, with permission, from USMLERx.com.

(A) Folate level
(B) Homocysteine level
(C) Methylmalonic acid level
(D) Serum B_{12} level
(E) Urine vitamin B_{12} level

7. While working in a microbiology laboratory, a researcher comes across an unlabeled cryotube in the –80° freezer. She deduces that it contains a strain of *Escherichia coli* and decides to test whether this strain has an intact lactose (*lac*) operon. After growing the cells in media containing both glucose and lactose, she observes that the β-galactosidase, encoded by the *lac* operon, is expressed. No protein products are produced when the *E coli* is grown only with glucose. Based on this observation, where is the mutation most likely located?

(A) Cyclic adenosine monophosphate-receptor protein
(B) Inducer-binding site
(C) Promoter
(D) Repressor
(E) RNA polymerase

8. A mother brings her 2-month-old infant to the emergency department because of lethargy, failure to thrive, and a fever of 39.2°C (102.6°F). Physical examination reveals increased head circumference and prominent hepatosplenomegaly. Screening laboratory tests reveal a profound anemia and leukopenia. Despite fluid resuscitation and initiation of antibiotic therapy, the child dies. On autopsy, histologic analysis of the child's bone marrow space reveals a marked infiltration of the medullary canal space by primary bony spongiose tissue. Which malfunctioning cells are the cause of this patient's disease process?

    (A) Hepatocytes
    (B) Lymphoid progenitor cells
    (C) Osteoblasts
    (D) Osteoclasts
    (E) Reticulocytes

9. A 7-year-old boy is brought to his pediatrician for evaluation of a rash. The boy's mother reports that the family moved to a new home in a forested area approximately one month prior to the onset of the rash. On questioning, the boy reports that he last played in the woods two days before the rash began. Which of the following is characteristic of the cells that mediate this boy's immune reaction?

    (A) Buffering of acid generated by tissue metabolism
    (B) Cell surface immunoglobulin receptor
    (C) Defense against parasitic disease
    (D) Degranulation and release of histamine
    (E) Interaction with antigen-MHC complex
    (F) Nonspecific phagocytosis and presentation of skin antigens
    (G) Phagocytosis of opsonized cells

10. A woman whose mother had cancer in both breasts develops breast cancer at age 26 years. The patient's identical twin sister decides to undergo genetic testing to determine her chances of developing breast cancer. What mechanism causes the genes that are most commonly tested for breast cancer to become tumorigenic?

    (A) Chromosomal rearrangement
    (B) Dominant negative effect
    (C) Gain of function
    (D) Loss of function
    (E) Viral insertion

11. A 45-year-old woman with a long history of menstrual irregularities and infertility presents with complaints of worsening vision. A thorough review of systems reveals the presence of constipation, cold intolerance, and increased pigmentation of skin. The physician performs basic visual field testing and maps the visual disturbance in the patient's chart. Which of the following visual field defects is most likely in this patient?

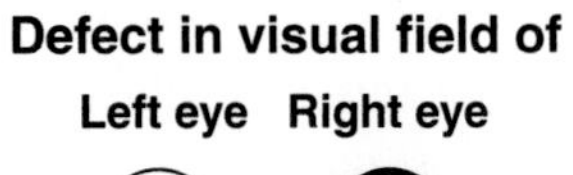

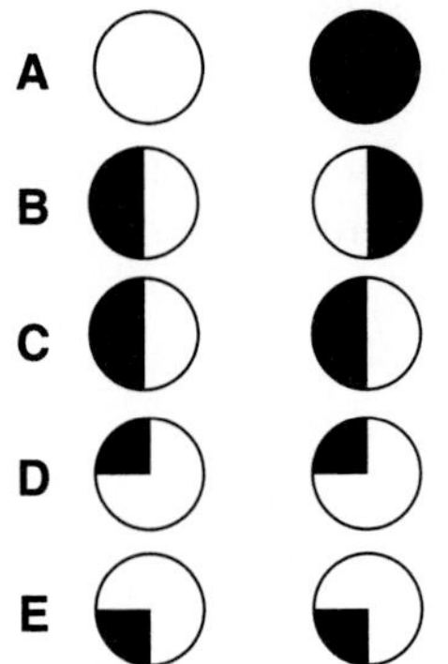

Reproduced, with permission, from USMLERx.com.

    (A) A
    (B) B
    (C) C
    (D) D
    (E) E

12. A 12-year-old boy is brought to the emergency department suffering from an acute asthma attack. The intern reaches for a drug used for the chronic prevention of asthma exacerbations rather than a drug needed for this acute attack. The intern likely reached for which of the following medications?

    (A) Cromolyn
    (B) Epinephrine

(C) Ipratropium
(D) Terbutaline
(E) Theophylline

13. A 44-year-old woman presents with worsening fatigue for the past two months. She recently overcame her battle with alcoholism and says her next goal is to improve her "horrible diet." Physical examination is unremarkable. Laboratory studies are significant for a hemoglobin level of 8 g/dL and a mean corpuscular volume of 110 fL. A folic acid deficiency is suspected. Which of the following is the most accurate description of the function of folic acid?

(A) Catalyzes γ-carboxylation of glutamic acid residues
(B) Hydroxylates prolyl and lysyl residues
(C) Increases intestinal calcium and phosphate absorption
(D) Makes up the constituents of the visual pigments
(E) Transfers one-carbon intermediates

14. ABO testing on a sample of B-positive blood and two unknown sample types (donor and recipient) is performed. Positive antibody-antigen interaction results in RBC agglutination. Five experiments are conducted for each sample, as shown in the image. Which of the following pairs represents the blood types for donor and recipient?

	Blood group		
	B+	Donor	Recipient
1. anti-A	No agglutination	No agglutination	Agglutination
2. anti-B	Agglutination	No agglutination	No agglutination
3. A cells	Agglutination	Agglutination	No agglutination
4. B cells	No agglutination	Agglutination	Agglutination
5. anti-D	Agglutination	No agglutination	Agglutination

Key: ○ No agglutination; ● Agglutination

Reproduced, with permission, from USMLERx.com.

(A) A-positive donor and O-negative recipient
(B) AB-negative donor and A-positive recipient
(C) AB-positive donor and B-negative recipient
(D) B-negative donor and AB-positive recipient
(E) O-negative donor and A-positive recipient
(F) O-positive donor and B-negative recipient

15. A 10-year-old boy with an X-linked immunodeficiency disease suffers from chronic recurrent gastrointestinal inflammation, which only moderately improves with cyclosporine therapy. The child has had previous laboratory evaluation that showed a negative reaction to the nitroblue tetrazolium test. The patient's father wants to know how his son can have both an immunodeficiency disease and an autoimmune disease. Deficiencies in which of the following provide a logical link between this child's immunodeficiency and his autoimmune gut inflammation?

(A) Antibodies
(B) IgA
(C) IgM
(D) Lysosomes
(E) Neutrophils

16. A 3-year-old girl presents to the emergency department with two weeks of abdominal pain. The mother denies any nausea, vomiting, or fever in the child. The child says that her hands feel "funny," and she apparently has been stumbling, while walking, more frequently over the past few months. Serum laboratory tests are normal. The child's peripheral blood smear reveals stippling of RBCs. Poisoning with which of the following substances is most likely?

(A) Arsenic
(B) Copper
(C) Iron
(D) Lead
(E) Mercury

17. A mother brings her 1-month-old infant to the pediatrician. She says the baby is crying more than usual, is vomiting, and does not want to eat. Physical examination reveals a bulging fontanel. Lumbar puncture shows:

Opening pressure: 240 mm H_2O (normal: 100-200 mm H_2O)
WBC count: 1200/mm^3
Protein: 200 mg/dL
Glucose: 30 mg/dL
Gram stain: gram-positive rods

Which of the following organisms is most likely responsible for this infant's presentation?

(A) *Escherichia coli*
(B) Herpes simplex virus
(C) *Listeria monocytogenes*
(D) *Neisseria meningitides*
(E) *Streptococcus agalactiae*

18. A 68-year-old man suffered from a resting tremor and postural instability during his last five years of life. The neuropathology shown in the image was observed during postmortem examination. Mutations in which protein are genetically linked to the disease from which this man suffered?

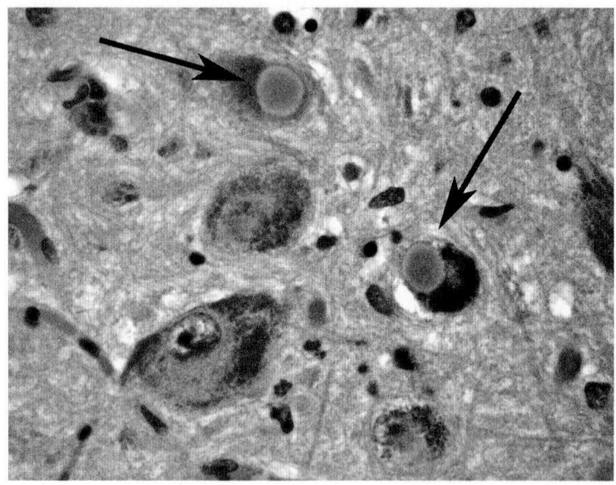

Reproduced, with permission, from USMLERx.com.

(A) α-Synuclein
(B) Dystrophin
(C) Huntingtin
(D) Presenilin
(E) Tau

19. A 60-year-old man is found to have advanced adenocarcinoma of the stomach. The tumor is centered at the pyloric zone just near the pyloric sphincter, on the lesser curvature. Which of the following signs and symptoms is most likely to be seen in this patient due to the mass effect of the tumor?

(A) Anemia
(B) Constipation
(C) Hoarseness
(D) Jaundice
(E) Periumbilical swelling

20. Kabuki make-up syndrome (KMS, or Niikawa-Kuroki syndrome) is a very rare genetic disorder of unknown cause that presents in neonates as mental retardation, unusual skin ridging in the hands, fingers, and toes, and an everted lower eyelid. Estimates of worldwide prevalence range from 1:100,000 to 1:10,000,000. If a new genetic test were developed that was positive in 99 neonates with KMS and negative in one neonate with KMS, and additional studies demonstrated that this test had a consistently high sensitivity and specificity, what can be expected for the positive predictive value of this test?

(A) It will be high because of a low prevalence
(B) It will be high because of high accuracy
(C) It will be low because of a bias
(D) It will be low because of a low prevalence
(E) It will be low because of low accuracy

21. A 35-year-old woman is brought to the emergency department because of diffuse muscle contractions. On examination she is unable to open her mouth. Her husband reports that last week she accidentally stuck her finger with a rusty nail. By which of the following mechanisms does this organism cause the symptoms associated with this disease?

(A) The organism produces a cytotoxin that damages colonic mucosa

(B) The organism produces a heat-labile toxin that stimulates adenylate cyclase
(C) The organism produces an exotoxin that blocks glycine release at spinal synapses
(D) The toxin blocks release of acetylcholine at spinal synapses
(E) The toxin produced is a superantigen that binds to MHC II protein and T lymphocyte receptors

22. A 62-year-old man comes to the physician complaining of a skin rash that is extremely painful. A picture of the rash is shown. A pathology specimen is obtained. Which of the following results would most likely be seen on biopsy?

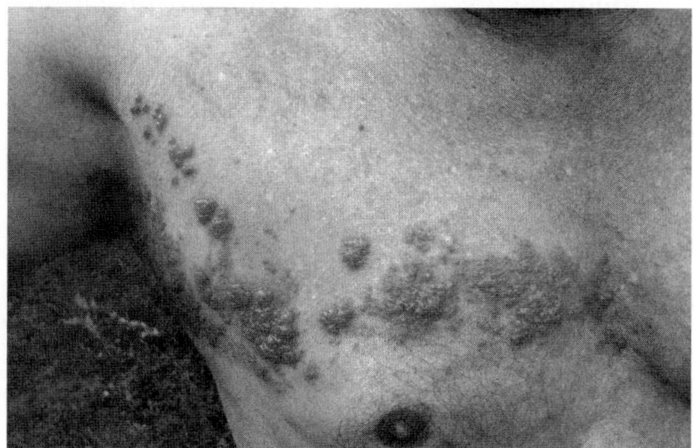

Courtesy of Wikipedia.

(A) Auer bodies
(B) Cabot ring bodies
(C) Call-Exner bodies
(D) Cowdry A inclusion bodies
(E) Mallory bodies

23. A 32-year-old woman with schizophrenia presents to the physician with amenorrhea and a milky discharge from both nipples. A pregnancy test is negative. Laboratory results show an increased serum prolactin level, a decreased serum gonadotropin level, and a normal thyroid stimulating hormone level. Which of the following medications is the most likely cause of this patient's presentation?

(A) Amantadine
(B) Bromocriptine
(C) Cabergoline
(D) Chlorpromazine
(E) Clozapine

24. A 20-year-old woman is referred to an endocrinologist for lack of menarche. Physical examination reveals normal breast tissue and external genitals. However, the vagina ends in a blind pouch. Laboratory studies show elevated levels of testosterone, estrogen, and luteinizing hormone. Which of the following is characteristic of this patient's condition?

(A) Deficiency of 5α-reductase
(B) Elevated 17-hydroxyprogesterone
(C) Excessive early gestational androgenic exposure
(D) Karyotype of 46,XX or 47,XXY
(E) Unresponsive testosterone receptors

25. A newborn initially is healthy but begins to have bilious emesis and fails to pass meconium during the first 48 hours of life. An emergent abdominal barium study is performed during this time and results are shown in the image. What is the pathophysiology of this disease?

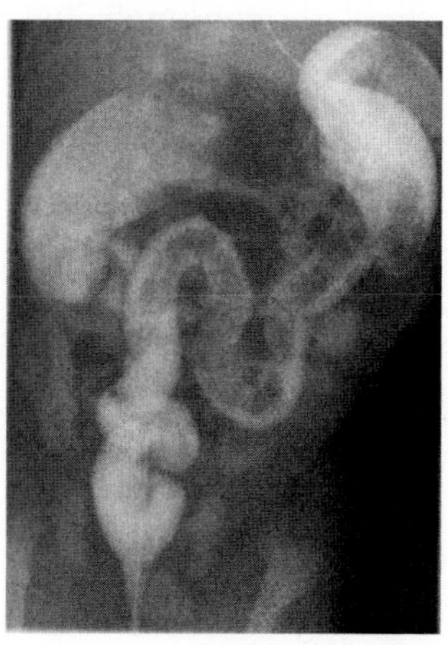

Reproduced, with permission, from USMLERx.com.

(A) Failure of neural crest cell migration
(B) Failure of neural tube closure
(C) Herniation of mucosal tissue
(D) Remnant portion of the vitelline duct
(E) Volvulus

26. An 18-year-old woman is brought to the pediatrician by her mother because of changes in her behavior. The mother states that her daughter has always been "a bit strange," often keeping to herself and reading books on witchcraft and UFOs. Recently her daughter has begun to wear only black clothing and plays the lute for many hours each day while wearing a cape and a witch's hat. The patient says she feels fine and just wants to be left alone, but the physician notes her speech is rather vague and shows little affect. She continues to perform well in school and has few friends, but is otherwise healthy. What personality type best describes this patient?

(A) Antisocial
(B) Avoidant
(C) Borderline
(D) Paranoid
(E) Schizotypal

27. A previously healthy 5-year-old boy is brought to the pediatrician with a three-day history of sore throat, conjunctivitis, rhinitis, and cough. His mother explains that more than 10 children in his class at school have similar symptoms, particularly conjunctivitis. No cultures are ordered, and the mother is assured that her son's illness will go away on its own. One week later, the mother reports that her son is healthy and back at school. Which of the following is the most likely causative agent in this child's illness?

(A) Adenovirus
(B) Coxsackie A virus
(C) Cytomegalovirus
(D) Herpes simplex virus type 1
(E) Rotavirus

28. A 40-year-old woman presents with progressive fatigue and bilateral joint inflammation characterized by pain, swelling, warmth, and morning stiffness. The patient says that the symptoms began in her hands over one year ago but have now begun to affect her knees. Which of the following agents would be most useful in her treatment?

(A) Ceftriaxone
(B) Cyclophosphamide
(C) Methotrexate
(D) Probenecid
(E) Tamoxifen

29. A 28-year-old man presents to the primary care clinic because his thinking has been "slow" recently, citing for example that he has had trouble remembering the names of his friends. The patient also mentions that he has been feeling depressed, and that he has recently lost a significant amount of weight. The patient reports no history of familial illnesses. Physical examination is notable for purplish skin lesions distributed across his torso. CT of the brain shows diffuse volume loss. Which of the following are most consistent with his current presentation?

(A) Ataxia, urinary incontinence, and seizures
(B) High fever, rigidity of the neck, and encapsulated yeasts in cerebrospinal fluid
(C) Involuntary, dance-like movements of the arms and gross cortical atrophy
(D) Paralysis and atrophy of muscles localized to the extremities
(E) Progressively decreased mental status and amyloid plaque formation in the brain

30. A 20-year-old mother is unsure of the paternity of her newborn son. To determine the father of her child, a genetic test based on DNA restriction fragment length polymorphism was performed. Blood was drawn from the four men suspected to be the father (F1, F2, F3, F4) as well as from the mother (M) and the infant (C). DNA extracted from the samples was amplified using polymerase chain reaction and then treated with the restriction enzyme EcoRI. The resulting fragments were separated with gel electrophoresis and a Southern blot analysis was performed. According to the Southern blot shown in the image, who is most likely the father of the child?

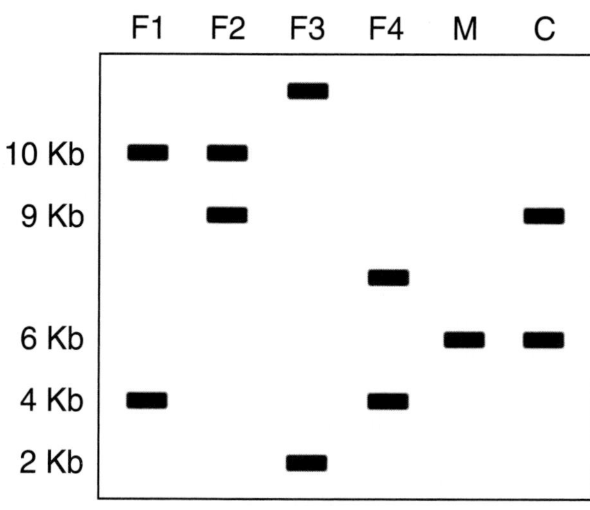

Reproduced, with permission, from USMLERx.com.

(A) F1
(B) F2
(C) F3
(D) F4

31. A 2-week-old premature male infant is examined in the neonatal intensive care unit, and shows a wide pulse pressure and a holosystolic and holodiastolic murmur. On echocardiography he has blood flow between the left pulmonary artery and the aorta. Which of the following symptoms would the mother have experienced during pregnancy to increase the risk of having a child with this disorder?

(A) A firm, nonpainful, red lesion on the outside of her vagina followed several weeks later by a maculopapular rash on her palms
(B) Maculopapular rash spreading from face to body
(C) Mild fever, sore throat, body aches, malaise, and swollen glands
(D) Prolonged, persistent paroxysmal cough
(E) Vaginal itching and mucopurulent discharge

32. A 53-year-old woman presents with irregular menstrual periods. She claims that she sometimes goes two-three months without a period. On further questioning, she also complains of vaginal dryness and occasional hot flashes. Blood tests reveal an estrogen level of 22 pg/mL (normal: 60-400 pg/mL), follicle-stimulating hormone (FSH) level of 100 mIU/L (normal: 1-26 mIU/L), and luteinizing hormone level of 50 mIU/mL (normal: 1-12 mIU/L), without surge. Which of the following is most likely the primary cause of this patient's symptoms?

(A) Decreased estrogen levels
(B) Decreased feedback on the anterior pituitary
(C) Increased FSH levels
(D) Increased progesterone levels
(E) Increased testosterone levels

33. A young couple presents to a fertility clinic, reporting that they have been attempting to conceive a child for 16 months without any success. The 25-year-old wife has undergone hormonal analysis, and it has been determined that she menstruates normally and her follicles are viable. The 27-year-old husband is 188 cm (6'2") tall and weighs 64.4 kg (142 lb). On examination, he has small testes. Karyotype analysis is performed, and reveals the presence of an extra sex chromosome. Which of the following laboratory results is most consistent with this man's condition?

(A) Decreased follicle-stimulating hormone level
(B) Decreased thyroid-stimulating hormone level
(C) Decreased gonadotropin-releasing hormone level
(D) Increased luteinizing hormone level
(E) Increased testosterone level

34. A G2P1 woman at 39 weeks' gestation is rushed to the hospital by her husband because she is in labor. She elects to have epidural anesthesia for the delivery. After injection of the anesthetic agent, the woman complains of palpitations and severe dizziness. ECG shows evidence of heart block. Upon investigation it is discovered that the resident did not ensure that the epidural needle did not pierce a vessel. Which of the following anesthetic agents was most likely administered for the procedure?

(A) Bupivacaine
(B) Fentanyl
(C) Halothane
(D) Ibuprofen
(E) Morphine

35. Comparing the oxygen-hemoglobin dissociation curves in the image, which of the following conditions represents curve B as compared to curve A?

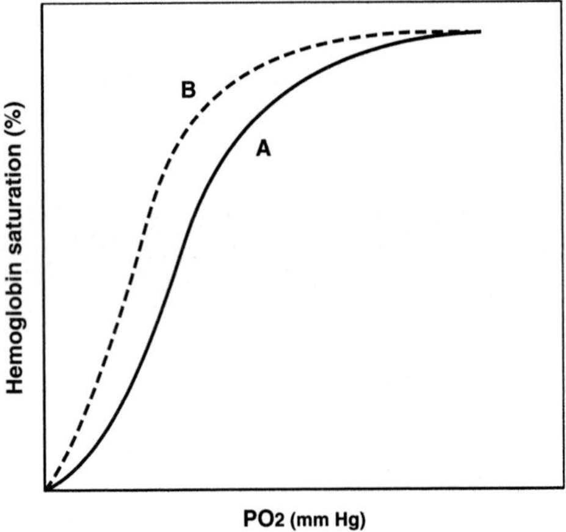

Reproduced, with permission, from USMLERx.com.

(A) A higher concentration of fetal hemoglobin
(B) An elevated concentration of adult hemoglobin
(C) Decreased pH
(D) High altitude
(E) Increased temperature

36. A 27-year-old woman is involuntarily committed to a psychiatric ward. Her physician notes persistently elevated blood pressure with a mean arterial pressure of 120 mm Hg, but she remains asymptomatic. Her physician would like to begin an antihypertensive agent but the patient refuses, fully understanding the risks, benefits, and outcomes that would result with or without treatment. What ethical principle has priority in the treatment of this patient?

(A) Beneficence
(B) Informed consent
(C) Justice
(D) Non-maleficence
(E) Patient autonomy

37. A 19-year-old woman with no significant past medical history presents to her primary care physician for a sports physical. Her examination is notable for a brachial artery pressure of 160/110 mm Hg and a weak femoral pulse. Prompted by the weak pulse, her physician measures her blood pressure in the lower extremity and finds it to be 80/40 mm Hg. An x-ray film of the chest shows rib notching. This woman is presenting with a congenital condition that places her at high risk for bacterial endocarditis and which of the following other conditions?

(A) Acute lymphocytic leukemia
(B) Boot-shaped heart
(C) Cerebral hemorrhage
(D) Cor pulmonale
(E) Eisenmenger syndrome

38. A 21-year-old man presents to a new primary care physician for routine physical examination. He demonstrates hyperextensible skin and reports a history of finger and shoulder dislocations, which he has reduced himself. He reports a history of easy bruising. He has no cardiac abnormalities. A defect in the synthesis of which molecule likely accounts for these symptoms?

(A) Collagen type I
(B) Collagen type II
(C) Collagen type III
(D) Collagen type IV
(E) Elastin

(F) Fibrillin
(G) Sphingomyelinase

39. A 56-year-old man who is undergoing chemotherapy for colorectal carcinoma develops profound nausea and vomiting four hours after receiving treatments. The drug most likely to relieve the patient's symptoms functions by which of the following mechanisms?

(A) Acetylcholine antagonist
(B) Dopamine agonist
(C) Norepinephrine reuptake inhibitor
(D) Serotonin agonist
(E) Serotonin antagonist

40. A 15-month-old boy is brought to the pediatrician by his parents because they have noticed that he has difficulty walking. On physical examination, the child exhibits a broad-based waddling gait. Laboratory studies show a serum calcium level of 6.0 mg/dL, a serum phosphate level of 2.0 mg/dL, and a serum alkaline phosphatase activity of 85 U/L. Which of the following is the most likely cause of this patient's condition?

(A) Decreased bone mineral density
(B) Diminished hydroxylation of proline and lysine in collagen synthesis
(C) Diminished intestinal absorption of calcium and phosphate
(D) Increased bone turnover
(E) Renal failure

41. A 24-year-old man who has smoked 1.5 packs per day for the past six years comes to the local emergency room complaining of sudden onset of unilateral pleuritic chest pain and shortness of breath. He is tall and thin. He has no personal or family history of medical illnesses and denies trauma prior to the onset of his pain. On examination, he is tachypneic and has decreased breath sounds at the right upper zone of the lung. Which of the following additional physical findings is likely to be present?

(A) Bilateral chest expansion
(B) Bronchial breath sounds
(C) Hyperresonance on percussion
(D) Increased tactile fremitus
(E) Tracheal deviation away from the affected lung

42. A 7-year-old girl with no significant medical history presents with a five-month history of persistent weakness despite taking vitamins and supplements. Physical examination is completely benign, with normal blood pressure and no peripheral edema. Laboratory studies show hyponatremia, hypokalemia, metabolic alkalosis, and an increased plasma renin level. Renal biopsy reveals juxtaglomerular cell hyperplasia. Which of the following diuretics acts at the same location as the defect in the patient's syndrome?

(A) Acetazolamide
(B) Furosemide
(C) Hydrochlorothiazide
(D) Spironolactone
(E) Triamterene

43. A 47-year-old man presents with diarrhea, abdominal pain, loss of appetite, weight loss, and fatigue. A jejunal biopsy is obtained and is shown in the image. Which of the following is the most likely diagnosis?

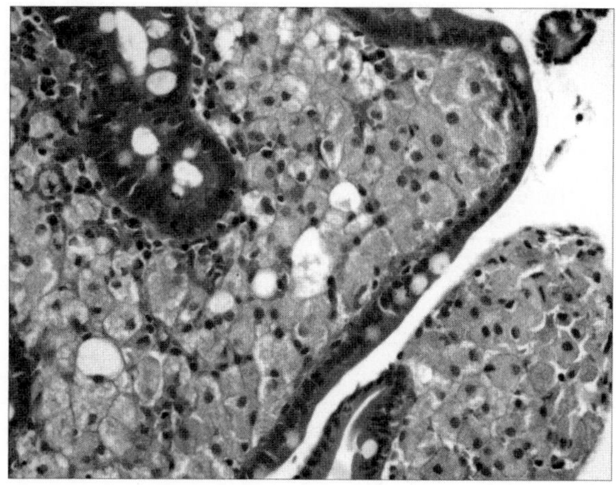

Reproduced, with permission, from USMLERx.com.

(A) Disaccharidase deficiency
(B) Chronic pancreatitis
(C) Infection by *Tropheryma whipplei*
(D) Tropical sprue
(E) Celiac sprue

44. A 28-year-old woman comes to the physician's office complaining of anxiety and a recent 4.5-kg (9.9-lb) weight loss. Her physical examination is significant for an inability to fully cover her eyes with her eyelids and swelling on the anterior surface of both legs. The skin of her anterior legs appears dry and waxy and has several diffuse, slightly pigmented papules. Laboratory studies show low levels of serum thyroid-stimulating hormone (TSH) and high levels of serum total thyroxine (T_4) and serum free T_4. The drug of choice for this disorder acts at what step in thyroid hormone synthesis?

(A) Active absorption of iodide from the blood
(B) Oxidation of I- to I_2
(C) Production of TSH
(D) Proteolysis of colloid to release T_4 and triiodothyronine
(E) Tyrosine iodination and coupling

45. A 61-year-old alcoholic presents to the emergency department with disorientation, confusion, and an unsteady gait. Horizontal nystagmus, pulmonary râles, and edematous lower extremities are noted on physical examination. On questioning, the patient states that he started drinking alcohol when he was a prisoner of war in Vietnam. His current alcohol level is within the legal limit, a toxicology screen is negative, and a stroke has been ruled out by imaging. Which of the following additional tests should be performed to estimate the extent of his disease?

(A) A lumbar puncture
(B) A transesophageal echocardiogram
(C) Coagulation studies
(D) Tissue pressure in the lower extremities
(E) Venous Doppler ultrasound imaging of the lower extremities

46. A 42-year-old man comes to the physician complaining of abdominal pain for the past three months. His pain is sharp, and is worse after meals and when lying down. He also mentions having black, tarry stools for the past month. Laboratory tests show:

Hemoglobin: 11.2 g/dL
Hematocrit: 35%
Mean corpuscular volume: 98 fL
WBCs: 7000/mm^3
Platelets: 260,000/mm^3

Endoscopy of the stomach reveals a small flat lesion on the fundus; it has smooth borders and is filled with exudate. Which of the following is a major risk factor for his condition?

(A) Bacterial infection
(B) Celecoxib usage
(C) Diabetes
(D) Hypertension
(E) Vegan diet

47. A patient with long-standing renal failure secondary to focal segmental glomerulosclerosis undergoes parathyroid biopsy that shows marked hyperplasia. On physical examination, tapping over the cheek elicits facial muscle spasm. Which of the following sets of laboratory values is most likely to be seen in this patient?

Choice	Parathyroid hormone	Serum Ca^{2+}	Serum phosphate	Alkaline phosphatase
A	↑	↑	↑	↑
B	↑	↑	↓	↑
C	↑	↓	↑	↑
D	↑	↓	↑	↓
E	↑	↓	↓	↑

Reproduced, with permission, from USMLERx.com.

(A) A
(B) B
(C) C
(D) D
(E) E

48. A 40-year-old woman presents with a persistent cough of two months' duration. She reports a 6.8-kg (15-lb) unintentional weight loss and general loss of appetite. She says she drinks wine occasionally but has never smoked cigarettes. X-ray of the chest reveals a subpleural mass. Which of the following is the most likely diagnosis?

(A) Adenocarcinoma of the lung
(B) Carcinoid tumor of the lung
(C) Metastases to lung from a primary tumor from another tissue type
(D) Small-cell carcinoma of the lung
(E) Squamous cell carcinoma of the lung

ANSWERS

1. **The correct answer is B.** This patient most likely has multiple endocrine neoplasia (MEN) type 2 (formerly known as type 2A), a genetic disorder characterized by tumors of the parathyroid gland, medullary carcinoma of the thyroid, and tumors of the adrenal medulla. All MEN syndromes follow an autosomal dominant mode of inheritance with incomplete penetrance. MEN 2 is thought to result from an activating mutation in the proto-oncogene *ret*. MEN type 1 involves parathyroid hyperplasia, pancreatic islet cell tumors, and pituitary adenomas, whereas MEN type 3 (formerly known as type 2B) involves medullary thyroid carcinomas, mucosal neuromas, and pheochromocytomas. Medullary carcinoma of the thyroid is a calcitonin-secreting tumor of parafollicular thyroid cells ("C cells"). Microscopically, the tumor consists of nests of tumor cells in an amyloid-filled stroma.

   Answer A is incorrect. Atrophic follicles with prominent germinal center formation and lymphocyte infiltrate are characteristic of Hashimoto thyroiditis.

   Answer C is incorrect. A papillary branching pattern of epithelial cells with ground-glass nuclei and psammoma bodies (laminated concentric calcified spherules) is seen in papillary carcinoma of the thyroid, the most common form of thyroid cancer and also the form with the best prognosis.

   Answer D is incorrect. Sheets of undifferentiated pleomorphic cells are seen in anaplastic, or undifferentiated, thyroid cancer. This form of thyroid cancer is more common in older patients and has a very poor prognosis.

   Answer E is incorrect. Follicular carcinoma of the thyroid can resemble normal thyroid tissue. It is composed of relatively uniform follicles lined with cells that are typically larger than those seen in a normal thyroid. Colloid is sparse.

2. **The correct answer is E.** The appointed durable power of attorney is truly durable and therefore supersedes even a living will. The patient, in good state of mind, believed that the friend would make decisions with which he would agree. It is always appropriate to facilitate a discussion between people involved in making end-of-life decisions, but it is unethical to try to sway the friend by making the choice for him or telling him to listen to the patient's son or the living will.

   Answer A is incorrect. The durable power of attorney should always make decisions consistent with what he believes the patient would want. The physician should not advise the friend to comply with the son's wishes, but rather remind them both as to the responsibilities of the durable power of attorney.

   Answer B is incorrect. Only the patient can change his/her power of attorney. If the patient is non-communicative, the power of attorney cannot be transferred. Many states acknowledge next of kin as durable power of attorney, unless it has been otherwise specifically assigned, as in this case.

   Answer C is incorrect. The durable power of attorney is the ultimate decision maker and their decision to withdraw life support will be upheld despite the existence of a living will.

   Answer D is incorrect. The durable power of attorney was appointed as such to make decisions in accordance with the patient's wishes. Input from family members is both important and appropriate, but is not legally necessary.

3. **The correct answer is C.** A presentation of fullness, fatigue, and weight loss along with splenomegaly immediately raises the clinician's suspicion of a possible slowly progressing hematopoietic neoplasm. Hairy cell leukemia is caused by malignant B lymphocytes that commonly show varying numbers of projections from cytoplasm, giving the cell a "hairy" or "ruffled" appearance as seen in the image above. It is four times more prevalent in men than in women, and patients usually complain of abdominal fullness, fatigue, and weight loss

but rarely of night sweats or fevers. Elevation of tartrate-resistant acid phosphatase in the B lymphocytes from bone marrow confirms the diagnosis of hairy cell leukemia. Think "hair trap."

Answer A is incorrect. Chronic lymphocytic leukemia is also a B lymphocyte-derived neoplasm whose presentation is very similar to that of hairy cell leukemia. Its B lymphocytes, however, would not typically demonstrate an elevation in tartrate-resistant acid phosphatase.

Answer B is incorrect. Follicular lymphomas are the most common type of indolent non-Hodgkin lymphomas and are characterized by an increase in number of normal-appearing germinal centers, which are not described here.

Answer D is incorrect. Mantle cell lymphoma is a B lymphocyte subtype of non-Hodgkin lymphoma that is characterized by small cells with cleaved nuclei resembling the cells in germinal centers. Although its clinical presentation can be similar to that of hairy cell leukemia, it lacks the "hairy" appearance histologically and does not show any increase in tartrate-resistant acid phosphatase.

Answer E is incorrect. All Hodgkin lymphoma variants are differentiated by the presence of Reed-Sternberg cells and commonly present clinically with night sweats, fevers, and weight loss. The nodular sclerosis variant is distinguished by a nodular pattern separated by areas of collagen banding and the presence of lacunar cells.

4. **The correct answer is D.** Myositis and rhabdomyolysis are potential complications of co-treatment with a statin drug and a fibric acid derivative. Although this combination is not explicitly contraindicated, the two drugs should be used together with caution. Statin drugs decrease LDL substantially but also pose a risk of myositis. Fibrates cause a decrease in triglyceride levels and an increase in HDL cholesterol levels by promoting lipolysis and decreasing the secretion of triglycerides by the liver, and are also associated with a risk of myositis. In combination, statins and fibrates have an additive risk of myositis.

Answer A is incorrect. The adverse effects of ezetimibe include diarrhea, abdominal discomfort, and arthralgias.

Answer B is incorrect. The adverse effects of fibrates include myositis and gastrointestinal (GI) discomfort. The combination of fibrates with statin medications has an additive effect that might more frequently result in myositis.

Answer C is incorrect. Simvastatin and ezetimibe combined can cause elevation in liver transaminases, so patients taking these drugs together should have periodic liver function tests.

Answer E is incorrect. Whereas statins can cause myositis, the most common adverse effects of niacin are flushing and GI upset.

5. **The correct answer is B.** A Bell palsy is a lesion of cranial nerve VII (facial nerve) and affects the muscles of facial expression. These muscles are derived from the second branchial (pharyngeal) arch. Patients with sarcoidosis, tumors, diabetes, AIDS, and Lyme disease are at increased risk for Bell palsy, although most cases are idiopathic. Important signs of Bell palsy are ptosis and facial droop. The second arch also gives rise to the posterior belly of the digastric, the stylohyoid, and the stapedius muscles.

Answer A is incorrect. The first branchial arch develops into the muscles of mastication, the mylohyoid, the anterior belly of the digastric, the tensor veli palatini, and the tensor tympani. These muscles are innervated by cranial nerve V and are not affected by Bell palsy.

Answer C is incorrect. The third branchial pouch develops into the inferior parathyroid glands and the thymus. It is implicated in DiGeorge syndrome but has no relation to Bell palsy.

Answer D is incorrect. The fourth branchial pouch develops into the superior parathyroid glands. It is implicated in DiGeorge syndrome but is not related to Bell palsy.

Answer E is incorrect. The thyroglossal duct connects the thyroid diverticulum to the foregut in the embryo but is obliterated during development. Its only remnant in the adult is the foramen cecum.

6. **The correct answer is B.** This patient has a macrocytic anemia with hypersegmented neutrophils, a condition most likely caused by either vitamin B_{12} deficiency or folate deficiency. Increased homocysteine levels are indicative of folate deficiency or vitamin B_{12} deficiency, but are not helpful in distinguishing between the two.

   Answer A is incorrect. Any patient with a macrocytic anemia and hypersegmented neutrophils could have a folate deficiency. However, this is highly unlikely in this patient who ingests a diet high in leafy green vegetables.

   Answer C is incorrect. This patient has a macrocytic anemia with hypersegmented neutrophils. Two causes of these findings on blood smear are vitamin B_{12} deficiency and folate deficiency. A primary dietary deficiency can often be seen in people who maintain a strict vegan diet for many years with no vitamin supplements, since vitamin B_{12} is primarily obtained from animal products. Foods rich in vitamin B_{12} include eggs, milk, fish, poultry, and meats. Using the blood levels of vitamin B_{12} as a clue to deficiency, however, can be misleading because a large fraction of this vitamin is bound to protein and therefore unavailable for other metabolic processes. Methylmalonic acid is a product of methylmalonyl CoA. In normal metabolism, methylmalonyl CoA is converted to succinyl CoA with the cofactor vitamin B_{12}. If there is not enough vitamin B_{12} present, methylmalonyl CoA is alternatively converted into methylmalonic acid. Therefore, vitamin B_{12} deficiencies can be diagnosed based on high methylmalonic acid levels.

   Answer D is incorrect. Although this patient has a macrocytic anemia with hypersegmented neutrophils, the serum vitamin B_{12} level is not the best test to determine whether the patient is deficient in folate or vitamin B_{12}. The blood levels of vitamin B_{12} can be misleading at times because a large fraction of vitamin B_{12} is bound to protein and therefore unavailable for other metabolic processes.

   Answer E is incorrect. Urine vitamin B_{12} levels are not normally measured.

7. **The correct answer is A.** The lactose (*lac*) operon is an example of an inducible operon. Glucose is the preferred energy source for the *E coli* bacterium and in the presence of glucose, *lac* operon transcription is inhibited by a repressor protein that binds to the operator region of the *lac* operon and blocks RNA polymerase. In the absence of glucose and the presence of lactose, lactose binds the repressor molecule and changes its shape so that it can no longer bind to the operator, allowing transcription to occur. Furthermore, as glucose levels decrease, cAMP levels rise and bind to the cAMP receptor protein (CRP). The CRP-cAMP complex binds to the operon and promotes the binding of RNA polymerase to the promoter. When the cells are exposed to both glucose and lactose, lactose does bind the repressor and release its repression. However, because the presence of glucose decreases levels of cAMP, the CRP-cAMP complex formation decreases consequently and RNA polymerase does not efficiently bind the promoter. Thus, under normal conditions, if the bacterium is grown in the presence of both lactose and glucose, the *lac* operon should be mostly inactive. In this vignette, glucose fails to suppress transcription of the *lac* operon. Therefore, the mutation is most likely located in the CRP.

   Answer B is incorrect. Lactose is the inducer of the lactose operon. Lactose binds tightly to the repressor so that the repressor can no longer bind to the operator and block the RNA polymerase from transcribing the products of the *lac* operon. If the inducer-binding site were mutated, the lactose operon would not be expressed in the presence of lactose.

   Answer C is incorrect. A mutation in the promoter of the lactose operon is not consistent with the above observation. If the promoter were mutated, the ability of RNA polymerase to bind to it would be altered regardless of the presence of glucose or lactose.

Answer D is incorrect. In the absence of lactose, the lactose operon repressor binds to the operator and halts transcription. In this case, a mutation in the repressor protein would either increase or decrease repressor binding to the operator, which would alter the amount of products produced. No such changes were observed, which makes it unlikely that the mutation is located in the repressor.

Answer E is incorrect. If RNA polymerase were mutated in these bacterial cells, all gene expression would be affected.

8. **The correct answer is D.** The most likely diagnosis for this child is osteopetrosis. This rare hereditary disorder occurs from a failure of the resorption and remodeling of bone due to malfunctioning osteoclasts. The skeleton becomes diffusely sclerotic and dense as new bony matrix is laid into the medullary canal, replacing the hematopoietic tissue. Patients compensate with extramedullary hematopoiesis, leading to hepatosplenomegaly. Despite the increased density, the bone is brittle and predisposed to fracture. There are two main types of the disease, characterized by their inheritance patterns. The autosomal-recessive form is more malignant and is often fatal in utero or in the neonatal period. The autosomal-dominant form is usually benign and may be discovered incidentally on x-ray.

   Answer A is incorrect. Osteopetrosis presents with hepatomegaly due to the need for extramedullary hematopoiesis, not a defect of the intrinsic cellular makeup of the liver.

   Answer B is incorrect. Despite finding leukopenia in osteopetrosis, the root cause is not a defect in the lymphoid progenitor cells. Their normal proliferation is prevented by the filling of the intramedullary space with bony tissue.

   Answer C is incorrect. In osteopetrosis, the function of the osteoblasts goes unchecked by malfunctioning osteoclasts. Though there is an excess of bony material, osteopetrosis is not a neoplastic process.

   Answer E is incorrect. Patients with osteopetrosis may often present with anemia. However, this is not due to a defect in RBC maturation. It is due to the crowding effect of limited intramedullary space.

9. **The correct answer is E.** The patient is experiencing a type IV, or delayed-type, hypersensitivity reaction. These immune reactions require prior exposure to the triggering antigen and typically manifest 24-48 hours after new contact with a trigger. Type IV hypersensitivity is mediated by the action of T lymphocytes, which secrete cytokines that, in turn, recruit additional inflammatory cells to the site of contact. T-lymphocyte activation depends on interaction between the cell surface T-lymphocyte receptor and an antigen-MHC complex on an antigen-presenting cell.

   Answer A is incorrect. RBCs are partially responsible for the transport and buffering of acid generated by tissue metabolism. RBC carbonic anhydrase converts carbon dioxide to carbonic acid, which rapidly dissociates into a proton and a bicarbonate ion. The bicarbonate ion is in turn exchanged across the RBC membrane in a process termed the physiologic chloride shift. None of these processes is involved in delayed-type hypersensitivity.

   Answer B is incorrect. Cell surface immunoglobulin receptors are characteristic of B lymphocytes. Through their production of antibodies, B lymphocytes are involved in types I, II, and III hypersensitivity, but are unrelated to the pathophysiology of delayed-type hypersensitivity.

   Answer C is incorrect. Eosinophils are especially important in the immune system's response to parasites and may also be associated with neoplastic processes. Eosinophils are not, however, involved in the physiology of delayed-type hypersensitivity.

   Answer D is incorrect. Degranulation and histamine release are characteristic of mast cells and basophils. Both are important in mediating type I hypersensitivity reactions via their cell surface IgE Fc receptors, but are not involved in delayed-type hypersensitivity.

Answer F is incorrect. Nonspecific phagocytosis in the epidermal layer is characteristic of Langerhans cells, a differentiated type of dendritic cell. They are found in lymph nodes, where they act as antigen-presenting cells.

Answer G is incorrect. Opsonization refers to the "marking" of foreign antigens either by antibody binding or by complement binding. In either case, certain phagocytic cells, predominately macrophages, can subsequently internalize and destroy the antigens. Although macrophages may be recruited by cytokines to the site of a delayed-type hypersensitivity reaction, it is the T lymphocyte that mediates the reaction.

10. **The correct answer is D.** *BRCA1* and *BRCA2* are tumor-suppressor genes whose protein products function in DNA repair. Frameshift or nonsense mutations commonly occur in *BRCA1* and *BRCA2* and produce truncated protein products. Mutations in these genes result in a gene product that has less or no function, and can lead to DNA instability and subsequent gene rearrangements. Both alleles of these tumor-suppressor genes must be inactivated to cause loss of function of these genes. Mutations to *BRCA* can increase the risk of many cancers aside from breast cancer.

Answer A is incorrect. The chromosomal alterations in human solid tumors are heterogeneous and complex, and allow for selection of the loss of tumor suppressor genes on the involved chromosome. However, in leukemias and lymphomas, the chromosomal alterations are often simple translocations, in which the breakpoints of chromosomal arms occur at the site of cellular oncogenes. For example, the Philadelphia chromosome in chronic lymphocytic leukemia is produced from a reciprocal translocation involving the *ABL* oncogene (a tyrosine kinase on chromosome 9) being placed in proximity to the *BCR* (breakpoint cluster region) on chromosome 22. The expression of the *BCR-ABL* gene product leads to tumorigenic growth.

Answer B is incorrect. Dominant negative effects occur when the loss of one allele leads to disease, because either the body cannot produce enough of the necessary protein product from just one functioning allele or the mutated allele produces an altered gene product that is antagonistic to the wild-type allele. An example of this is osteogenesis imperfecta, which caused by mutations in the *COL1A1* gene. The abnormal gene product from the mutated allele incorporates itself into the collagen matrix, weakening the structure.

Answer C is incorrect. Oncogenes acquire gain-of-function mutations that lead to increased activity of the gene product, which causes uninhibited cellular proliferation. This mutational event typically occurs in a single allele of the oncogene and acts in a dominant fashion. An example of this is the *c-Myc* gene, which is implicated in Burkitt lymphoma.

Answer E is incorrect. Viral insertion describes the process in which a viral gene is inserted into the host cell and promotes malignant transformation. Human papilloma virus inserts its genes into the cellular DNA. Several of the viral sequences act as oncogenes that promote tumor growth and may cause cervical and anal cancers. The *BRCA1* and *BRCA2* genes are tumor suppressor genes, and have not been shown to be inactivated by viral insertion.

11. **The correct answer is B.** The patient has bitemporal hemianopia secondary to a lesion compressing the optic chiasm. The history of menstrual irregularities, cold intolerance, constipation, and increased skin pigmentation suggests multiple endocrine disorders that can be attributed to dysfunction of the anterior pituitary. Due to the close anatomic relationship of the pituitary and the optic chiasm, expanding lesions of the pituitary can compress the optic chiasm, leading to visual loss in the temporal portions of the visual fields bilaterally. This is because only the nasal (or medial) retinal fibers for each eye cross in the optic chiasm, and the medial retinal fibers are responsible for the temporal (or lateral) hemifields as depicted in the drawing above. Common lesions leading to bitemporal hemianopia include pi-

tuitary adenoma, meningioma, craniopharyngioma and hypothalamic glioma.

Answer A is incorrect. This defect is monocular visual loss caused by complete destruction of the ipsilateral retina or ipsilateral optic nerve. A lesion in this area would not account for this patient's endocrine abnormalities.

Answer C is incorrect. This defect is contralateral homonymous hemianopia, which can be caused by lesions of the contralateral optic tract (in this case, the right optic tract), a lesion of the contralateral optic radiation, or lesions diffusely damaging the contralateral primary visual cortex. In general, retrochiasmal lesions (those distal to the optic chiasm including the optic tracts, lateral geniculate nucleus, optic radiations, or visual cortex) cause homonymous visual field defects (meaning the same regions of the fields for both eyes are involved). Lesions in these areas would not account for this patient's endocrine abnormalities.

Answer D is incorrect. This defect is contralateral superior quadrantanopia due to lesions in the contralateral Meyer's loop (or inferior optic radiations) through the temporal lobe. The inferior optic radiations carry information from the inferior retina or the superior visual field. Inferior optic radiations terminate in the inferior aspect of the primary visual cortex in the occipital lobe. Therefore, lesions of the contralateral inferior primary visual cortex could lead to contralateral superior quadrantanopia. However, lesions in these areas would not account for this patient's endocrine abnormalities.

Answer E is incorrect. This defect is contralateral inferior quadrantanopia due to lesions in the contralateral superior optic radiations that pass under the parietal lobe. The superior optic radiations carry information from the superior retina or the inferior visual field. Superior optic radiations terminate in the superior aspect of the primary visual cortex in the occipital lobe. Therefore, lesions of the contralateral superior primary visual cortex could lead to contralateral inferior quadrantanopia. However, lesions in these areas would not account for this patient's endocrine abnormalities.

12. **The correct answer is A.** Cromolyn is given by aerosol for the prophylactic treatment of asthma. The mechanism of action involves stabilization of mast cells and thus a decrease in the release of mediators (eg, leukotrienes and histamine) responsible for bronchoconstriction. These drugs are insoluble and thus have only local effects. They are used only in the prophylaxis of acute asthma, not during an attack.

    Answer B is incorrect. Epinephrine is an acceptable treatment and is often the drug of choice for a severe acute asthma attack. This autonomic activator relaxes smooth muscle, facilitating breathing during an acute attack.

    Answer C is incorrect. Ipratropium is an acceptable treatment for an acute asthma attack. It works as a competitive blocker of muscarinic receptors, preventing bronchoconstriction.

    Answer D is incorrect. Terbutaline is an acceptable treatment for an acute asthma attack. This drug relaxes bronchial smooth muscle.

    Answer E is incorrect. Theophylline is an acceptable treatment for an acute asthma attack. It likely causes bronchodilation by inhibiting phosphodiesterase, decreasing cAMP hydrolysis.

13. **The correct answer is E.** Folic acid plays a key role as a coenzyme for one-carbon transfer as seen in methylation reactions and is essential for the biosynthesis of purines and the pyrimidine thymidine. Deficiency of the vitamin is characterized by growth failure in children and macrocytic megaloblastic anemia. The anemia is a result of diminished DNA synthesis in erythropoietic stem cells. Large cells are seen with mean cell volumes of 100-150 fL and reduced levels of hemoglobin. Folic acid is a water-soluble vitamin stored in small amounts by the body; thus a continuous supply is needed from foods such as green, leafy vegetables, lima beans, and whole-grain cereals. Nutrient deficiency can commonly lead to folate deficiency. The deficiency is usually seen in pregnant women and alcoholics, and is the most common vitamin deficiency in the United States. Folic acid supplementation

by pregnant women reduces the incidence of neural tube defects.

Answer A is incorrect. Vitamin K serves as a coenzyme in the γ-carboxylation of glutamic acid residues in blood clotting proteins. A vitamin K deficiency is rarely seen because adequate amounts are generally produced by intestinal bacteria or easily obtained from the diet. Decreased bacterial production in the gut (as with antibiotics, for example) can lead to hypoprothrombinemia and, subsequently, hemorrhage. Newborns have sterile intestines and cannot initially synthesize vitamin K. Because human milk fails to provide the adequate daily requirement of vitamin K, it is recommended that all newborns receive a single dose of vitamin K as prophylaxis against hemorrhagic diseases.

Answer B is incorrect. Ascorbic acid (vitamin C) acts as a coenzyme in hydroxylation of prolyl- and lysyl- residues of collagen, allowing collagen fibers to crosslink and providing greater tensile strength to the assembled fiber. A deficiency of ascorbic acid results in scurvy, a disease characterized by sore, spongy gums, loose teeth, fragile blood vessels, swollen joints, anemia, and poor wound healing.

Answer C is incorrect. 1,25-Dihydroxycholecalciferol, the active molecule of vitamin D, produces its effect at the DNA level to produce proteins in intestinal cells that allow for greater calcium and phosphate absorption. Vitamin D deficiency causes a net demineralization of bone, resulting in rickets in children and osteomalacia in adults. Rickets is characterized by continuous formation of collagen matrix of bone but incomplete mineralization, resulting in soft, pliable bones. In osteomalacia, demineralization of preexisting bones increases their susceptibility to fracture.

Answer D is incorrect. Vitamin A (retinol) is a component of the visual pigments of rod and cone cells. This fat-soluble vitamin plays an essential role in vision, growth, maintenance of epithelial cells, and reproduction. Night blindness is one of the earliest signs of vitamin A deficiency as a result of a loss in the number of visual cells. Further deficiency can lead to dryness of conjunctiva and cornea, leading to corneal ulceration and ultimately blindness.

14. **The correct answer is E.** Because the donor's RBCs do not agglutinate with anti-A or anti-B antibodies, the donor blood type must be O. The fact that donor sera agglutinates both A cells and B cells confirms this, because type O serum contains both anti-A and anti-B antibodies. By similar reasoning, the recipient must be blood type A. Anti-D agglutination implies that RBCs in a sample have the Rh antigen. Thus the donor is Rh negative, and the recipient is Rh positive. Hence the correct pair is an O-negative donor and A-positive recipient. Donor and recipient blood should always be cross-matched, because pre-formed antibodies in the recipient can lyse donor RBCs and vice versa. This immunologic response can culminate in an acute hemolytic transfusion reaction with sequelae of shock, pyrexia, and both chest and flank pain.

Answer A is incorrect. Anti-A antibodies do not agglutinate donor RBCs. Thus the donor cannot be type A.

Answer B is incorrect. Anti-A and anti-B antibodies do not agglutinate donor RBCs. Thus the donor cannot be type AB.

Answer C is incorrect. Anti-A and anti-B antibodies do not agglutinate donor RBCs. Thus the donor cannot be blood type AB. No agglutination implies that the antigen is not present on the sample RBCs (hence this donor is type O). Both A and B RBCs are agglutinated in the donor serum, as expected, because anti-A and anti-B antibodies are generated in patients with blood type O.

Answer D is incorrect. Anti-B antibodies do not agglutinate donor RBCs. Thus the donor cannot be type B.

Answer F is incorrect. Donor RBCs do not agglutinate with either anti-A or anti-B antibody. Thus the donor blood type must be O. Because anti-D agglutination is negative, the donor must be Rh negative. The donor blood type is therefore O negative, not O positive.

15. **The correct answer is E.** Chronic granulomatous disease (CGD) is a disorder in which neutrophils are unable to completely eradicate certain phagocytosed bacteria and fungi. As a result, the chronic immune response to these lingering pathogens leads to the development of self-tissue damage. This answer provides a logical link between a correct description of CGD (a disorder of neutrophil production of nicotinamide adenine dinucleotide phosphatase [NADPH] oxidase, which results in neutrophils that are unable to completely eradicate certain phagocytosed bacteria and fungi) and the development of autoimmune disease. This answer points to theories questioning why 50% of patients with CGD suffer a chronic gut inflammation that is similar to Crohn disease.

    Answer A is incorrect. Common variable immunodeficiency, the most common symptomatic primary antibody deficiency syndrome, is a disorder characterized by differing degrees of deficiency of antibody production, leading to recurrent sinopulmonary and GI infections.

    Answer B is incorrect. This choice is not the correct immunologic deficiency of CGD. The disorder characterized by a deficiency of IgA antibodies is called IgA deficiency, the most common primary immunodeficiency disease in the Western hemisphere.

    Answer C is incorrect. Wiskott-Aldrich syndrome is an X-linked disorder that results in the body being unable to mount an IgM response to capsular polysaccharides or bacteria. It is associated with low levels of IgM, high levels of IgA, and normal levels of IgE.

    Answer D is incorrect. Chédiak-Higashi syndrome is an autosomal recessive disease affecting a lysosomal trafficking regulator gene; it leads to defective microtubular function and lysosomal emptying of phagocytic cells. This disease is characterized by a partial oculocutaneous albinism, abnormally large granules found in many different cell types, and recurrent pyogenic staphylococcal and/or streptococcal infections.

16. **The correct answer is D.** Toxicities associated with lead poisoning begin at blood lead levels of only 10 µg/dL. Toxic effects include abdominal pain, peripheral neuropathy, and basophilic RBC stippling. Additional findings might include lead lines along the gingival and cognitive impairment.

    Answer A is incorrect. Acute arsenic poisoning results in immediate GI distress. Cardiac instability, respiratory distress, and death sometimes follow.

    Answer B is incorrect. Wilson disease results from inadequate hepatic copper excretion and failure of copper to enter circulation as ceruloplasmin. It is characterized by asterixis, parkinsonian symptoms, dementia, and hemolytic anemia.

    Answer C is incorrect. Iron poisoning is characterized by vomiting, diarrhea, GI bleeding, cyanosis, and metabolic acidosis.

    Answer E is incorrect. Mercury toxicity is characterized by intention tremor, nephrotoxicity, and change in personality.

17. **The correct answer is C.** Increased irritability, feeding difficulty, and other general nonspecific signs along with a bulging fontanel characterize meningitis in infants. The cerebrospinal fluid (CSF) findings point toward a bacterial meningitis (increased protein and decreased glucose). In infants 0-3 months old, the most common organisms causing meningitis are *Listeria monocytogenes*, *Escherichia coli*, and Group B streptococci. *L monocytogenes* is the only gram-positive rod in the group.

    Answer A is incorrect. *Escherichia coli* can cause bacterial meningitis in infants, but a Gram stain of CSF would show gram-negative rods.

    Answer B is incorrect. Herpes simplex virus has also been shown to cause meningitis in infants. In viral meningitis, the CSF findings would show far fewer leukocytes (11-500/mm^3), protein levels between 50 and 200 mg/dL, and normal glucose levels; a Gram stain would not show any organisms.

    Answer D is incorrect. *Neisseria meningitidis* also causes bacterial meningitis but is commonly seen in older children. It is also a gram-negative diplococcus.

Answer E is incorrect. *Streptococcus agalactiae* can cause bacterial meningitis in infants, but a Gram stain of CSF would show gram-positive cocci.

18. **The correct answer is A.** This patient suffered from Parkinson disease (PD), a neurodegenerative disorder of the substantia nigra and locus ceruleus that is most often characterized by **T**remor, **R**igidity, **A**kinesia, and **P**ostural instability (**TRAP**). The photomicrograph shows several neurons from the substantial nigra stained with haematoxylin and eosin at 500 times magnification, at least two of which (arrows) exhibit large Lewy bodies (eosinophilic cytoplasmic inclusions that consist of a dense core surrounded by a halo of 10-nm wide radiating fibrils). These aggregates are the major pathological feature of PD, and are composed primarily of the protein α-synuclein. Some inherited forms of PD have been shown to be caused by mutations in the α-synuclein gene.

 Answer B is incorrect. Dystrophin is the gene disrupted in Duchenne muscular dystrophy. This disease is characterized by progressive muscle weakness and does not have any significant neuropathology.

 Answer C is incorrect. Trinucleotide repeat expansions inside the huntingtin protein cause Huntington disease (HD), a neurodegenerative disease that primarily affects the caudate nucleus and clinically presents with chorea and dementia. This patient's clinical symptoms and pathology are not consistent with HD.

 Answer D is incorrect. Mutations in the presenilin gene have been linked to early forms of Alzheimer disease (AD), the most common cause of dementia in the elderly. Neuropathologically, AD presents with darkly staining neurofibrillary tangles and extracellular amyloid plaques. Resting tremor and Lewy bodies are not associated with AD.

 Answer E is incorrect. Mutations in tau cause frontotemporal dementia with parkinsonism linked to chromosome 17 (FTDP-17). Several other neurodegenerative disorders including Alzheimer disease, Pick disease, and progressive supranuclear palsy present with abnormal cytoplasmic accumulations of tau protein. Lewy bodies are not associated with these neurodegenerative disorders.

19. **The correct answer is D.** This question tests the concept of mass effect of tumors, as well as anatomy. These two topics are inseparable and are necessary to understanding the etiology of some symptoms seen in the context of neoplasms. The adenocarcinoma impinges on the omental foramen, which is formed partly by the hepatoduodenal ligament. This ligament contains the common bile duct along with the hepatic artery proper and the hepatic portal vein. Obstruction of the common bile duct would lead to cholestasis and subsequently conjugated hyperbilirubinemia.

 Answer A is incorrect. Anemia may be a sign of GI bleeding (seen with stomach or colonic cancers) or that bone marrow is dysfunctional and/or being replaced with malignant cells. Although anemia may be seen in this patient due to bleeding into the stomach, anemia is not a direct result of mass effect of the tumor.

 Answer B is incorrect. Constipation may be a symptom of obstruction of the left colon.

 Answer C is incorrect. Persistent hoarseness could be a manifestation of impingement of the recurrent laryngeal nerve. This symptom may be seen with thyroid or lung cancer.

 Answer E is incorrect. Although the tumor can metastasize to the periumbilical region to form a subcutaneous nodule, known as a Sister Mary Joseph nodule, the direct mass effect of the tumor does not affect the periumbilical region.

20. **The correct answer is D.** As the disease prevalence decreases, the likelihood of a positive test being a true-positive decreases. In diseases with very low prevalence, a positive test is more likely a false-positive. In this case, if the prevalence was 1:1,000,000, and the sensitivity and specificity are both 99%, then performing the test on 100,000,000 people will yield 99

true-positives and 999,999 false-positives, for a positive predictive value of approximately 0.00009.

Answer A is incorrect. As disease prevalence decreases, the positive predictive value will decrease, not increase.

Answer B is incorrect. Accuracy measures validity and not reliability, but changes between different tests instead of between prevalences. Positive predictive value is a measure that changes as prevalence changes

Answer C is incorrect. There is no reason to suspect bias in this test. Bias would imply that the information given is inaccurate.

Answer E is incorrect. Accuracy measures validity and not reliability, but changes between different tests instead of between prevalences. Positive predictive value is a measure that changes as prevalence changes

21. **The correct answer is C.** Strong muscle contractions and trismus (contraction of the jaw muscles) are symptoms of tetanus. Tetanus is caused by *Clostridium tetani* spores that are found in soil. They usually enter the body through a puncture wound. The disease is caused by the exotoxin produced by the bacterium. The exotoxin blocks glycine and GABA release, preventing the inhibitory signal from reaching motor neurons downstream, thus predisposing motor neurons to tonic contraction, or tetanus.

    Answer A is incorrect. *Clostridium difficile* causes pseudomembranous colitis by producing a cytotoxin (the A-B toxin) that kills enterocytes and causes pseudomembranous colitis, not lockjaw.

    Answer B is incorrect. *Escherichia coli* produces a heat-labile toxin that stimulates adenylate cyclase by adenosine diphosphate ribosylation of G proteins, which then causes watery diarrhea.

    Answer D is incorrect. *Clostridium botulinum* causes botulism by producing a toxin that blocks the release of acetylcholine at spinal synapses and can cause anticholinergic symptoms. While cranial nerves are often the first to be affected, the paralysis is flaccid rather than contractile. Furthermore, the method of transmission is often through improperly canned goods and honey (in babies) rather than rusty nails.

    Answer E is incorrect. *Staphylococcus aureus* causes disease by producing a toxin that acts as a superantigen and binds to MHC II protein and T lymphocyte receptors. This leads to toxic shock characterized by fever, rash, and shock.

22. **The correct answer is D.** The image shows grouped vesicular lesions following the distribution of a dermatome unilaterally. This is the classic appearance of herpes zoster. Cowdry A inclusion bodies are seen in pathology preparations of herpes zoster skin rashes. They are intranuclear eosinophilic inclusions surrounded by a clear halo.

    Answer A is incorrect. Auer bodies, or Auer rods, are rod-shaped bodies in myeloid cells. They appear primarily in acute promyelocytic leukemia (M3) and are made of fused lysosomes. Care must be taken in treating these patients because release of Auer rods may lead to disseminated intravascular coagulation.

    Answer B is incorrect. Cabot ring bodies are ring-shaped structures found in RBCs in severe cases of megaloblastic anemia.

    Answer C is incorrect. Call-Exner bodies are spaces between granulosa cells in ovarian follicles and in granulosa cell tumors.

    Answer E is incorrect. Mallory bodies, or alcoholic hyaline bodies, are accumulations of eosinophilic material in the cytoplasm of damaged hepatic cells. They are commonly found in hepatocytes of patients with alcoholic hepatitis whose livers would also show cirrhosis and fatty change.

23. **The correct answer is D.** Chlorpromazine is an antipsychotic agent used to treat schizophrenia and psychosis. It acts by blocking dopamine D_2 receptors (some have posited that schizophrenia may result from aberrant do-

paminergic signal transduction). Because dopamine inhibits the secretion of prolactin, a dopamine antagonist such as chlorpromazine can cause hyperprolactinemia.

Answer A is incorrect. Amantadine is used for influenza A prophylaxis. It causes release of dopamine from intact nerve terminals, and thus is sometimes used to treat Parkinson disease. A relative excess of dopamine would not account for this woman's presentation, nor is there any suggestion that she might be taking amantadine.

Answer B is incorrect. Bromocriptine is a dopamine agonist that decreases (rather than increases) prolactin levels. It can actually be used to treat hyperprolactinemia.

Answer C is incorrect. Cabergoline, like bromocriptine, is a dopamine agonist that decreases prolactin levels.

Answer E is incorrect. One of the atypical antipsychotic agents, clozapine blocks both serotonin and dopamine receptors. It tends to have fewer extrapyramidal adverse effects (of which hyperprolactinemia is one example) than typical antipsychotics such as chlorpromazine. Patients taking clozapine, however, must be screened regularly for the development of agranulocytosis. Although clozapine might cause hyperprolactinemia, chlorpromazine is much more likely to do so.

24. **The correct answer is E.** This patient has testicular feminization syndrome (androgen insensitivity), which is due to unresponsiveness of the testosterone receptor protein to androgenic stimulation.

Answer A is incorrect. A deficiency of 5α-reductase presents with ambiguous genitals until puberty, when there is masculinization of the genitals. Testosterone and estrogen levels are normal.

Answer B is incorrect. 17-Hydroxyprogesterone is elevated in congenital adrenal hyperplasia (CAH) commonly as a result of a deficiency of 21α-hydroxylase, or 11α-hydroxylase enzymes necessary for proper steroid synthesis. Although there are many variants of CAH, patients often present in infancy as a result of ambiguous genitals and salt-wasting.

Answer C is incorrect. Excessive exposure to androgenic steroids during early gestation leads to female pseudohermaphroditism (XX), a condition in which ovaries are present, but the external genitalia are virilized.

Answer D is incorrect. Very rare true hermaphroditism is karyotype 46,XX or 47,XXY with ambiguous genitals.

25. **The correct answer is A.** Hirschsprung disease is characterized by a lack of Auerbach and Meissner plexuses, both of which are components of the nerve plexus in the large intestine. These plexuses are composed of cells that have migrated from the neural crest. Auerbach plexus is found between the outer circular and longitudinal muscle layers that are responsible for motility. Meissner plexus is in the submucosal layer. Failure of these plexuses to develop leads to the characteristic megacolon (colonic dilation) seen on this radiograph.

Answer B is incorrect. Failure of neural tube closure during embryogenesis leads to neural tube defects such as anencephaly and spina bifida, both of which would be obvious at birth. Folic acid supplementation by women prior to conception decreases the fetus' risk of developing neural tube defects, although folic acid's mechanism of action is unknown.

Answer C is incorrect. Herniation of mucosal and submucosal tissue at the cricopharyngeus muscle (junction of the pharynx and esophagus) describes Zenker diverticulum. This is a false diverticulum (does not involve the muscular layers) with presenting symptoms of halitosis (malodorous breath), dysphagia, and regurgitation of undigested food.

Answer D is incorrect. A remnant portion of the vitelline duct is describing Meckel diverticulum. It commonly is located in the antimesenteric border of the ileum, usually within 60 cm of the ileocecal valve. Meckel diverticulum can be remembered with the "**rule of 2s**": 2 inches long; 2 feet from the ileocecal valve; 2% of the population get it;

commonly presents in the first 2 years of life; and may have 2 types of epithelium (gastric and/or pancreatic). Ectopic acid-secreting gastric mucosa found in Meckel diverticulum can cause ulcers, which may bleed and result in bloody stool.

Answer E is incorrect. Volvulus occurs when a portion of the bowel rotates around its mesentery, leading to bowel obstruction, ischemia, and possible perforation with resultant peritonitis. Whereas midgut volvulus can occur in infants with congenital intestinal malrotation and in the cecum in young adults, volvulus is most common in redundant segments of the colon such as the sigmoid in elderly, debilitated patients.

26. **The correct answer is E.** Schizotypal patients are often described by others as odd. They display magical thinking, idiosyncratic thought processes, and unusual beliefs or behaviors. Schizotypal patients also manifest unusual perceptions, suspiciousness, constricted affect, lack of close relationships, and social anxiety. Patients with schizotypal personality disorder are at a higher-than-average risk of developing schizophrenia. Under stress, people with schizotypal personality may decompensate and have psychotic symptoms, but these are brief and fragmentary. Excessive social anxiety is associated with paranoid fears.

Answer A is incorrect. Antisocial patients have a disregard for the rights of others, are often in trouble with the law, and show a lack of remorse for wrongful acts.

Answer B is incorrect. Avoidant patients are socially inhibited, often have feelings of inadequacy, and are hypersensitive to criticism. Although both avoidant and schizoid patients have minimal social contacts, avoidant patients desire relationships but do not pursue them out of fear of rejection, whereas schizoid patients genuinely prefer solitude.

Answer C is incorrect. Borderline patients show instability in relationships, self-image, and emotions. They often manifest impulsive behaviors and parasuicidal behavior such as cutting themselves with a sharp object.

Answer D is incorrect. Paranoid patients have a pervasive mistrust and suspiciousness of others without odd behavior.

27. **The correct answer is A.** Adenovirus is a major cause of epidemic keratoconjunctivitis (pink eye). It is the fourth most common cause of childhood respiratory tract infections, after respiratory syncytial virus, parainfluenza, and rhinovirus. It is a naked, icosahedral, double-stranded linear DNA that results in a self-limited illness that requires no treatment.

Answer B is incorrect. Coxsackie A virus causes cold symptoms and rashes. It is also the causative agent of herpangina and hand, foot, and mouth disease.

Answer C is incorrect. Cytomegalovirus (CMV) can reactivate and cause a variety of illnesses in the immunocompromised but is usually asymptomatic in healthy individuals.

Answer D is incorrect. Herpes simplex virus type 1 causes gingivostomatitis, herpetic keratitis of the eye, and encephalitis.

Answer E is incorrect. Rotavirus is the most common cause of diarrhea in infants less than 3 years old.

28. **The correct answer is C.** This patient is presenting with signs suggestive of rheumatoid arthritis. Methotrexate, a folic acid analog antimetabolite that inhibits dihydrofolate reductase, is often used as treatment due to reduction of adenosine-mediated inflammatory changes. Methotrexate is used in a number of neoplastic conditions, including breast carcinoma, head and neck carcinoma, lung carcinoma, choriocarcinoma, acute lymphoblastic leukemia, and non-Hodgkin lymphoma. Other non-oncologic uses of methotrexate include ectopic pregnancy, psoriasis, and inflammatory bowel disease.

Answer A is incorrect. Ceftriaxone is a third-generation cephalosporin antibiotic that inhibits bacterial transpeptidase and cell wall synthesis. It is most commonly used to treat serious gram-negative infections, including meningitis and gonorrhea. Although gonorrhea can present with unilateral arthritis of the knee, this patient's clinical presentation is more consistent with rheumatoid arthritis. Ceftriaxone would therefore not be an effective treatment for this patient. Notably, tetracyclines *can* be used to inhibit the activity of metalloproteinases involved in joint destruction by the rheumatoid synovium, and are therefore effective agents in patients with early rheumatoid arthritis.

Answer B is incorrect. Cyclophosphamide is an alkylating agent that is useful in the treatment of non-Hodgkin lymphoma and breast and ovarian carcinomas. It is also used as an immunosuppressant in systemic lupus erythematosus, multiple sclerosis, and autoimmune hemolytic anemia. It is not generally used as a treatment for rheumatoid arthritis.

Answer D is incorrect. Probenecid is an organic acid that is used most commonly for the treatment of chronic tophaceous gout or increasingly frequent gouty attacks. The drug acts at the anionic transport sites in the renal tubule to inhibit the reabsorption of uric acid, promoting its secretion. Gout normally presents with intermittent acute inflammatory arthritis, most often at only one site. In more chronic disease, more joints become involved and the intervals between attacks become shorter. Advanced gout results in chronic arthropathy, characterized by persistent asymmetric and asynchronous joint inflammation accompanied by uric acid deposits known as tophi, and can occasionally resemble rheumatoid arthritis. Nevertheless, the progressive and steady nature of this patient's disease strongly suggests a diagnosis of rheumatoid arthritis rather than gout. Probenecid would therefore be an ineffective pharmacologic therapy.

Answer E is incorrect. Tamoxifen is an estrogen receptor mixed agonist-antagonist that is most useful against estrogen-sensitive breast cancers.

29. **The correct answer is A.** This patient's clinical description is consistent with AIDS, and his symptoms are consistent with AIDS complex dementia (ADC). Symptoms of ADC include slowed cognition, depressed mood, ataxia, seizures, and urinary and bowel incontinence later in the course of the disease. Symptoms result from HIV-induced demyelination of neurons in the central nervous system. The patient's recent weight loss supports the diagnosis of HIV infection, and purplish skin lesions are consistent with Kaposi sarcoma, a cancer that predominantly affects patients with AIDS.

    Answer B is incorrect. High fever, rigidity of the neck, and encapsulated yeasts in CSF are characteristic of meningitis caused by *Cryptococcus neoformans*. Although patients with AIDS are at higher risk for developing cryptococcal meningitis, the patient's current presentation does not suggest this etiology.

    Answer C is incorrect. Involuntary, dance-like movements of the extremities is descriptive of the chorea of Huntington disease, an autosomal dominant disorder that involves dementia, psychosis, and gross motor dysfunction, progressing to death. CT scan or autopsy often reveals gross cortical atrophy.

    Answer D is incorrect. Paralysis and atrophy of the extremities is characteristic of infection with poliovirus.

    Answer E is incorrect. Progressively decreased mental status and amyloid plaque formation are characteristic of Alzheimer disease. Given the patient's young age, absence of family history, and associated symptoms, there is no reason to suspect Alzheimer disease.

30. **The correct answer is B.** F2 is most likely the father of this child. Restriction site polymorphisms are characteristic sites on individual allele that are recognized by restriction enzymes. These sites can be inherited along with the chromosomes on which they reside. Therefore, every fragment in the child's Southern blot should be found in either the father's or the mother's profile. The child could have received the 6-kb fragment from the mother (M) and the 9-kb fragment from F2.

    Answer A is incorrect. F1 is unlikely to be the father of this child. The child could have received the 6-kb fragment from his mother (M), but he could not have received the 9-kb fragment from either the mother or F1.

Answer C is incorrect. F3 is unlikely to be the father of this child. The child could have received the 6-kb fragment from his mother (M), but he could not have received the 9-kb fragment from either the mother or F3.

Answer D is incorrect. F4 is unlikely to be the father of this child. The child could have received the 6-kb fragment from his mother (M), but he could not have received the 9-kb fragment from either the mother or F4.

31. **The correct answer is B.** The child has a patent ductus arteriosus (PDA), identified in this question by its role in fetal circulation. This causes exercise intolerance, a wide pulse pressure, and a continuous machine-like murmur. Indomethacin may be used to close PDA in the neonate, but older children will require surgery or catheter placement. An important risk factor for PDA is congenital rubella. Rubella is a mild, self-limited illness in adults, which manifests itself as a maculopapular rash beginning in the face and spreading down the body. It is one of the **ToRCHeS** (**To**xoplasmosis, **R**ubella, **C**ytomegalovirus, **He**rpesvirus/HIV, and **S**yphilis) organisms that can cross the placenta and cause congenital disease. There is no specific treatment for rubella, but a vaccine exists that can prevent maternal infection and thus significantly reduce the risk of congenital PDA. The Centers for Disease Control and Prevention warn that rubella vaccine should not be given to a pregnant woman because of a possible risk to the fetus. Administering the rubella vaccine to a woman before she becomes pregnant, however, would lower the risk of congenital PDA in any future offspring. Most ToRCHeS infections present as mild or asymptomatic infections in the mother, but can cause a variety of congenital defects when transmitted to the fetus.

Answer A is incorrect. A firm, non-painful, red genital lesion is suggestive of primary syphilis with the chancre at the site of treponemal entrance. This heals in three to six weeks regardless of whether or not the individual is treated. Secondary syphilis presents with skin lesions on the palms or soles, condylomata lata, and systemic symptoms of lymphadenopathy, fever, malaise, and weight loss. Syphilis is one of the ToRCHeS infections. Congenital syphilis classically manifests as Hutchinson's triad of notched central incisors, blindness, and deafness due to cranial nerve VIII injury. Maternal transmission most frequently occurs during the primary or secondary stage of syphilis.

Answer C is incorrect. These symptoms are nonspecific and are seen commonly in infectious mononucleosis. Although infectious mononucleosis is caused by Epstein-Barr virus, a similar picture can occur in some healthy individuals who are infected by CMV. CMV is one of the ToRCHeS organisms, but it typically causes mental retardation, microcephaly, and deafness; CMV does not commonly cause PDA.

Answer D is incorrect. These are symptoms of whooping cough, caused by *Bordetella pertussis*. Although a vaccine exists to prevent infection by *B pertussis*, this is not one of the organisms known to cause congenital disease and is not a risk factor for PDA.

Answer E is incorrect. These symptoms are suggestive of a gonococcal infection. Gonorrhea is an important cause of pelvic inflammatory disease, infertility, and ectopic pregnancies, but does not cross the placenta and is not associated with PDA.

32. **The correct answer is A.** Menopause is the cessation of estrogen production because of a loss of ovarian sensitivity to gonadotropin stimulation caused by ovarian dysfunction and a decreased number of available ovarian follicles. In the United States, the average age at onset of menopause is 51 years, with a normal range between 45-55 years. Remember, menopause causes **HAVOC**: **H**ot flashes, **A**trophy of the **V**agina, **O**steoporosis, and **C**oronary artery disease (CAD). Estrogen is necessary for the maintenance and development of the vagina and bone deposition, so a decrease leads to vaginal atrophy and osteoporosis. There is no direct link between estrogen and heart

disease, but the incidence of CAD following menopause is two to three times higher than in premenopausal women, suggesting some protective effect of endogenous estrogen. Hot flashes are related to changes in the ability of the hypothalamus to recognize body temperature. Because estrogen replacement therapy alleviates these symptoms, there may be a role for estrogen in body temperature regulation. The estrogen level in this patient is low (<100 pg/ml), and levels of follicle-stimulating hormone (FSH) and luteinizing hormone (LH) are elevated. FSH and LH levels are elevated in menopause because of decreased feedback inhibition from estrogen, but these levels are not the primary cause of menopause.

Answer B is incorrect. Decreased negative feedback on the pituitary occurs secondary to decreased levels of estrogen. A primary decrease in negative feedback would lead to increased levels of FSH and LH and therefore increased levels of estrogen. However, this patient shows symptoms of decreased estrogen.

Answer C is incorrect. Although increased FSH levels are found in menopause, this is secondary to decreased estrogen levels, which decrease negative feedback on the anterior pituitary. The increased FSH level itself is not known to be the cause of menopausal symptoms. The symptoms are due to low levels of estrogen.

Answer D is incorrect. High levels of progesterone may result in fatigue, depression, and vaginal dryness. However, this woman's symptoms are more characteristic of menopause, which is due to low levels of estrogen.

Answer E is incorrect. Increased testosterone levels in a woman are classically seen in congenital adrenal hyperplasia or polycystic ovarian syndrome and lead to masculine features such as hirsutism. Testosterone levels are typically low in menopause.

33. **The correct answer is D.** A common cause of male infertility is Klinefelter syndrome. It occurs in one out of about every 900 men. A patient with this condition has an extra X chromosome, and either the patient's mother or the father can contribute this extra chromosome, and the origin of the chromosome appears to make no difference. The patient's karyotype is 47,XXY. In Klinefelter syndrome, the testicles are nonfunctional, and therefore testosterone levels are decreased, resulting in a secondary increase in gonadotropin levels (FSH and LH) due to the lack of negative feedback. Patients with Klinefelter syndrome tend also to have the following signs: They are tall, long-limbed, and have a distribution pattern of fat and hair more typical of women. They also tend to have gynecomastia, or enlargement of the breasts.

    Answer A is incorrect. Because of testicular dysfunction, FSH secondarily becomes increased, not decreased, in Klinefelter syndrome.

    Answer B is incorrect. Thyroid-stimulating hormone (TSH), a measure of thyroid function, has no clinical application in diagnosing Klinefelter syndrome.

    Answer C is incorrect. Gonadotropin-releasing hormone will be increased secondary to the diminished testosterone level.

    Answer E is incorrect. Klinefelter syndrome causes testicular atrophy. This results in decreased, not increased, testosterone.

34. **The correct answer is A.** Bupivacaine is an amide-based local anesthetic. It has greater cardiotoxic effects than other drugs in this class and can thus produce arrhythmias and hypotension if used intravenously.

    Answer B is incorrect. Fentanyl is an opioid and thus its toxicity profile is similar to that of morphine. Adverse effects include constipation, nausea, vomiting, respiratory depression, and coma.

    Answer C is incorrect. Halothane is a gaseous anesthetic used for both its analgesic and muscle relaxant properties. It is hepatotoxic and may cause malignant hyperthermia in genetically predisposed patients or when used in conjunction with depolarizing paralytic agents such as succinylcholine. It also leads to a significant decrease in cardiac output and blood pressure.

Answer D is incorrect. Ibuprofen, a nonsteroidal anti-inflammatory drug (NSAID), may cause gastric ulceration and renal failure due to interaction with kidney autoregulation.

Answer E is incorrect. Morphine, an opioid, may cause constipation, nausea, vomiting, respiratory depression, and coma.

35. **The correct answer is A.** Curve B represents hemoglobin with greater affinity (lower partial pressure of oxygen at which the hemoglobin is 50% saturated) for oxygen compared to curve A. Of the answers provided, only increasing the concentration of $\alpha 2 \gamma 2$ hemoglobin (fetal hemoglobin, HbF) will shift the curve to the left. In adult hemoglobin (HbA), the two γ chains have been replaced with two β chains. The oxygen affinity of HbF is higher than that of HbA because of a lower affinity for 2,3-biphosphoglyceric acid (BPG) (from having a neutral serine in the BPG binding site compared to a positive histamine in HbA), enabling oxygen to be transferred from mother to fetus. Continued production of HbF in adults is seen in patients with β thalassemia due to a decreased or absent production of β chain.

Answer B is incorrect. Hemoglobin $\alpha 2 \beta 2$ is HbA, the normal HbA. Elevated hemoglobin increases the total oxygen content carried in blood, but it does not affect the affinity of hemoglobin for oxygen.

Answer C is incorrect. A decrease in pH, through the stabilization of deoxyhemoglobin by hydrogen, results in a shift of the curve to the right.

Answer D is incorrect. High altitude, through the increased concentration of 2,3-diphosphoglycerate in RBCs, results in a shift of the curve to the right.

Answer E is incorrect. Increased temperature promotes the offloading of oxygen in tissues by shifting the curve to the right.

36. **The correct answer is E.** Patient autonomy in a legally competent patient is paramount. Understanding the risks and benefits of a treatment, as well as outcomes with and without the treatment, are defining characteristics of competence. In a competent adult, a physician is obligated to respect patient autonomy over the principles of non-maleficence and beneficence. Beneficence and non-maleficence may take precedence with minors, those who are physically or mentally impaired, and in emergency situations. Patients are admitted involuntarily only for the treatment of psychiatric conditions. Even then, unless they pose a risk to themselves or others, competent patients can refuse psychiatric treatment. Therefore, the physician should respect the patient's wishes and refrain from treating the hypertension.

Answer A is incorrect. Beneficence implies that an intervention is in a patient's best interest. All interventions have this characteristic in modern medicine but cannot be instituted without patient consent.

Answer B is incorrect. Informed consent implies patient acknowledgment of the risks, benefits, and alternatives of a procedure or treatment, and also implies the patient's autonomous permission for the physician to intervene. Informed consent is generally obtained before a procedure, and is not applicable in this case.

Answer C is incorrect. The ethical principle of justice implies that the benefits and burdens placed on patients are distributed fairly among patients. By having offered the patient an established treatment for hypertension, the physician has followed the principle of justice. This answer is incorrect, because patient autonomy takes precedence to justice.

Answer D is incorrect. Non-maleficence is the principle that the physician will do no harm to the patient, and therefore implies that risks of a treatment are superseded by the benefits. Such a treatment can be offered by physicians but cannot be instituted without patient consent.

37. **The correct answer is C.** A blood pressure in the upper extremity significantly greater than in the lower extremity, a weak to nonexistent femoral pulse, and rib notching on chest x-ray are all consistent with postductal coarctation

of the aorta. This condition is associated with a high risk of bacterial endocarditis and cerebral hemorrhage. Postductal coarctation is caused by an abnormal constriction of the aorta distal to the ductus arteriosus during fetal development.

Answer A is incorrect. Acute lymphocytic leukemia is associated with Down syndrome, which is also associated with an increased risk of an atrial septal defect. However, this is not associated with coarctation of the aorta.

Answer B is incorrect. A boot-shaped heart refers to the cardiac silhouette produced in cases of isolated right ventricular hypertrophy, classically seen in tetralogy of Fallot. While aortic coarctation may theoretically lead to right ventricular hypertrophy, it will do so only after the left ventricle has hypertrophied and thus will not produce the boot-shaped silhouette.

Answer D is incorrect. Cor pulmonale is defined as heart failure secondary to lung disease. If lung disease produces pulmonary hypertension, it will lead to right-sided failure. Since aortic coarctation is not lung disease, it cannot be associated with cor pulmonale.

Answer E is incorrect. Eisenmenger syndrome is the secondary development of cyanosis in conditions that produce a left-to-right shunt, such as ventricular septal defects. The increased blood flow in the pulmonary circulation leads to pulmonary hypertension, which raises the pressure on the right side of the heart, eventually reversing the shunt. Because blood is now shunted right to left, avoiding the pulmonary circulation, cyanosis develops. Aortic coarctation does not produce a left-to-right shunt and thus does not lead to Eisenmenger syndrome.

38. **The correct answer is C.** Ehlers-Danlos syndrome is characterized by defects in the synthesis or structure of collagen type III. Accordingly, patients with this disorder have collagen that lacks tensile strength, and they demonstrate hyperextensible skin and hypermobile joints. Because of a defect in connective tissue, patients with this disorder are more susceptible to berry aneurysms.

Answer A is incorrect. Collagen type I is the primary component of bone, skin, tendon, dentin, fascia, cornea, and late wound repair. The most common form of osteogenesis imperfecta occurs as a result of an autosomal dominant defect in type I collagen. Osteogenesis imperfecta is characterized by multiple fractures, blue sclerae, hearing loss, and dental imperfections. Because of the multiple fractures, this disorder often is confused with child abuse.

Answer B is incorrect. Collagen type II is the primary component of cartilage (including hyaline), vitreous body, and the nucleus pulposus. Abnormalities in type II collagen result in a fatal form of osteogenesis imperfecta in utero or in the neonatal period.

Answer D is incorrect. Collagen type IV is the primary component of basement membranes or the basal lamina of the kidney, ears, and eyes. Alport syndrome, characterized by progressive hereditary nephritis and deafness, is identified most commonly as an X-linked recessive disorder.

Answer E is incorrect. Elastin is a stretchy protein within the lungs, large arteries, elastic ligaments, vocal cords, and ligamenta flava that is broken down by elastase. α_1-antitrypsin deficiency results in excess elastase activity, which is a major cause of emphysema.

Answer F is incorrect. Marfan syndrome results from a defect in fibrillin, the major component of microfibrils found in the extracellular matrix. These patients display bilateral lens subluxation or dislocation, distinctive skeletal abnormalities, and aortic aneurysms (dilation of the aortic ring resulting in aortic incompetence), as well as incompetent mitral and tricuspid valves.

Answer G is incorrect. Sphingomyelinase defects characterize Niemann-Pick disease. This disease is characterized by progressive neurodegeneration, hepatosplenomegaly and a characteristic cherry-red spot on the macula.

39. **The correct answer is E.** The first-line therapy for treating severe nausea and vomiting due to

chemotherapy is ondansetron. It is the strongest available antiemetic, surpassing more common agents, such as metoclopramide, in its ability to decrease symptoms. The mechanism of action of ondansetron is blockade of serotonin 5-HT_3 receptors. Adverse effects of ondansetron are headache and constipation.

Answer A is incorrect. Anticholinergic drugs include atropine, benztropine, scopolamine, and ipratropium. These drugs decrease parasympathetic activity by blocking muscarinic receptors. Scopolamine is commonly used to treat motion sickness but would not be the first-line therapy for chemotherapy-induced nausea and vomiting.

Answer B is incorrect. Dopamine agonists include bromocriptine, L-dopa, pramipexole, and amantadine. These drugs are mainly used for the treatment of Parkinson disease and are not indicated for nausea and vomiting.

Answer C is incorrect. Tricyclic antidepressants (TCAs) such as imipramine and amitriptyline act by inhibiting presynaptic reuptake of norepinephrine, thus augmenting their effect on postsynaptic receptors. TCAs are primarily used to treat depression. Their adverse effects include sedation, α-blocking effects, and anticholinergic properties.

Answer D is incorrect. Serotonin agonists include selective serotonin reuptake inhibitors such as paroxetine and sertraline, which are antidepressants.

40. **The correct answer is C.** The vignette describes a patient with rickets, the clinical syndrome that results from vitamin D deficiency. Hallmarks of this condition include a broad-based waddling gait, bending of long weight-bearing bones on radiographs, and hypocalcemia with low to normal serum phosphate levels and elevated serum alkaline phosphatase activity. Vitamin D functions in its active form, 1,25-dihydroxycholecalciferol, to increase intestinal absorption of calcium and phosphate. A deficiency in this nutrient will result in a deficiency in intestinal calcium and phosphate absorption. Note that 25-dihydroxycholecalciferol is synthesized initially in the liver and then is further hydroxylated to 1,25-dihydroxycholecalciferol in the kidney.

Answer A is incorrect. A decrease in bone mineral density is typical of osteoporosis. Patients with osteoporosis are usually older women, unlike the patient in this vignette. Patients with osteoporosis tend to suffer from fractures including vertebral compression fractures and hip fractures. Patients with osteoporosis will have normal serum levels of phosphate, calcium, and alkaline phosphatase.

Answer B is incorrect. A deficiency in the hydroxylation of proline and lysine in collagen synthesis is typically a result of ascorbic acid, or vitamin C, deficiency. This usually results in the clinical syndrome known as scurvy, which is not consistent with the clinical scenario described. Patients with scurvy may have bleeding gums and unhealed wounds. This vitamin deficiency is usually the result of insufficient dietary intake, the so-called "tea and toast" diet.

Answer D is incorrect. An increase in bone turnover is typical of Paget disease of bone. This disorder is marked by excessive bone resorption followed by excessive bone formation. It results in disorganized bone formation that is more likely to result in fracture than normal bone and may result in deafness through restructuring of the bony surroundings of the ear. Furthermore, patients are susceptible to the formation of sarcomas. In Paget disease of bone the serum alkaline phosphatase level is highly elevated. The patient in this vignette does not meet the clinical manifestations of Paget disease.

Answer E is incorrect. Although a patient with renal failure would also exhibit a deficiency of vitamin D (because it is synthesized in the kidneys), one would expect to see an elevated phosphate level due to decreased excretion. One would also expect to see a low calcium level due to diminished vitamin D (and hence, diminished intestinal absorption of calcium). Lastly, one would also expect to see elevated parathyroid hormone (PTH) levels as the body attempts to increase serum calcium.

41. **The correct answer is C.** Dyspnea and unilateral pleuritic chest pain in a young male smoker are highly suggestive of spontaneous pneumothorax. Risk factors include male sex, smoking, and a tall, thin stature. Because air is filling up the space previously occupied by the lung, there will be hyperresonance on percussion on the side with the lesion.

    Answer A is incorrect. Primary pneumothorax presents with unilateral chest expansion, indicating that one side is not being filled with air during inspiration. It may or may not be accompanied by tracheal deviation away from the affected lung.

    Answer B is incorrect. Lobar pneumonia may have bronchial breath sounds over the lesion, whereas pneumothorax will have decreased breath sounds over the lesion.

    Answer D is incorrect. Lobar pneumonia would present with increased tactile fremitus, whereas pneumothorax will have absent tactile fremitus.

    Answer E is incorrect. Tension pneumothorax will have tracheal deviation away from the side with the lesion. In spontaneous pneumothorax, there may or may not be any tracheal deviation. If it is present, a contralateral shift of the mediastinum will be seen on chest x-ray.

42. **The correct answer is B.** This is a classic description of a patient with Bartter syndrome, a defect in the ion channels of the thick ascending loop of Henle. Clinically, patients have low-to-normal blood pressure, with short stature and failure to thrive, and various lab abnormalities, including hypokalemia, metabolic alkalosis, and hyperaldosteronism. Depending on the extent of the metabolic derangements, patients may also have nonspecific symptoms such as nausea, vomiting, diarrhea, and muscle cramps. If the electrolyte abnormalities become severe, patients are at risk for seizures. Bartter syndrome has three variants, each affecting the sodium-potassium-chloride pump and each resulting in a different defective channel in the thick ascending limb of the loop of Henle, the site at which furosemide, a loop diuretic, acts.

    Answer A is incorrect. Acetazolamide acts at the proximal convoluted tubule, inhibiting carbonic anhydrase. It causes a reduction in total-body bicarbonate. Acetazolamide can result in type 2 renal tubular acidosis, but not Bartter syndrome.

    Answer C is incorrect. Hydrochlorothiazide is a thiazide diuretic that acts early in the distal tubule. Metabolic derangements seen with this drug include hypokalemic metabolic acidosis, hyponatremia, hyperglycemia, hyperlipidemia, hyperuricemia, and hypercalcemia.

    Answer D is incorrect. Spironolactone is a potassium-sparing diuretic that acts as a competitive aldosterone receptor antagonist in the cortical collecting tubule. Adverse effects include hyperkalemia and antiandrogenic effects, such as gynecomastia.

    Answer E is incorrect. Triamterene is a potassium-sparing diuretic that blocks sodium channels in the cortical collecting tubule.

43. **The correct answer is C.** This image shows numerous vacuolated macrophages crowding the lamina propria. On periodic acid-Schiff (PAS) stain, vacuoles of the macrophages within the lamina propria react intensely and appear purple, indicating the presence of glycoprotein. PAS-positive macrophages are seen in Whipple disease, which is caused by infection with *Tropheryma whippelii.* Whipple disease most commonly affects older white men. Although this disease can affect any part of the body (including the heart, lungs, brain, joints, and eyes), the most common presenting feature of Whipple disease is diarrhea due to malabsorption.

    Answer A is incorrect. The most common disaccharidase deficiency is lactase deficiency, which results in lactose intolerance. In patients with lactose intolerance, drinking milk can cause abdominal pain, diarrhea, and increased flatulence. PAS-positive macrophages, however, are not seen in lactase deficiency, and the villi appear normal.

    Answer B is incorrect. Chronic pancreatitis is characterized by malabsorption of protein, fat, and vitamins A, D, E, and K; thus steatorrhea is a common sign of chronic pancreatitis. PAS-positive macrophages, however, are not seen in this condition.

Answer D is incorrect. Similar to celiac sprue, tropical sprue is characterized by autoantibodies to gluten (gliadin) in wheat and other grains. Although its cause is unknown, it is likely due to infection. PAS-positive macrophages are not seen in sprue, however.

Answer E is incorrect. Histologic examination in celiac sprue reveals villus flattening and lymphocytic infiltrate. Antigliadin, anti-endomysial, and anti-tissue transglutaminase antibodies are present, resulting in malabsorption. PAS-positive macrophages are not seen in sprue.

44. **The correct answer is E.** This patient has Graves disease, an autoimmune disorder resulting from the presence of elevated levels of thyroid-stimulating immunoglobulin (TSI), an IgG that binds to and stimulates the TSH receptor of the thyroid gland. This causes an increase in the production and release of thyroid hormone. The presence of TSI is relatively specific for Graves disease. While the exact trigger for this autoimmune response is unknown, Graves disease is associated with the HLA-B8 subtype. The three classic findings associated with Graves disease are hyperthyroidism, ophthalmopathy (exophthalmos), and dermopathy/pretibial myxedema (ie, nonpitting edema on the anterior surface of both legs, with overlying skin that is dry and waxy and may have several diffuse, slightly pigmented papules). Propylthiouracil and methimazole are used to treat hyperthyroidism. They work by blocking tyrosine iodination (also known as organification) and coupling. Propylthiouracil also decreases peripheral conversion of thyronine to triiodothyronine (T_3). β-blockers are also used to control the cardiac abnormalities of thyrotoxicosis.

Answer A is incorrect. Active absorption of iodide is known as "trapping" and is the first step in thyroid hormone synthesis. However, it is not affected by propylthiouracil.

Answer B is incorrect. Iodide must be oxidized to iodine before it can be attached to thyroglobulin. This step is not affected by propylthiouracil.

Answer C is incorrect. TSH regulates many steps in the synthesis or thyroid hormone and is released from the anterior pituitary gland. Due to negative feedback, one would expect to see a low serum TSH level in this patient. Thus, blocking this step would not help a patient with Graves disease.

Answer D is incorrect. Colloid is the stored form of thyroid hormone and when stimulated by TSH, it is cleaved by proteases to release thyroxine and T_3 This step can be inhibited by iodide salts but is not commonly used as a first-line treatment.

45. **The correct answer is B.** This patient suffers from Wernicke-Korsakoff syndrome. Alcoholic patients often have reduced intake of calories other than from alcohol and become deficient in various nutrients, among them vitamin B_1 (thiamine). Thiamine is a needed cofactor in some of the key reactions in the Krebs cycle. Without it, cells are in a low-energy state that will eventually damage those cells with high-energy requirements (neurons and myocardium). Wernicke encephalopathy is an acute syndrome that is reversible with thiamine administration; it is characterized by mental status changes (disorientation, confusion, inattention), ophthalmoplegia, ataxia, and nystagmus. Korsakoff dementia is a chronic syndrome and is irreversible; it is characterized by symptoms of Wernicke encephalopathy, selective anterograde and retrograde amnesia, and confabulations (note that the patient is too young to have been in World War II). Additionally, peripheral neuropathy (dry beriberi) or dilated cardiomyopathy (wet beriberi) may develop, as in this patient. A transesophageal echocardiogram allows for assessment of the extent of the cardiomyopathy.

Answer A is incorrect. Lumbar puncture may be helpful in the case of meningitis. However, nothing in the patient's history points to meningitis (headache, stiff neck). Imaging is needed to assess the extent of cerebral atrophy.

Answer C is incorrect. Coagulation studies will most likely reveal prolonged times in this patient (ie, the patient is anticoagulated). This is commonly seen in patients with damaged livers. Although coagulation studies allow appreciation of the amount of liver dysfunction, they do not measure the extent of the patient's primary problem, which is the nutritional deficit of thiamine and its associated consequences.

Answer D is incorrect. Tissue pressures are a measure of the severity of compartment syndrome. Although compartment syndrome presents with edematous tissues, it is not associated with neurologic symptoms such as confusion and confabulation. Furthermore, the question stem does not describe any possible historical clues for compartment syndrome to develop (such as recent trauma).

Answer E is incorrect. Venous Doppler ultrasonography is used to diagnose deep venous thrombosis (DVT). Although a patient's legs may become edematous and pulmonary râles (in the case of embolization to the lung) may develop, DVT does not explain the neurologic status of this patient. The patient is too old for an inherited clotting disorder to appear (usually occurs before age 40), and no predisposing factors are listed in the question stem (eg, recent surgery, cancer, oral contraceptives). In fact, many alcoholics are somewhat anticoagulated, as a damaged liver produces fewer clotting factors.

46. **The correct answer is A.** This patient has peptic ulcer disease (PUD), which presents as a burning epigastric pain worsened by eating. Bleeding from the ulcer may lead to black, tarry stools and anemia. The gold standard for diagnosis is endoscopy. Benign lesions are flat and have smooth borders, unlike malignant lesions, which may protrude into the lumen and have irregular borders. *H pylori* infection is a major cause of PUD; >70% of patients with PUD have concurrent *H pylori* infection.

Answer B is incorrect. Although the use of NSAIDs is a risk factor associated with PUD, celecoxib spares cyclooxygenase isoform 1 found in gastric mucosa. Thus celecoxib use is not a risk factor for PUD.

Answer C is incorrect. Diabetes is not a risk factor for PUD.

Answer D is incorrect. Hypertension is not associated with PUD.

Answer E is incorrect. In the past, PUD was attributed to many factors, including stress, spicy foods, chewing gum, and poor eating habits. While some spicy foods might exacerbate the symptoms of PUD, poor eating habits do not cause PUD. A vegan diet might lead to megaloblastic anemia from a lack of vitamin B_{12}, but this patient's anemia is likely due to chronic blood loss.

47. **The correct answer is C.** The patient is suffering from hyperparathyroidism secondary to renal disease, also known as renal osteodystrophy. As the glomerular filtration rate decreases, excretion of phosphate also decreases, leading to hyperphosphatemia. Additionally, the diseased kidney no longer can produce adequate amounts of $1,25(OH)_2D_3$, which decreases the amount of calcium being absorbed from the gut, resulting in hypocalcemia. The hyperphosphatemia amplifies the fall in serum calcium and independently increases PTH secretion. The fall of serum calcium, low levels of $1,25(OH)_2D_3$ and the hyperphosphatemia combine to result in hyperparathyroidism. The hypocalcemia in this patient is demonstrated as a positive Chvostek sign, in which tapping on the hyperexcitable facial nerve causes temporary facial muscle spasms. The increase in PTH also activates osteoclasts, leading to bone resorption and increased levels of alkaline phosphatase.

Answer A is incorrect. Patients with renal disease have decreased serum calcium levels secondary to impaired activation of vitamin D to $1,25(OH)_2D_3$. Lack of biologically active vitamin D results in decreased absorption of calcium from the GI tract. Thus these lab values would not be consistent with this patient.

Answer B is incorrect. This set of lab values is characteristic of a patient with primary hyperparathyroidism. The major difference between the lab results for a patient with primary versus secondary hyperparathyroidism is the relationship between PTH and serum calcium. Patients with primary hyperparathyroidism will have a resultant increase in serum calcium levels, while those with secondary hyperparathyroidism have a decreased serum calcium level, which then leads to the increase in PTH.

Answer D is incorrect. Increased levels of PTH in patients with secondary hyperparathyroidism leads to osteoclast activation. This of course increases bone resorption and alkaline phosphatase.

Answer E is incorrect. Patients with renal disease have increased, not decreased, levels of phosphate.

48. **The correct answer is A.** Critical points to consider in this question are first, that the patient is a nonsmoker; second, that the lesion is localized peripherally (subpleural mass); and third, that the patient is a woman. About 95% of all lung cancers can be classified into one of two categories: small cell lung cancers make up 13%, and non-small cell lung cancers (consisting of adenocarcinoma, squamous cell carcinomas, and other histologic types) make up the rest. Adenocarcinoma is the most prevalent type of lung cancer, representing 38% of all diagnosed cases. Relative to squamous cell carcinoma (the second most prevalent subtype), adenocarcinoma is more often seen in nonsmokers than in smokers (62% vs 18%), and more often seen in women than in men irrespective of smoking status. Treatment interventions differ by type. Because adenocarcinomas are typically peripherally located (75%), they often are more amenable to surgical removal than other tumor types, although the success of treatment depends more on the stage of the tumor than the type. Adenocarcinoma often, but not always, presents as multiple masses.

Answer B is incorrect. Carcinoid tumors are found in major bronchi and may cause carcinoid syndrome (flushing due to excessive histamine release). They are of neuroendocrine origin and have no link with smoking.

Answer C is incorrect. Although metastases from other organs arise more commonly than primary lung tumors, they are most often multifocal, not a single peripheral nodule. Metastases to lung principally arise from primary tumors of the breast, colon, and kidney.

Answer D is incorrect. Small cell carcinoma of the lung is an undifferentiated tumor usually present in a central location. There is a strong association with smoking and it is more often seen in men. Small cell carcinoma metastasizes early and may secrete hormones such as ADH and ACTH. Small cell lung cancer is rarely resectable and is most often treated with combination chemotherapy and radiation.

Answer E is incorrect. Squamous cell carcinoma of the lung often presents as a centrally located hilar mass. This lung cancer subtype is more common in men, and it exhibits the strongest link to smoking.

Test Block 6

QUESTIONS

1. A 45-year-old man presents to his physician complaining of a five-month history of occasional burning mid-epigastric pain that improves when he eats food. He denies any history of recent travel or excessive use of nonsteroidal anti-inflammatory drugs. The physician begins a course of pharmacologic therapy to improve the patient's symptoms. Blockade of which of the following receptors would improve the patient's symptoms most significantly?

   (A) Cholecystokinin B
   (B) $Histamine_2$
   (C) $Muscarinic_3$
   (D) Norepinephrine
   (E) Secretin

2. A 27-year-old woman with a history of recurrent neurologic complaints (including temporary loss of vision, migrating areas of weakness and sensory deficits, and bladder incontinence) presents to her internist's office with a new neurologic complaint. She says her husband has noticed that her eyes have recently been "moving out of sync" with one another. She admits that at times she has double vision. A lesion of the right medial longitudinal fasciculus would result in which combination of eye movements?

   (A) Normal conjugate movement with attempted lateral gaze
   (B) Palsy of the left medial rectus with attempted left lateral gaze
   (C) Palsy of the left medial rectus with attempted right lateral gaze
   (D) Palsy of the right medial rectus with attempted left lateral gaze
   (E) Palsy of the right medial rectus with attempted right lateral gaze

3. A 22-year-old man comes to the physician complaining of difficulty walking up the stairs because he "can't catch his breath." Physical examination reveals moderate pitting edema in his lower extremities and a new S_3 gallop. The patient's history includes a recently treated severe upper respiratory infection that did not respond to antibiotics. The patient is not diabetic, hypertensive, or dyslipidemic, and all of his family members are healthy. Which of the following is the most likely cause of this patient's symptoms?

   (A) Adenovirus
   (B) *Brugia malayi*
   (C) Coxsackie B virus
   (D) *Haemophilus influenzae* type B
   (E) *Streptococcus pneumoniae*
   (F) *Wuchereria bancrofti*

4. A primigravida at 30 weeks' gestation has been diagnosed with diabetes mellitus. She is rushed to delivery because of signs of preeclampsia. After a cesarean section delivery, the newborn baby is noted to have signs of cyanosis, tachypnea, and dyspnea. Which of the following is a characteristic of the substance that is insufficient in the baby?

   (A) It consists primarily of sphingomyelin
   (B) It decreases compliance of small alveoli
   (C) It disrupts liquid intermolecular forces in alveoli
   (D) It increases the surface tension of alveoli
   (E) It is produced by type I pneumocytes in alveoli
   (F) It lines medium-sized bronchi, not alveoli

5. A 30-year-old African-American man presents to his primary care physician complaining of dizziness and lethargy. About a week ago he completed a 14-day course of antibiotics prescribed by his doctor for bacterial sinusitis. He is normally in good health, eats a diet full of fruits and vegetables, and exercises daily. He denies any changes in his diet and has not experienced any gastrointestinal distress, although he admits to tea-colored urine over the past three-four days. On physical examination he appears pale and uncomfortable, with icteric sclerae. His blood pressure is 100/70 mm Hg, pulse is 110/min, and respirations are 19/min. Laboratory studies show:

RBC count: 5300/mm³
WBC count: 9,500/mm³
Hemoglobin: 8 g/dL
Hematocrit: 24%
Mean corpuscular volume: 90 fL

Which of the following is the most likely cause of this patient's anemia?

(A) α-Thalassemia
(B) Blood donation
(C) Folic acid deficiency
(D) Glucose-6-phosphate dehydrogenase deficiency
(E) Intrinsic factor deficiency
(F) Iron deficiency
(G) Sickle cell disease

6. A 27-year-old man dies of acute respiratory distress syndrome one day after presenting to the hospital with shortness of breath and a fever of 38°C (100.4°F). On the second hospital day, he developed extreme pulmonary edema and hypotension before he died. His family says that he had recently gone hiking and caving in an area heavily populated with rodents. Which of the following is the most likely cause of death in this patient?

(A) Dengue virus
(B) Ebola virus
(C) Hantavirus
(D) Marburg virus
(E) Rhabdovirus

7. A 33-year-old refugee from Sudan presents to the emergency department with a history of increasing fever and fatigue over the past six months. A large mass on his left mandible is observed. Biopsy of the mass is shown in the image. Which of the following results supports the diagnosis?

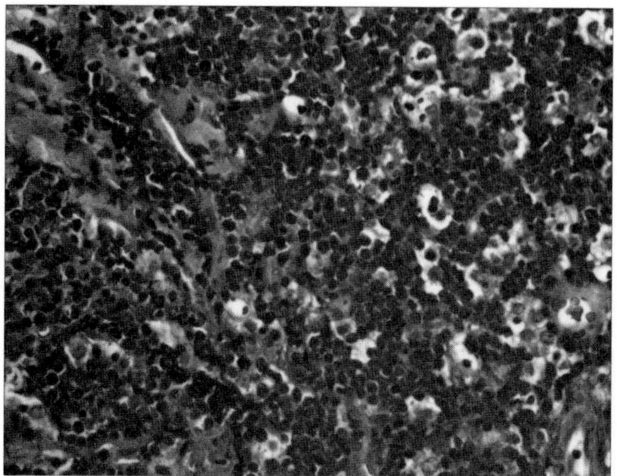

Reproduced, with permission, from USMLERx.com.

(A) Karyotypic analysis demonstrating t(8;14)
(B) Karyotypic analysis demonstrating t(9;22)
(C) Lymphocytes positive for interleukin-21 on flow cytometry
(D) Lymphocytes positive for terminal deoxynucleotidyl transferase on flow cytometry
(E) Physical examination that reveals bilateral orchitis

8. Intravenous administration of drug X to an anesthetized animal produces an increase in its systolic blood pressure. After administration of drug Y, readministration of drug X produces a decrease in the animal's systolic blood pressure. Which of the following pairs of drugs could produce this sequence of events?

(A) Drug X = acetylcholine; Drug Y = neostigmine
(B) Drug X = epinephrine; Drug Y = phentolamine
(C) Drug X = isoproterenol; Drug Y = atropine
(D) Drug X = norepinephrine; Drug Y = propranolol
(E) Drug X = phenylephrine; Drug Y = hexamethonium

9. An 82-year-old retired banker comes to the physician because of a three-week history of progressively worsening nonlocalizing, nonradicular low back pain that is not relieved by sitting or sleeping. He describes urinary hesitancy and a long history of benign prostatic hyperplasia that has recently worsened. He has been afebrile throughout this time. Physical examination is notable for perianal hyperesthesia with slightly decreased rectal tone, a uniformly enlarged prostate, and diminished ankle jerk reflexes bilaterally. No pain is elicited with straight leg raises in the supine position. X-ray films of the thoracic and lumbosacral spine show moderate osteoarthritis. Laboratory studies are unremarkable. Which of the following is the most likely cause of the patient's symptoms?

(A) Conus medullaris tumor
(B) Guillain-Barré syndrome
(C) L4-5 disc herniation
(D) Spinal epidural abscess
(E) Vertebral osteomyelitis

10. An 8-year-old girl presents to the clinic for a check-up required by her new school. She is a recent immigrant to the United States and did not have access to regular medical care growing up. Her mother reports that when her daughter was an infant she had swollen hands and feet as well as "something wrong with the sides of her neck." The patient's left arm is smaller than the right. When height and weight data are plotted on a growth curve, she is short for her age. What congenital cardiovascular anomaly does this patient most likely have?

(A) Postductal coarctation of the aorta
(B) Preductal coarctation of the aorta
(C) Subclavian steal syndrome
(D) Tetralogy of Fallot
(E) Transposition of the great vessels

11. A 6-year-old boy with recurrent otitis media was treated with ceftriaxone by his pediatrician. One week after beginning treatment, his father notices he has been bruising easily on his legs and bleeding heavily when he brushes his teeth. Examination reveals streaks of blood under the fingernails. Blood tests reveal an increased prothrombin time and partial thromboplastin time. Which of the following describes the function of the enzymes or cofactors most likely to be involved?

(A) Activation of antithrombin III
(B) Carboxylation of glutamic acid residues
(C) Cross-linking of fibrin polymers
(D) Hydrolyzation of fibrinogen
(E) Hydroxylation of proline residues

12. The inhaled anesthetic drugs A, B, C, and D have the properties indicated in the chart. Which of the following statements best describes the properties of these drugs?

	Minimum alveolar concentration	Blood solubility
Drug A	7.3	0.5
Drug B	3.1	1.0
Drug C	2.0	0.1
Drug D	4.4	0.15

Reproduced, with permission, from USMLERx.com.

(A) Drug A is more potent than drug D
(B) Drug B is less soluble in blood than drug C
(C) Drug C will have both the highest potency and the most rapid induction
(D) Drug D will induce anesthesia more rapidly than drug C
(E) Patients treated with drug B will recover more quickly from anesthesia than drug A

13. A 46-year-old man presents with a three-week history of burning substernal and epigastric pain that improves after meals. Medical history is significant for hypertension, which is controlled with exercise and diet. Medications include a daily vitamin supplement. He has no other complaints. Social history reveals that the patient was born in Cambodia, and lived

there until five years ago when he moved to the United States. A urease breath test performed in the office is positive. What is the recommended treatment for the patient?

(A) Ampicillin, clindamycin, and bismuth
(B) Bismuth, metronidazole, tetracycline, and omeprazole
(C) Imipenem and cilastatin
(D) Ranitidine, omeprazole, and bismuth
(E) Vancomycin, gentamicin, and aztreonam

14. A 34-year-old woman is brought to the emergency department in mid-August after collapsing during a picnic at a local park. She is hypotensive, tachycardic, and diaphoretic with cold extremities. Her oxygen saturation is 85% on room air. Physical examination reveals she is using accessory muscles to breathe. Which of the following is involved in the production of this patient's symptoms?

(A) C3a
(B) Granulocyte macrophage colony-stimulating factor
(C) IgA
(D) Interleukin-3
(E) Membrane attack complex

15. A 25-year-old woman presents to her primary care physician because she has been feeling fatigued. She states the fatigue has been getting progressively worse for the past three months and is not relieved by sleep, although she has been averaging 12-16 hours of sleep per night. She also complains of difficulty concentrating at work, poor appetite, a 4.5-kg (10-lb) weight loss, and reduced interest in socializing with her friends. Physical examination is normal. Laboratory tests reveal a negative Monospot test, normal liver function, and normal thyroid function. Serum iron, ferritin, total iron-binding capacity, vitamin B_{12}, and folate are all within normal limits. The patient is diagnosed with a major depressive episode and given a prescription for an antidepressant. Nortriptyline acts by which of the following mechanisms?

(A) Depleting the adrenergic nerve terminal of norepinephrine
(B) Inhibiting serotonin reuptake and acting as a partial serotonin agonist
(C) Inhibiting the presynaptic enzyme responsible for the breakdown of dopamine, norepinephrine, and serotonin
(D) Inhibiting the reuptake mechanism responsible for terminating the action of both norepinephrine and serotonin
(E) Inhibiting the reuptake mechanism responsible for terminating the action of serotonin only

16. A 13-year-old boy is brought to the physician because of swelling and pain in his right leg. He says he first noticed these symptoms about three months ago, but the pain has gotten much worse over the past few weeks. An x-ray film of the leg shows a large lytic lesion with an onion-skin appearance located midway along the femur. Malignancy is suspected, and a karyotype of the biopsied bone tumor cells is ordered. Which of the following chromosomal translocations would most likely be found in the karyotype of this patient?

(A) t(8;14)
(B) t(9;22)
(C) t(11;14)
(D) t(11;22)
(E) t(21;22)
(F) t(15;17)

17. A 19-year-old woman is brought to the emergency department after losing a substantial amount of blood in a motor vehicle collision. The patient requires large amounts of intravenous fluids, blood replacement, and medications to maintain her blood pressure. On the third day of hospitalization she becomes severely acidotic and has a tense, tender abdomen. Which of the following is most likely the cause of her abdominal pain?

(A) Cecum
(B) Hepatic flexure, large bowel
(C) Ileum
(D) Jejunum
(E) Splenic flexure, large bowel
(F) Stomach

18. The image shows a mutation that can cause hemoglobinopathy. This is an example of which type of mutation?

mRNA transcript of normal gene	UCU UCA CGU
mRNA transcript of mutation	UCU UAA

Reproduced, with permission, from USMLERx.com.

(A) Frameshift mutation
(B) Insertion mutation
(C) Missense mutation
(D) Nonsense mutation
(E) Silent mutation

19. A 35-year-old woman from Arizona comes to the physician with an x-ray film of her chest taken during a routine health insurance examination. The x-ray film shows bilateral hilar adenopathy. The patient is completely asymptomatic. Sarcoidosis is suspected. She was told that her serum levels of angiotensin-converting enzyme (ACE) were elevated. The sensitivity and specificity of using ACE levels to test for the disease in question are 80% and 50%, respectively. Assuming that sarcoidosis is highly prevalent among residents in the southwestern United States, how would the patient's place of residence affect the positive predictive value (PPV) and negative predictive value (NPV) of the test?

(A) In areas of higher prevalence, both the PPV and the NPV are higher
(B) In areas of higher prevalence, both the PPV and the NPV are lower
(C) In areas of higher prevalence, the PPV is higher and the NPV is lower
(D) In areas of higher prevalence, the PPV is lower and the NPV remains the same
(E) Regardless of the prevalence, both the PPV and the NPV are unchanged

20. A lanky 13-year-old boy presents to the emergency department complaining that he "can't see." He has many bruises. He says he is "double-jointed," and to demonstrate, touches his long thumb to his thin wrist. The ophthalmologic examination reveals that both lenses have been dislocated upward and outward. The boy's chest is sunken and he has a heart murmur. Which of the following is most likely deficient in this patient?

(A) Glycosylation of the pro-α chain
(B) Hydroxylation of preprocollagen
(C) Normal synthesis of type I collagen
(D) Synthesis of type III collagen
(E) Transcription of fibrillin

21. A 56-year-old heart transplant recipient presents to the emergency department with shortness of breath and dyspnea at rest. His cardiologist immediately observes that the patient has jugular venous distention and lower extremity edema. However, he eventually lapses into decompensated heart failure and dies. The appearance of his lung at autopsy is shown in the image. Compared to normal lung tissue, what cells are more prominent in this patient's lung?

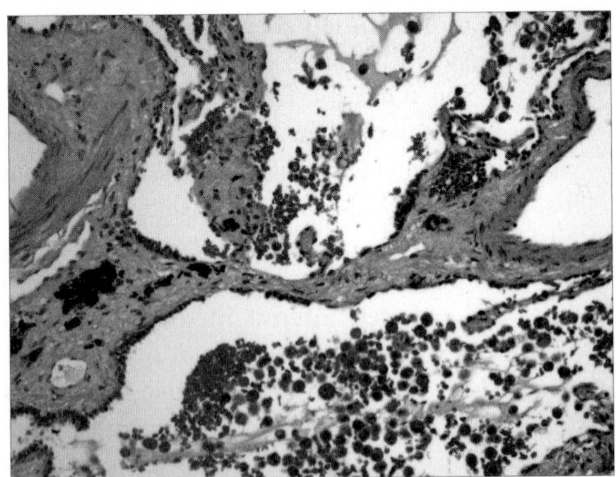

Reproduced, with permission, from USMLERx.com.

(A) Fluid-filled dendritic cells
(B) Hemosiderin-laden macrophages
(C) T-cells
(D) Type I pneumocytes
(E) Type II pneumocytes

22. A 64-year-old man with a history of type 2 diabetes mellitus comes to his primary care physician complaining of sweating, tremors, palpitations, and memory impairment since starting an oral medication to treat his diabetes. His doctor decides to change the patient's oral medication. Which of the following would be the best choice of medication with which to replace his current regimen?

(A) Glargine
(B) Glipizide
(C) Glyburide
(D) Pioglitazone
(E) Ultralente insulin

23. A 6-year-old boy is brought to the pediatrician by his mother, who is very concerned about his health. Physical examination shows an extensive erythematous reticular skin rash on the face trunk, and extremities (see image), along with swelling around his wrists that causes him pain on movement at the joint. He is in no acute distress, but his mother is very anxious. Which of the following is the next best step in treatment for this illness?

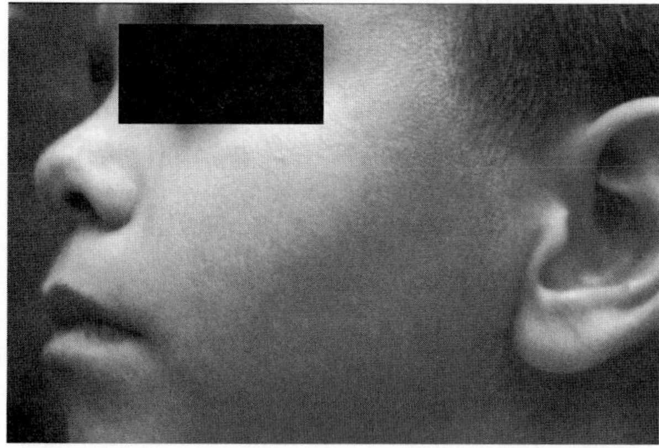

Courtesy of the Centers for Disease Control and Prevention.

(A) No treatment necessary; it is a self-limiting disease
(B) Prescribe a corticosteroid cream
(C) Prescribe an oral corticosteroid
(D) Prescribe the appropriate antibiotic cream
(E) Prescribe the appropriate oral antibiotic

24. A 47-year-old man complains of episodic diaphoresis, palpitations, and headache. These spells have been occurring more frequently and are lasting longer. Physical examination reveals a patient in obvious distress with facial pallor, sweating, tachycardia, and severe hypertension. Urinary and plasma catecholamine and metanephrine levels are increased. MRI of the abdomen reveals a mass. Which of the following is the embryologic origin of the cells that comprise this mass?

(A) Endoderm
(B) Mesoderm
(C) Neural crest
(D) Neuroectoderm
(E) Surface ectoderm

25. A 30-year-old man presents to the emergency department complaining of shortness of breath, dizziness, nausea, and vomiting. He also says that his heart feels "like it is jumping out of my chest." Two days ago, he passed a burning house and stopped to help the residents evacuate. He reports inhaling a significant amount of smoke, but declined medical assistance at the scene because he had no symptoms. The patient reports feeling very fatigued the day prior to presentation and stayed in bed for most of the day. On physical examination, his pulse is 90/min, blood pressure is 100/60 mm Hg, and respiratory rate is 30/min with deep, gasping respirations. The rest of the examination is unremarkable with the exception of bright red vessels in both of his eyes and a smell of bitter almonds on his breath. What is the mechanism of action of the toxic agent that resulted in this patient's symptoms?

(A) Decreased blood oxygen-carrying capacity
(B) Direct tissue injury
(C) Inhibition of cellular respiration
(D) Inhibition of cholinesterase
(E) Ribosome inhibition

26. The human leukocyte antigen complex is a 4-megabase region on chromosome 6 that is densely packed with expressed genes that lead to proteins critical for immunologic specificity and thus autoimmune diseases. Pedigree is shown in the image: Note that the two DR alleles possessed by the proband's grandparents are shown above their pedigree symbols. What combination of alleles that could be inherited by the proband would confer the greatest risk to the patient of contracting type 1diabetes?

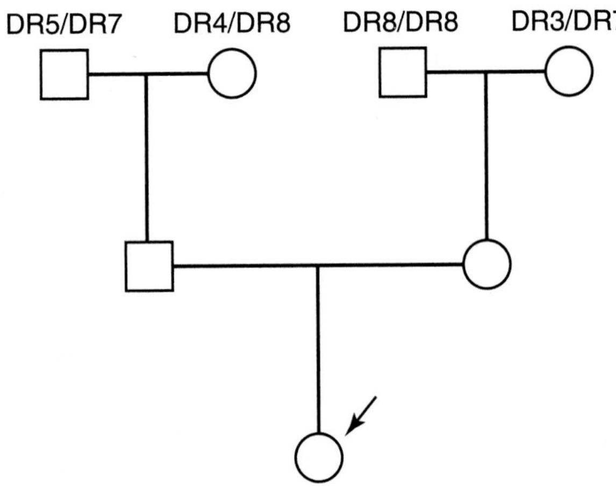

Reproduced, with permission, from USMLERx.com.

(A) DR3/DR3
(B) DR3/DR4
(C) DR5/DR3
(D) DR7/DR3
(E) DR8/DR8

27. A 26-year-old woman and her husband visit the clinic, because they have been trying to conceive for the past 14 months without success. An infertility work-up of the husband shows viable, healthy sperm capable of fertilization. After structural causes are ruled out in the woman, the physician and the couple decide to attempt in vitro fertilization. The physician utilizes a common oral medication to induce ovulation for egg collection and assessment. Which of the following is a common adverse effect of this medication?

(A) Esophagitis
(B) Nausea and vomiting
(C) Ovarian hyperstimulation
(D) Psychosis
(E) Weight gain

28. An intoxicated man is found unresponsive in the woods and is brought to the emergency department. He is found to have animal bite marks on his lower left extremity. He is unable to explain their existence. Which of the following is the most likely recommended, most appropriate next course of action?

(A) Administer human immune globulin immediately, and follow-up with injections of killed virus vaccine only if the patient develops symptoms
(B) Administer human immune globulin immediately, and give a series of five injections of killed virus vaccine
(C) Administer human immune globulin in a series of five doses
(D) Administer killed virus vaccine immediately, and follow-up with injections of human virus vaccine only if the patient develops symptoms
(E) Administer killed virus vaccine immediately, and give a series of five injections of human immune globulin
(F) Do nothing

29. An 82-year-old woman presents to the emergency department with a three-week history of fever, weight loss, and malaise in the setting of hip and shoulder girdle pain that is most severe in the morning. She also reports a one-week history of headaches and left-sided jaw pain that occurs at every meal. The patient's temperature is 38.2°C (100.8°F), her pulse is 104/min, and her blood pressure is 140/80 mm Hg. Laboratory studies show a hemoglobin level of 11.8 g/dL, a WBC count of 11,900/mm^3, and an erythrocyte sedimentation rate of 121 mm/h. Physical examination is unremarkable except for moderate synovitis of the ankles and wrist. Which of the following procedures is most likely to be diagnostic in this patient?

(A) Arthrocentesis
(B) Mesenteric angiogram

(C) Temporal artery biopsy
(D) Testing for anti-double-stranded DNA and antinuclear antibody levels
(E) Testing for rheumatoid factor and anti-cytidine cyclic phosphate levels

30. A 45-year-old man presents to his primary care physician with a blood pressure of 160/90 mm Hg that has failed to drop substantially after initiation of lifestyle changes. The patient is subsequently placed on a low dose of hydrochlorothiazide, which lowers his blood pressure to 128/86 mm Hg. Which of the following accurately represents the site of action of hydrochlorothiazide?

(A) Chloride-binding sites on the cytoplasmic surface of the early distal tubule
(B) Chloride-binding sites on the luminal surface of the early distal tubule
(C) Chloride-binding sites on the luminal surface of the thick ascending limb of the loop of Henle
(D) Sodium binding sites on the basolateral membrane of the thick ascending limb of the loop of Henle
(E) Sodium-binding sites on the luminal surface of the early distal tubule

31. The micrograph shown in the image was obtained from cerebrospinal fluid that demonstrated lymphocytosis, decreased glucose, and increased protein. Which of the following organisms is most likely responsible for the patient's symptoms?

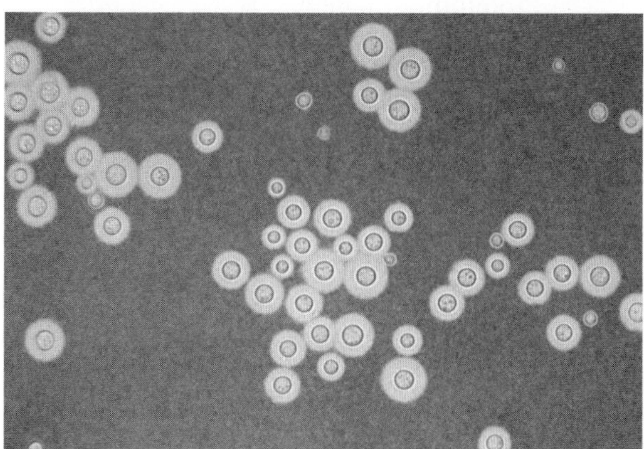

Courtesy of Dr. Leanor Haley, Centers for Disease Control and Prevention.

(A) *Aspergillus*
(B) *Cryptococcus*
(C) Echovirus
(D) *Haemophilus*
(E) *Neisseria*
(F) *Toxoplasma*
(G) *Treponema*

32. Oxygen unloading is increased when hemoglobin passes through active tissues. Which of the following is one reason for this phenomenon?

(A) Decreased temperature in the peripheral tissues shifts the hemoglobin dissociation curve to the left
(B) Decreased temperature in the peripheral tissues shifts the hemoglobin dissociation curve to the right
(C) Increased CO_2 and H^+ in the tissues shift the hemoglobin dissociation curve to the left
(D) Increased CO_2 and increased diphosphoglycerate shift the hemoglobin dissociation curve to the left
(E) Increased CO_2 and H^+ in the tissues shift the hemoglobin dissociation curve to the right

33. A 59-year-old man presents to the emergency department after waking up in the middle of the night with a very severe headache. When asked about the intensity of pain, the patient exclaims, "I feel like my head is going to explode." Emergent CT of the head demonstrates blood tracking down the sulci and following the contours of the pia. What is the most likely underlying pathophysiologic mechanism for this patient's condition?

(A) Arteriovenous malformation
(B) Atherosclerosis
(C) Cerebral contusion
(D) Hypertension
(E) Rupture of arterial aneurysm

34. A 39-year-old man was seen by a psychiatrist after reports that he had been locking himself in his apartment because "the devil is trying to put thoughts into my head." After three weeks of pharmacologic treatment, he begins to experience muscular rigidity, decreased perspiration, hyperthermia, and signs of autonomic instability. Which of the following drugs should be administered to the patient immediately?

(A) Dantrolene
(B) Diazepam
(C) Flumazenil
(D) Haloperidol
(E) Phenobarbital

35. The mother of a 3-year-old boy is referred to genetic counseling after her son is diagnosed with an enzyme deficiency. Recently, the mother noticed that her son has an abnormal facial appearance as well as pearly papular skin lesions over the scapulae and on the lateral upper arms and thighs, however, his corneas are clear bilaterally. She has also noticed that her son is hyperactive compared to other children of the same age. This patient carries a diagnosis of which of the following syndromes?

(A) Hunter syndrome
(B) Hurler syndrome
(C) Morquio syndrome
(D) Sanfilippo syndrome
(E) Sly syndrome

36. A 31-year-old man comes to the physician with a five-day history of shortness of breath. The patient says that he also has had a nonproductive cough in the same time period. X-ray film of the chest reveals bilateral diffuse infiltrates, and laboratory results show a WBC count of 2500/mm³. An enzyme-linked immunosorbent assay is positive for HIV infection, and methenamine silver stain shows the causative organism. The patient is started on sulfamethoxazole-trimethoprim. Which of the following is the mechanism of action of the antibiotic used to treat this patient's infection?

(A) Blockade of ergosterol synthesis
(B) Blockade of the pathway that utilizes pteridine and PABA in nucleotide formation
(C) Cell wall synthesis
(D) Inhibition of the 30S ribosomal subunit
(E) Inhibition of the 50S ribosomal subunit

37. A 30-year-old male drug user with a history of methylphenyltetrahydropyridine (MPTP) exposure presents to the clinic with a tremor at rest, cogwheel rigidity, and postural instability. Direct innervation from the site of the lesion to which nuclei has been damaged?

(A) Caudate and putamen (striatum)
(B) Globus pallidus externus
(C) Globus pallidus internus
(D) Lateral geniculate nucleus
(E) Subthalamic nucleus

38. A 25-year-old construction worker presents to his primary care physician complaining of abdominal pain and constipation. The pain is diffuse, and is neither better nor worse following a meal. He also reports fatigue and difficulty concentrating. His vital signs are within normal limits. His examination is remarkable only for darkened, painless gingival lesions, and a non-distended but tender abdomen. Which of the following is the most appropriate medical treatment for this patient?

(A) Deferoxamine
(B) Dimercaprol
(C) N-acetylcysteine
(D) Naloxone
(E) Protamine sulfate
(F) Thiosulfate

39. A 9-year-old boy with type 1 diabetes mellitus is brought to the emergency department because he has become delirious in the past hour. Earlier this afternoon, after his usual dose of insulin, the patient began complaining of abdominal pain and shortly thereafter he vomited. On further questioning his father says the boy has had a cough and fever for the past couple days. Blood is drawn for laboratory

studies, and the patient is immediately started on fluids with added potassium. Which of the following sets of laboratory parameters is most likely to be seen in this patient?

Choice	pH	Sodium	Potassium	Bicarbonate
A	↓	↓	↓	↓
B	↓	↓	↑	↓
C	↓	↑	↓	↓
D	↓	↑	↑	↑
E	↑	↑	↓	↓

Reproduced, with permission, from USMLERx.com.

(A) A
(B) B
(C) C
(D) D
(E) E

40. A 32-year-old man presents with a three-month history of arthralgias, weight loss, diarrhea with fatty stools, and abdominal pain. After careful observation and testing, his physician obtains a biopsy of the lamina propria of the small intestine, which shows periodic acid-Schiff-positive material, particularly in macrophages. What is the cause of this man's symptoms?

(A) Celiac sprue
(B) Crohn disease
(C) MALT lymphoma
(D) Ulcerative colitis
(E) Whipple disease

41. A pregnant woman comes to the physician for a check-up before the beginning of her third trimester. It is learned that she has been exposed to an infectious disease. Fortunately, the infectious disease caused no morbidity to the fetus, and the resulting pregnancy is uncomplicated. The woman later gives birth to a healthy child. To which of the following pathogens was the woman most likely exposed?

(A) Cytomegalovirus
(B) Epstein-Barr virus
(C) Herpes simplex virus
(D) HIV
(E) Rubella
(F) Syphilis
(G) Toxoplasmosis

42. A 67-year-old man with a history of prostate cancer presents for follow-up after surgical management. He has been having back pain that has awakened him at night for the past two months, and that responds poorly to ibuprofen. On x-ray, a significant lesion is found in the L2 vertebral body. A bone biopsy is obtained and reveals poorly differentiated cells with some resemblance to prostatic cells. The overexpression of what factor could allow the neoplastic cells to metastasize?

(A) γ-Glutamyl transpeptidase
(B) CD44
(C) Collagenase
(D) E-cadherin
(E) Keratin

43. A 41-year-old man comes to the physician complaining of crampy, bloating abdominal discomfort. He also reports changes in his bowel habits and recently noticed dark stool. His father, sister, and uncle died of colorectal cancer. At the physician's office, a fecal occult blood test is positive. Colonoscopy reveals 8-10 small flat polyps in the proximal colon. Which of the following is the most likely cause of these findings?

(A) A defect in mismatch repair
(B) A defect in nucleotide excision repair
(C) A translocation between chromosomes 15 and 17
(D) Exposure to benzo(a)pyrene
(E) The *bcr-abl* hybrid gene

44. A 75-year-old man comes to the physician because he recently began experiencing seizures. CT of the head shows an irregular, ring-enhancing lesion with central necrosis in his right cerebral hemisphere. Results of biopsy are shown in the image. Which of the following is the most likely diagnosis?

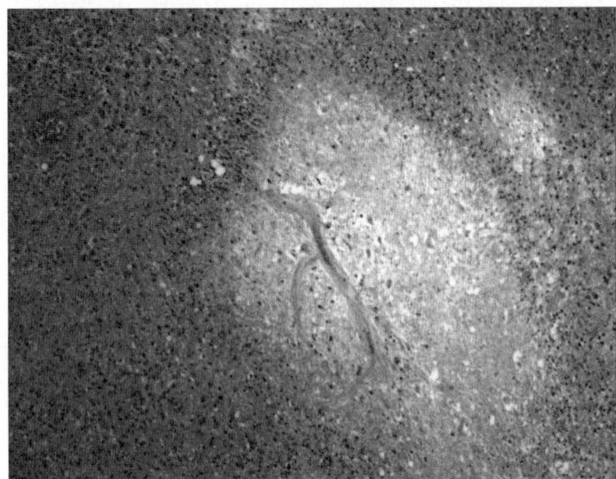

Reproduced, with permission, from USMLERx.com.

(A) Glioblastoma multiforme
(B) Medulloblastoma
(C) Meningioma
(D) Neurilemmoma
(E) Oligodendroglioma

45. A 19-year-old college student developed sore throat, palatal petechiae, splenomegaly, fever, and generalized lymphadenopathy after she began dating her first serious boyfriend. The symptoms were self-limiting and lasted approximately two-three weeks. Upon presentation at the campus health clinic, a blood sample tests positive for heterophil antibodies and she is diagnosed with symptomatic primary Epstein-Barr virus (EBV) infection. Which of the following innate immune cell types plays a direct and important role in controlling the early stages of the systemic response to EBV infection?

(A) Eosinophils
(B) Mast cells
(C) Megakaryocytes
(D) Microglia
(E) Natural killer cells
(F) Plasma cells
(G) Regulatory T lymphocytes

46. A 4-month-old girl who was born full-term presents to her pediatrician with an upper respiratory infection. Her mother notes that this is the fifth time her daughter has had an upper respiratory infection since birth. Her past medical history is significant for seizures shortly after birth. In addition to pulmonary findings, the physical examination is notable for oropharyngeal candidiasis that the patient's mother says has been occurring regularly. This child is presenting with a syndrome that is due to aberrant development of which of the following embryonic structures?

(A) First and second branchial arches
(B) First and second branchial pouches
(C) Fourth and sixth branchial arches
(D) Second and third branchial clefts
(E) Third and fourth branchial pouches

47. A 91-year-old man is brought to the emergency department by his daughter after being found unresponsive in his home. The patient's oral temperature is 39.8°C (103.6°F), blood pressure is 80/50 mm Hg, heart rate is 120/min, and respiratory rate is 26/min. Initial laboratory tests reveal leukocytosis and elevated lactate levels. The patient's blood pressure remains at 80/50 mm Hg despite adequate hydration. What is the expected hemodynamic pattern in this patient in terms of peripheral vascular resistance, cardiac output, and pulmonary capillary wedge pressure?

Choice	Peripheral vascular resistance	Cardiac output	Pulmonary capillary wedge pressure
A	↓	↓	↓
B	↓	↑	↓
C	↑	↓	↓
D	↑	↓	↑
E	↑	↑	↑

Reproduced, with permission, from USMLERx.com.

(A) A
(B) B
(C) C
(D) D
(E) E

48. A 67-year-old man presents to the emergency department with diaphoresis and crushing chest pain that radiates down his left arm. ECG shows ST-segment elevations and inverted T waves in leads II, III, and aVF. His troponin I level is high. He is taken to the cardiac catheterization unit, where he is diagnosed with an obstructive myocardial infarction due to occlusion of the right coronary artery. Assuming this man's coronary vasculature is right dominant, which of the following areas is most likely to be spared after this event?

(A) Anterior interventricular septum
(B) Atrioventricular node
(C) Posterior interventricular septum
(D) Right ventricle
(E) Sinoatrial node

ANSWERS

1. **The correct answer is B.** This patient's symptoms are consistent with those of a duodenal ulcer. A duodenal ulcer can be caused by hypersecretion of stomach acid, *Helicobacter pylori* infection, or the use of nonsteroidal anti-inflammatory drugs. Initial treatment of a duodenal ulcer involves a trial of a histamine$_2$ (H$_2$)-blocker such as cimetidine or a proton pump inhibitor such as omeprazole. Activation of H$_2$-receptors leads to increased gastric acid production. By inhibiting the H$_2$-receptor, gastric acid secretion is decreased, allowing the ulcer to heal. If a biopsy of the ulcer is positive for *H pylori*, appropriate treatment involves "triple therapy," commonly involving clarithromycin 500 mg twice a day, amoxicillin 1 g twice a day, and a proton pump inhibitor twice a day for 10-14 days.

   Answer A is incorrect. Gastrin is a gastrointestinal (GI) hormone secreted by the G cells of the stomach in response to small peptides and amino acids in the gut, stomach distention, and vagal stimulation. Gastrin causes an increase in gastric acid secretion, and whereas blockade of gastrin receptors (cholecystokinin B) would decrease gastric acid production slightly, alternative receptors would continue to stimulate gastric acid secretion.

   Answer C is incorrect. Acetylcholine is released by cholinergic neurons in the enteric nervous system, resulting in contraction of smooth muscle, relaxation of sphincters, increase in gastric secretion, and increase in pancreatic secretion. Blockade of the muscarinic$_3$-receptor would not lead to a significant decrease in acid production, which is necessary for this patient.

   Answer D is incorrect. Norepinephrine is released from adrenergic neurons in the enteric nervous system, resulting in relaxation of smooth muscle, contraction of sphincters, and increase in salivary secretion.

   Answer E is incorrect. Secretin is a GI hormone secreted by the S cells of the duodenum in response to acidification of the duodenum and the presence of fatty acids and bile in the duodenum. Secretin increases pancreatic and biliary bicarbonate secretion, and decreases gastric acid secretion. Blockade of secretin receptors potentially could increase the amount of acid produced as a result of loss of feedback inhibition.

2. **The correct answer is D.** Medial longitudinal fasciculus (MLF) syndrome (also known as internuclear ophthalmoplegia) is characteristic of multiple sclerosis (MS), from which this patient likely suffers. Normally, the right MLF connects the left nucleus of cranial nerve (CN) VI with the right subnucleus of CN III. Consequently, with left lateral gaze, the left nucleus of CN VI sends a signal via the right MLF to the right subnucleus of CN III, which stimulates contraction of the right medial rectus, preserving conjugate gaze. In MS, demyelination of the right MLF would prevent normal signal transmission, leading to a palsy of the right medial rectus with attempted left lateral gaze (horizontal nystagmus of the left eye will also likely be observed).

   Answer A is incorrect. Patients with MS who have lesions affecting either one or both of the medial longitudinal fasciculus tracts will have disconjugate gaze with attempted lateral gaze.

   Answer B is incorrect. Left lateral gaze requires contraction of the left lateral rectus, not the left medial rectus. To assess the function of the left medial rectus, the examiner should instruct the patient to attempt right lateral gaze.

   Answer C is incorrect. Palsy of the left medial rectus with attempted right lateral gaze would result from a lesion affecting the left medial longitudinal fasciculus.

   Answer E is incorrect. Right lateral gaze requires contraction of the right lateral rectus, not the right medial rectus. To assess the function of the right medial rectus, the examiner should instruct the patient to attempt left lateral gaze.

3. **The correct answer is C.** Based on the physical exam findings, the patient is likely experiencing congestive heart failure. Given his young age and lack of risk factors, a myocarditis should be high on the differential. Half of all viral cases of myocarditis are caused by coxsackie B. Coxsackie B, an icosahedral member of the Picornaviridae family, can cause a variety of illnesses, including meningitis, respiratory infections, and epidemic pleurodynia. However, it is important to note that while coxsackievirus is the most common cause, there are many different agents that can cause myocarditis, including other viruses (eg, adenovirus, HIV), bacteria (eg, *Haemophilus influenzae*, *Mycoplasma pneumoniae*, streptococcal infections), and protozoa (*Toxoplasma* and *Trypanosoma cruzi*).

   Answer A is incorrect. Adenoidal-pharyngeal-conjunctival viruses, also known as adenoviruses, can cause acute upper respiratory diseases, conjunctivitis, gastroenteritis, and hemorrhagic cystitis. While in rare cases it can be associated with infections of the heart, it is not the most common cause of myocarditis.

   Answer B is incorrect. *Brugia malayi* is a filarial worm that infects the lymphatics and subcutaneous tissues. It can cause lymphadenopathy, lymphatic destruction, and subsequent edema. Infection with this worm would not, however, explain the S_3 gallop.

   Answer D is incorrect. *Haemophilus influenzae* type B is a rod-shaped gram-negative bacterium that is responsible for respiratory infections and meningitis in childhood. It is currently recommended that all children receive the Hib vaccine, which is effective against this strain of bacteria. While it can be associated with infections of the heart, it is (1) not the most common cause of myocarditis, and (2) a bacterium, which would therefore respond to antibiotics.

   Answer E is incorrect. *Streptococcus pneumoniae* is a gram-positive diplococcus and the most common cause of lobar pneumonia worldwide. While it can be associated with infections of the heart, it is (1) not the most common cause of myocarditis, and (2) a bacterium, which would therefore respond to antibiotics.

   Answer F is incorrect. *Wuchereria bancrofti* is a filarial worm that produces symptoms similar to those of *Brugia malayi*. However, of all of the filariae, *W bancrofti* causes the overwhelming majority of genital lymphatic involvement.

4. **The correct answer is C.** This neonate is suffering from neonatal respiratory distress syndrome (NRDS) caused by a lack of surfactant. Surfactant is formed relatively late in fetal life (begins at 28 weeks and is produced most abundantly at 34 weeks). It reduces surface tension by disrupting the intermolecular forces (hydrogen bonds) between molecules of water. This prevents small alveoli from collapsing and increases compliance. Synthesis of surfactant is decreased by insulin. Thus, maternal diabetes is also a risk factor for RDS in infants, because fetal hyperglycemia stimulates an increased release of insulin. Cortisol increases synthesis of surfactant; therefore, women who have to deliver their babies prematurely typically receive glucocorticoids to help prevent RDS in their infants.

   Answer A is incorrect. Surfactant consists primarily of dipalmitoyl phosphatidylcholine (lecithin), the main lipid component, not sphingomyelin.

   Answer B is incorrect. Surfactant prevents small alveoli from collapsing by decreasing alveolar surface tension. The compliance in small alveoli is increased (not decreased), allowing the lung to inflate more easily and decreasing the work of breathing.

   Answer D is incorrect. Surfactant is a lipoprotein consisting of both a hydrophobic and hydrophilic region. It reduces alveolar surface tension by adsorbing to the air-water interface—the hydrophilic portion interfering with the hydrogen bonds between molecules of water and the hydrophilic portion facing the air. Decreasing surface tension prevents small alveoli from collapsing.

Answer E is incorrect. Type II pneumocytes secrete pulmonary surfactant and serve as precursors to both type I and type II pneumocytes. Type I pneumocytes make up 97% of the alveolar surface and are thin, squamous cells optimal for gas diffusion.

Answer F is incorrect. Surfactant lines alveoli, not larger airways.

5. **The correct answer is D.** Glucose-6-phosphate dehydrogenase (G6PD) deficiency is an X-linked recessive disorder that is particularly common in African-American males. Individuals of Mediterranean heritage are also affected. G6PD is the first enzyme in the pentose phosphate pathway, and it reduces oxidized nicotinamide adenine dinucelotide phosphate to reduced nicotinamide adenine dinucelotide phosphate (NADPH) as it oxidizes glucose-6-phosphate. NADPH is a necessary cofactor for the enzyme glutathione reductase, which generates reduced glutathione. Reduced glutathione, in turn, can reduce peroxides into less harmful substances such as water and alcohol. A deficiency of G6PD makes erythrocytes more susceptible to oxidative stress, resulting in a hemolytic anemia that can be triggered by antibiotics such as sulfa drugs or bacterial infections. Heinz bodies are a hallmark of G6PD deficiency; they represent accumulations of denatured hemoglobin in affected red blood cells.

   Answer A is incorrect. α-thalassemia is caused by a defect in one or more of the four α-globin chains of hemoglobin. Symptoms range in severity from silent carriers who have no detectable changes on a complete blood count to in utero fatalities. However, these are typically constant conditions that are not precipitated by infection or medications.

   Answer B is incorrect. Blood donation would not be expected to cause anemia in a healthy individual, and there is no reason to believe that this patient has recently donated blood.

   Answer C is incorrect. Folic acid deficiency can result in a megaloblastic anemia. This type of deficiency is often seen in alcoholics or individuals with poor nutrition, neither of which is present in this patient.

   Answer E is incorrect. Intrinsic factor (IF) deficiency causes pernicious anemia. IF is synthesized in the stomach, and a deficiency results from destruction of those cells. However, there is no reason to believe that this patient has suffered from any autoimmune attack on gastric cells. Pernicious anemia also causes a megaloblastic anemia, not seen here.

   Answer F is incorrect. Iron deficiency anemia is one of the most common causes of anemia but is not likely in this patient given the presentation. It is typically observed in menstruating women.

   Answer G is incorrect. Sickle cell disease is the result of a point mutation in the β-globin chain of hemoglobin. Symptoms typically present in childhood as severe joint pain with exertion and do not resemble the presentation of this patient.

6. **The correct answer is C.** Hantavirus pulmonary syndrome is a rare viral cause of acute respiratory distress syndrome (ARDS). Hantavirus is a Bunyavirus that has been found in rodents throughout the United States. It is thought to be transmitted via rodent droppings and saliva.

   Answer A is incorrect. Dengue virus is an *Aedes* mosquito-transmitted virus that causes a hemorrhagic fever. It is found in tropical regions of Asia and has spread to South and Central America. Patients present with rash and bleeding from mucous membranes.

   Answer B is incorrect. Ebola virus and Marburg virus are members of the *Filovirus* genus, which cause hemorrhagic fever. Both are found only in central and southern Africa. They have an animal reservoir that has not been found. Treatment is supportive, and symptoms include massive hemorrhage from the mucous membranes accompanied by high fevers.

   Answer D is incorrect. Ebola virus and Marburg virus are members of the *Filovirus* genus, which cause hemorrhagic fever. Both are found only in central and southern Africa. They have an animal reservoir that has not been found. Treatment is supportive, and symptoms include massive hemorrhage from the mucous membranes accompanied by high fevers.

Answer E is incorrect. Rhabdovirus is the causative agent of rabies. It is possible to become infected with rabies from a rodent; however, the incubation period is much longer (weeks to a year), and the later stages of the disease are classically acute encephalitis.

7. **The correct answer is A.** This is a case of Burkitt lymphoma. Burkitt lymphoma is associated with Epstein-Barr virus infection, resulting in a t(8;14) translocation. This frequently involves the mandible as well as the kidneys, ovaries, and adrenals. Histology typically demonstrates a characteristic "starry-sky" pattern; this pattern is produced by macrophages, which ingest tumor cells, producing light spots against a background of highly mitotic basophilic lymphoma cells. Burkitt lymphoma is among the most common cancers in Africa.

   Answer B is incorrect. Chronic myelogenous leukemia (CML) is characterized by a markedly elevated WBC count, fatigue, night sweats, low-grade fever, abdominal fullness secondary to splenomegaly, and sternal tenderness. CML is associated with the Philadelphia chromosome, t(9;22).

   Answer C is incorrect. The most common presentation of Hodgkin lymphoma includes constitutional symptoms including night sweats, fever, or weight loss, and mediastinal lymphadenopathy. Biopsy of the nodes demonstrates the characteristic Reed-Sternberg cells with reactive lymphocytes, which are large and bi-nucleate with a prominent nucleolus, giving the cell its "owl-eye" appearance. B cells associated with Hodgkin lymphoma may express the T-cell marker interleukin-21.

   Answer D is incorrect. Acute lymphoblastic lymphoma typically presents with circulating lymphoid blasts (leukemic phase) and a mediastinal mass. The symptoms include rapid-onset bone marrow suppression resulting in anemia, neutropenia, and thrombocytopenia. This condition is frequently diagnosed in children. Lymphoma cells typically are positive for immature B-cell marker terminal deoxynucleotidyl transferase.

   Answer E is incorrect. The symptoms of mumps virus include a prodromal stage of fever, malaise, and anorexia followed by tender swelling of the parotid glands that typically resolves within one week. Although this patient has a lesion on his mandible that is suggestive of parotitis, his symptoms of fatigue and malaise have lasted for six months, which is longer than the typical clinical course of mumps. Two clinically significant complications of mumps virus include orchitis and aseptic meningitis. Furthermore the histologic characterization of the tumor makes mumps virus less likely.

8. **The correct answer is B.** Epinephrine is an agonist at α_1, α_2, β_1, and β_2 receptors; phentolamine is an antagonist at α_1 and α_2 receptors. Therefore, after the administration of phentolamine, epinephrine administration stimulates only β receptors, which results in decreased blood pressure. This is called epinephrine reversal because epinephrine originally increased blood pressure and then produced the opposite effect after phentolamine administration.

   Answer A is incorrect. Acetylcholine stimulates the non-innervated muscarinic (M_3) receptors that are located on endothelial cells of the vasculature. Stimulation of these receptors releases endothelial-derived relaxing factor (nitric oxide), which produces a relaxation of the neighboring smooth muscle cells, leading to a decrease in blood pressure. Neostigmine, an acetylcholinesterase inhibitor, would simply prolong the action of acetylcholine at its receptors and would thus indirectly cause a decrease in blood pressure.

   Answer C is incorrect. Isoproterenol, a nonspecific β-agonist, decreases blood pressure by stimulation of β_2 receptors in the vasculature. Epinephrine, norepinephrine, and phenylephrine all increase blood pressure, so the remaining answers must be eliminated by examining the effects of drug Y on drug X.

Answer D is incorrect. Norepinephrine is an agonist at α_1, α_2, and β_1 receptors; propranolol is a nonselective β-antagonist. After administration of propranolol, norepinephrine can stimulate only α receptors, which will still cause vasoconstriction (primarily via α_1 stimulation in the vasculature) and therefore increase blood pressure.

Answer E is incorrect. Phenylephrine is an α_1 agonist, and hexamethonium is a nicotinic ganglionic blocker. Hexamethonium administration will eliminate the baroreceptor response after the second phenylephrine administration by blocking the peripheral ganglia. However, phenylephrine will still reach the α_1 receptors on the vasculature to produce an increase in blood pressure.

9. **The correct answer is A.** This patient is suffering from a cord compression syndrome due to a conus medullaris tumor. These tumors are relatively uncommon and can be very difficult to diagnose because they are difficult to differentiate from tumors of the cauda equina. Patients can manifest symptoms of one or both syndromes. Night and rest pain is an immediate red flag for metastatic disease, multiple myeloma, or spinal infections. The x-ray films and normal laboratory values help to make metastatic disease or myeloma less likely. The examination is consistent with conus medullaris syndrome because of the relatively rapid, bilateral onset of moderate back pain with a minimal radicular component and preserved ankle reflexes. These patients tend to have perianal numbness and urinary retention with an atonic rectal sphincter, as opposed to the saddle anesthesia more typically found in cauda equina syndrome. This patient's presentation warrants empiric steroids and emergent MRI.

Answer B is incorrect. Guillain-Barré syndrome is a symmetrical ascending weakness that commonly follows diarrheal or flu-like illness in young adults. It is not associated with focal neurological pain and is much less common in elderly patients.

Answer C is incorrect. The physical examination largely excludes the possibility of disc herniation as a cause of the patient's symptoms because of absent positive straight leg raises and pain that is neither aggravated by activity nor relieved by resting. Furthermore, the perianal region is innervated by sacral nerve roots that would not be impinged by a disc herniation at the L4-5 level.

Answer D is incorrect. The triad for spinal epidural abscess includes back pain, fever, and progressive weakness. This patient does not have the second two symptoms, making abscess a less likely possibility.

Answer E is incorrect. Vertebral osteomyelitis would most likely present in a patient that was suffering constitutional signs and symptoms, as opposed to the relatively focal findings presented in this case. Characteristically, a patient with osteomyelitis would have night sweats and fever. The patient would have symptoms that would point to the source of the hematogenous dissemination of the infectious agent to the spine (eg, urinary tract infection).

10. **The correct answer is B.** Turner syndrome is a chromosomal abnormality that results from the loss of all or part of one of the two X chromosomes (the absence of one set of genes from the short arm of one X chromosome) in a female fetus. This patient has the characteristic short stature and webbed neck often seen in Turner patients. Other clinical manifestations of Turner syndrome include a flat, shield-like chest (with widely spaced nipples), wide carrying angle at the elbows, and congenital lymphedema of hands and feet in neonates. Patients with Turner syndrome have a higher risk of cardiac abnormalities than their peers, the most common being coarctation of the aorta. Classically the coarctation is preductal, and can result in a small left arm due to compromised blood flow if the left subclavian artery is involved.

Answer A is incorrect. A postductal coarctation is not commonly found in patients with Turner syndrome. Furthermore, we would not expect a small left arm in a patient with a postductal coarctation because the left subclavian artery must be intact.

Answer C is incorrect. Subclavian steal syndrome refers to retrograde flow in a vertebral artery due to a stenosed subclavian artery associated with neurologic symptoms. This is not more common in patients with Turner syndrome than in their peers.

Answer D is incorrect. Patients with Turner syndrome do not have a higher incidence of tetralogy of Fallot than their peers.

Answer E is incorrect. Patients with Turner syndrome do not have a higher incidence of transposition of the great vessels than their peers.

11. **The correct answer is B.** Vitamin K-dependent γ-glutamyl carboxylase converts glutamic acid residues to γ-carboxyglutamic acid (GLA) residues on clotting factors II, VII, IX, and X, as well as proteins C and S. GLA residues function to bind calcium, which is required to activate the factors. Vitamin K deficiency is rare because it is synthesized by gut flora. This patient's deficiency is probably secondary to elimination of these organisms by oral antibiotics. This deficiency is also seen in neonates who have sterile guts and a relatively new liver. Easy bruising, melena, hematuria, and splinter hemorrhages can be seen with vitamin K deficiency.

    Answer A is incorrect. Activation of antithrombin III is the function of heparin, which inhibits serine proteases of the clotting cascade.

    Answer C is incorrect. The cross-linking of fibrin polymers is the function of factor XIIIa, which is activated by thrombin in the clotting cascade. This cross-linking functions to solidify the clot after the convergence of the intrinsic and extrinsic clotting cascades. Thrombin functions both to convert fibrinogen to fibrin and to activate factor XIIIa.

    Answer D is incorrect. The hydrolyzation of fibrinogen to form fibrin is the function of active thrombin, a serine protease in the clotting cascade. Thrombin also functions to activate factor XIIIa, which cross-links fibrin polymers and solidifies the clot.

    Answer E is incorrect. The hydroxylation of proline and lysine residues requires the coenzyme ascorbic acid, or vitamin C. Deficiency of vitamin C results in scurvy, a defective connective tissue syndrome that results in swollen gums, bruising, anemia, and poor wound healing. Vitamin C is a water-soluble vitamin; oral antibiotic use does not lead to its deficiency.

12. **The correct answer is C.** The potency of inhaled anesthetics is quantified as the minimum alveolar concentration (MAC). This is the concentration of inhaled gas that is needed to eliminate movement in 50% of patients who are challenged by surgical incision. For potent anesthetics, the MAC will be numerically small, meaning that it is inversely proportional to the anesthetic's potency. Drug C, which has the smallest MAC value, is thus the most potent. The blood solubility of an anesthetic is the physical property that determines both the speed of induction and time to recovery. Drugs with low blood solubility, such as nitrous oxide, will rapidly induce anesthesia, and patients will recover quickly. In contrast, an anesthetic gas with high blood solubility, such as halothane, will have a longer time to induction and a slower time to recovery. Therefore, drug C, which has the lowest blood solubility, will have the most rapid induction.

    Answer A is incorrect. The MAC for a drug is inversely related to its potency. Drug A has a larger MAC than drug D and will be less potent than drug D.

    Answer B is incorrect. Drug B, with a solubility of 1.0 (100% soluble in blood), will dissolve completely in the bloodstream, whereas drug C, with its solubility value of 0.1, will be only 10% dissolved in blood. Drug B is more soluble than Drug C.

    Answer D is incorrect. An anesthetic with greater blood solubility will have a slower induction time. Drug D, which is more soluble in blood than drug C, will therefore induce anesthesia less rapidly than drug C.

Answer E is incorrect. Recovery time from anesthesia is based on the blood solubility of a gas. Gases with high blood solubility result in slower recovery when compared with drugs that have lower blood solubility. Drug B has the highest blood solubility of all those that are listed and thus will have the slowest recovery time of all.

13. **The correct answer is B.** This patient most likely suffers from peptic ulcer disease caused by *Helicobacter pylori*, a bacterium that causes 70% of gastric ulcers and up to 90% of duodenal ulcers. Those from certain ethnic groups often have a higher rate of *H pylori* infection, especially if they grew up in areas with poor sanitation. Peptic ulcer disease typically presents with burning substernal epigastric pain. In the case of gastric ulcers, the pain increases after meals; for duodenal ulcers, the pain improves after eating. Infection with *H pylori* can be diagnosed with a urease breath test (*H pylori* contains the enzyme urease that cleaves urea to ammonia), or with biopsy that, on silver staining, demonstrates a spiral-shaped flagellated organism adherent to the mucosal epithelium. Treatment of *H pylori* involves therapy consisting of bismuth, metronidazole, omeprazole, and either tetracycline or amoxicillin; or metronidazole in combination with omeprazole and clarithromycin.

Answer A is incorrect. Ampicillin is an aminopenicillin antimicrobial with a wider spectrum than penicillin. It is penicillinase-sensitive but is often combined with clavulanic acid to enhance its spectrum. It is used to treat certain gram-positive and gram-negative infections, including *Haemophilus influenzae*, *Escherichia coli*, *Listeria*, *Proteus*, *Salmonella*, *enterococci*, and *Shigella*, but is not effective against *H pylori*. Clindamycin is a bacteriostatic antimicrobial that acts by blocking peptide bond formation at the 50S ribosomal subunit. It is used to treat anaerobic infections, including *Bacteroides fragilis* and *Clostridium perfringens*. It is not used in the treatment of *H pylori*.

Answer C is incorrect. Imipenem is a broad-spectrum, β-lactamase-resistant carbapenem. It is always administered with cilastatin, an inhibitor of the renal enzyme dihydropeptidase-I that otherwise inactivates imipenem in the renal tubules. Given its broad activity, imipenem is used clinically to treat infections caused by gram-positive cocci, gram-negative rods, and anaerobes. It is also the drug of choice for treatment of *Enterobacter* infection. It is not used in the treatment of *H pylori*.

Answer D is incorrect. Ranitidine is a histamine$_2$ blocker that decreases acid production and is used in the treatment of gastroesophageal reflux disease, peptic ulcers, and gastritis. Omeprazole is a proton pump inhibitor that decreases acid production and is used in the treatment of peptic ulcer disease, gastritis, esophageal reflux, and Zollinger-Ellison syndrome. Bismuth binds to the base of a gastric ulcer to provide physical protection to the gastric mucosa; it also allows bicarbonate secretion in order to re-establish the pH gradient in the mucous layer and stimulate ulcer healing. None of these medications effectively eradicates *H pylori*.

Answer E is incorrect. Vancomycin is an antimicrobial that acts by inhibiting cell wall mucopeptide formation by binding the D-alanyl-D-alanine portion of cell wall precursors. It is used for serious, gram-positive multidrug-resistant organisms, including *Staphylococcus aureus* and *Clostridium difficile*. It is not used in the treatment of *H pylori*. Gentamicin belongs to the antimicrobial family of aminoglycosides, which are bactericidal and act by inhibiting the formation of the initiation complex and causing misreading of mRNA. They require oxygen for uptake and are therefore ineffective against anaerobes. They are used to treat severe gram-negative rod infections, but are not used in the treatment of *H pylori*. Aztreonam is a monobactam antimicrobial that is resistant to β lactamases. It acts by inhibiting cell wall synthesis and is used clinically to treat gram-negative-rod infections. However, it is not used in the treatment of *H pylori*.

14. **The correct answer is A.** The clinical picture of hypotension (cold, clammy extremities, tachycardia, and hypotensive syncope) and respiratory compromise (hypoxia and use of ac-

cessory muscles to breathe) indicates that this woman is likely in anaphylactic shock. Given the setting of a picnic, the venom from a bee sting may have triggered the reaction. Anaphylactic shock may be mediated by binding of C3a and C5a to IgE, causing histamine release. C3 is converted to C3a and C3b by one of two C3 convertases. Similarly, C5 is converted to C5a and C5b by one of two C5 convertases. Both C3a and C5a circulate in the bloodstream and trigger anaphylaxis. Thus profuse release of C3a and C5a could lead to anaphylactic shock.

Answer B is incorrect. Granulocyte macrophage colony-stimulating factor triggers the growth and differentiation of granulocytes, monocytes, and megakaryocytes.

Answer C is incorrect. IgA is most abundant at mucous membranes and is responsible for defense against the attachment of bacteria and viruses. It has no role in anaphylaxis.

Answer D is incorrect. Interleukin-3 is secreted by activated T lymphocytes and functions similar to granulocyte macrophage colony-stimulating factor.

Answer E is incorrect. When C3 cleavage results in activation of C5, C6, C7, C8, and C9, these components form the membrane attack complex (MAC), which physically inserts into the membranes of target cells or bacteria and lyses them. Although important for the elimination of pathogens, the MAC is not involved in triggering anaphylaxis.

15. **The correct answer is D.** Nortriptyline is a tricyclic antidepressant that inhibits the reuptake of both norepinephrine and serotonin from the synaptic cleft of central nervous system (CNS) neurons. Serious adverse effects include arrhythmia, a prolonged QT interval, and seizures (remember the 3 **C**s: **C**oma, **C**onvulsions, and **C**ardiotoxicity). Anticholinergic adverse effects are common (eg, dry mouth and urinary retention).

Answer A is incorrect. Reserpine depletes presynaptic vesicles in the nerve terminal of their catecholamine and serotonin stores, which causes a drop in blood pressure as you would expect. Depletion of these neurochemicals can also cause depression.

Answer B is incorrect. Trazodone, a heterocyclic or second-generation antidepressant, works by inhibiting serotonin reuptake, and acting as a partial agonist at serotonin receptors. It is useful for the treatment of depression with insomnia. Male patients should be warned of its potential to cause priapism.

Answer C is incorrect. Monoamine oxidase (MAO) catabolizes monoamines such as dopamine, norepinephrine, and serotonin. Phenelzine, tranylcypromine, and selegiline are all examples of MAO inhibitors that increase the levels of these neurotransmitters in the brain. Selegiline is an MAO-B inhibitor also used to treat parkinsonism. These drugs can cause hypertensive crises when taken with substances high in tyramine such as red wine and cheese. When taken alone they can cause dose-related orthostatic hypotension.

Answer E is incorrect. Drugs such as fluoxetine, sertraline, and citalopram are selective serotonin reuptake inhibitors (SSRIs), and work by selectively blocking the reuptake of serotonin from the synaptic cleft. Adverse effects of SSRIs include nausea, headache, anxiety, insomnia, and sexual dysfunction (delayed ejaculation and anorgasmia). This last adverse effect is taken advantage of in the treatment of premature ejaculation. Their adverse effects can mimic the akathisia (subjective sense of restlessness) often seen with antipsychotics. A fatal serotonin syndrome can result from combining SSRIs with MAO inhibitors such as phenelzine.

16. **The correct answer is D.** This is a case of Ewing sarcoma, which can present with symptoms similar to those of an infection. The x-ray illustrates the classic location and appearance of the sarcoma. Ewing sarcoma is a small blue-cell tumor of childhood that most commonly arises in the medullary cavity in the diaphyses of long bones and the pelvis. It is found most often in boys <15 years of age.

Patients typically present with localized pain over the site of the tumor. The periosteal reaction results in reactive bone deposition in an onion-skin manner. The tumor cells carry the t(11;22) translocation 85% of the time, and this would be seen on karyotype. Positive staining for glycogen with periodic acid-Schiff is also seen. In all cases, there is a fusion of the *EWS* gene on 22q12 to a transcription factor.

Answer A is incorrect. t(8;14) is most commonly associated with Burkitt lymphoma.

Answer B is incorrect. t(9;22), the Philadelphia chromosome, is most commonly associated with chronic myeloid leukemia.

Answer C is incorrect. t(11;14) is associated with mantle cell lymphoma.

Answer E is incorrect. Although the translocation t(21;22) is seen in 5%-10% of cases of Ewing sarcomas, it is not as common as the t(11;22) translocation.

Answer F is incorrect. The translocation t(15;17) is associated with the M3 type of acute myeloid leukemia. This type is treatable by all-*trans* retinoic acid.

17. **The correct answer is E.** Given the patient's large blood loss and development of acidosis, ischemic bowel is the likely culprit. The splenic flexure of the large bowel is most vulnerable to ischemia from hypoperfusion because it lies at the junction of two vascular territories, the superior and inferior mesenteric arteries. (This watershed phenomenon also occurs in the brain in stroke.)

    Answer A is incorrect. The cecum is supplied by the superior mesenteric artery; it is not a watershed area.

    Answer B is incorrect. The hepatic flexure of the large bowel is supplied by the superior mesenteric artery; unlike the splenic flexure, it is not in a border zone between two vascular territories.

    Answer C is incorrect. The ileum is supplied by the superior mesenteric artery; it is not in a watershed area.

    Answer D is incorrect. The jejunum is supplies by the superior mesenteric artery; it is not a watershed area.

    Answer F is incorrect. The stomach is richly supplied by the celiac trunk; it is not a watershed area.

18. **The correct answer is D.** A nonsense mutation occurs when a single base substitution in DNA (in this case, cytosine to adenosine) results in a chain termination codon.

    Answer A is incorrect. A frameshift mutation involves a deletion or insertion that is not an exact multiple of three base pairs and therefore changes the reading frame of the gene downstream of the mutation.

    Answer B is incorrect. An insertion mutation is a chromosomal abnormality in which a DNA segment from one chromosome is inserted into a non-homologous chromosome, maintaining the appropriate reading frame.

    Answer C is incorrect. A missense mutation is a mutation that changes a codon specific for one amino acid to specify another amino acid.

    Answer E is incorrect. A silent mutation produces a mutant gene that has no detectable phenotypic effect. The mutation is usually a point mutation, often in the third position of the codon.

19. **The correct answer is C.** Sarcoidosis is a systemic granulomatous disease of unknown origin that particularly involves the lungs. The pathologic hallmark is the presence of noncaseating granulomas. Bilateral hilar adenopathy can be the presenting sign in asymptomatic patients with sarcoidosis. Sarcoidosis is associated with increased levels of angiotensin-converting enzyme (ACE), but testing serum ACE levels does not provide a definitive diagnosis of sarcoidosis because of the relatively low specificity and sensitivity of the test. Nevertheless, for any given test, the PPV (ie, the probability that a positive test result is truly positive for the disease one is looking for) increases and the NPV (ie, the probability that a negative test result is a truly negative for the disease one is looking

for) decreases as the prevalence of the disease increases. In the United States, sarcoidosis used to be strongly associated with residence in the southeastern United States; however, recent studies have suggested that the disease may be common in other areas as well.

Answer A is incorrect. For any given test, as the prevalence of the disease increases, the PPV increases and the NPV decreases.

Answer B is incorrect. For any given test, as the prevalence of the disease increases, the PPV increases and the NPV decreases.

Answer D is incorrect. For any given test, as the prevalence of the disease increases, the PPV increases and the NPV decreases.

Answer E is incorrect. For any given test, as the prevalence of the disease increases, the PPV increases and the NPV decreases.

20. **The correct answer is E.** Marfan syndrome and Ehlers-Danlos syndrome (EDS) both present with joint hyperextensibility. One form of EDS presents with vascular changes producing berry aneurysms that could result in a heart murmur. However, lens subluxation or dislocation (ectopia lentis) points strongly toward Marfan syndrome. Marfan develops as a result of an inherited autosomal-dominant defect in fibrillin. Fibrillin, the scaffolding for elastic fibers, is found abundantly in the aorta, ligaments, and the ciliary zonules of the lens.

Answer A is incorrect. In the endoplasmic reticulum, collagen synthesis is first translated, then hydroxylated, then glycosylated. Glycosylation is the attachment of carbohydrates to the newly bound hydroxy groups. The failure of glycosylation results in osteogenesis imperfecta, type I of which manifests clinically as brittle bones, blue sclerae (not lens dislocations), hearing deficits, and dental imperfections.

Answer B is incorrect. Scurvy is caused by a deficiency of vitamin C. Vitamin C is needed to complete the hydroxylation of preprocollagen in the endoplasmic reticulum. Without vitamin C, preprocollagen cannot achieve a stable helical formation for its hydroxylation, and remains un-cross-linked and weak. Scurvy manifests as hemorrhages, widening of the epiphyseal cartilage into bone, gingival swelling, and impaired wound healing.

Answer C is incorrect. Abnormalities in the synthesis of type I collagen result in osteogenesis imperfecta. This typically presents as an infant or child with multiple fractures at a young age.

Answer D is incorrect. EDS is clinically and genetically heterogenous. Each type affects collagen synthesis and structure. While Marfan syndrome can result in hyperextensible joints, EDS is more noted for its resulting in hyperextensible skin.

21. **The correct answer is B.** The patient experienced progressive left ventricular failure that eventually led to his decompensated heart failure. A fall in his forward cardiac output led to increased pulmonary venous congestion, pulmonary venous distention, and transudation of fluid into the lung. This backs up into the right heart, leading to symptoms of right heart failure (edema, distended jugular vein). The image shows intra-alveolar fluid, engorged capillaries, and hemosiderin-laden macrophages (also called "heart failure" cells), the hallmarks of pulmonary edema.

Answer A is incorrect. Dendritic cells are not prominent in lung tissue, and are not known to be affected in the lung secondary to pulmonary edema. Dendritic cells are antigen-presenting cells, located mainly in the skin and the inner lining of nose, lungs, and GI tract. They interact with T- and B-lymphocytes in lymphoid tissues.

Answer C is incorrect. Although inflammation from the pulmonary edema can cause an increase in the number of T-lymphocytes, hemosiderin-laden macrophages are much more characteristic.

Answer D is incorrect. Type I pneumocytes comprise 97% of the alveolar surfaces and line the alveoli. Their numbers are not increased in patients with pulmonary edema. Type I pneumocytes are thin cells that line the alveolar surface of the lung. They are responsible for gas exchange.

Answer E is incorrect. Type II pneumocytes produce pulmonary surfactant, which decreases the alveolar surface tension. They also serve as precursors to type I pneumocytes and other type II pneumocytes. However, they are not significantly increased in number in pulmonary edema.

22. **The correct answer is D.** This patient exhibits symptoms of hypoglycemia secondary to his current medication. Exogenous insulin and the sulfonylureas are effective treatments for type 2 diabetes, but they can cause hypoglycemia. The orally active antihyperglycemic drugs (metformin, rosiglitazone, and pioglitazone) are classified as such because they won't cause hypoglycemia in a euglycemic person or a patient with type 2 diabetes mellitus, but instead combat hyperglycemia via their mechanism of action. Pioglitazone is the only agent listed that doesn't have the potential for the hypoglycemic adverse effects described in the vignette.

    Answer A is incorrect. Glargine is a long-acting synthetic insulin that mimics the endogenous basal insulin levels. Like any other exogenous insulin (especially long-acting insulins), glargine may cause hypoglycemia in elderly patients who skip meals, thus leaving insulin relatively unopposed.

    Answer B is incorrect. Glipizide, a second-generation sulfonylurea, acts by blocking ATP-sensitive potassium channels, which depolarizes pancreatic β islet cells, causing the voltage-gated calcium channels to open. A rise in intracellular calcium activates phospholipase C, cleaving PIP_2 into IP_3 and DAG. IP_3 causes the sarcoplasmic reticulum to spill calcium intracellularly, which stimulating the release of insulin. This insulin release can be responsible for the symptoms of hypoglycemia seen in this patient.

    Answer C is incorrect. Glyburide, a second-generation sulfonylurea, acts by blocking ATP-sensitive potassium channels, which depolarizes pancreatic β islet cells, causing the voltage-gated calcium channels to open. A rise in intracellular calcium activates phospholipase C, cleaving PIP_2 into IP_3 and DAG. IP_3 causes the sarcoplasmic reticulum to spill calcium intracellularly, which stimulating the release of insulin. This insulin release can be responsible for the symptoms of hypoglycemia seen in this patient.

    Answer E is incorrect. Ultralente insulin is a long-acting insulin that has its peak effects around 16-28 hours after dosing and lasts around 18-24 hours. Like any other exogenous insulin (especially long-acting insulins), ultralente insulin may cause hypoglycemia in elderly patients who skip meals, thus leaving insulin relatively unopposed.

23. **The correct answer is A.** This description is classic for fifth disease, which is caused by parvovirus B19. It is a pediatric illness common in children 3-12 years old. The rash is called erythema infectiosum and develops after fever has resolved as a bright, blanchable erythema on the cheeks ("slapped cheeks") with perioral pallor. A more diffuse rash appears on the trunk and extremities and may wax and wane with temperature changes over three weeks. However, the disease itself is self-limiting, requiring no treatment.

    Answer B is incorrect. The rash seen in fifth disease will dissipate on its own after a few weeks and will not respond to corticosteroid cream.

    Answer C is incorrect. Although the rash of erythema infectiosum is a centrally distributed maculopapular eruption (like the rashes that accompany rickettsial illnesses, drug-induced eruptions, and Still's diseases), it is self-limiting, requiring no treatment.

    Answer D is incorrect. Erythema infectiosum is caused by infection with parvovirus B19 and will not respond to antibiotic treatment.

    Answer E is incorrect. Erythema infectiosum is caused by infection with parvovirus B19 and will not respond to antibiotic treatment.

24. **The correct answer is C.** The patient has a pheochromocytoma, a tumor of the adrenal

medulla. Pheochromocytomas can secrete catecholamines (norepinephrine, epinephrine, and dopamine), resulting in episodes characterized by headaches, diaphoresis, palpitations, and severe hypertension. Urinary catecholamine metabolites and plasma catecholamine levels are elevated in these patients. Most of these tumors are benign, unilateral, and located in the adrenal gland. Pheochromocytomas arise from the chromaffin cells of the adrenal medulla, which are derived from neural crest cells.

Answer A is incorrect. The chromaffin cells of the adrenal medulla are not of endodermal origin. Adult endoderm derivatives include the gut epithelium and its derivatives.

Answer B is incorrect. The adrenal cortex, which secretes aldosterone, glucocorticoids, and sex hormones, is derived from the mesoderm. The adrenal cortex does not secrete catecholamines, which are responsible for the hyperadrenergic episodes seen in patients with pheochromocytomas.

Answer D is incorrect. The chromaffin cells of the adrenal medulla are not of neuroectodermal origin. Adult neuroectoderm derivatives include the neurohypophysis, CNS neurons, oligodendrocytes, astrocytes, ependymal cells, and the pineal gland.

Answer E is incorrect. The chromaffin cells of the adrenal medulla are not derived from surface ectoderm. Surface ectoderm gives rise to the adenohypophysis, lens of the eye, epidermis, and the epithelial linings of the skin, ear, eye, and nose.

25. **The correct answer is C.** Cyanide is a very toxic compound that can be formed in the high-temperature combustion of many materials, such as polyurethane, acrylonitrile, nylon, wool, and cotton, thus making cyanide poisoning common in the setting of smoke inhalation. The most common cause of cyanide poisoning in industrialized countries is household fires. Cyanide modifies the iron within cytochrome oxidase (cytochrome aa_3) in the mitochondria, thereby abnormally interrupting the electron transport chain and halting cellular respiration. Tissues with the highest oxygen demands, such as the heart, brain, and liver, are most significantly affected because cyanide prevents oxygen from binding to cytochrome oxidase and serving as the final electron acceptor in the chain. On physical examination the retinal arteries and veins are bright red due to absent tissue oxygen extraction. Additionally, in some patients there is a smell of bitter almonds on the breath. These findings are not present with carbon monoxide inhalation, the other common toxin associated with smoke inhalation. Treatment includes induction of methemoglobinemia with a nitrite, then administration of a sulfate.

Answer A is incorrect. Carbon monoxide is a colorless, odorless, tasteless, nonirritating gas produced from the incomplete combustion of any carbon-containing material. Common sources include smoke inhalation in fires (as in this patient), automobile exhaust fumes, and poorly vented charcoal or gas stoves. Carbon monoxide binds to hemoglobin 250 times more strongly than oxygen, resulting in reduced oxyhemoglobin saturation and decreased blood oxygen-carrying capacity, as well as impairing oxygen delivery at the tissues. The majority of patients complain of headache, dizziness, and nausea; prolonged exposure results in impaired thinking, syncope, coma, convulsions, and death. While patients with carbon monoxide poisoning may have bright red venous blood, as seen in this patient, they do not have the smell of bitter almonds on their breath. Treatment is with 100% oxygen, either by rebreather or through an endotracheal tube; in severe cases a hyperbaric chamber may be used.

Answer B is incorrect. Substances such as ammonia or chlorine cause direct injury to exposed tissues. Symptoms include shortness of breath, severe throat pain, vomiting, and hemoptysis. The ocular symptoms in this patient are not characteristic of this type of poisoning.

Answer D is incorrect. Sarin gas irreversibly inhibits acetylcholinesterase, resulting in an overload of acetylcholine at synapses. As a result, the body experiences a parasympathetic overload and flaccid paralysis. Symptoms of sarin poisoning depend on the degree of exposure and the form of the toxin; they resemble some of the symptoms this patient is experiencing. However, the circumstances of his injury point to an adverse effect of smoke inhalation as opposed to poisoning with a biological warfare agent.

Answer E is incorrect. Ricin's toxic effects are the result of its ability to inhibit protein synthesis by stripping ribosomes of their purine bases. It is one of the most potent cytotoxins known, with a single ricin molecule able to affect 1500 ribosomes. Inhalation of ricin is characterized by a delay of clinical features for up to six hours, followed by fever, itchy eyes, cough, congestion, chest tightness, dyspnea, and nausea. Ricin is derived from the same plant that produces castor oil, and processing of castor plants has been associated with occupational disease.

26. **The correct answer is B.** Human leukocyte antigens (HLAs) DR4 and DR3 molecules are known to confer greater-than-average susceptibility to type 1 diabetes. In fact, epidemiologic studies suggest that a carrier of both HLA-DR4 and HLA-DR3 is 50 times more susceptible to type 1 diabetes than a non-carrier.

Answer A is incorrect. In would not be possible for the patient to inherit two HLA-DR3 alleles, as only one grandparent has it.

Answer C is incorrect. HLA-DR5 is associated with pernicious anemia and Hashimoto thyroiditis.

Answer D is incorrect. Although HLA-DR3 is associated with type 1 diabetes, HLA-DR7 is not and is associated with nephrotic syndrome.

Answer E is incorrect. HLA-DR8 is weakly associated with primary biliary cirrhosis.

27. **The correct answer is C.** Clomiphene is a selective estrogen receptor modulator, meaning that it acts as an estrogen receptor agonist in some tissues and as an estrogen receptor antagonist in others. Clomiphene treatment is one of the initial steps during in vitro fertilization, as it acts to induce ovulation for egg collection. It successfully treats women with anovulatory cycles but is not effective in women whose infertility is secondary to a pituitary abnormality. It induces ovulation by acting as a selective estrogen receptor antagonist in the hypothalamus and anterior pituitary, shielding the negative feedback of estrogen and disinhibiting gonadotropin-releasing hormone (GnRH) release. GnRH stimulates the anterior pituitary to release follicle-stimulating hormone and luteinizing hormone, which can in turn stimulate the ovary. A common adverse effect of clomiphene-induced ovulation is hyperstimulation of the ovaries and overrecruitment of follicles, producing a greater incidence of multiple births when compared with the general population. Clomiphene treatment can also cause menopausal symptoms because of the induced hypoestrogenic state. Clomiphene also acts as an estrogen agonist in the liver, stimulating protein synthesis; this increases clotting factors and thus increases the risk of deep venous thrombosis. Other adverse effects of clomiphene include ovarian enlargement, stillbirths, and temporary scintillating scotoma.

Answer A is incorrect. Esophagitis is a common adverse effect in postmenopausal women taking bisphosphonates such as alendronate and ibandronate to protect their bones against osteoporosis. To prevent esophagitis, patients taking bisphosphonates are directed to take the drug with water and to remain upright until after the first meal of the day.

Answer B is incorrect. Nausea and vomiting are common adverse effects of estrogen therapy, not anti-estrogen therapy. Estrogen therapy can be used as postmenopausal hormone therapy (to treat the symptoms of menopause and protect against osteoporosis) and for hypogonadism.

Answer D is incorrect. Psychosis, nasal congestion, orthostasis, nausea/vomiting, and headache may occur with cabergoline in the treatment of infertility due to hyperprolactinoma. Cabergoline is an ergoline derivative with potent inhibitory effects on prolactin secretion by dopamine receptor agonist activity.

Answer E is incorrect. Weight gain and fluid retention are adverse effects of gonadotropins, which can be used to increase ovarian follicular maturation.

28. **The correct answer is B.** This man may have been bitten by a rabid animal. The best prophylaxis for rabies infection is immediate administration of human rabies immune globulin to provide passive immunity, followed with a series of five injections of killed rabies virus vaccinations to develop active immunity. The idea is to provide immunity while the virus is still in the incubation period.

    Answer A is incorrect. If the patient develops symptoms, the disease will have progressed to an incurable stage.

    Answer C is incorrect. The administration of human rabies immune globulin is not the best course of action, because it does not provide long-term active immunity.

    Answer D is incorrect. If the patient develops symptoms, the disease will have progressed to an incurable stage.

    Answer E is incorrect. Providing the killed rabies virus vaccine first and following with a series of human rabies immune globulin does not give immediate passive immunity and is not the standard of care.

    Answer F is incorrect. Although rabies is not curable after symptoms develop, it is possible to provide immunity to a patient who has been exposed before the virus replicates enough to cause disease. Therefore doing nothing is not the appropriate response.

29. **The correct answer is C.** This patient has symptoms consistent with polymyalgia rheumatica (PMR) and giant cell arteritis (temporal arteritis). She requires immediate steroids for treatment and subsequent temporal artery biopsy to confirm the diagnosis. PMR occurs in 50% of patients with temporal arteritis and involves symmetrical aching of the proximal muscles and girdle stiffness. The elevated erythrocyte sedimentation rate indicates a generalized inflammatory process, and additional evidence is provided by the new-onset jaw claudication and constitutional symptoms that usually present in patients with temporal arteritis.

    Answer A is incorrect. Analysis of joint fluid would be neither diagnostic nor possible in this patient because she is only currently suffering from synovitis of her wrists and ankles.

    Answer B is incorrect. Mesenteric angiography is the primary imaging modality used to determine the presence of aneurysms and vessel narrowing in patients with polyarteritis nodosa (PAN). PAN is a necrotizing vasculitis that typically presents with constitutional signs as well as with myalgias, arthralgias, and fatigue. This patient's girdle stiffness and jaw claudication are not consistent with this diagnosis.

    Answer D is incorrect. Testing for anti-double-stranded DNA and antinuclear antibody levels would be appropriate to diagnose lupus, which is uncommon in patients this age and does not involve jaw claudication.

    Answer E is incorrect. Testing for rheumatoid factor and anti-cytidine cyclic phosphate levels would be appropriate to diagnose rheumatoid arthritis, which may produce symmetrical and proximal joint symptoms. However, rheumatoid arthritis does not cause jaw claudication and does not usually present for the first time in someone this elderly.

30. **The correct answer is B.** Thiazides work through binding to the chloride site of the sodium-chloride cotransporter on the luminal surface of the early distal tubule and inhibiting sodium-chloride reabsorption. Other thiazides include chlorothiazide, chlorthalidone, and metolazone.

    Answer A is incorrect. Most diuretic agents, including thiazides, loop diuretics, and most potassium-sparing diuretics, act at the luminal surface by inhibiting transporters. Exceptions are carbonic anhydrase inhibitors, which inhibit a cytoplasmic enzyme, and the potassium-sparing diuretic spironolactone, which inhibits steroid receptor function.

Answer C is incorrect. Loop diuretics such as furosemide, bumetanide, torsemide, and ethacrynic acid bind to the chloride-binding site of the sodium-potassium-chloride symporter of the thick ascending limb of the loop of Henle. Thiazides do not act at this site.

Answer D is incorrect. Aldosterone acts to increase the number of sodium-potassium exchange channels in the basolateral membrane at several sites, but especially in the collecting duct, effectively increasing sodium reabsorption and potassium excretion. Digitalis agents can act to inhibit the action of the sodium-potassium exchange pump, but are used as inotropes, not diuretics. Thiazides do not act on basolateral sodium channels or pumps.

Answer E is incorrect. Thiazides do bind to the luminal surface of the distal convoluted tubule, but to the chloride-binding sites.

31. **The correct answer is B.** This is a case of cryptococcal meningitis, which can be diagnosed if encapsulated yeast forms are seen on India ink stain of cerebrospinal fluid (CSF). *Cryptococcus* is the most common opportunistic cause of meningitis that presents in a subacute manner. Increased opening pressure on lumbar tap is present in most patients with cryptococcal meningitis. The CSF findings are typical of fungal or mycobacterial meningitis; the differentiating factor between bacterial and fungal/mycobacterial meningitis is the predominant cell type found in the CSF. Bacterial meningitis results in increased polymorphonuclear leukocytes, and fungal/tubercular meningitis results in lymphocytosis. Intravenous (IV) drug users are at increased risk of acquiring HIV and developing opportunistic infections such as cryptococcal meningitis.

Answer A is incorrect. *Aspergillus* is a filamentous fungus, so hyphae would be seen on staining of fungal culture from CSF.

Answer C is incorrect. Echovirus is also a cause of meningitis but is not diagnosed by staining of CSF. It is the most common cause of aseptic meningitis.

Answer D is incorrect. *Haemophilus* is a gram-negative coccobacillus that can be found in CSF if it is the cause of meningitis.

Answer E is incorrect. *Neisseria* meningitis can be demonstrated by finding gram-negative diplococci in bacterial culture of the CSF.

Answer F is incorrect. *Toxoplasma* is most commonly a cause of encephalitis in immunocompromised patients. It can, however, cause meningitis. If this were the case, *Toxoplasma* tachyzoites would be seen in CSF.

Answer G is incorrect. *Treponema*, the spirochete that causes syphilis, can also cause subacute meningitis, but this answer choice is inconsistent with the image shown.

32. **The correct answer is E.** Active tissues produce acid, CO_2, higher temperatures, and diphosphoglycerate (DPG). Each of these shifts the hemoglobin dissociation curve to the right, facilitating oxygen unloading. A shift of the curve to the right means that at the same partial pressure of oxygen, the percent saturation of hemoglobin is lower. A shift to the left means that at the same partial pressure of oxygen, the percent saturation of hemoglobin is higher, or hemoglobin affinity for oxygen is higher. A shift to the left occurs with low CO_2, low DPG, low temperature, and alkaline pH. A useful mnemonic is **CADET, face right!**: **C**O_2, **A**cid (or low pH), **D**PG, **E**xercise, and **T**emperature shift the curve to the **RIGHT**.

Answer A is incorrect. Temperatures are increased, not decreased, in active tissues and serve to shift the hemoglobin dissociation curve to the right to facilitate oxygen unloading.

Answer B is incorrect. Temperatures are increased, not decreased, in active tissues and serve to shift the hemoglobin dissociation curve to the right to facilitate oxygen unloading.

Answer C is incorrect. Increased CO_2 and H^+ are present in active tissues and serve to shift the hemoglobin dissociation curve to the right to facilitate oxygen unloading. A shift to the left would produce higher oxygen binding and would oppose oxygen unloading.

Answer D is incorrect. Increased CO_2 and increased diphosphoglycerate are present in active tissues and serve to shift the hemoglobin dissociation curve to the right to facilitate oxygen unloading. A shift to the left would produce higher oxygen binding and would oppose oxygen unloading.

33. **The correct answer is E.** The patient is likely suffering from a subarachnoid hemorrhage (SAH). Subarachnoid hemorrhages begin abruptly, occurring at night in 30% of cases, and are classically described as the "worst headache of my life." The headache is unilateral in approximately one-third of patients. The onset of the headache may or may not be associated with a brief loss of consciousness, seizure, nausea, vomiting, focal neurologic deficit, or stiff neck. There are usually no important focal neurologic signs at presentation unless bleeding occurs into the brain and CSF at the same time (meningocerebral hemorrhage). Rupture of arterial aneurysms represents the chief cause of SAH. Upon rupture, aneurysms release blood directly into the CSF under arterial pressure. The blood spreads quickly within the CSF, rapidly increasing intracranial pressure. Death or deep coma ensues if the bleeding continues. The bleeding usually lasts only a few seconds, but rebleeding is common. Risk factors for intracranial aneurysm include atherosclerotic disease, arteriovenous malformations (AVMs), adult polycystic kidney disease, and connective tissue disease. When present, risk factors for aneurysmal rupture include hypertension, smoking, alcohol, and situations causing sudden elevations in blood pressure. Other less common causes of SAH, including vascular malformations, bleeding diatheses, trauma, amyloid angiopathy, and illicit drug use, feature bleeding that is less abrupt and may continue over a longer period.

Answer A is incorrect. AVM is the cause of SAH in approximately 4%-5% of cases. AVMs are congenital anomalies in which there are abnormal direct connections between arteries and veins. Hemorrhage secondary to an AVM is usually intraparenchymal, but it can extend to the intraventricular or subarachnoid space at times.

Answer B is incorrect. Atherosclerosis is associated with ischemic strokes, not SAH.

Answer C is incorrect. Traumatic SAH is most often caused by bleeding into the CSF from damaged blood vessels associated with cerebral contusion. While traumatic SAH is more common than non-traumatic (spontaneous) SAH, there is no evidence of trauma in the case above. Indeed, the patient's pain began during sleep, a relatively common finding in cases of nontraumatic aneurysmal SAH.

Answer D is incorrect. While not the most common cause of SAH, hypertensive hemorrhage is the most common cause of nontraumatic intraparenchymal hemorrhage. The pathogenesis of hypertensive hemorrhage is unknown, but is believed to be related to chronic pathologic effects of hypertension on the small penetrating blood vessels.

34. **The correct answer is A.** This patient is likely suffering from neuroleptic malignant syndrome, a severe and potentially life-threatening extrapyramidal adverse effect of antipsychotic agents. Classic symptoms of this syndrome include hyperpyrexia, autonomic instability, and severe muscle rigidity. Treatment requires immediate discontinuation of all neuroleptics, supportive care, and the administration of dantrolene. Dantrolene uncouples muscle excitation-contraction coupling by binding to the ryanodine receptor, and preventing accumulation of intracellular calcium that is needed to sustain contraction.

Answer B is incorrect. Diazepam, a benzodiazepine, is not indicated for the treatment of neuroleptic malignant syndrome. It is first-line treatment for status epilepticus and is used in most alcohol withdrawal protocols.

Answer C is incorrect. Flumazenil, a competitive antagonist at the γ-aminobutyric acid receptor, is used to treat an overdose of benzodiazepines but is not indicated for the treatment of neuroleptic malignant syndrome.

Answer D is incorrect. Haloperidol, a neuroleptic agent, would worsen the symptoms of neuroleptic malignant syndrome and therefore should not be given.

Answer E is incorrect. Phenobarbital, a barbiturate, would not be helpful in a patient who is experiencing neuroleptic malignant syndrome. It is used as a third-line agent for status epilepticus when first- and second-line agents fail.

35. **The correct answer is A.** Hunter syndrome is an X-linked disorder that is caused by a deficiency of iduronate sulfatase. Although Hunter syndrome and Hurler syndrome are similar, Hunter syndrome is notable for the absence of corneal clouding, which is present in Hurler syndrome.

Answer B is incorrect. Hurler syndrome is a severe disorder with a broad spectrum of clinical findings. It is generally diagnosed within the first year of life and is characterized by a variety of musculoskeletal abnormalities, corneal clouding, hepatosplenomegaly, and severe mental retardation.

Answer C is incorrect. Morquio syndrome is typically diagnosed around the age of one year and is characterized primarily by short stature and joint laxity. Other musculoskeletal abnormalities are also associated with this autosomally transmitted disorder. Some patients demonstrate hepatosplenomegaly, mild corneal clouding, and valvular heart disease.

Answer D is incorrect. There are multiple enzyme deficiencies associated with Sanfilippo syndrome, but this class of disorders is primarily distinguished by the CNS symptoms in these patients. Some of the physical abnormalities seen in the other mucopolysaccharidoses are also observed in Sanfilippo patients, but the hallmarks of this disease are developmental delay and behavioral problems such as aggressive tendencies and hyperactivity that manifest in early childhood. Sleep disorders are also common in these patients, and the physical findings typically develop after the behavioral and sleep pattern abnormalities.

Answer E is incorrect. Patients with Sly syndrome have a defect in the beta-glucuronidase enzyme and are generally diagnosed as toddlers. The disorder is autosomal recessive, and the presentation can resemble that of Hurler syndrome. Mental retardation is not a significant component of Sly syndrome, although various musculoskeletal abnormalities are common.

36. **The correct answer is B.** The patient described is infected with *Pneumocystis jiroveci* pneumonia, which is commonly associated with AIDS and immunosuppression. It is diagnosed with methenamine silver stain of lung biopsy tissue. *P jiroveci* pneumonia is treated primarily with sulfamethoxazole-trimethoprim, but it can be treated with pentamidine or dapsone. Both sulfamethoxazole and trimethoprim inhibit the folate-synthesis pathway. In the folate synthesis pathway, pteridine and PABA are incorporated into folic acid, which is important in the formation of nucleic acids and certain amino acids.

Answer A is incorrect. Many antifungal agents inhibit ergosterol synthesis, including fluconazole and terbinafine. Although *Pneumocystis jiroveci* is a fungus, antifungals that block ergosterol synthesis are not effective in the treatment of this infection.

Answer C is incorrect. Cell wall synthesis is blocked by many antibiotics, including penicillins, cephalosporins, and vancomycin. Trimethoprim-sulfamethoxazole is the drug of choice for treating *P jiroveci* infection, and does not act on the cell wall synthesis pathway.

Answer D is incorrect. Inhibition of the small ribosomal subunit (30S) is the mechanism of action for many antibiotics, including aminoglycosides and tetracyclines. None of these antibiotics is used for *Pneumocystis jiroveci* pneumonia.

Answer E is incorrect. Inhibition of the larger ribosomal subunit (50S) is the mechanism of action of chloramphenicol, erythromycin, clindamycin, and linezolid. None of these is used to treat *Pneumocystis jiroveci* pneumonia.

37. **The correct answer is E.** The subthalamic nucleus is innervated by the globus pallidus externus in the indirect pathway of the basal ganglia. It is not directly innervated by the substantia nigra.

Answer A is incorrect. This patient has the classic signs of Parkinson disease (PD). Acute PD in young patients has been associated with drug users who have had exposure to MPTP, a contaminant in some illicit street drugs that causes damage to the substantia nigra and induces early-onset PD. The site of the lesion is the substantia nigra, which sends direct projections to the striatum. The striatum is composed of the caudate and putamen, which are involved in both direct and indirect motor pathways of the basal ganglia. The direct pathway, promoted by dopamine release from the substantia nigra, facilitates movement, and the indirect pathway, inhibited by dopamine release from the Sn, inhibits movement. When the substantia nigra is damaged in PD, dopamine is no longer released in adequate amounts, so the direct pathway is inhibited and the indirect pathway is unchecked, leading to the paucity of movement characteristic of PD.

Answer B is incorrect. The globus pallidus externus is innervated by the striatum in the indirect pathway of the basal ganglia. It is not directly innervated by the substantia nigra.

Answer C is incorrect. The globus pallidus internus is a downstream nucleus in both direct and indirect pathways of the basal ganglia. It is not directly innervated by the substantia nigra.

Answer D is incorrect. The lateral geniculate nucleus is a thalamic nuclei involved in visual processing. It is not part of the basal ganglia motor pathway and is not innervated by the Sn.

38. **The correct answer is B.** This patient presents with signs and symptoms of lead poisoning. Construction workers, especially those exposed to industrial paints (found on bridges), are at risk for lead toxicity that may manifest with wrist and foot drop, in addition to the symptoms described above. Blood smears reveal basophilic stippling of erythrocytes. Dimercaprol and ethylenediamine tetraacetic acid (EDTA) are first-line medical treatments for lead poisoning. Succimer is the preferable treatment for lead poisoning in children.

Answer A is incorrect. Deferoxamine is the treatment for iron toxicity. High levels of iron produce cellular damage through the formation of free radicals and lipid peroxidation. Early symptoms include abdominal pain, diarrhea, and GI bleeding. Later complications include cardiovascular dysfunction and liver failure.

Answer C is incorrect. *N*-acetylcysteine is the treatment for acetaminophen toxicity, which is often asymptomatic initially. Patients will occasionally present with nausea, vomiting, sweating, and lethargy. With continued exposure, signs of nephrotoxicity (oliguria and electrolyte abnormalities) develop.

Answer D is incorrect. Naloxone is the treatment for opioid overdose. Patients with opioid toxicity most commonly present with respiratory depression, depressed mental status, and constricted ("pinpoint") pupils.

Answer E is incorrect. Protamine sulfate is the treatment for heparin overdose.

Answer F is incorrect. Thiosulfate is one of the first-line treatments for cyanide poisoning. Symptoms of cyanide poisoning stem primarily from neurologic (headache, confusion, and seizure) and cardiovascular (tachycardia and hypertension) dysfunction.

39. **The correct answer is B.** The patient has type 1 diabetes and is suffering from diabetic ketoacidosis (DKA); his recent illness has prompted an increased need for insulin. Increased ketone production causes an anion gap metabolic acidosis, characterized by decreased pH and bicarbonate levels. The low insulin and hyperosmolarity cause an increase in serum potassium levels. Although the potassium levels are high initially, they fall rapidly with fluid administration and insulin therapy, thus supplementary IV potassium is needed. Hyperglycemia and the resulting fluid shift out of

the cells causes a dilution of the serum sodium level.

Answer A is incorrect. DKA causes initially high potassium levels.

Answer C is incorrect. DKA causes low sodium and initially high potassium levels.

Answer D is incorrect. DKA causes low sodium and bicarbonate levels.

Answer E is incorrect. DKA causes low pH and sodium levels and initially high potassium levels.

40. **The correct answer is E.** The cause of these four common symptoms (arthralgias, weight loss, diarrhea, and abdominal pain) is *Tropheryma whippelii*, which can exist throughout the intestinal tract, lymphoreticular system, and CNS as a result of exposure to soil microbes. This is a gram-positive, non-acid-fast, periodic acid-Schiff (PAS)-positive bacillus with a recognizable trilaminar plasma membrane. Biopsy of the lamina propria shows accumulation of macrophages with brightly stained PAS-positive intracellular material.

Answer A is incorrect. Celiac sprue is an autoimmune disorder of the small intestine. Patients with the disease make autoantibodies to the gluten in wheat and other grains (gliadin). Symptoms include chronic diarrhea, abdominal pain, and malabsorption. Biopsy of the small intestine in celiac sprue shows flattened villi, decreased brush border enzymes, and lymphocytic infiltration.

Answer B is incorrect. Crohn disease is a type of inflammatory bowel disease that has intestinal complications such as chronic diarrhea, malabsorption, and abdominal pain, as well as extra-intestinal symptoms such as rashes (erythema nodosum), arthritis, and uveitis. Major findings of intestinal biopsy in Crohn disease include focal ulcerations as well as acute and chronic inflammation.

Answer C is incorrect. Gastric MALT lymphoma (mucosa-associated lymphoid tissue tumor) is frequently associated with chronic infection with *Helicobacter pylori*. On biopsy, dense, monotonous, lymphoid infiltrate in the lamina propria and pale-staining marginal zone B cells surrounding the epithelium are apparent.

Answer D is incorrect. Ulcerative colitis is a type of irritable bowel disease that typically begins at the rectum (spares the anus) and spreads continuously up the colon. It can present with bloody diarrhea, abdominal pain, and extra-intestinal symptoms such as arthritis. Major findings of intestinal biopsy include crypt abscesses and chronic changes including branching of the crypts, atrophy of glands, and loss of mucin in goblet cells.

41. **The correct answer is B.** Epstein-Barr virus (EBV), the virus that causes infectious mononucleosis, is a rare cause of congenital defects. The other answer choices make up the ToRCHeS diseases, a collection of serious infections of pregnancy that are associated with morbidity and mortality of the fetus and newborn. **ToRCHeS** stands for **To**xoplasmosis, **R**ubella, **C**ytomegalovirus, **He**rpes/HIV, and **S**yphilis.

Answer A is incorrect. Congenital cytomegalovirus (CMV) can result in hepatosplenomegaly, jaundice, and brain calcifications.

Answer C is incorrect. Herpes simplex virus (HSV) can result in a variety of congenital defects, spontaneous abortion, and neonatal encephalitis.

Answer D is incorrect. Congenital HIV results in neonatal AIDS.

Answer E is incorrect. Congenital rubella infection can result in deafness, patent ductus arteriosus, pulmonary artery stenosis, cataracts, and microcephaly.

Answer F is incorrect. Congenital syphilis can result in cranial nerve VIII deafness, mulberry molars, saber shins, saddle nose, and Hutchinson's teeth.

Answer G is incorrect. Congenital toxoplasmosis infection can result in mental retardation and chorioretinitis.

42. **The correct answer is C.** Collagen is a major component of the basement membrane. Neoplastic cells bound to the basement membrane can potentially escape if they can break through it into the underlying tissue. Aberrant expression of collagenase and hydrolase can confer that ability, leading to an invasive neoplasm. Metastasis occurs when these cells escape the confines of the basement membrane, find their way to the lymph or bloodstream, and subsequently adhere to tissues in another part of the body.

    Answer A is incorrect. γ-glutamyl transpeptidase (GGT) participates in the transfer of amino acids across the cellular membrane and in the metabolism of glutathione. High concentrations are found in the liver, bile ducts, and kidney. A test for serum GGT is used to detect diseases of the liver, bile ducts, and kidney and to differentiate liver or bile duct (hepatobiliary) disorders from bone disease.

    Answer B is incorrect. CD44 is an adhesion molecule used by T lymphocytes to migrate to selective sites in lymphoid tissue. Although important in metastasis, it is not a factor in basement membrane invasion.

    Answer D is incorrect. E-cadherins keep the epithelial cells together and play a role in relaying signals between the cells. In several epithelial tumors, including adenocarcinoma of the colon and breast, E-cadherin expression is decreased, not increased.

    Answer E is incorrect. Keratin is a marker of epithelial differentiation and is not a factor in metastasis.

43. **The correct answer is A.** This patient has hereditary nonpolyposis colorectal cancer (HNPCC), which can be caused by an inherited mutation in one of the five DNA mismatch repair genes. The mismatch repair mechanism replaces segments of DNA that include mismatched bases. Without this proofreading function, errors can accumulate in crucial areas, such as inactivating mutations in cancer suppressor genes or activating mutations in proto-oncogenes. HNPCC is associated predominantly with an increased risk for cancers of the colorectum and endometrium, but cancers may also occur in the stomach, ovary, pancreas, ureter and renal pelvis, biliary tract, small bowel, and brain.

    Answer B is incorrect. A defect in nucleotide excision repair results in xeroderma pigmentosum, a disease characterized by extreme sensitivity to sunlight, skin damage, and a predisposition to malignancies such as melanoma.

    Answer C is incorrect. t(15;17) is characteristic of acute promyelocytic leukemia. This translocation causes the polymorphonuclear leukocytes and RAR α genes to fuse, arresting the development of myeloid lineage cells at the promyelocyte stage.

    Answer D is incorrect. Benzo(a)pyrene is a carcinogen found in cigarette smoke. This carcinogen binds to DNA and forms bulky adducts with guanine residues. Bulky lesions are repaired by nucleotide excision.

    Answer E is incorrect. The *bcr-abl* hybrid gene is the result of a translocation between chromosomes 9 and 22, t(9,22). Chronic myeloid leukemia is associated with t(9,22), or the Philadelphia chromosome.

44. **The correct answer is A.** Glioblastoma multiforme (GBM) is the most common primary intracranial neoplasm and is typically seen in older patients. The characteristic features shown in the image include a central area of necrosis surrounded by a hypercellular zone called pseudopallisading necrosis. Patients with GBM have a very poor prognosis regardless of management, which typically consists of chemotherapy, radiotherapy, and/or surgery.

    Answer B is incorrect. Medulloblastomas are tumors that preferentially affect children in the first decade of life. The cells have a characteristic blue appearance and crowd together to form perivascular rosettes or pseudorosettes. They arise from the cerebellum and commonly block the fourth ventricle, resulting in obstructive (noncommunicating) hydrocephalus.

    Answer C is incorrect. Meningiomas are the second most common primary intracranial tumor in adults and are typically benign, slow-growing, and resectable. They commonly affect people in the fourth and fifth decades of life but can affect younger adults as well. There is a female predominance and an association with neurofibromatosis type 2. Meningiomas arise from arachnoidal cells of the meninges and classically exhibit calcified whorls called psammoma bodies on histologic examination.

Answer D is incorrect. Neurilemmomas are benign tumors arising from Schwann cells associated with cranial nerve VIII (appropriately, they are also called acoustic schwannomas). They are the third most common primary intracranial tumor in adults and, if bilateral, are associated with neurofibromatosis type 2. The two typical patterns seen histologically are either compact palisading nuclei (Antoni A) or loose arrangement of cells (Antoni B).

Answer E is incorrect. Oligodendrogliomas are slow-growing tumors that arise from oligodendrocytes. They are the fourth most common primary intracranial tumors. Oligodendrogliomas typically have the appearance of fried eggs with interspersed capillaries that appear like chicken wire.

45. **The correct answer is E.** Natural killer (NK) cells are a component of the innate immune system. These cells have a battery of germline-encoded activating and inhibitory receptors that can detect and distinguish virally infected cells from uninfected cells. For example, virally infected cells often express less major histocompatibility complex class I on their surface, and this absence is detected by the NK cell. Detection of a virally infected cell signals the NK cell to release cytotoxic granules onto the infected cell; thus they play a direct and important role in controlling the early stages of systemic response to viral infection. NK cells express CD16 and CD56 among other markers. It should be noted that individuals with defective NK cell function are particularly susceptible to herpes virus infection. This suggests that NK cells play an important, nonredundant physiologic function in the control of this family of viral infections. EBV binds to CD21 on B lymphocytes, which become infected. In addition to the NK cell-mediated response, CD8+ T lymphocytes mediate the main cellular immune response to this infection.

Answer A is incorrect. Eosinophils are important effector cells in host defense against parasites.

Answer B is incorrect. Mast cells control the early inflammatory response by release of potent vasoactive granules.

Answer C is incorrect. Megakaryocytes are resident bone marrow cells that give rise to platelets.

Answer D is incorrect. Microglia are tissue macrophages located within the CNS and do not play as direct a role in the control of systemic viral infections as natural killer cells do.

Answer F is incorrect. Plasma cells are antibody-producing B lymphocytes and an important component of the adaptive immune system.

Answer G is incorrect. Regulatory T lymphocytes are components of the adaptive immune response that suppress effector T-lymphocyte functions in both an antigen-specific and antigen-nonspecific manner.

46. **The correct answer is E.** The child is presenting with DiGeorge syndrome, which is due to abnormal development of the third and fourth branchial (pharyngeal) pouches. This leads to hypoplasia of the thymus and parathyroid glands. Without a properly functioning thymus, T lymphocyte maturation fails, resulting in impaired cell-mediated immunity. Thus, patients with DiGeorge syndrome often present with recurrent viral and fungal infections, as in this patient. Without adequate production of parathyroid hormone, these patients are often hypocalcemic, leading to tetany and seizures. DiGeorge syndrome can be summarized by the mnemonic **CATCH-22**: **C**ardiac defects, **A**bnormal facies, **T**hymic hypoplasia, **C**left palate, and **H**ypocalcemia due to a microdeletion on chromosome **22**.

Answer A is incorrect. The first and second branchial arches play no role in DiGeorge syndrome. For first-arch derivatives, think "M": **M**andible, **M**alleus, spheno **M**andibular ligament; muscles of **M**astication (te**M**poralis, **M**asseter, **M**edial and lateral pterygoids). The first arch is associated with cranial nerve V. For second-arch derivatives, think "S": **S**tapes, **S**tyloid process, **S**tylohyoid ligament, muscles of facial expression, **S**tapedius, **S**tylohyoid. Cranial nerve VII is associated with the second arch.

Answer B is incorrect. The first branchial pouch arises in the pharynx and extends laterally and cephalad to contact the first branchial cleft, forming the eustachian tube. The second branchial pouch originates in the oropharynx and contributes to the middle ear and tonsils. They are not involved in DiGeorge syndrome.

Answer C is incorrect. The fourth and sixth pharyngeal arches do not play a role in DiGeorge syndrome. The fourth arch is responsible for muscles of the soft palate (but not the tensor veli palatini, a first arch derivative), the muscles of the pharynx (except the stylopharyngeus), the cricothyroid, and the aortic arch. Fourth-arch muscles are innervated by the superior laryngeal branch of cranial nerve X. The sixth arch produces the muscles of the larynx (except for the cricothyroid) as well as the pulmonary arteries. These muscles are innervated by the recurrent laryngeal branch of cranial nerve X.

Answer D is incorrect. The second through fourth branchial clefts form temporary sinuses but are obliterated before maturation. Thus, they have no derivatives in the adult.

47. **The correct answer is B.** This pattern of hemodynamic parameters is evident in septic shock. This patient's vital signs on presentation to the emergency department are consistent with a diagnosis of sepsis. The lack of blood pressure rise on fluid administration advances this patient's diagnosis to septic shock. Endotoxin, and the cytokines released in response, will cause vasodilation (decreased systemic vascular resistance [SVR]), increased cardiac output (CO), and decreased pulmonary capillary wedge pressure (PCWP).

Answer A is incorrect. Neurogenic shock follows CNS trauma. It is characterized by loss of vasomotor tone, decreased CO, and decreased PCWP.

Answer C is incorrect. Hypovolemic shock is a less likely diagnosis because this patient's blood pressure does not respond to fluid administration and he has an elevated WBC count. This form of shock is characterized by increased SVR, decreased CO, and decreased PCWP.

Answer D is incorrect. Cardiac shock is the result of decreased pump function. As such, it is characterized by increased SVR in an attempt to maintain blood pressure, decreased CO, and increased PCWP.

Answer E is incorrect. This pattern of parameters is not seen in the setting of any form of shock.

48. **The correct answer is A.** The right coronary artery (RCA) arises from the aortic sinus of the ascending aorta and runs along the right side of the pulmonary trunk in the coronary groove. It gives off a sinoatrial (SA) nodal branch, the acute marginal artery, and an atrioventricular (AV) nodal branch. About 80% of people have "right-dominant" circulation, meaning the RCA also gives off the posterior descending artery, which supplies the posterior and inferior ventricles and the posterior one-third of the interventricular septum. An acute occlusion of the RCA commonly manifests on ECG as ST-segment elevations in leads II, III, and aVF. These leads are called the "inferior leads" because they represent the inferior surface of the heart. ST-segment elevations in these leads suggest an occlusion of the RCA because the inferior surface is most commonly supplied by this vessel. The left anterior descending (LAD) artery branches from the left main coronary artery as it approaches the AV junction. It descends toward the apex on the anterior wall of the heart between the right and left ventricles and supplies the anterior wall of both ventricles and the anterior two-thirds of the inter-

ventricular septum, including the AV bundle. These areas of myocardium supplied by the LAD would be less affected by an occlusion of the RCA.

Answer B is incorrect. In 80% of people the AV node is supplied by AV nodal branches that come off the RCA, making it unlikely to be spared after an RCA occlusion. Note that in 20% of people the AV node is supplied by branches of the left main coronary artery.

Answer C is incorrect. In right-dominant individuals, the RCA courses around to the posterior wall of the heart and gives off the posterior descending artery. This vessel supplies the posterior regions of both the left and right ventricles, as well as the posterior one-third of the interventricular septum. Thus the posterior septum is less likely to be spared in an occlusion of the RCA. If this patient's coronary vessels were left-dominant (as occurs in 20% of people), the posterior descending artery would branch off the left circumflex artery and the posterior septum would not be affected by an RCA occlusion.

Answer D is incorrect. The right ventricle receives most of its blood supply from the acute marginal and posterior descending arteries, both of which are branches of the RCA in right-dominant individuals. The LAD, which runs in the interventricular groove, also provides some blood flow to portions of the right ventricle. However, the primary source of blood supply is from the RCA, so the right ventricle is less likely to be spared when the RCA becomes occluded.

Answer E is incorrect. In 60% of people the RCA gives off SA nodal branches near its origin that supply the SA node. Thus this area is less likely to be spared in an acute occlusion of the RCA. However, it is important to note that in the remaining 40% of people, the SA node is supplied by branches from the circumflex artery, which comes off the left main coronary artery.

Test Block 7

QUESTIONS

1. A 23-year-old G1P0 woman is 39 weeks' pregnant. For three days she experiences dysuria, polyuria, and fever, which she attributes to a recent urinary tract infection. Instead of consulting with her doctor, the woman decides to use the remaining pills from her old prescription to treat her symptoms. Three weeks later she gives birth to a mildly jaundiced boy who is otherwise healthy. Five days later, however, she brings the infant to the emergency department stating that the baby has become fussy, refuses feeding, and wails at a high pitch. He soon becomes extremely lethargic and stops producing urine. Which of the following medications did the mother most likely use during the last weeks of her pregnancy to treat what she believed to be a recurrence of her urinary tract infection?

    (A) Amoxicillin
    (B) Ampicillin
    (C) Nitrofurantoin
    (D) Ofloxacin
    (E) Trimethoprim-sulfamethoxazole

2. A 42-year-old woman presents with red papular lesions along her arm, some of which have ulcerated. She reports that the lesions appeared one week ago, a day after she worked in her garden. Initially there were only a couple of lesions on her right forearm. Since then, more lesions have appeared along her arm approaching her axilla. The physician cultures material from one of the lesions at 25°C, which grows the organism shown in the image. This patient is most likely infected with which of the following fungi?

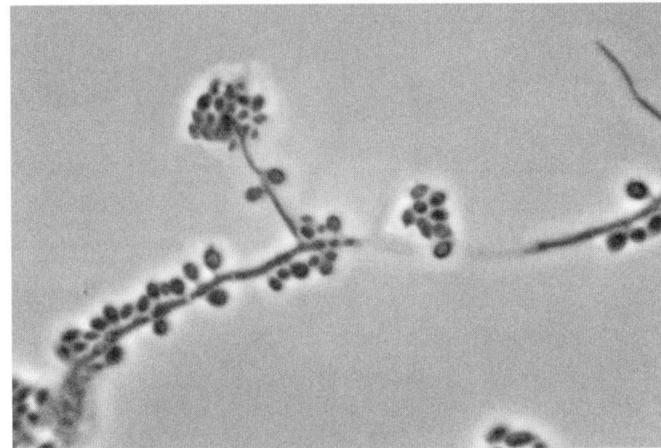

Courtesy of Dr. Libero Ajello, Centers for Disease Control and Prevention.

    (A) *Blastomyces* species
    (B) *Coccidioides* species
    (C) *Malassezia furfur*
    (D) *Pneumocystis jiroveci*
    (E) *Sporothrix schenckii*

3. A 9-year-old boy with no vaccine history presents with an erythematous maculopapular rash that erupted about five days after the onset of cough, conjunctivitis, coryza, high fever, and white spots on the buccal mucosa. The patient's immune system is activated to combat the infecting virus. Which of the following types of cells are the most capable of providing the two signals necessary for T lymphocyte activation?

    (A) Activated B lymphocytes, other T lymphocytes, and natural killer cells
    (B) Activated CD8+ T lymphocytes, B lymphocytes, and dendritic cells
    (C) Activated macrophages, epithelial cells, and B lymphocytes

(D) Activated macrophages, Langerhans cells, and B lymphocytes
(E) Activated macrophages, Langerhans cells, and natural killer cells

4. A 54-year-old white man presents for a routine preoperative assessment. Physical examination reveals that the man is unable to close his left eye completely or to seal the corner of his mouth on the left side. ECG reveals new atrioventricular heart block. The patient denies any recent changes in his health, but notes that he recently traveled to upstate New York for a camping trip. The patient is given a common medication to treat the underlying cause of his symptoms. What is a major adverse effect of this treatment in adults?

(A) Acute cholestatic hepatitis
(B) Discoloration of teeth
(C) Nephrotoxicity
(D) Ototoxicity
(E) Photosensitivity

5. A healthy 29-year-old, gravida 2 para 0 woman who is 36 weeks' pregnant presents to the emergency department experiencing contractions that are five minutes apart. She delivers an apparently healthy baby boy. On initial survey, the physician notes that the baby has good color and is crying loudly, but seems unable to move either of his legs very well and is not startled by loud noises. Radiography reveals healing fractures bilaterally in the femoral shaft and new fractures in the right tibia. The woman denies any significant abdominal trauma over the course of the pregnancy. The baby's condition is caused by which of the following?

(A) A mutation in *COL43A*, resulting in defective formation of type IV collagen
(B) A mutation in fibrillin-I, leading to reduced integrity of connective tissues
(C) A substitution of glycine by a bulky amino acid in type I collagen
(D) Maternal vitamin D deficiency

6. A medical oncologist is seeing a patient who has been diagnosed with breast cancer. As he begins to take the patient's history, she interrupts and states, "I can't stand Dr. Smith. He is a lousy surgeon and he doesn't know how to treat people. Next time you see him, tell him he has made his patients extremely angry and should learn how to become a better doctor." What would be the most suitable response to this patient?

(A) "Do you think I have treated you appropriately?"
(B) "I will bring up the issues with Dr. Smith in our next meeting."
(C) "Dr. Smith is an excellent doctor. He does a great job with all of my patients."
(D) "I understand you are upset, but I suggest you speak directly to Dr. Smith regarding your concerns."

7. A young woman comes to the her primary care physician complaining of eight weeks of fevers, chills, night sweats, fatigue, and weight loss. About three weeks ago she noticed a large bump around her clavicle. It is surgically removed and biopsied (see image). The type of cell shown in the image is a key to making which of the following diagnoses?

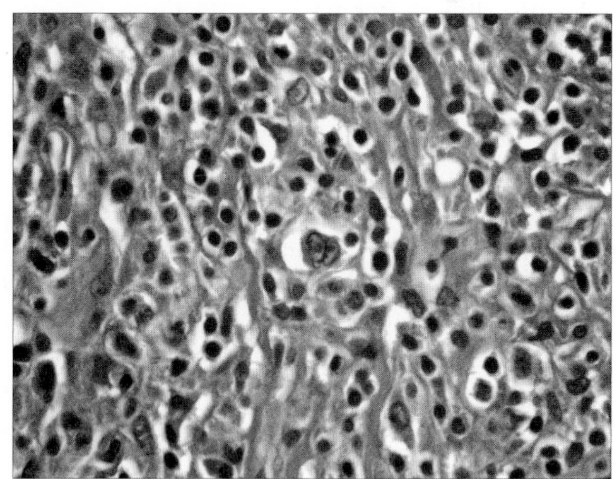

Reproduced, with permission, from USMLERx.com.

(A) Hodgkin lymphoma
(B) Infectious mononucleosis
(C) Leukemia
(D) Multiple myeloma
(E) Non-Hodgkin lymphoma

8. A 35-year-old woman comes to the emergency department after returning home from a trip to Mexico with a one-week history of intractable vomiting. Laboratory tests show a serum bicarbonate level of 50.9 mmol/L, pH of 7.61, serum sodium of 125 mEq/L, potassium of 1.8 mEq/L, and chloride of 55 mEq/L. She is treated aggressively with fluid, electrolytes, and a diuretic. Which of the following is the most appropriate diuretic to treat this patient?

   (A) Acetazolamide
   (B) Ethacrynic acid
   (C) Furosemide
   (D) Hydrochlorothiazide
   (E) Mannitol

9. A 54-year-old woman with breast cancer in her right breast recently underwent surgical lumpectomy with axillary lymph node dissection. Several weeks into her subsequent radiation treatment, she presents with a swollen right arm and fingers, right facial edema that is most pronounced around the orbit, and shortness of breath. X-ray of the chest reveals some accumulation of fluid in the right pleural cavity. Which of the following is the most likely cause of these findings?

   (A) Deep venous thrombosis of the right cephalic vein
   (B) Disruption of the right lymphatic duct
   (C) Disruption of the thoracic duct
   (D) Metastatic disease to the humerus
   (E) Normal adverse effect of radiation

10. A 36-year-old man with a history of depression is laid off from work. That evening he goes to the gym and plays a particularly vigorous game of basketball. Which defense mechanism is this man employing?

   (A) Displacement
   (B) Projection
   (C) Reaction formation
   (D) Sublimation
   (E) Suppression

11. A 60-year-old man who is being treated for multiple myeloma develops osteonecrosis of his maxilla. His presentation is significant for a molar tooth extraction site that has healed poorly four months after surgery. Localized swelling, exposed bone, erythema, and a purulent discharge are noted on intraoral examination. Which of the following drug classes is most likely associated with this lesion?

   (A) Angiotensin converting enzyme inhibitors
   (B) Bisphosphonates
   (C) Cephalosporins
   (D) Osmotic diuretics
   (E) Vinca alkaloids

12. A 12-year-old girl presents to her pediatrician because of recent onset of bruising. Her mother states that she has been healthy other than a recent infection that she developed on a trip to Guatemala, for which she received antibiotics while there. Physical examination is remarkable for non-blanching purple and yellow bruises on her legs. Complete blood cell count reveals pancytopenia. Bone marrow biopsy shows hypercellularity with fatty infiltration. Which of the following is the mechanism of action of the medication that most likely caused the findings in this patient?

   (A) Binding to the 50S ribosomal subunit
   (B) Binding to the 30S ribosomal subunit
   (C) Competitive inhibitor of dihydropteroate synthetase
   (D) Inhibition of DNA gyrase
   (E) Inhibition of formation of peptidoglycan cross-links in the cell wall

13. A 50-year-old white woman presents to her physician with pain that she has had for several years. She describes the pain as constant, located in her neck, lower back, and hips, and as interfering with her day-to-day activities. Over the years she has had extensive work-ups, including laboratory testing and multiple modalities of imaging, none of which led to an

explanation for her symptoms. She has had no history of trauma, but does report feeling "down" occasionally. Which treatment would be most appropriate for her at this time?

(A) A 14-day course of oral doxycycline
(B) Behavioral therapy
(C) Group therapy
(D) Low-dose fentanyl patch
(E) No treatment; her symptoms will resolve spontaneously with time

14. The image shows the gross pathology of a congenital abnormality that results from incomplete obliteration of the omphalomesenteric (vitelline) duct. From which of the following is the pictured tissue derived?

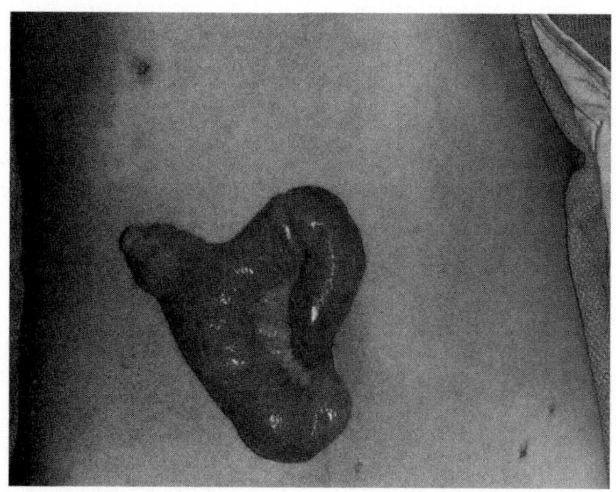

Reproduced, with permission, from F. Charles Brunicardi, et al. *Schwartz's Principles of Surgery*, Ninth Edition. New York: McGraw-Hill, 2010; Fig. 28-23.

(A) Dorsal mesentery
(B) Foregut
(C) Hindgut
(D) Mesonephric duct
(E) Midgut
(F) Neural crest cells

15. A 62-year-old woman with stage IV ovarian cancer presents with shortness of breath and chest pain. Diagnostic imaging indicates a fluid collection within the right pleural space. The physician prepares the patient for therapeutic thoracentesis, and she inserts the needle in the midaxillary line on the right side, in the lower margin of the ninth intercostal space. Which structure(s) does the physician aim to avoid by inserting the needle at this point?

(A) Ninth intercostal nerve, artery, and vein
(B) Parietal pleura
(C) Phrenic nerve
(D) Right pericardiophrenic artery and vein
(E) Tenth intercostal nerve, artery, and vein
(F) Visceral pleura

16. A 3-month-old girl is brought to her pediatrician because she has a high fever and cough. The patient is started on an antibiotic regimen. Over the next 24 hours, her condition deteriorates and she is taken to the emergency department. Further testing reveals a deficiency in the protein LFA-1. Which of the following best explains the etiology of the immunodeficiency syndrome from which the patient most likely suffers?

(A) There is a defect in the development of T and B lymphocytes
(B) There is a defect in an adhesion protein necessary for neutrophil migration
(C) There is a defect in the development of the third and fourth pharyngeal pouches
(D) There is a defect in the emptying of phagocytic cells
(E) There is a deficiency of NADPH oxidase in phagocytic cells

17. The statistical distribution of two studies is shown below. The mean is equal to the median and the mode in the first curve (labeled A). Which of the following correctly describes the mean, median, and mode in the second curve (labeled B)?

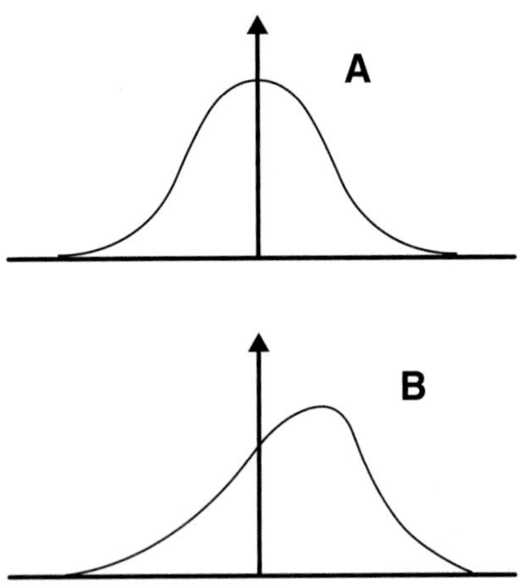

Reproduced, with permission, from USMLERx.com.

(A) Mean < median < mode
(B) Mean < mode < median
(C) Median < mean < mode
(D) Median < mode < mean
(E) Mode < mean < median
(F) Mode < median < mean

18. A 12-year-old boy with moderate mental retardation comes to the physician because of painful swollen joints. During the examination, the physician notices that the boy makes several uncontrolled spastic muscle movements. Past medical history includes a diagnosis of muscular hypotonia at five months of age. At age three, the patient was referred to a pediatric dentist for severe repetitive biting of his lip and tongue. Which of the following is the most likely cause of these findings?

(A) A deficiency of adenosine deaminase
(B) A deficiency of b-glucocerebroside
(C) A mutation of an enzyme in the de novo biosynthetic pathway
(D) Absence of hypoxanthine guanine phosphoribosyltransferase
(E) An excision repair enzyme deficiency

19. A 47-year-old woman visits her physician with complaints of having to use rewetting eye drops throughout the day. Physical examination and review of systems are unremarkable except for a low-grade fever and morning joint pain that has progressively worsened over the past four years. Which of the following additional conditions is this patient most at risk for developing?

(A) Dactylitis
(B) Dental caries
(C) Hyperglycemia
(D) Jaundice
(E) Septic joints

20. A biopsy of a lymph node from a 3-year-old who developed paralytic poliomyelitis following administration of a live attenuated polio vaccine is performed, revealing nodal architecture that lacks germinal centers (shown below). This patient would likely respond to treatment with which of the following therapies?

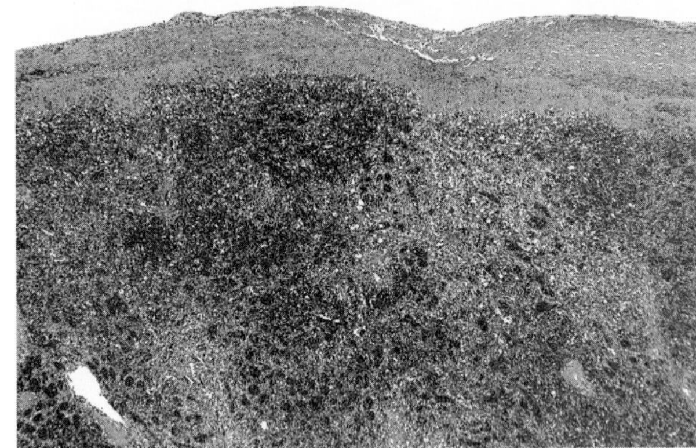

Courtesy of Wikipedia.

(A) Cyclosporine
(B) Regular intramuscular γ-globulin injections
(C) Sargramostim
(D) Tacrolimus
(E) Thrombopoietin

21. A study is designed to compare an experimental drug to a standard medication used in the treatment of psoriasis. One hundred patients are enrolled and randomized in the study. The study runs for 12 months, during which 30 participants drop out of the treatment group and 10 participants drop out of the control group. At the conclusion of the study, researchers decide to only analyze data from those who remained in the study. The results show that the experimental drug is better than the standard medication at treating psoriasis. The results of this study may be invalid because of what major issue?

(A) Procedural bias
(B) Recall bias
(C) Sampling bias
(D) Selection bias
(E) Small number of patients in the study

22. A 20-year-old man is an avid runner and sportsman. In his early 20s, however, he begins to smoke cigarettes, initially smoking one pack a day, escalating eventually to two-three packs per day. As he ages, his lung function gradually declines, and at age 60, he notices that he becomes tired easily and cannot climb a flight of stairs without having to catch his breath. He goes to see his primary care physician, who finds that his resting oxygen saturation is 90%. The physician performs in-office spirometry and makes a diagnosis of emphysema. Which of the following is responsible for this patient's decreased oxygen saturation?

(A) Decreased ability of hemoglobin to bind oxygen
(B) Decreased diffusion of oxygen across alveoli
(C) Decreased hemoglobin content of the blood
(D) Decreased perfusion to alveoli
(E) Decreased solubility of oxygen in the blood

23. A 71-year-old man presents to his physician because of a six-week history of progressive dyspnea, wheezing, and coughing. He has hypertension and a 60-pack-year history of smoking. The patient has difficulty speaking and is breathing using his accessory respiratory muscles. Neck vein distention and tongue swelling are evident. Which of the following is most likely diagnosis?

(A) Gastric adenocarcinoma
(B) Hodgkin lymphoma
(C) Hypertrophic cardiomyopathy
(D) Idiopathic pulmonary fibrosis
(E) Squamous cell carcinoma

24. A town with 1,000 citizens has a 10% prevalence of disease X. A screening test for disease X was just developed, with a sensitivity of 80% and a specificity of 70%. How many people without disease X will be falsely diagnosed positive by this screening test?

(A) 20
(B) 80
(C) 100
(D) 270
(E) 630

25. A 54-year-old woman has had longstanding rheumatoid arthritis. Her rheumatologist recently started her on methotrexate, a competitive inhibitor of dihydrofolate reductase. What effect does methotrexate have on dihydrofolate reductase (DHFR)?

(A) Methotrexate acts on DHFR by decreasing its Michaelis-Menten constant
(B) Methotrexate acts on DHFR by increasing its Michaelis-Menten constant
(C) Methotrexate does not affect DHFR's Michaelis-Menten constant
(D) The maximum reaction rate is decreased
(E) The maximum reaction rate is increased

26. An 80-year-old man is brought to the emergency department by his daughter after suffering a seizure. For months he has taken exceptionally short steps, unable to raise his legs. He is incontinent of urine and does not "know when to go." His recent memory is also impaired, and he denies having fallen despite evidence to the contrary. There is no history of stroke or intracranial mass lesions. On neurologic examination cranial nerves are intact, muscle strength is normal, and sensorium is normal. The patient sways during Romberg's test with eyes open or closed. A CT scan of the head is shown in the image. Cerebrospinal fluid pressure is normal. What is the most likely etiology of the dilated ventricles?

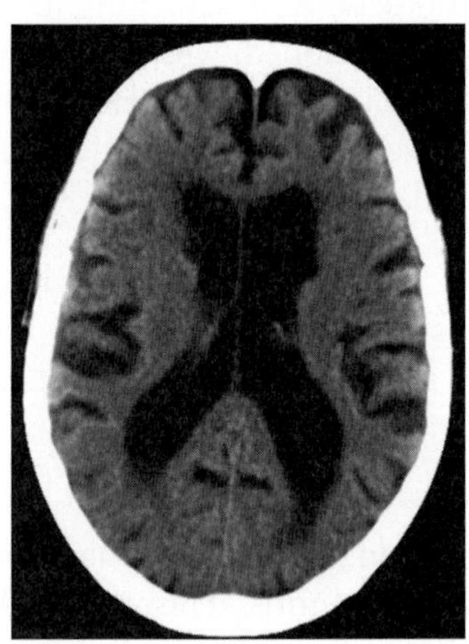

Reproduced, with permission, from USMLERx.com.

(A) Choroid plexus papilloma
(B) Communicating hydrocephalus
(C) Hydranencephaly
(D) Hypervitaminosis A
(E) Noncommunicating hydrocephalus

27. Parents bring their 8-year-old boy to the emergency department because his face appears swollen. The child recently completed a course of amoxicillin for pharyngitis. On further testing, he has a creatinine level of 1.4 mg/dL. What additional finding would we likely see based on this patient's history and symptoms?

(A) Epithelial cell casts
(B) Fatty casts
(C) Hyaline casts
(D) RBC casts
(E) WBC casts

28. A 66-year-old right-handed man with a history of atrial fibrillation is brought to the emergency department by his daughter, who reports that he began "talking funny" that morning. The man is unable to speak or write. However, he is able to respond to both verbal and written commands such as "close your eyes," and is visibly frustrated by his unsuccessful attempts to speak. In addition, the man has mild right-sided spastic paralysis of his face and arm. This man has a lesion that includes which of the following brain regions?

(A) Left inferior frontal gyrus
(B) Left postcentral gyrus (parietal lobe)
(C) Left superior temporal gyrus
(D) Right inferior frontal gyrus
(E) Right postcentral gyrus (parietal lobe)
(F) Right superior temporal gyrus

29. A 50-year-old Chinese immigrant presents to his primary care physician complaining of fever, night sweats, and blood-tinged sputum for the past three weeks. X-ray of the chest is remarkable for calcification in the right upper lobe. Which of the following adverse effects is commonly associated with a drug used in the treatment of this man's disease?

(A) Blue and yellow color blindness
(B) Myalgias
(C) Numbness and tingling
(D) Ophthalmoplegia
(E) Renal failure

30. A 76-year-old woman presents to the emergency department complaining of blurry vision and a headache that started five hours ago. She has a long history of hypertension and poorly-controlled asthma. She is afebrile with a heart rate of 75/min and blood pressure of 210/140 mm Hg. Fundoscopic examination shows swelling of the optic disks. Which of the following medications should be administered immediately?

(A) Captopril
(B) Hydrochlorothiazide
(C) Labetalol
(D) Losartan
(E) Sodium nitroprusside

31. A 35-year-old man presents to his primary care physician complaining of episodes of chest pain during exercise. Approximately one month ago he began running two miles on a treadmill three times a week. For the past two weeks he has experienced a severe, throbbing pain in his chest and felt dizzy after running for about 20 minutes, but claims that the pain stops immediately when he stops running. He is concerned because his younger brother, who is 32 years old, recently had a mild heart attack. In addition, both his father and his uncle died from complications after having heart attacks when they were 45 years old. The patient neither smokes nor drinks alcohol. Physical examination reveals the lesions shown in the image; lesions are also present on his arms and knees. His blood pressure is 130/80 mm Hg, pulse is 85/min, and respiratory rate is 12/min. Laboratory tests show a serum cholesterol level of 350 mg/dL, a serum LDL cholesterol level of 275 mg/dL, and a serum triglyceride level of 130 mg/dL. This patient's lipid disorder is characterized by a deficiency in which of the following?

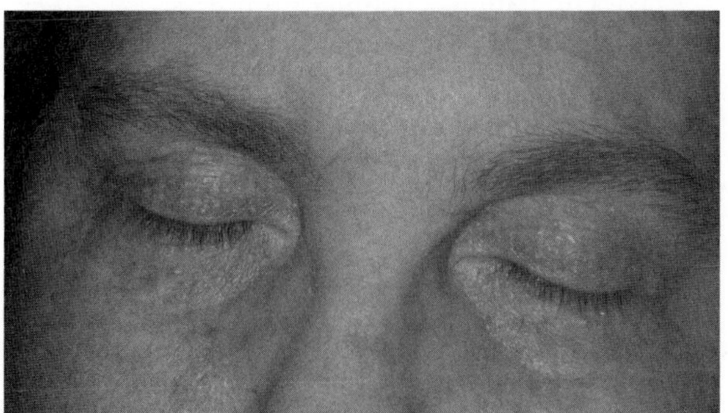

Reproduced, with permission, from USMLERx.com.

(A) 3-Hydroxy-3-methylglutaryl coenzyme A reductase
(B) 7α-Hydroxylase
(C) Apolipoprotein C-II
(D) Apolipoprotein E
(E) LDL cholesterol receptors
(F) Leptin receptors
(G) Lipoprotein lipase

32. A 15-year-old boy is brought to his pediatrician because he feels short of breath and has to stop and walk after brief runs. He underwent cardiac surgery when he was an infant for a congenital heart defect. An inspiratory chest x-ray shows an intact right hemidiaphragm that is much higher than the left one. This boy's exertional dyspnea is probably caused by which of the following conditions?

(A) Damaged left phrenic nerve
(B) Damaged right phrenic nerve
(C) Eisenmenger syndrome
(D) Left diaphragmatic hernia
(E) Right diaphragmatic hernia

33. Some fats and proteins are both produced by the body and consumed in the diet. Many other nutritional components, however, cannot be synthesized by the body and must be obtained in food. Which of the following substances can a healthy adult synthesize?

(A) The fatty acid linoleic acid
(B) The glucogenic amino acid histidine
(C) The ketogenic amino acid leucine
(D) The micronutrient folic acid
(E) The micronutrient vitamin K

34. A 52-year-old man presents with nocturia, dysuria, and crippling back pain. X-ray of the spine reveals lytic lesions in the lower spine. Laboratory studies are notable for a hemoglobin level of 10.2 mg/dL, calcium level of 13.1 mg/dL, and increased total protein. Which of the following is the most likely explanation of the increased total protein observed in this man?

(A) Inability to clear chylomicron particles from the blood
(B) Increased production of albumin
(C) Increased production of clotting factors and acute-phase reactants
(D) Increased production of IgG molecules
(E) Increased production of IgM molecules

35. A 33-year-old HIV-positive man is taken to the emergency department by his roommate. Initially the patient complained of generalized weakness and vision difficulties. Later, the patient lost his peripheral vision and became unable to talk or walk. Lumbar puncture reveals unremarkable cerebrospinal fluid. MRI of the brain reveals multiple, non-contrast-enhancing lesions in the white matter, primarily in the parietal and occipital lobes. What is the most likely diagnosis?

(A) Cryptococcal meningitis
(B) Guillain–Barré syndrome
(C) Herpes simplex meningitis
(D) Progressive multifocal leukoencephalopathy
(E) Syringomyelia

36. During a routine visit to his primary care physician, a 55-year-old man with no significant medical history is found to have a singular thyroid nodule. Work-up suggests the nodule to be neoplastic. A section of resected tissue is shown in the image. What type of thyroid malignancy has this patient developed?

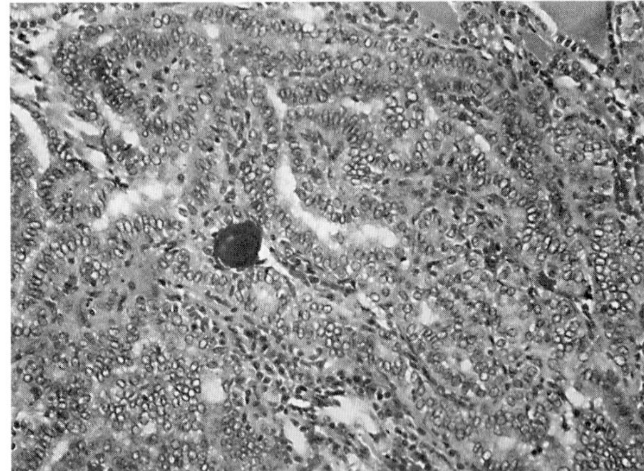

Courtesy of Dr. Edwin P. Ewing Jr, Centers for Disease Control and Prevention.

(A) Anaplastic carcinoma
(B) Follicular carcinoma of the thyroid
(C) Medullary carcinoma of the thyroid
(D) Thyroid lymphoma
(E) Papillary carcinoma

37. Oogenesis results in the production of one haploid ovum and three polar bodies in a process of meiotic cell division. Female gametogenesis involves two arrest phases that are released by ovulation and fertilization, respectively. What stage of the cell cycle do oocytes remain in from birth to ovulation?

(A) Anaphase I
(B) Anaphase II
(C) Metaphase I
(D) Metaphase II
(E) Prophase I
(F) Prophase II

38. In a discussion with his psychiatrist, a university student reveals an obsession with a fellow student. He also notes he intends to purchase a gun but does not clearly state why. Whom must the physician be sure is contacted?

(A) Law enforcement authorities only
(B) Law enforcement authorities and the fellow student
(C) No one; the physician is bound by confidentiality
(D) The fellow student only
(E) The patient's parents

39. A 28-year-old woman presents to the clinic concerned that she has begun growing hair on her upper lip and around her nipples. Physical examination reveals a 167 cm (5′6″) tall, 85.5-kg (188-lb) woman with coarse facial hair on her upper lip, chin, shoulders, nipples, and back. She says she has always been overweight, but has gained 9.1 kg (20 lb) in the past three months. Physical examination reveals hyper-

pigmented, velvety patches of skin on the nape of her neck and around her axillae. When questioned, she admits she never has been sexually active, and she always has had irregular, spotty menstrual periods, often missing them completely. Which laboratory finding is most closely associated with this patient's condition?

(A) Hypercalcemia
(B) Hyperinsulinemia
(C) Hypermagnesemia
(D) Hyperuricemia

40. To ascertain the specific genetic defect in patients with cystic fibrosis, scientists obtained buccal smears from several patients and isolated DNA from these cells. The DNA was amplified by polymerase chain reaction and then sequenced. The region of the sequencing gel where the normal gene differs from the mutated gene is shown in the image. Which of the following types of DNA mutations caused this disease?

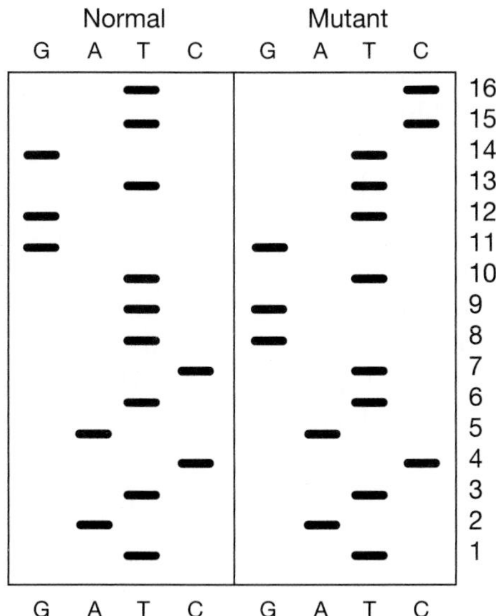

Reproduced, with permission, from USMLERx.com.

(A) Deletion mutation
(B) Frameshift mutation
(C) Insertion mutation
(D) Missense mutation
(E) Nonsense mutation
(F) Silent mutation
(G) Transition

41. A 4-year-old girl is transferred to the pediatric intensive care unit because of suspected bacterial sepsis secondary to a bout of *Clostridium difficile* enterocolitis. A course of antibiotic therapy is begun via infusion. Ten minutes later, the child begins crying inconsolably and scratching her face. Confluent, erythematous patches without exfoliation appear on her face, neck, and upper body, and she develops tachycardia and fever. Treatment is administered and the rash clears within three hours. This patient's reaction was most likely caused by administration of which of the following agents?

(A) Amoxicillin
(B) Chloramphenicol
(C) Clindamycin
(D) Metronidazole
(E) Vancomycin

42. A 25-year-old man is witnessed by his family to have a seizure of sudden onset. The seizure involved movement of all four of his extremities and was associated with loss of consciousness. When emergency personnel arrived at the home 35 minutes later, the patient continued to show signs of tonic-clonic activity without return to full consciousness. Which of the following agents is an effective medication to be given at this point?

(A) Carbamazepine
(B) Diazepam
(C) Ethosuximide
(D) Gabapentin
(E) Phenobarbital

43. A 45-year-old man comes to the physician because of a fever of 39.6° C (103.2° F) that developed suddenly the previous night. On physical examination, the physician notes a new-onset murmur along with white spots on the retina. The appearance of his nailbeds is shown in the image. Which agent, if used alone, is most likely to be used to treat this patient prior to the results of blood culture?

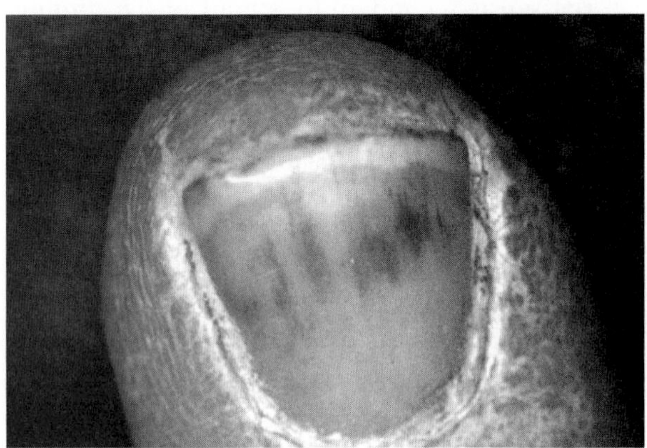

Reproduced, with permission, from USMLERx.com.

(A) Ceftriaxone
(B) Ciprofloxacin
(C) Erythromycin
(D) Gentamicin
(E) Vancomycin

44. A 5-year-old boy is in the intensive care unit because of an intraventricular hemorrhage sustained in a car accident. A blood sample is drawn from an intravenous line that has been kept patent by intermittent flushing with heparin. For accurate coagulation studies to be obtained, the first 5 mL of blood drawn from such lines must be discarded prior to blood collection. Which of the following laboratory results is most likely in this patient if the first 5 mL of blood are not discarded?

(A) Decreased activated partial thromboplastin time
(B) Decreased International Normalized Ratio
(C) Decreased prothrombin time
(D) Increased activated partial thromboplastin time
(E) Increased International Normalized Ratio
(F) Increased prothrombin time

45. A 43-year-old woman in a psychiatry ward is admitted from a medical floor after attempting suicide by overdosing on extra strength Tylenol. She states that she recently broke up (for the fifth time) with her boyfriend, who disapproves of her cocaine and marijuana use. She also states that she and her ex-boyfriend fight constantly, and that she has made "hundreds" of suicide attempts and has been hospitalized many times. Physical examination reveals reddened conjunctivae, an eroded nasal septum, and numerous small, uniformly sized punched-out skin lesions on the upper and lower extremities. Which of the following defense mechanisms is associated with this patient's condition?

(A) Denial
(B) Humor
(C) Reaction formation
(D) Splitting
(E) Sublimation

46. A 20-year-old man is brought to the emergency department by the police after being picked up in the streets for acting violently towards others. He was found in an agitated state, acting belligerently. On physical examination his temperature is 38.5°C (101.3°), heart rate is 115/min, blood pressure is 140/95 mm Hg, and he has vertical and horizontal nystagmus. Which of the following treatments should this patient receive?

(A) Benzodiazepines
(B) Flumazenil
(C) N-acetylcysteine
(D) Naloxone
(E) Sodium bicarbonate

47. A 70-year-old woman presents with fevers, chills, and a nonproductive cough. She has also been experiencing chest pain, and diarrhea. Gram stain and routine culture of induced sputum is unrevealing. A silver stain of an induced sputum specimen is shown in the image. Which of the following is the most likely diagnosis?

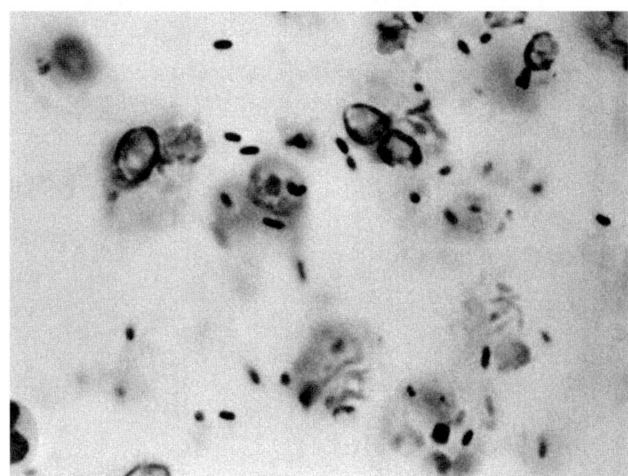

Courtesy of Dr. William Cherry, Centers for Disease Control and Prevention.

(A) Aspergillosis
(B) Brucellosis
(C) Legionnaire's disease
(D) *Mycoplasma* pneumonia
(E) *Pneumocystis jiroveci* pneumonia

48. A 64-year-old woman presents to the physician because of new onset postmenopausal bleeding. Ultrasonography reveals a small mass in the left adnexa, along with a thickened endometrial stripe. A biopsy of her left ovary reveals the presence of Call-Exner bodies. Which of the following is the most likely diagnosis?

(A) Endometrioid tumor
(B) Granulosa cell tumor
(C) Krukenberg tumor
(D) Serous cystadenocarcinoma
(E) Teratoma

ANSWERS

1. **The correct answer is E.** Trimethoprim-sulfamethoxazole (TMP-SMX) is one of the most commonly used treatments for simple urinary tract infections, most of which are caused by *Escherichia coli*. Sulfamethoxazole, as is the case with all sulfonamides, binds to and will displace unconjugated bilirubin from albumin. In a newborn this can lead to kernicterus, also known as bilirubin encephalopathy. The condition results from bilirubin deposition and accumulation in the brain because of an incompletely formed blood-brain barrier. The basal ganglia are particularly susceptible to injury. Early symptoms include lethargy, poor feeding, and an absent Moro reflex. Infants who survive can develop seizures, mental retardation, deafness, choreoathetoid movements, and decreased upward eye movements.

   Answer A is incorrect. Amoxicillin is not associated with kernicterus.

   Answer B is incorrect. Ampicillin is not associated with kernicterus.

   Answer C is incorrect. Nitrofurantoin, commonly used to treat urinary tract infections, is not associated with kernicterus.

   Answer D is incorrect. Ofloxacin is not associated with kernicterus.

2. **The correct answer is E.** When *Sporothrix schenckii* is introduced via inoculation of soil through the skin, usually by a thorn prick, a papule develops days to weeks later at the site of inoculation. The primary lesion can ulcerate or stay nodular, and similar lesions can be found along lymphatic channels (ascending lymphangitis). In an immunocompetent host, pain is generally mild and there are no systemic symptoms. *S schenckii* is a dimorphic fungus that produces septate hyphae and conidia when grown at 25°C (as shown in the image) and cigar-shaped yeast when grown at 37°C. Itraconazole or potassium iodide is used for the treatment of sporotrichosis.

   Answer A is incorrect. Blastomycosis can present with flu-like symptoms: fevers, chills, productive cough, myalgia, arthralgia, and pleuritic chest pain. It is most common in the upper Mississippi and Ohio River basins as well as around the Great Lakes. Diagnosis is made by use of potassium hydroxide prep to reveal big, broad, budding organisms in sputum or tissues. Some patients will fail to recover from an acute infection and progress to develop chronic pulmonary infection or widespread disseminated infection. Fluconazole or ketoconazole is used for the treatment of local blastomycosis, and amphotericin B is used for the treatment of systemic infections.

   Answer B is incorrect. Coccidioidomycosis is the second most common fungal infection encountered in the United States and is usually contracted in the Southwest. There are several cutaneous signs including erythema nodosum ("desert bumps"), erythema multiforme, and toxic erythema. Severe forms of the infection can present with blood-tinged sputum, loss of appetite, weight loss, a painful red rash on the legs, and change in mental status. Triazole antifungals are first-line drugs for most cases of coccidioidomycosis, but amphotericin B is used in severe cases.

   Answer C is incorrect. *Malassezia furfur* infection is the cause of tinea versicolor. Symptoms of this infection include hypo-pigmented skin lesions that occur in hot and humid conditions. *M furfur* has a "spaghetti and meatball" appearance on slides because of the short curved hyphae and yeast clusters, and is treated with topical miconazole or selenium sulfide.

   Answer D is incorrect. *Pneumocystis jiroveci* (formerly *carinii*) infection, like most fungal infections, does not present with any symptoms in the immunocompetent host. In children or patients afflicted with AIDS, cancer, or inherited immune deficiencies, *P jiroveci* can present with pneumonia. Symptoms begin suddenly in this form of pneumonia. The patient develops a fever and begins to cough and breathe abnormally fast. The diffuse interstitial pneumonia gives a ground-glass appearance on x-ray of the chest. *P jiroveci* infection is treated with TMP-SMX.

3. **The correct answer is D.** T-lymphocyte activation requires two signals: (1) T-lymphocyte receptor recognition of major histocompatibility complex/peptide, and (2) CD28-B7 interaction. Only professional antigen-presenting cells (APCs) are capable of delivering both of these signals. The three types of professional APCs are the dendritic cells, macrophages, and B lymphocytes. Langerhans cells are a type of dendritic cells present within the skin.

   Answer A is incorrect. T lymphocytes and natural killer cells are not professional antigen-presenting cells.

   Answer B is incorrect. T lymphocytes are not professional antigen-presenting cells.

   Answer C is incorrect. Epithelial cells are not professional antigen-presenting cells.

   Answer E is incorrect. Natural killer cells are not professional antigen-presenting cells.

4. **The correct answer is E.** This patient presents with stage 2 Lyme disease, which is marked by Bell palsy and evidence of a new heart block. Bell palsy results from a lower motor neuron lesion of the facial nerve, and manifests as an ipsilateral facial paralysis with the inability to close the eye or seal the corner of the mouth on the affected side. The patient most likely acquired Lyme disease from an *Ixodes* tick bite during his recent camping trip to upstate New York. The most common antibiotic used to treat Lyme disease is doxycycline. Photosensitivity, gastrointestinal (GI) distress, and the discoloration of teeth in children are common adverse effects of doxycycline.

   Answer A is incorrect. Acute cholestatic hepatitis is an adverse effect of macrolides.

   Answer B is incorrect. Discoloration of the teeth from doxycycline occurs among children who are <8 years old rather than in adults.

   Answer C is incorrect. Nephrotoxicity is an adverse effect associated with aminoglycosides and vancomycin.

   Answer D is incorrect. Ototoxicity is an adverse effect of aminoglycosides, vancomycin, and high doses of aspirin.

5. **The correct answer is C.** This child has osteogenesis imperfecta (OI), an inherited defect in collagen type I. The substitution of glycine by a bulky amino acid interferes with the formation of the triple helix. The spectrum of severity observed with OI ranges from prepubertal fractures with mild deformity and normal stature, to frequent childhood fractures, to even more severe in utero fractures that result in fetal death (Note that gravida 2 para 0 indicates a prior unsuccessful pregnancy). The most common form of the disease is an autosomal dominant mutation in the genes coding for collagen type I. Patients typically experience multiple fractures with minimal trauma, the first of which may occur during birth; blue sclera; conductive hearing loss due to deformities of the middle ear bones; and dental imperfections.

   Answer A is incorrect. Alport syndrome is another connective tissue disease that may present with hearing loss. However, it is not usually associated with in utero fractures. This disease is caused by a mutation in collagen type IV, which is found in the basement membrane of various organs. A defective basement membrane tends to cause problems in the kidney, inner eye, and ear. Patients with Alport syndrome typically have a history of glomerular nephritis and sensorineural hearing loss.

   Answer B is incorrect. Marfan syndrome involves an inherited defect in fibrillin, a glycoprotein that forms a sheath around elastin to ensure its proper function. The condition is characterized by ocular defect, arachnodactyly, and a predisposition to aortic dissection due to a weakened aortic wall.

   Answer D is incorrect. Vitamin D is necessary for ossification of the cartilaginous framework. Reduced availability of vitamin D leads to soft, bowed long bones. Clinically, this disease is referred to as "rickets" in children and "osteomalacia" in adults.

6. **The correct answer is D.** The appropriate response when a patient expresses concerns about another physician is to have the patient address those concerns with that physician directly. If the problem is with a member of your office staff, tell the patient you will speak to that individual.

   Answer A is incorrect. Although it is important to obtain feedback from patients, directly after a patient has expressed concerns about another physician is not the correct time to do so.

   Answer B is incorrect. It is not appropriate to mediate between your patient and another of their physicians, particularly when the issues are not directly related to concerns regarding the patient's treatment regimen.

   Answer C is incorrect. While you should avoid getting drawn into mediating between your patient and other physicians, it is important not to dismiss a patient's concern without acknowledging it.

7. **The correct answer is A.** This binucleated cell with prominent nucleoli and surrounded by lymphocytes is a classic picture of a Reed-Sternberg (RS) cell. Hodgkin lymphoma is a lymphoproliferative neoplasm that typically affects young adults, especially men, and presents with fever, night sweats, and weight loss. The presence of RS cells is essential in the diagnosis of any of the Hodgkin lymphoma variants. In addition, increasing numbers of RS cells correlate with a progressively poorer prognosis.

   Answer B is incorrect. Infectious mononucleosis is caused by Epstein-Barr virus and demonstrates characteristic atypical (reactive) lymphocytes on a blood smear. It is not characterized by the presence of Reed-Sternberg cells. Clinical characteristics include prominent sore throat, fever, fatigue, generalized lymphadenopathy, and often hepatosplenomegaly. The spleen is susceptible to traumatic rupture.

   Answer C is incorrect. Leukemias are an abnormal proliferation of cells arising from the bone marrow and are characterized by their lymphoid or hematopoietic lineage as well as by the level of differentiation seen. They are not characterized by the presence of Reed-Sternberg cells.

   Answer D is incorrect. Multiple myeloma is a blood dyscrasia characterized by a hyperproliferation of plasma cells, which are recognized by their off-center, clock-face nuclei. The RBCs can also take on a rouleaux formation resembling a stack of poker chips. Multiple myeloma usually affects older individuals and typically involves bone (lytic lesions). It is associated with prominent serum and urinary protein abnormalities (hyperglobulinemia and Bence Jones protein).

   Answer E is incorrect. Non-Hodgkin lymphoma is also a lymphoproliferative neoplasm that arises in the lymph nodes but is not characterized by the presence of Reed-Sternberg cells.

8. **The correct answer is A.** This patient has two primary disturbances. She is dehydrated due to excessive vomiting and she has a metabolic alkalosis from loss of HCl and hypokalemia. Acetazolamide inhibits the enzyme carbonic anhydrase, which is important in the reabsorption of sodium, bicarbonate, and chloride in the proximal tubule. Since it promotes the loss of HCO_3^- in the urine, it will create a metabolic acidosis that will help balance the patient's metabolic alkalosis.

   Answer B is incorrect. Ethacrynic acid is a phenoxyacetic acid derivative that essentially has the same action as furosemide. It is used in patients who are likely to be allergic to furosemide, and it is contraindicated in this patient because it will worsen her metabolic alkalosis.

   Answer C is incorrect. Furosemide is a sulfonamide loop diuretic that also causes a metabolic alkalosis. Furosemide is a strong diuretic that inhibits the $Na^+/K^+/2Cl^-$ cotransporter of the thick ascending loop of Henle and, like the thiazides, is contraindicated in this patient because it will worsen her metabolic alkalosis.

Answer D is incorrect. Hydrochlorothiazide inhibits sodium chloride reabsorption in the early distal tubule. It is contraindicated in this patient because it leads to hypokalemic metabolic alkalosis, which would only worsen her acid-base balance.

Answer E is incorrect. Mannitol is an osmotic diuretic that will only remove fluids and will not be beneficial in correcting the patient's metabolic alkalosis.

9. **The correct answer is B.** Most of the lymph in the body is drained via the thoracic duct. It passes through the diaphragm with the aorta and azygous vein posteriorly at the level of T12. The right chest, back, arm, neck, and head, however, are drained via the right lymphatic duct, which empties into the angle between the internal jugular and subclavian veins. With symptoms of swelling in the right upper quadrant of the body, one must consider disruption of this structure, especially in a patient with a history of surgery and/or radiation in the right breast and axilla.

   Answer A is incorrect. Symptoms of deep venous thrombosis (DVT) include swelling, redness, and tenderness of the areas distal to the thrombosis. DVTs can develop in the axillary or subclavian veins, most commonly as a complication of venous catheters in these sites, and may present with unilateral swelling. Patients with cancer have an increased risk of DVTs, since malignancies cause a prothrombotic state. A DVT in the cephalic vein, however, does not explain the facial edema.

   Answer C is incorrect. The thoracic duct drains all of the lymph in the body except that from the right upper quadrant, which includes the right arm and right side of the face. Therefore, a lesion of the thoracic duct could not explain the edema in this patient.

   Answer D is incorrect. Metastatic disease to bone is common in advanced breast cancer, and most metastatic disease occurs in the central skeleton (vertebrae, pelvis, ribs, upper legs, and upper arms). Bone metastases may cause pain and pathologic fractures, but do not best explain this patient's symptoms of swelling and edema in the face and arm.

   Answer E is incorrect. Radiation has many adverse effects, including systemic effects, such as decreased WBC count, as well as local effects, such as skin irritation. Local radiation to the right breast, however, does not explain this patient's edema of the arm and face. These symptoms should prompt a more thorough work-up.

10. **The correct answer is D.** Sublimation occurs when one replaces an unacceptable impulse with a course of action that is similar to the impulse but does not conflict with one's value system. This method is considered one of the four mature defense mechanisms, along with altruism, humor, and suppression.

    Answer A is incorrect. Displacement is an immature defense mechanism in which avoided ideas and feelings are transferred to a neutral person or object. An example of this is a woman who is angry at her boss and instead yells at her sister on the phone.

    Answer B is incorrect. Projection is an immature defense mechanism in which an unacceptable internal impulse is attributed to an external source. An example of this is a man who is attracted to another woman and accuses his wife of cheating on him.

    Answer C is incorrect. Reaction formation is an immature defense mechanism in which a warded-off idea or feeling is replaced by an unconsciously derived emphasis on its opposite. An example of this is a patient with libidinous thoughts entering a monastery.

    Answer E is incorrect. Suppression is another mature defense mechanism in which unwanted feelings are voluntarily (unlike other defenses) withheld from conscious awareness. An example of this is a patient with pancreatic cancer who decides that he will only think about his illness 15 minutes per day.

11. **The correct answer is B.** Osteonecrosis of the jaw (avascular necrosis of the jaw) has been associated with dental extraction, local

infection, pathologic fracture of the jaw, and chronic bisphosphonate therapy. Bisphosphonates, such as alendronate and risedronate, are used to treat metastatic bone diseases and osteoporosis. Multiple myeloma causes bone destruction due to increased osteoclast activity. Bisphosphonates decrease pain and fractures by reducing the number and activity of osteoclasts and inhibiting bone resorption. GI toxicity and hypocalcemia have also been reported in patients taking bisphosphonates.

Answer A is incorrect. Angiotensin converting enzyme (ACE) inhibitors, such as enalapril, inhibit angiotensin-converting enzyme and are utilized in the treatment of hypertension. ACE inhibitor toxicity can include cough, angioedema, proteinuria, taste changes, rash, and hyperkalemia. Osteonecrosis is not associated with use of ACE inhibitors.

Answer C is incorrect. Cephalosporins are β-lactam antibiotics used to treat infections caused by gram-positive and gram-negative bacteria. Use of cephalosporins does not cause osteonecrosis.

Answer D is incorrect. Osmotic diuretics such as mannitol are used to treat shock and drug overdose. Osmotic diuretics are not associated with osteonecrosis.

Answer E is incorrect. The vinca alkaloids, such as vincristine and vinblastine, are microtubule inhibitors used in the treatment of testicular carcinoma and Hodgkin and non-Hodgkin lymphomas. Vinca alkaloids are not associated with osteonecrosis.

12. **The correct answer is A.** Despite its potent bacteriostatic activity, chloramphenicol is now used rarely because of its toxicities (gray baby syndrome and aplastic anemia). Aplastic anemia with chloramphenicol use is a dose-dependent adverse event that can occur after only a short course of therapy and can be fatal. Because it is inexpensive, chloramphenicol is often used in resource-limited settings overseas. Chloramphenicol acts by binding to and inhibiting the 50S ribosomal subunit.

Answer B is incorrect. Gentamicin binds to the 30S subunit and is associated with nephrotoxicity and ototoxicity with prolonged use.

Answer C is incorrect. Erythromycin is associated with cholestatic hepatitis, eosinophilia, and skin rashes. Azithromycin, a related macrolide, is better tolerated and results in fewer adverse events. The sulfonamides act by inhibiting dihydropteroate synthetase, an enzyme involved in folate synthesis. They can cause serious allergic reactions, urinary tract disorders, and porphyria. Although the sulfonamides can cause aplastic anemia, it occurs far less frequently than with chloramphenicol.

Answer D is incorrect. Ciprofloxacin, an inhibitor of DNA gyrase, is associated with superinfections, skin rashes, headache, and dizziness. The more unique complications include tendonitis and tendon rupture in adults, and cartilage malformation in children and in the developing fetus.

Answer E is incorrect. Clindamycin is classically associated with intestinal colonization by *Clostridium difficile*. This leads to pseudomembranous colitis, in which patients usually present with cramping, watery diarrhea, and a low-grade fever. The penicillin drugs act by inhibiting peptidoglycan cross-linking. The most serious adverse effect is the possibility of an anaphylactic reaction.

13. **The correct answer is B.** This patient is presenting with pain disorder. This is characterized by pain symptoms that are inconsistent with physiological processes. There is typically a close temporal relationship with psychological factors, and such disorders are seen more commonly in females than males. Peak onset is at age 40-50, and it may be associated with depression. Treatment typically includes rehabilitation, such as behavioral therapy, physical therapy, and psychotherapy. Analgesia is usually not helpful. Tricyclic antidepressants (TCAs) and venlafaxine may be therapeutic.

Answer A is incorrect. Doxycycline is the standard treatment for Lyme disease. Lyme disease in advanced stages can present with joint pain and fatigue. However, the patient has had extensive laboratory and clinical assessments, with no indication of an infectious process.

Answer C is incorrect. Group therapy is helpful for many psychiatric conditions, including hypochondriasis. In this disorder there is preoccupation with or fear of having a serious disease despite medical reassurance. This leads to significant distress and impairment, and often involves a history of prior physical disease. Men and women are equally affected, and the onset typically occurs in adulthood. Hypochondriasis is managed with group therapy and regularly scheduled appointments with the patient's primary caregiver. This patient has not described a preoccupation about her illness, so it is unlikely that she is suffering from hypochondriasis.

Answer D is incorrect. Analgesia, including opioid treatment, is generally not indicated for pain disorder. Physical therapy, TCAs and venlafaxine are more appropriate therapy.

Answer E is incorrect. This answer is incorrect because there are standard treatments for pain disorder. Moreover, pain disorder may not resolve on its own once it has been persistent for several years. In contrast, conversion disorder often resolves spontaneously. Patients with conversion disorder present with symptoms or deficits of voluntary or sensory function (eg, blindness, seizure, or paralysis). These symptoms often occur in close temporal relationship to stress or intense emotion. Conversion disorder is more common in young females, less-educated people, and those from lower socioeconomic classes.

14. **The correct answer is E.** The image shows a Meckel diverticulum, the result of the persistence of a portion of the vitelline duct. This manifests as a blind pouch that protrudes from the ileum. The ileum is derived from the midgut, a portion of the primitive gut tube that gives rise to the intestinal tract from the distal duodenum to the proximal two-thirds of the transverse colon. Meckel diverticulum is characterized by the "**rule of 2s**": it is 2 inches long, 2 feet from the ileocecal valve, occurs in 2% of the population, presents in first 2 years of life, and may have 2 types of epithelium (gastric and pancreatic). Occasionally acid secreted from the gastric mucosa in a Meckel diverticulum may cause local ulceration and bleeding.

Answer A is incorrect. The dorsal mesentery gives rise to, among other things, the spleen. Meckel diverticulum, however, arises from the midgut.

Answer B is incorrect. The foregut gives rise to the GI tract from the esophagus through the upper duodenum, as well as the liver, gallbladder, and pancreas. These structures are proximal to the region that would be affected by a Meckel diverticulum.

Answer C is incorrect. The hindgut gives rise to the GI tract from the distal third of the transverse colon to the upper anal canal. This is distal to the region where a Meckel diverticulum would appear.

Answer D is incorrect. The mesonephric (Wolffian) duct gives rise to male internal reproductive organs: seminal vesicles, epididymis, ejaculatory duct, and ductus deferens. It is not related to Meckel diverticulum.

Answer F is incorrect. Neural crest cells give rise to many structures in the body, including the intestinal ganglia affected in Hirschsprung disease. However, this image shows a Meckel diverticulum, a midgut malformation that does not arise directly from neural crest cells.

15. **The correct answer is A.** This patient presents with a pleural effusion, the accumulation of excess fluid in the pleural space. Pleural effusions can have a number of etiologies, including pneumonia, congestive heart failure, and cancer. Therapeutic thoracentesis can be performed to relieve symptoms and improve respiratory function. The intercostal vein, artery, and nerve run in the intercostal groove on the inferior surface of each rib. When thoracentesis is performed, the needle is always inserted at the most inferior aspect of an intercostal space to avoid these structures running along the superior aspect of the space.

Answer B is incorrect. The parietal pleura is the outer layer of the pleura and is attached to the chest wall. When performing a therapeutic thoracentesis, it is necessary to pierce the parietal pleura in order to access the pleural space.

Answer C is incorrect. The phrenic nerve is found deep in the thorax, running along the mediastinum and pericardium; it is too deep to be injured by thoracentesis.

Answer D is incorrect. The pericardiophrenic vessels travel with the phrenic nerve along the mediastinum and pericardium. These vessels are too deep to be injured by this procedure.

Answer E is incorrect. The needle here is inserted above the tenth rib, in the ninth intercostal space. The tenth intercostal vessels and nerve run below the tenth rib, in the tenth intercostal space.

Answer F is incorrect. The visceral pleura is the inner layer of pleura that covers the lungs and adjoining structures in the thorax. It is important to avoid piercing the visceral pleura because of its association with the lung. Avoidance of this structure, however, is not strongly dependent on inserting the needle at the inferior aspect of the intercostal space. This is instead best aided by asking patients to hold their breath.

16. **The correct answer is B.** This patient most likely has leukocyte adhesion deficiency (LAD) syndrome, which is caused by a deficiency of the β_2-integrin subunit and subsequent defects in several proteins, including LFA-1. LFA-1 is an adhesion protein on the surface of neutrophils. The disease usually presents with marked leukocytosis and localized bacterial infections that are difficult to detect until they have progressed to an extensive, life-threatening level. Because neutrophils are unable to adhere to the endothelium and transmigrate into tissues, infections in patients with LAD syndrome act similarly to those observed in neutropenic patients.

    Answer A is incorrect. A defect in the development and differentiation of T and B lymphocytes is characteristic of the severe combined immunodeficiency syndromes (SCIDs), which can have many causes. Their typical presentation includes recurrent bacterial, viral, protozoal, and fungal infections. SCIDs are not associated with a deficiency of LFA-1.

    Answer C is incorrect. A defect in the development of the third and fourth pharyngeal pouches is the cause of thymic aplasia (commonly in DiGeorge syndrome), in which the thymus and parathyroid glands fail to develop. The disease often presents with congenital defects such as cardiac abnormalities, cleft palate, and abnormal facies, but it is not associated with delayed umbilical separation. Thymic aplasia also can present with tetany due to hypocalcemia.

    Answer D is incorrect. A defect in the emptying of phagocytic cells, due to microtubular dysfunction, is the cause of Chédiak-Higashi disease, an autosomal recessive condition that presents with recurrent streptococcal and staphylococcal infections. It is not associated with a deficiency of LFA-1.

    Answer E is incorrect. A deficiency of NADPH oxidase is characteristic of chronic granulomatous disease, which presents with an increased susceptibility to infections by microbes that produce their own catalase (eg, *Staphylococcus*). A negative nitroblue tetrazolium dye reduction test confirms the diagnosis of chronic granulomatous disease.

17. **The correct answer is A.** The first curve, with mean = median = mode, represents a normal Gaussian distribution. The second curve represents a negative skew. The mean is equal to the center of the graph. The mode is equal to the most common result. This is represented at the top of the curve. The median is the middle value if the value were ordered sequentially. It turns out that during either a positive skew or a negative skew, the median is in between the mean and the mode. Therefore, mean < median < mode.

    Answer B is incorrect. In Gaussian distributions, the median is always between the mode and the mean.

Answer C is incorrect. In Gaussian distributions, the median is always between the mode and the mean.

Answer D is incorrect. In Gaussian distributions, the median is always between the mode and the mean.

Answer E is incorrect. In Gaussian distributions, the median is always between the mode and the mean.

Answer F is incorrect. This would be the case in a positively skewed data distribution, rather than a negative skew.

18. **The correct answer is D.** Lesch-Nyhan syndrome is an X-linked recessive disorder caused by a deficiency in the production of hypoxanthine guanine phosphoribosyltransferase that leads to the overproduction of purine and the accumulation of uric acid. This rare biochemical disorder is characterized clinically by hyperuricemia, excessive production of uric acid, and certain characteristic neurologic features, including self-mutilation, choreoathetosis, spasticity, and mental retardation.

    Answer A is incorrect. A deficiency of adenosine deaminase would result in SCID, which prevents development of both the humoral and cell-mediated immune systems. Therefore individuals with SCID are faced with recurrent devastating bacterial, viral, and fungal infections.

    Answer B is incorrect. A deficiency of b-glucocerebroside would result in Gaucher disease. There are several types of Gaucher disease based on the type of mutation, but most forms are marked by lipid-laden macrophages (termed Gaucher cells) that invade the bone marrow and cortex, leading to bone infarction, vertebral collapse, and anemia and thrombocytopenia.

    Answer C is incorrect. This boy's findings can best be explained by Lesch-Nyhan syndrome, which is caused by a deficiency in the production of hypoxanthine guanine phosphoribosyltransferase, not a mutation of an enzyme in the de novo biosynthetic pathway, which would result in deficiencies in nucleotides needed for DNA synthesis. Symptoms may resemble conditions in which dietary deficiencies impede de novo nucleotide synthesis, such as megaloblastic anemia due to folic acid and/or vitamin B_{12} deficiency.

    Answer E is incorrect. An excision repair enzyme deficiency would result in xeroderma pigmentosum, which is marked by dry and hyperpigmented skin that is extremely sensitive to exposure to ultraviolet radiation. Therefore, individuals with this disease are at increased risk for severe sunburns and skin cancer.

19. **The correct answer is B.** The patient's complaints of dry eyes (xerophthalmia) and associated joint pain are consistent with the clinical presentation of Sjögren syndrome; this condition can also present with dry mouth (xerostomia). Sjögren syndrome results from autoimmune destruction of the lacrimal and salivary glands. It can occur as an isolated disorder or in association with another autoimmune disease (secondary form). Among associated disorders, rheumatoid arthritis is the most common, explaining the joint pain and fever in this patient. Because patients with Sjögren syndrome have decreased salivary secretions, the defense against pathogenic bacteria that cause dental caries is compromised.

    Answer A is incorrect. Dactylitis (inflammation of an entire finger or toe) is a common condition associated with psoriatic arthritis. Psoriatic arthritis is a member of the seronegative (rheumatoid factor negative) spondyloarthropathies and is strongly associated with HLA-B27 and with male gender. Without a long history of multiple plaques over the skin or immunosuppressive treatment, psoriatic arthritis is very unlikely.

    Answer C is incorrect. Hyperglycemia is most commonly associated with insulin resistance and/or absence of insulin production associated with diabetes mellitus. It is not a common phenomenon in Sjögren syndrome, although there is a suggested association between Sjögren syndrome and type 1 diabetes, both of which are autoimmune diseases.

Answer D is incorrect. Jaundice is usually associated with pathologic processes involving liver or hemolytic anemias. These pathologies are relatively uncommon in Sjögren syndrome.

Answer E is incorrect. Septic joints are usually a consequence of an infectious process, whereas the arthritis in Sjögren syndrome is an inflammatory arthritis. Septic joints are usually acute onset monoarticular arthritides that produce warm and tender joints on physical exam.

20. **The correct answer is B.** This patient's histologic section demonstrates a lymph node lacking germinal centers. Activation of the B-lymphocyte response occurs in the follicular zone in the outer cortex of the lymph node. Proliferating B cells form clusters, termed germinal centers, where somatic hypermutation and affinity maturation take place. Lack of germinal centers and the clinical scenario of disease following vaccination with live pathogen suggest a B-lymphocyte immunodeficiency. Thus, the most helpful treatment would be administration of immunoglobulins.

    Answer A is incorrect. Cyclosporine is an immunosuppressant that increases susceptibility to infection and is contraindicated in this patient.

    Answer C is incorrect. Granulocyte-macrophage colony-stimulating factor (GM-CSF) is used to speed recovery of bone marrow granulocytes and monocytes.

    Answer D is incorrect. Like cyclosporine, tacrolimus is an immunosuppressive agent and is not the appropriate treatment for a patient suffering from immunodeficiency.

    Answer E is incorrect. Used clinically to increase platelet counts, thrombopoietin would not be a useful treatment option for this patient.

21. **The correct answer is D.** Selection bias can occur when the researcher decides to not use data obtained from patients who have dropped out of the study, especially if there is a difference in outcome between the group that dropped out and the group that continued treatment. It can also occur with nonrandom assignment of participants to study groups, such as when the subject chooses whether to enter a drug group or a placebo group rather than being randomly assigned, or when the investigator purposely chooses to put a subject in a drug or placebo group. In this experiment, for example, one possible result of selection bias is that people reacting poorly to the experimental drug may choose to drop out. Thus, when we account for these patients, we may see that the experimental drug actually has worse effects on psoriasis, causing patients to drop out of the study. Researchers need to account for dropout data in order to detect the actual difference between the two treatments.

    Answer A is incorrect. Procedural bias is the same as recall bias.

    Answer B is incorrect. In recall bias, knowledge of the presence of disorders alters the way subjects remember their histories. It is most common in retrospective studies when patients are asked to recall information. For example, those who develop a cold are more likely to identify their exposure than those who do not. They may recall being sneezed on, for example, while those who do not develop a cold do not.

    Answer C is incorrect. Sampling bias describes when volunteer subjects in a study are not representative of the population being studied, and as a consequence, the results of the study may not be applicable to the entire population. This is also referred to as external validity.

    Answer E is incorrect. Although larger sample sizes increase the power of a study, a study can be valid even with a relatively small number of subjects depending on the magnitude of differences in outcomes between the two groups and the variance of outcome measures among individuals within groups.

22. **The correct answer is B.** This patient is suffering from emphysema, an obstructive lung disease. Smoking leads to increased neutro-

phil elastase activity in alveoli in the lungs, and over time this results in destruction of the alveolar walls. This destruction results in decreased diffusion of oxygen into the alveolar walls, resulting in improper oxygenation of the blood running through the capillaries that supply these alveoli. This results in the oxygenation of the pulmonary circulation changing from perfusion-limited (as it is normally) to diffusion-limited. The oxygen-carrying capacity of the blood is now limited by the rate at which oxygen can diffuse into the capillaries. Since there is now pathologic destruction of alveolar walls, there is not enough surface area for oxygen to properly diffuse across.

Answer A is incorrect. Decreased ability of hemoglobin to bind oxygen would have to be the result of a defect in the hemoglobin molecule itself, which would most likely have been of congenital origin, or carbon monoxide poisoning. This man clearly is not affected with carbon monoxide poisoning, and has no history of any sort of problem with oxygen-carrying capacity of his blood. Emphysema is a problem of ventilation-perfusion mismatch, not a defect in hemoglobin.

Answer C is incorrect. The hemoglobin content of the blood will never affect a patient's oxygen saturation levels. Saturation levels are always a reflection of oxygen's ability to get into the bloodstream, not the amount of hemoglobin in the blood, since hemoglobin (assuming it is normal, which it is in this case) always has the same binding capacity and affinity for oxygen. However, patients with chronic diseases such as emphysema, who have chronically low oxygen saturation levels, typically have blood with higher levels of hemoglobin to attempt to compensate for the inability of blood to properly oxygenate in the lungs.

Answer D is incorrect. In emphysema, blood oxygenation in the pulmonary circulation is diffusion-limited. However, there is no impairment of perfusion to the alveoli. Rather, it is the decreased surface area of oxygenation over all alveoli that results in inadequate diffusion of oxygen into the bloodstream, leading to less available oxygen to bind to hemoglobin and low oxygen saturation.

Answer E is incorrect. The solubility of oxygen in the blood is dependent on the chemical properties of blood as a liquid and oxygen as a component of the air. Emphysema does not affect these basic chemical properties.

23. **The correct answer is E.** Lung cancer is the leading malignant cause of superior vena cava syndrome (SVCS), as seen in this patient. Compression of the superior vena cava leads to dilation of the venous collateral circulation and to head and neck edema. Although other malignancies can lead to SVCS, the patient's age and history of smoking make squamous cell carcinoma of the lung the most likely etiology. Squamous cell lung carcinoma and small-cell lung carcinoma demonstrate strong associations with smoking of 90% and 99%, respectively. Of note, the most common type of lung cancer in nonsmokers is adenocarcinoma of the lung.

Answer A is incorrect. Most cases of SVCS are attributed to mediastinal tumors or lymphomas, not to GI cancers such as gastric adenocarcinoma.

Answer B is incorrect. Lymphoma, particularly Hodgkin lymphoma, is the leading cause of SVCS in young adults. However, the age and medical history of this patient make this diagnosis unlikely.

Answer C is incorrect. Hypertrophic cardiomyopathy (HCM) can present as sudden death in young athletes as a result of expansion of the interventricular septum and obstruction of the outflow tract. Although dyspnea can be a presenting symptom of HCM, this patient has additional clinical signs suggestive of SVCS, and his smoking history and age make it more likely that lung cancer is the etiology.

Answer D is incorrect. Idiopathic pulmonary fibrosis (IPF) is a form of interstitial lung disease that causes progressive dyspnea on exertion and, in some cases, a nonproductive dry cough. Common chest radiographic findings are increased lung markings at the bases and a honeycombing pattern. However, the head and neck edema, in addition to the smoking history, in this patient suggest SVCS secondary to lung cancer rather than IPF.

24. **The correct answer is D.** The question is asking for the number of false-positives. Specificity = true-negatives/(true-negatives + false-positives). False-positive signifies the number of people without disease X who will be falsely diagnosed by the screening test. In this case, 900 people do not have the disease, represented by true-negatives + false-positives. Using a specificity of 70%, the number of true-negatives is 630, while the number of false-positives is 270. Thus, 270 people without disease X will be falsely diagnosed with this screening test (ie, they will be false-positives).

    Answer A is incorrect. The figure 20 is the number of people with the disease who will have an incorrect negative screening test result (ie, false-negatives).

    Answer B is incorrect. The figure 80 is the number of people who will have a correct positive screening test result (ie, true-positives).

    Answer C is incorrect. The figure 100 is the number of people in the town with disease X (ie, the prevalence of disease X).

    Answer E is incorrect. The figure 630 is the number of people who will have a correct negative screening test result (ie, true-negatives).

25. **The correct answer is B.** The Michaelis-Menten constant (K_m) of an enzyme such as DHFR reflects the enzyme's affinity for a particular substrate [S], such as methotrexate, in an inverse fashion. The K_m of an enzyme is the concentration of substrate required to achieve a reaction velocity equal to half of the maximum reaction rate (V_{max}). A competitive inhibitor binds reversibly to the same site that the substrate would normally occupy and thus competes with the substrate for that site. Therefore, in the presence of a competitive inhibitor, the concentration of methotrexate required to achieve half of V_{max} will be increased.

    Answer A is incorrect. The Michaelis-Menten constant of an enzyme is increased by a competitive inhibitor.

    Answer C is incorrect. The Michaelis-Menten constant of an enzyme is increased by a competitive inhibitor.

    Answer D is incorrect. The maximum reaction rate of an enzyme is unchanged by a competitive inhibitor.

    Answer E is incorrect. The V_{max} is the maximum rate or velocity in which substrate molecules are converted to product per unit time. At high substrate concentrations, the reaction rate levels off, reflecting the saturation of all available binding sites with substrate. At a sufficiently high substrate concentration, the reaction velocity reaches the V_{max} observed in the absence of inhibitor. Thus, the V_{max} of an enzyme is unchanged by a competitive inhibitor, as an increase in substrate outcompetes this type of inhibitor.

26. **The correct answer is B.** This patient has normal-pressure hydrocephalus (NPH), which is a condition of the elderly characterized by chronically dilated ventricles. Patients with NPH typically present with the following clinical triad: urinary incontinence, gait difficulties, and mental decline (remember the mnemonic: "wet, wobbly, and wacky"). Although the exact mechanism is not known, NPH is believed to be a form of communicating hydrocephalus in which cerebrospinal fluid (CSF) reabsorption is impaired at the arachnoid villi.

    Answer A is incorrect. Choroid plexus papilloma is a rare cause of hydrocephalus from excess CSF production. If our patient had this lesion, we would expect to see an enhancing mass in the lateral ventricle. A choroid plexus papillomas usually presents in patients under age 10, so it is unlikely in this case.

    Answer C is incorrect. Hydranencephaly is the absence of cerebral hemispheres, which have been replaced by fluid-filled sacs lined by leptomeninges. The skull and its brain cavities are normal. This patient clearly has cerebral hemispheres.

Answer D is incorrect. Excessive ingestion of vitamin A can increase secretion of CSF and/or increase permeability of the blood-brain barrier, leading to hydrocephalus. However, there is no reason to believe in this case that the patient is taking (or being given) excess vitamin A.

Answer E is incorrect. Non-communicating hydrocephalus is caused by obstruction of CSF flow within the ventricular system. Obstruction can be secondary to tumors, intraparenchymal hemorrhage, other masses, and congenital malformations. This patients CT was negative for these abnormalities.

27. **The correct answer is D.** This patient is suffering from poststreptococcal glomerulonephritis (PSG), and RBC casts are pathognomonic of glomerulonephritis. Symptoms in PSG usually develop one-three weeks after acute infection with specific nephritogenic strains of group A β-hemolytic streptococcus. The incidence of glomerulonephritis is approximately 5%-10% in persons with pharyngitis and 25% in those with skin infections during an epidemic of infection caused by group A β-hemolytic streptococcus. Some other examples of glomerulonephritis include diffuse proliferative glomerulonephritis and rapidly progressive crescentic glomerulonephritis.

Answer A is incorrect. The epithelial cell cast is formed by inclusion or adhesion of desquamated epithelial cells of the tubule lining. These casts can be seen in acute tubular necrosis and toxic ingestion (eg, mercury, diethylene glycol, or salicylate).

Answer B is incorrect. Fatty casts are products of breakdown of lipid-rich epithelial cells. They resemble hyaline casts with fat globule, yellowish-tan in color. These casts are found in various disorders, including nephrotic syndrome, and diabetic or lupus nephropathy.

Answer C is incorrect. Hyaline casts are the most common type of cast. They are formed from the tubular epithelial cells of individual nephrons. Contributing factors include low urine flow, concentrated urine, or an acidic environment. They may be seen in normal individuals during dehydration or vigorous exercise.

Answer E is incorrect. WBC casts are indicative of inflammation or infection. Thus WBC casts strongly suggest pyelonephritis. They also may be seen in inflammatory states such as acute allergic interstitial nephritis, nephrotic syndrome, or poststreptococcal acute glomerulonephritis.

28. **The correct answer is A.** This patient has a lesion affecting Broca area (Brodmann area 44) in the inferior frontal gyrus, causing an expressive aphasia characterized by decreased fluency of spontaneous speech with intact comprehension. Broca's aphasia is often caused by an infarction of the areas supplied by the superior division of the middle cerebral artery, which often includes both Broca area and the primary motor cortex, leading to an expressive aphasia and right-sided spastic paralysis. The majority of people (about 95% of right-handed and 70% of left-handed) have language lateralized to the left hemisphere.

Answer B is incorrect. The primary somatosensory cortex corresponding to the right side of the body is located in the left postcentral gyrus. A lesion of this area would cause right-sided sensory defects, which are not relevant to this case as this patient presents with aphasia and motor defects.

Answer C is incorrect. Wernicke area (Brodmann area 22) is located in the posterior two-thirds of the superior temporal gyrus in the dominant hemisphere. Assuming that this patient has a left-dominant hemisphere for language, a lesion of this area would lead to a receptive aphasia with impaired comprehension and meaningless, empty speech (Wernicke aphasia). Such a lesion could be caused by an infarct of the inferior division of the left middle cerebral artery. This patient, however, has an expressive aphasia and thus the inferior frontal gyrus (Broca area), not the superior temporal gyrus (Wernicke area), is likely to be involved.

Answer D is incorrect. About 30%-40% of left-handed individuals and <5% of right-handed individuals will have a right-dominant hemisphere for language. However, this patient's right-sided paralysis and right-handedness are indications that the lesion is in the left, not right, hemisphere.

Answer E is incorrect. The primary somatosensory cortex corresponding to the left side of the body is located in the right postcentral gyrus (parietal lobe). A lesion to the right postcentral gyrus would cause left-sided sensory deficits, but not aphasia or motor defects as in this patient.

Answer F is incorrect. In right hemisphere-dominant individuals, a lesion of the right superior temporal gyrus would lead to a receptive aphasia, but this patient is most likely left-hemisphere dominant for language and has an expressive, not a receptive, aphasia. Thus, the inferior frontal gyrus, and not the superior temporal gyrus, is likely to be involved.

29. **The correct answer is C.** This patient's symptoms of fever, night sweats, and hemoptysis are consistent with tuberculosis (TB). The calcification in the right upper lobe is a Ghon complex, which is the TB granuloma (Ghon focus), with surrounding lobar and perihilar lymph node involvement. TB is caused by *Mycobacterium tuberculosis*, which can be visualized with an acid-fast stain. The current treatment for active TB is a multidrug regimen, including rifampin, isoniazid (INH), pyrazinamide, and ethambutol. Of the adverse effects listed, only numbness and tingling (peripheral neuropathy) are commonly associated with INH and ethambutol. INH-associated peripheral neuropathy may be prevented or reversed with vitamin B_6 supplementation.

Answer A is incorrect. Blue and yellow color blindness is not an adverse effect associated with any of the anti-tuberculosis drugs. Red and green color blindness is associated with ethambutol. Other adverse effects of ethambutol include optic neuritis, peripheral neuropathy, arthralgia, and vertical nystagmus.

Answer B is incorrect. Arthralgias, not myalgias, are associated with ethambutol and pyrazinamide.

Answer D is incorrect. Optic neuritis, not ophthalmoplegia, is associated with ethambutol. Optic neuritis is inflammation of the optic nerve, which can cause abrupt partial or complete loss of vision.

Answer E is incorrect. Renal failure is not a common adverse effect of any of the four drugs listed. Hepatotoxicity is associated with INH, rifampin, and pyrazinamide.

30. **The correct answer is E.** This patient is having a hypertensive emergency, defined as a systolic blood pressure >210 mm Hg and/or a diastolic blood pressure >120 mm Hg. In addition, she is exhibiting the signs and symptoms of end-organ involvement: blurry vision and headache, as well as papilledema. Sodium nitroprusside, a first-line medication for hypertensive emergencies, acts by direct vasodilation of both arteries and veins. Adverse effects of nitroprusside include reflex tachycardia as well as cyanide toxicity, especially in patients with liver disease.

Answer A is incorrect. Captopril, an ACE inhibitor, is an extremely effective medication in controlling chronic hypertension. However, it is not useful in acute hypertensive emergencies because its mechanism of action is too slow.

Answer B is incorrect. Hydrochlorothiazide is an effective diuretic medication used for the treatment of chronic essential hypertension. Because of its mechanism of action, it does not cause a reduction in blood pressure rapid enough to be useful in an emergent situation such as the one described here.

Answer C is incorrect. β-blockers such as the nonselective agent labetalol are also first-line agents in managing hypertensive emergencies, although their mechanism is not completely understood. With first-time emergent use, the antihypertensive action of labetalol is thought to result from a decrease in cardiac output. However, this patient's history of asthma makes labetalol a suboptimal choice, as adrenergic blockade in the airways could precipitate bronchospasm.

Answer D is incorrect. As an angiotensin receptor blocker, losartan is a useful drug with which to control chronic hypertension. It has no role in the acute management of hypertensive emergency because of its slow onset of effect.

31. **The correct answer is E.** This is a case of familial hypercholesterolemia (FH), a genetic deficiency of LDL cholesterol receptors. As a result of this condition, serum LDL and total cholesterol levels are grossly elevated, although levels of other lipids may be within normal limits. Patients with FH often have a family history significant for myocardial infarctions before the age of 40 years. In addition, xanthomas (cholesterol deposits) are sometimes seen within the eyelids (shown) as well as the skin of the upper and lower extremities (not shown).

Answer A is incorrect. A deficiency in 3-hydroxy-3-methylglutaryl coenzyme A reductase (HMG CoA reductase) would result in extremely low levels of cholesterol, since this is the rate-limiting enzyme in cholesterol synthesis. Statin drugs block HMG CoA reductase in order to lower LDL cholesterol levels in patients with hypercholesterolemia.

Answer B is incorrect. 7α-hydroxylase is the rate-limiting enzyme in bile acid synthesis. A defect in this enzyme would not result in hypercholesterolemia.

Answer C is incorrect. Apolipoprotein C-II is a cofactor for lipoprotein lipase. A defect in apolipoprotein C-II would thus result in hyperchylomicronemia due to the inability to activate lipoprotein lipase.

Answer D is incorrect. A defect in apolipoprotein E would result in hyperchylomicronemia and elevated levels of triglycerides and VLDL cholesterol. However, serum triglycerides are within normal limits in this patient, making an apolipoprotein E defect less likely.

Answer F is incorrect. Defective leptin receptors would result in high serum levels of HDL cholesterol, not LDL cholesterol. The recent discovery of the scavenger receptor BI has led researchers to a better understanding of the role of leptin in the proper uptake of HDL cholesterol.

Answer G is incorrect. A deficiency in lipoprotein lipase would result in hyperchylomicronemia but would not produce an elevated cholesterol level. Lipoprotein lipase is required for the hydrolysis of triglycerides in chylomicrons and VLDL cholesterol. Genetic deficiency of lipoprotein lipase results in impaired lipolysis and profound elevations in plasma chylomicron levels. Although these patients also have elevations in plasma VLDL cholesterol levels, chylomicronemia predominates.

32. **The correct answer is B.** An x-ray film of the chest indicates that the boy has a paralyzed right hemidiaphragm. It is possible for the phrenic nerve to become damaged during heart surgery, since it runs along the pericardium. It is not unusual for a patient to remain asymptomatic until starting to run long distances.

Answer A is incorrect. When a patient holds his or her breath during a chest x-ray, a contracted diaphragm will move downward, and a paralyzed diaphragm will paradoxically move upward because of the negative pressure generated on the left side of the thorax pulling the mediastinal structures towards the left.

Answer C is incorrect. Eisenmenger syndrome is the cyanosis and symptoms that occur when a prior left-to-right shunt reverses and becomes a right-to-left shunt. Cyanosis does not occur in a left-to-right shunt because oxygenated arterial blood simply reenters the pulmonary circulation. After years of arterial blood overloading the right side of the heart, however, pulmonary pressures can increase above systemic pressures and the shunt reverses. When this occurs, deoxygenated blood enters systemic circulation and cyanosis results. Although the question states that this patient had a cardiac defect repaired in infancy, there is no evidence of cyanosis, which is the hallmark of Eisenmenger syndrome.

Answer D is incorrect. An x-ray film of a left diaphragmatic hernia would also reveal abdominal viscera in the thoracic cavity, which is not reported in this scenario.

Answer E is incorrect. An x-ray film of a right diaphragmatic hernia would also reveal abdominal viscera in the thoracic cavity, which is not reported in this scenario.

33. **The correct answer is B.** Histidine is an important and "essential" glucogenic amino acid in times of intense anabolic states such as infancy, growth spurts, and recovery from infection; however, it is usually categorized as a nonessential amino acid because it can be synthesized by the healthy adult. The eight essential amino acids are leucine, lysine, isoleucine, phenylalanine, tryptophan, methionine, threonine, and valine; these must be obtained exogenously from the diet.

    Answer A is incorrect. The essential fatty acids are linoleic and linolenic acid. They cannot be synthesized by healthy adults but are ubiquitous in natural diets.

    Answer C is incorrect. Leucine and lysine are essential ketogenic amino acids; they cannot be synthesized by the healthy adult. Glucogenic amino acids can be converted into glucose through gluconeogenesis. Ketogenic amino acids can only be converted to ketone bodies (not glucose) through ketogenesis. Both of these processes occur in the liver.

    Answer D is incorrect. Folic acid is produced by symbiotic bacteria from the precursor p-aminobenzoic acid. This production is inhibited by sulfa antibiotics. Folic acid cannot be produced through cellular metabolism. Folic acid is also obtained from leafy vegetables and cereal. Supplementation is recommended for pregnant women to prevent congenital neural tube defects.

    Answer E is incorrect. The healthy adult relies on microflora in the gut to synthesize vitamin K. This vitamin is also found in green, leafy vegetables. Patients taking warfarin or broad-spectrum antibiotics should be advised to maintain a stable intake of these vegetables from day to day, in order to prevent bleeding complications.

34. **The correct answer is D.** This question describes the most common symptoms of multiple myeloma. The increased total protein could be studied further by ordering a serum protein electrophoresis, which would show increased gamma-globulin fraction. Multiple myeloma is a neoplastic proliferation of plasma cells, which produce immunoglobulins. The molecule most commonly produced by the plasma cells is IgG.

    Answer A is incorrect. The inability to clear chylomicron molecules from the blood is the primary pathologic process in type I family dyslipidemias. However, these typically present at a young age with increased lipids, not increased total protein.

    Answer B is incorrect. The production of albumin typically is normal in multiple myeloma.

    Answer C is incorrect. There can be increased clotting factors and acute-phase reactants in a variety of conditions, but these are not the main cause of increased total protein in multiple myeloma.

    Answer E is incorrect. IgM molecules are produced in Waldenström macroglobulinemia, a condition related to multiple myeloma. Waldenström typically presents with hyperviscosity syndrome, adenopathy, and hepatosplenomegaly. Hypercalcemia, lytic lesions, and renal insufficiency are much less common in this condition.

35. **The correct answer is D.** This patient most likely now has AIDS and progressive multifocal leukoencephalopathy (PML), an opportunistic infection that affects the central nervous system (CNS). PML is the result of the reactivation of latent JC papovavirus, usually after the patient's CD4 count falls to less than 200/mm^3. Approximately 75% of all humans have been exposed to the JC virus. PML is a fatal CNS disease that causes demyelination of the white matter. Disease progression is subacute, and it is initially marked by visual field deficits, mental status changes, and weakness. The disease progresses to blindness, dementia, coma, and death, typically within six months. CSF

analysis is usually unremarkable, although the fact that PML does not enhance on MRI with contrast is a key feature.

Answer A is incorrect. Cryptococcal meningitis is classically associated with the acute onset of a severe headache, fever, nuchal rigidity, a change in mental status, focal neurologic signs, and high intracranial pressures with papilledema. The clinical presentation described is more consistent with progressive multifocal leukoencephalopathy than cryptococcal meninigitis.

Answer B is incorrect. Guillain-Barré syndrome (GBS) generally causes symmetric weakness that begins in the distal extremities and that ascends to affect the proximal extremities and the trunk. It is associated with recent infections of the upper respiratory and GI tracts. The classic CSF finding is albuminocytologic dissociation, which involves increased protein without increased WBCs. GBS is caused by immune reaction against epitopes in Schwann cell surface membrane as a result of molecular mimicry. The most commonly described precipitant of GBS is *Campylobacter jejuni*. GBS is also seen in patients with HIV infection.

Answer C is incorrect. Herpes simplex virus (HSV) may cause meningitis and encephalitis and is usually characterized by a necrotic temporal lobe lesion. Classic symptoms include fever, headache, altered mental status, olfactory hallucinations, seizures, and vomiting. CSF analysis typically reveals an increased number of lymphocytes and an elevated protein level. The clinical course is usually acute or subacute.

Answer E is incorrect. Syringomyelia, or the enlargement of the central canal of the spinal cord, causes bilateral sensory deficits in the upper extremities in a cape-like distribution. It is generally a congenital condition, and it is not associated with HIV.

36. **The correct answer is E.** The patient has papillary adenocarcinoma of the thyroid, which accounts for approximately 80% of thyroid carcinomas. Papillary thyroid carcinoma usually can be cured by resection of the primary tumor. Diagnosis is often made by fine-needle biopsy. The histologic finding in the image is a psammoma body (a structure with laminated, concentric, calcified spherules), which is found in approximately 50% of papillary adenocarcinomas of the thyroid. Psammoma bodies are also found in serous papillary cystadenocarcinomas of the ovary, meningiomas, and malignant mesotheliomas.

Answer A is incorrect. Anaplastic carcinoma is a poorly differentiated and aggressive type of thyroid cancer with a poor prognosis. Psammoma bodies are not seen.

Answer B is incorrect. Follicular carcinomas of the thyroid are less common but more malignant than papillary carcinomas of the thyroid. Unlike papillary carcinoma, in which hematogenous metastasis is rare, follicular carcinomas commonly metastasize via the blood to lungs or bones. Histologically, follicular carcinomas tend to form acini or follicles lined with cells that are larger than those found in normal thyroid. Psammoma bodies are not found in follicular carcinoma.

Answer C is incorrect. Medullary carcinoma of the thyroid arises from the C cells of the thyroid, which produce calcitonin. It is a rare cancer of the thyroid and can be associated with multiple endocrine neoplasia types II and III. Histologic examination of a medullary carcinoma would reveal sheets of tumor cells in an amyloid stroma. Psammoma bodies are not found in these tumors.

Answer D is incorrect. Thyroid lymphomas often arise in the setting of Hashimoto, but would not have a psammoma body.

37. **The correct answer is E.** Primary oocytes enter meiosis I during fetal life. At birth, all oocytes are arrested in prophase of meiosis I, and remain that way just prior to ovulation of the graafian follicle. After ovulation, the oocyte progresses through meiosis I and is arrested in metaphase II until after fertilization occurs, at which point the egg will complete the second meiotic division, followed by mitotic growth of the embryo.

Answer A is incorrect. Prior to ovulation, oocytes are arrested at prophase I, not anaphase I.

Answer B is incorrect. Prior to ovulation, oocytes are arrested at prophase I, not anaphase II.

Answer C is incorrect. Prior to ovulation, oocytes are arrested at prophase I, not metaphase I.

Answer D is incorrect. Prior to ovulation, oocytes are arrested at prophase I, not metaphase II. Once ovulation occurs the oocyte re-enters meiosis and progresses to metaphase II. The oocyte then remains in metaphase II until fertilization.

Answer F is incorrect. Prior to ovulation, oocytes are arrested at prophase I, not prophase II.

38. **The correct answer is B.** Patients entrust their physicians with highly personal information, and a physician who discloses such information without consent can be held liable. However, there are exceptions to the legal protection of confidentiality, such as the need to report certain infectious diseases or to warn third parties known to be at risk of harm. The information presented in this question is based on *Tarasoff v. Regents of the University of California* (1976), in which a student was murdered by a patient who implied his intentions to his psychiatrist. The Supreme Court ruled in a rehearing that "confidentiality ends with public peril" and that third parties must be informed in such cases.

Answer A is incorrect. The physician must also make sure the potential victim is notified.

Answer C is incorrect. This choice is perhaps the most seductive but is also the most frankly inappropriate. A physician has a legal obligation to protect the public from "peril" according to the Supreme Court of the United States, regardless of the breach of confidentiality required to do so.

Answer D is incorrect. The physician must also make sure law enforcement officials are notified.

Answer E is incorrect. Notifying the patient's parents is unnecessary and would be an unwarranted breach in patient confidentiality.

39. **The correct answer is B.** This patient has the clinical stigmata of polycystic ovary syndrome (PCOS). PCOS results from hormone derangements (luteinizing hormone hypersecretion is the hallmark of PCOS) that manifest as obesity, hirsutism, oligomenorrhea or amenorrhea, and acanthosis nigricans (the velvety hyperpigmentation described). PCOS often is associated with insulin resistance, hyperglycemia, and hyperlipidemia. Diagnosis is made by ultrasound of the ovaries, which will reveal >10 follicles per ovary as well as bilateral ovarian enlargement. Oral contraceptive pills often are used to reduce the levels of circulating androgens that result in the hirsutism, and to help regulate ovulation. Another commonly used treatment is clomiphene for women who desire pregnancy.

Answer A is incorrect. Although acanthosis nigricans sometimes is seen in occult visceral malignancies, which are associated with hypercalcemia, this patient does not exhibit any of the clinical signs or symptoms of hypercalcemia ("stones, bones, groans, and moans").

Answer C is incorrect. Hypermagnesemia frequently is associated with hospitalized patients in renal failure and not with PCOS. Magnesium levels rise as the renal failure worsens because the only regulatory method of magnesium is through renal excretion. Magnesium levels of 2-4 mEq/L are associated with nausea, vomiting, and lightheadedness; higher levels are associated with depressed consciousness, respiratory depression, and cardiac arrest.

Answer D is incorrect. Hyperuricemia is not associated with PCOS, but rather with gout. Patients with gout typically have a history of extremely painful monoarticular arthritis, hyperuricemia, and subcortical bone cysts (tophi). Definitive diagnosis is made using polarized microscopy that demonstrates negatively birefringent (yellow and parallel) monosodium urate crystals from the aspirated joint fluid.

This woman's history is not consistent with gout or an acute gouty arthritis attack.

40. **The correct answer is A.** This is a deletion mutation. Bases 7-9 of the normal gene have been deleted in the mutant gene, resulting in the subsequent loss of one amino acid. Because three nucleotides were deleted, there is no change in the reading frame. The most common cystic fibrosis mutation, ΔF508, does in fact yield gene product three nucleotides shorter than the normal gene product.

    Answer B is incorrect. A frameshift mutation is an insertion or deletion of nucleotides that results in a misreading of all codons downstream. Deletions or insertions in multiples of three do not cause a shift in the reading frame.

    Answer C is incorrect. An insertion mutation is an addition of one or more nucleotides to the DNA.

    Answer D is incorrect. A missense mutation occurs when a point mutation causes one amino acid in a protein to be replaced by a different amino acid.

    Answer E is incorrect. A nonsense mutation occurs when a point mutation results in an early stop codon. This type of mutation causes a truncated protein.

    Answer F is incorrect. A silent mutation occurs when a point mutation does not change the amino acid sequence of the protein. The point mutation is often in the third position of the codon.

    Answer G is incorrect. A transition is a mutation in which a nucleotide is replaced by another nucleotide of the same type (ie, purine for purine, or pyrimidine for pyrimidine). Purine-for-pyrimidine and pyrimidine-for-purine substitutions are called transversions.

41. **The correct answer is E.** Rapid administration of vancomycin can cause an anaphylactoid reaction mediated by IgE that leads to histamine release, causing redness of the face, neck, upper body, back, and arms as well as tachycardia, hypotension, and nausea. The rash produced is distinct from other types of drug-induced erythroderma because of the rapid onset after administration of the drug and lack of skin exfoliation. This reaction bears the unfortunate name "red man syndrome." The histamine release can be prevented with and treated by administration of diphenhydramine, a first-generation H_1- receptor antagonist. Diphenhydramine is a member of the ethanolamine family, and as such can cause marked sedation. These agents are also used as antiemetics.

    Answer A is incorrect. Amoxicillin would not cause a rash such as that described. However, it is known to produce a generalized rash in patients who are infected with the Epstein-Barr virus.

    Answer B is incorrect. Chloramphenicol is most often used to treat meningitis. Adverse effects include aplastic anemia and gray baby syndrome.

    Answer C is incorrect. Clindamycin is used to treat anaerobic infections. Its most common adverse effect is pseudomembranous colitis. Antibiotic-induced enterocolitis is often treated with vancomycin.

    Answer D is incorrect. Metronidazole is used to treat infection with anaerobic organisms and protozoa. It can cause a disulfiram-like reaction when taken with alcohol. However, it does not typically cause the hypersensitivity reaction seen in this patient.

42. **The correct answer is B.** A person is said to be in status epilepticus when seizure activity has continued for more than 30 minutes without regaining consciousness between episodes. The drug of choice for the treatment of status epilepticus is the benzodiazepine diazepam, due to its short duration of action. Benzodiazepines act by increasing the opening frequency of the chloride channel associated with the γ-aminobutyric acid (GABA) receptor, which inhibits further neuronal firing. When administered intravenously, diazepam's onset of action is virtually immediate. Of note, diazepam is often more readily available in the pre-hospital setting, as the drug does not require refrigeration and can be administered either intrave-

nously or per rectum. Generally, in a hospital setting lorazepam is the initial drug of choice for antiseizure therapy.

Answer A is incorrect. Carbamazepine is effective for the treatment of partial and generalized tonic-clonic seizures; however, it is not used for the treatment of status epilepticus. Carbamazepine blocks repetitive activation of sodium channels.

Answer C is incorrect. Ethosuximide is primarily used in the treatment of absence seizures and is not effective in the treatment of status epilepticus. Ethosuximide blocks low-threshold T-type calcium channels.

Answer D is incorrect. Gabapentin, an analog of the neurotransmitter GABA, is used for the treatment of simple or complex partial seizures, but is not used to treat status epilepticus. Gabapentin blocks H-current modulators.

Answer E is incorrect. Phenobarbital is used as a second-line agent to treat simple partial and generalized tonic-clonic seizures, and can also be used for febrile seizures in children. Phenobarbital is a very effective anticonvulsant, but is not first-line treatment for status epilepticus because it requires a longer time to administer, and is associated with a higher incidence of respiratory depression compared to benzodiazepines. Phenobarbital increases the duration of chloride channel opening.

43. **The correct answer is E.** *Staphylococcus aureus* causes acute bacterial endocarditis, which presents with an acute onset of high fever, other flu-like symptoms, new-onset murmur, petechiae, Roth's spots (white spots on the retina formed by microemboli), Janeway lesions (painless macules on the palms or soles), Osler's nodes (small, painful nodules on the pads of the fingers or toes), and nail bed (subungual) hemorrhages. The bacteria can attack healthy valves and result in vegetations that are much larger than those of subacute bacterial endocarditis. Vancomycin is typically used to treat S *aureus* endocarditis, and provides coverage in the case of methicillin-resistant S *aureus*.

Answer A is incorrect. Ceftriaxone is not used to treat *Staphylococcus aureus* endocarditis.

Answer B is incorrect. Ciprofloxacin is not used to treat *Staphylococcus aureus* endocarditis.

Answer C is incorrect. Erythromycin is not used to treat *Staphylococcus aureus* endocarditis.

Answer D is incorrect. Gentamicin may be used in combination with vancomycin to treat *Staphylococcus aureus* endocarditis, but not alone.

44. **The correct answer is D.** Heparin is used therapeutically for thromboembolism prophylaxis and treatment. Heparin also can be flushed through an intravenous line (IV) that has been disconnected temporarily from its source to prevent clogging and obstruction of the tubing; such an IV may be referred to as "hep-locked." Heparin primarily acts on the intrinsic pathway of coagulation, accelerating the action of anti-thrombin III, which inactivates thrombin and factors IXa, Xa, XIa, and XIIa. Therefore, intentionally or contaminated heparinized blood will show a delayed partial thromboplastin time (PTT).

Answer A is incorrect. Heparin primarily acts on the intrinsic pathway of coagulation, accelerating the action of anti-thrombin III, which inactivates thrombin and factors IXa, Xa, XIa, and XIIa. Therefore, heparin prolongs, rather than shortens, the PTT.

Answer B is incorrect. The International Normalized Ratio (INR) is a standardized measure of PT adjusted for the particular assay type and the machine used to measure the PT. INR is increased if PT is increased. Because heparin exerts little effect on the extrinsic pathway, the INR may not be changed significantly by the presence of heparin.

Answer C is incorrect. Heparin facilitates inactivation of intrinsic and common pathway factors, measured by PTT, more than extrinsic factors, which are measured by PT. Thus PT is less affected than the PTT in clotting studies of heparin-containing blood samples. In sufficiently high doses, heparin prolongs, rather than shortens, the PT.

Answer E is incorrect. The INR is a standardized measure of PT adjusted for the particular assay type and the machine used to measure the PT. INR is increased if PT is increased. Because heparin exerts little effect on the extrinsic pathway, the INR may not be changed significantly by the presence of heparin.

Answer F is incorrect. Heparin facilitates inactivation of factor Xa and thrombin, both of which are part of the common pathway of coagulation. Thus prothrombin time (PT) may be prolonged in blood samples containing heparin. However, the PT prolongation is minimal and may even be normal compared to prolongation of the PTT. PTT is influenced by intrinsic pathway factors, which makes it the preferred marker of heparin anticoagulant activity.

45. **The correct answer is D.** Splitting is a defense mechanism associated with borderline personality disorder (BPD). Patients with BPD often engage in self-destructive behaviors such as cutting or burning themselves with cigarettes. They have extremely labile moods and unstable relationships. Splitting involves the either/or categorization of things as all good or all bad. The patient might state that the male resident is the only doctor who has ever understood her, and that all the other doctors are ignorant. Or she might view the nursing staff as wonderful and the medical staff as abominable.

Answer A is incorrect. Denial involves the refusal to accept a reality that a person deems unsettling. For instance, a person may write off persistent negative job performance reviews rather than accepting that his work abilities are deficient.

Answer B is incorrect. Humor is a mature defense mechanism, which involves expressing uncomfortable emotions in a comfortable way (ie, as funny): an overweight patient might make jokes about "fat people."

Answer C is incorrect. Reaction formation has been called unconscious hypocrisy. The person adopts opposite attitudes to unconscious emotions. A burnt out doctor who dislikes medicine may spend his time encouraging medical students in their professional development.

Answer E is incorrect. Sublimation is a mature defense mechanism that involves the expression of uncomfortable emotions (anger) in a socially useful way, such as becoming an advocate for social justice. In reaction formation, the person unconsciously replaces the uncomfortable emotion with actions that are opposite his/her true emotion.

46. **The correct answer is A.** This patient is presenting with phencyclidine (PCP) intoxication. Patients often display assaultive behavior, belligerence, psychosis, violence, impulsiveness, psychomotor agitation, fever, tachycardia, vertical and horizontal nystagmus, hypertension, impaired judgment, ataxia, seizures, and delirium. The most dangerous aspect of PCP use is the reckless behavior it precipitates. The treatment is typically benzodiazepines or haloperidol for severe symptoms. Reassurance is also important in calming the patient.

Answer B is incorrect. Flumazenil is the antidote to benzodiazepine overdose. Benzodiazepines have an effect on the body quite similar to alcohol, and overdose can cause amnesia, ataxia, somnolence, and mild respiratory depression. Flumazenil reverses the effects of benzodiazepines by competitive inhibition at the benzodiazepine-binding site on the $GABA_A$ receptor.

Answer C is incorrect. N-acetylcysteine is used as an antidote to acetaminophen overdose. Symptoms of acetaminophen overdose include abdominal pain, nausea, vomiting, convulsions, diarrhea, jaundice, and occasionally convulsions and coma. Excessive use can damage multiple organs, especially the liver and kidney. In both organs, toxicity is not from the drug itself, but from one of its metabolites, N-acetyl-p-benzoquinoneimine (NAPQI). In the liver, the cytochrome P450 enzymes

CYP2E1 and CYP3A4 are primarily responsible for the conversion of acetaminophen to NAPQI. In the kidney, cyclooxygenases are the principal route by which acetaminophen is converted to NAPQI. Overdose leads to the accumulation of NAPQI, which undergoes conjugation with glutathione. Conjugation depletes glutathione, a natural antioxidant. This, in combination with direct cellular injury by NAPQI, leads to cell damage and death. Acetaminophen overdose is one of the most common causes of acute liver failure. If untreated, overdose can lead to liver failure and death within days. Treatment is aimed at removing acetaminophen from the body and replacing glutathione stores. Activated charcoal can be used to decrease absorption of paracetamol if the patient presents for treatment soon after the overdose. While the antidote, N-acetylcysteine, acts as a precursor for glutathione and helps the body regenerate enough to prevent damage to the liver, a liver transplant is often required if damage to the liver becomes severe.

Answer D is incorrect. Naloxone is a remedy for opioid intoxication (heroin). Patients with opioid intoxication present with euphoria that often progresses to apathy, CNS depression, constipation, papillary constriction, and respiratory depression that can be life-threatening in overdose. Naloxone/naltrexone block opioid receptors and reverse the depressant effects.

Answer E is incorrect. Sodium bicarbonate is used to treat TCA overdose, and it helps narrow the QRS complex, which is widened in this toxicity. Remember the 3 Cs: Coma, Convulsions, and Cardiac toxicity, for TCA overdose. Diazepam or lorazepam should be administered if the patient is seizing, and there should be cardiac monitoring for arrhythmias.

47. **The correct answer is C.** Legionnaire's disease, which is also known as legionellosis, is a form of pneumonia. Most infections with this disease occur in elderly people. Symptoms include fever, chills, and a nonproductive cough. Other symptoms include muscle aches, headache, malaise, fatigue, shortness of breath, chest pain, diarrhea, and ataxia. Legionnaire's disease is confirmed by laboratory tests that detect the presence of the bacterium *Legionella pneumophila*. The bacterium Gram stains poorly, so silver stain is used to visualize the rods. Transmission does not occur from person to person; rather, it occurs by aerosol transmission from an environmental water source such as an air conditioner.are most often found on the upper pole of the testes adjacent to the tunica vaginalis.

Answer A is incorrect. Aspergillosis is caused by the fungus *Aspergillus*. Symptoms include fever and a productive cough. Invasive infection often occurs in an immunocompromised host. Aspergilloma (fungus ball) often occurs in a TB cavity. Silver stain of *Aspergillus* would show septate hyphae that branch into a V shape.

Answer B is incorrect. Brucellosis is caused by bacteria of the genus *Brucella*. Humans become infected by coming in contact with animals or animal products that are contaminated with these bacteria. Brucellosis can cause a range of symptoms that may include fever, sweats, headaches, back pains, and physical weakness. Severe infections of the CNS or of the endocardium may occur.

Answer D is incorrect. *Mycoplasma* pneumonia is a common, mild pneumonia that usually affects people <40 years old. Its symptoms are very similar to those of Legionnaire's disease, with the exception of diarrhea. Additionally, silver stain would not be used to diagnose *Mycoplasma pneumoniae* infection. Instead, serology, cold agglutinins, or polymerase chain reaction testing for mycoplasma would be in order.

Answer E is incorrect. *Pneumocystis jiroveci* (formerly *carinii*) pneumonia presents with fever, shortness of breath, and nonproductive cough. It targets mainly immunocompromised patients (eg, those with AIDS), and it is identified by immunofluorescent staining of sputum or lavage fluid. Silver stain is also used, but would show cysts, not the rod-shaped bacteria seen in this image.

48. **The correct answer is B.** The classic histologic finding in a granulosa cell tumor of the ovary is the presence of Call-Exner bodies, which are follicles with granulosa cells haphazardly arranged around a space containing eosinophilic secretions. The clinical presentation also supports this diagnosis. About two-thirds of ovarian granulosa cell tumors occur in postmenopausal women (average age at menopause in the United States is 51 years). Granulosa cell tumors are usually estrogen-secreting, but occasionally produce androgens leading to virilization. Estrogen-secreting tumors in children and adolescents can cause precocious puberty. In adults they are often associated with endometrial hyperplasia, cystic breast disease, and endometrial carcinoma. Up to 15% of patients with estrogen-secreting tumors develop an endometrial carcinoma. Evidence of increased endometrial thickness (revealing hyperplasia or carcinoma) is found in this patient as a thickened endometrial stripe on ultrasonography. The endometrial stripe is an area of the endometrium with differing echogenicity, allowing the thickness to be measured. This increased risk of endometrial hyperplasia and carcinoma is due to the unopposed estrogen secretion by the tumor, which stimulates growth of the endometrium. This abnormal endometrial growth leads to subsequent sloughing off, resulting in abnormal vaginal bleeding, a common presentation of endometrial abnormalities.

Answer A is incorrect. An endometrioid tumor, as the name suggests, histologically resembles endometrium. It does not have Call-Exner bodies on histologic examination, and because it does not secrete estrogen, it would not present with vaginal bleeding and a thickened endometrial stripe.

Answer C is incorrect. Krukenberg tumors are tumors that are metastatic to the ovaries from the GI system, most commonly the stomach. The classic histologic finding is a mucin-secreting signet-ring cell, not a Call-Exner body.

Answer D is incorrect. Call-Exner bodies would not be found in serous cystadenocarcinoma. Instead, one would expect to see a tumor lined with epithelium resembling that of the fallopian tube and psammoma bodies (concentric rings of calcification). These types of tumors are very common and account for >50% of ovarian carcinomas. Because they do not secrete estrogen, they do not classically present with vaginal bleeding and would not cause a thickened endometrial stripe.

Answer E is incorrect. A teratoma contains tissue derived from at least two different embryonic layers. For example, thyroid tissue, neural tissue, muscle tissue, bone, and even teeth may be present. Immature teratomas are more aggressive and are always malignant, while mature teratomas are well differentiated and benign. One would not expect to see Call-Exner bodies or vaginal bleeding with a teratoma.

Common Laboratory Values

* = Included in the Biochemical Profile (SMA-12)

Blood, Plasma, Serum	Reference Range	SI Reference Intervals
*Alanine aminotransferase (ALT, GPT at 30°C)	8–20 U/L	8–20 U/L
Amylase, serum	25–125 U/L	25–125 U/L
*Aspartate aminotransferase (AST, GOT at 30°C)	8–20 U/L	8–20 U/L
Bilirubin, serum (adult) Total // Direct	 0.1–1.0 mg/dL // 0.0–0.3 mg/dL	 2–17 μmol/L // 0–5 μmol/L
*Calcium, serum (Total)	8.4–10.2 mg/dL	2.1–2.8 mmol/L
*Cholesterol, serum	140–250 mg/dL	3.6–6.5 mmol/L
*Creatinine, serum (Total)	0.6–1.2 mg/dL	53–106 μmol/L
Electrolytes, serum Sodium Chloride * Potassium Bicarbonate	 135–147 mEq/L 95–105 mEq/L 3.5–5.0 mEq/L 22–28 mEq/L	 135–147 mmol/L 95–105 mmol/L 3.5–5.0 mmol/L 22–28 mmol/L
Gases, arterial blood (room air) P_{O_2} P_{CO_2} pH	 75–105 mmHg 33–44 mmHg 7.35–7.45	 10.0–14.0 kPa 4.4–5.9 kPa $[H^+]$ 36–44 nmol/L
*Glucose, serum	Fasting: 70–110 mg/dL 2-h postprandial: < 120 mg/dL	3.8–6.1 mmol/L < 6.6 mmol/L
Growth hormone – arginine stimulation	Fasting: < 5 ng/mL provocative stimuli: > 7 ng/mL	< 5 μg/L > 7 μg/L
Osmolality, serum	275–295 mOsm/kg	275–295 mOsm/kg
*Phosphatase (alkaline), serum (p-NPP at 30°C)	20–70 U/L	20–70 U/L
*Phosphorus (inorganic), serum	3.0–4.5 mg/dL	1.0–1.5 mmol/L
*Proteins, serum Total (recumbent) Albumin Globulins	 6.0–7.8 g/dL 3.5–5.5 g/dL 2.3–3.5 g/dL	 60–78 g/L 35–55 g/L 23–35 g/L
*Urea nitrogen, serum (BUN)	7–18 mg/dL	1.2–3.0 mmol urea/L
*Uric acid, serum	3.0–8.2 mg/dL	0.18–0.48 mmol/L

(continues)

Cerebrospinal Fluid		
Glucose	40–70 mg/dL	2.2–3.9 mmol/L
Hematologic		
Erythrocyte count	Male: 4.3–5.9 million/mm^3 Female: 3.5–5.5 million/mm^3	4.3–5.9 × 10^{12}/L 3.5–5.5 × 10^{12}/L
Hematocrit	Male: 41–53% Female: 36–46%	0.41–0.53 0.36–0.46
Hemoglobin, blood	Male: 13.5–17.5 g/dL Female: 12.0–16.0 g/dL	2.09–2.71 mmol/L 1.86–2.48 mmol/L
Hemoglobin, plasma	1–4 mg/dL	0.16–0.62 μmol/L
Leukocyte count and differential		
Leukocyte count	4500–11,000/mm^3	4.5–11.0 × 10^9/L
Segmented neutrophils	54–62%	0.54–0.62
Band forms	3–5%	0.03–0.05
Eosinophils	1–3%	0.01–0.03
Basophils	0–0.75%	0–0.0075
Lymphocytes	25–33%	0.25–0.33
Monocytes	3–7%	0.03–0.07
Mean corpuscular hemoglobin	25.4–34.6 pg/cell	0.39–0.54 fmol/cell
Platelet count	150,000–400,000/mm^3	150–400 × 10^9/L
Prothrombin time	11–15 seconds	11–15 seconds
Reticulocyte count	0.5–1.5% of red cells	0.005–0.015
Sedimentation rate, erythrocyte (Westergren)	Male: 0–15 mm/h Female: 0–20 mm/h	0–15 mm/h 0–20 mm/h
Proteins, total	< 150 mg/24 h	< 0.15 g/24 h

Index

C

D

E

F

G

H

I

J

K

L

M

O

P

Q

R

S

T

W

X

Y

Z

ABOUT THE SENIOR EDITORS

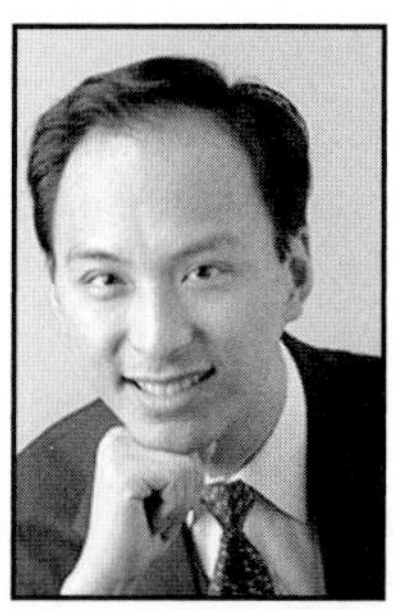

Tao Le, MD, MHS

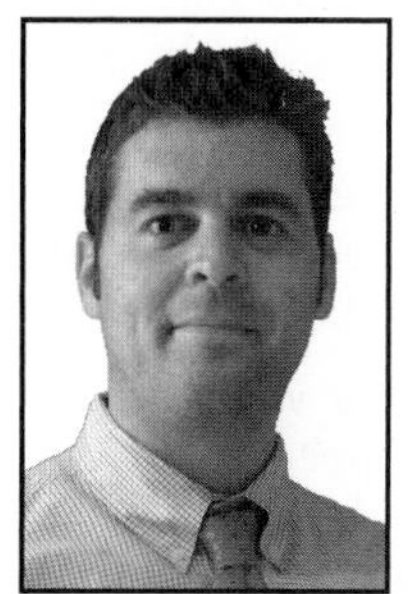

James A. Feinstein, MD

Tao Le, MD, MHS

Tao has been a well-recognized figure in medical education for the past 20 years. As senior editor, he led the expansion of *First Aid* into a global educational series. In addition, he is the founder and editor-in-chief of the *USMLERx* online test bank series as well as a co-founder of the *Underground Clinical Vignettes* series. As a medical student, he was editor-in-chief of the University of California, San Francisco *Synapse,* a university newspaper with a weekly circulation of 9000. Tao earned his medical degree from the University of California, San Francisco in 1996 and completed his residency training in internal medicine at Yale University and fellowship training at Johns Hopkins University in allergy and immunology. In addition, he earned a Master of Health Science degree at the Johns Hopkins Bloomberg School of Public Health. At Yale, he was a regular guest lecturer on the USMLE review courses and an adviser to the Yale School of Medicine curriculum committee. Tao subsequently went on to co-found Medsn and served as its chief medical officer. He is currently pursuing research in asthma education at the University of Louisville.

James A. Feinstein, MD

James is a practicing pediatrician and pediatric health services researcher. He attends in the Special Care Clinic at The Children's Hospital Colorado, where he provides care to children with complex medical issues and special healthcare needs. He is also a research fellow at the University of Colorado School of Medicine, where he is obtaining a graduate degree in biostatistics. His research is focused on improving the outpatient care delivered to children with complex, chronic illnesses. He attended Dartmouth College, the University of Pennsylvania School of Medicine, and completed residency at the Children's Hospital of Philadelphia. Outside of medicine, James writes (www.shortwhitecoat.com) and he absolutely loves to run up (and then down) various Rocky mountains.

ABOUT THE EDITORS

Mark W. Ball, MD

Mark hails from Harlan, Kentucky. He is an alumnus of Centre College, where he majored in biochemistry and molecular biology, the Johns Hopkins School of Medicine, and the Halsted General Surgery Internship at Johns Hopkins Hospital. He is currently a urological surgery resident at the Brady Urological Institute at Johns Hopkins Hospital. Mark's academic interests include the detection and treatment of malignancies of the bladder, prostate, and kidney. In his free time, he enjoys spending time with his wife, cooking, running, and exploring the outdoors.

Annie Dude, MD

Annie hails from Milwaukee, Wisconsin, but has been proud to call Chicago home for almost ten years now. Annie graduated from the University of Chicago Pritzker School of Medicine in June and then began residency training in obstetrics and gynecology at Duke University Medical Center. She enjoys spending time with her husband, six-month-old daughter, dog, family, and friends, as well as hiking, running, and traveling.

Rebecca L. Hoffman, MD

Rebecca is currently a resident in the general surgery program at the Hospital of the University of Pennsylvania. She grew up in a small town in central Pennsylvania and then attended Haverford College, majoring in chemistry. Before starting medical school at the University of Pennsylvania, she spent a year doing clinical research in the Division of Orthopaedic Surgery at The Children's Hospital of Philadelphia. When she isn't taking care of patients or operating, Rebecca loves to write, edit, teach, travel, and spend time in the outdoors.

Mark Robert Jensen

Mark is a fourth-year student at the University of Rochester School of Medicine. He plays ice hockey in his spare time and does his best to stay out of the penalty box. Off the ice, he tutors inner city students in math and science and likes to travel when he can get away. He has always loved writing and has published articles on bone sclerosis, dry eye disorder, the utility of CT in evaluation of the left ventricular assist device, and the development of radical Islam in London. He plans to follow his father and grandfather's footsteps into anesthesia, and to hopefully, someday, publish a book of his own.

Kimberly Kallianos

Originally from Atlanta, Georgia, Kim attended the University of North Carolina at Chapel Hill where she earned a Bachelor of Science degree in biology. She is currently a fifth-year student at Harvard Medical School and will begin her radiology residency at the University of California, San Francisco in 2012.

Cesar Raudel Padilla

Cesar was raised in the San Francisco Bay area and is a first-generation Mexican American. He dropped out of high school but managed to get a scholarship to a community college and ultimately graduated from the University of San Francisco with a degree in biological sciences. He plans to become an anesthesiologist and specialize in critical care. Cesar hopes to serve the Latino community in California as well as in Guadalajara, Mexico, where he has spent his summers since childhood. He has helped the University of Rochester School of Medicine reach out to the local Latino community by coordinating mock interviews with Spanish-speaking standardized patients. Cesar is an avid *fútbol* fan and enjoys spending time with his wife and daughter Elena.

Lauren Rothkopf, MD

Lauren attended Johns Hopkins University, earning a Bachelor of Arts degree in English with a minor in psychology. She graduated from Temple University School of Medicine in 2007 and completed her internship year in internal medicine at Beth Israel Deaconess Medical Center in Boston. She is currently pursuing a Master's degree in public health while raising her 1-year-old son.

James Yeh, MD

James is a clinical fellow in medicine at Harvard Medical School and a resident physician at the Cambridge Hospital/Cambridge Health Alliance. He is a graduate of Boston University School of Medicine, where he received the Henry J. Bakst Award in community medicine and was an Albert Schweitzer Fellow. He completed his undergraduate and graduate degrees at the University of California, Berkeley and Harvard University. He has extensive basic science and clinical research background and has received multiple grants and awards. James has wide-ranging experiences in tutoring and teaching, and he has been working with *First Aid* and USMLERx since 2009. In his spare time, he enjoys traveling around the world, exploring new places and museums, cooking/eating, playing guitar, riding his bike, and photography.

ABOUT THE AUTHORS

Kirsten Austad

Kirsten graduated from the University of Wisconsin-Madison with degrees in English literature and medical microbiology & immunology. She is currently taking a year off after completing two years at Harvard Medical School to be a fellow at the Edmond J. Safra Center for Ethics at Harvard University. Her work looks at how to improve physician-pharmaceutical industry interactions, and she will soon start her third year in Cambridge Hospital's Integrated Clerkship. Kirsten plans to remain involved in medical education as well as practice community-based primary care with underserved populations in the U.S. or abroad and work to link health care to poverty reduction and community empowerment.

Eike Blohm

Eike grew up in Germany and came to the U.S. to study medicine. He worked as a paramedic and ICU tech before starting his studies at Johns Hopkins. Now at the end of his third year in medical school, Eike is starting the application process for a residency seat in emergency medicine. In his free time, he is an avid marathoner, competing in five marathons this year alone.

Benjamin Caplan, MD

Ben is a family medicine resident at Boston Medical Center. After earning his undergraduate degree in psychology at Williams College, Ben worked as a staff researcher at the UCLA Brain Mapping Center, where he authored several neuroscience publications and helped launch the international Human Brain Project. Apart from the medical world, he is a concert cellist of 25 years, a world traveler, and a performance magician of 18 years.

Po-Hao Chen

Po-Hao is completing his medical training at Harvard Medical School and is a joint-degree student at Harvard Business School to learn more about health policy and hospital administration. After graduation, he would like to enter a radiology residency program while continuing to participate in medical education and research. Ultimately, Po-Hao wishes to hold a leadership position at a hospital as well as be involved in medical innovation to develop ways physicians can organize increasing amounts of patient information more effectively.

Lauren de Leon, MD

Lauren is a recent graduate of the Alpert Medical School of Brown University. She is finishing her internship year in internal medicine and loving it. She enjoys traveling, cooking, and searching for the perfect dumpling. In terms of her medical career, Lauren is debating between gastroenterology and palliative/end of life care.

Philip Eye

Philip grew up in Baldwin, New York. Four years after being accepted into Boston University's seven-year medical program, he graduated with a Bachelor of Science degree in economics and medical sciences. Phil is currently a Second Lieutenant in the United States Army and a medical student at Boston University School of Medicine. He plans to pursue a residency in neurology upon graduation in 2012. In his spare time, Phil both studies and teaches kung fu.

Jim Griffin, MD

Jim is originally from Waynesboro, Georgia, and attended the University of Georgia, where he majored in biochemistry and molecular biology. After graduating from Johns Hopkins School of Medicine in May 2011, he began a general surgery internship at the Johns Hopkins Hospital and plans to pursue a career in surgical oncology.

John Hegde
John was born in Philadelphia and grew up in Carmel, Indiana. He graduated from Indiana University and is currently a third-year student at Harvard Medical School. He is still undecided about which medical specialty to pursue, although he is considering a career in either radiation oncology or radiology. John enjoys reading, watching movies, traveling, and cheering on all Philly sports teams.

Emily Heikamp
Emily is currently working in the MD/PhD program at Johns Hopkins. She is originally from New Orleans, Louisiana, and she attended Duke University as an undergraduate. Before coming to Hopkins, Emily earned a Master's degree in medical oncology from Oxford University. Her clinical and research interests include tumor immunology and autoimmunity.

Thomas Robert Hickey, MD
Originally from central New York, Tom recently graduated from Harvard Medical School and is currently pursuing an anesthesia residency at Brigham and Women's Hospital.

Henry R. Kramer, MD
Henry attended Cornell University, where he studied biology and psychology. He earned his medical degree from the Johns Hopkins University School of Medicine. He is now a resident in internal medicine at the Massachusetts General Hospital. Henry enjoys running with his dog, cooking, wine, craft beer, and bourbon.

Thomas Lardaro
Thomas is originally from Peace Dale, Rhode Island. After graduating summa cum laude from the University of Connecticut, he worked for two years researching molecular neurobiology at Harvard Medical School. Thomas has since enrolled at the Johns Hopkins University School of Medicine, where he has taken an additional year of study as part of a funded clinical research training program. He will graduate with MD/MPH degrees in the spring of 2012. In his free time, Thomas enjoys playing soccer, traveling, and being outdoors.

Katherine Latimer
Katherine is a third-year medical student at Johns Hopkins University School of Medicine. She is originally from Bethesda, Maryland, and earned her Bachelor of Science degree from Georgetown University. She plans to pursue a career in obstetrics and gynecology.

Joseph Liao
Joey is from sunny Ventura, California. He earned a degree in biology from MIT and has been living in New England ever since. He is currently a third-year student at Boston University School of Medicine, and plans to go into radiology. As a second-year, Joey formed a rock band with two of his college buddies, proving that there is indeed time during medical school to have fun. He also enjoys photography.

Jerry Loo
Jerry did his undergraduate studies in microbiology, immunology & molecular genetics at UCLA. He is currently finishing his fourth year at the USC Keck School of Medicine and will be continuing his training there as a radiology resident in 2012. In his free time, Jerry enjoys playing piano, computer programming, basketball, and the occasional death match on PlayStation 3.

Aya Michaels, MD
After graduating from Columbia University in 2007 with a Bachelor of Arts degree in biochemistry, Aya entered Harvard Medical School. She graduated in May 2011 and is excited to start her training as a radiologist at Brigham and Women's Hospital in Boston.

Somala Muhammed, MD
Somala recently graduated from Harvard Medical School and is excited to return to her hometown of Houston for a general surgery residency at Baylor College of Medicine. She hopes to specialize in surgical oncology or pediatric surgery.

Behrouz Namdari, MD
Behrouz earned his medical degree from Chicago Medical School and is currently a resident in psychiatry at Duke University. In his nonmedical time, he is often found on the golf course or basketball court.

Tashera Perry, MD
Tashera hails from Westfield, New Jersey. She studied biology at Mary Baldwin College and completed a two-year postbaccalaureate Intramural Research Training fellowship at the National Heart, Lung, and Blood Institute prior to attending the University of Chicago Pritzker School of Medicine. She began residency training in obstetrics and gynecology at the University of Illinois at Chicago College of Medicine in June 2011. Aside from medicine, Tashera's interests include art history, mountain biking, and bikram yoga.

Christopher Roxbury
Christopher is currently a third-year medical student at Johns Hopkins University. He hails from Bridgewater, New Jersey, and attended Johns Hopkins University as an undergraduate, majoring in molecular and cellular biology and Spanish. After completing medical school, he plans to pursue a career in otolaryngology—head and neck surgery.

Neepa Shah
Neepa is from Toronto, Canada and is a third-year medical student at Boston University. She plans to pursue a career in ophthalmology, with a focus on academics and teaching. Her hobbies include traveling, baking, and Indian classical dance.

Bethany Strong
Bethany is originally from Oklahoma City, Oklahoma. She completed her undergraduate education at Spelman College, where she studied biology and biochemistry. As a participant in the five-year MD/PhD program at Harvard Medical School, she spent an additional year of training completing clinical rotations at McCord Hospital in Durban, South Africa and conducting research at the Centers for Disease Control and Prevention in Atlanta. She plans to complete a residency program in general surgery, focusing her career on global health and medical student education.

Seenu Susarla, MD, DMD, MPH
Seenu is from Vestal, New York, and graduated with a degree in chemistry from Princeton University. After graduating college, Seenu decided that being a degree-collector would be an interesting career. As such, he earned his Master of Public Health, Doctor of Dental Medicine, and Doctor of Medicine degrees from Harvard University. He is currently a resident in the combined general surgery/oral & maxillofacial surgery residency program at Massachusetts General Hospital.

Jeffrey Tosoian
Jeff is originally from Farmington, Michigan, and attended the University of Michigan in Ann Arbor, where he majored in cellular and molecular biology. Jeff graduated from the Johns Hopkins Bloomberg School of Public Health in May 2011 with a Master of Public Health degree in biostatistics and epidemiology. After completing medical school in 2012, Jeff plans to pursue a career in urological surgery with a focus in genitourinary cancers.

Jackson Vane, MD
Jackson is from Whittier, California. He attended California State University, Los Angeles to earn his undergraduate degree in biology in 2005. He then ventured out of the sunny confines of Southern California to Chicago, where he attended Rosalind Franklin University of Medicine and Science and earned his Master of Science degree in applied physiology in 2006. He then attended Chicago Medical School and graduated in 2010. He is currently at the University of California, Irvine doing his residency in pediatrics. In his free time, Jackson enjoys wandering aimlessly in his new surroundings, riding his bike, playing poker, trying all sorts of new restaurants, and catching up on the many movies he has missed over the years.

Daniel J. Verdini, MD
After graduating Boston College with degrees in biology and economics, Dan worked as an investment analyst before deciding to embark on a career in medicine. After graduating from Ross University, Dan spent a year at Massachusetts General Hospital as a research fellow in cardiac imaging and will be starting a radiology residency at the University of Texas in San Antonio after completing a year in preliminary medicine at the University of Nevada School of Medicine in Reno.

Marc E. Walker
Marc is an MD/MBA student at Harvard Medical School and Harvard Business School. On the business side, Marc is interested in health care delivery systems development and innovation and entrepreneurship in medicine and surgery. He will be dedicating the upcoming year to the pursuit of his research interests in plastic surgery and plans to graduate in May 2012 with the intent of entering a surgical residency thereafter.